S0-BOT-836

BIOPROCESS ENGINEERING

BIOPROCESS ENGINEERING

KINETICS, BIOSYSTEMS, SUSTAINABILITY, AND REACTOR DESIGN

Shijie Liu
SUNY ESF
Department of Paper and Bioprocess Engineering,
Syracuse, NY 13210, USA

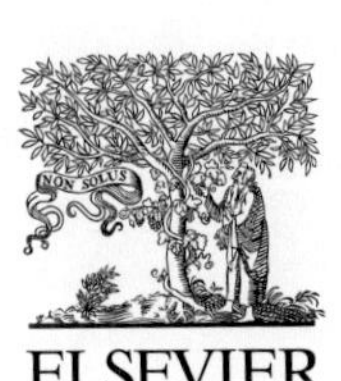

ELSEVIER
AMSTERDAM • BOSTON • HEIDELBERG • LONDON • NEW YORK • OXFORD
PARIS • SAN DIEGO • SAN FRANCISCO • SYDNEY • TOKYO

Elsevier

Radarweg 29, PO Box 211, 1000 AE Amsterdam, The Netherlands
The Boulevard, Langford Lane, Kidlington, Oxford OX5 1GB, UK

First edition 2013

British Library Cataloguing in Publication Data
A catalogue record for this book is available from the British Library

Library of Congress Cataloging-in-Publication Data
A catalog record for this book is available from the Library of Congress

ISBN: 978-0-444-59525-6

Printed and bound in Spain.

12 13 14 15 16 10 9 8 7 6 5 4 3 2 1

Contents

Preface

All I know is just what I read in the papers.
Will Rogers

The quote above is quite intriguing to me and reflective of this text. Everything in this text can be found either directly or with "extrapolation" or "deduction" from the books and papers one can find to date. The most influential books to this time are the "*Biochemical Engineering Fundamentals*" by J.E. Bailey and D.F. Ollis, "*Elements of Chemical Reaction Engineering*" by H.S. Fogler, "*The Engineering of Chemical Reactions*" by L.D. Schmidt, "*Chemical Reaction Engineering*" by O. Levenspiel, "*Bioprocess Engineering—Basic Concepts*" by M.L. Shuler and F. Kargi, and many others. All these texts and others have formed part of this text. In no intention this text is compiled to replace all these great textbooks of the time. A mere rearrangement and/or compiling is made in this text to give you the reader an opportunity to understand some of the basic principles of chemical and biological transformations in bioprocess engineering.

The computer age has truly revolutionized the literature, beyond the literature revolution brought about by the mass production or availability of paper and distribution of books via library. The explosion of the shear amount of literature, birth of interdisciplines and disciplines or subject areas in the past decades has been phenomenal. Bioprocess Engineering is one that born of biotechnology and chemical engineering. With the maturing of Bioprocess Engineering as a discipline, it evolves from an interdisciplinary subject area of Biology and Chemical Engineering, to a discipline that covers the engineering and engineering science aspects of biotechnology, green chemistry, and biomass or renewable resources engineering. As such, textbooks in the area are needed to cover the needs of educating the new generation of fine bioprocess engineers, not just by converting well-versed chemical engineers and engineering-savvy biologists to bioprocess engineers. I hope that this textbook can fill this gap and brings the maturity of bioprocess engineering. Yet, some of the materials in this text are deep in analyses that are suited for graduate work and/or research reference.

The key aspect that makes Bioprocess Engineering special is that Bioprocess Engineering as a discipline is centered around solving problems of transformation stemmed from cellular functions and biological and/or chemical conversions concerning the sustainable use of renewable biomass. The mechanism, rate, dynamic behavior, transformation performance and manipulations of bioprocess systems are the main topics of this text.

Chapter 1 is an introduction of bioprocess engineering profession including green chemistry, sustainability considerations and regulatory constraints. Chapter 2 is an overview of biological basics or cell chemistry including cells, viruses, stem cell, amino acids, proteins, carbohydrates and various biomass components, and fermentation media. In Chapter 3, a survey of chemical reaction analysis is introduced. The basic knowledge of reaction rates, conversion, yield, stoichiometry and energy regularity for bioreactions are reviewed. The concepts of approximate and coupled reactions are introduced, providing the basis of understanding for the metabolic pathway representations later in the book. Mass and energy balances for reactor analyses, as well as the definitions of ideal reactors and commonly known bioreactors are introduced before an introduction to reactor system analyses. The biological basics and chemical reaction basics are followed by the reactor analysis basics in Chapters 4 and 5, including the effect of reaction kinetics, flow contact patterns and reactor system optimizations. Gasification (of coal and biomass) is also introduced in Chapter 5. How the ideal reactors are selected, what flow reactor to choose and what feed strategy to use are all covered in Chapter 5.

Chapters 6, 7, 8, 9, 10 and 11 are studies on bioprocess kinetics. In Chapter 6, you will learn the collision theory for reaction kinetics and approximations commonly employed to arrive at simple reaction rate relations. Kinetics of acid hydrolysis, of an important unit operation in biomass conversion, is introduced as a case study. In Chapter 7, we turn to discuss the techniques for estimating kinetic parameters from experimental data, breaking away from the traditional straight line approaches developed before the computer age. You can learn how to use modern tools to extract kinetic parameters reliably and quickly without complex manipulation of the data. In Chapters 8 and 9, we discuss the application of kinetic theory to catalytic systems. Enzymes, enzymatic reactions and application of enzymes are examined in Chapter 8, while adsorption and solid catalysis are discussed in Chapter 9. The derivation of simplified reaction rate relations, such as the Michaelis–Menten equation for enzymatic reaction and LHHW for solid catalysis, is demonstrated. The applicability of these simple kinetic relations is discussed. In Chapter 9, you will learn both ideal and non-ideal adsorption kinetics and adsorption isotherms. Is multilayer adsorption the trademark for physisorption? The heterogeneous kinetic analysis theory is applied to reactions involving woody biomass where the solid phase is not catalytic in §9.5. Chapter 10 discusses the cellular genetics and metabolism. The replication of genetic information, protein production, substrate uptake, and major metabolic pathways are discussed, hinting at the application of kinetic theory in complicated systems. In Chapter 11, you will learn how cell grows: cellular material quantifications, batch growth pattern, cell maintenance and endogenous needs, medium and environmental conditions, and kinetic models. Reactor analyses are also presented in Chapters 8 and 11.

In Chapters 12 and 13, we discuss the controlled cell cultivation. Continuous culture and wastewater treatment are discussed in Chapter 12. Exponential growth is realized in continuous culturing. An emphasis is placed on the reactor performance analyses, using mostly Monod growth model in examples, in both Chapters. Chapter 13 introduces fed-batch operations and their analyses. Fed batch can mimic exponential growth in a controlled manner as opposed to the batch operations where no control (on growth) is asserted besides environmental conditions.

Chapter 14 discusses the evolution and genetic engineering, with an emphasis on biotechnological applications. You will learn how cells transform, how cells are manipulated, and what some of the applications of cellular transformation and recombinant cells are. Chapter 15 introduces the sustainability perspectives. Bioprocess engineering principles are applied to examine the sustainability of biomass economy and atmospheric CO_2. Is geothermal energy a sustainable or renewable energy source? Chapter 16 discusses the stability of catalysts: activity of chemical catalyst, genetic stability of cells and mixed cultures, as well as the stability of reactor systems. Sustainability and stability of bioprocess operations are discussed. A stable process is sustainable. Multiple steady states, approach to steady state, conditions for stable operations and predator–prey interactions are discussed. Continuous culture is challenged by stability of cell biomass. In ecological applications, sustainability of a bioprocess is desirable. For industrial applications, the ability of the bioprocess system to return to the previous set point after a minor disturbance is an expectation. In Chapter 17, the effect of mass transfer on the reactor performance, in particular with biocatalysis, is discussed. Both external mass transfer, e.g. suspended media, and internal mass transfer, e.g. immobilized systems are discussed, as well as temperature effects. The detailed numerical solutions can be avoided or greatly simplified by following directly from the examples. It is recommended that examples be covered in classroom, rather than the reading material. Chapter 18 discusses the reactor design and operation. Reactor selection, mixing scheme, scale-up, and sterilization and aseptic operations are discussed.

Shijie Liu

Nomenclature

a	Catalyst activity
a	Specific surface or interfacial area, m^2/m^3
a	Thermodynamic activity
a_d	Dimensionless dispersion coefficient
a	Constant
A	Chemical species
A	Adenine
A	Constant
A	Heat transfer area, m^2
Ac	Acetyl
ADP	Adenosine diphosphate
AMP	Adenosine monophosphate
ATP	Adenosine triphosphate
B	Chemical species
B	Constant
BOD	Biological oxygen demand
BOD_5	Biological oxygen demand measured for 5 days
c	constant
C	Chemical species
C	Concentration, mol/L or kg/m^3
C	Constant
C	Cytosine
C_P	Heat capacity, J/(mol·K), or kJ/(kg·K)
CoA	Coenzyme A
CHO	Chinese hamster ovary cell
COD	Chemical oxygen demand
CSTR	Continuously stirred tank reactor
d	Diameter, m
D	Diameter, m
D	Diffusivity, m^2/s
D	Dilution rate, s^{-1}
D–	Chirality or optical isomers: right-hand rule applies
DO	Concentration of dissolved oxygen, g/L
DNA	Deoxyribonucleic acid
e	electron
E	Enzyme
E	Energy, kJ/mol
EMP	Embden-Meyerhof-Parnas
f	Fractional conversion
f	Fanning friction factor
F	Flow rate, kg/s or kmol/s
F	Farady constant
FAD	Flavin adenine dinucleotide in oxidized form
FADH	Flavin adenine dinucleotide in reduced form
FDA	Food and Drug administration
FES	Fast equilibrium step (hypothesis)
g	Gravitational acceleration, 9.80665 m^2/s
G	Gibbs free energy, kJ/mol
G	Guanine
GRAS	Generally regarded as safe
GMP	Good manufacture practice
GTP	Guanosine triphosphate
h	height or length
H	Enthalpy, kJ/mol or kJ/kg
H_C	Harvesting cost
HMP	Hexose Monophosphate (pathway)
J	Total transfer flux, kmol/s or kg/s

J	Transfer flux, kmol/(m^2·s) or kg/(m^2·s)
k	Kinetic rate constant
k	Mass transfer coefficient, m/s
K	Thermodynamic equilibrium constant
K	Saturation constant, mol/L or kg/L
K_L	Overall mass transfer coefficient (from gas to liquid)
L	Length
L-	Chirality or optical isomers: left hand rule applies
m	Amount of mass, kg
$\dot{m}$	Mass flow rate, kg/s
m_S	Maintenance coefficient
M	Molecular weight, Darton (D) or kg/kmol
MC	Molar (or mass) consumption rate
MG	Mass generation rate
MR	Mass removal rate
MS	Molar or Mass supply rate
MSS	Multiple steady state
n	Total matters in number of moles
N	Mass transfer rate, kJ/(m^2·s) or kg/(m^2·s)
N	Number of species
NAD	Nicotinamide adenine dinucleotide
NADP	Nicotinamide adenine dinucleotide phosphate
O_R	Order of reaction
OTR	Oxygen transfer rate
OUR	Oxygen utilization rate
p	Pressure
P	Probability
P	Pressure
P	Product, or Product concentration, kg/m^3, or g/L, or mol/L
P	Power (of stirrer input)
P_X	Productivity or production rate of biomass
P_0	Probability of the vanishing of the entire population
P_1	Probability of the entire population not vanishing
PCR	Polymerase chain reaction
PEP	Phosphoenol pyruvate
PFR	Plug flow reactor
PP	Pentose phosphate (pathway)
PSSH	Pseudo-steady-state hypothesis
P/O	ATP formation per oxygen consumption
q	Thermal flux, J/s or W
Q	Volumetric flow rate, m^3/s
$\dot{Q}$	Thermal energy transfer rate into the system
r	Radial direction
r	Rate of reaction, mol/(m^3·s) or kg/(L·s)
R	Correlation coefficient
R	Ideal gas constant, 8.314 J/(mol·K)
R	Product, or product concentration
R	Recycle ratio
Re	Reynolds number
RNA	Ribonucleic acid
s	Selectivity
S	Entropy
S	Overall selectivity
S	Substrate (or reactant)
S	Substrate concentration, g/L
S	Surface area, m^2
Sh	Sherwood number
SMG	Specific mass generation rate
SMR	Specific mass removal rate
t	Time, s
T	Temperature, K
T	Thymine

TCA	Tricarboxylic acid
u	superficial velocity, m/s
U	Average velocity or volumetric flux
U	Internal energy
U	Overall heat transfer coefficient, kJ/m^2
U	Uracil
CoQ_n	Co-Enzyme ubiquinone
v	Molar volume, $m^3/kmol$
V	Volume, m^3
$\dot{W}$	Rate of work input to the system
$\dot{W}_s$	Rate of shaft work done by the system
x	Variable
x	Axial direction
X	Cell or biomass
X	Cell biomass concentration, L^{-1}, or g/L
X_{SU}	Biomass storage for managed forest
X_{SU}	Biomass storage for undisturbed unmanaged forest
y	Mole fraction
y	Variable
Y	Yields
YF	Yield factor, or ratio of stoichiometric coefficients
z	Vertical direction
z	Variable
Z	Collision frequency
Z	Valence of ionic species

Greek Symbols

α	Constant
α	Chirality or optical isomers: two chiral centers with different hand gestures
β	Heat of reaction parameter
β	Constant
β	Chirality or optical isomers: two chiral centers with the same hand gestures
χ	Fraction
γ	Thermodynamic activity coefficient
γ	Activation energy parameter
γ_{DR}	Degree of reduction
δ	Thickness or distance
Δ	Difference
ε	Void ratio
ϕ	Thiele modulus
η	Effectiveness factor
θ	Fractional coverage (on available active sites)
μ	Specific rate of formation, or rate of reaction normalized by the catalyst or cell biomass concentration, s^{-1} or $g \cdot g^{-1} \cdot s^{-1}$
μ	Specific biomass growth rate, s^{-1} or $g \cdot g^{-1} \cdot s^{-1}$
μ_f	Dynamic viscosity of fluid, Pa·s
ν	Stoichiometric coefficient
ν_f	Kinematic viscosity of fluid or medium, m^2/s
ρ	Density, kg/m^3
σ	Active site
σ	Variance
τ	Space time, s
ω	Mass fraction
ω	Rotational speed
ω	Weighting factor

Subscript

ads	Adsorption
app	Apparent
A	Species A
b	reverse reaction
B	Batch
c	Combustion

cat	Catalyst
C	Species C
C	Cold stream
C	Concentration based
C	Calculated based on model
d	Death
d	Doubling
des	Desorption
D	Diffusion coefficient related
e	Endogenous (growth needs)
e	External (mass transfer)
e	In effluent stream
eq	Equilibrium
eff	Effective
f	Final or at end
f	Fluid or medium
f	Formation
f	Forward reaction
F	In feed stream
G	Growth
H	Heat of reaction
H	Hot stream
i	Reaction i
i	Initial
i	Impeller
in	Inlet
I	Inhibition
j	Species j
m	Maximum
max	Maximum
net	Net
OPT	Optimum
obs	Observed
out	Outlet
p	Particle
P	Product
P	Preparation
R	Reaction; Reactor
R	Reference; Reduced
s	Solid
S	Sterilization
S	Saturation
S	Substrate
S	Surface
S	Total species
t	Tube, or reactor
T	Tube
T	Total
U	Unloading
0	Initial
0	In feed
0	Pre-exponential
+	Plasmid-containing
−	Plasmid-free
∞	maximum or at far field
Σ	Total or sum

Superscript

0	(Thermodynamic) Standard conditions
*	Equilibrium
*	Based on transitional state
′	Catalyst mass based
′	Variant

CHAPTER

1

Introduction

OUTLINE

1.1. BIOLOGICAL CYCLE

Figure 1.1 illustrates the natural biological processes occurring on Earth. Living systems consist of plants, animals and microorganisms. Sunlight is used by plants to convert CO_2 and H_2O into carbohydrates and other organic matter, releasing O_2. Animals consume plant matter, converting plant materials into animal cells, and using the chemical energy from oxidizing plant matter into CO_2 and H_2O (H_2O also serves as a key substrate for animals), finishing the cycle. Microorganisms further convert dead animal and/or plant biomass into other form of organic substances fertilizing the growth of plants, releasing CO_2 and H_2O, and the cycle is repeated. Energy from the Sun is used to form molecules and organisms that we call life. Materials or matter participating in the biological cycle are renewable so long as the cycle is maintained. Bioprocess engineers manipulate and make use of this cycle by designing processes to make desired products, either by training microorganisms, plants, and animals or via direct chemical conversions.

Bioprocess Engineering
http://dx.doi.org/10.1016/B978-0-444-59525-6.00001-9

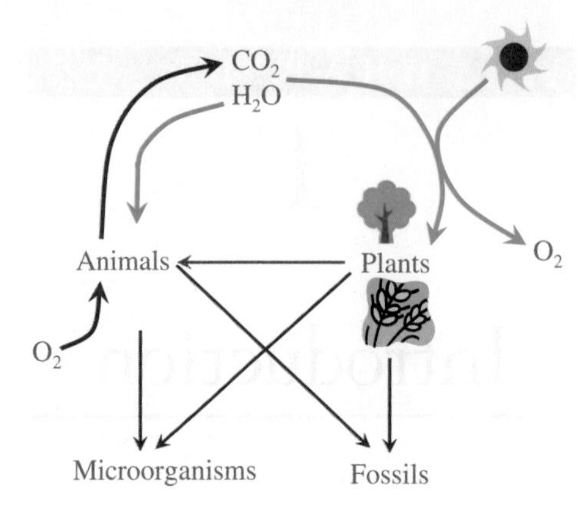

FIGURE 1.1 The natural biological processes.

The reactor is the heart of any chemical and/or biochemical processes. With reactors, bioprocesses turn inexpensive sustainably renewable chemicals, such as carbohydrates, into valuable ones that humans need. As such, bioprocesses are chemical processes that use biological substrates and/or catalysts. While not limited to such, we tend to refer to bioprocesses as 1) biologically converting inexpensive "chemicals" or materials into valuable chemicals or materials and 2) manipulating biological organisms to serve as "catalyst" for conversion or production of products that human need. Bioprocess engineers are the only people technically trained to understand, design, and efficiently handle bioreactors. Bioprocess engineering ensures that a favorable sustainable state or predictable outcome of a bioprocess is achieved. This is equivalent to saying that bioprocess engineers are engineers with, differentiating from other engineers, training in biological sciences, especially quantitative and analytical biological sciences and green chemistry.

If one thinks of science as a dream, engineering is making the dream a reality. The maturing of Chemical Engineering to a major discipline and as one of the very few well-defined disciplines in the 1950s has led to the ease in the mass production of commodity chemicals and completely changed the economics or value structure of materials and chemicals, thanks to the vastly available what were then "waste" and "toxic" materials: fossil resources. Food and materials can be manufactured from the cheap fossil materials. Our living standards improved significantly. Today, chemical reactors and chemical processes are not built by *trial-and-error* but by design. The performance of a chemical reactor can be predicted, not just found to happen that way; the differences between large and small reactors are largely solved. Once a dream for the visional pioneers, it can now be achieved at ease. Fossil chemical and energy sources have provided much of our needs for advancing and maintaining the living standards of today. With the dwindling of fossil resources, we are facing yet another value structure change. The dream has been shifted to realizing a society that is built upon renewable and sustainable resources. Fossil sources will no longer be abundant for human use. Sustainability becomes the primary concern. Who is going to make this dream come true?

On a somewhat different scale, we can now manipulate life at its most basic level: the genetic. For thousands of years, people have practiced genetic engineering at the level of selection and breeding or directed evolution. But now it can be done in a purposeful, predetermined manner with the molecular-level manipulation of DNA, at a quantum leap level (as compared with directed evolution) or by design. We now have tools to probe the mysteries of life in a way unimaginable prior to the 1970s. With this intellectual revolution emerges new visions and new hopes: new medicines, semisynthetic organs, abundant and nutritious foods, computers based on biological molecules rather than silicon chips, organisms to degrade pollutants and clean up decades of unintentional damage to the environment, zero harmful chemical leakage to the environment while producing a wide array of consumer products, and revolutionized industrial processes. Our aim of comfortable living standards is ever higher.

Without hard work, these dreams will remain merely dreams. Engineers will play an essential role in converting these visions into reality. Biosystems are very complex and beautifully constructed, but they must obey the rules of chemistry and physics and they are susceptible to engineering analysis. Living cells are predictable, and processes to use them can be methodically constructed on commercial scales. There lies a great task: analysis, design, and control of biosystems to the greater benefit of a sustainable humanity. This is the job of the bioprocess engineer.

This text is organized such that you can learn bioprocess engineering without requiring a profound background in reaction engineering and biotechnology. To limit the scope of the text, we have left out the product purification technologies, while focusing on the production generation. We attempt to bridge molecular-level understandings to industrial applications. It is our hope that this will help you to strengthen your desire and ability to participate in the intellectual revolution and to make an important contribution to the human society.

1.2. GREEN CHEMISTRY

Green chemistry, also called sustainable chemistry, is a philosophy of chemical research and engineering that encourages the design of products and processes that minimize the use and generation of hazardous substances while maximizing the efficiency of the desired product generation. Whereas environmental chemistry is the chemistry of the natural environment, and of pollutant chemicals in nature, green chemistry seeks to reduce and prevent pollution at its source. In 1990, the Pollution Prevention Act was passed in the United States. This act helped create a *modus operandi* for dealing with pollution in an original and innovative way. It aims to avoid problems before they happen.

Examples of green chemistry starts with the choice of solvent for a process: water, carbon dioxide, dry media, and nonvolatile (ionic) liquids, which are some of the excellent choices. These solvents are not harmful to the environment as either emission can easily be avoided or they are ubiquitous in nature.

Paul Anastas, then of the United States Environmental Protection Agency, and John C. Warner developed 12 principles of green chemistry, which help to explain what the definition means in practice. The principles cover such concepts as: a) the design of processes to maximize the amount of (all) raw material that ends up in the product; b) the use of safe, environment-benign substances, including solvents, whenever possible; c) the design of energy efficient processes; and d) the best form of waste disposal: not to create it in the first place. The 12 principles are:

(1) It is better to prevent waste than to treat or clean up waste after it is formed.
(2) Synthetic methods should be designed to maximize "atom efficiency."
(3) Wherever practicable, synthetic methodologies should be designed to use and generate substances that possess little or no toxicity to human health and the environment.
(4) Chemical products should be designed to preserve efficacy of function while reducing toxicity.
(5) The use of auxiliary substances (e.g. solvents, separation agents, etc.) should be made unnecessary wherever possible and innocuous when used.
(6) Energy requirements should be recognized for their environmental and economic impacts and should be minimized. Synthetic methods should be conducted at ambient temperature and pressure.
(7) A raw material or feedstock should be renewable rather than depleting wherever technically and economically practicable.
(8) Reduce derivatives—Unnecessary derivatization (blocking group, protection/deprotection, and temporary modification) should be avoided whenever possible.
(9) Catalytic reagents (as selective as possible) are superior to stoichiometric reagents.
(10) Chemical products should be designed so that at the end of their function they do not persist in the environment and break down into innocuous degradation products.
(11) Analytical methodologies need to be further developed to allow for real-time, in-process monitoring and control prior to the formation of hazardous substances.
(12) Substances and the form of a substance used in a chemical process should be chosen to minimize potential for chemical accidents, including releases, explosions, and fires.

One example of green chemistry achievements is the polylactic acid (or PLA). In 2002, Cargill Dow (now NatureWorks) won the Greener Reaction Conditions Award for their improved PLA polymerization process. Lactic acid is produced by fermenting corn and converted to lactide, the cyclic dimmer ester of lactic acid using an efficient, tin-catalyzed cyclization. The L,L-lactide enantiomers are isolated by distillation and polymerized in the melt to make a crystallizable polymer, which is used in many applications including textiles and apparel, cutlery, and food packaging. Wal-Mart has announced that it is using/will use PLA for its produce packaging. The NatureWorks PLA process substitutes renewable materials for petroleum feedstocks, does not require the use of hazardous organic solvents typical in other PLA processes and results in a high-quality polymer that is recyclable and compostable.

Understanding the concept of green chemistry holds a special position for bioprocess engineers. Processes we design and operate must have minimal potential environmental impacts while optimized for maximum benefit. Basic steps for green chemistry that are what bioprocess engineering do include:

(1) Developing products and processes based on renewable resources, such as plant biomass.
(2) Design processes that bypass dangerous/toxic chemical intermediates.
(3) Design processes that avoid dangerous/toxic solvent use.

(4) Reducing chemical processing steps but demands high efficiency.
(5) Promoting biochemical processes to reduce chemical processing steps or toxic chemical utilization.
(6) Design milder (closer to atmosphere temperature and pressure) processes and multiple product recovery routes.
(7) Bypassing chemical equilibrium with innovative reactor design, and biocatalysis, rather than adding intermediate steps.
(8) Avoid production of unwanted products other than H_2O and CO_2.

1.3. SUSTAINABILITY

Sustainability is the capacity to endure or maintain at the longest timescale permissible. In other words, sustainability is the ability to maintain continuum. In ecology, the word describes how biological systems remain diverse and productive over time. Long-lived and healthy wetlands and forests are examples of sustainable biological systems. For humans, sustainability is the potential for long-term maintenance of well being, which has environmental, economic, and social dimensions.

Healthy ecosystems and environments provide vital goods and services to humans and other organisms. Utilization and release of substances at a rate that is harmonious with a steady state nature is the key for sustainability. This naturally leads to a carrying capacity for each substance or species with which humans interact. The sustainable state can be influenced by (process conditions or) how we interact with nature. There are two major ways of reducing negative human impact and enhancing ecosystem services. The first is environmental management; this approach is based largely on information gained from earth science, environmental science, and conservation biology. The second approach is management of human consumption of resources, which is based largely on information gained from economics. Practice of these major steps can ensure a more favorable sustainable state to be evolved into.

Sustainability interfaces with economics through the social and ecological consequences of economic activity. Sustainable economics involves ecological economics where social, cultural, health-related, and monetary/financial aspects are integrated. Moving toward sustainability is also a social challenge that entails international and national law, urban planning and transport, local and individual lifestyles, and ethical consumerism. Ways of living more sustainably can take many forms from reorganizing living conditions (e.g. ecovillages, eco-municipalities, and sustainable cities), reappraising economic sectors (permaculture, green building, and sustainable agriculture), or work practices (sustainable architecture), using science to develop new technologies (green technologies and renewable energy) to adjustments in individual lifestyles that conserve natural resources. These exercises reduce our reliance or demand on disturbing the environment. To make all these concepts come to light, bioprocess engineers will be at the forefront of developing and implementing the technologies needed. On a grand scale, maintaining renewability or looking for a favorable predictable steady state on everything we touch or interact is the key to sustainability (Fig. 1.2). This falls right in the arena of bioprocess engineering.

Are you ready for the challenge of designing processes that meets sustainability demands?

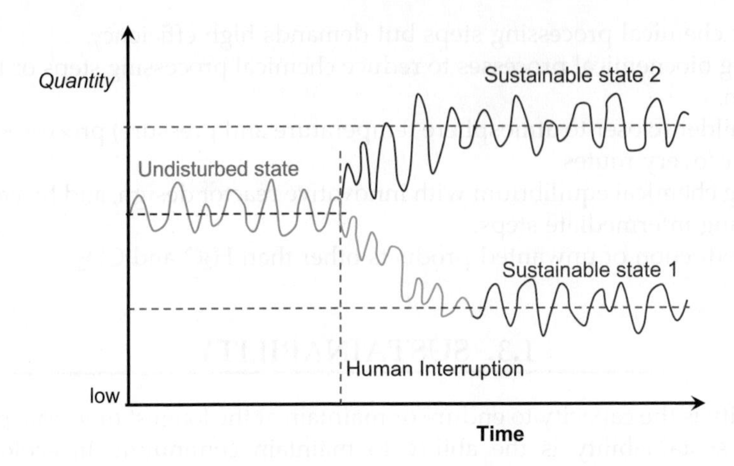

FIGURE 1.2 Change of sustainable state owing to human interruption.

1.4. BIOREFINERY

On a grand scale, sustainability is the basis of nature. Enforcing sustainability at the timescale of humanity is an insurance of our way of life to continue. Prior to the 1900s, agriculture and forestry were the predominant sources of raw materials for energy, food and a wide range of everyday commodities, and the human civilization depended almost entirely on renewable materials. Humanity was restricted by the sustainable supply inefficiently harvested from the biomass, which drew energy from the sun. The industrial revolution has brought a leap in the human civilization. Mass production of goods by machines dominates our daily life. The industrial revolution was brought to mature by the development of combustion engines and subsequent development of fossil energy and chemical industry. Besides the more than doubling of useful biomass production/harvest, mankind has increasingly taped into the large fossil energy reserves. At first the fossil chemicals were regarded as waste and thus any use was welcomed. It soon became the cheapest chemical and energy sources for the industrial revolution. As a result, our living standards have seen a leap. There is no turning back to the primitive way of life in the past. However, fossil energy and chemical sources are depleting. There is a critical need to change the current industry and human civilization to a sustainable manner, assuring that our way of life today continues on the path of improvement after the depletion of fossil sources. Our way of life exists only if sustainability is maintained on a timescale no longer than our life span.

Biorefinery is a concept in analogous to a petroleum refinery whereby a raw material feed (in this case, plant lignocellulosic biomass instead of petroleum) is refined to a potpourri of products (on demand). In a biorefinery, lignocellulosic biomass is converted to chemicals, materials, and energy that runs on the human civilization, replacing the needs of petroleum, coal, natural gas, and other nonrenewable energy and chemical sources. Lignocellulosic biomass is renewable as shown in Fig. 1.1, in that plant synthesizes chemicals by drawing energy from the sun, and carbon dioxide and water from the environment, while releasing oxygen. Combustion of biomass releases energy, carbon dioxide, and water. Therefore, biorefinery plays a key role in ensuring the cycle of biomass production and consumption included satisfying human needs for energy and chemicals.

A biorefinery integrates a variety of conversion processes to produce multiple product streams such as transportation liquid fuels, steam/heat, electricity, and chemicals from lignocellulosic biomass. Biorefinery has been identified as the most promising route to the creation of a sustainable bio-based economy. Biorefinery is a collection of the essential technologies to transform biological raw materials into a range of industrially useful intermediates. By producing multiple products, a biorefinery maximizes the value derived from a lignocellulosic biomass feedstock. A biorefinery could produce one or more low-volume high-value chemical products together with a low-value, high-volume liquid transportation fuel, while generating electricity and process heat for its own use and/or export.

Figure 1.3 shows a schematic of various biorefinery processes. There are two major categories or approaches in biorefining: biochemical or systematical disassembling processes and thermochemical processes. In biochemical processes, the lignocellulosic biomass is commonly disassembled to individual components systematically for optimal conversions that followed. The basic approach is based on a systematical disassembling and conversion to desired chemicals. The biochemical processes depend heavily on separation and/or physical fractionation of the intermediates as well as the final desired products. Biological conversions are preferred over chemical conversions due to their selectivity or green chemistry concepts. However, owing to the complexity of the lignocellulosic biomass, a multitude of

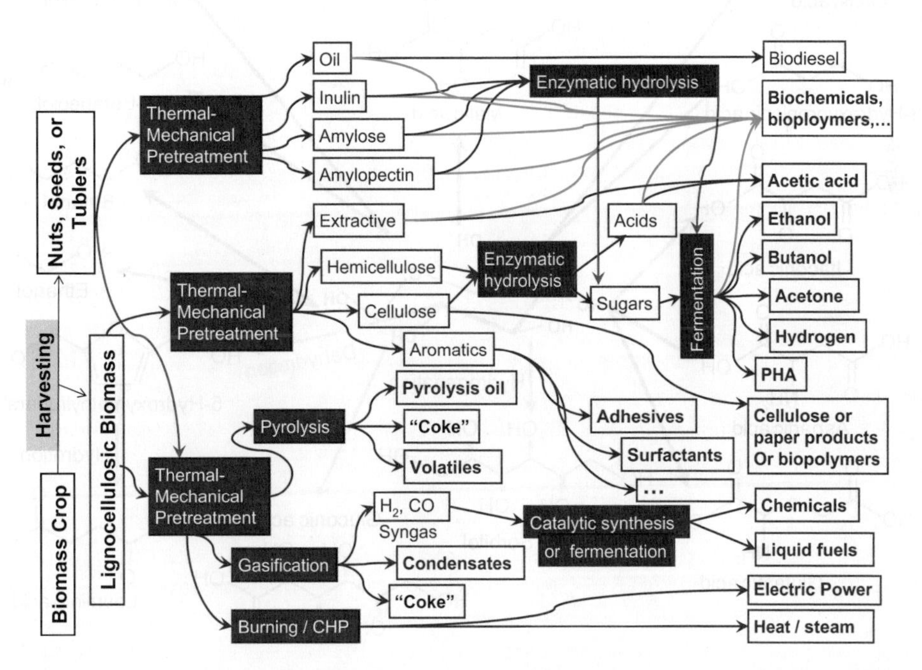

FIGURE 1.3 A schematic of various biorefinery processes (with permission: S. Liu, Z. Zhang, and G.M. Scott. 2010 "The Biorefinery: Sustainably Renewable Route to Commodity Chemicals, Energy, and Materials", J. Biotech. Adv. 28:542).

biological processes is required for optimal operations. The biological reactions are also very slow and thus require larger facility footprints.

Pyrolysis resembles more closely to the refinery, whereby the products can be controlled in a more systematical manner. It may be classified as systematical disassembling as well. However, there are restrictions on the type of products the process can produce. Gasification as shown in Fig. 1.3 is at the extreme side of conversion technology, whereby the lignocellulosic biomass is disassembled to the basic building block for hydrocarbons: H_2 and CO and then reassembled to desired products as desired. The final products can be more easily tailored from syn gas or $CO + H_2$. For example, Fischer–Tropsch process can turn $CO + H_2$ into higher alcohol, alkenes, and many other products. Syn gas (together with air: mixture of N_2 and O_2) is also the starting point for ammonia synthesis, from which nitrogen fertilizers and many other products are produced. However, all thermochemical processes suffer from selectivity. During the disassembling process, "coke" or "carbon" is produced especially at high temperatures and thus reduces the conversion efficiency if H_2 and CO are the desired intermediates. Thermal–chemical processes are generally considered

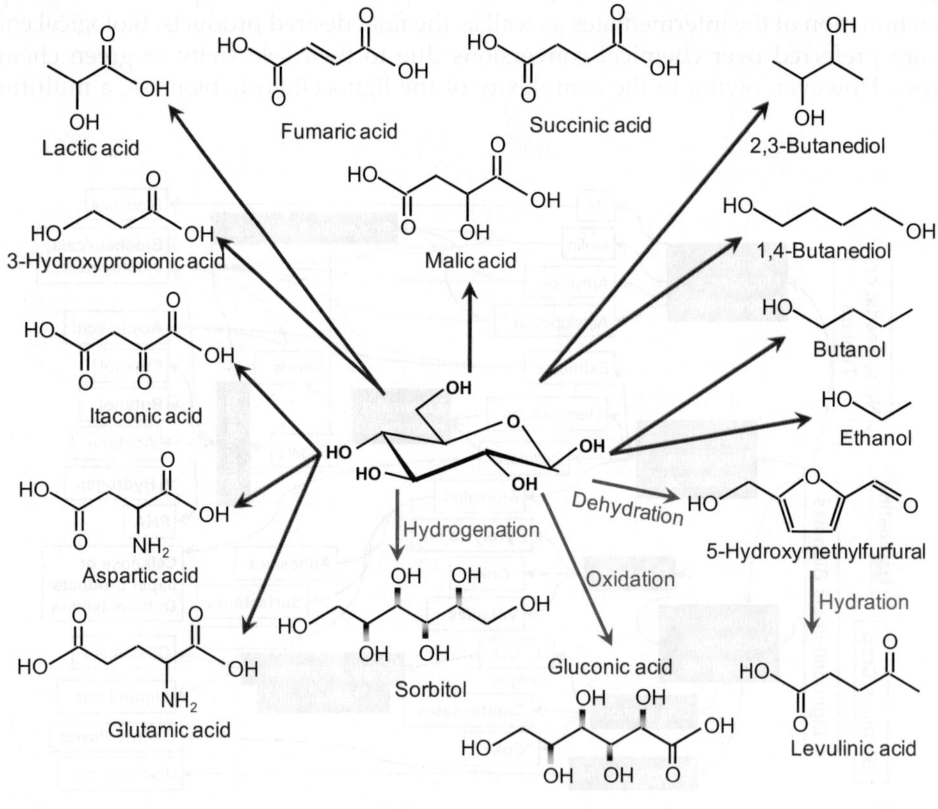

FIGURE 1.4 The platform chemicals derived from glucose (the molecule in the center of the diagram). Most of these chemicals are produced via fermentation (or biotransformation), while a few of them are produced via chemical reaction (or chemical transformation) as indicated.

less "green" than biological and other sequential disassembling processes due to their severe operating conditions, poor selectivity or by-products generation, and thermodynamic restrictions.

The promise of a biorefinery to supply the products human needs is shown in Fig. 1.4 for the various examples of building blocks or platform chemicals that sugar (a specific example of glucose) can produce, besides the very basic building blocks of CO and H_2. For example, glucose can be fermented to ethanol by yeast and bacteria anaerobically, and lactic acid can be produced by lacto bacteria. As shown in Fig. 1.4, each arrow radiates from the glucose in the center represents a route of biotransformation (or fermentation) by default, whereas chemical transformations are shown with labeled arrows. For example, glucose can be dehydrated to 5-hydroxymethylfurfural catalyzed with an acid, which can be further decomposed to levulinic acid by hydration. All these chemicals shown in Fig. 1.4 are examples of important platform (or intermediate) chemicals, as well as commodity chemicals. For example, ethanol is well known for its use as a liquid transportation fuel. Ethanol can be dehydrated to ethylene, which is the monomer for polyethylene or dehydrognated and dehydrated to make 1,3-butadiene, monomer for the synthetic rubber. Ethanol can also be employed to produce higher alcohols and alkenes.

Are you prepared to be at the forefront of developing, designing, and operating these processes for the sustainability and comfortability in humanity?

1.5. BIOTECHNOLOGY AND BIOPROCESS ENGINEERING

Biotechnology is the use or development of methods of direct genetic manipulation for a socially desirable goal. Such a goal might be the production of a particular chemical, but it may also involve the production of better plants or seeds, gene therapy, or the use of specially designed organisms to degrade wastes. The key element is the use of sophisticated techniques outside the cell for genetic manipulation. Biotechnology is applied biology; it bridges biology to bioprocess engineering, just like applied chemistry or chemical technology bridges chemistry to chemical engineering.

Many terms have been used to describe engineers working with biotechnology. The two terms that are considered general: *Biological Engineering* and *Bioengineering* come from the two major fields of applications that require deep understanding of biology: agriculture and medicine. *Bioengineering* is a broad title including work on industrial, medical, and agricultural systems; its practitioners include agricultural, electrical, mechanical, industrial, environmental and chemical engineers, and others. As such, *Bioengineering* is not a well-defined term and usually it refers to biotechnology applications that are not easily categorized or in medical fields. *Biological Engineering* stems from engineering of biology which is also a general term. However, the term *Biological Engineering* is initially used by agricultural engineers for the engineering applications to or manipulation of plants and animals and is thus specific. For example, the Institute of Biological Engineering has a base in, although not limited to, agricultural engineering. ABET (Accreditation Board for Engineering and Technology, Inc.) brands Biological Engineering together with Agricultural Engineering when accrediting BS (Bachelor of Science) and MS (Master of Science) in engineering and technology educational programs. On the other hand, the Society for Biological Engineers was created within

American Institute of Chemical Engineers. Therefore, *biological engineering* is also regarded as not a well-defined term and can at times refer to biotechnology applications in agricultural fields. While not exclusive, most relate biological engineering to agricultural engineering or more specifically applications of agriculture sciences. *Biochemical engineering* has usually meant the extension of chemical engineering principles to systems using a biological catalyst to bring about desired chemical transformations. It is often subdivided into bioreaction engineering and bioseparations. *Biomedical engineering* has traditionally been considered totally separate from biochemical engineering, although the boundary between the two is increasingly vague, particularly in the areas of cell surface receptors and animal cell culture. Another relevant term is *biomolecular engineering*, which has been defined by the National Institutes of Health as "...research at the interface of biology and chemical engineering and is focused at the molecular level." In all, a strong background in quantitative analysis, kinetic/dynamic behaviors, and equilibrium behaviors are strongly desirable. Increasingly, these bio-related engineering fields have become interrelated, although the names are restricting.

Bioprocess engineering is a broader and at the same time a narrower field than the commonly used terms referred above: biological engineering, biochemical engineering, biomedical engineering, and biomolecular engineering. Bioprocess Engineering is a profession than spans all the bio-related engineering fields as mentioned above. It is a profession that has emerged to stand alone, as compared to the interdisciplinary profession once it was. Unlike the term Bioengineering, the term Bioprocess Engineering is specific and well defined. *Bioprocess engineering* emphasizes the engineering and sciences of industrial processes that are biobased: 1) biomass feedstock conversion for a sustainable society or biorefinery; 2) biocatalysis-based processing; and 3) manipulation of microorganisms for a sustainable and socially desirable goal. Bioprocess engineering is neither product-based nor is substrate based. Therefore, bioprocess engineering deals with biological and chemical processes involved in all areas, not just for a particular substrate or species (of feedstock or intermediate), outcome, or product. Thus, *bioprocess engineering* intercepts chemical, mechanical, electrical, environmental, medical, and industrial engineering fields, applying the principles to designing and analysis of processes based on using living cells or subcomponents of such cells, as well as nonliving matters. Bioprocess engineering deals with both microscale (cellular/molecular) and large-scale (systemwide/industrial) designs and analyses. Science and engineering of processes converting biomass materials to chemicals, materials, and energy are therefore part of bioprocess engineering by extension. Predicting and modeling system behaviors, detailed equipment and process design, sensor development, control algorithms, and manufacturing or operating strategies are just some of the challenges facing bioprocess engineers. At the heart of bioprocess engineering lays the process kinetics, reactor design, and analysis for biosystems, which forms the basis for this text.

We will focus primarily on the kinetics, dynamics, and reaction engineering involved in the bioprocess engineering. A key component is the application of engineering principles to systems containing biological catalysts and/or biomass as feedstock, but with an emphasis on those systems making use of biotechnology and green chemistry. The rapidly increasing ability to determine the complete sequence of genes in an organism offers new opportunities for bioprocess engineers in the design and monitoring of bioprocesses. The cell, itself, is now a designable component of the overall process.

For practitioners working in the bioprocess engineering, some of the journals and periodicals provide the latest developments in the field. Here, we name a few:

Biochemical Engineering Journal
Journal of Biological Engineering
Journal of Biomass Conversion and Biorefinery
Journal of Bioprocess Engineering and Biorefinery
Journal of Bioprocess and Biosystems Engineering
Journal of Biotechnology
Journal of Biotechnology Advances
Journal of Biotechnology and Bioprocess Engineering

1.6. MATHEMATICS, BIOLOGY, AND ENGINEERING

Mathematical modeling holds the key for engineers. Physics at its fundamental level examines forces and motion; one can view it as applied mathematics. In turn, chemistry examines molecules and their interactions. Since physics examines the motions of atoms, nuclei, and electrons, at the basis of molecules, one can view chemistry as applied physics. This directly connects chemistry to mathematics at a fundamental level. Indeed, most physicists and chemists rely extensively on mathematical modeling. While one can view biology as applied chemistry through the connection of chemicals and molecules, the fundamental trainings of biologists today and engineers are distinctly different. In the development of knowledge in the life sciences, unlike chemistry and physics, mathematical theories and quantitative methods (except statistics) have played a secondary role. Most progress has been due to improvements in experimental tools. Results are qualitative and descriptive models are formulated and tested. Consequently, biologists often have incomplete backgrounds in mathematics but are very strong with respect to laboratory tools and, more importantly, with respect to the interpretation of laboratory data from complex systems.

Engineers usually possess a very good background in the physical and mathematical sciences. Often a theory leads to mathematical formulations, and the validity of the theory is tested by comparing predicted responses to those in experiments. Quantitative models and approaches, even to complex systems, are strengths. Biologists are usually better at the formation of testable hypotheses, experimental design, and data interpretation from complex systems. At the dawn of the biotechnology era, engineers were typically unfamiliar with the experimental techniques and strategies used by life scientists. However, today bioprocess engineers have entered even more sophisticated experimental techniques and strategies in life sciences (than biologists) due to the understanding and progress in the prediction and modeling of living cells.

The well groundedness in mathematical modeling gives bioprocess engineers an edge and responsibility in enforcing sustainability demands. In practice, the sustainable (or steady) state can be different from what we know today or when no human interruption is imposed. The sustainable state could even be fluctuating with a noticeable degree. Engineers hold great responsibility to convincing environmentalists and the public what to expect by accurately predicting the dynamic outcomes without speculating on the potential dramatic changes ahead.

The skills of the engineer and of the life scientist are complementary. To convert the promises of molecular biology into new processes to make new products requires the integration of these skills. To function at this level, the engineer needs a solid understanding of biology and its experimental tools. In this book, we provide sufficient biological background for you to understand the chapters on applying engineering principles to biosystems. However, if you are serious about becoming a bioprocess engineer, it is desirable if you had taken courses in microbiology, biochemistry, and cell biology, as you would appreciate more of the engineering principles in this text.

1.7. THE STORY OF PENICILLIN: THE DAWN OF BIOPROCESS ENGINEERING

Penicillin is an antibiotic of significant importance. The familiar story of penicillin was well presented by Kargi and Shuler in their text "Bioprocess Engineering—Basic Concepts." As you would expect, the discovery of the chemical was accidental and the production of the chemical is elaborate. In September 1928, Alexander Fleming at St. Mary's Hospital in London was trying to isolate the bacterium, *Staphylococcus aureus*, which causes boils. The technique in use was to grow the bacterium on the surface of a nutrient solution. One Friday, the basement window was accidently left open overnight. The experiments were carried out in the basement and one of the dishes had been contaminated inadvertently with a foreign particle. Normally, such a contaminated plate would be tossed out. However, Fleming noticed that no bacteria grew near the invading substance.

Fleming's genius was to realize that this observation was meaningful and not a "failed" experiment. Fleming recognized that the cell killing must be due to an antibacterial agent. He recovered the foreign particle and found that it was a common mold of the *Penicillium* genus (later identified as *Penicillium notatum)*. Fleming nurtured the mold to grow and, using the crude extraction methods then available, managed to obtain a tiny quantity of secreted material. He then demonstrated that this material had powerful antimicrobial properties and named the product penicillin. Fleming carefully preserved the culture, but the discovery lay essentially dormant for over a decade.

World War II provided the impetus to resurrect the discovery. Sulfa drugs have a rather restricted range of activity, and an antibiotic with minimal side effects and broader applicability was desperately needed. In 1939, Howard Florey and Ernst Chain of Oxford decided to build on Fleming's observations. Norman Heatley played the key role in producing sufficient material for Chain and Florey to test the effectiveness of penicillin. Heatley, trained as a biochemist, performed as a bioprocess engineer. He developed an assay to monitor the amount of penicillin made so as to determine the kinetics of the fermentation, developed a culture technique that could be implemented easily, and devised a novel back-extraction process to recover the very delicate product. After months of immense effort, they produced enough penicillin to treat some laboratory animals.

Eighteen months after starting on the project, they began to treat a London policeman for a blood infection. The penicillin worked wonders initially and brought the patient to the point of recovery. Most unfortunately, the supply of penicillin was exhausted and the man relapsed and died. Nonetheless, Florey and Chain had demonstrated the great potential for penicillin, if it could be made in sufficient amount. To make large amounts of penicillin would require a process, and for such a process development, engineers would be needed, in addition to microbial physiologists and other life scientists.

The war further complicated the situation. Great Britain's industrial facilities were already totally devoted to the war. Florey and his associates approached pharmaceutical firms in the United States to persuade them to develop the capacity to produce penicillin, since the United States was not at war at that time. Many companies and government laboratories, assisted by many universities, took up the challenge. Particularly prominent were Merck, Pfizer, Squibb, and the USDA Northern Regional Research Laboratory in Peoria, Illinois.

The first efforts with fermentation were modest. A large effort went into attempts to chemically synthesize penicillin. This effort involved hundreds of chemists. Consequently, many companies were at first reluctant to commit to the fermentation process, beyond the pilot plant stage. It was thought that the pilot plant fermentation system could produce sufficient penicillin to meet the needs of clinical testing, but large-scale production would soon be done by chemical synthesis. At that time, U.S. companies had achieved a great deal of success with chemical synthesis of other drugs, which gave the companies a great deal of control over the drug's production. The chemical synthesis of penicillin proved to be exceedingly difficult. (It was accomplished in the 1950s, and the synthesis route is still not competitive with fermentation.) However, in 1940, fermentation for the production of a pharmaceutical was an unproved approach, and most companies were betting on chemical synthesis to ultimately dominate.

The early clinical successes were so dramatic that in 1943 the War Production Board appointed A. L. Elder to coordinate the activities of producers to greatly increase the supply of penicillin. The fermentation route was chosen. As Elder recalls, "I was ridiculed by some of my closest scientific friends for allowing myself to become associated with what obviously was to be a flop-namely, the commercial production of penicillin by a fermentation process" (from Elder, 1970). The problems facing the fermentation process were indeed very formidable.

The problem was typical of most new fermentation processes: a valuable product made at very low levels. The low rate of production per unit volume would necessitate very large and inefficient reactors, and the low concentration (titer) made product recovery and purification very difficult. In 1939, the final concentration in a typical penicillin fermentation broth was one part per million (ca. 0.001 g/L); gold is more plentiful in seawater. Furthermore, penicillin is a fragile and unstable product, which places significant constraints on the approaches used for recovery and purification.

Life scientists at the Northern Regional Research Laboratory made many major contributions to the penicillin program. One was the development of a corn steep liquor-lactose-based medium. Andrew J. Moyer succeeded to increase productivity about tenfold with this medium in November 26, 1941. A worldwide search by the laboratory for better producer strains of *Penicillium* led to the isolation of a *Penicillium chrysogenum* strain. This strain, isolated from a moldy cantaloupe at a Peoria fruit market, proved superior to hundreds of other isolates tested. Its progeny have been used in almost all commercial penicillin fermentations.

The other hurdle was to decide on a manufacturing process. One method involved the growth of the mold on the surface of moist bran. This bran method was discarded because of difficulties in temperature control, sterilization, and equipment size. The surface method involved the growth of the mold on top of a quiescent medium. The surface method used a variety of containers, including milk bottles, and the term "bottle plant" indicated such a manufacturing technique. The surface method gave relatively high yields but had a long growing cycle and was very labor intensive. The first manufacturing plants were bottle plants because the method worked and could be implemented quickly. However, it was clear that the surface method would not meet the full need for penicillin. If the goal of the War Production Board was met by bottle plants, it was estimated that the necessary bottles would fill a row stretching from New York City to San Francisco. Engineers generally favored a submerged tank process. The submerged process presented challenges in terms of both mold physiology and tank design and operation. Large volumes of absolutely clean, oil- and dirt-free sterile air were required. What were then very large agitators were required, and the mechanical seal for the agitator shaft had to be designed to prevent the entry of organisms. Even today, problems of oxygen supply and heat removal are important constraints on antibiotic fermenter design. Contamination by foreign organisms could degrade the product as fast as it was formed, consume nutrients before they were converted to penicillin, or produce toxins.

In addition to these challenges in reactor design, there were similar hurdles in product recovery and purification. The very fragile nature of penicillin required the development of special techniques. A combination of pH shifts and rapid liquid–liquid extraction proved useful.

Soon processes using tanks of about 10,000 gal were built. Pfizer completed in less than 6 months the first plant for commercial production of penicillin by submerged fermentation (Hobby, 1985). The plant had 14 tanks each of 7000-gal capacity. By a combination of good luck and hard work, the United States had the capacity by the end of World War II to produce enough penicillin for almost 100,000 patients per year. A schematic of the process is shown in Fig. 1.5.

This accomplishment required a high level of multidisciplinary work. For example, Merck realized that men who understood both engineering and biology were not available. Merck assigned a chemical engineer and microbiologist together to each aspect of the problem. They planned, executed, and analyzed the experimental program jointly, "almost as if they were one man" (see the chapter by Silcox in Elder, 1970).

Progress with penicillin fermentation has continued, as has the need for the interaction of biologists and engineers. From 1939 to now, the yield of penicillin has gone from 0.001 g/L to over 50 g/L of fermentation broth. Progress has involved better understanding of mold physiology, metabolic pathways, penicillin structure, methods of mutation and selection of mold genetics, process control, and reactor design.

Before the penicillin process, almost no chemical engineers sought specialized training in the life sciences. With the advent of modem antibiotics, the concept of the bioprocess engineering was born. The penicillin process also established a paradigm for bioprocess development and biochemical engineering. This paradigm still guides much of our profession's thinking. The mindset of bioprocess engineers was cast by the penicillin experience. It is for this reason that we have focused on the penicillin story, rather than on an example for production of a protein from a genetically engineered organism. Although many parallels can be made between the penicillin process and our efforts to use recombinant DNA, no similar paradigm has yet emerged from our experience with genetically engineered cells.

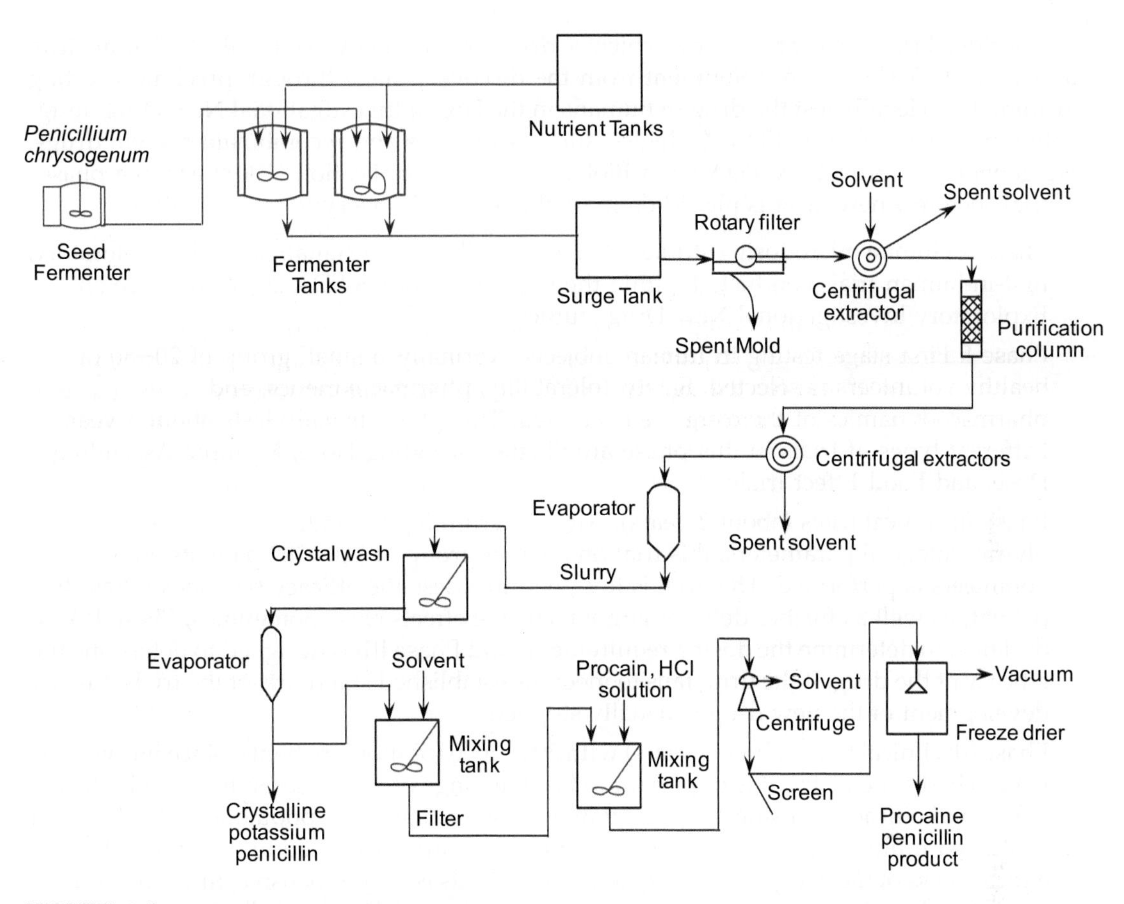

FIGURE 1.5 Schematic of penicillin production process.

We must continually reexamine the prejudices the field has inherited from the penicillin experience.

It is you, the student, who will best be able to challenge these prejudices.

1.8. BIOPROCESSES: REGULATORY CONSTRAINTS

To be an effective in bioprocess engineering, you must understand the regulatory climate in which many bioprocess engineers work. The U.S. Food and Drug Administration (FDA) and its equivalents in other countries must ensure the safety and efficacy of food and medicines. For bioprocess engineers working in the pharmaceutical industry, the primary concern is not reduction of manufacturing cost (although that is still a very desirable goal), but the production of a product of consistently high-quality in amounts to satisfy the medical needs of the population.

Consider briefly the process by which a drug obtains FDA approval. A typical drug undergoes 6–7 years of development from the discovery stage through preclinical testing in animals. To legally test the drug in humans in the US, an Investigational New Drug designation must be issued by FDA. Biologics, such as vaccines and recombinant protein drugs, are generally approved by FDA via a Biologic License Application. There are five phases of trials before a new drug is placed on market after its discovery:

Phase 0: Human microdosing studies (1–3 years). This is a designation for the exploratory, first-in-human trials conducted within the regulations of US-FDA 2006 Guidance on Exploratory Investigational New Drug studies.

Phase I: First stage testing in human subjects. Normally, a small group of 20–80 of healthy volunteers is selected. Safety, tolerability, pharmacokinetics, and pharmacodynamics of the drug are evaluated. This phase usually lasts about 1 year. Different types of trials in this phase are Single Ascending Dose, Multiple Ascending Dose, and Food Effect trials.

Phase II: clinical trials (about 2 years). After determining the initial safety and pharmacological parameters, this trial on a larger group of 100–300 patients and volunteers is performed. This trial is designed to assess the efficacy (i.e. does it help the patient) as well as further determining which side effects exist. Sometimes, Phase IIA is designed to determine the dosing requirements and Phase IIB is designed to determine the efficacy of the drug. If the drug fails to meet the established standards of the trials, further development of the new drug is usually stopped.

Phase III: clinical trials (about 3 years) with 300–3000 (or more) patients. Since individuals vary in body chemistry, it is important to test the range of responses in terms of both side effects and efficacy by using a representative cross-section of the population. Randomized controlled multicenter trials on large patient groups are conducted to determine the effectiveness of the drug. This phase of the clinic trials is very expensive, time-consuming, and difficult to design and run, especially in therapies for chronic medical conditions. It is common practice that certain Phase III trials will continue while the regulatory submission is pending at the appropriate regulatory agency. This allows patients to continue to receive possibly life-saving drugs until the drug is available in the market for distribution. These trials also provide additional safety data and support for marketing claims for the drug. Data from the clinical trials is presented to the FDA for review (2 months to 3 years). The review document presented to the FDA clearly shows the trial results combined with the description of the methods and results of human and animal studies, manufacturing procedures, formulation details, and shelf life. If the clinical trials are well designed and demonstrated statistically significant improvements in health with acceptable side effects, the drug is likely to be approved.

Phase IV: Post Marketing Surveillance Trial. Continue safety surveillance (pharmacovigilance) and technical support of a drug after receiving permission to be put on the market.

The whole discovery-through-approval process takes 5–10 years for a conventional small molecule drug and 12–15 years for a new biological drug to make it to the market. It takes about $800 million to $2000 million to send a new drug to the market. Only one in ten drugs that enter human clinical trials receive approval. Recent FDA reforms have decreased the time to obtain approval for life-saving drugs in treatment of diseases such as cancer and AIDS, but the overall process is still lengthy.

This process greatly affects a bioprocess engineer. FDA approval is for the product *and* the process together. There have been tragic examples where a small process change has allowed a toxic trace compound to form or become incorporated in the final product, resulting in severe side effects, including death. Thus, process changes may require new clinical trials to test the safety of the resulting product. Since clinical trials are very expensive, process improvements are made under a limited set of circumstances. Even during clinical trials it is difficult to make major process changes.

Drugs sold on the market or used in clinical trials must come from facilities that are certified as GMP or cGMP and must follow the appropriate Code of Federal Regulations. GMP stands for *(current) good manufacturing practice*. GMP concerns the actual manufacturing facility design and layout, the equipment and procedures, training of production personnel, control of process inputs (e.g. raw materials and cultures), and handling of product. The plant layout and design must prevent contamination of the product and dictate the flow of material, personnel, and air. Equipment and procedures must be *validated*. Procedures include not only operation of a piece of equipment but also cleaning and sterilization. Computer software used to monitor and control the process must be validated. Off-line assays done in laboratories must satisfy *good laboratory practice*. Procedures are documented by *standard operating procedures*.

The GMP guidelines stress the need for documented procedures to validate performance. "Process validation is establishing documented evidence which provides a high degree of assurance that a specific process will consistently produce a product meeting its predetermined specifications and quality characteristics" and "There shall be written procedures for production and process control to assure that products have the identity, strength, quality, and purity they purport or are represented to possess."

The actual process of validation is often complex, particularly when a whole facility design is considered. The FDA provides extensive information and guidelines that are updated regularly. If students become involved in biomanufacturing for pharmaceuticals, they will need to consult these sources. However, certain key concepts do not change. These concepts are written documentation, consistency of procedures, consistency of product, and demonstrable measures of product quality, particularly purity and safety. These tasks are demanding and require careful attention to detail. Bioprocess engineers will often find that much of their effort will be to satisfy these regulatory requirements. The key point is that process changes cannot be made without considering their considerable regulatory impact.

1.9. THE PILLARS OF BIOPROCESS KINETICS AND SYSTEMS ENGINEERING

As a profession, Bioprocess Engineers must be well versed in thermodynamics, transport phenomena, colloids, bioseparations, microbiology, bioprocess kinetics and systems engineering, and process simulation and design. This text deals with the core of bioprocess engineering. Unlike earlier texts in this subject area, this text integrates bioprocess engineering

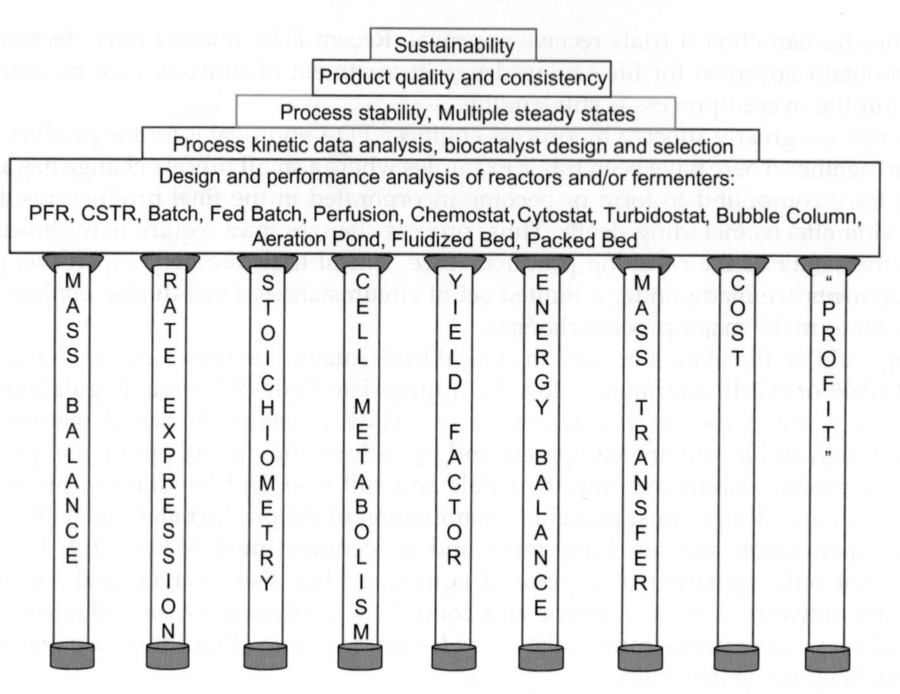

FIGURE 1.6 The pillars of bioprocess kinetics and system engineering.

principles, in particular bioprocess kinetics and transformation or reaction engineering principles together. Chemical reaction engineering is not a prerequisite before taking on this text. Figure. 1.6 shows the pillars of this text. The sustainability on this pillar is narrowly defined as having the net benefit to the human society and/or benign environmental effects.

As shown in Fig. 1.6, the fundamental knowledge of engineering science you will learn or expect in this text is among the "pillars": mass balance, rate expression, stoichiometry, cell metabolism, yield factor, energy balance, mass transfer, cost, and profit analyses. These engineering science fundamentals form the basis or foundation for the design and performance analysis of reactors and/or fermenters. In turn, process kinetic data analysis, biocatalyst design and selection can be learned from the reactor performance, and applied to the design and performance analysis of reactors and/or bioprocess systems. Process stability usually stems from multiplicity of the process, which controls the product quality and consistency. Finally, the design and control of bioprocess systems must obey the greater law of nature: sustainability.

1.10. SUMMARY

Sustainability and green chemistry are important to the practice of bioprocess engineers. Biorefinery is a desired approach to provide the products of human needs, putting the human needs into the biological cycle. Both biotransformation and chemical transformations are important to biorefinery.

Genetic manipulations and biotransformation are important to the bioprocess engineering profession. Because of the fundamental impact genetic manipulation and biotransformation can have on the cycle of life, ethics, and regulations are critical to the practice of bioprocess engineers.

It is the intention that this text can be used as a senior and/or graduate text for bioprocess engineering students. It may also be served as a reference and/or graduate text for chemical kinetics, chemical reactor analysis, and bioprocess systems engineering. At the same time, we have inserted materials, more advanced analysis, or complex systems in the text as an extension to the introductory material. It is our aim that this text can serve equally as a reference or resource for further research or development.

Further Reading

A. Green Chemistry

Anatas, P.C., Warner, J.C., 1988. Green Chemistry: Theory and Practice. Oxford University Press, New York.

Linthorst, J.A., 2010. An Overview: Origins and Development of Green Chemistry. *Foundations of Chemistry* 12 (1), 55–68.

Wilson, M., Schwarzman, M., 2009. Toward a New U.S. Chemicals Policy: Rebuilding the Foundation to Advance New Science. Green Chemistry, and Environmental Health 117 (8), 1202–1209 and A358.

www.epa.gov/greenchemistry/.

B. Sustainability

Adams, W.M., Jeanrenaud, S.J., 2008. *Transition to Sustainability: Towards a Humane and Diverse World.* IUCN, Gland, Switzerland, p. 108.

Atkinson, G., Dietz, S., Neumayer, E., 2007. *Handbook of Sustainable Development.* Edward Elgar, Cheltenham.

Blackburn, W.R., 2007. *The Sustainability Handbook.* Earthscan, London.

Blewitt, J., 2008. *Understanding Sustainable Development.* Earthscan, London.

Costanza, R., Graumlich, L.J., Steffen, W. (Eds.), 2007. *Sustainability or Collapse? An Integrated History and Future of People on Earth.* MIT Press, Cambridge, MA.

Norton, B., 2005. *Sustainability, a Philosophy of Adaptive Ecosystem Management.* The University of Chicago Press, Chicago.

Soederbaum, P., 2008. *Understanding Sustainability Economics.* Earthscan, London.

C. Biorefinery

Liu, S., Lu, H., Hu, R., Shupe, A., Lin, L., Liang, L., 2012. A Sustainable Woody Biomass Biorefinery. J. Biotech. Adv http://dx.doi.org/10.1016/j.biotechadv.2012.01.013.

FitzPatrick, M., Champagne, P., Cunningham, M.F., Whitney, R.A., 2010. A biorefinery processing perspective: treatment of lignocellulosic materials for the production of value-added products. *Bioresour. Technol.* 101 (23), 8915–8922.

Kaparaju, P., Serrano, M., Thomsen, A.B., Kongjan, P., Angelidaki, I., 2009. Bioethanol, biohydrogen and biogas production from wheat straw in a biorefinery concept. *Bioresour. Technol.* 100 (9), 2562–2568.

Koutinas, A.A., Arifeen, N., Wang, R., Webb, C., 2007. Cereal-based biorefinery development: integrated enzyme production for cereal flour hydrolysis. *Biotechn. Bioeng.* 97 (1), 61–72.

Liu, S., Amidon, T.E., Francis, R.C., Ramarao, B.V., Lai, Y.-Z., Scott, G.M., 2006. From forest biomass to chemicals and energy: biorefinery initiative in New York. *Ind. Biotech.* 2 (2), 113–120.

Ohara, H., 2003. Biorefinery. *Appl. Micobiol. Biotechn.* 62 (5–6), 474–477.

D. History of Penicillin

Elder, A.L. (Ed.), 1970. *The History of Penicillin Production,* Chem. Eng. Prog. Symp. Ser. 66 (#100). American Institute of Chemical Engineers, New York.

Hobby, G.L., 1985. *Penicillin. Meeting the Challenge.* Yale University Press, New Haven, CT.

Mateles, R.I., 1998. *Penicillin: A Paradigm for Biotechnology.* Candida Corp., Chicago, IL.
Moberg, C.L., 1991. Penicillin's forgotten man: Norman Heatley. *Science* 253, 734–735.
Sheehan, J.C., 1982. *The Enchanted Ring. The Untold Story of Penicillin.* MIT Press, Cambridge, MA.

E. Regulatory Issues

Currey, B., Klemic, P.A., 2008. A new Phase in Pharmaceutical Regulation. DRI Drug and Medical Device and Product Liability Committee, O'Melveny & Myers LLP.
Durfor, C.N., Andscribner, C.L., 1992. An FDA perspective of manufacturing changes for products in human use. *Ann. NY Acad. Sci.* 665, 356–363.
Naglak, T.J., Keith, M.G., Omstead, D.R., 1994. Validation of fermentation processes. *Biophann* (July/Aug.) 28–36.
Reisman, H.B., 1993. Problems in scale-up of biotechnology production processes. *Crit. Rev. Biotechnol.* 13, 195–253.
Wechsler, J. Science and Safety. Magazine: Pharmaceutial Excutive – Washington Report, Oct., 2009.
http://www.FDA.gov
http://www.FDAreview.org/approval_process

PROBLEMS

1.1. Why are renewable materials preferred?
1.2. What is green chemistry?
1.3. What is sustainability?
1.4. What is a biorefinery?
1.5. Why is ethanol an important platform chemical?
1.6. An uninformed researcher is questioning the sustainability of biomass cultivation and utilization, arguing that fertilizer and fuels for heavy machinery must be produced with fossil energy and thus not renewable. Research into the basis of the arguments and dismiss the notion of unsustainable biomass use.
1.7. What is GMP and how does it relate to the regulatory process for pharmaceuticals?
1.8. When the FDA approves a process, it requires *validation* of the process. Explain what validation means in the FDA context.
1.9. Why does the FDA approve the process and product together?
1.10. What is biotransformation? What is chemical transformation?

CHAPTER

2

An Overview of Biological Basics

OUTLINE

Bioprocess engineers seek chemicals and materials for human needs in a sustainable manner. It is the chemicals and materials from biological origin that can sustain the needs of humans. Microorganism also provides a tool for bioprocess engineers to manipulate the chemicals and materials so that they can meet the needs of humanity. Therefore, we shall first review some of the biological basics to learn how living organisms (more specific: microorganisms) function and what their important chemicals and materials are.

2.1. CELLS AND ORGANISMS

The *cell* is the basic structural and functional unit of all known living organisms. Cells are to living organisms as like atoms are to molecules. It is the smallest unit of life that is

Bioprocess Engineering
http://dx.doi.org/10.1016/B978-0-444-59525-6.00002-0

classified as a living thing, and so is often called the building block of life. Some organisms, such as most bacteria, are unicellular (consist of a single cell). Other organisms, such as humans, are multicellular. (Humans have an estimated 100 trillion or 10^{14} cells; a typical cell size is 10 μm; a typical cell mass is 1 ng.) The largest known cell is an unfertilized ostrich egg cell. An average ostrich egg is an oval about 15 cm × 13 cm and weighs 1.4 kg.

In 1835, before modern cell theory was developed, Jan Evangelista Purkyně observed small "granules" while looking at plant tissue through a microscope. The cell theory, first developed in 1839 by Matthias Jakob Schleiden and Theodor Schwann, states that all organisms are composed of one or more cells, that all cells come from preexisting cells, that vital functions of an organism occur within cells, and that all cells contain the hereditary information necessary for regulating cell functions and for transmitting information to the next generation of cells.

Each cell is at least somewhat self-contained and self-maintaining: it can take in nutrients, convert these nutrients into energy, carry out specialized functions, and reproduce as necessary. Each cell stores its own set of instructions for carrying out each of these activities.

2.1.1. Microbial Diversity

Life is very tenacious and can exist in extreme environments. Living cells can be found almost anywhere that water is in the liquid state. The right temperature, pH, and moisture levels vary from one organism to another. Some cells can grow at −20 °C (in a brine to prevent freezing), while others can grow at 120 °C (where water is under high enough pressure to prevent boiling). Cells that grow best at low temperatures (below 20 °C) are usually called *psychrophiles*, while those with temperature optima in the range of 20°−50 °C are *mesophiles*. Organisms that grow best at temperatures greater than 50 °C are *thermophiles*.

Many organisms have pH optima far from neutrality; some prefer in an environment with a pH value down to 1 or 2, while others may grow well at pH 9. Some organisms can grow at both low pH values and high temperatures.

Although most organisms can grow only with the presence of liquid water, others can grow on barely moist solid surfaces or in solutions with high-salt concentrations.

Some cells require oxygen for growth and metabolism. Such organisms can be termed *aerobic*. Other organisms are inhibited by the presence of oxygen and grow only *anaerobically*. Some organisms can switch metabolic pathways to allow them to grow under either circumstance. Such organisms are *facultative*.

Often, organisms can grow in environments with almost no obvious source of nutrients. Some *cyanobacteria* (formerly called blue-green algae) can grow in an environment with only a little moisture and a few dissolved minerals. These bacteria are photosynthetic and can convert CO_2 from the atmosphere into the organic compounds necessary for life. They can also convert N_2 into NH_3 for use in making the essential building blocks of life.

$$CO_2 + H_2O \rightarrow CH_2O + O_2$$

$$N_2 + 3\,H_2O \rightarrow 2\,NH_3 + 3/2O_2$$

Cyanobacteria are important in colonizing nutrient-deficient environments. Organisms from these extreme environments (*extremophiles*) often provide humanity with important tools for processes to make useful chemicals and medicinals. They are also key to the maintenance of natural cycles and can be used in the recovery of metals from low-grade ores or in the desulfurization of coal or other fuels. The fact that organisms can develop a capacity to exist and multiply in almost any environment on Earth is extremely useful.

Not only do organisms occupy a wide variety of habitats, but they also come in a wide range of sizes and shapes. Spherical, cylindrical, ellipsoidal, spiral, and pleomorphic cells exist. Special names are used to describe the shape of bacteria. A cell with a spherical or elliptical shape is often called a *coccus* (plural, *cocci*); a cylindrical cell is a rod or *bacillus* (plural, *bacilli*); a spiral-shaped cell is a *spirillum* (plural, *spirilla*). Some cells may change shape in response to changes in their local environment. Pleomorphic cells take on at least two different forms or shapes during their life cycle.

Thus, organisms can be found in the most extreme environments and have evolved a wondrous array of shapes, sizes, and metabolic capabilities. This great diversity provides the engineer with an immense variety of potential tools. We have barely begun to learn how to manipulate these tools.

2.1.2. How Cells are Named

The naming of cells is complicated by the large variety of organisms. A systematic approach to classifying these organisms is an essential aid to their intelligent use. *Taxonomy* is the development of approaches to organize and summarize our knowledge about the variety of organisms that exist. Although knowledge of taxonomy may seem remote from the needs of an engineer, it is necessary for efficient communication among engineers and scientists working with living cells. Taxonomy can also play a critical role in patent litigation involving bioprocesses.

While taxonomy is concerned with approaches to classification, *nomenclature* refers to the actual naming of organisms. For microorganisms, we use a dual name (binary nomenclature). The names are given in Latin or are Latinized. A genus is a group of related species, while a species includes organisms that are sufficiently alike to reproduce. A common well-documented gut organism is *Escherichia coli*. *Escherichia* is the genus and *coli* the species. When writing a report or paper, it is common practice to give the full name when the organism is first mentioned, but to abbreviate the *genus* to the first letter in subsequent discussion, e.g. *E. coli*. Although organisms that belong to the same species all share the same major characteristics, there are subtle and often technologically important variations within species. A strain of *E. coli* used in one laboratory may differ from that used in another. Thus, various strains and substrains are designated by the addition of letters and numbers. For example, *E. coli* fBr5 will differ in growth and physiological properties from *E. coli* K01.

Now that we know how to name organisms, we could consider broader classification up to the level of kingdoms. There is no universal agreement on how to classify microorganisms at this level. Such classification is rather arbitrary and need not concern us. However, we must be aware that there are two primary cell types: *eukaryotic* and *prokaryotic*. The primary difference between them is the presence or absence of a membrane around the cell's genetic information.

Prokaryotes have a simple structure with a single chromosome (Fig. 2.1). Prokaryotic cells have no nuclear membrane and no organelles (such as mitochondria and endoplasmic

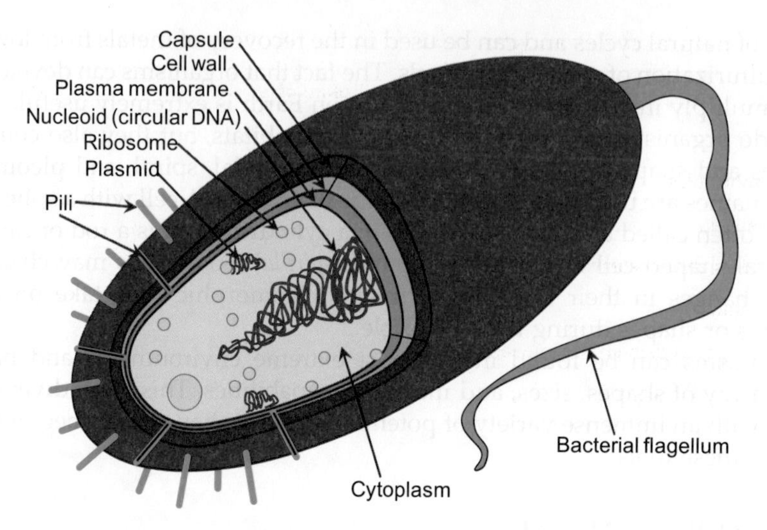

FIGURE 2.1 A schematic of a typical prokaryotic cell.

reticulum). Eukaryotes have a more complex internal structure, with more than one chromosome (DNA molecule) in the nucleus. Eukaryotic cells have a true nuclear membrane and may contain a variety of specialized organelles such as mitochondria, endoplasmic reticulum, and Golgi apparatus (Fig. 2.2). A detailed comparison of prokaryotes and eukaryotes is presented in Table 2.1. Structural differences between prokaryotes and eukaryotes are discussed later.

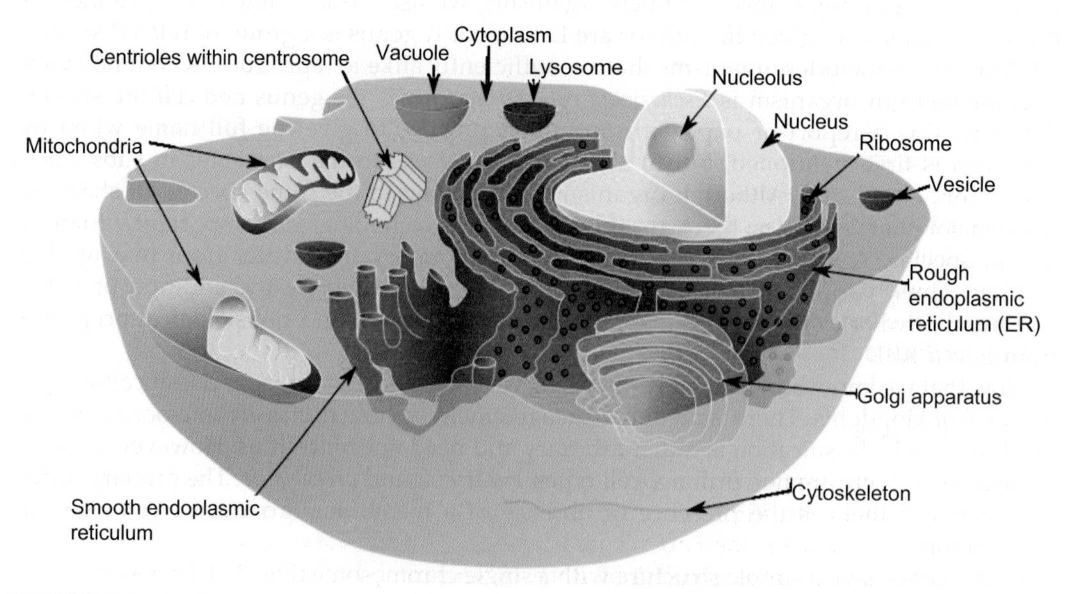

FIGURE 2.2 A schematic of a typical eukaryotic cell.

TABLE 2.1 A comparison of Prokaryotes with Eukaryotes

Characteristic	Prokaryotes	Eukaryotes
Genome		
No. of DNA molecules	One	More than one
DNA in organelles	No	Yes
DNA observed as chromosomes	No	Yes
Nuclear membrane	No	Yes
Mitotic and meiotic division of the nucleus	No	Yes
Formation of partial diploid	Yes	No
Organelles		
Mitochondria	No	Yes
Endoplasmic reticulum	No	Yes
Golgi apparatus	No	Yes
Photosynthetic apparatus	Chromosomes	Chloroplasts
Flagella	Single protein, simple structure	Complex structure, with microtubules
Spores	Endospores	Endo- and exospores
Heat resistance	High	Low

Source: Millis NF in Comprehensive Biotechnology, *M. Moo-Young, ed., Vol. I, Elsevier Science, 1985.*

Evidence suggests that a common or universal ancestor gave rise to three distinctive branches of life: eukaryotes, eubacteria (or "true" bacteria), and archaebacteria. Table 2.2 summarizes some of the distinctive features of these groups. The ability to sequence the genes of whole organisms will have a great impact on our understanding of how these families evolved and are related.

The cellular organisms summarized in Table 2.2 are free-living organisms and are all DNA based. Viruses cannot be classified under any of these categories, as they are not independent (or free-living) organisms. Still, viruses are all nucleic acid (either DNA or RNA) based. Prions, on the other hand, are not even nucleic acid based. Let's consider first some of the characteristics of these rather simple "organisms."

2.1.3. Viruses

Viruses are very small and are obligate parasites of other cells, such as bacterial, yeast, plant, and animal cells. Viruses cannot capture or store free energy and are not functionally active except when inside their host cells. The sizes of viruses vary from 30 to 200 nm. Viruses contain either DNA (DNA viruses) or RNA (RNA viruses) as genetic material. DNA and RNA molecules will be discussed in §2.3.6 in more detail. In free-living cells, all genetic

TABLE 2.2 Primary Subdivisions of Cellular Organisms that Have Been Recognized

Group	Cell morphology	Properties	Constituent groups
Eukaryotes	Eukaryotic	Multicellular; extensive differentiation of cells and tissues Unicellular, coenocytic or mycelial; little or no tissue differentiation	Plants (seed plants, ferns, mosses) Animals (vertebrates, invertebrates) Protists (algae, fungi, protozoa, slime molds)
Eubacteria	Prokaryotic	Cell chemistry similar to eukaryotes	Most bacteria
Archaea	Prokaryotic	Distinctive cell chemistry	Crenarchaeota (sulfolobus, therofilum, thermopteus, pyrobaculum, haloquadratum walsbyi) Nanoarchaeota Euryarchaeota (methanogens, halophiles, thermoacidophiles) Korarchaeota

information is contained in the DNA, whereas viruses can use either RNA or DNA to encode such information. This nuclear material is covered by a protein coat called a *capsid*. Some viruses have an outer envelope of a lipoprotein and some do not.

Almost all cell types are susceptible to viral infections. Viruses infecting bacteria are called *bacteriophages*. The most common type of bacteriophage has a hexagonal head, tail, and tail fibers as shown in Fig. 2.3. Bacteriophages attach to the cell wall of a host cell with tail fibers,

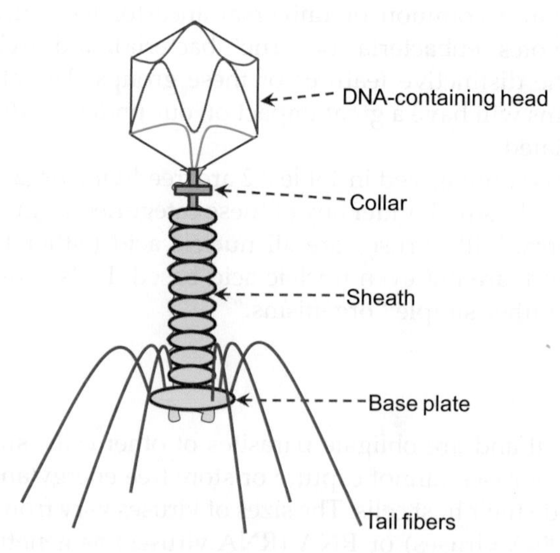

FIGURE 2.3 The structure of a typical bacteriophage.

alter the cell wall of the host cell, and inject the viral nuclear material into the host cell. Figure 2.4 describes the attachment of a virus onto a host cell. Bacteriophage nucleic acids reproduce inside the host cells to produce more phages. At a certain stage of viral reproduction, host cells lyse or break apart and the new phages are released, which can infect new host cells. This mode of reproduction of viruses is called the *lytic cycle.* In some cases, phage DNA may be incorporated into the host DNA, and the host may continue to multiply in this state, which is called the *lysogenic cycle.*

Viruses are the cause of many diseases, and antiviral agents are important targets for drug discovery. However, viruses are also important to bioprocess technology. For example, a phage attack on an *E. coli* fermentation to make a recombinant protein product can be extremely destructive, causing the loss of the whole culture in vessels of many thousands of liters. However, phages can be used as agents to move desired genetic material into *E. coli.* Modified animal viruses can be used as vectors to genetically engineer animal cells to produce proteins from recombinant DNA technology. In some cases, a killed virus preparation can be used as a vaccine. Genetic engineering allows the production of virus-like units that are empty shells; the shell is the capsid and all nucleic acid is removed. Such units can be used as vaccines without fear of viral infection or replication, since all of the genetic material has been removed. For gene therapy, one approach is to use a virus where viral genetic material has been replaced with the desired gene to be inserted into the patient. The viral capsid can act as a Trojan Horse to protect the desired gene in a hostile environment and then to

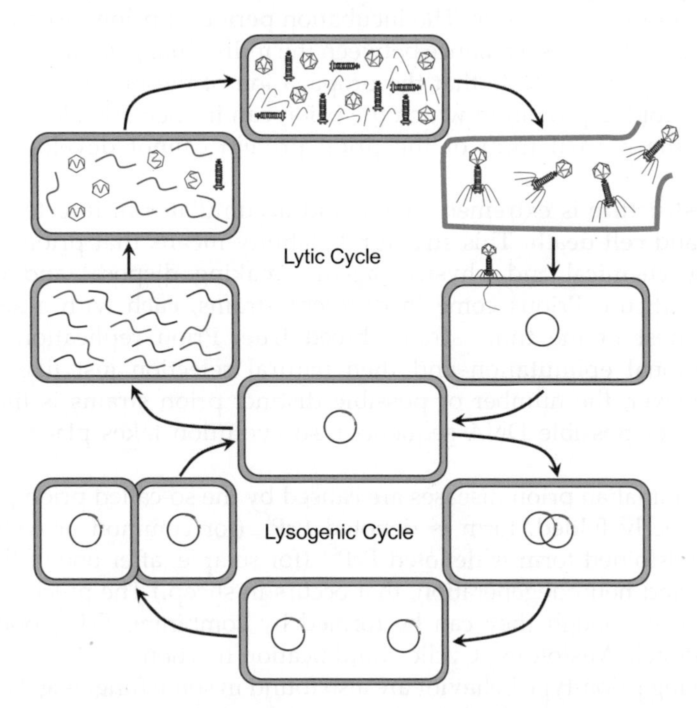

FIGURE 2.4 Replication of a virulent bacteriophage. A virulent phage undergoes a lytic cycle to produce new phage particles within a bacterial cell. *Cell lysis* releases new phage particles that can infect more bacteria.

deliver it selectively to a particular cell type. Thus, viruses can do great harm but can also be important biotechnological tools.

2.1.4. Prions

A prion is an infectious agent composed of protein in a misfolded form. This is in contrast to all other known infectious agents that must contain nucleic acids (either DNA, RNA, or both). The word prion, coined in 1982 by Stanley B. Prusiner, is a portmanteau derived from the words protein and infection. Prions are responsible for the transmissible spongiform encephalopathies in a variety of mammals, including bovine spongiform encephalopathy (also known as "mad cow disease") in cattle and Creutzfeldt–Jakob disease in humans. All known prion diseases affect the structure of the brain or other neural tissue and all are currently untreatable and universally fatal.

Prions propagate by transmitting a misfolded protein state. When a prion enters a healthy organism, it induces existing, properly folded proteins to convert into the disease-associated, prion form; the prion acts as a template to guide the misfolding of more protein into prion form. The newly formed prions can continue to convert more proteins themselves; this triggers a chain reaction that produces large amounts of the prion form. All known prions induce the formation of an amyloid fold, in which the protein polymerizes into an aggregate consisting of tightly packed beta sheets. Amyloid aggregates are fibrils, growing at their ends, and replicating when breakage causes two growing ends to become four growing ends. The incubation period of prion diseases is determined by prion replication, which is a balance between the individual prior aggregate growth and the breakage of aggregates. Note that the propagation of the prion depends on the presence of normally folded protein in which the prion can induce misfolding, animals which do not express the normal form of the prion protein cannot develop or transmit the disease.

This altered structure is extremely stable and accumulates in infected tissue, causing tissue damage and cell death. This structural stability means that prions are resistant to denaturation by chemical and physical agents, making disposal and containment of these particles difficult. Prions come in different strains, each with a slightly different structure, and most of the time, strains breed true. Prion replication is nevertheless subject to occasional epimutation and then natural selection just like other forms of replication. However, the number of possible distinct prion strains is likely far smaller than the number of possible DNA sequences, so evolution takes place within a limited space.

All known mammalian prion diseases are caused by the so-called prion protein, PrP. The endogenous, properly folded, form is denoted PrP^{C} (for common or cellular) while the disease-linked, misfolded form is denoted PrP^{Sc} (for scrapie, after one of the diseases first linked to prions and neurodegeneration, that occurs in sheep.) The precise structure of the prion is not known, though they can be formed by combining PrP^{C}, polyadenylic acid, and lipids in a Protein Misfolding Cyclic Amplification reaction.

Proteins showing prion-type behavior are also found in some fungi (e.g. *Saccharomyces cerevisiae* and *Podospora anserine*), which has been useful in helping to understand mammalian prions. Interestingly, fungal prions do not appear to cause disease in their hosts.

2.1.5. Prokaryotes

The sizes of most prokaryotes vary from 0.5 to 3 μm in equivalent radius. Different species have different shapes, such as spherical or coccus (e.g. *Staphylococci*), cylindrical or bacillus (*E. coli*), or spiral or spirillum (*Rhodospirillum*). Prokaryotic cells grow rapidly, with typical doubling times of half an hour to several hours. Also, prokaryotes can utilize a variety of nutrients as carbon sources, including carbohydrates, hydrocarbons, proteins, and CO_2.

2.1.5.1. Eubacteria

The Eubacteria can be divided into several different groups. One distinction is based on the gram stain (developed by Hans Christian Gram in 1884). The staining procedure first requires fixing the cells by heating. The basic dye, crystal violet, is added; all bacteria will stain purple. Next, iodine is added, followed by the addition of ethanol. *Gram-positive* cells remain purple, while *gram-negative* cells become colorless. Finally, counterstaining with safranin leaves gram-positive cells purple, while gram-negative cells turn red. Cell reactions to the gram stain reveal intrinsic differences in the structure of the cell envelope.

A typical gram-negative cell is *E. coli*. It has an *outer membrane* supported by a thin peptidoglycan layer, as shown in Fig. 2.5. *Peptidoglycan* is a complex polysaccharide with amino acids and forms a structure somewhat analogous to a chain-link fence. A second membrane (the inner or *cytoplasmic membrane*) exists and is separated from the outer membrane by the *periplasmic space*. The cytoplasmic membrane contains about 50% protein, 30% lipids, and 20% carbohydrates. The cell envelope serves to retain important cellular compounds and to preferentially exclude undesirable compounds in the environment. Loss of membrane integrity leads to *cell lysis* (cells breaking open) and cell death. The cell envelope is crucial to the transport of selected material in and out of the cell.

A typical gram-positive cell is *Bacillus subtilis*. Gram-positive cells do not have an outer membrane. Rather, they have a very thick, rigid cell wall with multiple layers of peptidoglycan. Gram-positive cells also contain *teichoic acids* covalently bonded to the peptidoglycan. Because gram-positive bacteria have only a cytoplasmic membrane, they are better suited to excretion of proteins. Excretion is technologically advantageous when the protein is a desired product.

Some bacteria are neither gram-positive nor gram-negative. For example, *Mycoplasma* has no cell walls. These bacteria are important not only clinically (e.g. primary atypical pneumonia) but also because they commonly contaminate media used industrially for animal cell culture.

Actinomycetes are bacteria but morphologically resemble molds with their long and highly branched hyphae. However, the lack of a nuclear membrane and the composition of the cell wall require classification as bacteria. Actinomycetes are important sources of antibiotics. Certain Actinomycetes possess amylolytic and cellulolytic enzymes and are effective in the enzymatic hydrolysis of starch and cellulose. *Actinomyces*, *Thermomonospora*, and *Streptomyces* are examples of genera belonging to this group.

Other distinctions within the eubacteria can be made based on cellular nutrition and energy metabolism. One important example is photosynthesis. Cyanobacteria (formerly called blue-green algae) have chlorophyll and fix CO_2 into sugars. Anoxygenic photosynthetic bacteria (the purple and green bacteria) have light-gathering pigments called *bacteriochlorophyll*. Unlike true photosynthesis, the purple and green bacteria do not obtain reduction energy from the splitting of water and do not form oxygen.

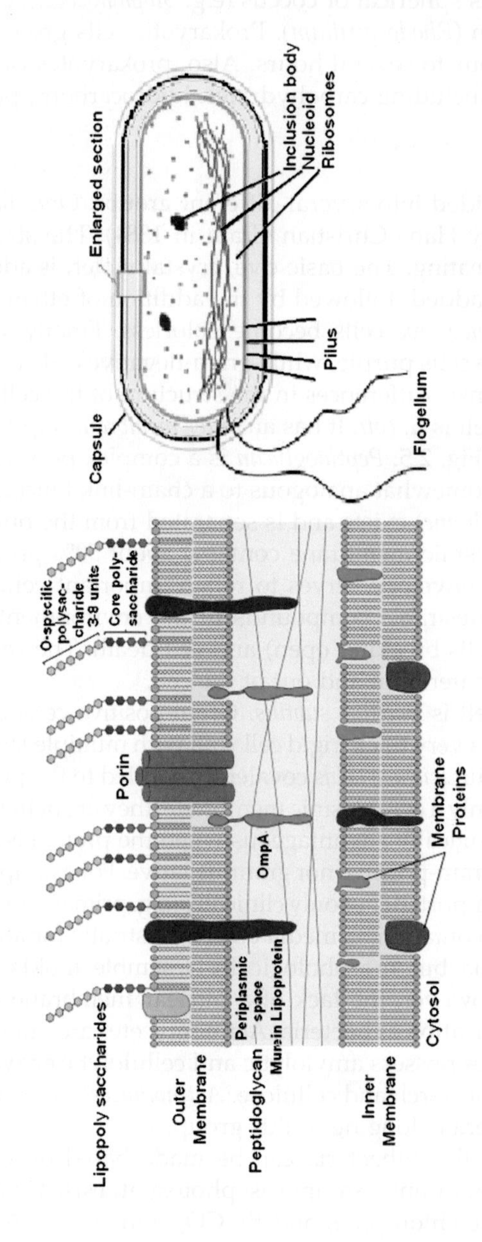

FIGURE 2.5 Schematic of a typical gram-negative bacterium. A gram-positive cell is similar, except that it has no outer membrane, its peptidoglycan layer is thicker, and the chemical composition of the cell wall differs significantly from the outer envelope of the gram-negative cell.

When stained properly, the area occupied by a prokaryotic cell's DNA can be easily seen. Prokaryotes may also have other visible structures when viewed under the microscope, such as *ribosomes*, *storage granules*, *spores*, and *volutins*. Ribosomes are the site of protein synthesis. A typical bacterial cell contains approximately 10,000 ribosomes per cell, although this number can vary greatly with growth rate. The size of a typical ribosome is 10–20 nm and consists of approximately 63% RNA and 37% protein. Storage granules (which are not present in every bacterium) can be used as a source of key metabolites and often contain polysaccharides, lipids, and sulfur granules. The sizes of storage granules vary between 0.5 and 1 μm. Some bacteria make intracellular spores (often called endospores in bacteria). Bacterial spores are produced as a resistance to adverse conditions such as high temperature, radiation, and toxic chemicals. The usual concentration is 1 spore per cell, with a spore size of about 1 μm. Spores can germinate under favorable growth conditions to yield actively growing bacteria.

Volutin is another granular intracellular structure, made of inorganic polymetaphosphates, that is present in some species. Some photosynthetic bacteria, such as *Rhodospirillum*, have chromatophores that are large inclusion bodies (50–100 nm) utilized in photosynthesis for the absorption of light.

Extracellular products can adhere to or become incorporated within the surface of the cell. Certain bacteria have a coating or outside cell wall called *capsule*, which is usually a polysaccharide or sometimes a polypeptide. Extracellular polymers are important to biofilm formation and response to environmental challenges (e.g. viruses). Table 2.3 summarizes the architecture of most bacteria.

2.1.5.2. Archaebacteria

Under the microscope, archaebacteria appear to be nearly identical to eubacteria. However, these cells differ greatly at the molecular level. In many ways, the archaebacteria are as similar to the eukaryotes as they are to the eubacteria. Some examples of differences between archaebacteria and eubacteria are as follows:

(1) Archaebacteria have no peptidoglycan.
(2) Nucleotide sequences in ribosomal RNA are similar within the archaebacteria but distinctly different from those of eubacteria.
(3) The lipid composition of the cytoplasmic membrane is very different for the two groups.

Archaebacteria usually live in extreme environments and possess unusual metabolism. Methanogens, which are methane-producing bacteria, belong to this group, as well as thermoacidophiles, which can grow at high temperatures and low pH values. Halobacteria, which can live only in very strong salt solutions, are also members of this group. These organisms are important sources for catalytically active proteins (enzymes) with novel properties.

2.1.6. Eukaryotes

Fungi (yeasts and molds), algae, protozoa, and animal and plant cells constitute the eukaryotes. Eukaryotes are five to ten times larger than prokaryotes in diameter (e.g. yeast about 5 μm, animal cells about 10 μm, and plants about 20 μm). Eukaryotes have a true

TABLE 2.3 Characteristics of Various Components of Bacteria

Part	Size	Composition and comments
SLIME LAYER		
Microcapsule	5–10 nm	Protein–polysaccharide–lipid complex responsible for the specific antigens of enteric bacteria and other species.
Capsule	0.5–2.0 μm	Mainly polysaccharides (e.g. *Streptococcus*); sometimes polypeptides (e.g. *Bacillus anthracis*).
Slime	Indefinite	Mainly polysaccharides (e.g. *Leuconostoc*); sometimes polypeptides (e.g. *Bacillus subtilis*).
CELL WALL		
Gram-positive species	10–20 nm	Confers shape and rigidity upon the cell. 20% dry weight of the cell. Consists mainly of macromolecules of a mixed polymer of *N*-acetyl muramic peptide, teichoic acids, and polysaccharides.
Gram-negative species	10–20 nm	Consists mostly of a protein–polysaccharide–lipid complex with a small amount of the muramic polymer.
Cell membrane	5–10 nm	Semipermeable barrier to nutrients. 5–10% dry weight of the cell, consisting of 50% protein, 28% lipid, and 15–20% carbohydrate in a double-layered membrane.
Flagellum	10–20 nm by 4–12 μm	Protein of the myosin–keratin–fibrinogen class, MW of 40,000. Arises from the cell membrane and is responsible for motility.
Pilus (fimbria)	5–10 nm by 0.5–2.0 μm	Rigid protein projections from the cell. Especially long ones are formed by *Escherichia coli.*
INCLUSIONS		
Spore	1.0–1.5 μm by 1.6–2.0 μm	One spore is formed per cell intracellularly. Spores show great resistance to heat, dryness, and antibacterial agents.
Storage granule	0.5–2.0 μm	Glycogen like, sulfur, or lipid granules may be found in some species.
Chromatophore	50–100 nm	Organelles in photosynthetic species. *Rhodospirillum rubrum* contains about 6000 per cell.
Ribosome	10–30 nm	Organelles for synthesis of protein. About 10,000 ribosomes per cell. They contain 63% RNA and 37% protein.
Volutin	0.5–1.0 μm	Inorganic polymetaphosphates that stain metachromatically.
Nuclear material		Composed of DNA that functions genetically as if the genes were arranged linearly on a single endless chromosome but that appears by light microscopy as irregular patches with no nuclear membrane or distinguishable chromosomes. Autoradiography confirms the linear arrangement of DNA and suggests an MW of at least 10^9.

Source: S. Aiba, A. E. Humphrey, and N. F. Millis, Biochemical Engineering, *2d ed., University of Tokyo Press, Tokyo, 1973.*

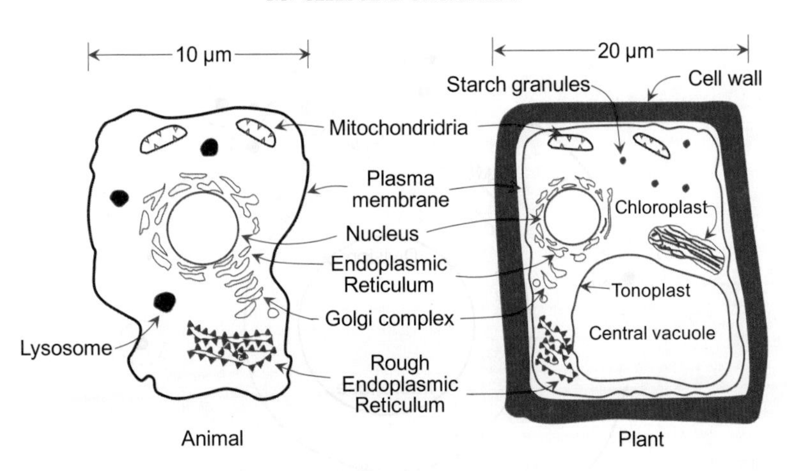

FIGURE 2.6 Sketches of the two primary types of higher eukaryotic cells. Neither sketch is complete, but each summarizes the principal differences and similarities of such cells.

nucleus and a number of cellular organelles inside the cytoplasm. Figure 2.6 is a schematic of two typical eukaryotic cells.

In cell wall and cell membrane structure, eukaryotes are similar to prokaryotes. The plasma membrane is made of proteins and phospholipids that form a bilayer structure. Major proteins of the membrane are hydrophobic and are embedded in the phospholipid matrix. One major difference is the presence of sterols in the cytoplasmic membrane of eukaryotes. Sterols strengthen the structure and make the membrane less flexible. The cell wall of eukaryotic cells shows considerable variations. Some eukaryotes have a peptidoglycan layer in their cell wall; some have polysaccharides and cellulose (e.g. algae). The plant cell wall is composed of cellulose fibers embedded in pectin aggregates, which impart strength to the cell wall. Animal cells do not have a cell wall but only a cytoplasmic membrane. For this reason, animal cells are very shear-sensitive and fragile. This factor significantly complicates the design of large-scale bioreactors for animal cells.

The *nucleus* of eukaryotic cells contains *chromosomes* as nuclear material (DNA molecules with some closely associated small proteins), surrounded by a membrane. The nuclear membrane consists of a pair of concentric and porous membranes. The nucleolus is an area in the nucleus that stains differently and is the site of ribosome synthesis. Many chromosomes contain small amounts of RNA and basic proteins called *histones* attached to the DNA. Each chromosome contains a single linear DNA molecule on which the histones are attached.

Cell division (asexual) in eukaryotes involves several major steps: DNA synthesis, nuclear division, cell division, and cell separation. Sexual reproduction in eukaryotic cells involves the conjugation of two cells called *gametes* (egg and sperm cells). The single cell formed from the conjugation of gametes is called a *zygote.* The zygote has twice as many chromosomes as the gamete. Gametes are *haploid* cells, while zygotes are *diploid.* For humans, a haploid cell contains 23 chromosomes, and diploid cells have 46. The cell-division cycle (asexual reproduction) in a eukaryotic cell is depicted in Fig. 2.7.

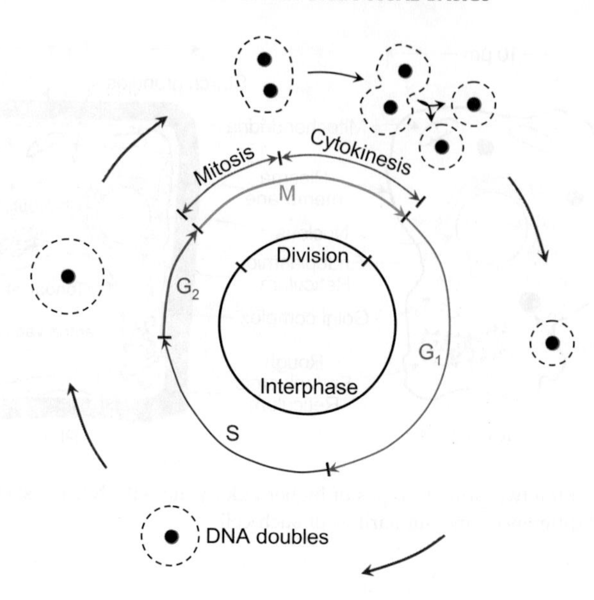

FIGURE 2.7 Schematic of cell-division cycle in a eukaryote. (See text for details.)

The cell-division cycle is divided into four phases. The M phase consists of *mitosis* where the nucleus divides, and *cytokinesis* where the cell splits into separate daughter cells. All of the phases between one M phase and the next are known collectively as *interphase.* The interphase is divided into three phases: G_1, S, and G_2.The cell increases in size during the interphase. In the S phase, the cell replicates its nuclear DNA. There are key checkpoints in the cycle when the cell machinery must commit to entry to the next phase. Checkpoints exist for entry into the S and M phases and exit from the M phase. Cells may also be in a G_0 state, which is a resting state without growth.

Mitochondria are the powerhouses of a eukaryotic cell, where respiration and oxidative phosphorylation take place. Mitochondria have a nearly cylindrical shape 1 μm in diameter and 2−3 μm in length. A typical structure of a mitochondrion is shown in Fig. 2.8. The external membrane is made of a phospholipid bilayer with proteins embedded in the lipid matrix. Mitochondria contain a complex system of inner membranes called *cristae.* A gel-like matrix containing large amounts of protein fills the space inside the cristae. Some enzymes of oxidative respiration are bound to the cristae. A mitochondrion has its own DNA and protein-synthesizing machinery and reproduces independently.

The *endoplasmic reticulum* is a complex, convoluted membrane system leading from the cell membrane into the cell. The rough endoplasmic reticulum contains ribosomes on the inner surfaces and is the site of protein synthesis and modifications of protein structure after synthesis. The smooth endoplasmic reticulum is more involved with lipid synthesis.

Lysosomes are very small membrane-bound particles that contain and release digestive enzymes. Lysosomes contribute to the digestion of nutrients and invading substances. *Peroxisomes* are similar to lysosomes in their structure but not in function. Peroxisomes carry out

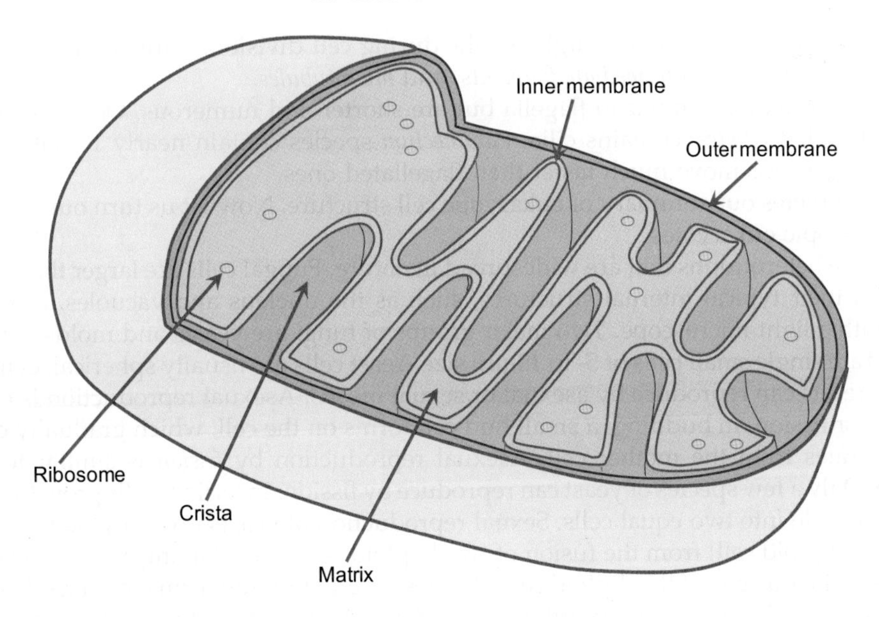

FIGURE 2.8 Diagram of a mitochondrion.

oxidative reactions that produce hydrogen peroxide. *Glyoxysomes* are also very small membrane-bound particles that contain the enzymes of the glyoxylate cycle.

Golgi bodies are very small particles composed of membrane aggregates and are responsible for the secretion of certain proteins. Golgi bodies are sites where proteins are modified by the addition of various sugars in a process called *glycosylation*. Such modifications are important to protein function in the body.

Vacuoles are membrane-bound organelles of low density and are responsible for food digestion, osmotic regulation, and waste product storage. Vacuoles may occupy a large fraction of the cell volume (up to 90% in plant cells).

Chloroplasts are relatively large green organelles containing chlorophyll that are responsible for photosynthesis in photosynthetic eukaryotes, such as algae and plant cells. Every chloroplast contains an outer membrane and a large number of inner membranes called *thylakoids*. Chlorophyll molecules are associated with thylakoids, which have a regular membrane structure with lipid bilayers. Chloroplasts are autonomous units containing their own DNA and protein-synthesizing machinery.

Certain prokaryotic and eukaryotic organisms contain flagella—long, filamentous structures that are attached to one end of the cell and are responsible for the motion of the cell. Eukaryotic flagella contain two central fibers surrounded by 18 peripheral fibers, which exist in duplets. These fibers are arranged in a tube structure called a *microtubule* and are composed of proteins called tubulin. The whole fiber assembly is embedded in an organic matrix and is surrounded by a membrane.

The *cytoskeleton* (in eukaryotic cells) refers to filaments that provide an internal framework to organize the cell's internal activities and control its shape. These filaments are critical to cell movement, transduction of mechanical forces into biological responses, and separation of chromosomes into the two daughter cells during cell division. Three types of fibers are present: *actin filaments*, *intermediate filaments*, and *microtubules*.

Cilia are structures similar to flagella but are shorter and numerous. Only one group of protozoa, called *ciliates*, contains cilia. *Paramecium* species contain nearly 10^4 cilia per cell. Ciliated organisms move much faster than flagellated ones.

This completes our summary of eukaryotic cell structure. Now let us turn our attention to the microscopic eukaryotes.

Fungi are heterotrophs that are widespread in nature. Fungal cells are larger than bacterial cells, and their typical internal structures, such as the nucleus and vacuoles, can be seen easily with a light microscope. Two major groups of fungi are yeasts and molds.

Yeasts are single small cells of 5- to 10-μm size. Yeast cells are usually spherical, cylindrical, or oval. Yeasts can reproduce by asexual or sexual means. Asexual reproduction is by either budding or fission. In budding, a small bud cell forms on the cell, which gradually enlarges and separates from the mother cell. Asexual reproduction by *fission* is similar to that of bacteria. Only a few species of yeast can reproduce by fission. In fission, cells grow to a certain size and divide into two equal cells. Sexual reproduction of yeasts involves the formation of a *zygote* (a diploid cell) from the fusion of two haploid cells, each having a single set of chromosomes. The nucleus of the diploid cells divides several times to form *ascospores*. Each ascospore eventually becomes a new haploid cell and may reproduce by budding and fission. The life cycle of a typical yeast cell is presented in Fig. 2.9.

The classification of yeasts is based on reproductive modes (e.g. budding or fission) and the nutritional requirements of cells. The most widely used yeast, *S. cerevisiae*, is used in alcohol formation under anaerobic conditions (e.g. in wine, beer, and whiskey making) and also for baker's yeast production under aerobic conditions.

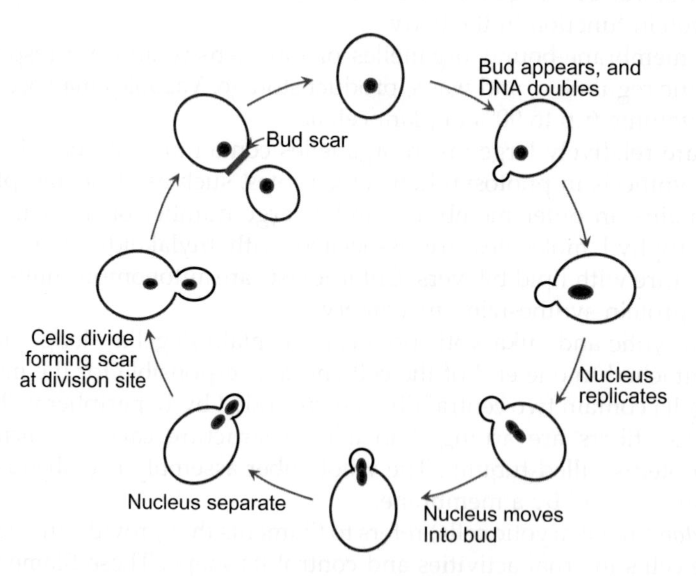

FIGURE 2.9 Cell-division cycle of a typical yeast, *Saccharomyces cerevisiae*.

Molds are filamentous fungi and have a mycelial structure. The *mycelium* is a highly branched system of tubes that contains mobile cytoplasm with many nuclei. Long, thin filaments on the mycelium are called *hyphae*. Certain branches of mycelium may grow in the air, and asexual spores called *conidia* are formed on these aerial branches. Conidia are nearly spherical in structure and are often pigmented. Some molds reproduce by sexual means and form sexual spores. These spores provide resistance against heat, freezing, drying, and some chemical agents. Both sexual and asexual spores of molds can germinate and form new hyphae. Figure 2.10 describes the structure and asexual reproduction of molds.

Molds usually form long, highly branched cells and easily grow on moist, solid nutrient surfaces. The typical size of a filamentous mold is 5–20 μm. When grown in submerged culture, molds often form cell aggregates and pellets. The typical size of a mold pellet varies between 50 μm and 1 mm, depending on the type of mold and growth conditions. Pellet formation can cause some nutrient-transfer (mainly oxygen) problems inside the pellet. However, pellet formation reduces broth viscosity, which can improve bulk oxygen transfer.

On the basis of their mode of sexual reproduction, fungi are grouped into four classes.

(1) The phycomycetes are algalike fungi; however, they do not possess chlorophyll and cannot photosynthesize. Aquatic and terrestrial molds belong to this category.

(2) The ascomycetes form sexual spores called ascospores, which are contained within a sac (a capsule structure). Some molds of the genera *Neurospora* and *Aspergillus* and yeasts belong to this category.

(3) The basidiomycetes reproduce by basidiospores, which are extended from the stalks of specialized cells called the basidia. Mushrooms are basidiomycetes.

(4) The deuteromycetes (*Fungi imperfecti*) cannot reproduce by sexual means. Only asexually reproducing molds belong to this category. Some pathogenic fungi, such as *Trichophyton*, which causes athlete's foot, belong to the deuteromycetes.

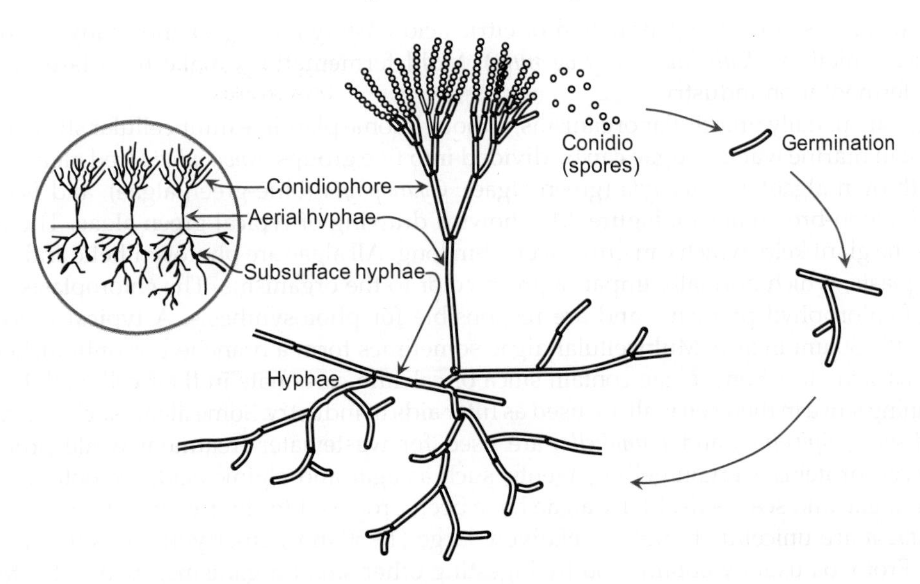

FIGURE 2.10 Structure and asexual reproduction of molds.

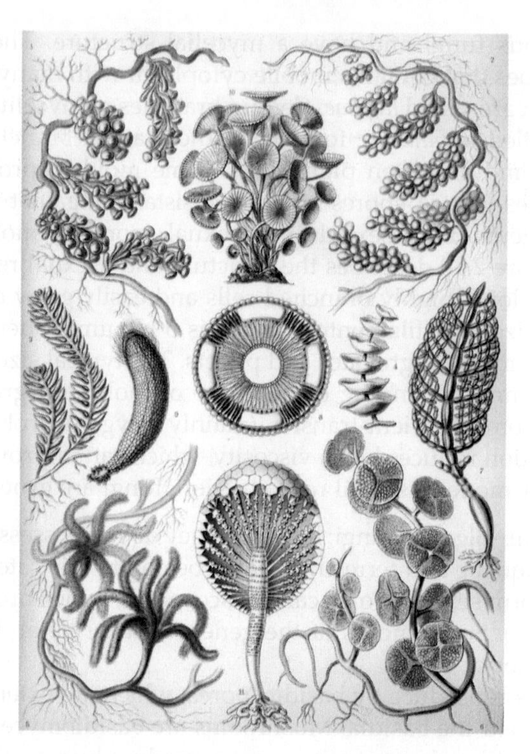

FIGURE 2.11 A sketch of green algae. *Source: "Siphoneae", Ernst Haecket, Kunstformen der Natur, 1904.*

Molds are used for the production of citric acid (*Aspergillus niger*) and many antibiotics, such as penicillin (*Penicillium chrysogenum*). Mold fermentations make up a large fraction of the fermentation industry.

Algae are usually unicellular organisms, although some plantlike multicellular structures are present in marine waters. Algae can be divided into five groups: *Rhodophyta* (red algae), *Phaeophyta* (brown algae), *Chlorophyta* (green algae), *Cyanophyta* (blue-green algae), and *Bacillariophyta* (golden-brown algae). Figure 2.11 shows a drawing of typical green algae. The largest alga is the giant kelp, which can grow over 60-m long. All algae are photosynthetic and contain chloroplasts, which normally impart a green color to the organisms. The chloroplasts are the sites of chlorophyll pigments and are responsible for photosynthesis. A typical unicellular alga is 10−30 μm in size. Multicellular algae sometimes form a branched or unbranched filamentous structure. Some algae contain silica or calcium carbonate in their cell wall. Diatoms containing silica in their cell wall are used as filter aids in industry. Some algae, such as *Chlorella*, *Scenedesmus*, *Spirulina*, and *Dunaliella*, are used for wastewater treatment while producing single-cell proteins. Certain gelling agents, such as agar and alginic acid, are obtained from marine algae and seaweeds. Many algae have been proposed for biofuel production.

Protozoa are unicellular, motile, relatively large (1−50 mm) eukaryotic cells that lack cell walls. Protozoa usually obtain food by ingesting other small organisms, such as bacteria or other food particles. Protozoa are usually uninucleate and reproduce by sexual or asexual means. They are classified on the basis of their motion. The *amoebae* move through ameboid motion, whereby the cytoplasm of the cell flows forward to form a pseudopodium (false foot), and the rest of the cell flows toward this lobe. The *flagellates* move using their flagella. *Trypanosomes* move by flagella and cause a number of diseases in humans. The *ciliates* move through motion of a large number of small appendages on the cell surface called *cilia*. The *sporozoans* are nonmotile and contain members that are human and animal parasites. These protozoa do not engulf food particles but absorb dissolved food components through their membranes. Protozoa cause some diseases, such as malaria and dysentery. Protozoa may have a beneficial role in removing bacteria in biological wastewater treatment processes.

2.2. STEM CELL

Stem cells are unspecialized cells (in multicellular organisms) that have two defining properties: 1) potency or the ability to differentiate into diverse specialized cells including differentiated stem cells and 2) reproductivity or the ability to duplicate.

Stem cells are found in all multicellular organisms. In mammals, there are two broad types of stem cells: embryonic stem cells and adult stem cells. Adult stem cells, also known as somatic (from Greek, "of the body") stem cells and germline (giving rise to gametes) stem cells, are found in various tissues and in children as well as adults. In adult organisms, stem cells and progenitor cells act as a repair system for the body, replenishing adult tissues. Embryonic stem cells are isolated from the inner cell mass of blastocysts. In a developing embryo, stem cells can differentiate into all the specialized cells (these are called pluripotent cells) but also maintain the normal turnover of regenerative organs, such as blood, skin, or intestinal tissues.

The ability to differentiate is the potential to develop into other cell types. Table 2.4 shows the potency of the stem cells. In a normal development of a multicellular organism, a totipotent stem cell (e.g. spores and fertilized egg) is the stem cell having the highest potency, which can differentiate into all cell types including the embryonic membranes, pluripotent cells,

TABLE 2.4 Potency or the Differentiation Potential of the Stem Cell

Stem cell type	Potency: types of stem cells can be produced.
Totipotent (or omnipotent)	Can differentiate into embryonic and extraembryonic cell types. Such cells can construct a complete, viable multicellular organism, for example, spores and fertilized egg. These cells are produced from the fusion of an egg and sperm cell. Cells produced by the first few divisions of the fertilized egg are also totipotent.
Pluripotent	Descendants of totipotent cells. Can differentiate into nearly all cells, i.e., cells derived from any of the three germ layers.
Multipotent	Can differentiate into a number of stem cell types, but only those of a closely related family of cells.
Oligopotent	Can differentiate into only a few stem cell types, such as lymphoid or myeloid stem cells.
Unipotent	Can produce only one stem cell type, their own, but have the property of self-renewal, which distinguishes them from nonstem cells (e.g. muscle stem cells).

multipotent cells, oligopotent cells, unipotent cells, and terminal cells. A pluripotent stem cell can develop into cells from all three germinal layers (e.g. cells from the inner cell mass). Other cells can be oligopotent, bipotent, or unipotent depending on their ability to differentiate into few, two or one other cell type(s). Stem cell's differentiation is regulated in a feedback mechanism. In normal developments, stem cell differentiation observe strict lineage, that is, cells in general do not "differentiate" back to their "parent" cell type(s), nor their "cousin" types.

Reproductivity is the ability of stem cells to divide and produce more stem cells of the same type without differentiation. During early development, the cell division is symmetrical, i.e. each cell divides to two daughter cells each with the same potential. Later in development, the cell divides asymmetrically to two cells with one of the daughter cells preserving the stem cell type and the other a more differentiated cell.

Stem cells can be artificially grown and transformed into specialized cell types with characteristics consistent with cells of various tissues such as muscles or nerves through cell culture. Highly plastic adult stem cells are routinely used in medical therapies. Stem cells can be taken from a variety of sources, including umbilical cord blood and bone marrow.

To ensure reproductivity, stem cells undergo two types of cell divisions. Symmetric division gives rise to two identical daughter cells both endowed with the same stem cell properties (or potency). For example, one cell of totipotency divides to two cells of totipotency. Asymmetric division, on the other hand, produces only one stem cell (of the same potency) and a progenitor cell with limited self-renewal potential (or lower potency). Progenitors can go through several rounds of cell division before terminally differentiating into a mature cell. Most adult stem cells are lineage-restricted (multipotent), i.e. they do not produce cells of higher potency. It is possible that the molecular distinction between symmetric and asymmetric divisions lies in differential segregation of cell membrane proteins (such as receptors) between the daughter cells.

Stem cell division is regulated by a feedback mechanism. Stem cells remain undifferentiated due to environmental cues in their particular niche. Stem cells differentiate when they leave that niche or no longer receive those signals to reproduce their own type. For example, studies in *Drosophila* germarium have identified the signals *dpp* and adherens junctions that prevent germarium stem cells from differentiating.

The signal pathways that lead to reprogramming of cells to an embryonic-like state have been found to include several transcription factors including the oncogene c-Myc. Initial studies indicated that transformation of mice cells with a combination of these antidifferentiation signals can reverse differentiation and may allow adult cells to become pluripotent. However, the need to transform these cells with an oncogene may prevent the use of this approach in therapy.

Challenging the integrity of lineage commitment, researchers have been attempting to alter fermentation conditions to affect different outcomes. The somatic expression of combined transcription factors were found to directly induce other defined somatic cell fates; researchers identified three neural-lineage-specific transcription factors that could directly convert mouse fibroblasts (skin cells) into fully functional neurons. This "induced neurons" (iN) cell research inspires the researchers to induce other cell types implies that *all* cells are totipotent: with the proper tools or environmental conditions, all cells may form all kinds of tissue.

The nature of stems makes them unique in medical applications. Since stem cells can differentiate into cells that had been damaged or not regeneratable naturally, one can artificially apply stems to grow new cells of desire to heal damaged cells.

2.3. CELL CHEMISTRY

Living cells are composed of high molecular-weight polymeric compounds such as proteins, nucleic acids, polysaccharides, lipids, and other storage materials (fats, polyhydroxybutyrate, and glycogen). These biopolymers constitute the major structural elements of living cells. For example, a typical bacterial cell wall contains polysaccharides, proteins, and lipids; cell cytoplasm contains proteins mostly in the form of enzymes; in eukaryotes, the cell nucleus contains nucleic acids mostly in the form of DNA. In addition to these biopolymers, cells contain other metabolites in the form of inorganic salts (e.g. NH_3^+, PO_4^{3-}, K^+, Ca^{2+}, Na^+, SO_4^{2-}), metabolic intermediates (e.g. pyruvate, acetate), and vitamins. The elemental composition of a typical bacterial cell is 50% carbon, 20% oxygen, 14% nitrogen, 8% hydrogen, 3% phosphorus, and 1% sulfur, with small amounts of K^+, Na^+, Ca^{2+}, Mg^{2+}, Cl^-, and vitamins.

Cellular macromolecules are functional only when in the proper three-dimensional configuration. The interactions among them are very complicated. Each macromolecule is part of an intracellular organelle and functions in its unique microenvironment. Information transfer from one organelle to another (e.g. from the nucleus to ribosomes) is mediated by special molecules (e.g. messenger RNA). Most of the enzymes and metabolic intermediates are present in the cytoplasm. However, other organelles, such as mitochondria, contain enzymes and other metabolites. A living cell can be visualized as a very complex reactor in which more than 2000 reactions take place. These reactions (metabolic pathways) are interrelated and are controlled in a complicated fashion.

Despite all their complexity, an understanding of biological systems can be simplified by analyzing the system at several different levels: the molecular level (molecular biology, biochemistry), the cellular level (cell biology, microbiology), the population (microbiology, ecology), and production (bioprocess engineering). This section is devoted mainly to the structure and function of biological molecules.

2.3.1. Amino Acids and Proteins

Proteins are the most abundant organic molecules in living cells, constituting 40–70% of their dry weight. Proteins are polymers built from amino acid monomers. Proteins typically have molecular weights (MWs) of 6000 to several hundred thousand. The α-amino acids are the building blocks of proteins and contain at least one carboxyl group and one α-amino group, but they differ from each other in the structure of their R groups or side chains.

$$H_2N-\overset{\displaystyle H}{\underset{\displaystyle R}{C}}-COOH$$

L-α-amino acid

$$HOOC-\overset{\displaystyle H}{\underset{\displaystyle R}{C}}-NH_2$$

D-α-amino acid

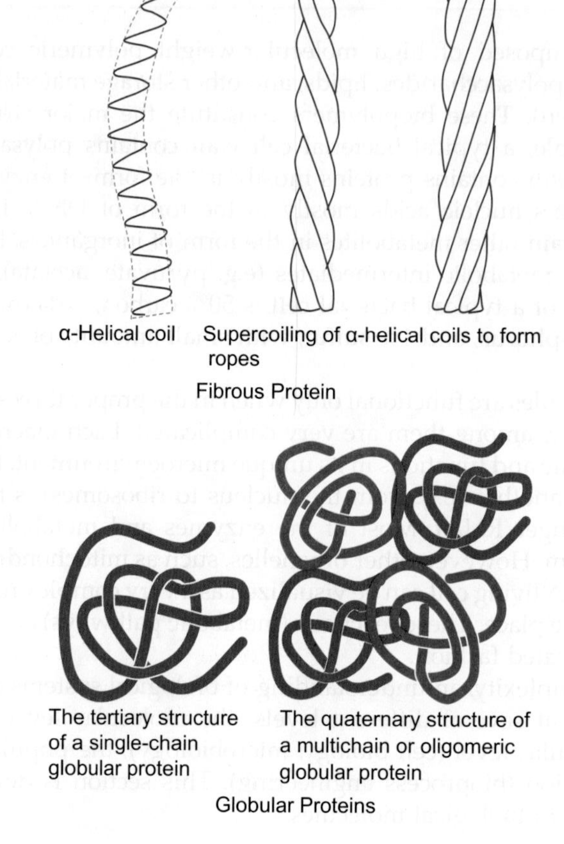

FIGURE 2.12 Fibrous and globular proteins.

Although the sequence of amino acids determines a protein's *primary* structure, the *secondary* and *tertiary* structures are determined by the weak interactions among the various side groups. The ultimate three-dimensional structure is critical to the biological activity of the protein. Two major types of protein conformation are (1) fibrous proteins and (2) globular proteins. Figure 2.12 depicts examples of fibrous and globular proteins. Proteins have diverse biological functions, which can be classified into five major categories:

(1) Structural proteins: glycoproteins, collagen, keratin.
(2) Catalytic proteins: enzymes.
(3) Transport proteins: hemoglobin, serum albumin.
(4) Regulatory proteins: hormones (insulin, growth hormone).
(5) Protective proteins: antibodies, thrombin.

Enzymes represent the largest class of proteins. Over 2000 different kinds of enzymes are known. Enzymes are highly specific in their function and have extraordinary catalytic power.

Each enzyme's molecule contains an *active site* to which its specific substrate is bound during catalysis. Some enzymes are regulated and are called *regulatory* enzymes. Most enzymes are globular proteins.

The building blocks of proteins are α-amino acids, and there are 20 common amino acids. Amino acids are named on the basis of the side (R) group attached to the α-carbon. Amino acids are optically active and occur in two chiral isomeric forms. Only L-amino acids are found in proteins. D-amino acids are rare; only found in the cell walls of some microorganisms and in some antibiotics.

Amino acids have acidic (−COOH) and basic ($-NH_2$) groups. The acidic group is neutral at low pH (−COOH) and negatively charged at high pH ($-COO^-$). At intermediate pH values, an amino acid has positively and negatively charged groups, becoming a dipolar molecule called a *zwitterion.*

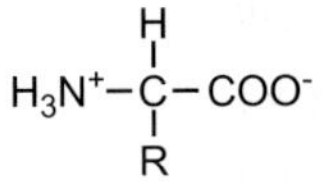

$$H_3N^+-\underset{R}{\overset{H}{\underset{|}{\overset{|}{C}}}}-COO^-$$

zwitterion

The pH value at which amino acids have no net charge is called the *isoelectric point*, which varies depending on the R group of amino acids. At its isoelectric point, an amino acid does not migrate under the influence of an electric field. Knowledge of the isoelectric point can be used in developing processes for protein purification. A list of 20 amino acids and one common type of derivatives that are commonly found in proteins is given in Table 2.5. In the structural drawings of R groups, every node has a carbon atom if no other atom is explicitly shown. All the carbon atoms have four bonds, with hydrogen H's as the default if no other atom is explicitly shown. This is the convention to be used throughout this text. For example, the −R group for Tyrosine (TYR),

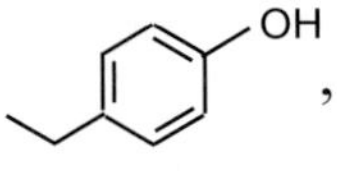

OH ,

is $-CH_2-C_6H_5-OH$.

Proteins are amino acid chains. The condensation reaction between two amino acids results in the formation of a *peptide bond* as depicted below

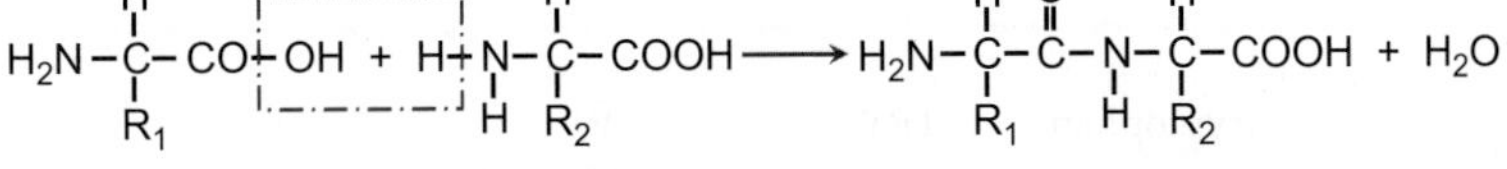

$$H_2N-\underset{R_1}{\overset{H}{\underset{|}{\overset{|}{C}}}}-CO\text{-}OH + H\text{-}\underset{H}{\underset{|}{N}}-\underset{R_2}{\overset{H}{\underset{|}{\overset{|}{C}}}}-COOH \longrightarrow H_2N-\underset{R_1}{\overset{H}{\underset{|}{\overset{|}{C}}}}-\overset{O}{\overset{\|}{C}}-\underset{H}{\underset{|}{N}}-\underset{R_2}{\overset{H}{\underset{|}{\overset{|}{C}}}}-COOH + H_2O$$

The peptide bond is planar. Peptides contain two or more amino acids linked by peptide bonds. Polypeptides usually contain fewer than 50 amino acids. Larger amino acid chains are called *proteins.* Many proteins contain organic and/or inorganic components other than amino acids. These components are called *prosthetic groups,* and the proteins containing prosthetic groups are named *conjugated proteins.* Hemoglobin is

TABLE 2.5 Chemical Structure of 20 Amino Acids of the General Structure $H_2N-\underset{R}{\overset{H}{C}}-COOH$

–R Group or whole	Name	Abbreviation	Symbol	Class
–H	Glycine	GLY	G	Aliphatic
$-CH_3$	Alanine	ALA	A	
$-CH(CH_3)_2$	Valine	VAL	V	
$-CH_2CH(CH_3)_2$	Leucine	LEU	L	
$-CH(CH_3)CH_2CH_3$	Isoleucine	ILE	I	
$-CH_2OH$	Serine	SER	S	Hydroxyl or sulfur containing
$-CH(OH)CH_3$	Threonine	THR	T	
$-CH_2SH$	Cysteine	CYS	C	
$-CH_2CH_2SCH_3$	Methionine	MET	M	
$-CH_2COOH$	Aspartic acid	ASP	D	Acids and corresponding amides
$-CH_2CONH_2$	Asparagine	ASN	N	
$-CH_2CH_2COOH$	Glutamic acid	GLU	E	
$-CH_2CH_2CONH_2$	Glutamine	GLN	Q	
$-CH_2CH_2CH_2CH_2NH_2$	Lysine	LYS	K	
$-CH_2CH_2CH_2NHCNHNH_2$	Arginine	ARG	R	Basic
	Histidine	HIS	H	
	Phenylalanine	PHE	F	Aromatic
	Tyrosine	TYR	Y	
	Tryptophan	TRY	W	

(*Continued*)

TABLE 2.5 Chemical Structure of 20 Amino Acids of the General Structure —*Cont'd*

–R Group or whole	Name	Abbreviation	Symbol	Class
	Proline	PRO	P	
$—CH_2SSCH_2—$	Cystine	Disulfide, a derivative of cysteine		

a conjugated protein and has four heme groups, which are iron-containing organometallic complexes.

The three-dimensional structure of proteins can be described at four different levels.

(1) *Primary structure*: The primary structure of a protein is its linear sequence of amino acids. Each protein has not only a definite amino acid composition, but also a unique sequence. The one-dimensional structure of proteins (the amino acid sequence) has a profound effect on the resulting three-dimensional structure and, therefore, on the function of proteins.

(2) *Secondary structure*: This is the way the polypeptide chain is extended and is a result of hydrogen bonding between residues not widely separated. Two major types of secondary structure are helixes and sheets. Helical structure can be either α-helical or triple helix. In an α-helical structure, hydrogen bonding can occur between the α-carboxyl group of one residue and the -NH group of its neighbor four units down the chain, as shown in Fig. 2.13. The triple-helix structure present in collagen consists of three α-helixes intertwined in a superhelix. The triple-helix structure is rigid and stretch-resistant. The α-helical structure can be easily disturbed, since H bonds are not highly stable. However, the sheet structure (β-pleated sheet) is more stable. The hydrogen bonds between parallel chains stabilize the sheet structure and provide resistance to stretching (Fig. 2.14).

(3) *Tertiary structure*: This is a result of interactions between R groups widely separated along the chain. The folding or bending of an amino acid chain induced by interaction between R groups determines the tertiary structure of proteins. R groups may interact by covalent, disulfide, or hydrogen bonds. Hydrophobic and hydrophilic interactions may also be present among R groups. The disulfide bond can cross-link two polypeptide chains (for example, insulin). Disulfide bonds are also critical in proper chain folding, as shown in Fig. 2.16. The tertiary structure of a protein has a profound effect on its function.

(4) *Quaternary structure*: Only proteins with more than one polypeptide chain have quaternary structure. Interactions among polypeptide chains determine the quaternary structure (Fig. 2.15). Hemoglobin has four subunits (oligomeric), and interaction among these

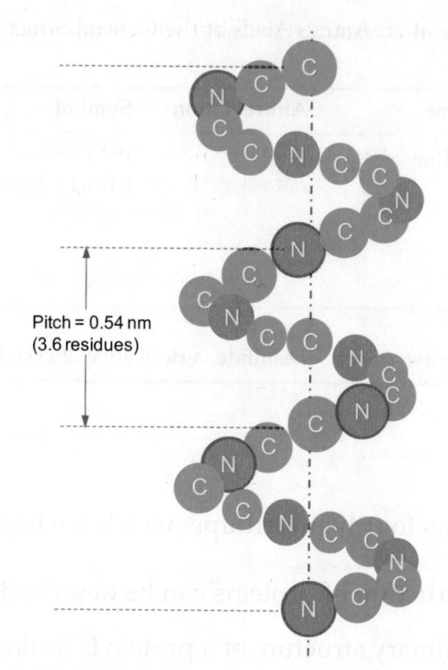

FIGURE 2.13 The α-helical structure of fibrous proteins.

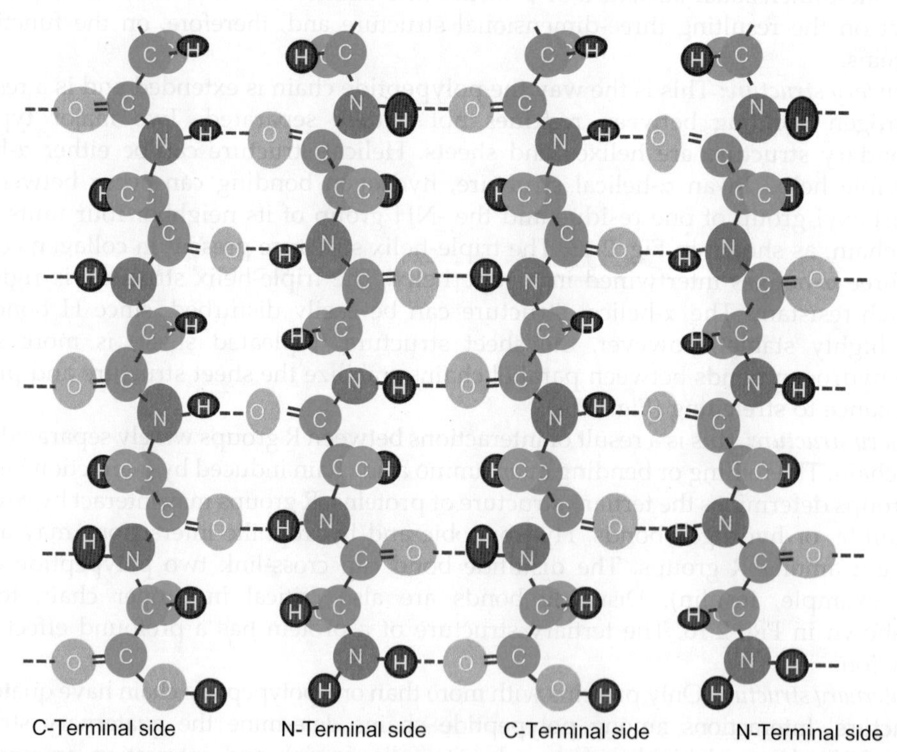

FIGURE 2.14 Representation of an antiparallel β-pleated sheet. Dashed lines indicate hydrogen bonds between strands.

subunits results in a quaternary structure. The forces between polypeptide chains can be disulfide bonds or other weak interactions. The subunit structure of enzymes has an important role in the control of their catalytic activity.

Antibodies or *immunoglobulins* are proteins that bind to particular molecules or portions of large molecules with a high degree of specificity. Antibody (Ab) molecules appear in the

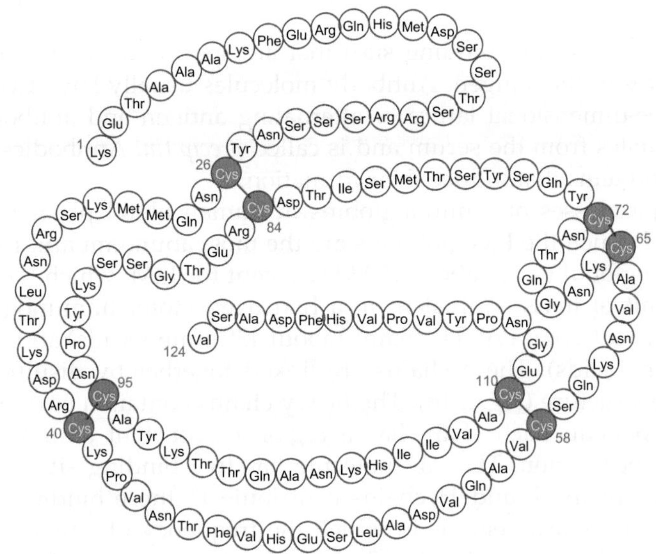

(a) Primary amino acid sequence, showing how sulfur-sulfur bonds between cysteine residues cause folding of the chain.

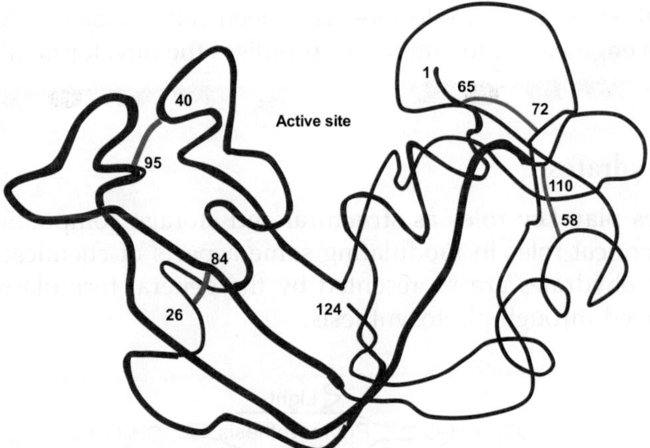

(b) The three-dimensional structure of ribonuclease, showing how the macromolecule folds so that a site of enzymatic activity is formed, the active site.

FIGURE 2.15 Structure of the enzyme ribonuclease. (a) Primary amino acid sequence, showing how sulfur–sulfur bonds between cysteine residues cause folding of the chain. (b) The three-dimensional structure of ribonuclease, showing how the macromolecule folds so that a site of enzymatic activity is formed, the active site.

blood serum and in certain cells of a vertebrate in response to foreign macromolecules. The foreign macromolecule is called the *antigen* (*Ag*). The specific antibody molecules can combine with the antigen to form an *antigen–antibody complex*. The complex formation between Ag and Ab is called the *immune response*. In addition to their obvious clinical importance, antibodies are important industrial products for use in diagnostic kits and protein separation schemes. Antibodies may also become a key element in the delivery of some anticancer drugs. Antibodies have emerged as one of the most important products of biotechnology.

Antibody molecules have binding sites that are specific for and complementary to the structural features of the antigen. Antibody molecules usually have two binding sites and can form a three-dimensional lattice of alternating antigen and antibody molecules. This complex precipitates from the serum and is called *precipitin*. Antibodies are highly specific for the foreign proteins that induce their formation.

The five major classes of immunoglobins in human blood plasma are IgG, IgA, IgD, IgM, and IgE, of which the IgG globulins are the most abundant and the best understood. MWs of immunoglobulins are about 150 kDa except for IgM, which has a MW of 900 kDa. A *dalton* is a unit of mass equivalent to a hydrogen atom. Immunoglobulins have four polypeptide chains: two heavy (H) chains (about 430 amino acids) and two light (L) chains (about 214 amino acids). These chains are linked together by disulfide bonds into a Y-shaped, flexible structure (Fig. 2.16). The heavy chains contain a covalently bonded oligosaccharide component. Each chain has a region of constant amino acid sequence and a variable-sequence region. The Ab molecule has two binding sites for the antigen; the variable portions of the L and H chains contribute to these binding sites. The variable sections have *hypervariable* regions in which the frequency of amino acid replacement is high. The study of how cells develop and produce antibodies is being actively pursued worldwide. Recent developments have also led to insights on how to impart catalytic activities to antibodies. These molecules have been called *abzymes*. Appling new developments in protein engineering to antibodies promises the development of extremely specific catalytic agents.

2.3.2. Carbohydrates

Carbohydrates play key roles as structural and storage compounds in cells. They also appear to play critical roles in modulating some aspects of chemical signaling in animals and plants. Carbohydrates are represented by the general formula $(CH_2O)_n$, where $n \geq 3$ and are synthesized through photosynthesis.

$$CO_2 + H_2O \underset{\text{Respiration}}{\overset{\text{Light, Photosynthesis}}{\rightleftharpoons}} CH_2O + O_2$$

The gases CO_2 and H_2O are converted through photosynthesis into sugars in the presence of sunlight and are then polymerized to yield polysaccharides, such as cellulose or starch.

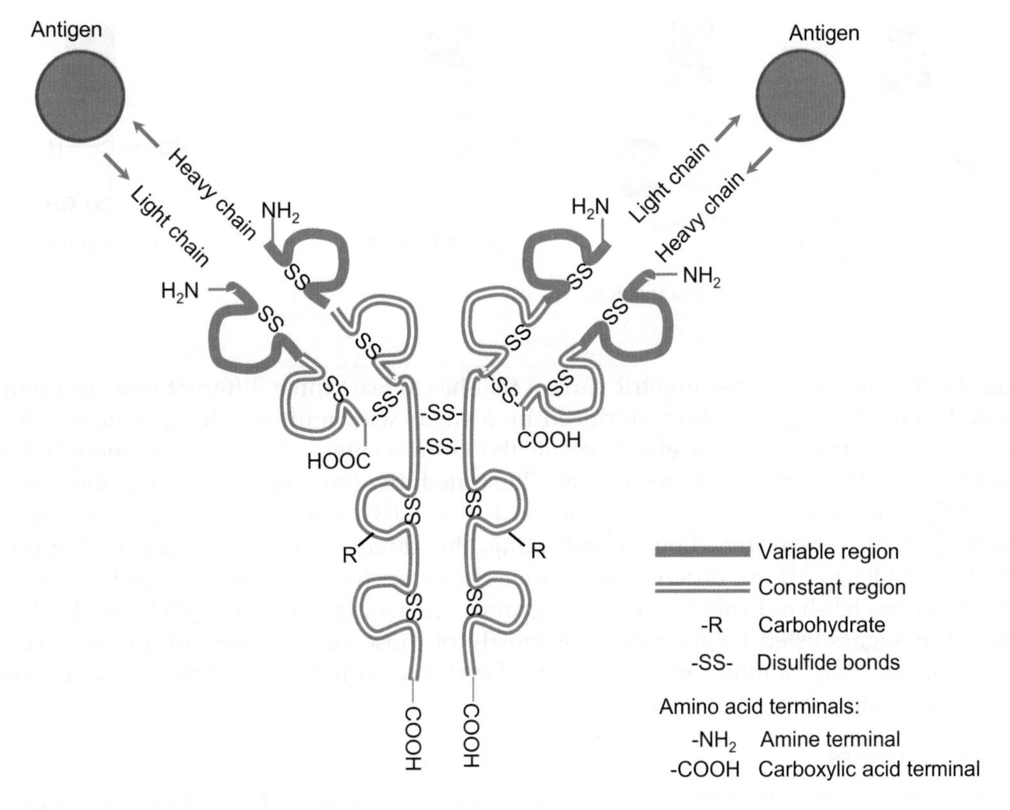

FIGURE 2.16 Structure of immunoglobulin G (IgG). Structure showing disulfide linkages within and between chains and antigen-binding site.

2.3.2.1. Monosaccharides

Monosaccharides are the smallest carbohydrates and contain three to nine carbon atoms. Common monosaccharides are presented below. Common monosaccharides are aldehydes and ketones. For example, glucose is an aldohexose. Glucose may be present in the form of a linear or ring structure. In solution, D-glucose is in the form of a ring (pyranose, or 6-membered) structure. Pyranose (a 6-member ring-structured sugar) is more stable than furanose (a 5-member ring-structured sugar). Pyranose can have four conformations: chair, boat, skew boat, and half-chair. The chair conformation is most stable and energetic as it is free from steric interactions. The D-forms (or D-enantiomers) and L-forms (L-enantiomers) of the monosaccharides are based on the chiral center farthest away from the reducing end group as illustrated in Fig. 2.17. The difference in structure is the side (left or right; or up or down) of the OH group connected to the second last carbon in sugar molecular representations (for example, D-arabinose and L-arabinose). The L-enantiomers cause polarized light to rotate counter-clockwise, whereas the D-enantiomers cause polarized light to rotate clockwise. One should note that this polarized light effect applies only to simple sugars

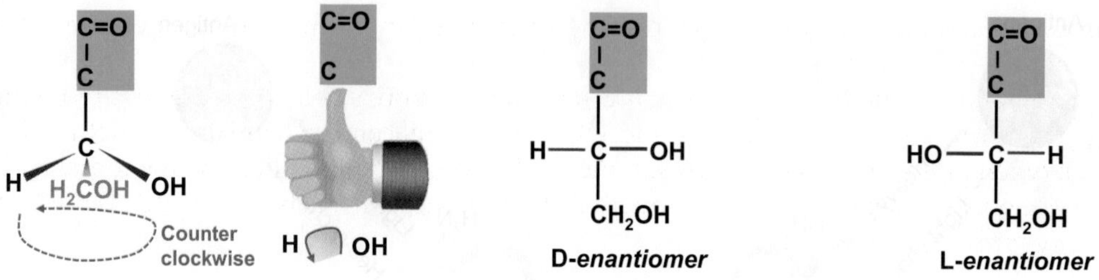

FIGURE 2.17 Representation of enantiomers.

(one chiral center, or one asymmetric carbon that has at least three different units or groups bonded to it). The light rotation produced by a sugar with multiple chiral centers will be determined by the combined effects of all the chiral centers. The D-enantiomers is best described by the right-hand gesture as illustrated by the two figures on the left in Fig. 2.17, where the thumb points toward the CHO end group, and the natural bending of the other four fingers indicating the direction in which the end groups (OH to CH_2OH to H) are ordered as counter-clockwise (opposite to polarized light). For L-enantiomers, left-hand rule applies (end groups are arranged OH, CH_2OH, and H clockwise). The sugars listed below consist of mostly of those sugars naturally present. The L form generally plays a minor role in biological systems, with the exceptions of L-arabinose, L-rhamnose, and L-fucose.

2.3.2.1.1. ALDOSES

An aldose is a sugar having a reducing end group: CHO. The C=O double bond is located on the last (or first) carbon when the sugar molecule is represented linearly.

a. D-hexoses

These sugars (hexoses) all have the same chemical formula ($C_6H_{12}O_6$) and even the same number, type, and sequence of bonds. They only differ by the spatial arrangement about one single carbon atom in the chain. They are epimers. In the above, the only difference is one of the orientations of the OH (hydroxyl) groups (left or right). Although most epimers' physical and chemical properties are the same, their biological activities can be quite different.

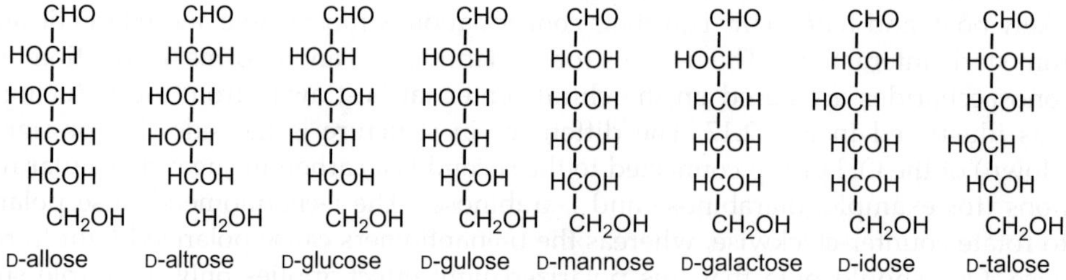

In aqueous solutions, the sugars form ring structures. For example, glucose can have three different forms as shown on the right:

The pyranose structure (6-member ring structure) is more stable than furanose (5-member ring structure). The carbon atom around which the hemiacetal or hemiketal structure forms (two oxygen atoms each with a single bond with one carbon) is called the anomeric carbon atom or anomeric center. One may note that there is only one such carbon atom attached to two oxygen atoms in the ring.

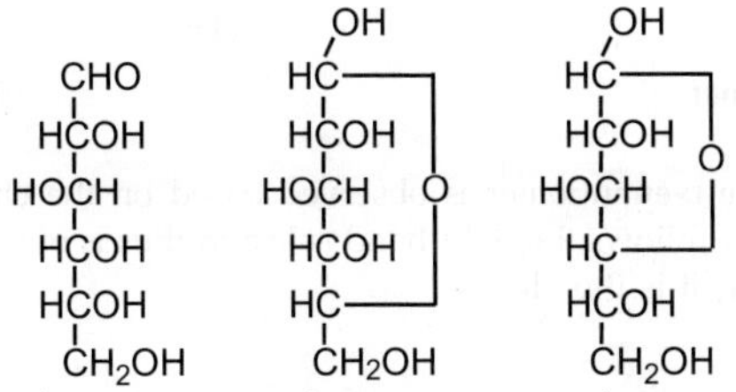

D-glucose, linear structure

D-glucose, pyranose structure

D-glucose, furanose structure

Pyranose can exist in four different configurations: chair, boat, half-chair, and inverted boat. Again, the chair form is the most energetic. Here are some sample hexoses in ring structure:

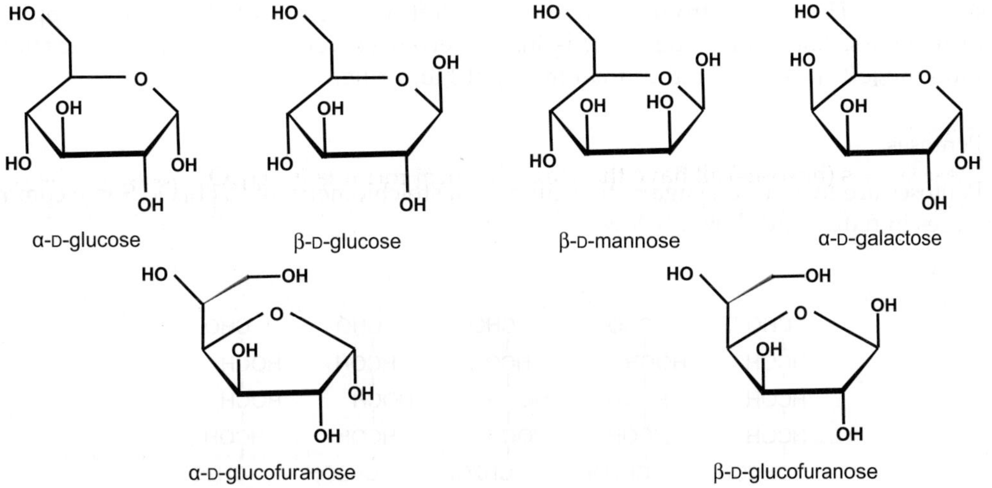

α-D-glucose

β-D-glucose

β-D-mannose

α-D-galactose

α-D-glucofuranose

β-D-glucofuranose

Notice that in the ring structure, the hydroxyl group attached to the anomeric center (two oxygen atoms attached to the one carbon atom center) is either pointing downward or upward. OH (of the anomeric center) attached from above the ring is β-anomer (OH on the thumb of the right hand with ring being the circle form by the hand—right-hand gesture), whereas the α-anomer has the anomeric OH group attached from below the

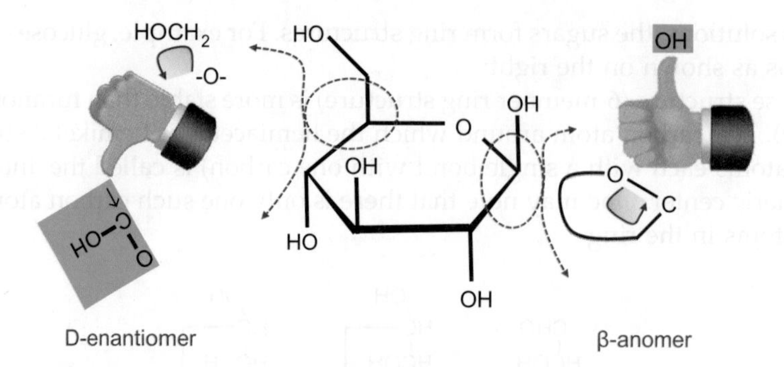

FIGURE 2.18 β-D-glucose. The D-enantiomer is observed based on the chiral center furthest away from the reducing end. The C-5 chiral center follows the right-hand rule and thus is of the D-form. The anomeric OH follows also the right-hand rule. Therefore, it is β-D-glucose.

ring (left-hand gesture). Figure 2.18 shows the configuration of β-D-glucose, where both right-hand rule applied for the D-enantiomer and β-anomer (OH). When the enantiomer and anomeric OH follow the same hand rule, the anomer is a β-anomer, whereas when different hand rules apply the anomer is an α-anomer. One can also interpret it with the anomeric proton (H-atom), which is omitted from the ring presentations. α-anomer has the anomeric proton attached from above the ring (H on the thumb of the right hand with ring being the circle form by the hand—right hand gesture), whereas β-anomer has anomeric H attached from below the ring (left-hand gesture). These rules apply for D-form sugars. For L-form sugars, it is just reversed (α versus β) because L-enantiomer follows the left-hand rule, rather than the right-hand rule.

b. Pentoses

Pentoses are five carbon sugars, they all have a stoichiometry of $C_5H_{10}O_5$. Some common pentoses in nature are shown below:

D-ribose	D-arabinose	L-arabinose	D-xylose	D-lyxose
CHO	CHO	CHO	CHO	CHO
HCOH	HOCH	HCOH	HCOH	HOCH
HCOH	HCOH	HOCH	HOCH	HOCH
HCOH	HCOH	HOCH	HCOH	HCOH
CH2OH	CH2OH	CH2OH	CH2OH	CH2OH

D-arabinose and L-arabinose are mirror image of one another. These are known as enantiomers. D-form sugars are more common in nature. There are only a few L-form sugars in nature and L-arabinose is one of them.

Some pentoses are shown below in ring structure:

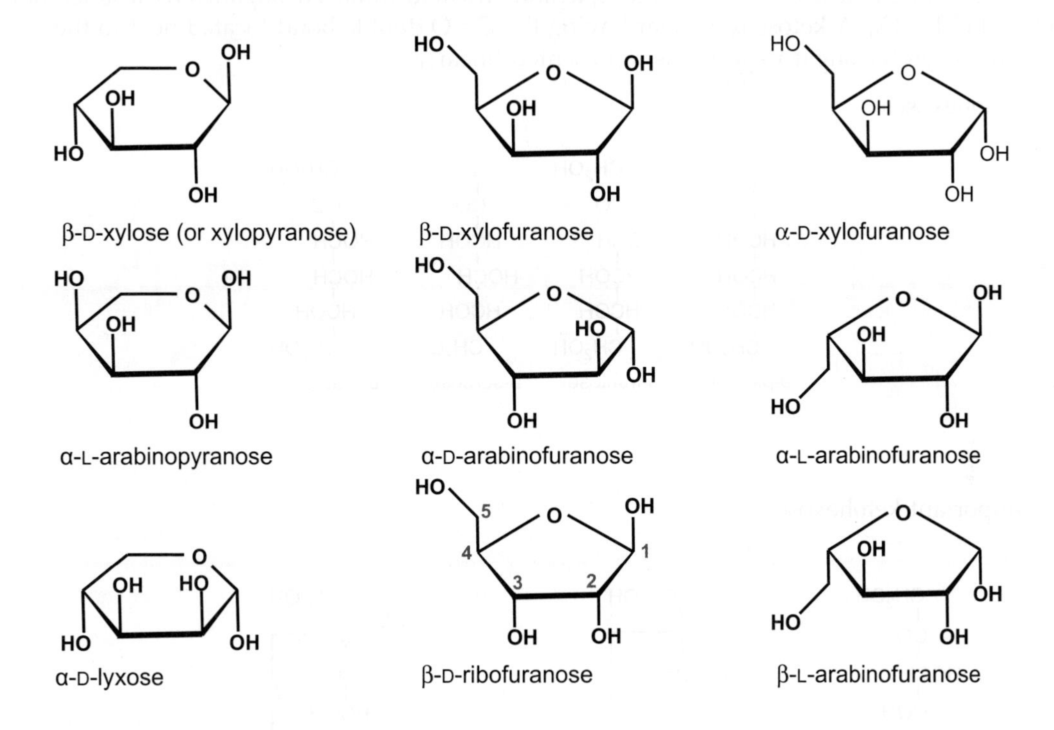

c. D-tetroses

Tetroses are four carbon sugars, there are two common in nature. These sugars all have a stoichiometry of $C_4H_8O_4$. They are shown below in linear form (left) and ring form (right):

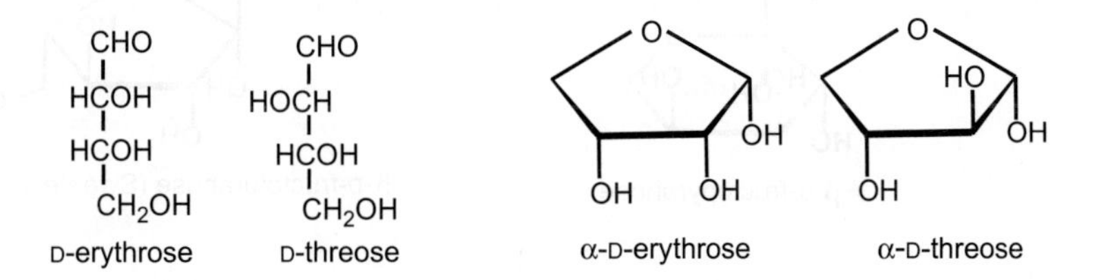

d. D-trioses

Trioses are three carbon sugars and they have a stoichiometry of $C_3H_6O_3$. The common one in nature is D-glyceraldehyde as shown below:

CHO
|
HCOH
|
CH_2OH

D-glyceraldehyde

2.3.2.1.2. KETOSES

Ketoses and aldoses share the same stoichiometrical formula. All sugars have a stoichiometry of $C_nH_{2n}O_n$. A ketose is a sugar having the C=O double bond located next to the end carbon when the sugar molecule is represented linearly.

a. Ketohexoses

D-psicose	D-fructose	D-sorbose	D-toatose
CH_2OH	CH_2OH	CH_2OH	CH_2OH
CO	CO	CO	CO
HCOH	HOCH	HCOH	HOCH
HCOH	HCOH	HOCH	HOCH
HCOH	HCOH	HCOH	HCOH
CH_2OH	CH_2OH	CH_2OH	CH_2OH

Important ketohexoses:

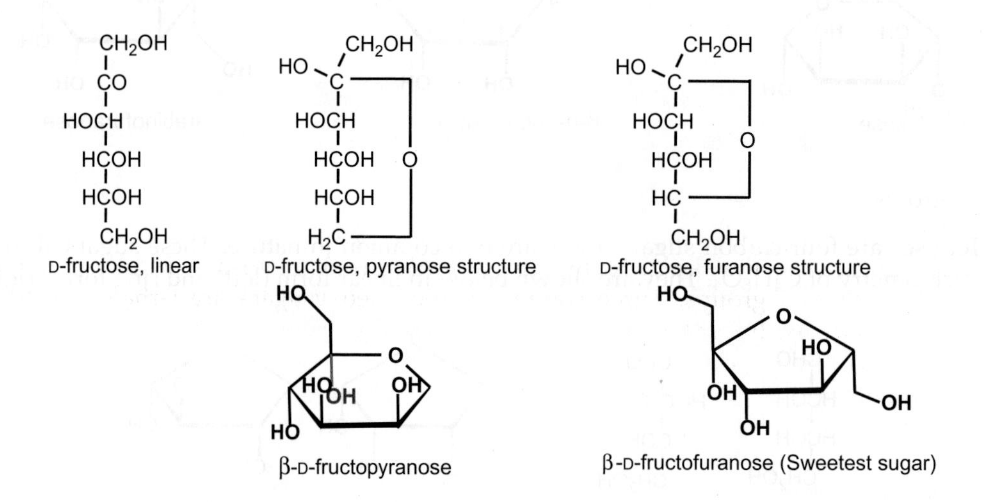

b. Ketopentoses

D-ribulose	D-xylulose
CH_2OH	CH_2OH
CO	CO
HCOH	HOCH
HCOH	HCOH
CH_2OH	CH_2OH

In ring structure, ketopentoses look similar to ribofuranose (D-ribulose) and xylofuranose (D-xylose), except the hydroxyl group next to the ester O.

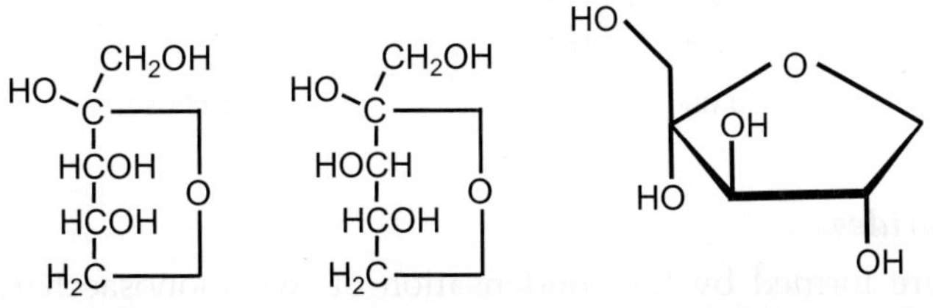

D-ribulose D-xylulose β-D-xylulose

c. Ketotetroses

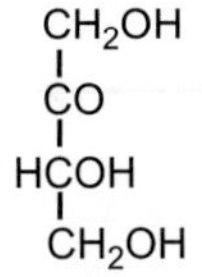

D-erythrulose

d. Ketotriose

There is only one common ketotriose in nature, that is, CH_2OH–CO–CH_2OH or Dihydroxyacetone.

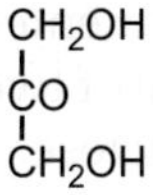

2.3.2.1.3. DEOXYSUGARS

Deoxysugars are the sugars shown above with one or more oxygen atoms removed from the hydroxyl groups. Three commonly seen deoxysugars are L-rhamnose (deoxy mannose or methyl lyxose), L-fucose (deoxy galactose or methyl arabinose), and D-deoxyribose. Both rhamnose and fucose are deoxyhexoses, while deoxyribose is a deoxypentose.

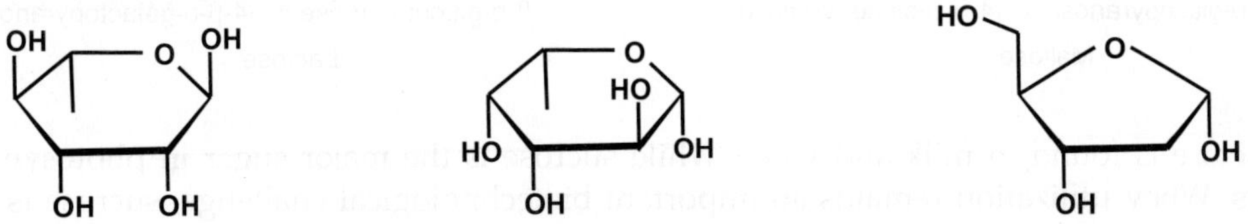

α-L-rhamnose β-L-fucose α-D-deoxyribose

Particularly important monosaccharides are D-ribose and deoxyribose. These five carbon ring-structured sugar molecules are essential components of DNA and RNA.

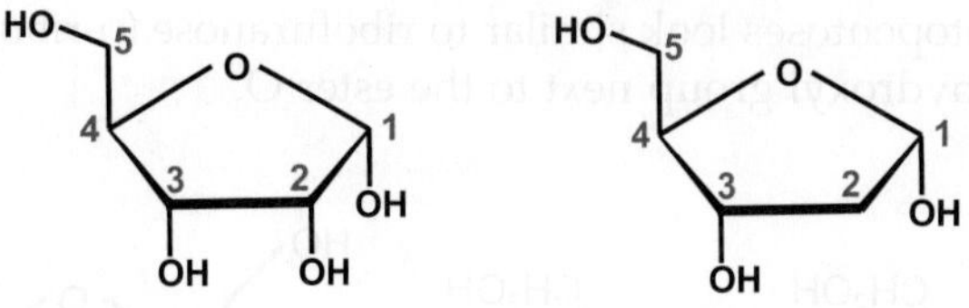

D-ribose Deoxyribose

2.3.2.2. *Disaccharides*

Disaccharides are formed by the condensation of two monosaccharides. For example, sucrose is formed by the condensation of one (α-D-) glucose molecule and one (β-D-) fructose molecule via α-1,4 glycosidic linkage (or α-1-O-4). This can be illustrated as follows:

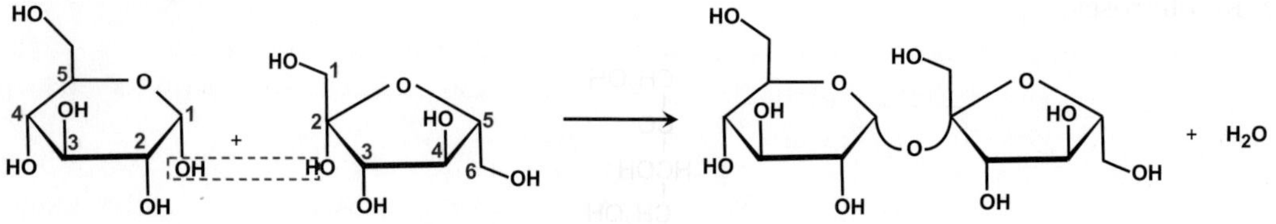

α-D-glucose β-D-fructose Sucrose

Sucrose can also be represented as α-D-glucopyranose-1→2-β-D-fructofuranose.

Maltose is a disaccharide of two identical α-D-glucose molecules. Lactose is a disaccharide of β-D-glucose and β-D-galactose. The stereo structures of these two disaccharides are shown below:

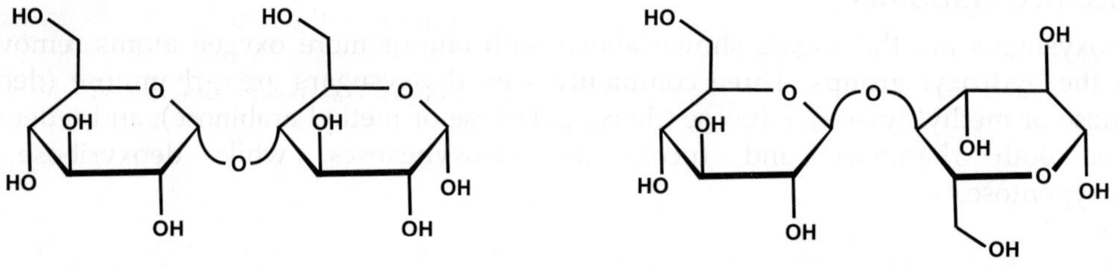

α-D-glucopyranose-1→4-α-D-glucopyranose

Maltose

β-D-glucopyranose-1→4-β-D-galactopyranose

Lactose

Lactose is found in milk and whey, while sucrose is the major sugar in photosynthetic plants. Whey utilization remains an important biotechnological challenge; sucrose is often a major component in artificial growth media.

2.3.2.3. *Polysaccharides*

Polysaccharides are formed by the condensation of two or more monosaccharides by glycosidic bonds. The polysaccharide processing industry makes extensive use of enzymatic processing and biochemical engineering.

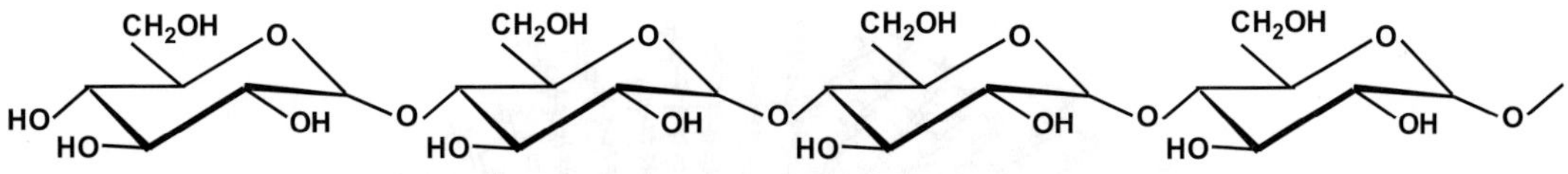

FIGURE 2.19 Structure of amylose.

2.3.2.3.1. STARCH

Starch consists of two types of polysaccharides: amylose and amylopectin. Amylose is a straight linear chain of glucose molecules linked by α-1,4 glycosidic linkages as shown in Fig. 2.19, in the same manner as in the disaccharide maltose. Maltose is a dimmer usually derived from amylose (by hydrolysis). The MW of amylose varies between several thousand and one-half million daltons. Amylose is water insoluble and constitutes about 20% of starch.

Amylopectin is a branched chain of α-D-glucose molecules, as illustrated in Fig. 2.20. Branching occurs between the glycosidic-OH of one chain and the 6th carbon of another glucose, which is called α-1,6 glycosidic linkage.

Amylopectin molecules are much larger than those of amylose, with an MW of 1−2 million daltons. Amylopectin is water soluble. Partial hydrolysis of starch (acidic or enzymatic) yields glucose, maltose, and dextrins, which are branched sections of amylopectin. Dextrins are used as thickeners.

2.3.2.3.2. GLYCOGEN

Glycogen is a branched chain of glucose molecules that resembles amylopectin. It is similar to starch but is produced by animals as secondary long-term energy storage. Glycogen is highly branched and contains about 12 glucose units in straight-chained segments. Glycogen is found in the form of granules in the cytosol of many cell types. The MW of a typical glycogen molecule is less than 5×10^6 Da. An illustration of a glycogen molecule is shown in Fig. 2.21, with the connections clearly shown in Fig. 2.22.

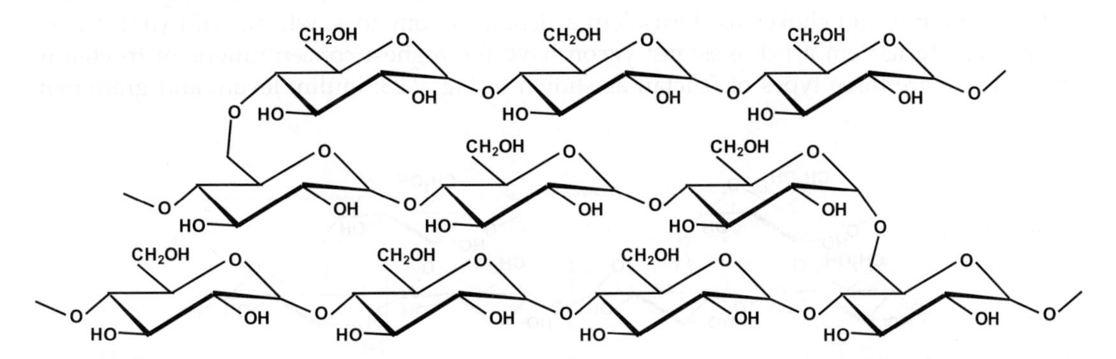

FIGURE 2.20 An illustration of the structure of amylopectin. Amylopectin is a branched homopolymer of α-D-glucose. Each straight chain is of an amylose chain. The branches occur on the 6th carbon of the α-D-glucose units.

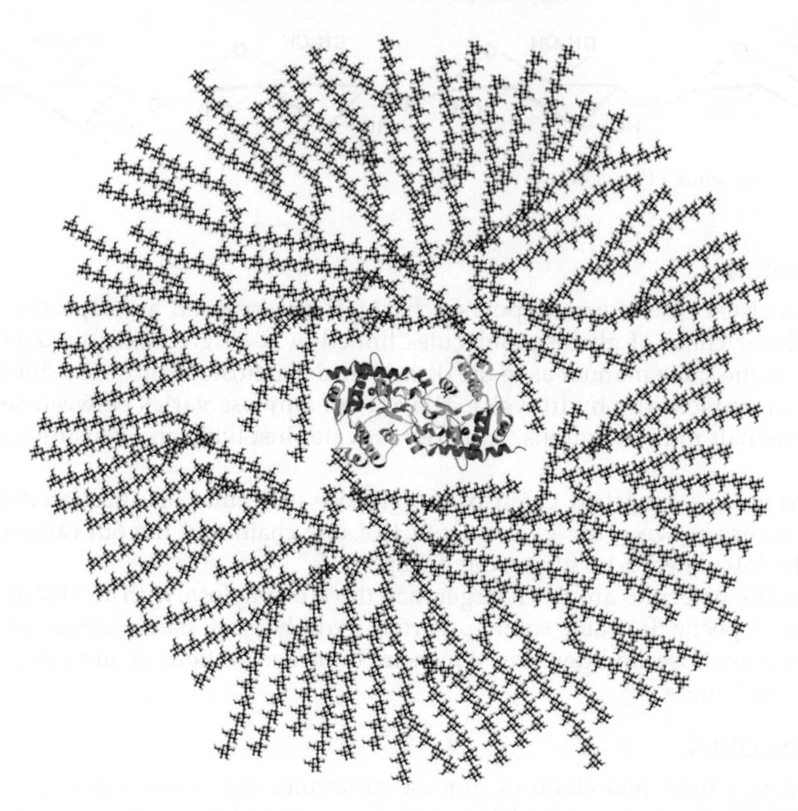

FIGURE 2.21 An illustration of a glycogen macromolecule. The core is a glycogenic protein. The entire globular granule may contain approximately 30,000 glucose units.

2.3.2.3.3. FRUCTAN

The second-most abundant easily digestible polysaccharide found naturally is fructan. Fructan is a polymer of β-D-fructofuranose. Fructan appears in agaves, artichokes, asparagus, bananas, barley, burdock, camas, chicory root, dandelion, elecampane, garlic, green beans, leeks, onion, rye, sun chokes (or Jerusalem artichokes), tomatoes, wheat, wild yam, yacon, yicama, etc. Jerusalem artichokes and yacon have the highest concentrations of fructan in crops. There are three types of fructan as shown in Fig. 2.23: inulin, levan, and graminan.

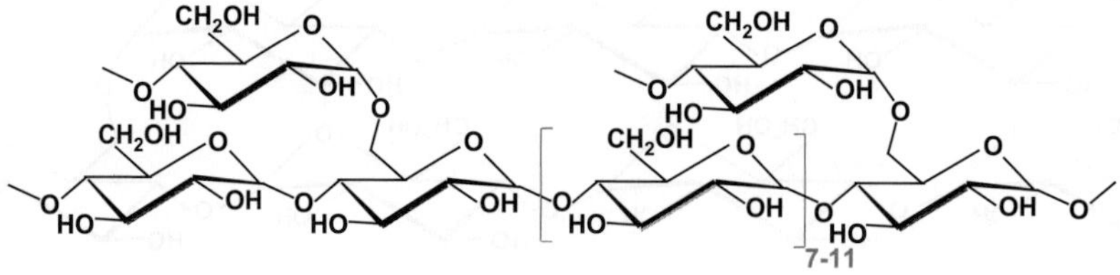

FIGURE 2.22 Glycogen structural segment. The straight chain may have 8–12 units in each section, which is connected by α1-O-4, while the branching occurs via α1-O-6.

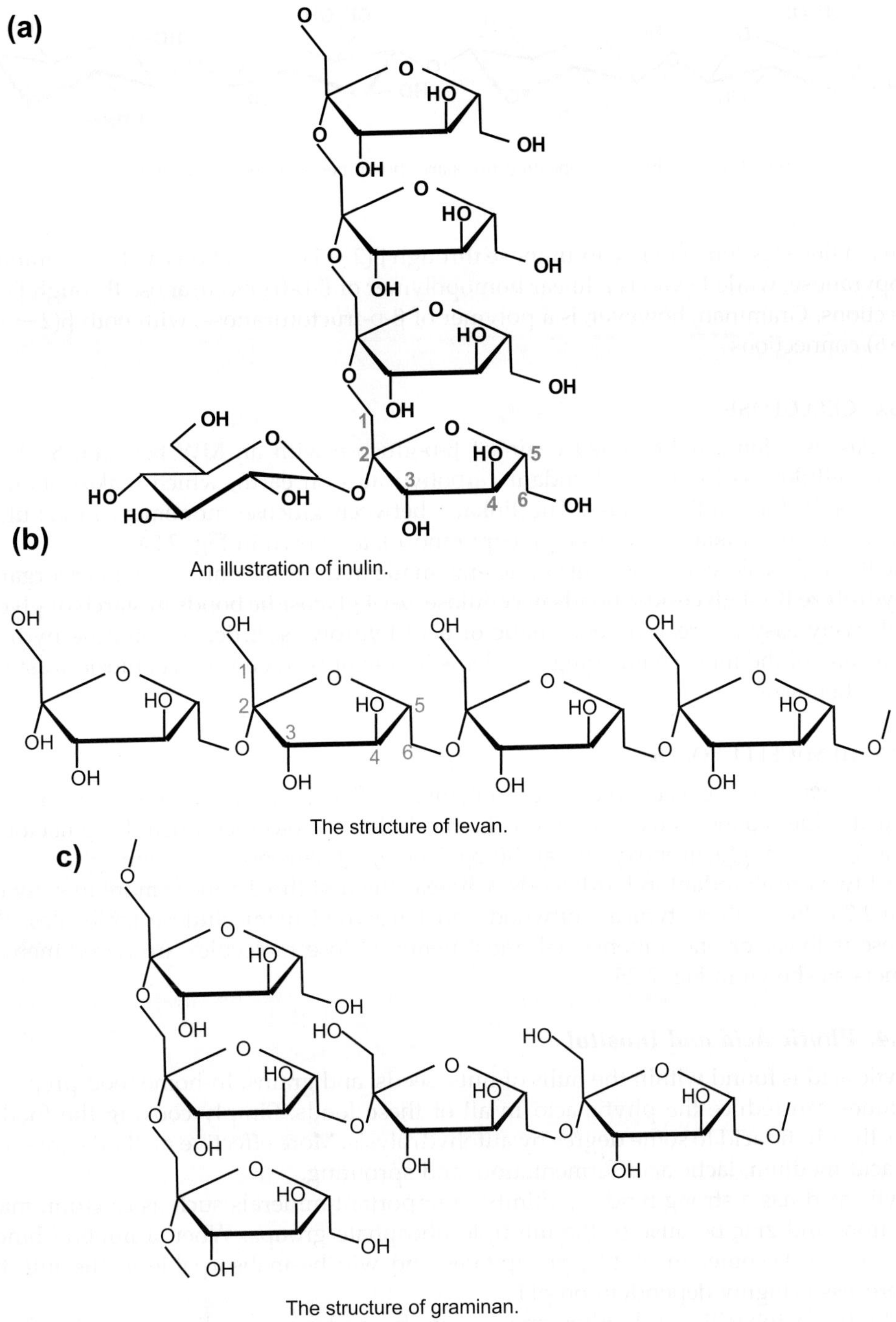

(a)

An illustration of inulin.

(b)

The structure of levan.

c)

The structure of graminan.

FIGURE 2.23 The principle structures of fructan.

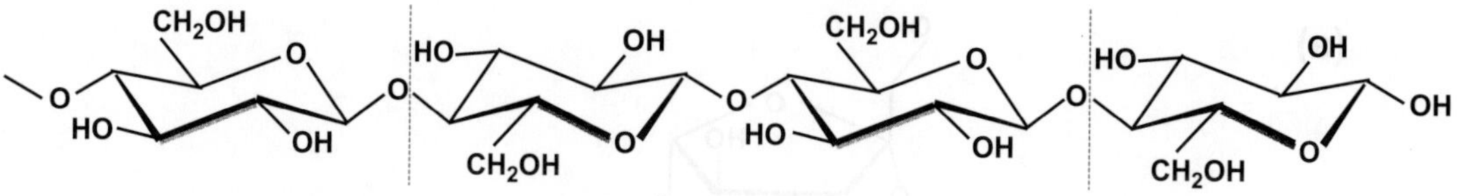

FIGURE 2.24 Structure of cellulose. Repeating units are shown between the two dashed lines.

Inulin is a linear polymer of fructofuranose through β(2→1) connections, with a terminal α-D-glucopyranose, while Levan is a linear homopolymer of β-D-fructofuranose through β(2→6) connections. Graminan, however, is a polymer of β-D-fructofuranose, with both β(2→1) and β(2→6) connections.

2.3.2.3.4. CELLULOSE

Cellulose is a long, unbranched chain of β-D-glucose with an MW between 50,000 and 10^6 Da. Cellulose is the most abundant carbohydrates on earth, which makes about 40% of the woody (or pant) biomass. The linkage between glucose monomers in cellulose is a β-1,4 glycosidic linkage (β-1→4-D-glucopyranose), as shown in Fig. 2.24.

The β-1,4 glycosidic bond is resistant to enzymatic hydrolysis: only a few microorganisms can hydrolyze β-1,4 glycosidic bonds in cellulose. α-1,4 glycosidic bonds in starch or glycogen are relatively easy to break by enzymatic or acid hydrolysis. Efficient cellulose hydrolysis remains one of the most challenging problems in attempts to convert cellulosic wastes into fuels or chemicals.

2.3.2.3.5. HEMICELLULOSES

Hemicelluloses are a collection of heteropolymers of five- and six-carbon sugars with short-branched side connections. Common hemicellulose molecules include galactoglucomannans, arabinoglucuronoxylan, arabinogalactan, glucuronoxylan, and glucomannan. The last two are abundant in hardwoods, whereas the first three appear more in softwoods. Figure 2.25 shows these typical softwood and hardwood hemicellulose molecules. While cellulose is linear or one-dimensional, most hemicellulose molecules are two-dimensional polymers as shown in Fig. 2.25.

2.3.2.4. *Phytic Acid and Inositol*

Phytic acid is found within the hulls of nuts, seeds, and grains. In-home food preparation techniques can reduce the phytic acid in all of these foods. Simply cooking the food will reduce the phytic acid to some degree by autohydrolysis. More effective methods are soaking in an acid medium, lactic acid fermentation, and sprouting.

Phytic acid has a strong binding affinity to important minerals such as calcium, magnesium, iron, and zinc because of the multiple phosphate groups. When a mineral binds to phytic acid, it becomes insoluble, precipitates and will be inabsorpable in the intestines. This process is highly dependent on pH.

Probiotic lactobacilli, and other species of the endogenous digestive microflora as well, are an important source of the enzyme phytase which catalyzes the release of

(a)

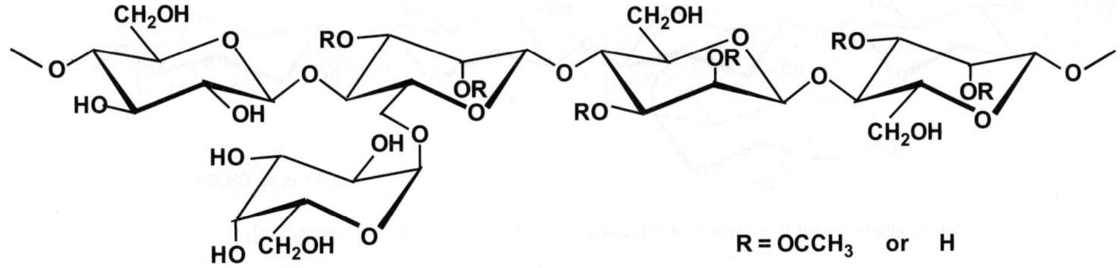

$R = OCCH_3$ or H

→4-β-D-glucose-1→4-β-D-mannose(2 or 3←Acetyl)-1→4-β-D-mannose(2 or 3←Acetyl)-1→4-β-D-mannose(2 or 3←Acetyl)-1→
6
↑
1
α-D-galactose

Principle structure of galactoglucomannans. The OH groups in the mannose units were partially substituted by O-acetyl groups on the C-2 or C-3 positions, i.e. $R = CH_3CO$ or R = H.

(b)

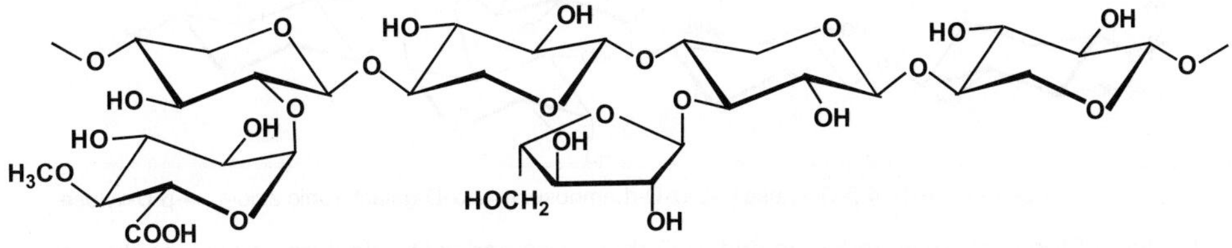

→4-β-D-xylose-1→[4-β-D-xylose-1→(6 ↑ 1 4-methoxyl-α-D-glucuronic acid)]$_2$ 4-β-D-xylose-1→ 4-β-D-xylose-1→ [4-β-D-xylose-1→]$_5$
(3 ↑ 1 α-L-arabinofuranose)

Principle structure of arabinoglucuronoxylan. α-L-arabinofuranose units are present among the β-D-xylose units and 4-methoxyl-α-D-glucouronic acid residues.

(c)

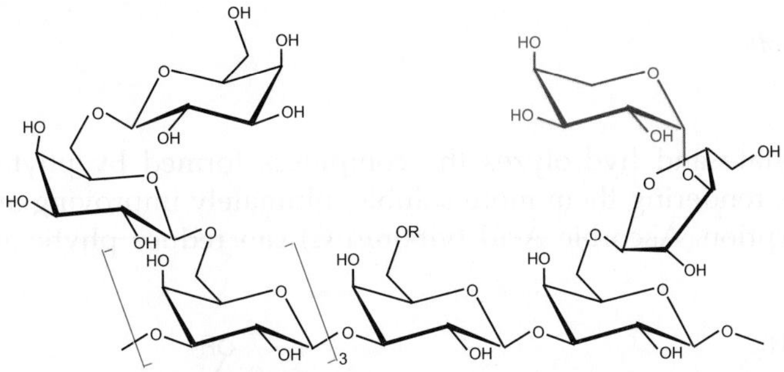

Principle structure of arabinogalactan, where R is β-D-galactopyranose, or less frequently α-L-arabinofuranose, or β-D-glucuronic acid residue.

FIGURE 2.25 Stereochemical structure of common softwood and hardwood hemicelluloses molecules.

(d)

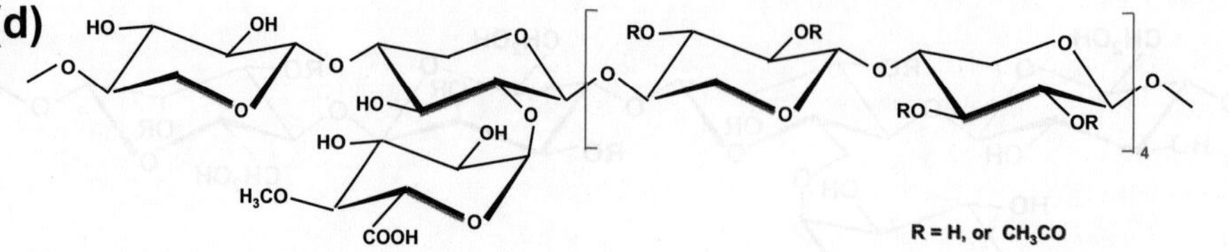

HO OH O O RO OR O O O O HO O O RO OR HO OH H_3CO O COOH 4

R = H, or CH_3CO

→4-β-D-xylose-1→4-β-D-xylose-1→4-β-D-xylose-1[→ 4-β-D-xylose (2 or 3←acetyl) -1]$_7$→

2
↑
1
4-methoxyl-α-glucuronic acid

Stereochemical structure of a common hardwood hemicellulose: glucuronoxylan. For every 10 xylose units, about 7 of them were partially acetylated on the C-2 or C-3 positions.

(e)

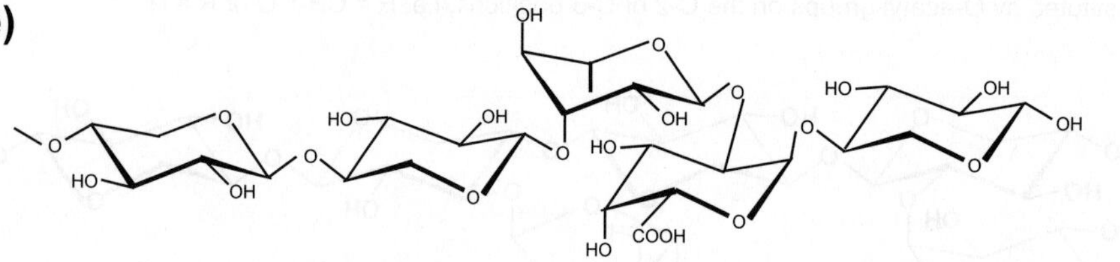

OH O O HO OH O HO OH OH O O HO O O HO OH O O HO COOH O

→4-β-D-xylose-1→4-β-D-xylose1→3-α-D-rhamnose-1→2-α-D-galacturonic acid-1→4-β-D-xylose

Structure of the birch xylan reducing end. α-D-rhamnose and α-D-galacturonic acid residues are present just prior to the reducing end β-D-xylose unit.

(f)

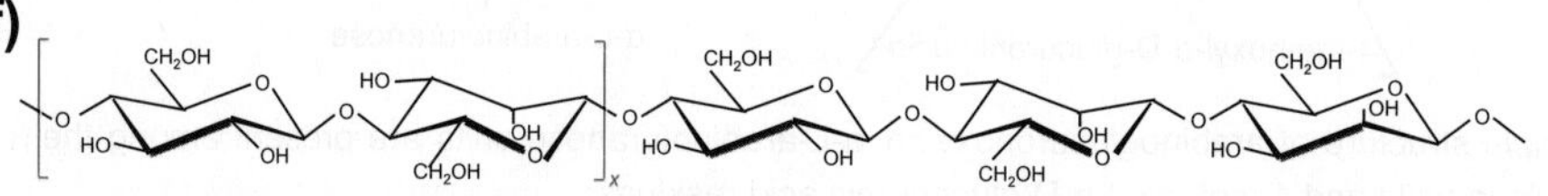

CH_2OH O HO O HO OH OH O CH_2OH x CH_2OH O HO O HO OH OH O CH_2OH CH_2OH O OH HO O

Hardwood hemicelluloses: glucomannan, $x \geq 0$. For every β-D-glucose unit, there are one to two β-D mannose units depending on the wood species.

FIGURE 2.25 *(Continued).*

phosphate from phytate and hydrolyzes the complexes formed by phytate and metal ions or other cations, rendering them more soluble, ultimately improving and facilitating their intestinal absorption. Ascorbic Acid (vitamin C) can reduce phytic acid effects on iron.

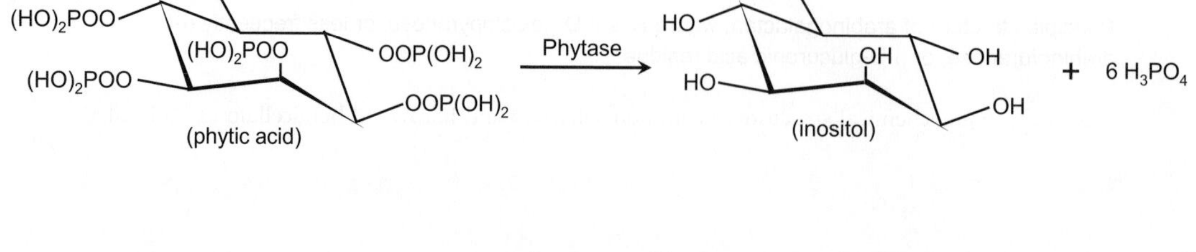

$OOP(OH)_2$ $(HO)_2POO$ $(HO)_2POO$ $OOP(OH)_2$ $(HO)_2POO$ $OOP(OH)_2$ (phytic acid) —Phytase→ OH HO OH OH HO OH (inositol) + 6 H_3PO_4

2.3.3. Chitin and Chitosan

Chitin is a polysaccharide constituted of *N*-acetylglucosamine, which forms a hard, semi-transparent biomaterial found throughout the natural world. Chitin is the main component of the exoskeletons of crabs, lobsters, and shrimps. Chitin is also found in insects (e.g. ants, beetles, and butterflies), cephalopods (e.g. squids and octopuses), and even in fungi. Nevertheless, the industrial source of chitin is mainly crustaceans.

Because of its similarity to the cellulose structure, chitin may be described as cellulose with one hydroxyl group on each monomer replaced by an acetylamine group. This allows for increased hydrogen bonding between adjacent polymers, giving the polymer increased strength.

Chitin's properties as a tough and strong material make it favorable as surgical thread. Additionally, its biodegradability means it wears away with time as the wound heals. Moreover, chitin has some unusual properties that accelerate healing of wounds in humans. Chitin has even been used as a stand-alone wound-healing agent.

Industrial separation membranes and ion-exchange resins can be made from chitin, especially for water purification. Chitin is also used industrially as an additive to thicken and stabilize foods and pharmaceuticals. Since it can be shaped into fibers, the textile industry has made extensive use of chitin, especially for socks, as it is claimed that chitin fabrics are naturally antibacterial and antiodor *(www.solstitch.net)*. Chitin also acts as a binding agent in dyes, fabrics, and adhesives. Some processes to size and strengthen paper employ chitin.

Chitosan is produced commercially by deacetylation of chitin. It is a linear polysaccharide composed of randomly distributed, β-(1,4)-linked D-glucosamine units (deacetylated) and *N* -acetyl-D-glucosamine units (acetylated). The degree of deacetylation in commercial chitosans is in the range of 60–100% (Fig. 2.26).

The amino group in chitosan has a pKa value of about 6.5. Therefore, chitosan is positively charged and soluble in acidic to neutral solutions with a charge density dependent on pH and the deacetylation extent. In other words, chitosan readily binds to negatively charged surfaces such as mucosal membranes. Chitosan enhances the transport of polar drugs across epithelial surfaces and is biocompatible and biodegradable. Purified qualities of chitosan are available for biomedical applications.

Chitosan possesses flocculating properties, which are used in water processing engineering as a part of the filtration process. It may remove phosphorus, heavy minerals, and oils from the water. In the same manner, it is used to clarify wine and beer (as a substitute for egg albumin).

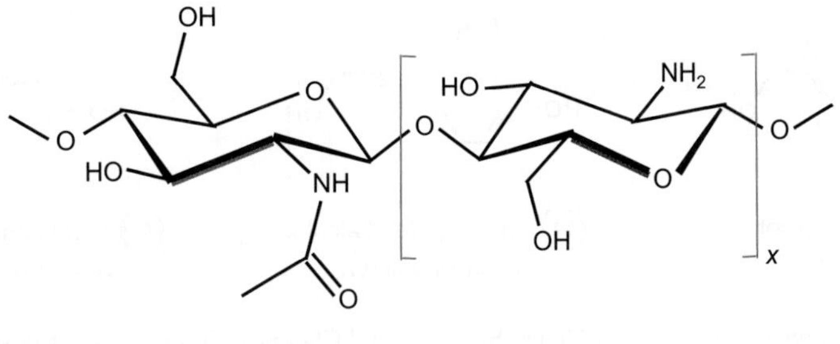

FIGURE 2.26 General formula for chitosan ($x \geq 1.5$) and chitin ($x = 0$).

2.3.4. Lignin

Lignin is a heteropolymer composed primarily of methoxylated phenylpropylene alcohol monomeric units interconnected by a variety of stable carbon–carbon and carbon–oxygen–carbon (ethers and esters) linkages (Dence and Lin, 1992). Structurally, lignin is a three-dimensional macromolecule. While the lignin of gymnosperms (also called softwoods, conifers, needle trees or evergreens) is primarily an enzyme-mediated dehydrogenative polymerization product of coniferyl alcohol (Fengel and Wegener, 1989), the lignin of angiosperms (also hardwoods, deciduous or broad-leaved trees, and grasses) is derived primarily from a mixture of coniferyl and sinapyl alcohols. Figure 2.27 shows the three cinnamyl alcohols, the lignin precursors. The oxygen to carbon ratio in the lignin precursors (Fig. 2.27) is less than 4/11. One can infer that lignin is much less oxygenated than carbohydrates, where approximately each carbon atom is accompanied by one oxygen atom as shown in the previous subsections. The aromatic ring structure also provides excellent functional chemical sources when depolymerized.

The phenylpropane units in lignin are linked together by different bonds, as shown in Fig. 2.28. The β-O-4 interunit linkages are the most abundant in lignin, estimated to be as high as 50% in softwoods and almost 60% in hardwoods (Sjöström, 1993). More than two-thirds of the phenylpropane units are linked by ether bonds, the rest by carbon–carbon bonds.

Lignins can be divided into several classes according to their structural elements. Guaiacyl–syringyl lignin (GS-lignin) found in hardwoods is a copolymer of coniferyl and synapyl alcohols (precursors of G- and S-units, respectively) with the G/S ratio varying from 4:1 to 1:2. Guaiacyl lignin (G-lignin), occurring in almost all softwoods, is largely a polymerization product of coniferyl alcohol. Different contributions of p-hydroxycinnamyl alcohols in the biosynthesis of hardwood and softwood lignins causes significant differences in their structure, including the contents of different types of bonds and main functional groups, for example, methoxyl (OMe), phenolic hydroxyl (PhOH), aliphatic hydroxyl, carbonyl, and carboxyl groups. Softwood lignin is more condensed than hardwood lignin due to the difference in substitution of lignin precursors (substituted C_3 and unsubstituted C_5 in coniferyl alcohol versus substituted C_3 and C_5 in synapyl alcohol). Significant differences observed between the hardwood and softwood lignin structure indicate different physical and chemical properties of these two lignin types.

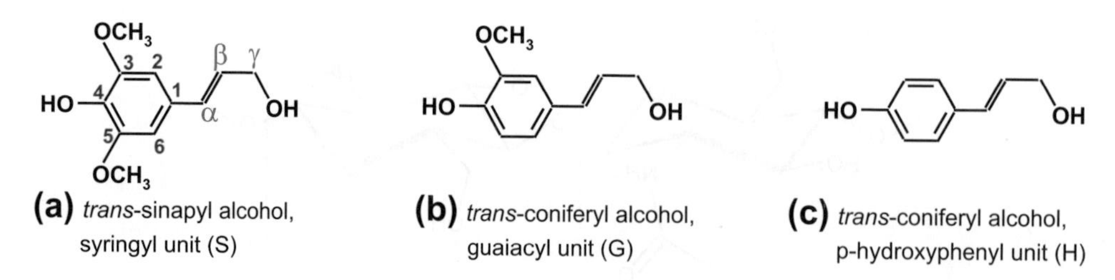

FIGURE 2.27 The precursors of lignin (Alén R. Structure and Chemical Composition of Wood. In: Glullichsen J., Paulapuro H., editors, Forest Products Chemistry. Jyväskylä.Finland Oy 2000).

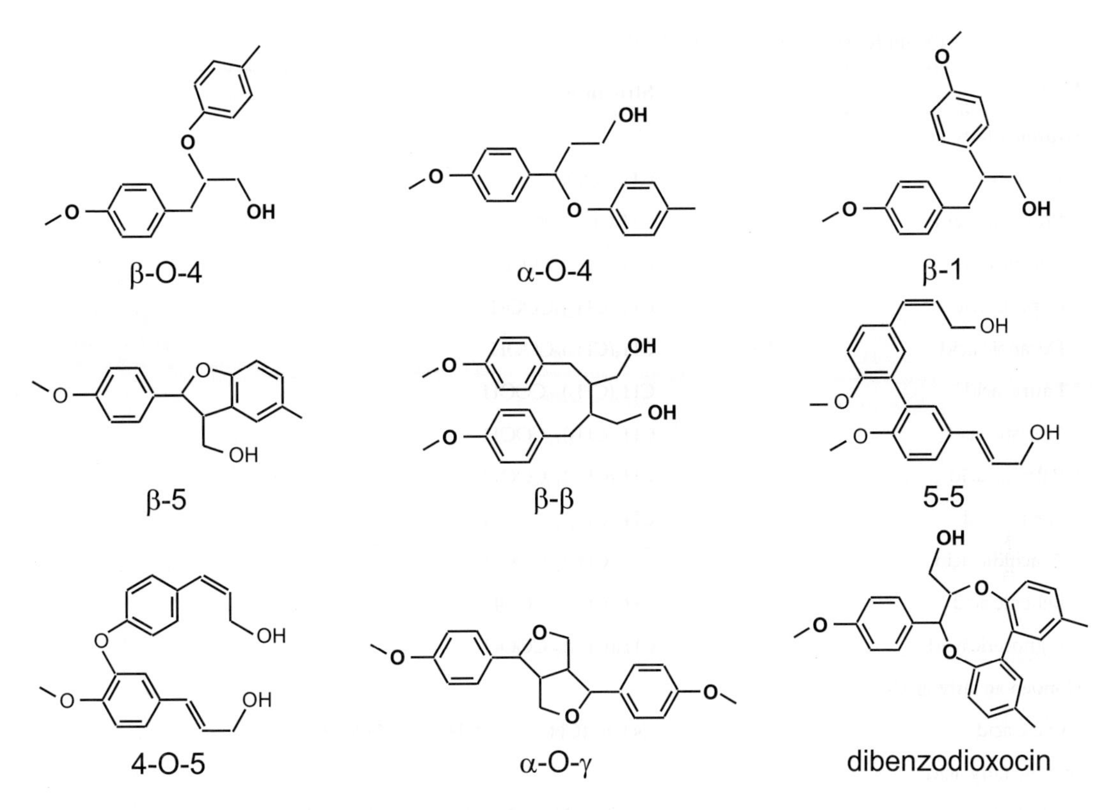

FIGURE 2.28 Common linkages between phenylpropane units in lignin.

2.3.5. Lipids, Fats, and Steroids

Lipids are hydrophobic biological compounds that are insoluble in water but soluble in nonpolar solvents such as benzene, chloroform, and ether. They are usually present in nonaqueous biological phases, such as plasma membranes. Fats are lipids that can serve as biological fuel-storage molecules. Lipoproteins and lipopolysaccharides are other types of lipids, which appear in the biological membranes of cells. Cells can alter the composition of lipids in their membranes to compensate (at least partially) for changes in temperature or to increase their tolerance to the presence of chemical agents such as ethanol.

The major component in most lipids is *fatty acids*. A list of common fatty acids is presented in Table 2.6. The hydrocarbon chain of a fatty acid is hydrophobic (water insoluble), but the carboxyl group is hydrophilic (water soluble). A typical fatty acid can be represented as

$$CH_3(CH_2)_nCOOH$$

TABLE 2.6 Examples of Common Fatty Acids

Acid	Structure
Saturated fatty acids	
Acetic acid	CH_3COOH
Propionic acid	CH_3CH_2COOH
Butyric acid	$CH_3(CH_2)_2COOH$
Caproic acid	$CH_3(CH_2)_4COOH$
Decanoic acid	$CH_3(CH_2)_8COOH$
Lauric acid	$CH_3(CH_2)_{10}COOH$
Myristic acid	$CH_3(CH_2)_{12}COOH$
Palmitic acid	$CH_3(CH_2)_{14}COOH$
Stearic acid	$CH_3(CH_2)_{26}COOH$
Arachidic acid	$CH_3(CH_2)_{18}COOH$
Behenic acid	$CH_3(CH_2)_{20}COOH$
Lignoceric acid	$CH_3(CH_2)_{22}COOH$
Monoenoic fatty acids	
Oleic acid	*cis* $CH_3(CH_2)_7CH{=}CH(CH_2)_7COOH$
Dienoic fatty acid	
Linoleic acid	*cis - cis* $CH_3(CH_2)_4(CH{=}CHCH_2)_2(CH_2)_6COOH$
Trienoic fatty acids	
α-Linolenic acid	*cis - cis - cis* $CH_3CH_2(CH{=}CHCH_2)_3(CH_2)_6COOH$
γ-Linolenic acid	*cis - cis - cis* $CH_3(CH_2)_4(CH{=}CHCH_2)_3(CH_2)_3COOH$
Tetraenoic fatty acid	
Arachidonic acid	*cis - cis - cis - cis* $CH_3(CH_2)_4(CH{=}CHCH_2)_4(CH_2)_2COOH$
Unusual fatty acids	
Tariric acid	$CH_3(CH_2)_{10}C{\equiv}C(CH_2)_4COOH$
Lactobacillic acid	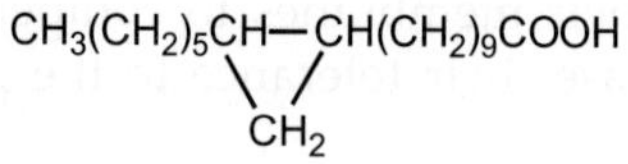 $CH_3(CH_2)_5CH{-}CH(CH_2)_9COOH$ CH_2
Prostaglandin	
PGE_1	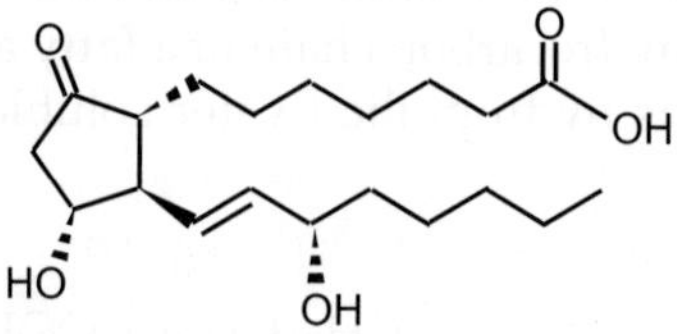 O O OH HO OH

(*Continued*)

TABLE 2.6 Examples of Common Fatty Acids—*Cont'd*

Acid	Structure
PGE_2	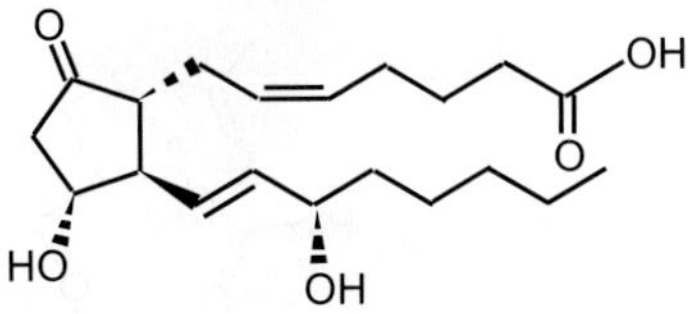 O, OH, O, HO, OH

The value of n is typically between 12 and 20. Unsaturated fatty acids contain double –C=C– bonds, such as oleic acid.

$$\text{Oleic acid}: \ CH_3(CH_2)_7CH{=}CH(CH_2)_7COOH$$

Sometimes, the location of the double bond nearest to the end opposite to the carboxyl group is of interest. For example, oleic acid's double bound is at the 9th carbon (opposite to COOH) and it is an ω-9 fatty acid.

Fats are esters of fatty acids with glycerol. The formation of a fat molecule can be represented by the following reaction:

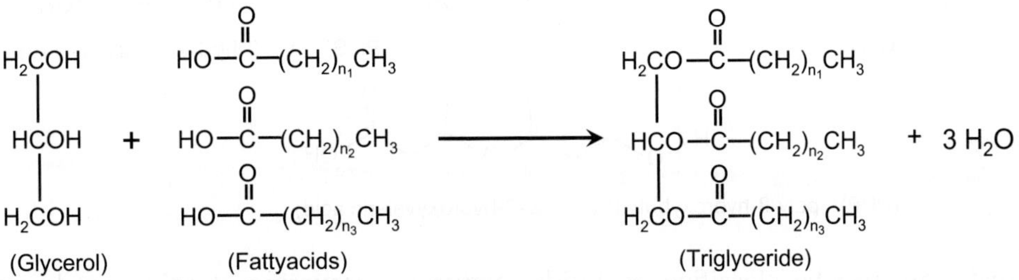

$$\begin{array}{c} H_2COH \\ | \\ HCOH \\ | \\ H_2COH \\ \text{(Glycerol)} \end{array} + \begin{array}{c} HO{-}C({=}O){-}(CH_2)_{n_1}CH_3 \\ HO{-}C({=}O){-}(CH_2)_{n_2}CH_3 \\ HO{-}C({=}O){-}(CH_2)_{n_3}CH_3 \\ \text{(Fattyacids)} \end{array} \longrightarrow \begin{array}{c} H_2CO{-}C({=}O){-}(CH_2)_{n_1}CH_3 \\ | \\ HCO{-}C({=}O){-}(CH_2)_{n_2}CH_3 \\ | \\ H_2CO{-}C({=}O){-}(CH_2)_{n_3}CH_3 \\ \text{(Triglyceride)} \end{array} + 3\,H_2O$$

Phosphoglycerides have similar structures to fats, the only difference being that phosphoric acid replaces a fatty acid and is esterified at one end to glycerol.

Membranes with selective permeability are key to life. Cells must control the entry and exit of molecules. *Phospholipids* are key components, but membranes contain large amounts of proteins. Biological membranes are based on a lipid bilayer. The hydrophobic tails of the phospholipids associate with each other in the core of the membrane. The hydrophilic heads form the outsides of the membrane and associate with the aqueous cytosol or the aqueous extracellular fluid. Some proteins span across the membrane, while others are attached to one of the surfaces. Membranes are dynamic structures, and lipids and proteins can diffuse rapidly. Typical membrane phospholipids include phosphatidylcholine, phosphatidylserine, phosphatidyl glycerol, and phosphatidyl inositol. The phosphatidyl group is shown below, which has two fatty acid groups, one glycerol group, and one phosphate group.

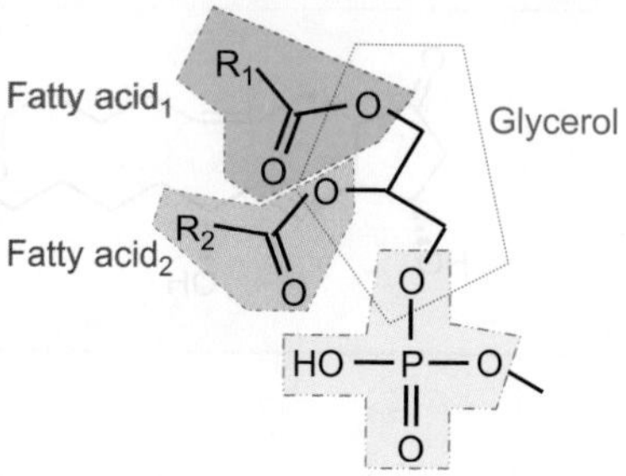

Fatty acid$_1$
Glycerol
Fatty acid$_2$

Stero structure of phospholipids

Another class of lipids of increasing technological importance is the polyhydroxyalkanoates (PHA). PHA's are polyesters formed by ester bonds end-to-end with hydroxyl group and carboxylic acid group. This natural polymer can be developed to replace existing polymers. In particular, *polyhydroxybutyrate* (PHB) is a good example of PHA. It can be used to form a clear, biodegradable polymeric sheet. Polymers with a variety of PHAs are being commercially developed. In some cells, PHB is formed as a storage product, much like fat in animals.

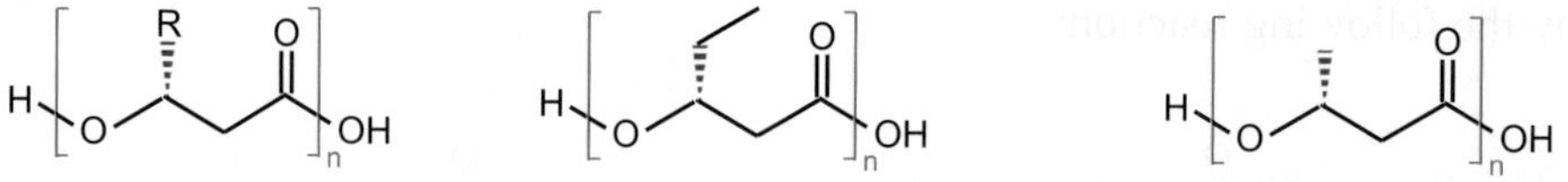

(PHA) (PHV) (PHB: poly-3-hydroxybutyric acid)

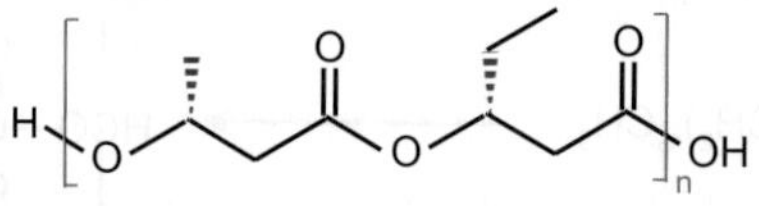

(PHBV: poly-3-hydroxybutyric acid-co-3-hydroxyvaleric acid)

Steroids can also be classified as lipids. Naturally occurring steroids are hormones that are important regulators of animal development and metabolism at very low concentrations (for example, 10^{-8} mol/L). A well-known steroid, cholesterol, is present in membranes of animal tissues. Figure 2.29 depicts the structures of some important steroids. Cortisone is an anti-inflammatory used to treat rheumatoid arthritis and some skin diseases. Derivatives of estrogens and progesterone are used as contraceptives. The commercial production of steroids is very important and depends on microbial conversions. Because of the large number of asymmetric centers, the total synthesis of steroids is difficult. Plants provide a source of abundant lipid precursors for these steroids, but the highly specific hydroxylation of these substrates at positions 11 (and 16) or dehydrogenations at position 1 are necessary to convert the precursors into compounds similar to those made in the adrenal gland. This cannot be done easily with chemical means and is done commercially using microbes that contain enzymes mediating specific hydroxylations or dehydrogenations.

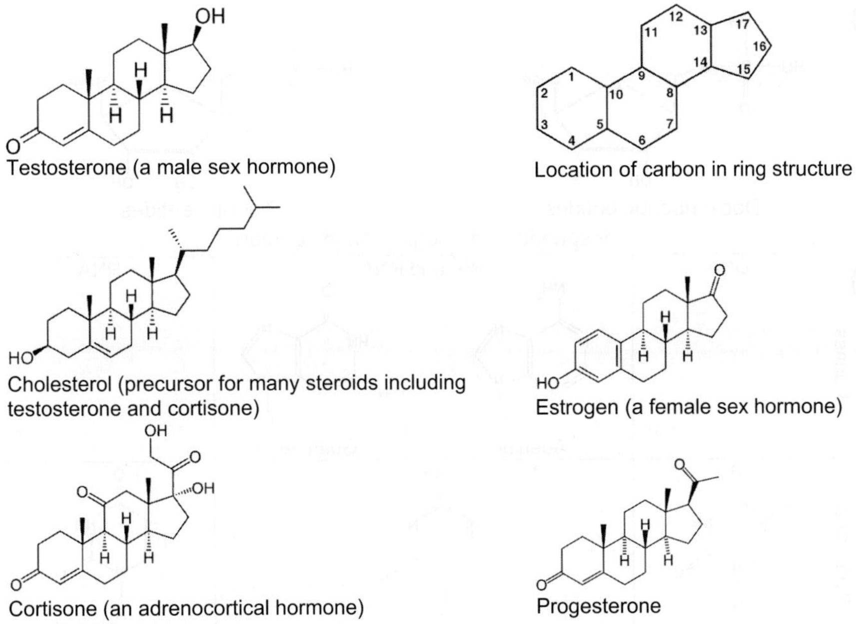

Testosterone (a male sex hormone)

Location of carbon in ring structure

Cholesterol (precursor for many steroids including testosterone and cortisone)

Estrogen (a female sex hormone)

Cortisone (an adrenocortical hormone)

Progesterone

FIGURE 2.29 Examples of important steroids. The basic numbering of the carbon atoms in these molecules is also shown.

2.3.6. Nucleic Acids, RNA, and DNA

Nucleic acids play a central role in the reproduction of living cells. DNA stores and preserves genetic information. RNA plays a central role in protein synthesis. Both DNA and RNA are large polymers made of their corresponding nucleotides.

Nucleotides are the building blocks of DNA and RNA and also serve as molecules to store energy and reducing power. The three major components in all nucleotides are phosphoric acid, pentose (ribose or deoxyribose), and a base (purine or pyrimidine). Figure 2.30 depicts the structure of nucleotides and purine–pyrimidine bases. Two major purines present in nucleotides are adenine (A) and guanine (G), and three major pyrimidines are thymine (T), cytosine (C), and uracil (U). DNA contains A, T, G, and C, and RNA contains A, U, G, and C as bases. It is the base sequence in DNA that carries genetic information for protein synthesis. This information is expressed in its owner and passed on from one generation to another.

The triphosphates of adenosine (and, to a lesser extent, guanosine) are the primary energy currency of the cell. The phosphate bonds in *adenosine triphosphate* (*ATP*) and *guanosine triphosphate* (*GTP*) are high-energy bonds. The formation of these phosphate bonds and their hydrolysis is the primary means by which cellular energy is stored and used. For example, the synthesis of a compound that is thermodynamically unfavorable can be accomplished in conjunction with ATP hydrolysis to ADP (adenosine diphosphate) or to AMP (adenosine monophosphate).

The coupled reactions can proceed to a much greater extent, since the free-energy change becomes much more negative. In reactions that release energy (for example, oxidation of

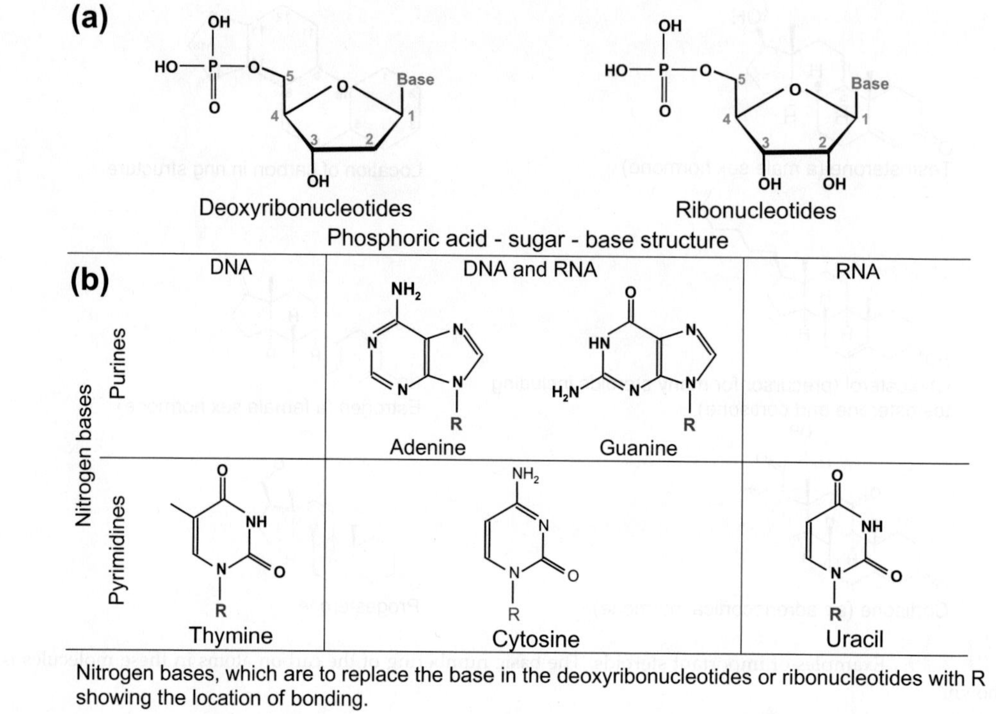

(a)

Deoxyribonucleotides Ribonucleotides

Phosphoric acid - sugar - base structure

(b)

Nitrogen bases	DNA	DNA and RNA	RNA
Purines		Adenine, Guanine	
Pyrimidines	Thymine	Cytosine	Uracil

Nitrogen bases, which are to replace the base in the deoxyribonucleotides or ribonucleotides with R showing the location of bonding.

FIGURE 2.30 (a) General structure of ribonucleotides and deoxyribonucleotides. (b) Five nitrogenous bases found in DNA and RNA.

a sugar), the energy is captured and stored by the formation of a phosphate bond in a coupled reaction where ADP is converted into ATP. In Chapter 10, we will discuss further the role of nucleotides in cellular energetics.

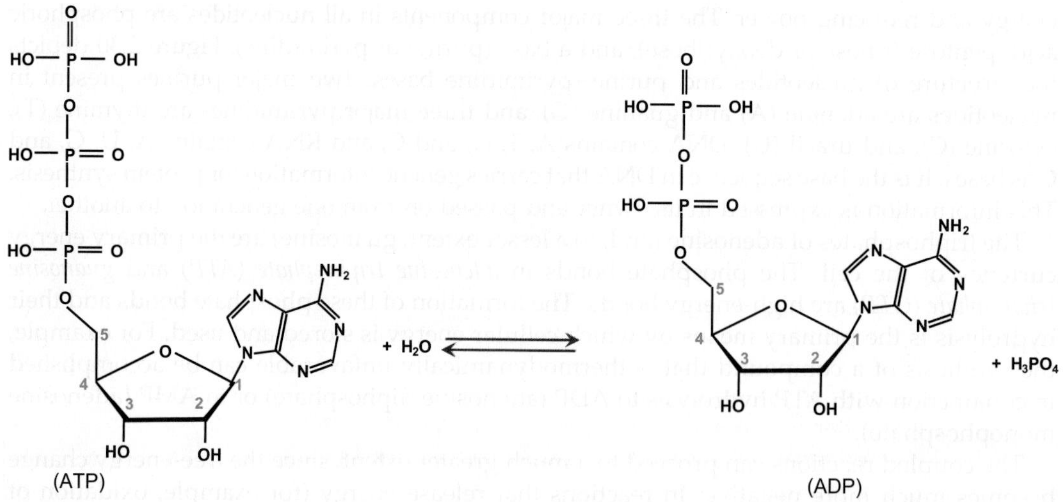

$$\text{(ATP)} + H_2O \rightleftharpoons \text{(ADP)} + H_3PO_4$$

In addition to using ATP to store energy, the cell stores and releases hydrogen atoms from biological oxidation–reduction reactions by using nucleotide derivatives. The two most common carriers of reducing power are *nicotinamide adenine dinucleotide* (*NAD*) and *nicotinamide adenine dinucleotide phosphate (NADP).*

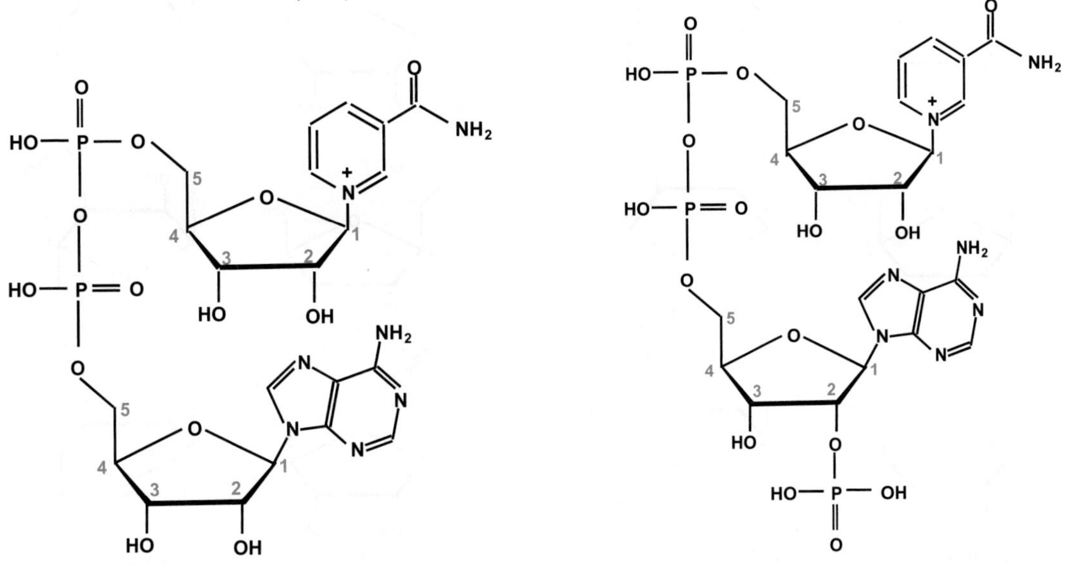

(NAD)

(NADP)

In addition to this important role in cellular energetics, the nucleotides are important monomers. Polynucleotides (DNA and RNA) are formed by the condensation of nucleotides. Nucleotides are linked together between the 3 and 5 carbons' successive sugar rings by phosphodiester bonds. The structures of DNA and RNA are illustrated in Fig. 2.31.

DNA is a very large threadlike macromolecule (MW of 2×10^9 Da in *E. coli*) and has the three-dimensional structure of a double-helix. The sequence of bases (purines and pyrimidines) in DNA carries genetic information, whereas sugar and phosphate groups perform a structural role. The base sequence of DNA is written in the 5 → 3 direction (starting at the 5th carbon in one sugar unit and moving toward the 3rd carbon in another sugar unit as shown in Fig. 2.30), e.g. pAGCT (p represents the terminal phosphate group, situated before the 3rd carbon of the new sugar unit). The double-helical structure of DNA is depicted in Fig. 2.32. In this structure, two helical polynucleotide chains (strands) are coiled around a common axis to form a double-helical DNA, and the chains run in opposite directions, 5 → 3 and 3 ← 5. The main features of the double-helical DNA structure are as follows:

(1) The phosphate and deoxyribose units are on the outer surface, but the bases point toward the chain center. The planes of the bases are perpendicular to the helix axis.

(2) The diameter of the helix is 2 nm. The helical structure repeats after ten residues on each chain, at intervals of 3.4 nm.

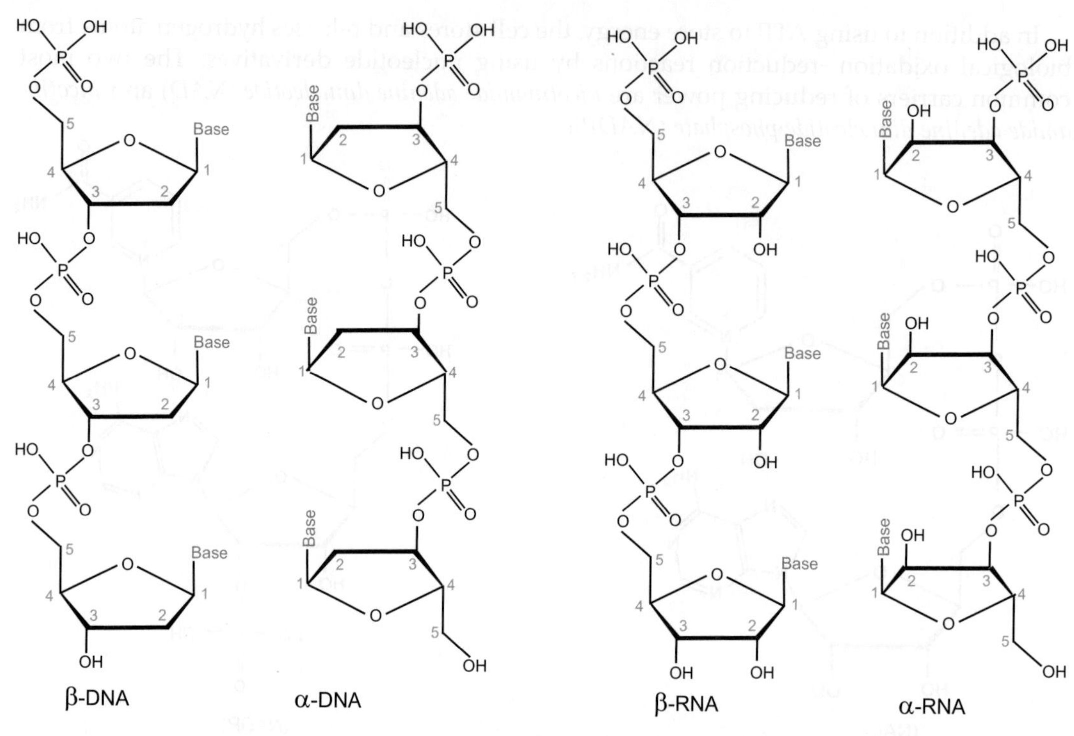

FIGURE 2.31 Structure of DNA and RNA chains. Only short chain (three-unit) segments are shown. Both α-anomers and β-anomers form strands uniformly by phosphodiester bonds formed between the 3rd and 5th carbon atoms of two sugar units. Since nucleotides and ribonucleotides all have phosphate connected on the 5th carbon, we say that DNA and RNA strands all run from 5 (th carbon) to 3 (rd carbon of the next sugar unit). However, β-strands and α-strands run opposite in directions, i.e. 5 → 3 for β strand and 3 ← 5 for α strand. The two strands (α and β) always pair together (with "head" and "tail" opposite each other).

(3) The two chains are held together by hydrogen bonding between pairs of bases. *Adenine is always paired with thymine* (two H bonds); guanine is always paired with cytosine (three H bonds). *This feature is essential to the genetic role of DNA.*

(4) The sequence of bases along a polynucleotide is not restricted in any way, although each strand must be complementary to the other. The precise sequence of bases carries the genetic information.

The large number of H bonds formed between base pairs provides molecular stabilization, as shown in Fig. 2.33. Regeneration of DNA from original DNA segments is known as *DNA replication.* When DNA segments are replicated, one strand of the new DNA segment comes directly from the parent DNA, and the other strand is newly synthesized using the parent DNA segment as a template. Therefore, DNA replication is semiconservative, as depicted in Fig. 2.34. The replication of DNA is discussed in more detail in Chapter 10.

Some cells contain circular DNA segments in cytoplasm called *plasmids.* Plasmids are nonchromosomal, autonomous, replicating DNA segments. Plasmids are easily moved in and out of cells and are often used for genetic engineering. Naturally occurring plasmids

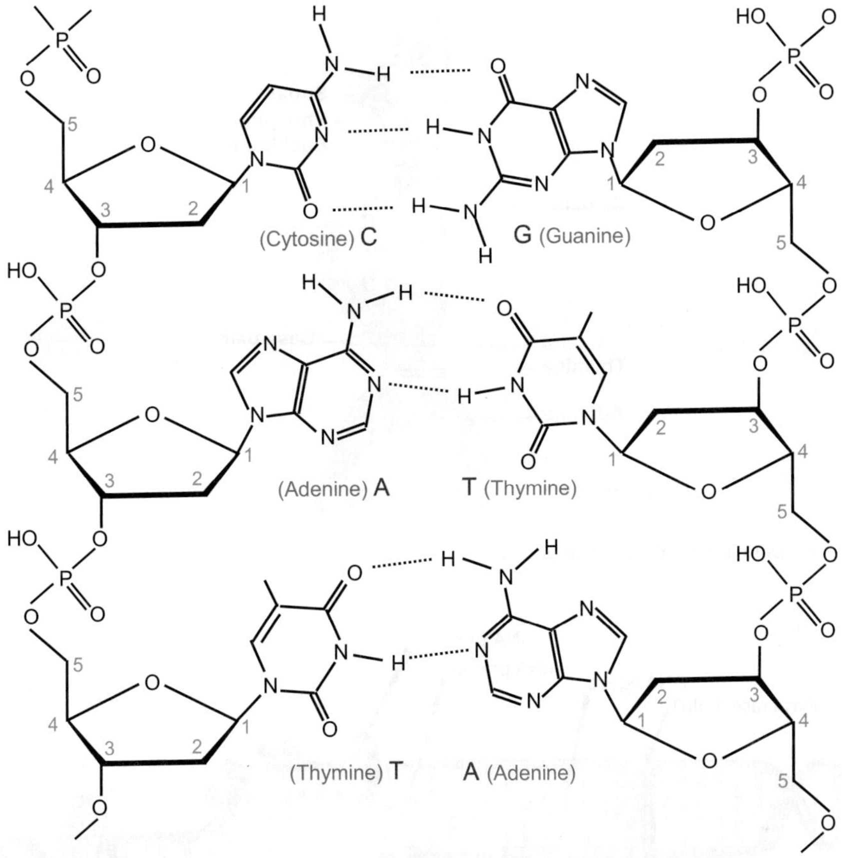

FIGURE 2.32 Molecular structure of DNA. The β-strand (left) and the α-strand (right) are linked to form double strands through hydrogen bonds between base units. The hydrogen bonds bring extra stability to the double strands. The pairing of the bases are (T–A), (A–T), (C–G), and (G–C). While bases bonded to the β-strand are mirror images of those bonded to the α-strand, the deoxyribose sugar backbones are not mirror images of one another between the β-strand and the α-strand.

can encode factors that protect cells from antibiotics or harmful chemicals. Linear rather than circular plasmids can be found in some yeasts and other organisms.

The major function of DNA is to carry genetic information in its base sequence. The genetic information in DNA is first transcribed into RNA molecules and then translated in protein synthesis. The templates for RNA synthesis are DNA molecules, and RNA molecules are the templates for protein synthesis. The formation of RNA molecules from DNA is known as DNA *transcription*, and the formation of peptides and proteins from RNA is called *translation*.

Certain RNA molecules function as intermediates carrying genetic information in protein synthesis (*messenger* or *mRNA*), whereas other RNA molecules (*transfer tRNA* and *ribosomal rRNA*) are part of the machinery of protein synthesis. The rRNA is located in *ribosomes* which

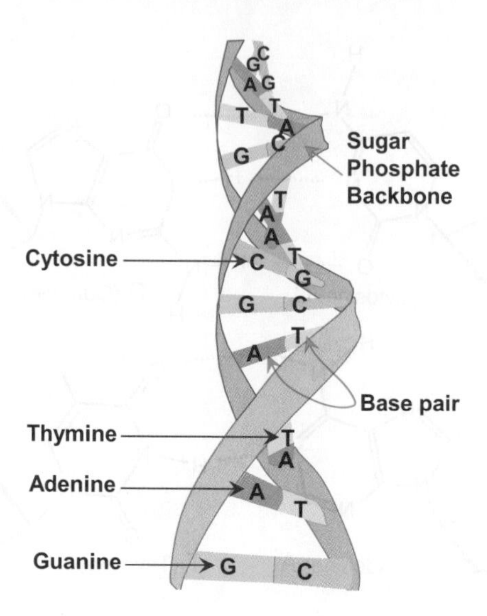

FIGURE 2.33 Double-helical structure of DNA.

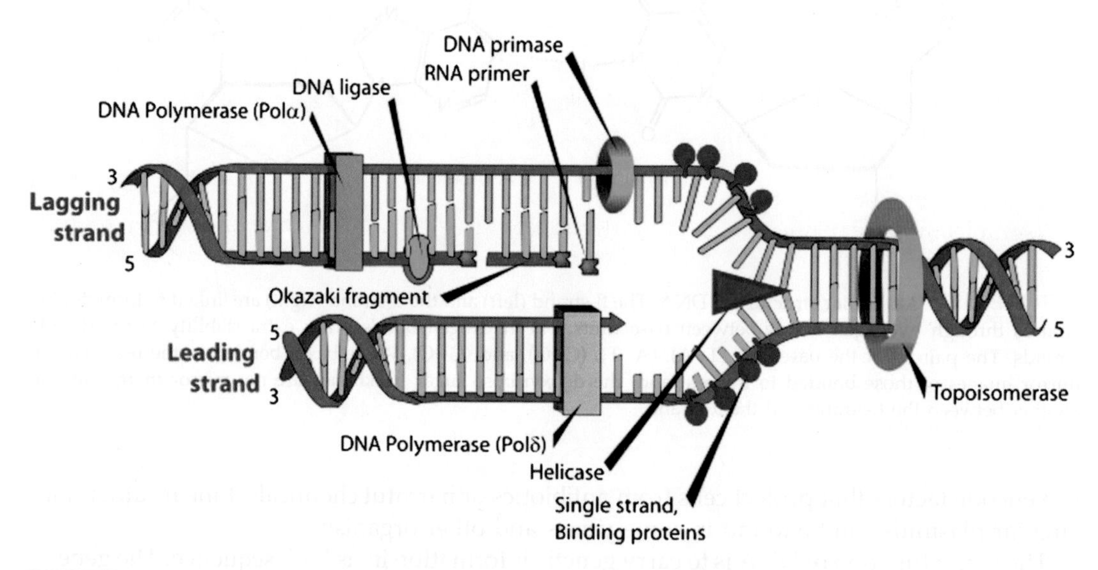

FIGURE 2.34 Overall process of replication by complementary base pairing.

are small particles made of protein and RNA. *Ribosomes* are cytoplasmic organelles (usually attached to the inner surfaces of endoplasmic reticulum in eukaryotes) and are the sites of protein synthesis.

RNA is a long, unbranched macromolecule consisting of nucleotides joined by 5-3 phosphodiester bonds. An RNA molecule may contain from 70 to several thousand nucleotides.

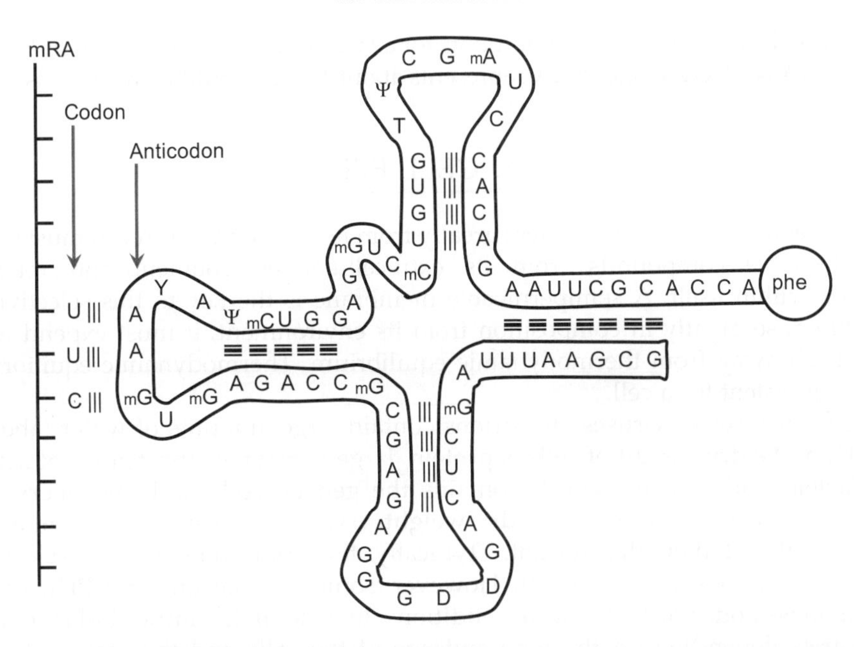

FIGURE 2.35 The structure of the tRNA molecule and the manner in which the anticodon of tRNA associates with the codon on mRNA by complementary base pairing. The amino acid corresponding to this codon (UUC) is phenylalanine that is bonded to the opposite end of the tRNA molecule. Many tRNA molecules contain unusual bases, such as methyl cytosine (mC) and pseudouridine (Ψ).

RNA molecules are usually single-stranded, except for certain viral RNA molecules containing regions of double-helical structure, resembling hairpin loops. Figure 2.35 describes the cloverleaf structure of transfer RNA (tRNA). In double-helical regions of tRNA, adenine (A) base pairs with uracil (U) and guanine base (G) pairs with cytosine (C). The RNA content of cells is usually two to six times higher than the DNA content.

Let us summarize the roles of each class of RNA:

Messenger RNA (mRNA) is synthesized in the chromosome in the nucleolus and carries genetic information from the chromosome for synthesis of a particular protein to the ribosomes. The mRNA molecule is a large one with a short half-life.

Transfer RNA (t-RNA) is a relatively small and stable molecule that carries a specific amino acid from the cytoplasm to the site of protein synthesis on ribosomes. tRNA is an adapter molecule composed of RNA, typically of 73–93 nucleotides in length, that is used to bridge the four-letter genetic code in mRNA with the twenty-letter code of amino acids in protein. Each of the 20 amino acids has at least one corresponding type of tRNA molecule.

Ribosomal RNA (rRNA) is the major component of ribosomes, constituting nearly 65%. The remainder is various ribosomal proteins. Three distinct types of rRNAs present in the *E. coli* ribosome are specified as 23S, 16S, and 5S, respectively, on the basis of their sedimentation coefficients, determined in a centrifuge (the symbol S denotes a Svedberg unit). The MWs are 35 kD for 5S, 550 kD for 16S, and 1100 kD for 23S. These three rRNA types differ in their base sequences and ratios. Eukaryotic cells have larger ribosomes and four different types of rRNAs:

5S, 7S, 18S, and 28S. Ribosomal RNA accounts for a large fraction of total RNA. In *E. coli*, about 85% of all RNA is rRNA, while tRNA represents about 12% and mRNA represents 2–3%.

2.4. CELL FEED

A cell's chemical composition differs greatly from its environment. A cell must selectively remove desirable compounds from its extracellular environment and retain other compounds within itself. A semipermeable membrane is the key to this selectivity. Since the cell differs so greatly in composition from its environment, it must expend energy to maintain itself away from thermodynamic equilibrium. Thermodynamic equilibrium and death are equivalent for a cell.

All organisms except viruses and prions contain large amounts of water (about 80%). About 50% of the dry weight of cells is protein, largely enzymes (proteins that act as catalysts). Nucleic acid content (which contains the genetic code and machinery to make proteins) varies from 10% to 20% of dry weight. (However, viruses may contain nucleic acids up to 50% of their dry weight.) Typically, the lipid content of most cells varies between 5% and 15% of dry weight. However, some cells accumulate PHB up to 90% of the total mass under certain culture conditions. In general, the intracellular composition of cells varies depending on the type and age of the cells and the composition of the nutrient media. Typical compositions for major groups of organisms are summarized in Table 2.7.

Most of the products formed by cells are produced as a result of their response to environmental conditions, such as nutrients, growth hormones, and ions. The qualitative and

TABLE 2.7 Chemical Analyses, Dry Weights, and the Populations of Different Microorganisms Obtained in Culture

	Composition, % dry weight					
Organism	**Protein**	**Nucleic acid**	**Lipid**	**Typical population in culture, numbers/l**	**Typical dry weight of the culture, g/l**	**Comments**
Viruses	50–90	50–50	<1	10^{11}–10^{12}	0.005*	Viruses with a lipoprotein sheath may contain 25% lipid.
Bacteria	40–70	13–34	10–15	2×10^{11} -2×10^{12}	0.2–29	PHB content may reach 90%.
Filamentous fungi	10–25	1–3	2–7		30–50	Some *Aspergillus* and *Penicillium* sp. contain 50% lipid.
Yeast	40–50	4–10	1–6	$1–4 \times 10^{11}$	10–50	Some *Rhodotorula* and *Candida* sp. contain 50% lipid.
Small unicellular algae	10–60 (50)	1–5 (3)	4–80 (10)	$4–8 \times 10^{10}$	4–9	Figures in ( ) are commonly found values but the composition varies with the growth conditions.

* *For a virus of 200 nm diameter.*

Source: S. Aiba, A. E. Humphrey, and N. F. Millis, Biochemical Engineering, *2d ed., University of Tokyo Press, Tokyo, 1973.*

quantitative nutritional requirements of cells need to be determined to optimize growth and product formation. Nutrients required by cells can be classified into two categories:

(1) *Macronutrients* are needed in concentrations larger than 10^{-4} mol/L. Carbon, nitrogen, oxygen, hydrogen, sulfur, phosphorus, Mg^{2+}, and K^{+} are nutrients.
(2) *Micronutrients* are needed in concentrations of less than 10^{-4} mol/L. Trace elements such as Mo^{+}, Zn^{2+}, Cu^{2+}, Mn^{2+}, Ca^{2+}, Na^{+}, vitamins, growth hormones, and metabolic precursors are micronutrients.

2.4.1. Macronutrients

Carbon compounds are major sources of cellular carbon and energy. Microorganisms are classified into two categories on the basis of their carbon source: 1) *heterotrophs* use organic compounds such as carbohydrates, lipids, and hydrocarbons as a carbon and energy source; 2) *autotrophs* use carbon dioxide as a carbon source. Mixotrophs concomitantly grow under both autotrophic and heterotrophic conditions; however, autotrophic growth is stimulated by certain organic compounds. Facultative autotrophs normally grow under autotrophic conditions; however, they can grow under heterotrophic conditions in the absence of CO_2 and inorganic energy sources. *Chemoautotrophs* utilize CO_2 as a carbon source and obtain energy from the oxidation of inorganic compounds. *Photoautotrophs* use CO_2 as a carbon source and utilize light as an energy source.

The most common carbon sources in industrial fermentations are molasses (sucrose), starch (glucose, dextrin), corn syrup, and waste sulfite liquor (glucose). In laboratory fermentations, glucose, sucrose, and fructose are the most common carbon sources. Methanol, ethanol, and methane also constitute cheap carbon sources for some fermentations. In aerobic fermentations, about 50% of substrate carbon is incorporated into cells and about 50% of it is used as an energy source. In anaerobic fermentations, a large fraction of substrate carbon is converted to products and a smaller fraction is converted to cell mass (less than 30%).

Nitrogen constitutes about 10–14% of cell dry weight. The most widely used nitrogen sources are ammonia or the ammonium salts [NH_4Cl, $(NH_4)_2SO_4$, NH_4NO_3], proteins, peptides, and amino acids. Nitrogen is incorporated into cell mass in the form of proteins and nucleic acids. Some organisms such as *Azotobacter* spp. and the cyanobacteria fix nitrogen from the atmosphere to form ammonium. Urea may also be used as a nitrogen source by some organisms. Organic nitrogen sources such as yeast extract and peptone are expensive compared to ammonium salts. Some carbon and nitrogen sources utilized by the fermentation industry are summarized in Table 2.8.

Oxygen is present in all organic cell components and cellular water and constitutes about 20% of the dry weight of cells. Molecular oxygen is required as a terminal electron acceptor in the aerobic metabolism of carbon compounds. Gaseous oxygen is introduced into growth media by sparging air or by surface aeration.

Hydrogen constitutes about 8% of cellular dry weight and is derived primarily from carbon compounds, such as carbohydrates. Some bacteria such as methanogens can utilize hydrogen as an energy source.

Phosphorus constitutes about 3% of cellular dry weight and is present in nucleic acids and in the cell wall of some gram-positive bacteria such as teichoic acids. Inorganic phosphate

TABLE 2.8 Some Carbon and Nitrogen Sources Utilized by the Fermentation Industry

Carbon sources	Nitrogen sources
Starch waste (maize and potato)	Soya meal
Molasses (cane and beet)	Yeast extract
Whey	Distillers solubles
n-Alkanes	Cottonseed extract
Gas oil	Dried blood
Sulfite waste liquor	Corn steep liquor
Domestic sewage	Fish solubles and meal
Cellulose waste	Groundnut meal
Carbon bean	

Source: G. M. Dunn in Comprehensive Biotechnology, *M. Moo-Young, ed., Vol. 1, Elsevier Science, 1985.*

salts, such as KH_2PO_4 and K_2HPO_4 are the most common phosphate salts. Glycerophosphates can also be used as organic phosphate sources. Phosphorus is a key element in the regulation of cell metabolism. The phosphate level in cell growth media should be less than 1 mmol/L for the formation of many secondary metabolites such as antibiotics.

Sulfur constitutes nearly 1% of cellular dry weight and is present in proteins and some coenzymes. Sulfate salts such as $(NH_4)_2SO_4$ are the most common sulfur source. Sulfur containing amino acids can also be used as a sulfur source. Certain autotrophs utilize S^{2+} and S^0 as energy sources.

Potassium is a cofactor for some enzymes and is required in carbohydrate metabolism. Cells tend to actively take up K^+ and Mg^{2+} and exclude Na^+ and Ca^{2+}. The most commonly used potassium salts are K_2HPO_4, KH_2PO_4, and K_3PO_4.

Magnesium is a cofactor for some enzymes and is present in cell walls and membranes. Ribosomes specifically require Mg^{2+} ions. Magnesium is usually supplied as $MgSO_4 \cdot 7H_2O$ or $MgCl_2$.

Table 2.9 lists the eight major macronutrients and their physiological roles.

2.4.2. Micronutrients

Trace elements are essential to microbial nutrition. A lack of essential trace elements increases the lag phase (the time from inoculation to active cell replication in batch culture) and may decrease the specific growth rate and yield. The three major categories of micronutrients are discussed below.

(1) The most widely needed trace elements are Fe, Zn, and Mn. Iron (Fe) is present in ferredoxin and cytochrome and is an important cofactor. Iron also plays a regulatory role in some fermentation processes (e.g. iron deficiency is required for the excretion of riboflavin by *Ashbya gossypii* and iron concentration regulates penicillin production by *Penicillium chrysogenum*). Zinc (Zn) is a cofactor for some enzymes and also regulates some

TABLE 2.9 The Eight Macronutrient Elements and Some Physiological Functions and Growth Requirements

Element	Physiological function	Required concentration, mol/L
Carbon	Constituent of organic cellular material. Often the energy source.	$>10^{-2}$
Nitrogen	Constituent of proteins, nucleic acids, and coenzymes.	10^{-3}
Hydrogen	Organic cellular material and water.	
Oxygen	Organic cellular material and water. Required for aerobic respiration.	
Sulfur	Constituent of proteins and certain coenzymes.	10^{-4}
Phosphorus	Constituent of nucleic acids, phospholipids, nucleotides, and certain coenzymes.	10^{-4}–10^{-3}
Potassium	Principal inorganic cation in the cell and cofactor for some enzymes.	10^{-4}–10^{-3}
Magnesium	Cofactor for many enzymes and chlorophylls (photosynthetic microbes) and present in cell walls and membranes.	10^{-4}–10^{-3}

Source: G. M. Dunn in Comprehensive Biotechnology, *M. Moo-Young, ed., Vol. 1, Elsevier Science, 1985.*

fermentation process, such as penicillin. Manganese (Mn) is also an enzyme cofactor and plays a role in the regulation of secondary metabolism and the excretion of primary metabolites.

(2) Trace elements needed under specific growth conditions are Cu, Co, Mo, Ca, Na, Cl, Ni, and Se. Copper (Cu) is present in certain respiratory-chain components and enzymes. Copper deficiency stimulates penicillin and citric acid production. Cobalt (Co) is present in corrinoid compounds such as vitamin Bu. Propionic bacteria and certain methanogens require cobalt. Molybdenum (Mo) is a cofactor of nitrate reductase and nitrogenase and is required for growth on NO_3 and N_2 as the sole source of nitrogen. Calcium (Ca) is a cofactor for amylases and some proteases and is also present in some bacterial spores and in the cell walls of some cells, such as plant cells.

Sodium (Na) is needed in trace amounts by some bacteria, especially by methanogens for ion balance. Sodium is important in the transport of charged species in eukaryotic cells. Chloride (Cl^-) is needed by some halobacteria and marine microbes, which require Na^+, too. Nickel (Ni) is required by some methanogens as a cofactor and Selenium (Se) is required in formate metabolism of some organisms.

(3) Trace elements that are rarely required are B, Al, Si, Cr, V, Sn, Be, F, Ti, Ga, Ge, Br, Zr, W, Li, and I. These elements are required in concentrations of less than 10^{-6} mol/L and are toxic at high concentrations, such as 10^{-4} mol/L.

Some ions such as Mg^{2+}, Fe^{3+}, and PO_4^{3-} may precipitate in nutrient medium and become unavailable to the cells. *Chelating agents* are used to form soluble compounds with the precipitating ions. Chelating agents have certain groups termed *ligands* that bind to metal ions to form soluble complexes. Major ligands are carboxyl (−COOH), amine ($-NH_2$), and mercapto (−SH) groups. Citric acid, EDTA (ethylene diamine tetra-acetic acid), polyphosphates, histidine, tyrosine, and cysteine are the most commonly used chelating agents. Na_2 EDTA is the most common chelating agent. EDTA may remove some metal ion components of the cell wall, such as Ca^{2+}, Mg^{2+}, and Zn^{2+} and may cause cell wall disintegration. Citric acid can be metabolized by some bacteria. Chelating agents are included in media in low concentrations (e.g. 1 mmol/L).

Growth factors stimulate the growth and synthesis of some metabolites. Vitamins, hormones, and amino acids are major growth factors. Vitamins usually function as coenzymes. Some commonly required vitamins are thiamine (B_1), riboflavin (B_2), pyridoxine (B_6), biotin, cyanocobalamin (B_{12}), folic acid, lipoic acid, p-amino benzoic acid, and vitamin K. Vitamins are required at a concentration range of 10^{-6}–10^{-12} mol/L. Depending on the organism, some or all of the amino acids may need to be supplied externally in concentrations from 10^{-6}–10^{-13} mol/L. Some fatty acids, such as oleic acid and sterols, are also needed in small quantities by some organisms. Higher forms of life, such as animal and plant cells, require hormones to regulate their metabolism. Insulin is a common hormone for animal cells, and auxin and cytokinins are plant-growth hormones.

2.4.3. Growth Media

The two types of growth media are defined media and complex media. *Defined media* contain specific amounts of pure chemical compounds with known chemical compositions.

TABLE 2.10 Compositions of Typical Defined Media

Constituent	Purpose	Concentration, g/L
GROUP A		
Glucose	C, energy	30
KH_2PO_4	K, P	1.5
$MgSO_4 \cdot 7H_2O$	Mg, S	0.6
$CaCl_2$	Ca	0.05
$Fe_2(SO_4)_3$	Fe	1.5×10^{-4}
$ZnSO_4 \cdot 7H_2O$	Zn	6×10^{-4}
$CuSO_4 \cdot 5H_2O$	Cu	6×10^{-4}
$MnSO_4 \cdot H_2O$	Mn	6×10^{-4}
GROUP B		
$(NH_4)_2HPO_4$	N, P	6
$NH_4H_2PO_4$	N, P	5
GROUP C		
$C_6H_5Na_3O_7 \cdot 2H_2O$	Chelator	4
GROUP D		
Na_2HPO_4	Buffer	20
KH_2PO_4	Buffer	10

A medium containing glucose, $(NH_4)_2SO_4$, KH_2PO_4, and $MgCl_2$ is a defined medium. *Complex media* contain natural compounds whose chemical composition is not exactly known. A medium containing yeast extracts, peptone, molasses, or corn steep liquor is a complex medium. A complex medium usually can provide the necessary growth factors, vitamins, hormones, and trace elements, often resulting in higher cell yields, compared to the defined medium. Often, complex media are less expensive than defined media. The primary advantage of defined media is that the results are more reproducible and the operator has better control of the fermentation. Further, recovery and purification of a product is often easier and cheaper in defined media. Table 2.10 summarizes typical defined and complex media.

2.5. SUMMARY

Cells are the basic unit of living organisms. Living organisms can be single celled (unicellular) or multicellular. Therefore, living organisms are commonly cellular. The exception to the cellular living organism is a prion, which consists of protein only. Cells are usually very small, but big ones exist and can weigh over a kilogram. There are rich varieties of chemicals and materials associated with cells. These chemicals and materials present opportunities for bioprocess engineers to make sustainable products that meet the needs of humanity.

Microbes are tiny living organisms. Most microbes belong to one of the four major groups: bacteria, viruses, fungi, or protozoa. Microbes can grow over an immense range of conditions: at temperatures above boiling and below freezing; in high-salt concentrations; under high pressures (>1000 atm) and in strong acidic or caustic environments (pH at about 1–10). Cells that must use oxygen are known as *aerobic*. Cells that find oxygen toxic are *anaerobic*. Cells that can adapt to growth either with or without oxygen are *facultative*. The diversity of the microbes provides bioprocess engineers adaptable tools to the every bioprocess conditions needed.

The two major groups of cells are *prokaryotic* and *eukaryotic*. Eukaryotic cells are more complex. The essential demarcation is the absence (in prokaryotes) or presence (in eukaryotes) of a membrane around the chromosomal or genetic material. The prokaryotes can be further divided into two groups: the *eubacteria* and the *archaebacteria*. The archaebacteria are a group of ancient organisms; subdivisions include methanogens (methane-producing organisms), halobacteria (which live in high-salt environments), and thermoacidophiles (which grow best under conditions of high temperature and high acidity). Most eubacteria can be separated into gram-positive and gram-negative cells. *Gram-positive* cells have both an inner membrane and strong cell wall. *Gram-negative* cells have an inner membrane and an outer membrane. The outer membrane is supported by cell wall material but is less rigid than in gram-positive cells. The *cyanobacteria* (blue-green algae) are photosynthetic prokaryotes classified as a subdivision of the eubacteria. The eukaryotes contain both unicellular and multicellular organisms. The fungi and yeasts, most algae species, and the protozoa are all examples of unicellular eukaryotes. Plants and animals are multicellular eukaryotes.

Viruses are replicating particles that are obligate parasites. Some viruses use DNA to store genetic information, while others use RNA. Viruses specific to bacteria are called *bacteriophages* or phages. A prion is an infectious agent composed of protein in a misfolded form, in contrast to all other known infectious agents that contain nucleic acids (either DNA, RNA, or both). Prion is not able to reproduce but produced by inducing proteins to misfold.

Stem cells are unspecialized cells that have two defining properties: 1) potency, or the ability to differentiate into diverse specialized cells (different cell types) including differentiated stem cells and 2) reproductivity or the ability to self-regenerate (same cell type).

All cells contain at least one of the three macromolecules: *protein*, *RNA*, and *DNA*. Other essential components of these cells are constructed from lipids and carbohydrates.

Proteins are polymers of amino acids; typically, 20 different amino acids are used. Each amino acid has a distinctive side group. The sequence of amino acids determines the *primary structure* of the protein. Interactions among the side groups of the amino acids (hydrogen bonding, disulfide bonds, and hydrophobic or hydrophilic regions) determine the *secondary* and *tertiary structure* of the molecule. Separate polypeptide chains can associate to form the final structure, which termed *quaternary*. The 3D shape of a protein is critical to its function.

DNA and RNA are polymers of nucleotides. DNA contains the cell's genetic information. RNA is involved in transcribing and translating that information into real proteins. mRNA transcribes the code, tRNA is an adapter molecule that transports a specific amino acid to the reaction site for protein synthesis, and ribosomal RNA is an essential component of ribosomes, which are the structures responsible for protein synthesis. In addition to their roles as monomers for DNA and RNA synthesis, nucleotides play important roles in cellular energetics. The *high-energy phosphate bonds* in *ATP* can store energy. The hydrolysis of ATP when coupled with otherwise energetically unfavorable reactions can drive the reaction toward completion. *NAD* and *NAPH* are important carriers of *reducing power*.

Carbohydrates consist of sugars, and the polymerized products of sugars are called *polysaccharides*. Sugars represent convenient molecules for the rapid oxidation and release of energy. The polysaccharides play an important structural and stability roles (such as cellulose, hemicelluloses, and lignin) and can be used as a cellular reserve of carbon and energy (as in glycogen, PHA, starch and fructan).

Lipids and related compounds are critical in the construction of cellular membranes. Some fats also form reserve sources. A number of growth factors or hormones involve lipid materials. *Phospholipids* are the primary components of biological membranes.

The maintenance of cellular integrity requires the selective uptake of nutrients. One class of nutrients is the *macronutrients*, which are used in large amounts. *Micronutrients* and trace nutrients are used in low concentrations; some of these compounds become toxic if present at high levels.

In a *defined medium*, all components added to the medium are identifiable. In a *complex medium*, one or more components are not chemically defined (e.g. yeast extract). Complex media are commonly mixtures obtained from cell culture or natural sources without (complete) componentwise separation/purification.

Further Reading

Alberts, B., Bray, D., Johnson, A., Lewis, I., Raff, M., Roberts, K., and Walter, P., 1998. *Essential Cell Biology: An Introduction to the Molecular Biology of the Cell*, Garland Publ., Inc., New York.

Beckmann, J., Scheitza, S., Wernet, P., Fischer, J.C., Giebel, B., 2007. "Asymmetric cell division within the human hematopoietic stem and progenitor cell compartment: identification of asymmetrically segregating proteins". *Blood* **109** (12): 5494-501. http://dx.doi.org/10.1182/blood-2006-11-055921. PMID 17332245.

Black, J.G., 1996. *Microbiology: Principles and Applications*, third ed. Prentice Hall, Upper Saddle River, NJ.

Dence, C.W., and Lin, S.Y., 1992. Introduction. In Dence, C.W., and Lin, S.Y. (Eds.), *Methods in Lignin Chemistry.* Berlin Heidelberg: Springer-Verlag.

Fengel, D., and Wegener, G., 1989. *Wood Chemistry, Ultrastructure, Reactions.* Walter deGruyter, Berlin.

Moran, L.A., Scrimgeourh, K.G., Horton, R., Ochs, R.S., and Rawn, J.D., 1994. *Biochemistry,* Second ed. Prentice Hall, Upper Saddle River, NJ.

Shuler, M.L. and F. Kargi., 2006. Bioprocess Engineering - Basic Concepts, Second ed. Prentice Hall, Upper Saddle River, NJ.

Sjöström, E., 1993. *Wood Chemistry - Fundamentals and Applications,* Second ed., Academic Press, San Diego, CA.

Song, X., Zhu, C., Doan, C., Xie, T., 2002. "Germline stem cells anchored by adherens junctions in the Drosophila ovary niches". *Science* **296** (5574): 1855-7. doi:10.1126.

Takahashi, K., Yamanaka, S., 2006. "Induction of pluripotent stem cells from mouse embryonic and adult fibroblast cultures by defined factors". *Cell* **126** (4): 663-76. http://dx.doi.org/10.1016/j.cell.2006.07.024. PMID 16904174.

Vierbuchen, T., Ostermeier, A., Pang, Z.P., Kokubu, Y., Südhof, T.C., Wernig, M., 2010-02-25. "Direct conversion of fibroblasts to functional neurons by defined factors". *Nature* **463** (7284): 1035-41. doi:10.1038/nature08797. PMC 2829121. PMID 20107439.

PROBLEMS

2.1. What makes a living cell?

2.2. Briefly compare prokaryotes with eukaryotes in terms of internal structure and functions.

2.3. What is a virus cell? What is a prion?

2.4. What are the major classes of fungi? Cite the differences among these classes briefly.

2.5. What are the major classes of algae? Cite the differences among these classes and their potential applications.

2.6. Briefly describe distinct features of actinomycetes and their important products.

2.7. Briefly compare protozoa with algae in terms of their cellular structures and functions.

2.8. What is a stem cell?

2.9. What are major sources of carbon, nitrogen, and phosphorus in industrial fermentations?

2.10. Explain the functions of the following trace elements in microbial metabolism: Fe, Zn, Cu, Co, Ni, Mn, vitamins.

2.11. What are chelating agents? Explain their function with an example.

2.12. Cite five major biological functions of proteins.

2.13. Briefly describe the primary, secondary, tertiary, and quaternary structure of proteins. What could happen if you substituted a tyrosine for a cysteine in the active site? What might happen if the substitution occurred elsewhere?

2.14. Contrast DNA and RNA. Cite at least four differences.

2.15. Why are phosphates being added in a fermentation medium?

2.16. Contrast the advantages and disadvantages of chemically defined and complex media.

2.17. You are asked to develop a medium for production of an antibiotic. The antibiotic is to be made in large amounts (ten 100,000 L fermenters) and is relatively inexpensive. The host cell is a soil isolate of a fungal species, and the nutritional requirements for rapid growth are uncertain. Will you try to develop a defined or complex medium? Why?

2.18. You wish to produce a high-value protein using recombinant DNA technology. Would you try to develop a chemical-defined medium or a complex medium? Why?

2.19. Explain what semiconservative replication means.

2.20. Give characteristic dimensions for each of these cells: *E. coli*, yeast (*S. cerevisiae*), liver cell (hepatocyte), plant cell.

2.21. What are the differences in the cell envelope structure between gram-negative and gram-positive bacteria? These differences become important if you wish to genetically engineer bacteria to excrete proteins into the extracellular fluid.

2.22. True or False:

a. An organism that can grow using oxygen as an electron acceptor and can also grow and metabolize in the absence of oxygen is called facultative.

b. Yeasts are prokaryotes.

c. A bacteriophage is a virus that infects bacteria.

d. When you supplement growth media with amino acids, you should use the D-form.

2.23. Summarize the argument that all chemical energy sources are derived from solar energy. What is a reasonable definition of renewable and nonrenewable energy sources?

2.24. What is the difference between cellulose and hemicelluloses? What are the similarities and differences between starch, cellulose and fructan?

CHAPTER

3

An Overview of Chemical Reaction Analysis

OUTLINE

Chapter 2 has been an introduction and review of microbiology and chemistry. In this chapter, we turn to a quick survey of chemical engineering, with applications in bioprocesses.

Bioprocess Engineering
http://dx.doi.org/10.1016/B978-0-444-59525-6.00003-2

3.1. CHEMICAL SPECIES

We begin our study by performing mole balances on each chemical species in the system. Here, the term *chemical species* refers to any chemical compound, element, or living organism with a given identity. The identity of a chemical species is determined by the *kind, number,* and *configuration* of that species' atoms. For example, the species penicillin V ($C_{16}H_{18}O_4N_2S$, an antibiotic) is made up of a fixed number of specific elements in a definite molecular arrangement or configuration. The structure shown illustrates the kind, number, and configuration of the species penicillin V on a molecular level.

Penicillin V

Chemical species are commonly represented by elemental formula (NH_3 for ammonia, N_2 for nitrogen, H_2O for water, $C_{16}H_{18}O_4N_2S$ for penicillin V, and so on) and Roel's formula. Roel's formula is elemental formula normalized by carbon (Table 3.1). For example, penicillin V is represented by $CH_{1.125}O_{0.25}N_{0.125}S_{0.0625}$.

Even though two chemical compounds have exactly the same number of atoms of each element, they could still be different species because of different configurations. For example, glucose and fructose both have six carbon atoms, 12 hydrogen atoms, and six oxygen atoms; however, the atoms in the two compounds are arranged differently.

As a consequence of the different configurations, these two isomers display different chemical and physical properties. Therefore, we consider them as two different species even though each has the same number of atoms of each element.

3.2. CHEMICAL REACTIONS

We say that a *chemical reaction* has taken place when a detectable number of molecules of one or more species have assumed a new form by a change in the kind or number of atoms in the compound and/or by a change in structure or configuration of these atoms. To begin, let us look at one particular reaction in the production of soft drinks. Soft drinks are essentially sweetened water with a small amount of flavoring added (usually synthetic). The natural sugar in sugarcane and sugar beets is primarily sucrose,

TABLE 3.1 Chemical Species and Their Representation

Chemical species: chemical compound, element, or living system.

Water; Nitrogen; Corn; *Escherichia coli*

Elemental formula: elemental chemical composition of species

H_2O—water

N_2—nitrogen

Isomeric species (**isomers**): same stoichiometrical formula but different sterostructure

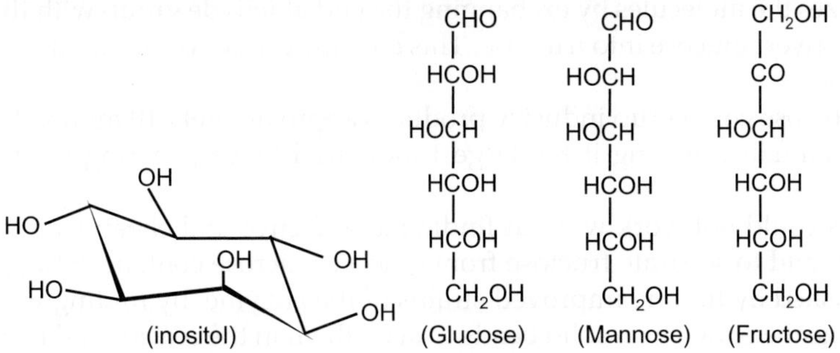

(inositol)	(Glucose)	(Mannose)	(Fructose)
HO, HO, OH, OH, OH, OH	CHO	CHO	CH_2OH
	HCOH	HOCH	CO
	HOCH	HOCH	HOCH
	HCOH	HCOH	HCOH
	HCOH	HCOH	HCOH
	CH_2OH	CH_2OH	CH_2OH

all share the same stoichiometrical formula $C_6H_{12}O_6$

Roel's formula: stoichiometrical formula normalized based on carbon

Sugar:	CH_2O
Xylan $H(C_5H_8O_4)_{200}OH$:	$CH_{1.602}O_{0.801}$

a disaccharide composed of one glucose residue and one fructose residue. Plants form these molecules as food reserves for themselves; we harvest the plants and extract sucrose from them in water solution. We have also bred strains of cane and beets that produce much more sucrose than wild strains.

Sucrose is rapidly dissociated into glucose and fructose by the enzymes in your mouth and in your stomach, and your taste receptors sense sweetness. In aqueous solution, fructose presents in two different isomers: D-fructopyranose (70%) and D-fructofuranose (30%). The more desired isomer is D-fructofuranose; it tastes five times as sweet as glucose and D-fructopyranose. Both sugars have the same calories, and the soft drink companies want to advertise lower calories for an acceptable sweetness.

Chemical engineers figured out how to run the reaction to convert glucose into fructose

$$\text{glucose} \rightleftharpoons \text{fructose} \tag{3.1}$$

which is drawn out in Eqn (3.2) (the fructose shown is D-fructofuranose):

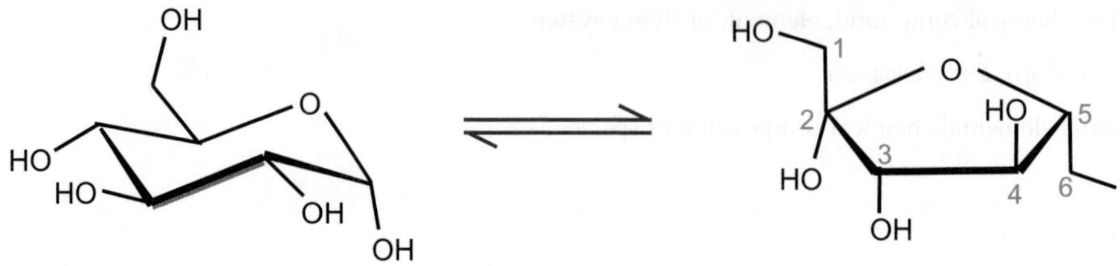

$$\text{glucose (pyranose)} \rightleftharpoons \text{fructose (furanose)} \tag{3.2}$$

The equilibrium in this isomerization reaction is 58% fructose (40.6% fructopyranose and 17.4% fructofuranose) and 42% glucose. An enzyme was discovered called *glucose isomerase*, which isomerizes the molecules by exchanging the end aldehyde group with the neighboring OH group to convert glucose into fructose. This enzyme cannot isomerize any other bonds in these molecules.

The high-fructose corn syrup industry produces approximately 10 million tons of fructose from glucose annually, making it the largest industrial bioengineering processes today, at least in volume.

This process could not work without finding an effective and cheap way to run this biological reaction and to separate fructose from glucose (sucrose contains 50% glucose). These were accomplished by finding improved strains of the enzyme, by finding ways to immobilize and stabilize the enzyme on solid beads to keep them in the reactor and by finding adsorbents to separate fructose from glucose.

These are accomplished in large fermentors in chemical plants, mostly in the Midwest. The cheapest feedstock is starch rather than sugar (other enzymes convert starch to glucose), and corn from the Midwest is the cheapest source of starch.

Artificial sweeteners have also been developed to give the taste of sweetness without the calories. These chemicals have sweetness many times that of sugar, so they sell for high prices as low-calorie sweeteners. Many artificial flavors have also been developed to replace natural biological flavors. In all cases, we search for processes that convert inexpensive raw materials into chemicals that taste or smell like natural chemicals, either by producing the same chemical synthetically or by producing a different chemical that can replace the natural chemical.

The glucose to fructose isomerization reaction can be written as

$$A \rightleftharpoons B \tag{3.3}$$

which is reversible. In other words, the reaction is both $A \rightarrow B$ and $B \rightarrow A$. When the reaction is far away from equilibrium, e.g. if we start out from pure glucose and in the short time when the reaction begins, we can regard the reaction as irreversible or

$$A \rightarrow B \tag{3.4}$$

Consider the isomerization reaction of cyclopropane to propylene,

$$\text{cyclo-}C_3H_6 \rightarrow C_3H_6 \tag{3.5}$$

or in symbols

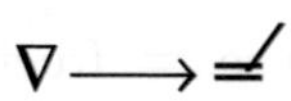

$$\triangledown \longrightarrow \text{=\!/} \tag{3.6}$$

Propylene will not significantly transform back to cyclopropane, and we call this reaction *irreversible*. The irreversible first-order reaction

$$A \rightarrow B \tag{3.7}$$

is the most used example in chemical kinetics, and we will use it throughout this book as the prototype of a "simple" reaction. However, the ring opening of cyclopropane to form propylene (which has absolutely no industrial significance) is one of only a handful of irreversible isomerization reactions of the type $A \rightarrow B$.

Next consider the formation of nitric oxide from air:

$$N_2 + O_2 \rightarrow 2\,NO \tag{3.8}$$

This extremely important reaction is the source of air pollution from automobiles. It is responsible for all NO_x formation in the atmosphere (the brown color of the air over large cities) as well as nitric acid and acid rain. This reaction only occurs in high-temperature combustion processes and in lightning bolts, and it occurs in automobile engines by free radical chain reaction steps. It is removed from the automobile exhaust in the automotive catalytic converter. The above reaction can also be written as

$$\tfrac{1}{2}N_2 + \tfrac{1}{2}O_2 \rightarrow NO \tag{3.9}$$

We could generalize these reactions as

$$\tfrac{1}{2}A + \tfrac{1}{2}B \rightarrow C \tag{3.10}$$

or

$$A + B \rightarrow 2C \tag{3.11}$$

with $A = N_2$, $B = O_2$, and $C = NO$. The coefficients of the chemical symbols in a reaction are termed *stoichiometric coefficients* and can be multiplied by a constant factor and still preserving mass conservation.

We need to generalize stoichiometric coefficients both of reactants and products. For this we move all terms to the left with appropriate signs, so that the preceding reaction becomes

$$-A - B + 2C = 0 \tag{3.12}$$

Note that convention negates the sign of coefficients for reactants. Further, since the alphabet is limited, we will increase our capacity for naming chemicals by naming a species j as A_j, so that this reaction is

$$-A_1 - A_2 + 2A_3 = 0 \tag{3.13}$$

with $A_1 = N_2$, $A_2 = O_2$, and $A_3 = NO$. In this notation, the *generalized single reaction* becomes

$$\sum_{j=1}^{N_S} \nu_j A_j = 0 \tag{3.14}$$

where N_S denotes the total number of species involved in the system. Most chemical process of practical interest forms several products (some undesired) and involves *multiple reactions*.

Consider next the reaction system

$$N_2 + O_2 \rightarrow 2\,NO \tag{3.15}$$

$$2NO + O_2 \rightarrow 2\,NO_2 \tag{3.16}$$

In NO_x smog formation (NO_x is a mixture of NO, N_2O, NO_2, N_2O_4, and N_2O_5), the NO is produced by the reaction of N_2 and O_2 at the high temperatures of combustion in automobiles and fossil fuel power plants, and NO_2 and the other NO_x species are produced by subsequent low-temperature oxidation of NO in air. NO is colorless, but NO_2 absorbs visible radiation and produces brown haze. We write these reactions as a set of two reactions among four species,

$$-A_l - A_2 + 2A_3 = 0 \tag{3.17}$$

$$-2A_3 - A_2 + 2A_4 = 0 \tag{3.18}$$

where A_l is N_2, A_2 is O_2, etc. This is a simplification of all the possible reactions involving N and O atoms, since we have not included stable molecules such as N_2O, N_2O_2, NO_3, and N_2O_5.

We can generalize this notation to any set of reactions as

$$\sum_{j=1}^{N_S} \nu_{ij} A_j = 0, \quad i = 1, 2, \ldots, N_R \tag{3.19}$$

or

$$\begin{bmatrix} \nu_{11} & \nu_{12} & \cdots & \nu_{1j} & \cdots & \nu_{1N_S} \\ \nu_{21} & \nu_{22} & \cdots & \nu_{2j} & \cdots & \nu_{2N_S} \\ \vdots & \vdots & \ddots & \vdots & \ddots & \vdots \\ \nu_{i1} & \nu_{i2} & \cdots & \nu_{ij} & \cdots & \nu_{iN_S} \\ \vdots & \vdots & \ddots & \vdots & \ddots & \vdots \\ \nu_{N_R1} & \nu_{N_R2} & \cdots & \nu_{N_Rj} & \cdots & \nu_{N_RN_S} \end{bmatrix} \begin{bmatrix} A_1 \\ A_2 \\ \vdots \\ A_j \\ \vdots \\ A_{N_S} \end{bmatrix} = \begin{bmatrix} 0 \\ 0 \\ \vdots \\ 0 \\ \vdots \\ 0 \end{bmatrix}$$

as a set of N_R reactions among N_S species, with j (=1 to N_S) the index of chemical species and i (=1 to N_R) the index of the reaction. Thus, we call v_{ij} the stoichiometric coefficient of species j in reaction i. We will use this standard notation throughout this book, and we suggest that you always give the i's and j's these meanings and never reverse them.

3.3. REACTION RATES

Reaction kinetics and reactor design are at the heart of producing almost all industrial chemicals and biologics. It is primarily a knowledge of reaction kinetics and reactor design that distinguishes the bioprocess (or chemical) engineer from other engineers. The selection of the reaction system that operates in the safest and most efficient manner can be the key to the economic success or failure of a chemical plant or biological facility. For example, if a reaction system produced a large amount of undesirable by-product, subsequent purification and separation of the desired product could make the entire process economically unfeasible. The reaction kinetic principles learned here, in addition to the production of chemicals, can be applied in areas such as living systems, waste treatment, and air and water pollution.

Reaction engineering is concerned with the rate at which reactions take place, together with the mechanism and rate-limiting steps that control the reaction process. The sizing of reactors to achieve production goals is an important element. How materials behave within reactors, either chemically, physically, or biologically, are significant to the designer of a bio-process, as is how the data from reactors should be recorded, processed, and interpreted.

3.3.1. Definition of the Rate of Reaction, r_A

As we have discussed earlier, we say that a *chemical reaction* has taken place when a detectable number of molecules of one or more species has assumed a new form by a change in the kind or number of atoms in the compound and/or by a change in structure or configuration of these atoms. In this classical approach to chemical change, it is assumed that the total mass is neither created nor destroyed when a chemical reaction occurs. The mass referred to is the total collective mass of all the different species in the system. However, when considering the individual species involved in a particular reaction, we do speak of the rate of formation of a particular species. The rate of formation of a species, say species A, is the number of A molecules being generated (from consuming other species) per unit time per volume, that is,

$$r_A = \frac{\text{Number of moles of species A formed}}{\text{Time} \times \text{Volume}} \tag{3.20}$$

As such, the reaction rate is defined and measured within a small volume (approaching zero) and at an instant (or small interval) in time. Concentration is defined in the same manner:

$$C_A = \frac{\text{Number of moles of species A}}{\text{Volume}} \tag{3.21}$$

This would give the concentration C_A units of moles per liter, mol/L (formerly, M as in molarity) or $kmol/m^3$.

The concentration can be defined in other units as well. One of the more common ones is

$$C_A = \frac{\text{Mass of species A}}{\text{Volume}} \tag{3.22}$$

which would give C_A units of kg/m^3. Therefore, units are important to engineers.

In biological, enzymatic, and heterogeneous reaction systems, the rate of reaction is usually expressed in measures other than the volume of the culture (total volume of the reaction mixture). For example,

$$r'_A = \frac{\text{Number of moles of species A formed}}{\text{Time} \times \text{Mass of Catalyst}} \tag{3.23}$$

The catalyst in a biological system is usually of biomass or cells. The biomass concentration is normally expressed in gram per liter, that is

$$X = \frac{m_X}{V} \tag{3.24}$$

where X is the biomass concentration, m_X is the dry weight of the biomass, and V is the volume of the culture. Thus,

$$r'_A = \frac{r_A}{X} \tag{3.25}$$

One commonly used rate in bioprocess engineering is the specific reaction rate or

$$\mu_A = \frac{\text{Mass of species A formed}}{\text{Time} \times \text{Mass of Catalyst}} \tag{3.26}$$

That is,

$$\mu_A = r'_A M_A = \frac{r_A M_A}{X} \tag{3.27}$$

where M_A is the molecular mass of species A.

The specific reaction rate is commonly used in biological reactions due to the complexity of the molecules involved, whereby the number of moles is not easy to measure or compute. For example, the exact numbers of all the atoms in the living cells or microorganisms are not easily available and can differ from one particular cell to another at various stages of their life. Counting the number of cells is not very easy, but it can be done. The lack of exact composition of all the cells, however, hinders chemical analysis if the number of cells is used. Mass, on the other hand, can be measured more easily by weighing. Therefore, the specific rate as defined by Eqn (3.26) is commonly used in cases where biological reactions are involved.

Example 3-1. Is sodium hydroxide reacting?

The reaction rate is defined by Eqn (3.20). If we notice that the concentration, Eqn (3.21), takes care of both number of moles and volume, we can further simplify the rate definition to

$$r_A = \frac{dC_A}{dt} \tag{E3-1.1}$$

In fact, you could find many books define the reaction rate this way. Before we discuss whether this definition is correct, let us consider the following operation as illustrated in Fig. 3.1.

Sodium hydroxide and fat (triglycerides) are continuously fed to a heated stirred tank in which they react to form soap (sodium fatty acetate) and glycerol:

$$3\,NaOH + fat \rightarrow 3\,soap + HOCH_2CH(OH)CH_2OH \tag{E3-1.2}$$

One triglyceride (fat) molecule reacts with three sodium hydroxide (NaOH) molecules produces three sodium fatty acid salt (soap) molecules and one glycerol molecule. The product stream, containing soap and glycerol, together with the unreacted sodium hydroxide and fat, is continuously withdrawn from the tank at a rate equal to the total feed rate. The contents of the tank in which this reaction is taking place may be considered to be perfectly mixed. Because the system operates at steady state, if we were to withdraw liquid samples at some location in the tank at various times and analyze them chemically, we would find that the concentrations of the individual species in the different samples were identical. That is,

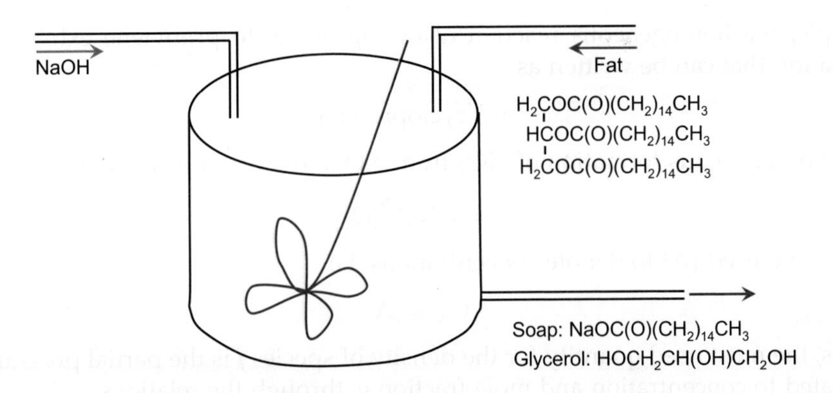

FIGURE 3.1 Well-mixed reaction vessel for soap production.

the concentration of the sample taken at 8 am is the same as that of the sample taken at 2 pm. Because the species concentrations are constant and therefore do not change with time,

$$\frac{dC_j}{dt} = 0 \tag{E3-1.3}$$

for any four species involved. Substitution of E(3-1.2) into (E3-1.1), however, would lead to

$$r_j = 0 \tag{E3-1.4}$$

which is incorrect because glycerol and soap *are* being formed from NaOH and fat at finite rates. Consequently, the rate of reaction as defined by Eqn (E3-1.1) cannot apply to a flow system and is incorrect if it is *defined* in this manner.

Example 3.1 has touched on the issue of reaction rate for different species involved in the same reaction. One can imagine that all the rates are related as there is only one reaction; in this example, the rate of formation of ethanol should be the same as the rate of formation of sodium acetate. In general, the rates can be related through stoichiometry, i.e. atom balance involving the reaction system. For convenience and clarity, we define a reaction rate specific form based on a given stoichiometry by

$$r = \frac{r_j}{\nu_j} \tag{3.28}$$

To avoid confusion in multiple reaction systems, the reaction rate for each reaction is given by

$$r_i = \frac{r_{ij}}{\nu_{ij}} \tag{3.29}$$

While r_j or r_{ij} does not change, r or r_i does change with stoichiometry. In other words, how you write the reaction will influence the stoichiometry-based rate form.

3.3.2. Rate of a Single Irreversible Reaction

It is found by experiment that rates almost always have power-law dependences on the densities (such as concentration, density on a surface, or partial pressure) of chemical species.

For example, the homogeneous reaction of cyclopropane to propylene exhibits a rate of decomposition that can be written as

$$r = k[\text{cyclopropane}] \tag{3.30}$$

while the homogeneous formation of NO_2 from NO and oxygen has a rate

$$r = k[\text{NO}]^2[\text{O}_2] \tag{3.31}$$

where we have used [A] to denote concentrations, i.e.

$$C_A = [A] \tag{3.32}$$

In gases, the most used quantity for the density of species j is the partial pressure P_j. This can be related to concentration and mole fraction y_j through the relations

$$y_j = \frac{n_j}{\sum n_j} = \frac{n_j}{n} \tag{3.33}$$

and

$$p_j = y_j P = C_j RT \tag{3.34}$$

where P is the total pressure and n is the total number of moles in the system. In this equation, we assume ideal gases ($PV = nRT$) to relate partial pressure to concentration, while for nonideal gases (not considered here), we would need an equation of state to describe the density of each chemical species.

For an irreversible reaction, we can frequently describe the rate to a good approximation as

$$r = k \prod_{j=1}^{N_S} C_j^{O_{Rj}} \tag{3.35}$$

where O_{Rj} is the order of the reaction with respect to the jth species and the product extends over all species in the reaction with $O_{Rj} = 0$ for species that do not affect the rate of reaction. If the rate is proportional to the concentration of a species raised to a power (O_{Rj}), we say that this form of the rate expression is described by "power-law kinetics." This empirical function is frequently used to describe reaction rates, but is frequently inaccurate, especially with surface- or enzyme-catalyzed reactions, which are of the main topic of discussion in this book.

3.3.3. Rate of an Elementary Reaction

The rate expression (3.35) has been found particularly helpful in many cases although it is overly simplified. To continue our discussion, let us define an elementary reaction. An elementary reaction is a reaction whereby the reactants (or reacting molecules) react stoichiometrically in each and every instance. For example, if the reaction

$$A + B \rightarrow C \tag{3.36}$$

is elementary, when A and B meet they can automatically get converted to C without going through any additional steps. Therefore, elementary reactions are idealized reactions or reaction steps. As such, the reaction rate form for elementary reactions strictly follow Eqn (3.35), with the order of reaction $O_{Rj} = -\nu_j$ for reactants and $O_{Rj} = 0$ for products. Since a fraction of a molecule cannot react with other species in an elementary reaction, the order of reaction for elementary reactions is always integer and positive. Therefore, how you write the reaction can even influence whether the reaction could be elementary or not.

3.3.4. Rate of a Reversible Reaction

One can rewrite a reversible reaction into two simultaneous reactions. For example,

$$(-\upsilon_A)A + (-\upsilon_B)B \rightleftharpoons \upsilon_C C \rightarrow r \tag{3.37}$$

is considered to be two reactions occurring simultaneously.

$$(-\upsilon_A)A + (-\upsilon_B)B \rightarrow \upsilon_C C \rightarrow r_f \tag{3.38}$$

$$\upsilon_C C \rightarrow (-\upsilon_A)A + (-\upsilon_B)B \rightarrow r_b \tag{3.39}$$

The rate expression is simply a combination of the two reactions. Because the stoichiometric coefficients are the same in the two reactions (only differing by sign), the same rate is applicable to every species involved, leading to a directly additive rate expression. That is,

$$r = r_f - r_b \tag{3.40}$$

3.3.5. Rates of Multiple Reactions

We also need to describe the rates of multiple reaction systems. We do this in the same way as for single reactions, with each reaction i in the set of N_R reactions being described by a rate r_i, rate coefficient k_i, order of the forward reaction O_{Rij} with respect to species j, etc.

Again, the procedure we follow is first to write the reaction steps with a consistent stoichiometry and then to express the rate of each reaction to be consistent with that stoichiometry. Thus, if we write a reaction step by multiplying each stoichiometric coefficient by two, the rate of that reaction would be smaller by a factor of two, and if we reverse the reaction, the forward and reverse rates would be switched.

For a multiple reaction system with reversible reactions, we can describe each of the N_R reactions through a reaction rate r_i,

$$r_i = r_{if} - r_{ib} \tag{3.41}$$

where $i = 1, 2, 3, \ldots, N_R$.

3.4. APPROXIMATE REACTIONS

Consider the hydrolysis or saponification of an *ester* (ethyl acetate) into an alcohol (ethanol) and an acid (acetic acid),

$$CH_3COOC_2H_5 + H_2O \rightleftharpoons CH_3COOH + C_2H_5OH \tag{3.42}$$

This reaction and its reverse take place readily in basic aqueous solution. This reaction follows the form

$$A + B \rightleftharpoons C + D \tag{3.43}$$

Next, consider the addition of water to an olefin to form an alcohol,

$$RCH = CH_2 + H_2O \rightleftharpoons RCH_2CH_2OH \tag{3.44}$$

which can be written as

$$A + B \rightleftharpoons C \tag{3.45}$$

In many situations, we carry out these reactions in dilute aqueous solutions, where there is a large excess of water. The concentration of pure liquid water is 55 mol/L, and the concentration of water in liquid aqueous solutions is nearly constant even when the above solutes are added up to fairly high concentrations. The reaction is essentially forward and the reverse reaction is negligible. The rates of these forward reactions are

$$r = k[CH_3COOC_2H_5][H_2O] \tag{3.46}$$

and

$$r = k[RCH = CH_2][H_2O] \tag{3.47}$$

respectively. However, since change in the concentration of water $[H_2O]$ is usually immeasurably small whenever water is a solvent, we may simplify these reactions to

$$CH_3COOC_2H_5 \rightarrow CH_3COOH + C_2H_5OH, \quad r = k[CH_3COOC_2H_5] \tag{3.48}$$

and

$$RCH = CH_2 \rightarrow RCH_2CH_2OH, \quad r = k[RCH = CH_2] \tag{3.49}$$

These reactions do not satisfy total mass conservation because the mole of water is omitted as a reactant. We have also redefined a new rate coefficient as $k = k[H_2O]$ by grouping the nearly constant $[H_2O]$ with k. After grouping the concentration of the solvent $[H_2O]$ into the rate coefficient, we say that we have a pseudo first-order rate expression.

It is fairly common to write reactions in this fashion, omitting H_2O from the chemical equation and the rate, so these reactions become of the type

$$A \rightarrow C + D, \; r = kC_A \tag{3.50}$$

and

$$A \rightarrow C, \; r = kC_A \tag{3.51}$$

respectively. Thus, in addition to isomerization, there are in fact a number of reactions that we write approximately as A → B or A → products, so our use of these simple rate expressions is in fact appropriate for a large number of reaction systems.

Reaction rate expressions are always empirical, which means that we use whatever expression gives an accurate enough description of the problem at hand. No reactions are as simple as these expressions predict if we need them to be correct to many decimal places. Further, all reaction systems in fact involve multiple reactions, and there is no such thing as a truly irreversible reaction if we measure all species to sufficient accuracy. If we need a product with impurities at the parts per billion (ppb) levels, then all reactions are in fact reversible and involve many reactions.

Process engineers are paid to make whatever approximations are reasonable to find answers at the level of sophistication required for the problem at hand. If this were easy, our salaries would be lower.

3.5. RATE COEFFICIENTS

We next consider the k's in the above rate expressions. We will generally call these the *rate coefficients* (the coefficient of the concentration dependences in r). They are sometimes called *rate constants* since they are independent of concentrations; however, rate coefficients are almost always strong functions of temperature. Figure 3.2 shows the free and internal energy G change during a reaction. As the reactants start to undergo structural changes at the onset of reaction, their free energy increases owing to the movement away from stable state and so is the internal energy. They reach a point having a maximum value of G at which the change becomes less reversible, i.e. more likely to move away from their original state than moving toward their original state, the structural changes cascade down to a new stable state, whereby new product is formed. This state of maximum G reactants (substrates) developed is commonly known as the Transitional State. From the viewpoint of nonequilibrium thermodynamics, the driving force for the change is the free energy. Therefore, the reaction rate may be correlated to the change in free energy, that is,

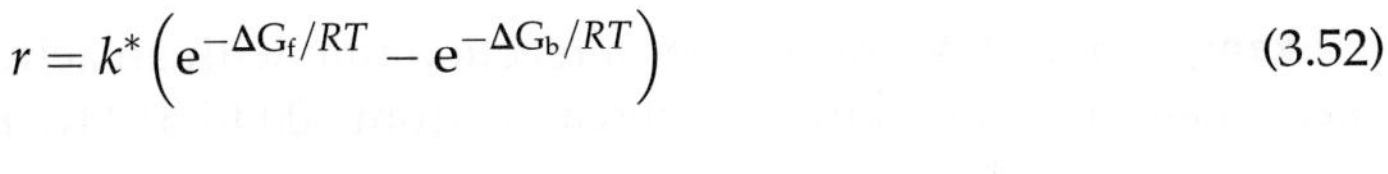

$$r = k^* \left(e^{-\Delta G_f/RT} - e^{-\Delta G_b/RT} \right) \tag{3.52}$$

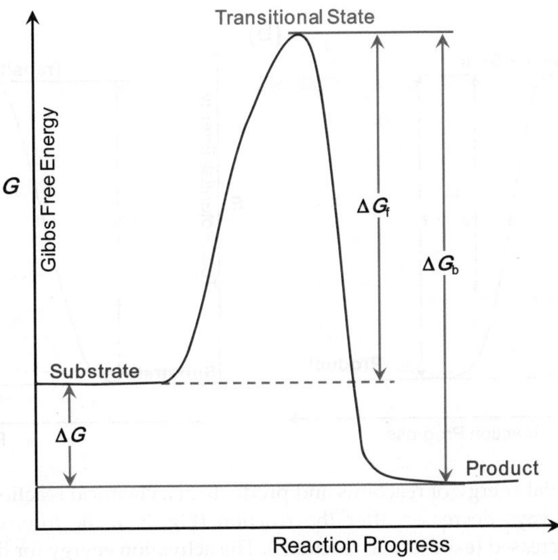

FIGURE 3.2 Plot of free energy of reactants and products in a chemical reaction vs the reaction coordinate. The free energy always decreases after the reaction and the energy barrier determines the rate of reaction.

where k^* is a constant. While this approach has its merit, we have three unknowns: k^*, ΔG_f, and ΔG_b, all of which may be dependent on the reaction path.

It is found empirically that the reaction rate coefficients frequently depend on temperature as

$$k(T) = k_0 e^{-E/RT} \tag{3.53}$$

where E is called the *activation energy* for the reaction and k_0 is called the *pre-exponential factor.* This relation is credited to Svante Arrhenius and is called the *Arrhenius law.* Arrhenius was mainly concerned with thermodynamics and chemical equilibrium. Some time later, Michael Polanyi and Eugene Wigner showed that simple molecular arguments lead to this temperature dependence, and so this form of the rate is frequently called the *Polanyi–Wigner relation.* They described chemical reactions as the process of crossing a potential energy surface between reactants and products (see Figs 3.2 and 3.3), where E_f and E_b are the energy barriers for the forward and reverse reactions, ΔH_R is the heat of the reaction (to be discussed later), and the horizontal scale is called the *reaction coordinate,* the loosely defined distance that molecules must travel to convert from reactants to products. Polanyi and Wigner first showed from statistical mechanics that the rates should be described by expressions of the form given in Eqn (3.53) by a Boltzmann factor, $\exp(-E/RT)$, which is the probability of crossing a potential energy barrier between product and reactant molecules. In fact, it is very rare ever to find reaction rate coefficients that cannot be described with fair accuracy by expressions of this form.

This functional form of $k(T)$ predicts a very strong dependence of reaction rates on temperature, and this fact is central in describing the complexities of chemical reactions, as we will see throughout this book.

Example 3-2. How much does a reaction rate with an activation energy of 15,000 cal/mol vary when the temperature is increased from 300 to 310 K? From 300 to 400 K?

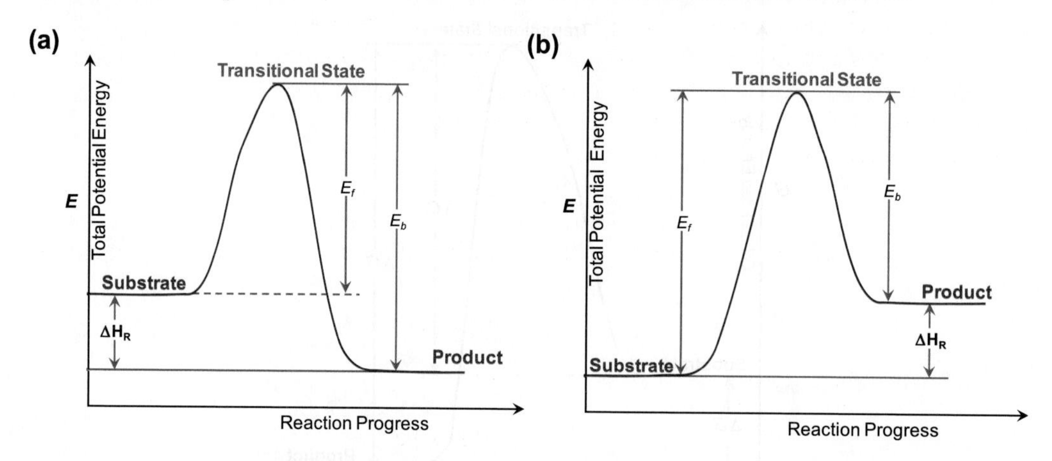

FIGURE 3.3 Plot of potential energy of reactants and products in a chemical reaction vs the reaction coordinate. Although the free energy always decreases after the reaction (Fig. 3.2), the internal energy can be increased (endothermic reactions) or decreased (exothermic reactions). The activation energy for the forward reaction is E_f and for the back reaction E_b. The heat of the reaction is $\Delta H_R = E_f - E_b$. (a). Potential energy variation for an exothermic reaction based on 1 mol of substrate. (b). Potential energy variation for an endothermic reaction based on 1 mol of substrate.

Solution: The ratio of the rate of this reaction at 310 K to that at 300 K,

$$\frac{k_{310}}{k_{300}} = \frac{e^{-E/RT_1}}{e^{-E/RT_2}} = \exp\left[\frac{E}{R}\left(\frac{1}{T_2} - \frac{1}{T_1}\right)\right] = \exp\left[\frac{15000}{1.9872}\left(\frac{1}{300} - \frac{1}{310}\right)\right] = 2.252$$

Between 300 and 400 K, this ratio is very large,

$$\frac{k_{400}}{k_{300}} = \frac{e^{-E/RT_1}}{e^{-E/RT_2}} = \exp\left[\frac{E}{R}\left(\frac{1}{T_2} - \frac{1}{T_1}\right)\right] = \exp\left[\frac{15000}{1.9872}\left(\frac{1}{300} - \frac{1}{400}\right)\right] = 539.29$$

This shows that for this activation energy an increase in temperature of 10 K approximately doubles the rate and an increase of 100 K increases it by a factor of more than 500.

Example 3-2 shows why temperature is so important in chemical reactions. For many nonreacting situations, a 10 K increase in T is insignificant, but for our example it would decrease by a factor of two the size of the reactor required for a given conversion. A decrease in temperature of 100 K would change the rate so much that it would appear to be zero, and an increase of this amount would make the rate so high that the process would be difficult or impossible to handle.

Let us consider finally the units of k. We choose units to make the rate (in moles/liter/time) dimensionally correct. For $r = k\, C_A^{O_{RA}}$, k has units of liter$^{O_{RA}-1}$·mole$^{1-O_{RA}}$·time^{-1}, which gives k units of time^{-1} for $O_{RA} = 1$ and k of liters/mole time for $O_{RA} = 2$.

3.6. STOICHIOMETRY

When a chemical reaction is written (for a given set of stoichiometric coefficients), we need to balance the number of each atom species (if nuclear reaction is absent).

Molecules are lost and formed by reaction, and mass conservation requires that amounts of species be related. In a closed (batch) system, the change in the numbers of moles of all molecular species n_j is related by reaction stoichiometry.

For our NO decomposition example,

$$NO \rightarrow \tfrac{1}{2}N_2 + \tfrac{1}{2}O_2,$$

from an O atom balance, we see that the total number of moles of the oxygen atoms in the system is

$$n_{NO} + 2n_{O_2} = \text{constant}_1 \tag{3.54}$$

while an N atom balance gives

$$n_{NO} + 2n_{N_2} = \text{constant}_2 \tag{3.55}$$

Subtracting these, we obtain

$$n_{N_2} - n_{O_2} = \text{constant}_3 \tag{3.56}$$

in a closed system. The stoichiometry of the molecules requires that the moles of these species be related by these relations.

These equations become more illustrative if we consider the initial values (subscript 0) before the reaction takes place. Equation (3.55) leads to

$$n_{NO} + 2n_{N_2} = n_{NO,0} + 2n_{N_2,0} \tag{3.57}$$

which can be rearranged to give

$$-(n_{NO} - n_{NO,0}) = 2(n_{N_2} - n_{N_2,0}) \tag{3.58}$$

or

$$\frac{n_{NO} - n_{NO,0}}{-1} = \frac{n_{N_2} - n_{N_2,0}}{1/2} \tag{3.59}$$

or

$$\frac{\Delta n_{NO}}{\nu_{NO}} = \frac{\Delta n_{N_2}}{\nu_{N_2}} \tag{3.60}$$

In general, for any single reaction, we can write

$$\frac{\Delta n_j}{\nu_j} = n_{ext}, \quad \forall j \tag{3.61}$$

and we can write $N_S - 1$ independent combinations of these relations among N_S chemical species in a reaction to relate the changes in the number of moles of all species to each other.

There is therefore always a *single composition variable* that describes the relationship among all species in a single reaction. In the preceding Eqn (3.61), we defined n_{ext} as the relation between the n_j's,

$$n_j = n_{j,0} + \upsilon_j n_{ext} \tag{3.62}$$

We call the quantity n_{ext} the *number of moles extent*.

For simple problems, we most commonly use one of the reactants as the concentration variable to work with and label that species A to use C_A as the variable representing composition changes during reaction. We also make the stoichiometric coefficient of that species $\upsilon_A = -1$.

Another way of representing a single reaction is the *fractional conversion f*, a dimensionless quantity ranging from 0, before reaction, to 1, when the reaction is complete. We define f through the relation

$$n_A = n_{A0}(1 - f_A) \tag{3.63}$$

To make $0 \le f_A \le 1$, we have to choose species A as the *limiting reactant* so that this reactant disappears and f_A approaches unity when the reaction is complete. We can then define all species through the relation

$$\frac{\Delta n_j}{\nu_j} = n_{A0} f_A, \quad \forall j \tag{3.64}$$

For multiple reactions, we need a variable to describe each reaction. Furthermore, we cannot in general find a single key reactant to call species A in the definition of f_A. However, it is straightforward to use the number of moles extent $n_{\text{ext},i}$ for each of the N_R reactions. Thus, we can define the change in the number of moles of species j through the relation

$$n_j = n_{j0} + \sum_{i=1}^{N_R} \nu_{ij} n_{\text{ext},i} \tag{3.65}$$

To summarize, we can always find a *single concentration variable* that describes the change in all species for a single reaction, and for N_R simultaneous reactions, there must be N_R independent variables to describe concentration changes. For a single reaction, this problem is simple (use either C_A or f_A), but for a multiple reaction system, one must set up the notation quite carefully in terms of a suitably chosen set of N_R concentrations or conversions (f_i's) or $n_{\text{ext},i}$'s.

Finally, the rate of reaction for a given species j in a set of N_R reactions can be computed via

$$r_j = \sum_{i=1}^{N_R} \nu_{ij} r_i \tag{3.66}$$

The rate of reaction for any given species is the summation of its reaction rates in all the reactions.

Example 3-3. Elemental balance. Consider the fermentation of carbon monoxide in aqueous solution using the bacterium *Methylotrophicum* to produce acetic acid, butyric acid, and additional cells. Based on the reported yields, stoichiometry is given by

$$\begin{aligned} &CO + (-\upsilon_{O_2})O_2 + (-\upsilon_{N_2})N_2 + (-\upsilon_{H_2O})H_2O \rightarrow \\ &0.52\,CO_2 + 0.21\,CH_3COOH + 0.006\,CH_3CH_2CH_2COOH + \upsilon_X X \end{aligned}$$

where X represents the *Methylotrophicum* cells. Assuming that cells produced in this reaction can be represented by the Roel's average biomass (that is, 1 C-mol cells $= CH_{1.8}O_{0.5}N_{0.2}$), determine all the remaining stoichiometric coefficients.

Solution: Let $X = CH_{1.8}O_{0.5}N_{0.2}$. To find the remaining stoichiometric coefficients, we need to perform atom balances individually. In this reaction, we have four atoms involved: C, O, N, and H. Four balance equations can be written independently.

C-mole balance:

$$1 - 0\upsilon_{O_2} - 0\upsilon_{N_2} - 0\upsilon_{H_2O} = 0.52 + 0.21 \times 2 + 0.006 \times 4 + \upsilon_X \tag{E3-3.1}$$

O-mole balance:

$$1 - 2\,0\upsilon_{O_2} - 0\,\upsilon_{N_2} - \upsilon_{H_2O} = 0.52 \times 2 + 0.21 \times 2 + 0.006 \times 2 + 0.5\,\upsilon_X \tag{E3-3.2}$$

N-mole balance:

$$0 - 0\,\upsilon_{O_2} - 2\,\upsilon_{N_2} - 0\,\upsilon_{H_2O} = 0.52 \times 0 + 0.21 \times 0 + 0.006 \times 0 + 0.2\,\upsilon_X \tag{E3-3.3}$$

H-mole balance:

$$0 - 0\,\upsilon_{O_2} - 0\,\upsilon_{N_2} - 2\,\upsilon_{H_2O} = 0.52 \times 0 + 0.21 \times 4 + 0.006 \times 8 + 1.8\,\upsilon_X \tag{E3-3.4}$$

Equations (E3-3.1) through (E3-3.4) need to be solved simultaneously to find all the stoichiometric coefficients.

From Eqn (E3-3.1), we obtain

$$\upsilon_X = 1 - 0.52 - 0.21 \times 2 - 0.006 \times 4 = 0.036 \tag{E3-3.5}$$

Using Eqn (E3-3.4), we have

$$\upsilon_{H_2O} = (0.21 \times 4 + 0.006 \times 8 + 1.8\ v_X) \div (-2) = -0.4764 \tag{E3-3.6}$$

Equation (E3-3.3) leads to

$$\upsilon_{N_2} = 0.2\ v_X \div (-2) = -0.0036 \tag{E3-3.7}$$

Equation (E3-3.2) can be rearranged to yield

$$\upsilon_{O_2} = (1 - \upsilon_{H_2O} - 0.52 \times 2 - 0.21 \times 2 - 0.006 \times 2 - 0.5\upsilon_X)/2 = -0.0068 \tag{E3-3.8}$$

This concludes the determination. The final stoichiometry is given by

$$CO + 0.0068\ O_2 + 0.0036\ N_2 + 0.476\ H_2O \rightarrow$$

$$0.52\ CO_2 + 0.21\ CH_3COOH + 0.006\ CH_3CH_2CH_2COOH + 0.036\ CH_{1.8}O_{0.5}NO_{0.2}$$

3.7. YIELD AND YIELD FACTOR

In the previous section, we found that for each (independent) reaction, there is one independent concentration related variable in the stoichiometry. We have defined the numbers of mole extent and fractional conversion. The fractional conversion is a visual quantity that examines the fraction of a key reactant being converted by the reaction. In this section, we will define new parameters that describe the product formed.

With many chemical and biochemical processes, we would like to know the ratio of a reactant that is converted to a particular product. This leads to the concept of yield. We know that the fractional conversion has a value between 0 and 1, which is easy to visualize and conceptually accepted. For the yield, we would like to retain the same range. It is easy for anyone to understand that a yield between 0 and 100%. However, in order for us to restrict the number range and make sense, we would need to have the right basis. For example, when two different molecules (species) combine to form a third molecule (species), it would be delicate to restrict the yield to be within unity. The yield is thus commonly defined based on given element of group of elements as

$$Y_{P/A/R} = \frac{\text{\#-moles of R in all the P formed}}{\text{\#-moles of R in all the A in the raw materials}} \tag{3.67}$$

Here R is the basis or element or groups of elements that is fully contained in both P and A.

In bioreactions, the natural reference (R) is carbon (C) as in most cases we use a carbon source and carbon is the key component of interest. In this case, Eqn (3.67) can be rewritten as

$$Y_{P/A/C} = \frac{\text{\#-C-moles of P formed}}{\text{\#-C-moles of A initially}} \tag{3.68a}$$

or simply

$$Y_{P/A} = \frac{\text{\#-C-moles of P formed}}{\text{\#-C-moles of A initially}} \tag{3.68b}$$

as carbon is implied.

One can observe from the above definitions, yield is for a desired product and is the fraction of all the particular reactant that is converted to the desired product. In many cases, we do not know the extent of reaction and thus yield becomes not convenient to use. One parameter used quite a bit in biochemical engineering is the yield factor. Yield factor is defined as the maximum fractional yield, and thus a state parameter, which is independent of the reaction kinetics. That is,

$$YF_{P/A} = \frac{\text{\#-C-moles of P that could be formed}}{\text{\#-C-moles of A}} = \frac{|\nu_P|}{|\nu_A|} \tag{3.69}$$

which is then only specific to the stoichiometry of the reactions involved. One often extends this yield factor definition to include reactants as well; in that case, the amount of species change in the definition is always defined as the absolute value in the net change (either increase or decrease). Still, A in Eqn (3.69) needs not be restricted to as reactant.

Sometimes, one can find that the yield factor defined above is not convenient to use. For example, counting the number of biomass or cells is not an easy task. We often use another definition,

$$YF_{P/A} = \frac{\text{Mass of P that could be produced}}{\text{Mass of A}} \tag{3.70a}$$

or

$$YF_{P/A} = \frac{\text{Total number of moles of P that could be produced}}{\text{Total number of moles of A}} \tag{3.70b}$$

The definition used in Eqn (3.70) can however push the yield factor out of the normal range (0,1) as the total masses (or moles) of P that could be produced and A are used in Eqn (3.70).

While the yield factor is the maximum fractional yield which has no units, one must be careful on the basis used. That is, either C-mole-P/C-mole-A, kg-P/kg-A, or mole-P/mole-A. They can have very different values. Therefore, it is recommended that units be retained.

We will learn later that the mass ratios are more convenient for biological reactions. The yield factors can be efficiently used in part to relate the specific reaction rates (μ's) instead of using the stoichiometric coefficients (ν's) for systems with a single reaction.

Example 3-4. Yield factors. Continue on Example 3-3, find the yield factors of biomass (X) and oxygen (O_2) over the substrate carbon monoxide (CO).

Solution. Based on the solution from Example 3-3

$$CO + 0.0068\ O_2 + 0.0036\ N_2 + 0.476\ H_2O \rightarrow$$

$$0.52\ CO_2 + 0.21\ CH_3COOH + 0.006\ CH_3CH_2CH_2COOH + 0.036\ CH_{1.8}O_{0.5}NO_{0.2}$$

One can find that

$$YF_{X/CO} = \frac{\text{#-C-moles of X that could be formed}}{\text{#-C-moles of CO}} = \frac{\nu_X}{-\nu_{CO}} = \frac{0.036}{1} \frac{\text{C} - \text{mole X}}{\text{C} - \text{mole CO}}$$

$$= 0.036 \frac{\text{C} - \text{mole X}}{\text{C} - \text{mole CO}}$$

or

$$YF_{X/CO} = \frac{\text{Mass of X that coule be produced}}{\text{Mass of CO}} = \frac{\nu_X M_X}{-\nu_{CO} M_{CO}}$$

$$= \frac{0.036 \times (12.011 + 1.8 \times 1.00794 + 0.5 \times 15.9994 + 0.2 \times 14.00674)}{1 \times (12.011 + 15.9994)} \frac{\text{kg-X}}{\text{kg-CO}}$$

$$= 0.03165 \frac{\text{kg-X}}{\text{kg-CO}}$$

One can observe that the yield factor is different when different basis (C-mole or kg) is used. For the yield factor of oxygen, we have

$$YF_{O_2/CO} = \frac{\text{#-moles of } O_2 \text{ that could be consumed}}{\text{#-C-moles of CO}} = \frac{-\nu_{O_2}}{-\nu_{CO}} = \frac{0.0068}{1} \frac{\text{mole } O_2}{\text{C} - \text{mole CO}}$$

$$= 0.0068 \frac{\text{mole } O_2}{\text{C} - \text{mole CO}}$$

or

$$YF_{O_2/CO} = \frac{\text{Mass of } O_2 \text{ that could be consumed}}{\text{Mass of CO}} = \frac{-\nu_{O_2} M_{O_2}}{-\nu_{CO} M_{CO}}$$

$$= \frac{0.068 \times (2 \times 15.9994)}{1 \times (12.011 + 15.9994)} \frac{\text{kg-}O_2}{\text{kg-CO}} = 0.007768 \frac{\text{kg-}O_2}{\text{kg-CO}}$$

3.8. REACTION RATES NEAR EQUILIBRIUM

Figure 3.2 shows the Gibbs free energy variation during a chemical reaction. Nonequilibrium thermodynamics stipulates that the flux of change is governed by the change of Gibbs free energy, i.e. Eqn (3.52) for a reaction,

$$r = k^* \left(e^{-\Delta G_f/RT} - e^{-\Delta G_b/RT} \right) \tag{3.52}$$

where ΔG's change with the contents of the reaction mixture, temperature, and other conditions.

More theoretically founded, in thermodynamics, we learned how to describe the composition of molecules in chemical equilibrium. For the generalized single reaction

$$\sum_{j=1}^{N_S} \nu_j A_j = 0 \tag{3.14}$$

It can be shown that the free energy change in a system of chemically interacting species is related to the chemical potentials $\overline{G}_j$ of each species through the relationship

$$\Delta G = \sum_{j=1}^{N_S} \nu_j G_j = \sum_{j=1}^{N_S} \nu_j \overline{G}_j \tag{3.71}$$

where G_j is the Gibbs free energy per mole of species j and ΔG is the Gibbs free energy change per mole in the reaction, as illustrated in Fig. 3.2. We call $\overline{G}_j = \partial G/\partial n_j$ the *chemical potential* of species j which is actually the partial molar free energy. The chemical potential of species j is related to its chemical potential in the standard state (the state in which the activity a_j of species j is unity) by the relation

$$\overline{G}_j = \overline{G}_j^0 + RT \ln a_j \tag{3.72}$$

At chemical equilibrium, at constant temperature and pressure, the Gibbs free energy of the system is a minimum and $\Delta G = 0$. Therefore, we have

$$0 = \Delta G = \sum_{j=1}^{N_S} \nu_j \overline{G}_j = \sum_{j=1}^{N_S} \nu_j \overline{G}_j^0 + \sum_{j=1}^{N_S} \nu_j RT \ln a_j \tag{3.73}$$

at chemical equilibrium. In this expression a_j is the activity of species j, which is a measure of the amount of a species defined such that $a_j = 1$ in the standard state where $\overline{G}_j = \overline{G}_j^0$. For gases, the standard state is usually defined as the ideal gas state at 1 bar (1 bar = 1.023 atm), while for liquids, it may be either the pure material or the material in a solution at a concentration of 1 mol/L. The definitions of standard state and activity are somewhat arbitrary, but they are uniquely related by the definition of unit activity in the standard state. Once the standard state is defined, the situation is well defined. Typical standard states are listed in Table 3.2. In all, one can observe that the activity is dimensionless.

Next, dividing the preceding equation by RT and taking exponentials on both sides, we obtain

$$\exp\left(-\frac{1}{RT} \sum_{j=1}^{N_S} \nu_j \overline{G}_j^0 \right) = \prod_{j=1}^{N_S} a_j^{\nu_j} \tag{3.74}$$

Since we define $\sum_{j=1}^{N_S} \nu_j \overline{G}_j^0 = \Delta G_R^0$, the Gibbs free energy change of the reaction in the standard state, we obtain

$$\prod_{j=1}^{N_S} a_j^{\nu_j} = \exp\left(-\frac{\Delta G_R^0}{RT} \right) = K_{eq} \tag{3.75}$$

where K_{eq} is the equilibrium constant as defined by this equation. [We note in passing that this notation is misleading in that the "equilibrium constant" is constant only for fixed temperature, and it usually varies strongly with temperature. To be consistent with our definition of the "rate coefficient", we should use "equilibrium coefficient" for the equilibrium constant, but the former designation has become the accepted one.]

TABLE 3.2 Species Activity Based on Different Choices of Standard-State Activity

State at (T, P)	Standard state at (T, P = 1 bar)	At low and moderate pressures
Pure gas	Pure gas $\overline{G}_j^0$	$a_j \approx \frac{P}{1\text{ bar}}$
Species in a gaseous mixture	Pure gas $\overline{G}_j^0$	$a_j \approx \frac{p_j}{1\text{ bar}}$
Pure liquid	Pure liquid $\overline{G}_j^0$	$a_j \approx 1$
Species in a liquid mixture	Pure liquid $\overline{G}_j^0$	$a_j \approx \frac{C_j}{C}\gamma_j,\quad \gamma_j \to 1 \text{ as } \frac{C_j}{C} \to 1$
	$\overline{G}_j^0 = \overline{G}_j(T, P = 1\text{ bar}, C_j = 1\text{ M})$	$a_j \approx \frac{C_j\gamma_j}{1\text{ M}},\quad \gamma_j \to 1 \text{ as } C_j \to 0$
	$\overline{G}_j^0 = \overline{G}_j\left(T, P = 1\text{ bar}, \frac{C_j}{C} = 1\right)$	$a_j \approx \frac{C_j}{C}\gamma_j,\quad \gamma_j \to 1 \text{ as } C_j \to 0$
Pure solid	Pure solid $\overline{G}_j^0$	$a_j \approx 1$
Species in a solid mixture	Pure solid $\overline{G}_j^0$	$a_j \approx 1$
Dissolved electrolyte in solution $A_j = \nu_+ A_{j+} + \nu_- A_{j-}$	$\overline{G}_j^0 = \nu_+\overline{G}_{j+}(T,\ P = 1\text{ bar},\ C_{j+} = 1\text{ M}) + \nu_-\overline{G}_{j-}(T,\ P = 1\text{ bar},\ C_{j-} = 1\text{ M})$	$a_j \approx \frac{C_{j+}^{\nu_+}C_{j-}^{\nu_-}}{(1\text{ M})^{\nu_+ + \nu_-}}(\gamma_\pm)^{\nu_+ + \nu_-}$

We define the standard state of a liquid as $a_j = 1$ and for gases as an ideal gas pressure of 1 bar, $p_j = 1$. For ideal liquid solutions (activity coefficients of unity), we write

$$a_j = \frac{C_j}{C_j^0} \tag{3.76}$$

where C_j^0 is either the total concentration or 1 mol/L (as shown in Table 3-1). At chemical equilibrium

$$K_{eq} = \exp\left(-\frac{\Delta G_R^0}{RT}\right) = \prod_{j=1}^{N_S}\left(\frac{C_j}{C_j^0}\right)^{\nu_j} \tag{3.77}$$

and for gases

$$K_{eq} = \exp\left(-\frac{\Delta G_R^0}{RT}\right) = \prod_{j=1}^{N_S} p_j^{\nu_j} \tag{3.78}$$

In these expressions, K_{eq} is dimensionless, while p_j has dimensions; this equation is still correct because we implicitly write each partial pressure as $p_j/1$ bar which is dimensionless.

We can now return to our reaction system and examine the situation near chemical equilibrium. Assuming the simple power-law rate expressions and for a reversible reaction we have

$$0 = r = r_f - r_b = k_f \prod_{j=1}^{N_S} C_j^{O_{fRj}} - k_b \prod_{j=1}^{N_S} C_j^{O_{bRj}} \tag{3.79}$$

because the rate is zero at chemical equilibrium. This is consistent with the arguments based on nonequilibrium thermodynamics, Eqn (3.52), as well. Rearranging this equation, we obtain

$$\frac{k_f}{k_b} = \frac{\prod_{j=1}^{N_S} C_j^{O_{bRj}}}{\prod_{j=1}^{N_S} C_j^{O_{fRj}}} = \prod_{j=1}^{N_S} C_j^{O_{bRj} - O_{fRj}} \tag{3.80}$$

Since we just noted that

$$K_{eq} = \exp\left(-\frac{\Delta G_R^0}{RT}\right) = \prod_{j=1}^{N_S} \left(\frac{C_j}{C_j^0}\right)^{\nu_j} \tag{3.81}$$

We can immediately identify terms in these equations,

$$K_{eq} \prod_{j=1}^{N_S} \left(C_j^0\right)^{\nu_j} = \frac{k_f}{k_b} \tag{3.82}$$

and

$$\nu_j = O_{bRj} - O_{fRj} \tag{3.83}$$

at equilibrium.

From the preceding equations it can be seen that the rate coefficients and the equilibrium constant are related. Recall from thermodynamics that

$$\Delta G_R^0 = \Delta H_R^0 - T \Delta S_R^0 \tag{3.84}$$

where ΔH_R^0 is the standard state enthalpy change and ΔS_R^0 is the standard state entropy change in the reaction. Both ΔH_R^0 and ΔS_R^0 are only weakly dependent on temperature. We can therefore write

$$K_{eq} = \exp(-\Delta G_R^0 / RT) = \exp(\Delta S_R^0 / R) \exp(-\Delta H_R^0 / RT) \tag{3.85}$$

Noting that Arrhenius law can be applied to the reaction rate constants:

$$\frac{k_f}{k_b} \prod_{j=1}^{N_S} \left(C_j^0\right)^{-\nu_j} = \frac{k_{f0}}{k_{b0}} \prod_{j=1}^{N_S} \left(C_j^0\right)^{-\nu_j} \exp\left[-\left(E_f - E_b\right) \big/ RT\right] \tag{3.86}$$

Therefore, we can identify

$$E_f - E_b = \Delta H_R^0 \tag{3.87}$$

and

$$\frac{k_{f0}}{k_{b0}} = \exp(\Delta S_R^0/R) \prod_{j=1}^{N_S} \left(C_j^0\right)^{\nu_j} \tag{3.88}$$

These relationships require that reactions be elementary, and it is always true that *near equilibrium* all reactions obey elementary kinetics. However, we caution once again that in general kinetics is empirically determined. These arguments show that near equilibrium the kinetics of reactions must be consistent with thermodynamic equilibrium requirements.

Note also that the description of a reaction as irreversible simply means that the equilibrium constant is so large that $r_f \gg r_b$. The notion of an irreversible reaction is an operational one, assuming that the reverse reaction rate is sufficiently small compared to the forward reaction so that it can be neglected. It is frequently a good approximation to assume a reaction to be irreversible when $\Delta G_R^0 \ll 0$.

Returning to the energy diagrams, Fig. 3.3, we see that the difference between E_f and E_b is the energy difference between reactants and products, which is the heat of the reaction ΔH_R^0. The heat of reaction is given by the relation

$$\Delta H_R^0 = \sum_{j=1}^{N_S} \nu_j \Delta H_{fj}^0 \tag{3.89}$$

where ΔH_{fj}^0 is the heat of formation of species j. We necessarily described the energy scale loosely, but it can be identified with the enthalpy difference ΔH_R^0 in a reaction system at constant pressure, an expression similar to that derived from classical thermodynamics.

These relations can be used to estimate rate parameters for a back reaction in a reversible reaction if we know the rate parameters of the forward reaction and the equilibrium properties ΔG_{fj}^0 and ΔH_{fj}^0.

We emphasize several cautions about the relationships between kinetics and thermodynamic equilibrium. First, the relations given apply only for a reaction that is close to equilibrium and what is "close" is not always easy to specify. A second caution is that kinetics describes the rate with which a reaction approaches thermodynamic equilibrium, and this rate cannot be predicted from its deviation from the equilibrium composition, i.e. using arguments from nonequilibrium thermodynamics.

A fundamental principle of bioprocess engineering is that we may be able to find a suitable catalyst that will accelerate a desired reaction while leaving others unchanged or an inhibitor that will slow reaction rates. We note the following important points about the relations between thermodynamics and kinetics:

(1) Thermodynamic equilibrium requires that we cannot go from one side of the equilibrium composition to the other in a single process.

(2) Kinetics predicts the rates of reactions and which reactions will go rapidly or slowly toward equilibrium.

One never should try to make a process violate the Second Law of Thermodynamics ($\Delta G \leq 0$ and the entropy generation $\Delta S \geq 0$), but one should never assume that ΔG_{fj}^0 alone predicts what will happen in a chemical reactor.

Reaction rate and concentration or activity. At this point, one may wonder if activity should be used in the reaction rate expressions rather than the concentrations. Based on arguments from nonequilibrium thermodynamics, Eqn (3.52) should be used to compute the reaction rate. This suspicion is also founded due to the equilibrium constant relationships and the reaction rate constants regulations arrived at thermodynamic equilibrium, Eqns (3.78) and (3.79). Thermodynamically, the chemical activity can be thought of as the effective concentration and therefore it can find uses in many places where (apparent) concentration appears. However, for reaction rates, the chemical activity should not be used in place of concentration. This conclusion is rather empirical than theoretical. (But again, nonequilibrium thermodynamics is also empirical; one could alter the arguments for nonequilibrium thermodynamics to fit the chemical kinetic behaviors.)

Figure 3.4 shows the variation of standard Gibbs free energy variation during a reaction. In these illustrations, the concentration effects have been removed. Therefore, Fig. 3.4 shows the energetics of the reaction. Using arguments similar to nonequilibrium thermodynamics, Eqn (3.52), and assuming that the chemical acitivity coefficient is independent of the concentrations, one can readily arrive at that

$$k_{\mathrm{f}} = k^{*}\exp\left(-\frac{\Delta G_{\mathrm{f}}^{o}}{RT}\right) = k * \exp\left(\frac{\Delta S_{\mathrm{f}}^{o}}{R} - \frac{E_{\mathrm{f}}}{RT}\right) \tag{3.90}$$

and

$$k_{\mathrm{b}} = k^{*}\exp\left(-\frac{\Delta G_{\mathrm{b}}^{o}}{RT}\right) = k * \exp\left(\frac{\Delta S_{\mathrm{b}}^{o}}{R} - \frac{E_{\mathrm{b}}}{RT}\right) \tag{3.91}$$

which forms the mathematical basis for the *Transitional State Theory* of chemical reaction kinetics. To this point, we have established the relationship between properties of state (enthalpy change, entropy change, and Gibbs free energy variation) with the reaction rate.

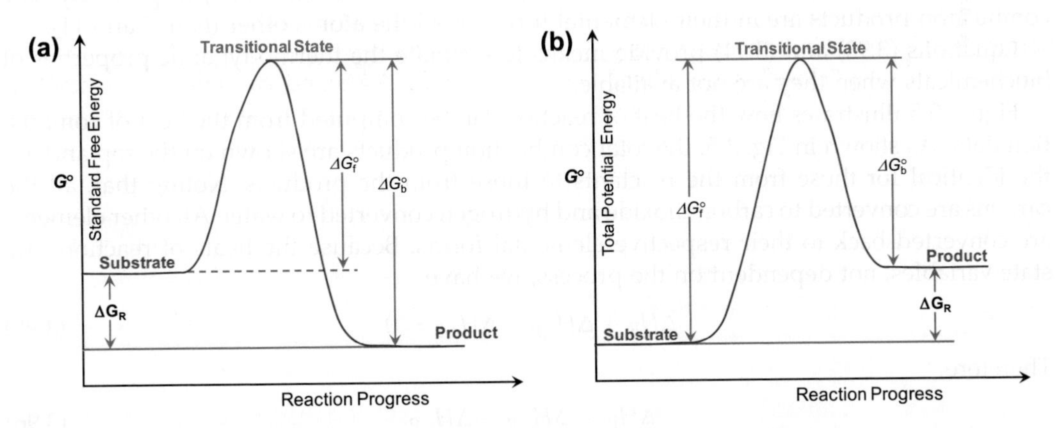

FIGURE 3.4 Plot of standard Gibbs free energy of reactants and products in a chemical reaction vs the reaction coordinate. Although the overall (total) free energy always decreases after the reaction (Fig. 3.2), the standard free energy can be increased or decreased. The reaction rate constants may be estimated via the standard Gibbs free energy barriers. (a) Standard free energy variation for an energetic reaction. (b) Standard free energy variation for an energy acquiring reaction.

3.9. ENERGY REGULARITY

In the preceding section, we have reviewed the thermodynamic limitations. For bioreactions, the chemicals involved often consist of carbon and hydrogen atoms. The lack of detailed information about most living cells and complex molecules has limited our ability to carry out thermodynamic estimations. Limiting on the carbon and hydrogen containing chemicals, biochemical engineers have empirically formulated relations that are of interests to biochemicals. The general degree of reduction is one of the parameters used in the correlations.

The generalized degree of reduction is defined as the number of electrons a molecule can give off to reach the usual state for every atom involved in the molecule. For a carbon and hydrogen containing molecule, this is given as

$$\gamma_{DR} = 4\nu_C + \nu_H - 2\nu_O \tag{3.92}$$

where ν_C is the number of carbon atoms in the molecule, ν_H is the number of hydrogen atoms in the molecule, and ν_O is the number of oxygen atoms in the molecule. The degree of reduction for oxygen (O_2) gas is set at zero, although a -2 is set for oxygen atom in a molecule as shown in Eqn (3.92). The degree of reduction has a unit of moles of electrons per mole.

Correlating on the organic compounds, the heats and Gibbs free energy of combustion (producing gaseous CO_2 and liquid H_2O) have been found to relate to the degree of reduction via (Sandler S.I., Chemical, Biochemical, and Engineering Thermodynamics, 4th Ed., John Wiley & Sons, Inc., 2006).

$$\Delta G_C^0 = -112\ \gamma_{DR}\ \text{kJ/mole} \tag{3.93}$$

and

$$\Delta H_C^0 = -110.9\ \gamma_{DR}\ \text{kJ/mole} \tag{3.94}$$

Where ΔG_C^0 and ΔH_C^0 are the Gibbs free energy and heat of combustion, respectively. The combustion products are in their elemental form for all the atoms other than C and H_2.

Equations (3.93) and (3.94) provide means to estimate the thermodynamic properties of biochemicals when they are not available.

Figure 3.5 illustrates how the heat of reaction can be computed from the heat of combustion data. As shown in Fig. 3.5, the total combustion products are shown on the top and are the identical for those from the reactants to those from the products. Noting that, all the carbons are converted to carbon dioxide and hydrogen converted to water. All other elements are converted back to their respective elemental forms. Because the heats of reactions are state variables, not dependent on the process, we have

$$\Delta H_R + \Delta H_{c,P} - \Delta H_{c,R} = 0 \tag{3.95}$$

Therefore,

$$\Delta H_R = \Delta H_{c,R} - \Delta H_{c,P} \tag{3.96}$$

We note also that

$$\Delta H_{C,R} = \sum_{j=\text{reactants}} \left(-\nu_j\right) \Delta H_{c,j} \tag{3.97}$$

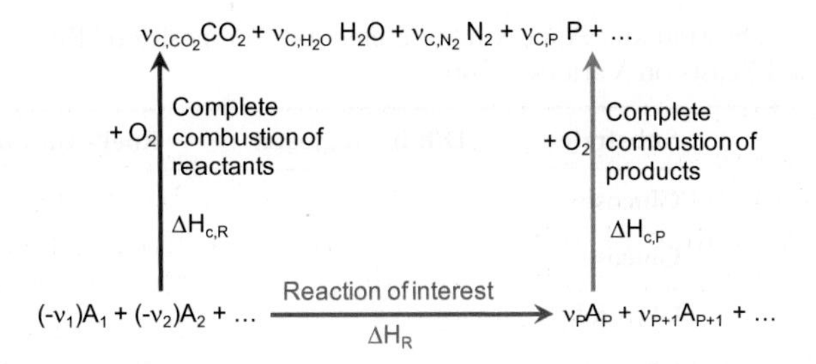

FIGURE 3.5 Relationship between reaction of interests and the complete combustion state of the species involved.

and

$$\Delta H_{\mathrm{c,P}} = \sum_{j=\mathrm{products}} \nu_j \Delta H_{\mathrm{c},j} \tag{3.98}$$

Substituting Eqns (97) and (98) into Eqn (96), we obtain

$$\Delta H_{\mathrm{R}} = \sum_{j=\mathrm{reactants}} \left(-\nu_j\right)\Delta H_{\mathrm{c},j} - \sum_{j=\mathrm{products}} \nu_j \Delta H_{\mathrm{c},j} = -\sum_{j=1}^{N_S} \nu_j \Delta H_{\mathrm{c},j} \tag{3.99}$$

Similarly, we can compute the Gibbs free energy change for the interested reaction from the combustion data:

$$\Delta G_{\mathrm{R}} = \Delta G_{\mathrm{c,R}} - \Delta G_{\mathrm{c,P}} = -\sum_{j=1}^{N_S} \nu_j \Delta G_{\mathrm{c},j} \tag{3.100}$$

Therefore, both heat of reaction and Gibbs free energy change can be computed from the combustion data. The energy regularity relationships can be applied to compute the thermodynamic properties when these data are not available. In bioprocess analysis, one often defines the yield factor on the heat generation along the same line as the yield factor by:

$$YF_{\mathrm{H}/j} = \frac{\Delta H_{\mathrm{R}}}{|\nu_j|} \tag{3.101}$$

Table 3.3 shows the heats of combustion and approximate elemental compositions (or Roel's formula) for some bacteria and yeasts.

3.10. CLASSIFICATION OF MULTIPLE REACTIONS AND SELECTIVITY

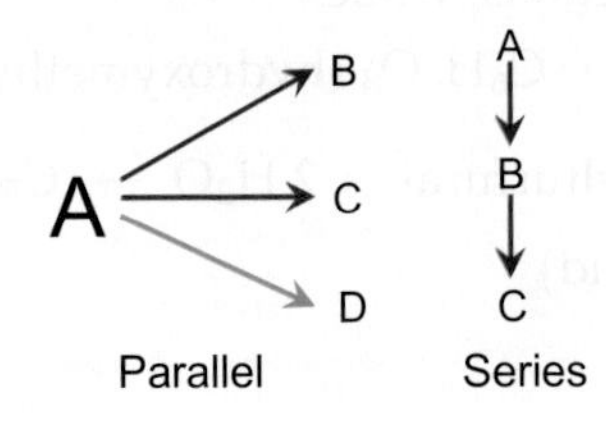

TABLE 3.3 Heats of Combustion and Approximate Elemental Composition (Roel's Formula) of Some Bacteria and Yeasts on Various Substrates

Strain	Substrate	D/h if chemostat	Roel's formula	ΔH_C, kJ/g
Bacillus thuringiensis	Glucose			22.08 ± 0.03
Enterobacter cloacae	Glucose			23.22 ± 0.14
	Glycerol			23.39 ± 0.12
E. coli	Glucose		$CH_{1.70}O_{0.424}N_{0.25}$	23.04 ± 0.06
	Glycerol			22.83 ± 0.07
Methylophilus methylotrophus	Method		$CH_{1.72}O_{0.400}N_{0.247}$	23.82 ± 0.06
Candida boidinii	Glucose			20.41 ± 0.18
	Ethanol			20.40 ± 0.14
	Methanol			21.52 ± 0.09
Candida lipolytica	Glucose			21.34 ± 0.16
Kluyveromyces fragilis	Lactose		$CH_{1.78}O_{0.575}N_{0.159}$	21.54 ± 0.07
	Galactose		$CH_{1.75}O_{0.530}N_{0.166}$	21.78 ± 0.10
	Glucose		$CH_{1.75}O_{0.517}N_{0.153}$	21.66 ± 0.19
	Glucose	0.036		21.07 ± 0.07
		0.061		21.30 ± 0.10
		0.158		20.66 ± 0.26
		0.227		21.22 ± 0.14

Data from Cordier J-C, Butsch BM, Birou B, and von Stockar U. "The relationship between elemental composition and heat of combustion of microbial biomass", Appl. Microbiol. Biotechnol. 1987, 25:305–312.

Frequently, chemical reactions do occur simultaneously in a given system. The reactions are said to be parallel if one reactant participates in reactions that generate different products. Series reactions on the other hand are product(s) of one reaction which further react to produce different products. For example,

$$CH_2O(\text{sugar}) + {}^1/_2 O_2 \rightarrow CO + H_2O$$

$$CH_2O(\text{sugar}) + {}^1/_2 O_2 \rightarrow CO_2 + H_2$$

$$CH_2O(\text{sugar}) + O_2 \rightarrow CO_2 + H_2O$$

is a set (or system) of parallel reactions, while

$$C_6H_{12}O_6(\text{glucose}) \rightarrow C_6H_6O_3\ (\text{hydroxymethylfufural}) + 3\,H_2O$$

$$C_6H_6O_3\ (\text{hydroxymethylfurfural}) + 2\,H_2O \rightarrow C_5H_8O_3\ (\text{levulinic acid}) + HCOOH\ (\text{formic acid})$$

is a set of series reactions.

A reaction system that contains both parallel and series reactions are called mixed reaction system. For example, the three-reaction system:

$$C_2H_5OH \rightarrow C_2H_4 + H_2O$$

$$C_2H_5OH \rightarrow CH_3CHO + H_2$$

$$C_2H_4 + CH_3CHO \rightarrow C_4H_6 + H_2O$$

is a mixed reaction system. The first two reactions are parallel reactions, and the third reaction is a series reaction of both the first and the second reactions.

Selectivity is defined as the fraction of a key reactant that is turned into the desired product, i.e.

$$S_{D/A} = \frac{\text{\#moles of A converted to D}}{\text{\#moles of A reacted}} \tag{3.102}$$

Correspondingly, an instantaneous selectivity can be defined as

$$s_{D/A} = \frac{d(\text{\#moles of A converted to D})}{d(\text{\#moles of A reacted})} = \frac{-r_A|_{\text{forming D}}}{-r_A} \tag{3.103}$$

One of the goals in using catalysts is to increase the selectivity of a desired product. Comparing Eqns (3.102), (3.69), and (3.70), we can see the similarity between selectivity and the less well-defined yield factor. However, selectivity is an especially useful concept for multiple reactions.

3.11. COUPLED REACTIONS

Chemical and biochemical engineers often simplify reactions for ease of understanding in applications. However, the integrity of stoichiometry is preserved when you add the omitted species. Coupled reactions are dependent reactions, meaning a reaction written may not occur if another reaction does not occur. Typical example is shown in Fig. 3.6 for the electrolysis of NaCl in water to produce Cl_2. This is an important reaction from which Cl_2 and NaOH are produced. The reaction occurring on the anode is given by

$$2\,Cl^- \rightarrow Cl_2 + 2\,e \tag{3.104}$$

which requires the reaction on the cathode to occur simultaneously:

$$2\,H^+ + 2\,e \rightarrow H_2 \tag{3.105}$$

such that the electron can be balanced. These two reactions are coupled. The ionization reactions of NaCl and H_2O are occurring in the aqueous solution, providing Cl^- and H^+. The electrochemical reactions are perfect examples of coupled reactions.

In bioprocess engineering, approximation and simplification are commonly used. For example, the approximate reaction (§ 3.4) is one that omitted species whose concentration

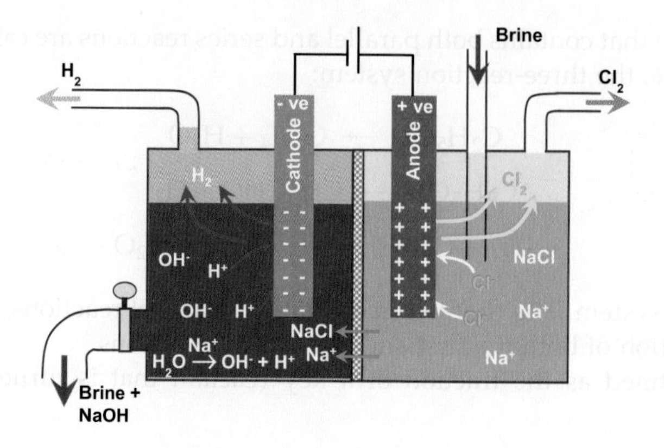

FIGURE 3.6 Electrolysis of sodium chloride in water to produce Cl_2 and sodium hydroxide.

change in the reaction mixture is expected to be negligible or minimal, otherwise the stoichiometry is intact. One example is the aqueous reaction:

$$C_6H_{12}O_6(\text{glucose}) \rightarrow C_6H_6O_3(\text{hydroxymethylfufural}) + 3\,H_2O \tag{3.106}$$

that occurs in many bioprocesses. This reaction can be represented by

$$C_6H_{12}O_6(\text{glucose}) \rightarrow C_6H_6O_3(\text{hydroxymethylfufural}) \tag{3.107}$$

Since H_2O is the solvent and in excess in the reaction mixture, generation of water amounts to negligible change in the total amount of water in the reaction mixture.

In this section, we shall discuss another type of simplifications often used by bioprocess engineers, in analogy to the coupled reactions used in electrochemical reactions. In some occasions, we need to show only part of the (complete) reaction for ease of understanding. For example, if we want to show how glucose (a renewable substrate) can be converted butene (intermediate for polymers, jet fuels, etc.):

$$C_6H_{12}O_6 + H_2 \rightarrow C_4H_8 + HCOOH + CO_2 + 2\,H_2O \tag{3.108}$$

This overall reaction does not mean much except seeing that stoichiometrically it is possible. This reaction is usually achieved in four steps:

$$C_6H_{12}O_6 \rightarrow C_6H_6O_3 + 3\,H_2O \tag{3.109}$$

$$C_6H_6O_3(\text{hydroxymethylfufural}) + 2\,H_2O \rightarrow C_5H_8O_3(\text{levulinic acid}) + HCOOH(\text{formic acid}) \tag{3.110}$$

$$C_5H_8O_3 + H_2 \longrightarrow \text{(}\gamma\text{-lactone ring: } H_2C{-}C({=}O){-}O{-}CH(CH_3){-}H_2C\text{)} + H_2O \tag{3.111}$$

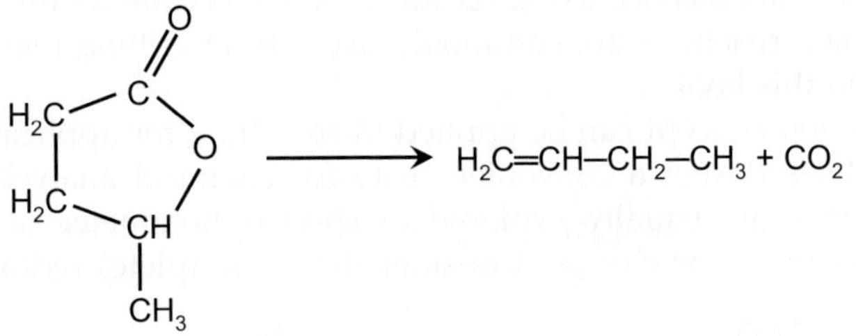

$$\text{(γ-valerolactone: } H_2C(-C(=O)-O-)-H_2C-CH(CH_3)\text{, ring)} \longrightarrow H_2C{=}CH{-}CH_2{-}CH_3 + CO_2 \quad (3.112)$$

To illustrate the reaction in a more easily readable fashion, we write

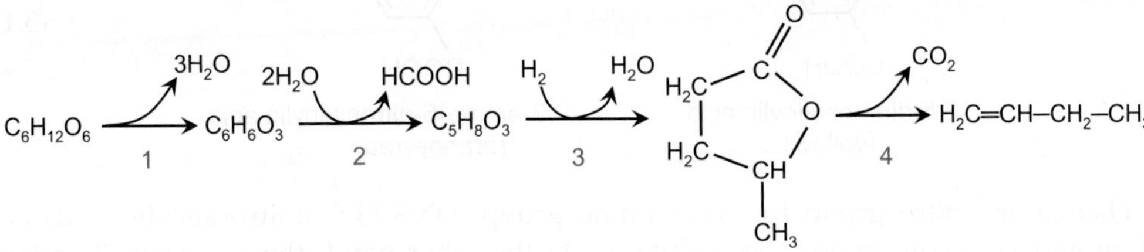

$$C_6H_{12}O_6 \xrightarrow[1]{\;-3H_2O\;} C_6H_6O_3 \xrightarrow[2]{\;2H_2O \rightarrow HCOOH\;} C_5H_8O_3 \xrightarrow[3]{\;H_2 \rightarrow H_2O\;} \text{(γ-valerolactone)} \xrightarrow[4]{\;-CO_2\;} H_2C{=}CH{-}CH_2{-}CH_3 \quad (3.113)$$

In this case, one can follow easily from glucose to butene. Sometimes, we even omit the side branches (species) shown above the horizontal arrow making it more simplified. In so doing, we only showed part of a reaction in each step. This is different from the approximate reactions as the side species may or may not be in excess in the reaction mixture that we can understand. As it stands, one can read carefully to discover that the stoichiometry is preserved in each step. However, our focus may not be on the complete reaction. For example, in step 2, our focus is on the (incomplete) reaction:

$$C_6H_6O_3(\text{hydroxymethylfufural}) \rightarrow C_5H_8O_3(\text{levulinic acid}) \quad (3.114)$$

This reaction as shown is incomplete, neither carbon nor hydrogen are balanced. In order for this (incomplete) reaction to occur, one C needs to be removed and two H need to be added. One can consider that this reaction is coupled with another reaction that can provide two H and remove one C. This coupled reaction is shown above the horizontal arrow in step 2, that is

$$2\,H_2O \rightarrow HCOOH(\text{formic acid}) \quad (3.115)$$

which by itself is not a complete reaction either. However, when we add these two reactions:

$$C_6H_6O_3 \longrightarrow C_5H_8O_3$$

$$2H_2O \longrightarrow HCOOH \qquad (+$$

$$C_6H_6O_3 + 2\,H_2O \longrightarrow C_5H_8O_3 + HCOOH$$

The resulting reaction is stoichiometrically correct. Therefore, for simplicity and brevity in describing complex reaction networks, we may write incomplete reactions to illustrate steps following a key substrate. However, each step will need to be coupled with another incomplete reaction in order to occur. We call the pair of (incomplete) reactions "coupled reactions," the same way as the reactions occurring on the anode and cathode for the electrochemical reactions. The coupled reactions are commonly used in describing metabolic pathways as we will learn later in this book.

The coupled reaction concept can be applied in searching for application of redox pairs, for example. When we design a convenient way for chemical analysis, color changes of certain substance pairs are usually explored as spectrophotometer can be brought in to quantitatively detect the color change. Consider the (incomplete) redox reaction:

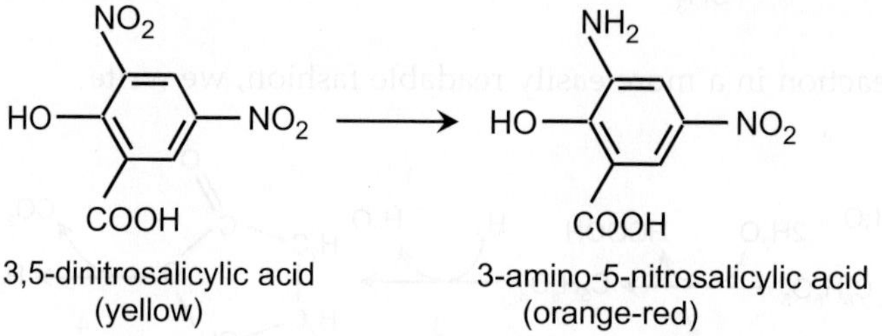

NO_2, HO, NO_2, COOH → NH_2, HO, NO_2, COOH (3.116)

3,5-dinitrosalicylic acid (yellow) → 3-amino-5-nitrosalicylic acid (orange-red)

that change one nitro group into one amino group. DNS (3,5-dinitrosalicylic acid) is an oxidant and is yellow in aqueous solution. On the other hand, the reductant 3-amino-5-nitrosalicylic acid is orange-red in aqueous solution. Examining the two substances, we found that (1) the reaction is only complete if two O are removed and two H are added in the above reaction; (2) the change in the degree of reduction: $\Delta\gamma_{DR} = \gamma_{DR\ 3,5\text{-dinitrosalicylic acid}} - \gamma_{DR\ 3\text{-amino-5-nitrosalicylic acid}} = 2\,\gamma_{DR,\,O} - 2\,\gamma_{DR,\,H} = -6$, which represents an oxidation power of six electrons. DNS is found to be able to oxidize the aldehyde end groups (R-CHO) to corresponding carboxylic acid groups (R-COOH). Each sugar (as one can recall from Chapter 2) molecule contains one aldehyde group. Therefore, DNS has been devised to estimate sugar concentrations (R. Hu, L. Lin, T. Liu, P. Ouyang, B. He, S. Liu 2008 "Reducing sugar content in hemicellulose hydrolysate by DNS method: A revist", JBMBE, 2: 156–161). For each molecule of aldehyde converted to carboxylic acid, there is only a net one O consumed. The oxidation power needed for oxidizing sugar to carboxylic acid is two electrons. Therefore, the DNS sugar pair works, by coupling the DNS (incomplete) redox reaction with

$$3\,\text{R–CHO} + H_2O \rightarrow 3\,\text{R–COOH} \tag{3.117}$$

as H_2O is abundant in an aqueous solution.

3.12. REACTOR MASS BALANCES

We need reaction rate expressions to insert into species mass balance equations for a particular reactor. These are the equations from which we can obtain compositions and other quantities that we need to describe a chemical process. In introductory chemistry courses, students are introduced to first-order irreversible reactions in the batch reactor, and the impression is sometimes left that this is the only mass balance that is important in chemical reactions. In practical situations, the mass balance becomes more complicated.

We will write all reactor mass balances as

$$\text{Accumulation} = \text{flow in} - \text{flow out} + \text{generation by reaction} \tag{3.118}$$

which is an expression we will see many times in mass and/or mole balances throughout this book. It is very simple mathematically and in words, yet it takes a life to learn and master.

We must formulate and solve many mass balance equations in reactor analyses. We strongly encourage the student not to memorize anything except the basic defining relations. We stress that you should be able to derive every equation from these definitions as needed. This is because (1) only by being able to do this will you understand the principles of the subject; and (2) we need to make many different approximations, and remembering the wrong equation is disastrous.

To begin apply this equation, one should always start with identifying the control volume or system of interest. This can be the whole reactor if it is well mixed or a differential volume at a given or arbitrary location inside a vessel. Let us consider a general case whereby the volume of the system (control volume) under consideration is V as shown in Fig. 3.7 where for a given chemical species j, its feed rate, withdrawing rate, and number of moles inside the system are shown. The mole balance equation can thus be written mathematically as

$$\frac{dn_j}{dt} = F_{j0} - F_j + r_j V \tag{3.119}$$

which corresponds term by term to the literal expression (3.118). Therefore, one could consider Eqn (3.119) as the general mass balance equation.

Example 3-5: Fermented Rice

Two kilograms of rice is cooked in 2 kg-water. The cooked rice and water mixture are cooled to 30 °C and mixed with 10 g of yeast. The rice-water-yeast mixture is sealed in a vessel undergoing anaerobic fermentation for 48 h at 30 °C. The final mixture (solids, water, and alcohol) can be eaten as alcoholic food. Assuming that the chemical formulas for rice is the same as starch or $HO(C_6H_{10}O_5)_nH$ and that the alcohol content in the final mixture is 5% (after gas released), find the total mass of the fermented rice mixture.

Solution: Figure E3-5 on the right shows a sketch to illustrate the problem. Drawing a sketch helps us to collect the thoughts together before tackling the problem. Assuming that all the hydrolyzed starch is converted to ethanol, the stoichiometry is then given by

$$HO(C_6H_{10}O_5)nH + (n-1)H_2O \rightarrow \underset{2n \times 46.07}{2n\, C_2H_5OH} + \underset{2n \times 44.01}{2n\, CO_2}$$

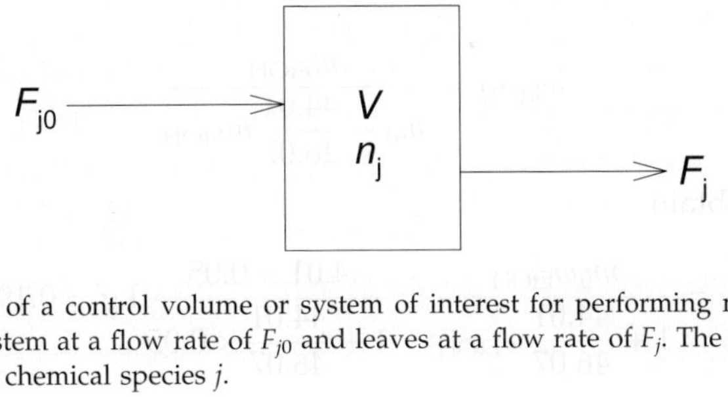

F_{j0} → V, n_j → F_j

FIGURE 3.7 Schematic of a control volume or system of interest for performing mass balances. A chemical species j enters into the system at a flow rate of F_{j0} and leaves at a flow rate of F_j. The volume of the system is V, which contains n_j moles of chemical species j.

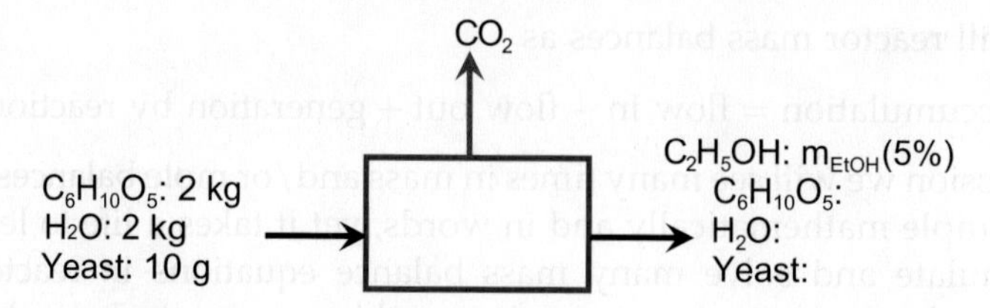

FIGURE E3-5 Schematic diagram showing the control volume or system of interest for mass balance.

To produce 1 mol of alcohol, 1 mol of CO_2 is also produced and released, while half a mole of glucose-equivalent of starch is consumed.

$$46.07 : m_{EtOH} = 44.01 : m_{CO_2}$$

$$m_{CO_2} = 44.01 \times \frac{m_{EtOH}}{46.07}$$

$$= \frac{44.01}{46.07} m_{EtOH}$$

Overall mass balance, Eqn (3.96):

$$\text{In} - \text{Out} + \overset{0}{\text{Generation}} = \overset{0}{\text{Accumulation}}$$

Which leads to: $m_0 = 2 + 2 + 0.01\ \text{kg} = \text{In} = \text{Out} = m_{CO_2} + m_{mix}$

Therefore:

$$m_{mix} = m_0 - m_{CO_2} = 4.01 - \frac{44.01}{46.07} m_{EtOH}$$

We also know that

$$5\% = \omega_{EtOH} = \frac{m_{EtOH}}{m_{mix}}$$

It then leads to:

$$\omega_{EtOH} = \frac{m_{EtOH}}{m_0 - \dfrac{44.01}{46.07} m_{EtOH}}$$

Solve for m_{EtOH}, we obtain

$$m_{EtOH} = \frac{m_0 \omega_{EtOH}}{1 + \dfrac{44.01}{46.07} \omega_{EtOH}} = \frac{4.01 \times 0.05}{1 + \dfrac{44.01}{46.07} \times 0.05}\ \text{kg} = 0.1914\ \text{kg}$$

Carbon dioxide released:

$$m_{CO_2} = \frac{44.01}{46.07} m_{EtOH} = \frac{44.01}{46.07} \times 0.1914 \text{ kg} = 0.1828 \text{ kg}$$

Thus:

$$m_{mix} = m_0 - m_{CO_2} = 4.01 - 0.1828 \text{ kg} = 3.8272 \text{ kg}$$

3.13. REACTION ENERGY BALANCES

We will write all reactor energy balances as

$$\text{energy accumulation} = \text{energy flow in} - \text{energy flow out} \tag{3.120}$$

which is the first law of thermodynamics.

Like the mass balance equation in the previous section, the equation is very simple mathematically and in words as it appears. However, due to the difficulty in defining energy, or rather relating energy to easily measurable quantities in a system, the situation is more complicated than the mass balance. As such, this equation is also only valid if no nuclear reaction occurs. The first law of thermodynamics states that energy cannot be created or destroyed (even chemical and/or biological reactions occur).

We must formulate and solve many energy balance equations in reactor analyses (simultaneously with mass balance equations). Therefore, it would be more convenient if we can translate this literal expression into a mathematical equation.

Figure 3.8 shows a schematic of a system in general where flow streams in and out exist, there is heat exchange between the surroundings occurring at a known rate and there is work

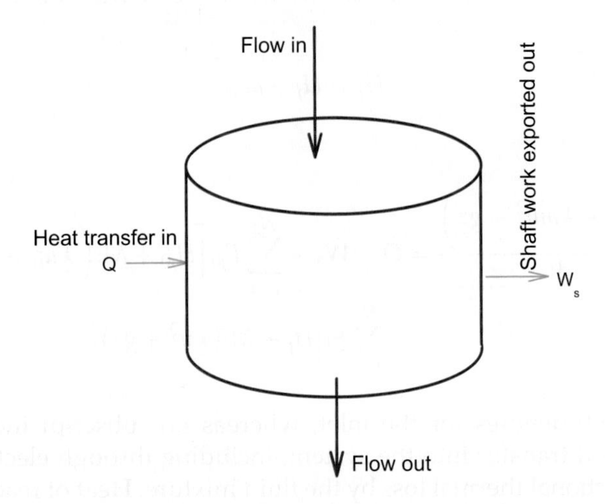

FIGURE 3.8 Schematic of a control volume or system of interest for performing energy balances.

done to the surroundings by the system. Mathematically, the first law of thermodynamics can be expressed for an open system (this concept of system or control volume comes into use again) as

$$\frac{d(E \cdot n)}{dt} = \dot{Q} - \dot{W} + F_{in}E_{in} - F_{out}E_{out} \tag{3.121}$$

where E is energy per mole of substance, $\dot{Q}$ is the rate of heat or thermal energy acquired by the system (flow in), $\dot{W}$ is the rate of work done by the system to the surroundings (energy flow out), and F is the molar flow rate. The total work done to the surroundings consists of two parts, one is due to the fluid streams flowing in and out of the system, and another is the energy exchange with the surroundings due to the shaft work imported from or exported to the surroundings. Thus,

$$\dot{W} = -\left[\sum_{j=1}^{N_S} F_j P v_j\right]_{in} + \left[\sum_{j=1}^{N_S} F_j P v_j\right]_{out} + \dot{W}_s \tag{3.122}$$

Here p is pressure, v is molar volume, and $\dot{W}_s$ is the shaft work done to the surroundings (for example, by a turbine). Thus,

$$\frac{d\sum_{j=1}^{N_S} n_j E_j}{dt} = \dot{Q} - \dot{W}_s + \left[\sum_{j=1}^{N_S} F_j(E_j + pv_j)\right]_{in} - \left[\sum_{j=1}^{N_S} F_j(E_j + pv_j)\right]_{out} \tag{3.123}$$

Noting that:

$$E_j = U_j + M_j \frac{u^2}{2} + M_j g z \tag{3.124}$$

where U is internal energy, u is average flow velocity, M is molecular mass, g is the gravitational acceleration, and z is the vertical distance from a reference point. And the enthalpy is defined as

$$H_j = U_j + pv_j \tag{3.125}$$

Therefore:

$$\begin{aligned} \frac{d\left(nU + \frac{1}{2}mu^2 + gz\right)}{dt} &= \dot{Q} - \dot{W}_s + \sum_{j=1}^{N_S} F_{j0}\left[H_{j0} + M_j\left(\tfrac{1}{2}u_0^2 + gz_0\right)\right] \\ &\quad - \sum_{j=1}^{N_S} F_j\left[H_j + M_j\left(\tfrac{1}{2}u^2 + gz\right)\right] \end{aligned} \tag{3.126}$$

where the subscript 0 denotes for the inlet, whereas no subscript indicating the outlet. Note: $\dot{Q}$ is the net heat transfer into the system, including through electric conversion and subtraction of the frictional thermal loss by the fluid mixture. Heat of reaction is not in either $\dot{Q}$ or $\dot{W}_s$.

In most cases, $E_j \approx U_j$, other than in an electro-hydro facility, or for simple flow loop calculations. Thus, Eqn (3.123) can be simplified to

$$\frac{d(nU)}{dt} = \dot{Q} - \dot{W}_s + \sum_{j=1}^{N_S} F_{j0}H_{j0} - \sum_{j=1}^{N_S} F_jH_j \tag{3.127}$$

The energy balance equation for open system is reduced to that for closed system if there is no flow in or out of the system, i.e. $F = 0$. When chemical reaction occurs, internal energy changes and so are the enthalpies according to the species change.

Since

$$nU = nH - pV = \sum_{j=1}^{N_S} H_jn_j - pV \tag{3.128}$$

and enthalpy is only a function of temperature for ideal gases and nearly so for condensed matters (i.e. liquids or solids),

$$\frac{dH_j}{dt} = C_{Pj}\frac{dT}{dt} \tag{3.129}$$

where C_{Pj} is the molar heat capacity of species j. Differentiating both sides of Eqn (3.108) and substituting Eqn (3.129) as needed, we obtain

$$\frac{d(nU)}{dt} = \sum_{j=1}^{N_S} C_{Pj}n_j\frac{dT}{dt} + \sum_{j=1}^{N_S} H_j\frac{dn_j}{dt} - \frac{d(pV)}{dt} \tag{3.130}$$

which expresses how the left hand side of Eqn (3.126) can be evaluated. Next, we apply the general mole balance equation,

$$F_{j0} - F_j + \sum_{i=1}^{N_R} \nu_{ji}r_iV = \frac{dn_j}{dt} \tag{3.131}$$

Equation (3.127) can be rearranged to give

$$F_jH_j = F_{j0}H_j + V\sum_{i=1}^{N_R} \nu_{ji}r_iH_j - \frac{dn_j}{dt}H_j \tag{3.132}$$

Thus,

$$\begin{aligned}\sum_{j=1}^{N_S} F_{j0}H_{j0} - \sum_{j=1}^{N_S} F_jH_j &= \sum_{j=1}^{N_S} F_{j0}H_{j0} - \sum_{j=1}^{N_S} F_{j0}H_j - V\sum_{i=1}^{N_R} r_i \sum_{j=1}^{N_S} \nu_{ji}H_j + \sum_{j=1}^{N_S} \frac{dn_j}{dt}H_j \\ &= \sum_{j=1}^{N_S} F_{j0}\left(H_{j0} - H_j\right) - V\sum_{i=1}^{N_R} r_i\Delta H_{Ri} + \sum_{j=1}^{N_S} \frac{dn_j}{dt}H_j\end{aligned} \tag{3.133}$$

Substituting Eqns (3.129) and (3.132) into Eqn (3.126), we obtain

$$\sum_{j=1}^{N_S} F_{j0}\left(H_j - H_{j0}\right) + V\sum_{i=1}^{N_R} r_i \Delta H_{Ri} + \sum_{j=1}^{N_S} C_{Pj} n_j \frac{dT}{dt} - \frac{d(pV)}{dt} = \dot{Q} - \dot{W}_s \tag{3.134}$$

which is the general energy balance equation. It is applicable to both flow (i.e. open) and batch (closed) systems. The assumptions we have made to obtain this equation are that the elevation and kinetic energy change can be neglected and that the contents in the control volume (or system) are either condensed matters (solids and/or liquids) or ideal gases. Therefore, Eqn (3.134) is valid in almost all the situations where reactors are used. On the left hand side of Eqn (3.134), the first term resembles the enthalpy change; the second term can be thought of as the heat of generation due to reaction; the third and the fourth terms together can be thought of as the accumulation of energy (which is not exactly true). On the right hand side of Eqn (3.134), they are the net energy rate being transferred to the system. Therefore, the interpretation can help us remember the general energy equation.

Example 3-6: Cooling of fermentation medium

A fermentation medium at 121 °C is pumped at a rate of 1000 kg/h through a heat exchanger to be cooled to 30 °C. The waste cold water used to cool this medium enters at 20 °C and leaves at 85 °C. The average heat capacity of the fermentation medium is 4.06 kJ/(kg·K) and that for water is 4.21 kJ/(kg·K). The fermentation stream and the wastewater stream are separated by a metal surface through which heat is transferred and do not physically mix with each other. Make a complete heat balance on the system. Calculate the water flow and the amount of heat removed from the fermentation medium assuming no heat losses. The process flow is shown in Fig. E3-6.

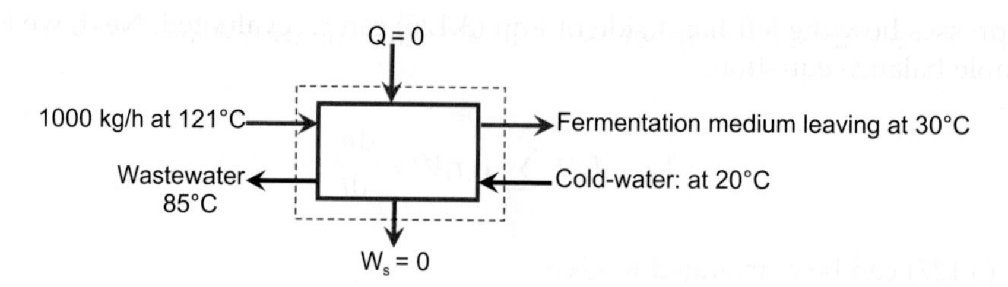

FIGURE E3-6 A schematic of flow streams in and out of a heat exchanger in adiabatic operations.

Solution: Overall energy balance over the system shown as enclosed by the dashed box:

$$\frac{d(U\cdot m)}{dt} = \dot{Q} - \dot{W}_s + \left[\sum_{j=1}^{N_S} \dot{m}_j H_j\right]_{in} - \left[\sum_{j=1}^{N_S} \dot{m}_j H_j\right]_{out} \tag{3.135}$$

0 Steady state; 0 no heat losses; 0 no work done

which is a direct translation Eqn (3.120) based on the mass in the system rather than number of moles. Therefore:

$$0 = \sum_{j=1}^{N_S} \dot{m}_j \left(H_{j,\text{out}} - H_{j,\text{in}} \right)$$

Because there are no changes in flow rates. (1) no phase change and (2) no reaction occurring.

$$\text{Since } \Delta H = \int C_P dT = \overline{C}_P \Delta T, \Rightarrow 0 = \sum_{j=1}^{N_S} \dot{m}_j \overline{C}_{Pj} \left(T_{j,\text{out}} - T_{j,\text{in}} \right)$$

Thus,

$$\dot{m}_H \overline{C}_{PH} \left(T_{H,\text{out}} - T_{H,\text{in}} \right) + \dot{m}_C \overline{C}_{PC} \left(T_{C,\text{out}} - T_{C,\text{in}} \right) = 0$$

$$q_H = \dot{m}_H \overline{C}_{PH} \left(T_{H,\text{in}} - T_{H,\text{out}} \right) = \dot{m}_C \overline{C}_{PC} \left(T_{C,\text{out}} - T_{C,\text{in}} \right) = q_C$$

For example, q_H can be understood by performing an energy balance just over the hot stream (in the heat exchanger) as illustrated in Fig. E3-6a.

$$\frac{d(U \cdot m)}{dt} = \dot{Q} - \dot{W}_s + \left[\sum_{j=1}^{N_S} \dot{m}_j H_j \right]_{\text{in}} - \left[\sum_{j=1}^{N_S} \dot{m}_j H_j \right]_{\text{out}}$$

$\frac{d(U \cdot m)}{dt} \rightarrow 0$ (Steady state); $\dot{Q} \rightarrow -q_H$ (heat loss to cold stream); $\dot{W}_s \rightarrow 0$ (no work done)

Therefore:

$$-q_H + \dot{m}_H \left(H_{H,\text{in}} - H_{H,\text{out}} \right) = 0$$

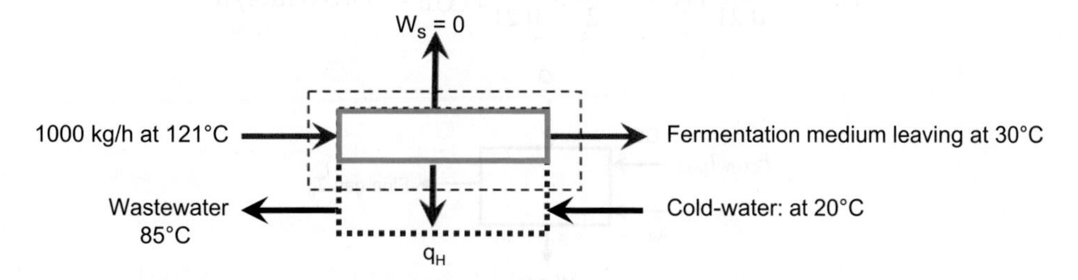

FIGURE E3-6A Schematic diagram of a control volume (or system) around the hot stream passing through the heat exchanger.

Similarly, q_C is defined. Thus, we have

$$q_H = \dot{m}_H \overline{C}_{PH}(T_{H,in} - T_{H,out}) = \frac{1000}{3600} \times 4.06 \times (121 - 30) \text{ kJ/s} = 102.628 \text{ kW}$$

$$\dot{m}_C = \frac{q_C}{C_{PC}(T_{C,out} - T_{C,in})} = \frac{102.628}{4.21 \times (85 - 20)} \text{kg/s} = 0.375 \text{ kg/s} = 1350.1 \text{ kg/h}$$

Example 3-7: Heat and material balances in combustion

The waste gas from a process of 1000 mol/h of CO at 473 K is burned at 1 atm pressure in a furnace using air at 373 K. The combustion is complete and 90% excess air is used. The flue gas leaves the furnace at 1273 K. Calculate the heat removed in the furnace.

Solution: A schematic diagram is shown in Fig. E3-7.Combustion stoichiometry

$$CO + {}^{1}\!/_{2}\, O_2 \rightarrow CO_2$$

Heats of formation can be found as

$\Delta H^0_{f,298} = -110.523 \times 10^3$ kJ/kmol for CO and -393.513×10^3 kJ/kmol for CO_2.

$$\Delta H^0_{R,298} = H^0_{CO_2,298} - H^0_{CO,298} - \frac{1}{2} H^0_{O_2,298}$$
$$= \Delta H^0_{fCO_2,298} - \Delta H^0_{fCO,298} - \Delta H^0_{fO_2,298}$$
$$\Delta H^0_{R,298} = -282.990 \times 10^3 \text{kJ/kmol}$$

From stoichiometry, 1 mol of CO requires half a mole of O_2 to produce 1 mol of CO_2 at complete combustion. Therefore, the minimum O_2 in feed is half of that of CO.

$$F_{O_2,min} = \frac{1}{2} F_{CO,0}$$

and

$$F_{O_2,0} = 1.9 F_{O_2,min} = \frac{1.9}{2} F_{CO,0} = 950 \text{ mol/h}.$$

The O_2 is supplied by air. In air, there are about 21% mole percent of O_2 and 79% mole percent of N_2. Thus, the requirement of O_2 brings N_2 along from the air. That is,

$$F_{N_2,0} = \frac{0.79}{0.21} F_{O_2,0} = \frac{1.9}{2} \times \frac{0.79}{0.21} F_{CO,0} = 3573.8 \text{ mol/h}$$

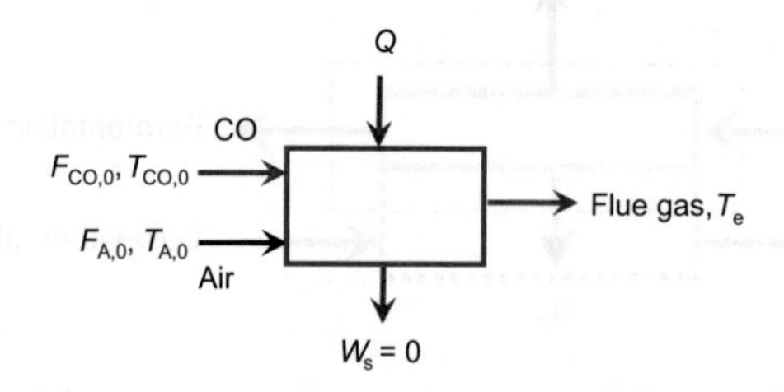

FIGURE E3-7 A schematic flow diagram of a flue gas combustion furnace.

In the flue gas,

$$F_{N_2,e} = F_{N_2,0} = 3573.8 \text{ mol/h};$$

$$F_{CO_2,e} = F_{CO,0} = 1000 \text{ mol/h};$$

$$F_{O_2,e} = F_{O_2,0} - F_{O_2,\min} = 0.45F_{CO,0} = 450 \text{ mol/h};$$

Energy balance over the system:

$$\underbrace{\frac{d(U \cdot n)}{dt}}_{\substack{0 \\ \text{Steady state}}} = Q - \underbrace{W_s}_{\substack{0 \\ \text{no work done}}} + \left[\sum_{j=1}^{N_S} F_j H_j\right]_{\text{in}} - \left[\sum_{j=1}^{N_S} F_j H_j\right]_{\text{out}}$$

Therefore:

$$Q = \sum_{j=1}^{N_S} \left(F_{j,\text{out}}\, H_{j,\text{out}} - F_{j,\text{in}}\, H_{j,\text{in}}\right)$$

Since the pressure is constant (at standard pressure), we have:

$$H_{j,T} = \Delta H^0_{fj,298} + \int_{298}^{T} C_{Pj} dT = \Delta H^0_{fj,298} + \overline{C}_{Pj}(T - 298)$$

Remark: if a table of C_P vs T is tabulated, numerical integration will be needed. If a correlation equation is known, then direct integration can be applied.

$$Q = \sum_{j=1}^{N_S} \left(F_{j,\text{out}}\, H_{j,\text{out}} - F_{j,\text{in}}\, H_{j,\text{in}}\right)$$

$$= \sum_{j=1}^{N_S} \left\{F_{j,e}\left[H^0_{j,298} + \overline{C}_{Pj,e}\left(T_{j,e} - 298\right)\right] - F_{j,0}\left[H^0_{j,298} + \overline{C}_{Pj,0}\left(T_{j,0} - 298\right)\right]\right\}$$

$$Q = \sum_{j=1}^{N_S} \left(F_{j,e} - F_{j,0}\right) H^0_{j,298} + \sum_{j=1}^{N_S} \left[F_{j,e}\overline{C}_{Pj,e}\left(T_{j,e} - 298\right) - F_{j,0}\overline{C}_{Pj,0}\left(T_{j,0} - 298\right)\right]$$

$$= F_{CO,0}\Delta H_{R,298} + \sum_{j=1}^{N_S} \left[F_{j,e}\overline{C}_{Pj,e}\left(T_{j,e} - 298\right) - F_{j,0}\overline{C}_{Pj,0}\left(T_{j,0} - 298\right)\right]$$

$$Q = 1000 \times (-282.990 \times 10^3) + (3573.8 \times 31.47 + 1000 \times 49.91 + 450 \times 33.25)$$

$$\times (1273 - 298) - [3573.8 \times 31.47 \times (373 - 298) + 1000 \times 39.38$$

$$\times (473 - 298) + 950 \times 29.66 \times (373 - 298) \text{ J/h} = -127523350 \text{ J/h}$$

$$= -1.2752 \times 10^8 \text{ J/h} = -35.42 \text{ kW}$$

From these two examples, one can observe that the energy balance equation can be further reduced for a reacting system. Noting that for ideal systems where the enthalpy is only a function of temperature,

$$H_j = \Delta H_{fj}^0 + \int_{T_R}^{T} C_{Pj} \mathrm{d}T \tag{3.136}$$

and

$$U_j = \Delta U_{fj}^0 + \int_{T_R}^{T} C_{Vj} \mathrm{d}T \tag{3.137}$$

For ideal gases,

$$\Delta U_{fj}^0 = \Delta H_{fj}^0 - RT_R \tag{3.138}$$

and for liquids,

$$\Delta U_{fj}^0 \approx \Delta H_{fj}^0 \tag{3.139}$$

These equations can be applied to compute the enthalpy and internal energy terms in the energy balance equations.

3.14. REACTOR MOMENTUM BALANCE

As we have learned in Fluid Mechanics, the flow of a fluid mixture is governed by the Navier–Stokes equation or the conservation of momentum equations. For a thorough analysis of a reactor, the solution coupling with the Navier–Stokes equation may be needed. However, for chemical reactor analysis, we normally simplify the analysis and avoiding the direct use of the Navier–Stokes equations. For example, in bioprocesses, most of the time we are dealing with liquid-phase reactions. The concentration of a component in liquid phase is rarely influenced by the fluid pressure, which is the driving force for flow. Therefore, the momentum equation is usually neglected in solving reactor problems. Still, in some cases, the momentum equation can be important, for example, in gas-phase reactions.

The Navier–Stokes equation can be significantly simplified in simple cases, such steady flow through a straight pipe (tubular reactor), flow through packed beds, and flow through fluidized beds. For flow through a pipe or column, the momentum equation is reduced to

$$-\frac{\mathrm{d}P}{\mathrm{d}z} = \rho u \frac{\mathrm{d}u}{\mathrm{d}z} + 2f_c \frac{1}{D_t} \rho u^2 \tag{3.140}$$

Where f_c is the Fanning friction factor, ρ is the density of the fluid, D_t is the diameter of the pipe and flow Reynolds number (or velocity, u). For fully turbulent flow, f_c is taken as constant. In laminar flow, however, the friction factor is inversely proportional to the velocity.

When the column is packed with particles of diameter d_p, the friction factor is a function of the particle flow Reynolds number as shown in Fig. 3.9. When the flow Reynolds number is

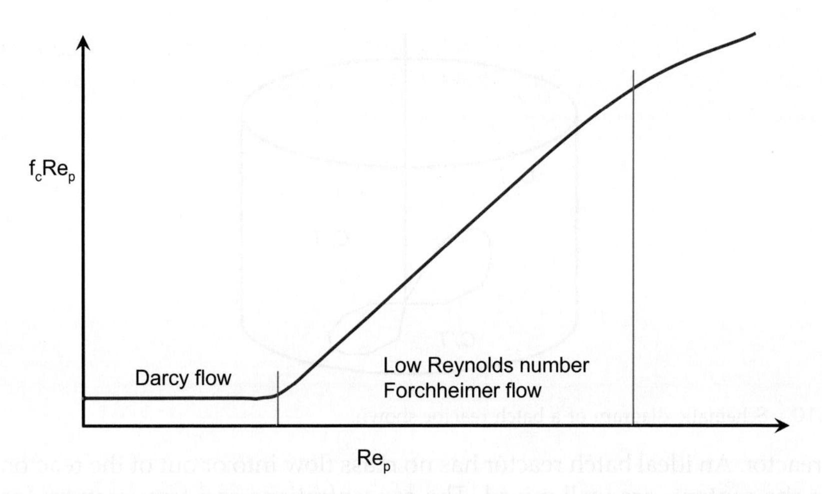

FIGURE 3.9 Friction factor for flow through a packed bed as a function of the particle Reynolds number. At low to intermediate Reynolds number region, there is a transition from Darcy's flow where the friction factor is inversely proportional to the flow rate, to inertial dominant flow (or Forchheimer flow) where the friction factor is constant.

high, the effect of the Darcy's region can be simplified and Ergun equation is commonly used to compute the pressure drop, i.e.

$$f_c = \frac{D_t}{2d_p}\frac{1-\varepsilon}{\varepsilon^3}\left[1.75 + 150(1-\varepsilon)\frac{\mu_f}{d_p \rho u}\right] \tag{3.141}$$

where ε is the bed voidage or porosity and μ_f is the dynamic viscosity of the fluid mixture. Noting that the flow transition exists in flow through packed beds, Liu et al. (Liu, S., Afacan, A. and Masliyah, J.H. 1994 "Steady Incompressible Laminar Flow in Porous Media", Chem. Eng. Sci., 49, 3565–3586) proposed a modified equation for the friction factor,

$$f_c = \frac{D_t}{2d_p}\frac{(1-\varepsilon)^2}{\varepsilon^{11/3}}\frac{\mu_f}{\rho d_p u}\left[85.2 + 0.69\frac{\mathrm{Re}_p^2}{16^2 + \mathrm{Re}_p^2}\right] \tag{3.142}$$

where Re_p is a particle Reynolds number defined by

$$\mathrm{Re}_p = \frac{1 + (1-\varepsilon^{1/2})^{1/2}}{(1-\varepsilon)\varepsilon^{1/6}}\frac{\rho d_p u}{\mu_f} \tag{3.143}$$

Equation (3.142) can describe the first two regions shown in Fig. 3.9 quite well, including the transition from the Darcy's flow to the Forchheimer flow.

3.15. IDEAL REACTORS

Reactors are "units" in which reaction occurs. Reactors can be operated in batch (no mass flow into or out of the reactor) or flow modes. Flow reactors can operate between limits of completely segregated (or unmixed) and completely mixed. Therefore, for simplicity in analysis, we define three types of idealized reactors based on the conditions of mixing and flow.

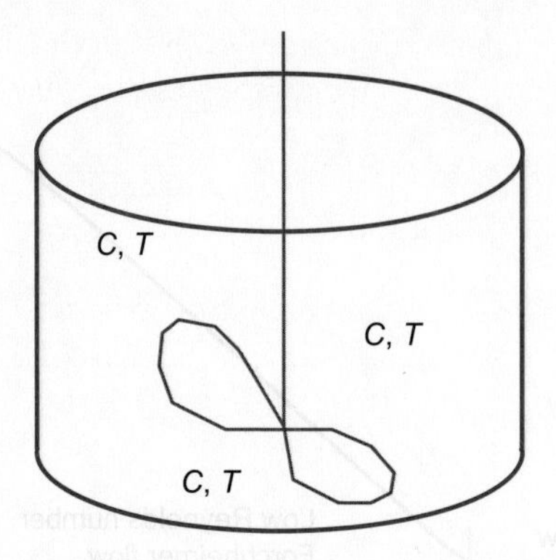

FIGURE 3.10 Schematic diagram of a batch reactor shown.

(1) Batch reactor. An ideal batch reactor has no mass flow into or out of the reactor. Inside the reactor, the contents are well mixed. The concentrations and temperature, for example, are identical everywhere inside the reactor at any given instant in time. However, they can vary with time. Figure 3.10 shows an illustration of a batch reactor.

(2) Plug flow reactor or in short PFR. A PFR is a completely segregated flow reactor, in which the contents are completely mixed transversely at any given location on the axial (flow direction) location. However, along the direction of flow, there is absolutely no mixing. Therefore, the concentrations and temperature can vary along the axial (flow) direction but not transversely or on the plane perpendicular to the direction of flow. PFR is an idealization of a tubular reactor. Figure 3.11 shows an illustration of a PFR.

(3) Continuous stirred-tank reactor, CSTR, or chemostat. A CSTR has mass flow into and out of the reactor that is otherwise a batch reactor. Therefore, the contents in a CSTR are well mixed. The concentrations and temperature are identical anywhere inside the reactor, which are also the same as those in the effluent. However, the feed stream can have different values. Figure 3.12 shows an illustration of a CSTR.

The well mixedness of a CSTR gives rise to unique properties for the reactor operation. Often, when the term CSTR is used, we refer to the steady state operation of a CSTR. In this case, the concentrations of any given species in the effluent and the same as those inside the reactor are constant, also independent of time. For any bioprocesses, the production of products is usually catalyzed by biological cells and/or catalysts. As we will learn later in the book,

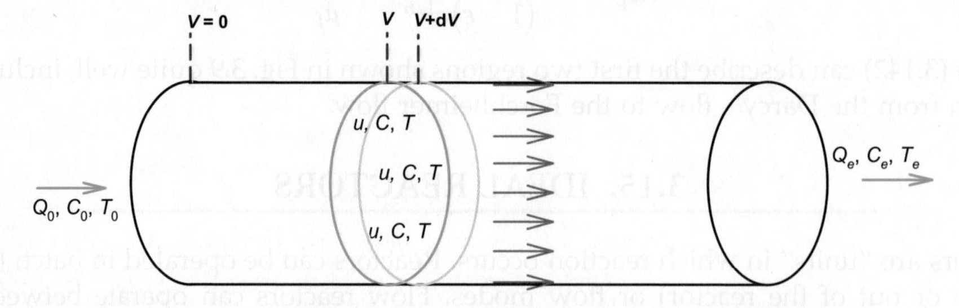

FIGURE 3.11 Schematic diagram of a PFR. It can be thought if as a tubular reactor with the velocity (u), concentrations (C), and temperature (T) uniform at any given plane along the axial direction.

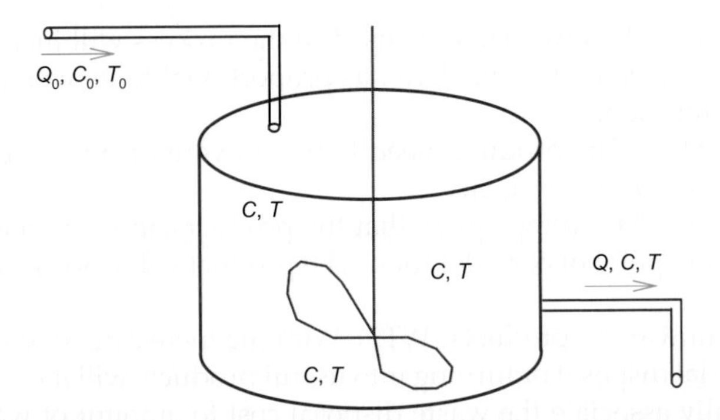

FIGURE 3.12 Schematic diagram of a CSTR or chemostat showing one stream flowing in and one stream flowing out of the reactor, with proper volumetric flow rates, temperature, and concentrations.

in Chapters 9, 14, and 16, that catalysts and/or microorganisms could change with time after extended time of exposure in the reactor. *Nonideality* can arise despite the conditions of flow and mixing being ideal. Therefore, controlling the flow rate alone cannot maintain all the parameters to be invariant with time for a *CSTR* operation in practice. Especially for bio-reactions, the variation of some parameters or quantities can be significant. Therefore, depending on the different set goals of maintaining different parameters in the reactor and/or in the effluent, different terminologies of "steady" bioreactor are used. For example, the commonly used term *chemostat* stands for "chemical environment being static." Other examples include

Turbidostat—Turbidity being static. If chemical species do not change, the change of turbidity is associated with the change of cell biomass concentration. Therefore, tubidostat is intended for an operation of steady cell biomass.
Cytostat—Cell biomass being static in the reactor.
pH-auxostat—pH values being static in the reactor.
Productostat—The concentration of a key metabolic product being static in the reactor.

3.16. BIOPROCESS SYSTEMS OPTIMIZATION

We have covered the reactor mass and energy balances so far. Next, we consider the overall economic performance as it will dictate how or whether the bioprocess will be in operation. At least in a short-time scale, a process that makes money or a profit is a process that creates value. Therefore, every process engineer would like to make sure the process he/she is working on is making a profit. The profit is a net accumulation of value from a process. The profitability of a process is strongly dependent on

(1) Reactor operating cost (RO\$). This includes the utility (solvent use, energy, equipment depreciation, etc.) cost and labor cost that associated with operating the reactor or reactors. For bioprocess operations, we normally related the reactor operating cost to the size of the reactor, the throughput, and the intended temperature of operation, i.e. $OP\$ = f(V, Q_0, T)$. Here is Q_0 the volumetric flow rate of raw material feed into the reactor.

(2) Material cost (RM$). All raw materials used in the process will incur a cost. The cost to raw materials can usually be considered as proportional to its weight or amount and quality or concentration.
(3) Separation cost (SC$). The products need to be recovered from the product stream and the catalyst needs to recovered, etc.
(4) Product value (P$). The average price that the product can fetch in an open market is usually the starting point of consideration. The product value is normally assigned based on the amount.
(5) Cost to dispose unwanted products (WT$). With the increasing environmental concerns, unwanted material disposal or turning into useful products will incur a cost to the overall plan. We normally associate the waste disposal cost to amount of waste material that needs further process.
(6) Cost to marketing the products (CM$). The products have no value if not claimed by their intended users. There is a cost to make the products known to their intended users and helping the intended users to claim the products.
(7) Transportation cost of the product before delivery (DC$). The price of a product is sometimes for a delivery at certain point. Transportation cost is proportional to the amount of goods to be delivered as well as the distance between the plant and the delivering point.
(8) Taxes (TX$). For any operations or plants, the governments will collect taxes over site coordination, utilities, land use, water and air disturbances, etc.
(9) Indirect cost (IC$).

Mathematically, one can write the profit as

$$\text{Profit} = \text{P\$} - \text{RO\$} - \text{RM\$} - \text{SC\$} - \text{WT\$} - \text{CM\$} - \text{DC\$} - \text{TX\$} - \text{IC\$} \tag{3.144}$$

Therefore as a bioprocess engineer, we want to make sure that the process we are dealing with makes a profit. The overall goal of the Bioprocess Systems Engineering is to maximize this profit.

As one can notice from Eqn (3.144) that the estimation of profit involves many details that may or may not be always available. As a bioprocess engineer, we frequently base our analysis on readily available data. We next define the gross profit (GP$) and gross operation cost (GC$):

$$\text{GP\$} = \text{P\$} - \text{RO\$} - \text{SC\$} - \text{RM\$} - \text{WT\$} \tag{3.145}$$

$$\text{GC\$} = \text{RO\$} + \text{SC\$} + \text{RM\$} + \text{WT\$} \tag{3.146}$$

These two parameters are frequently used to guide the design and operational performance analyses of bioprocesses. Depends on the amount of knowledge we know associate with the process, we normally start with maximizing the profit if possible. When not all the information is available, we examine the process by maximizing the gross profit (GP$) or minimizing the gross operation cost (GC$) or minimizing the reactor operating cost (RO$).

Example 3-8: Economic Analysis

We wish to produce R isothermally from the reaction

$$\text{A} \rightarrow \text{R}, \quad r_1 = k_1 C_\text{A} \tag{E3-8.1}$$

Unfortunately, A also decomposes into Q at the condition where R is formed:

$$A \rightarrow Q, \quad r_2 = k_2 C_A \tag{E3-8.2}$$

A costs \$0.05/lb, R sells for \$0.10/lb, and Q costs \$0.03/lb to dispose. Assume that cost to the reactor and operation is negligible.

(a) What relation between the k's will give a positive cash flow?
(b) What relation between the k's will give a 30% profit on sales?

Solution:

This is a system of first-order parallel reactions. The instantaneous selectivity of R is given by, Equation (3.103),

$$s_{R/A} = \frac{d(\#\text{moles of A converted to R})}{d(\#\text{moles of A reacted})} = \frac{-r_A|_{\text{forming R}}}{-r_A} = \frac{r_1}{r_1 + r_2} = \frac{k_1}{k_1 + k_2} \tag{E3-8.3}$$

which is constant. Therefore, one can conclude that the conversion of A into R is always a fraction of the total A reacted. This can simplify our computations (before we even know how to perform reactor analysis). The fraction of A converted to R is $s_{R/A}$ and the fraction of A converted to Q is $1 - s_{R/A}$. Therefore, for every pound of A reacted,

$$\text{Profit per lb of A reacted} = \$0.10 \times \frac{k_1}{k_1 + k_2} - \$0.03 \times \left(1 - \frac{k_1}{k_1 + k_2}\right) - \$0.05 \tag{E3-8.4}$$

(a) For the process to give a positive cash flow, it is equivalent to require:

$$0 < \text{Profit per lb of A reacted} = \$0.10 \times \frac{k_1}{k_1 + k_2} - \$0.03 \times \left(1 - \frac{k_1}{k_1 + k_2}\right) - \$0.05 \tag{E3-8.5}$$

That is to say

$$\frac{10k_1}{k_1 + k_2} - 3 \times \left(1 - \frac{k_1}{k_1 + k_2}\right) > 5 \tag{E3-8.6}$$

or

$$\frac{13k_1}{k_1 + k_2} > 8 \tag{E3-8.7}$$

which can be reduced to

$$\boxed{\frac{k_2}{k_1} < \frac{5}{8} = 0.625} \tag{E3-8.8}$$

(b) To make 30% profit on sales is equivalent to say that the profit is 30% of the value of R produced. Thus,

$$\$0.10 \times \frac{k_1}{k_1 + k_2} - \$0.03 \times \left(1 - \frac{k_1}{k_1 + k_2}\right) - \$0.05 = 30\% \times \$0.10 \times \frac{k_1}{k_1 + k_2} \tag{E3-8.5}$$

which can be reduced to

$$\frac{10k_1}{k_1 + k_2} = 8 \tag{E3-8.6}$$

or

$$\frac{k_2}{k_1} = \frac{2}{8} = 0.25 \tag{E3-8.7}$$

This concludes the example.

3.17. SUMMARY

Chemical reactions can be written as

$$\sum_{j=1}^{N_S} \nu_{ij} A_j = 0, \quad i = 1, 2, \ldots, N_R \tag{3.19}$$

with ν_{ij} being the stoichiometric coefficient for species A_j in reaction i. Stoichiometry leads to the relationships among the rates of reaction for each species,

$$r_i = \frac{r_{ij}}{\nu_{ij}} \tag{3.29}$$

And the rate of reaction for a given species j in a set of N_R reactions can be computed via

$$r_j = \sum_{i=1}^{N_R} \nu_{ij} r_i \tag{3.66}$$

That is, the rate of reaction for a given species is the sum of its reaction rates in all the reactions.

There is one independent reaction rate expression for each reaction. For a single reaction,

$$\frac{\Delta n_j}{\nu_j} = n_{\text{ext}}, \quad \forall j \tag{3.61}$$

where n_{ext} is the extent of reaction. Equation (3.61) governs the change for a species due to reactions. The fractional conversion is usually defined instead of using the extent of reaction:

$$n_A = n_{A0}(1 - f_A) \tag{3.60}$$

which is convenient for single reaction systems. For multiple reactions, one needs to define one conversion for each reaction.

The rate of formation of a species, say species A, is the number of A molecules being generated (from consuming other species) per unit time per volume, that is

$$r_A = \frac{\text{Number of moles of species A formed}}{\text{Time} \times \text{Volume}} \tag{3.20}$$

which is the definition of reaction rate. Bioprocess engineers should be proficient in relating the change of species in a reactor via mass balance. The direct use of

$$\times \quad r_A = \frac{dC_A}{dt} \tag{E3-1.1}$$

for reaction rate is discouraged. The reaction rate is to be obtained from kinetic studies and the relation of reaction rate to change is obtained by mass or mole balance:

$$\frac{dn_j}{dt} = F_{j0} - F_j + r_j V \tag{3.119}$$

where F_{j0} is the rate of species j being added to the reactor and F_j is the rate of species j being withdrawn from the reactor.

For bioreactions, reaction rates are normally expressed as the specific rates:

$$r'_A = \frac{r_A}{X} \tag{3.25}$$

where X is the mass concentration of biomass or cells.

$$\mu_A = r'_A M_A = \frac{r_A M_A}{X} \tag{3.27}$$

where M_A is molecular mass of species A.

For an irreversible homogeneous phase reaction, one frequently describes the rate to a good approximation as

$$r = k \prod_{j=1}^{N_S} C_j^{O_{Rj}} \tag{3.35}$$

where O_{Rj} is the order of the reaction with respect to the jth species and the product extends over all species in the reaction with $O_{Rj} = 0$ for species that do not affect the rate of reaction. If the rate is proportional to the concentration of a species raised to a power (O_{Rj}), we say that this form of the rate expression is described by "power-law kinetics". This empirical function is frequently used to describe reaction rates, but it frequently is not accurate, especially with surface or enzyme-catalyzed reactions, which are of the main topic of discussion in this book.

A reaction is said to be elementary if the rate of reaction follows Eqn (3.35) with the orders of reaction the same as the stoichiometric coefficients or

$$O_{Rj} = \text{Max}\left\{ -\upsilon_j, 0 \right\}$$

A reversible reaction can be decoupled into two reactions, one forward and the other backward. The rate of reaction is the summation (or subtraction as the two reactions move against each other) of the two rates.

The rate of reaction does not follow with the nonequilibrium thermodynamic theory as the rate expression in Eqn (3.35) is found to be dependent on the concentration not on the chemical activity. However, one may still be able to correlate the reaction rate constants through nonequilibrium thermodynamic arguments or via the standard Gibbs free energy change.

The reaction rate constants are functions of temperature only for a given system. The rate dependence on temperature is governed by the Arrhenius law or

$$k(T) = k_0 e^{-E/RT} \tag{3.53}$$

where E is called the *activation energy* for the reaction and k_0 is called (unimaginatively) the *pre-exponential factor*. For reversible reactions, the difference between the activation energy of the forward and backward reactions is the heat of reaction. The ratio of the forward reaction rate constant over the backward reaction rate constant is directly related to the equilibrium constant.

The degree of reduction is defined as the number of electrons a molecule can potentially give off when reacting with other molecules. The generalized degree of reduction for a carbon and hydrogen containing molecule is given as

$$\gamma_{DR} = 4\nu_C + \nu_H - 2\nu_O \tag{3.92}$$

where υ_C, υ_H, and υ_O are the numbers of carbon, hydrogen, and oxygen atoms, respectively, in the molecule. The degree of reduction for oxygen (O_2) gas is set at zero, although a -2 is set for oxygen atom in a molecule as shown in Eqn (3.92).

The heats and Gibbs free energy of combustion (producing gaseous CO_2 and liquid H_2O) have been found to relate to the degree of reduction via

$$\Delta G_C^0 = \Delta G_\gamma \gamma_{DR} = -112\ \gamma_{DR}\ \text{kJ/mole} \tag{3.93}$$

and

$$\Delta H_C^0 = \Delta H_\gamma \gamma_{DR} = -110.9\ \gamma_{DR}\ \text{kJ/mole} \tag{3.94}$$

Where ΔG_C^0 and ΔH_C^0 are the Gibbs free energy and heat of combustion, respectively. The combustion products are in their elemental form if other than C and H_2.

Yield is an important parameter in reactor analysis. The yield is defined as

$$Y_{P/A/R} = \frac{\text{\#-moles of R in all the P formed}}{\text{\#-moles of R in all the A initially}} \tag{3.67}$$

where R is a key element of group of elements present entirely in both P and A.

In bioreactions, the natural reference (R) is carbon (C) as most cases we use a carbon source and carbon is the key component of interest. In this case, Eqn (3.67) can be rewritten as

$$Y_{P/A/C} = \frac{\text{\#-C-moles of P formed}}{\text{\#-C-moles of A initially}} \tag{3.68a}$$

or simply

$$Y_{P/A} = \frac{\text{\#-C-moles of P formed}}{\text{\#-C-moles of A initially}} \tag{3.68b}$$

as carbon is implied. Yield is dependent on the extent of reaction and thus is not a thermodynamic (or equilibrium) parameter.

Yield factor is the maximum fractional yield and is defined as

$$YF_{P/A} = \frac{\text{\#-C-moles of P that could be formed}}{\text{\#-C-moles of A}} = \frac{|\nu_P|}{|\nu_A|} \tag{3.69}$$

which is then only specific to the stoichiometry of the reactions involved. One often extends this yield factor definition to include reactants as well, in that case, the amount of species change in the definition is always defined as the absolute value in the net change (either increase or decrease). One often extends this yield factor definition to include reactants as well, in that case, the amount of species change in the definition is always defined as the absolute value in the net change (either increase or different).

Sometimes, one can find that the yield factor defined above is not convenient to use. For example, counting the number of biomass or cells is not an easy task. We often use another definition,

$$YF_{P/A} = \frac{\text{Mass of P that could be produced}}{\text{Mass of A}} \tag{3.70}$$

Because of the various forms of yield or fractional yield are used, it is recommended that the units being always associated with the yield given. In bioprocess analysis, one often defines the yield factor on the heat generation along the same line as the yield factor by

$$YF_{H/j} = \frac{\Delta H_R}{|\nu_j|} \tag{3.101}$$

Another factor of importance is the selectivity for multiple reactions. Selectivity is defined as the fraction of a key reactant that is turned into the desired product, i.e.

$$S_{D/A} = \frac{\text{\#moles of A converted to D}}{\text{\#moles of A reacted}} \tag{3.102}$$

Correspondingly, an instantaneous selectivity can be defined as

$$s_{D/A} = \frac{d(\text{\#moles of A converted to D})}{d(\text{\#moles of A reacted})} = \frac{-r_A|_{\text{forming D}}}{-r_A} \tag{3.103}$$

One of the goals in using catalysts is to increase the selectivity of a desired product.

One cannot overemphasize the importance of mass (or mole) balance in reactor analysis. It is the most used concept in bioprocess engineering:

$$\boxed{\text{Accumulation} = \text{flow in} - \text{flow out} + \text{generation by reaction}} \tag{3.118}$$

It is very simple mathematically and in words, yet it takes a life to learn and master. A mathematical translation is given by

$$\frac{dn_j}{dt} = F_{j0} - F_j + r_j V \tag{3.119}$$

Energy balance is performed through the first law of thermodynamics. Energy cannot be generated nor destroyed, which is different from a particular species in a reaction mixture. Energy balance leads to

$$\begin{aligned}\frac{d\left(nU + \frac{1}{2}mu^2 + gz\right)}{dt} &= \dot{Q} - \dot{W}_s + \sum_{j=1}^{N_S} F_{j0}\left[H_{j0} + M_j\left(\tfrac{1}{2}u_0^2 + gz_0\right)\right] \\ &\quad - \sum_{j=1}^{N_S} F_j\left[H_j + M_j\left(\tfrac{1}{2}u^2 + gz\right)\right]\end{aligned} \tag{3.126}$$

where the subscript 0 denotes for the inlet, whereas no subscript indicating the outlet. Note: $\dot{Q}$ is the net heat transfer into the system, including through electric conversion and subtraction of the frictional thermal loss by the fluid mixture. Heat of reaction is not in either $\dot{Q}$ or $\dot{W}_s$.

In most cases, the kinetic energy and gravitational energy can be neglected, other than in an electro-hydro facility, or for simple flow loop calculations. Thus, Eqn (3.126) can be simplified to

$$\frac{d(nU)}{dt} = \dot{Q} - \dot{W}_s + \sum_{j=1}^{N_S} F_{j0}H_{j0} - \sum_{j=1}^{N_S} F_jH_j \tag{3.127}$$

The energy balance equation for an open system is reduced to that for closed system if there is no flow in or out of the system, i.e. $F = 0$. When chemical reaction occurs, internal energy changes and so are the enthalpies according to the species change. Equation (3.127) can be simplified as

$$\sum_{j=1}^{N_S} F_{j0}\left(H_j - H_{j0}\right) + V\sum_{i=1}^{N_R} r_i\Delta H_{Ri} + \sum_{j=1}^{N_S} C_{Pj}n_j\frac{dT}{dt} - \frac{d(pV)}{dt} = \dot{Q} - \dot{W}_s \tag{3.134}$$

which is the general energy balance equation. It is applicable to both flow (i.e. open) and batch (closed) systems. The assumptions we have made to obtain this equation are that the elevation and kinetic energy change can be neglected, and that the contents in the control volume (or system) are either condensed matters (solids and/or liquids) or ideal gases. Therefore, Eqn (3.134) is valid in almost all the situations where reactors are used. On the left hand side of Eqn (3.134), the first term resembles the enthalpy change; the second term can be thought of as the heat of generation due to reaction; the third and the fourth terms together can be thought of as the accumulation of energy (which is not exactly true). On the right hand side of Eqn (3.134), they are the net energy rate being transferred to the system. Therefore, the interpretation can help us remember the general energy equation.

Ideal reactors are defined as well mixed, i.e. no concentration, pressure, or temperature gradients in the reactor, except along the axial direction of a tubular reactor or PFR where absolutely no mixing is assumed. The idealization is meant to simplify the reactor analysis, thus obtaining an estimate quicker. There are three types of ideal reactors: batch, PFR, and CSTR. A batch reactor is a reactor, in which the contents are only changing with time. While CSTR has a similar appearance as a batch reactor, its contents are not changing with time at all with constant feed and withdrawing that were absent in a batch reactor. PFR is like a tubular reactor, the contents are changing only along the direction of flow.

Bioprocess engineers are commonly faced with problems of optimizing a facility or a process equipment. We often approach the problem by either maximizing the profit or minimizing the cost of operation.

Further Reading

Fogler, H. S. (2006). *Elements of Chemical Reaction Engineering* (4th ed.). Prentice-Hall.
Levenspiel, O. (1999). *Chemical Reaction Engineering* (3rd ed.). New York: John Wiley & Sons.
Sandler, S. I. (2006). *Chemical, Biochemical, and Engineering Thermodynamics* (4th ed.). New York: John Wiley & Sons.
Schmidt, L. D. (2005). *The Engineering of Chemical Reactions* (2nd ed.). New York: Oxford University Press.

PROBLEMS

3.1. Our ancestors have learned to make vinegar by aerobic bacterial fermentation of alcohol, which is derived by anaerobic fermentation of sugar. Vinegar can also be made by carbonylation of methanol, which is derived by reaction of synthesis gas, which can be obtained by steam reforming of methane. Write out these reactions.

3.2. What is an elementary reaction?

3.3. What is an approximate reaction? In what sense an approximate reaction should stoichiometry be held? How does approximate reaction differ from coupled reaction?

3.4. For the complex reaction with stoichiometry $A + 3B \rightarrow 2R + P$ and with second-order rate expression: $r_P = k\, C_A C_B$ are the reaction rates related by $r_A = r_B = r_R = r_P$? If the rates are not so related, then how are they related?

3.5. Given the reaction $2\ NO_2 + ½\ O_2 ==== N_2O_5$, what is the relationship between the rates of formation of N_2O_5 and disappearance of the two reactants?

3.6. We have a process that reacts 67% CH_4 in O_2 at 10 atm to form syngas ($\Delta H_R = -8.5$ kcal/mol-CH_4).

(a) Estimate the adiabatic reactor temperature at completion if we produce 100% syngas with a feed temperature of 400 °C. Assume $C_p = 7/2$ and $R = 7$ cal/(mol·K).

(b) Estimate the adiabatic reactor temperature if we suddenly begin producing 100% total combustion products ($\Delta H_R = -192$ kcal/mol).

(c) What do we have to be concerned with regarding reactor construction materials and pressure relief capabilities to design for this possibility?

3.7. Methanol is synthesized commercially from CO and H_2 by the reaction

$$CO + 2H_2 \rightleftharpoons CH_3OH$$

over a Cu/ZnO catalyst at ~350 °C at 50–100 atm. The standard-state thermodynamic data on this reaction are $\Delta H^\circ_{R,\,298} = -90.64$ kJ/mol and $\Delta G^\circ_{R,298} = -24.2$ kJ/mol.

(a) What is the equilibrium conversion of a stoichiometric mixture of CO and H_2 to methanol at 298 K at 1 atm?

(b) Assuming ΔH_R independent of T, what are K_{eq} and the equilibrium conversion at 1 atm and 350 °C?

(c) K_{eq} at 350 °C is measured to be 1.94×10^{-4}. How large is the error assuming constant ΔH_R?

(d) At what pressure will the equilibrium conversion be 50% at 350 °C?

3.8. The maximum allowable temperature for a reactor to maintain integrity is 800 K. At present, our operating set point is 780 K, the 20-K margin of safety to guard against fluctuating feed, sluggish controls, etc. With a more sophisticated control system, we could be able to raise our set point to 792 K without sacrificing the safety limits we have now. By how much can the reaction rate, hence, production rate, be raised by this change if the reaction taking place in the reactor has an activation energy of 200 kJ/mol?

3.9. The pyrolysis of ethane proceeds with an activation energy of about 300 kJ/mol. How much faster is the decomposition at 625 °C than at 525 °C?

3.10. At 1100 K n-nonane thermally cracks 20 times as rapidly as at 1000 K. Find the activation energy for this decomposition.

3.11. The growth of baker's yeast (*Saccharomyces cerevisiae*) on glucose may be simply described by the following equation:

$$C_6H_{12}O_6 + 3\ O_2 + 0.48\ NH_3 \rightarrow 0.48\ C_6H_{10}NO_3(\text{yeast}) + 4.32\ H_2O + 3.12\ CO_2$$

In a batch reactor of volume 10^5 L, the final desired yeast concentration is 50 g/L. Using the above reaction stoichiometry:

(a) Determine the concentration and total amount of glucose and $(NH_4)_2SO_4$ in the medium.
(b) Determine the yield factors $YF_{X/S}$ (biomass/glucose) and $YF_{X/O2}$ (biomass/oxygen).
(c) Determine the total amount of oxygen required.
(d) If the rate of growth at exponential phase is $r_X = 0.7$ g/(L·h), determine the rate of oxygen consumption, g-O_2/(L·h).
(e) Calculate the heat-removal requirements for the reactor.

3.12. The growth of *S. cerevisiae* on glucose under anaerobic conditions can be described by the following overall reaction:

$$C_6H_{12}O_6 - \upsilon_N\ NH_3 \rightarrow 0.59\ CH_{1.74}N_{0.2}O_{0.45}(\text{biomass}) + 0.43\ C_3H_8O_3 + 1.54\ CO_2 + \upsilon_{EtOH}\ C_2H_5OH + \upsilon_W\ H_2O$$

(a) Determine the biomass yield factor: $YF_{X/S}$.
(b) Determine the product yield factor: $YF_{EtOH/S}$, $YF_{CO_2/S}$, and $YF_{C_3H_8O_3/S}$.
(c) Determine the coefficient υ_N.

3.13. Aerobic growth of *S. cerevisiae* on ethanol is simply described by the following overall reaction:

$$C_2H_5OH - \upsilon_{O_2}\ O_2 - \upsilon_{NH_3}\ NH_3 \rightarrow \upsilon_X\ CH_{1.704}N_{0.149}O_{0.408} + \upsilon_{CO_2}\ CO_2 + \upsilon_W\ H_2O$$

(a) Determine the coefficients υ_{O_2}, υ_{NH_3}, υ_X, and υ_{CO_2}, where the respiratory quotient $RQ = \upsilon_{CO_2}/(-\upsilon_{O_2}) = 0.66$.
(b) Determine the biomass yield factor, $YF_{X/S}$, and oxygen yield factor, YF_{X/O_2} (g-X/g-O_2).

3.14. Aerobic degradation of benzoic acid by a mixed culture of microorganisms can be represented by the following reaction.

$$C_6H_5COOH\ (\text{substrate}) - \upsilon_{O_2}\ O_2 - \upsilon_{NH_3}\ NH_3 \rightarrow \upsilon_X\ C_5H_7NO_2(\text{biomass}) + \upsilon_W\ H_2O + \upsilon_{CO_2}\ CO_2$$

(a) Determine υ_{O2}, υ_{NH3}, υ_X, υ_W, and υ_{CO2} if the respiratory quotient $RQ = \upsilon_{CO_2}/(-\upsilon_{O_2}) = 0.9$.
(b) Determine the yield factors, $YF_{X/S}$ and YF_{X/O_2}.
(c) Determine degree of reduction for the substrate and bacteria.

3.15. Aerobic degradation of an organic compound by a mixed culture of organisms in wastewater can be represented by the following reaction.

$$C_3H_6O_3 - \upsilon_{O_2}\ O_2 - \upsilon_{NH_3}\ NH_3 \rightarrow \upsilon_X\ C_5H_7NO_2 + \upsilon_W\ H_2O + \upsilon_{CO_2}\ CO_2$$

(a) Determine υ_{O_2}, υ_{NH_3}, υ_X, υ_W, and υ_{CO_2}, if $YF_{X/S} = 0.4$ g-X/g-S.
(b) Determine the yield factors YF_{X/O_2} and YF_{X/NH_3}.
(c) Determine the degree of reductions for the substrate, bacteria, and the respiratory quotient $RQ = \upsilon_{CO_2}/(-\upsilon_{O_2})$ for the organisms.

3.16. Biological denitrification of nitrate-containing wastewaters can be described by the following overall reaction.

$$NO_3^- - \upsilon_{MeOH}CH_3OH + H^+ \rightarrow \upsilon_X\, C_5H_7NO_2 + \upsilon_{N_2}N_2 + \upsilon_W H_2O + \upsilon_{CO_2}\, CO_2$$

Determine υ_{MeOH}, υ_X, υ_{N_2}, υ_W, and υ_{CO_2}, if $YF_{X/S} = 0.5$ mol-X/mol-N-Substrate.

3.17. Polyhydroxyalkanoates (PHAs) are a family of polyesters synthesized by numerous bacteria as an intracellular carbon and energy storage compound, especially when one of the essential nutrients is lacking preventing the cells from multiplication. One important class of PHA: PHBV, is produced from sugars. PHBV synthesis reaction during anaerobic fermentation is given by:

$$-\upsilon_S\, CH_2O \rightarrow \upsilon_{PHA}[-OCH(CH_3)CH_2C(O)-] + CO_2 + 3\,H_2O$$

(a) Determine the stoichiometrical coefficients: υ_S and υ_{PHA}.
(b) Determine the PHA yield factor $Y_{PHA/S}$.

3.18. It has been reported that when bacteria *K. fragilis* is used in the aerobic fermentation of glucose using dissolved ammonia as a nitrogen source produces a biomass of atomic composition $CH_{1.75}O_{0.52}N_{0.15}$ and ethanol C_2H_5OH. The following yield factors have been reported: $YF_{X/S} = 0.569$ C-mol/C-mol and $YF_{CO_2/S} = 0.407$ C-mol/C-mol. Determine the other yield factors for this fermentation. What fraction of the carbon atoms present in glucose is converted to ethanol?

3.19. When the bacterium *Zymomonas mobilis* is used to produce ethanol from glucose in an anaerobic process with ammonia as the nitrogen source, it is found that bacteria biomass is produced to the extent of 0.06 C-mol per C-mole of glucose. The biomass has an elemental composition of $CH_{1.8}O_{0.5}N_{0.2}$. What are the fractional yield of ethanol, the amount of ammonia used, and the amount of carbon dioxide produced per C-mole of glucose consumed?

3.20. A considerable amount of methane is produced in Norway from its North Sea oil and gas wells. Some of this methane is converted to methanol by partial oxidation and then biochemically converted to biomass that is used as animal feed. The reported stoichiometry for the biochemical reaction is

$$CH_3OH + 0.731O_2 + 0.146\, NH_3 \rightarrow 0.269\, CO_2 + 0.731\, X$$

What is the atomic composition of the biomass produced?

3.21. Ethane costs $0.05/lb and ethylene sells for $0.18/lb. A typical ethylene plant produces 1 billion pounds/year.
(a) What are the annual sales?
(b) If we had a perfect process, what must be the cost of producing ethylene if we want a profit of 10% of sales?

(c) The actual process produces about 0.8 mol of ethylene per mole of ethane fed (the yield of the process is 80%). What is the cash flow of the process? What must be the cost of producing ethylene if we want a profit of 10% of sales?

3.22. Estimate the amount of CO_2 you will produce every time you fill your gasoline tank. Assume 55 L of octane with a density of 680 kg/m^3. How much CO_2 does your car liberate into the atmosphere each year assuming one fill-up every 2 weeks? Would it make any difference to the environment if you switch to a fuel that is produced from wheat straw and why?

3.23. We wish to produce B in the reaction system

$$A \rightarrow B + C, \; r_1 = k_1 c_A$$

$$2\,A \rightarrow D, \; r_2 = k_2 c_A$$

(a) What is the rate of formation of B?
(b) What is the disappearance rate of A?
(c) What operating parameters (temperature, pressure, feed rate, and feed concentrations) can one change to optimize the system?
(d) If A costs \$0.10/mol, B sells for \$0.25/mol, C and D cost \$0.05/mol to dispose, what relation of the k's will give a 20% profit on sales? Neglect the cost to reactor and operation.

3.24. We wish to produce B from the reaction:

$$A \rightarrow B, \quad r_1 = k_1 c_A$$

Unfortunately, A also decomposes to form a by-product C

$$A \rightarrow 2C, \quad r_2 = k_2 c_A$$

A costs \$1.00/lb, B sells for \$3.00/lb, and C costs \$0.80/lb to dispose. Neglect the reactor and operating costs.

(a) What relation between the *k's* will give a positive cash flow?
(b) What relation between the *k's* will give a 25% profit on sales?

3.25. We wish to produce R from the reaction:

$$2\,A \rightarrow R + P, \quad r_1 = k_1 c_A^{1.5}$$

Unfortunately, A also reacts to produce a by-product Q

$$A \rightarrow Q, \quad r_2 = k_2 c_A^{1.5}$$

A costs \$1.00/mol, R sells for \$3.80/mol, while P and Q cost \$0.50/mol to dispose. Neglect the reactor and operating costs.
(a) What relation between the *k's* will give a positive cash flow?
(b) What relation between the *k's* will give a 50% profit on sales?

CHAPTER

4

Batch Reactor

OUTLINE

The batch reactor is the generic term for a type of vessel widely used in the process industries. Batch reactors are used for a variety of process operations such as solid dissolution, product mixing, chemical reactions, crystallization, liquid/liquid extraction, and polymerization. In some cases, they are not referred to as reactors but have a name that reflects the role they perform (such as crystallizer or bioreactor).

A typical batch reactor consists of a tank with an agitator and integral heating/cooling system. These vessels may vary in size from less than 1 L to more than 15,000 L. They are usually fabricated in steel, stainless steel, alloys, glass lined steel, glass, Plexiglas, china, brick, cement, plastics, and even wood. Liquids and solids are usually charged via connections on the top cover of the reactor. Vapors and gases also discharge through connections on the top. Liquids and solids are usually discharged out of the bottom.

The advantages of the batch reactor lie with its versatility. A single vessel can carry out a sequence of different operations without the need to break containment. This is particularly useful when processing multiple feedstocks, toxic, or highly potent compounds or producing different unrelated products.

Commonly seen batch reactors are pots (in the kitchen – cooking), frying pans, pickling jars, beakers and test tubes (in chemistry laboratories), anaerobic digestion pits, to name a few. Batch reactor is an idealized reactor such that there are no inlets to or outlets from the reactor. Furthermore, in this text, we assume that the reaction mixture is well mixed all the time inside a batch reactor. Therefore, the temperature and concentrations are uniform

Bioprocess Engineering
http://dx.doi.org/10.1016/B978-0-444-59525-6.00004-4

inside the reactor at any given instant in time. However, the concentration and/or temperature can vary with time. This idealization makes the batch reactor analysis far simpler as now one need not to consider the locality of contents inside the reactor. This is one type of reactor that is frequently used in laboratories and classrooms.

4.1. ISOTHERMAL BATCH REACTORS

Figure 4.1 shows a schematic of a batch reactor. Mole balance for a given species j inside the reactor leads to

$$0 - 0 + r_j V = \frac{dn_j}{dt} \tag{4.1}$$

which leads to

$$r_j V = \frac{dn_j}{dt} \tag{4.2}$$

which is the general mole balance equation for a batch reactor.

For a single reaction that is carried out in a batch reactor, there is only one independent concentration or reaction mixture content variable and all other concentrations can be related through stoichiometry as shown in Chapter 3. Without loss of generosity, let us use component A as the key component of consideration. Equation (4.3) applied to species A gives

$$r_A V = \frac{dn_A}{dt} \tag{4.3}$$

If we use fractional conversion as the independent variable, Eqn (4.3) is reduced to

$$r_A V = -n_{A0} \frac{df_A}{dt} \tag{4.4}$$

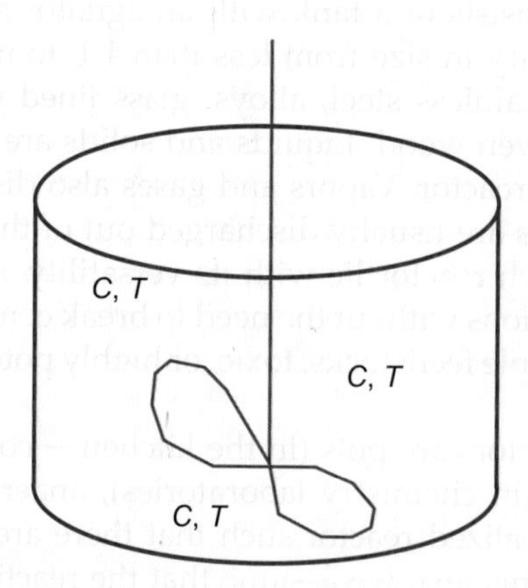

FIGURE 4.1 Schematic diagram of a batch reactor.

which can be rearranged to yield

$$dt = C_{A0}\frac{V_0}{V}\frac{df_A}{-r_A} \tag{4.5}$$

Since the total amount of mass is not changing with reaction or temperature and mass = ρV, we have

$$dt = C_{A0}\frac{\rho}{\rho_0}\frac{df_A}{-r_A} \tag{4.6}$$

The density is a function temperature and pressure. For condensed phase reactions, the density can be considered as constant. As we encounter liquid or liquid–gas phase reactions quite often, constant density or constant volume batch reactors have been studied extensively.

For a single-phase reaction mixture or for a condensed reaction mixture, if the effective reactor volume or density is constant, Eqn (4.3) can be reduced to

$$r_A = \frac{dC_A}{dt} \tag{4.7}$$

which is a commonly used equation. In fact, Eqn (4.7) has been abused in many situations by many people unintentionally. Now we know that this equation is only valid for constant density or constant volume batch reactors.

In order to solve for a batch reactor problem, one needs to solve for a differential equation like Eqns (4.3), (4.6), or (4.7). For example, Eqn (4.6) can be integrated to yield

$$t_f = C_{A0}\int_0^{f_{Af}}\frac{\rho}{\rho_0}\frac{df_A}{-r_A} \tag{4.8}$$

In general, the rate of reaction is a function of concentration and temperature. From Chapter 3, we learned that the stoichiometry can be applied to relate the amount of every species in the reaction mixture. The amount change of a component participating in the reaction divided by its stoichiometric coefficient is the universal extent of reaction for a single reaction. The stoichiometry can be written in a batch reactor as

$$\frac{dn_j}{\nu_j} = \frac{dn_A}{\nu_A} = rV \tag{4.9}$$

Equation (4.9) can be integrated to give

$$\frac{n_j - n_{j0}}{\nu_j} = \frac{n_A - n_{A0}}{\nu_A} \tag{4.10}$$

As the stoichiometrical coefficients are true constants for a given reaction, the total number of moles in the reactor can be computed by adding the number of moles for all the components (species) up. That is

$$n = \sum_{j=1}^{N_S} n_j = \sum_{j=1}^{N_S}\left(n_{j0} + \nu_j \frac{n_A - n_{A0}}{\nu_A}\right)$$
$$= n_0 + \frac{n_A - n_{A0}}{\nu_A}\sum_{j=1}^{N_S}\nu_j \tag{4.11}$$

Letting ν_Σ be the total stoichiometric coefficients, i.e.

$$\nu_\Sigma = \sum_{j=1}^{N_S}\nu_j \tag{4.12}$$

We obtain

$$n = n_0 + \frac{\nu_\Sigma}{\nu_A}(n_A - n_{A0}) \tag{4.13}$$

While the above derivation is concise, we often tabularize the stoichiometry to gain a thorough understanding of the stoichiometry for every species, either be those involved in the reaction or those that are not participating in the actual reaction. The stoichiometry is shown in Table 4.1.

The concentration can be related to the number of moles in the reactor through

$$C_j = \frac{n_j}{V} = \frac{n_{j0} + \frac{\nu_j}{\nu_A}(n_A - n_{A0})}{V} \tag{4.14}$$

which can be further reduced to

$$C_j = \frac{\rho}{\rho_0}C_{j0} + \frac{\nu_j}{\nu_A}\left(C_A - \frac{\rho}{\rho_0}C_{A0}\right) \tag{4.15}$$

TABLE 4.1 Stoichiometry of a Reaction System in a Batch Reactor

Species	Initial	Change	At time t
A	n_{A0}	$n_A - n_{A0}$	n_A
j	n_{j0}	$n_j - n_{j0} = \nu_j \frac{n_A - n_{A0}}{\nu_A}$	$n_j = n_{j0} + \nu_j \frac{n_A - n_{A0}}{\nu_A}$
…	…	…	…
Total	n_0	$\sum_{j=1}^{N_S}(n_j - n_{j0}) = \nu_\Sigma \frac{n_A - n_{A0}}{\nu_A}$	$\sum_{j=1}^{N_S} n_j = n_0 + \nu_\Sigma \frac{n_A - n_{A0}}{\nu_A}$

The reaction mixture density is a function of temperature, pressure, and concentration/composition. For isothermal operations, ρ is constant for reactions involving condensed matter (liquid or solid) only. For ideal gas, the reactor volume, pressure, and temperature are related through the ideal gas law

$$pV = nRT \tag{4.16}$$

That is

$$V = \frac{RT}{p}n = \frac{RT}{p}\left[n_0 + \frac{\nu_\Sigma}{\nu_A}(n_A - n_{A0})\right] \tag{4.17}$$

Using the fractional conversion f_A, Eqns (4.14) and (4.17), respectively, are reduced to

$$C_j = \frac{n_{j0} - \frac{\nu_j}{\nu_A}n_{A0}f_A}{V} \tag{4.18}$$

$$V = \frac{RT}{p}\left(n_0 - \frac{\nu_\Sigma}{\nu_A}n_{A0}f_A\right) \tag{4.19}$$

Therefore, one can conveniently working with n_A, C_A, or f_A in solving batch reactor problems.

For constant volume batch reactors,

$$t_f = \int_{C_{A0}}^{C_{Af}} \frac{dC_A}{r_A} = \int_{C_{Af}}^{C_{A0}} \frac{dC_A}{-r_A} = C_{A0}\int_0^{f_{Af}} \frac{df_A}{-r_A} \tag{4.20}$$

We see in this chapter that isothermal constant density reactions are more easily solved than other types of reactions.

Example 4-1. A reaction,

$$A \longrightarrow \text{products} \qquad r = kC_A^{O_{RA}} \tag{E4-1.1}$$

is being carried out isothermally in a constant volume batch reactor. Initially, the reactor is charged with A at a concentration of C_{A0}. Determine the concentration of A in the reactor as a function of time.

Solution. To start, let us draw a sketch to illustrate the problem as shown in Fig. E4-1.1. Mole balance of reactant A inside the reactor leads to

$$\overset{0}{\text{In}} - \overset{0}{\text{Out}} + \text{Generation} = \text{Accumulation}$$

$$r_A V = \frac{dn_A}{dt} \tag{E4-1.2}$$

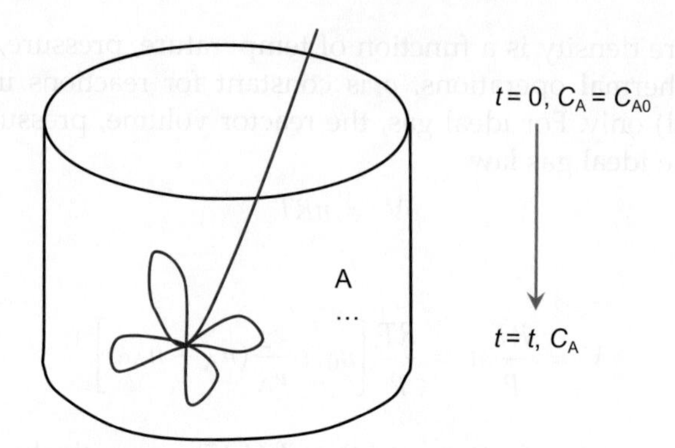

FIGURE E4-1.1 A schematic diagram of the batch reactor.

Since the volume is constant (constant volume batch reactor), Eqn (E4-1.2) is reduced to

$$\frac{dC_A}{dt} = r_A \tag{E4-1.3}$$

Applying the rate law,

$$r_A = \nu_A r = -kC_A^{O_{RA}} \tag{E4-1.4}$$

Substitute the rate expression, Eqn (E4-1.4), into the reduced mole balance Eqn (E4.1-3), one obtains

$$\frac{dC_A}{dt} = r_A = -kC_A^{O_{RA}} \tag{E4-1.5}$$

Separation of variables,

$$\frac{dC_A}{C_A^{O_{RA}}} = -kdt \tag{E4-1.6}$$

And integrate:

$$\int_{C_{A0}}^{C_A} \frac{dC_A}{C_A^{O_{RA}}} = -\int_0^t kdt \tag{E4-1.7}$$

If $O_{RA} = 1$, i.e. for a first-order reaction, we have

$$\int_{C_{A0}}^{C_A} \frac{dC_A}{C_A} = -\int_0^t kdt \tag{E4-1.8}$$

which can be integrated to yield

$$\ln C_A \Big|_{C_{A0}}^{C_A} = -kt\Big|_0^t \tag{E4-1.9}$$

Thus,

$$\ln C_A - \ln C_{A0} = -kt \tag{E4-1.10}$$

Equation (E4-1.10) can be rearranged to yield

$$C_A = C_{A0}\exp(-kt) \tag{E4-1.11}$$

That is, the concentration of A decreases exponentially in a batch reactor for a first-order reaction.

If $O_{RA} \neq 1$, Eqn (E4-1.7) is integrated to yield

$$\left.\frac{C_A^{1-O_{RA}}}{1-O_{RA}}\right|_{C_{A0}}^{C_A} = -kt|_0^t \tag{E4-1.12}$$

Thus,

$$C_A^{1-O_{RA}} - C_{A0}^{1-O_{RA}} = -(1-O_{RA})kt \tag{E4-1.13}$$

Equation (E4-1.13) can be rearranged to yield

$$C_A = \left[C_{A0}^{1-O_{RA}} - (1-O_{RA})kt\right]^{\frac{1}{1-O_{RA}}} \tag{E4-1.14}$$

That is, the concentration of A decreases following a hyperbolic path for an O_{RA}th-order reaction.

Fig. E4-1.2 shows the plots for the concentration of A as a function of time. One can observe that the concentration drops down quicker for a lower order reaction than a higher order reaction. This is due to the fact that at low concentrations, higher order reactions are slower than lower order reactions.

Example 4-2. Variable Volume Batch Reactor. A gaseous reaction

$$A \longrightarrow B + C \quad r = kC_A^2,$$

with $k = 0.1\ \text{mol}^{-1}\cdot\text{L}\cdot\text{s}^{-1}$

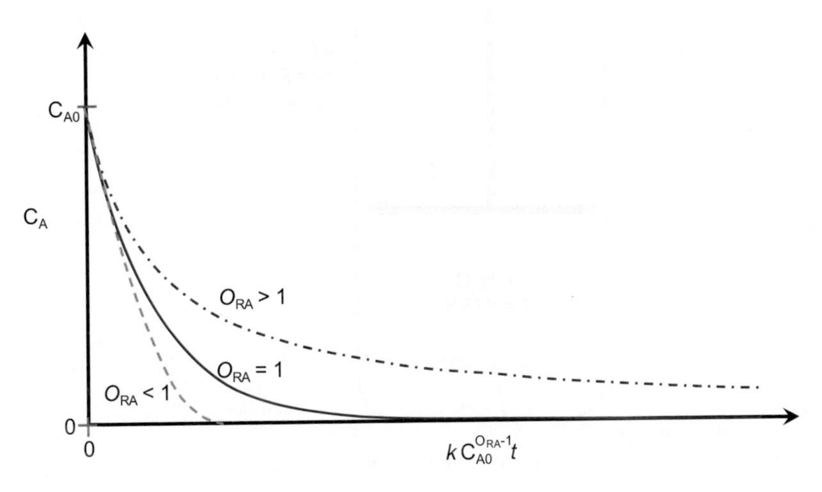

FIGURE E4-1.2 Concentration of A as a function time t for an O_{RA}th-order reaction in a constant volume batch reactor.

is occurring in an isothermal constant pressure batch reactor. The reactor is charged initially with pure A at 1 bar and 373 K. Determine the time required for the reaction volume to expand by 50%, i.e. $V/V_0 = 1.5$.

Solution. A sketch of the batch reactor is shown in Fig. E4-2.1. The stoichiometry of the reaction system is given by

$$\begin{array}{lccccl} & A & \longrightarrow & B & + C & \\ t=0: & n_{A0} & 0 & & 0 & +)=n_{A0} \\ t=t: & n_A & n_B & & n_C & +)=n_T \\ & n_A & n_{A0}-n_A & & n_{A0}-n_A & +)=2n_{A0}-n_A \end{array}$$

Assume ideal gas law applies. The volume of the reaction mixture and concentration of A in the reactor are given by

$$V = \frac{n_T RT}{P} = \frac{2n_{A0} - n_A}{n_{A0}} V_0 \tag{E4-2.1}$$

$$C_A = \frac{p_A}{RT} = \frac{n_A}{n_T}\frac{P}{RT} = \frac{n_A}{2n_{A0} - n_A} C_{A0} \tag{E4-2.2}$$

Based on Eqn (E4-2.1), we obtain

$$\frac{n_A}{n_{A0}} = 2 - \frac{V}{V_0} \tag{E4-2.3}$$

Thus, the extent of reaction is dependent on the volume expansion. Mole balance of A in the reactor gives

$$0 - 0 + r_A V = \frac{dn_A}{dt} \tag{E4-2.4}$$

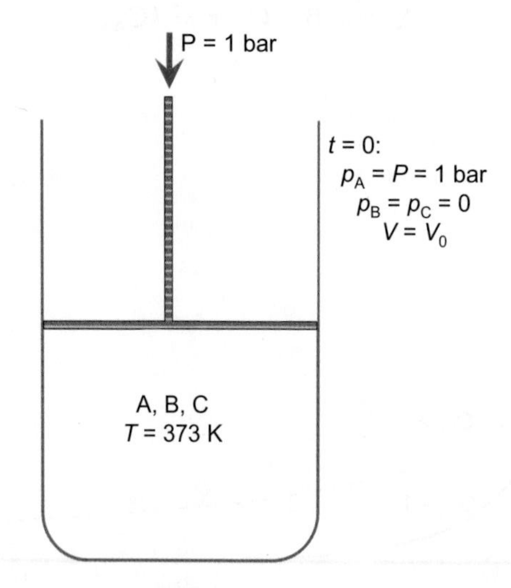

FIGURE E4-2.1 A schematic diagram of a constant pressure batch reactor.

Substituting the rate expression into the mole balance equation, we obtain

$$\frac{dn_A}{dt} = r_A V = -kC_A^2 V = kC_A n_A \tag{E4-2.5}$$

Substituting Eqn (E4-2.2) into Eqn (E4-2.4), we obtain

$$\frac{dn_A}{dt} = -kC_{A0}\frac{n_A^2}{2n_{A0} - n_A} \tag{E4-2.6}$$

Separation of variables,

$$\frac{2n_{A0} - n_A}{n_A^2} dn_A = -kC_{A0}dt \tag{E4-2.7}$$

Integration between $t = 0$ and $t = t$, we obtain

$$-\frac{2n_{A0}}{n_A} + \frac{2n_{A0}}{n_{A0}} - \ln\frac{n_A}{n_{A0}} = -kC_{A0}t \tag{E4-2.8}$$

which is reduced to

$$kC_{A0}t = 2\frac{n_{A0}}{n_A} - 2 - \ln\frac{n_{A0}}{n_A} \tag{E4-2.9}$$

Substituting Eqn (E4-2.3) into Eqn (E4-2.9), we obtain

$$t = \frac{\dfrac{2}{2 - V/V_0} - 2 + \ln\left(2 - \dfrac{V}{V_0}\right)}{kC_{A0}} \tag{E4-2.10}$$

Thus, the time required for 50% expansion of the reactor volume is given by

$$t = \frac{\dfrac{2}{2 - V/V_0} - 2 + \ln\left(2 - \dfrac{V}{V_0}\right)}{kC_{A0}} = \frac{\dfrac{2}{2 - V/V_0} - 2 + \ln\left(2 - \dfrac{V}{V_0}\right)}{k\dfrac{P}{RT}}$$

$$= \frac{\dfrac{2}{2 - 1.5} - 2 + \ln(2 - 1.5)}{0.1 \times 10^{-3} \times \dfrac{1 \times 10^5}{8.314 \times 373}} s = 405.3 \text{ s}$$

Therefore, it takes 405.3 s for the reactor volume to expand 50%.

Example 4-3. Concentration profile for a series reaction. For the following elementary reaction system

$$A \xrightarrow{k_1} B \xrightarrow{k_2} C$$

Find the change of concentrations of A, B, and C as a function of time starting with pure A initially at $C_A = C_{A0}$ in a constant volume isothermal batch reactor.

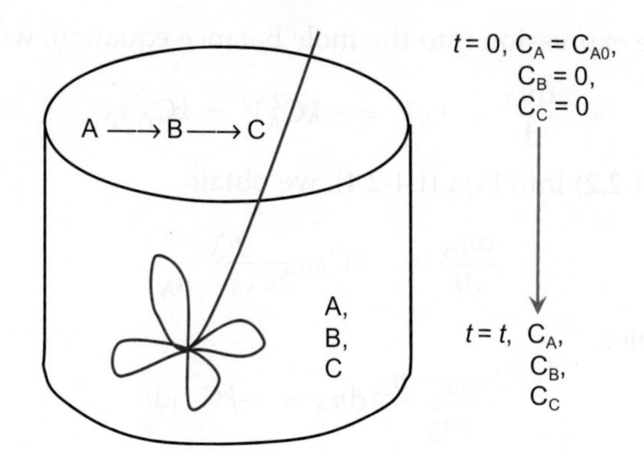

FIGURE E4-3.1 A schematic diagram of the batch reactor.

Solution. This is a set of two reactions occurring in series. Figure E4-3.1 shows a sketch of the reactor system. Mole balance for species j leads to

$$\frac{\mathrm{d}n_j}{\mathrm{d}t} = r_j V \tag{E4-3.1}$$

Since the volume is constant, we have

$$\frac{\mathrm{dC}_j}{\mathrm{d}t} = r_j \tag{E4-3.2}$$

We next find the rates of reaction. Applying Eqn (3.66), we obtain

$$\begin{aligned} r_\mathrm{A} &= \nu_{1\mathrm{A}} r_1 + \nu_{2\mathrm{A}} r_2 \\ &= -r_1 = k_1 \mathrm{C_A} \end{aligned} \tag{E4-3.3}$$

$$\begin{aligned} r_\mathrm{B} &= \nu_{1\mathrm{B}} r_1 + \nu_{2\mathrm{B}} r_2 \\ &= r_1 - r_2 = k_1 \mathrm{C_A} - k_2 \mathrm{C_B} \end{aligned} \tag{E4-3.4}$$

$$\begin{aligned} r_\mathrm{C} &= \nu_{1\mathrm{C}} r_1 + \nu_{2\mathrm{C}} r_2 \\ &= r_2 = k_2 \mathrm{C_B} \end{aligned} \tag{E4-3.5}$$

Substituting Eqn (E4-3.3) into Eqn (E4-3.2), we obtain

$$\frac{\mathrm{dC_A}}{\mathrm{d}t} = r_\mathrm{A} = -k_1 \mathrm{C_A} \tag{E4-3.6}$$

Separation of variables and integration,

$$\int_{\mathrm{C_{A0}}}^{\mathrm{C_A}} \frac{\mathrm{dC_A}}{\mathrm{C_A}} = \int_0^t -k_1 \mathrm{d}t \tag{E4-3.7}$$

We obtain

$$\ln \frac{\mathrm{C_A}}{\mathrm{C_{A0}}} = -k_1 t \tag{E4-3.8}$$

or

$$\boxed{C_A = C_{A0} \exp(-k_1 t)} \tag{E4-3.9}$$

Substituting Eqns (E4-3.9) and (E4-3.4) into Eqn (E4-3.2), we obtain

$$\frac{dC_B}{dt} = r_B = k_1 C_A - k_2 C_B = k_1 C_{A0} e^{-k_1 t} - k_2 C_B \tag{E4-3.10}$$

which can be rearranged to yield

$$e^{k_2 t}\left(dC_B + k_2 C_B dt\right) = e^{k_2 t} k_1 C_{A0} e^{-k_1 t} dt \tag{E4-3.11}$$

or

$$e^{k_2 t} dC_B + C_B de^{k_2 t} = d\left(C_B e^{k_2 t}\right) = k_1 C_{A0} e^{(k_2 - k_1)t} dt \tag{E4-3.12}$$

Integration of Eqn (E4-3.12) yields

$$C_B e^{k_2 t} = \begin{cases} \dfrac{k_1}{k_2 - k_1} C_{A0}[e^{(k_2 - k_1)t} - 1], & k_2 \neq k_1 \\ k_1 C_{A0} t, & k_2 = k_1 \end{cases} \tag{E4-3.13}$$

Thus, the concentration of *B* in the isothermal constant volume reactor is given by

$$\boxed{C_B = \begin{cases} \dfrac{k_1}{k_2 - k_1} C_{A0}(e^{-k_1 t} - e^{-k_2 t}), & k_2 \neq k_1 \\ k_1 C_{A0} t e^{-k_1 t}, & k_2 = k_1 \end{cases}} \tag{E4-3.14}$$

The concentration of **C** can be obtained either by substituting Eqns (E4-3.14) and (E4-3.5) into Eqn (E4-3.2) or via stoichiometry. Since there is only A in the reactor initially, the total concentration of A, B, and C is not going to change with time based on the stoichiometry as given by the series reaction (all the stoichiometry coefficients are unity). Thus,

$$C_C = C_{A0} - C_A - C_B \tag{E4-3.15}$$

which gives

$$C_C = C_{A0} - \frac{k_1 e^{-k_2 t} - k_2 e^{-k_1 t}}{k_1 - k_2} C_{A0} \tag{E4-3.16}$$

Figure E4-3.2 shows the change of concentrations with time based on Eqns (E4-3.9), (E4-3.14), and (E4-3.16). One can observe that there is a maximum for concentration C_B that changes with k_1 and k_2. This maximum can be obtained by setting

$$\begin{aligned} 0 = \left.\frac{dC_B}{dt}\right|_{t_m} &= r_B = k_1 C_A - k_2 C_B \\ &= k_1 C_{A0} e^{-k_1 t_m} - k_2 \frac{k_1}{k_2 - k_1} C_{A0}(e^{-k_1 t_m} - e^{-k_2 t_m}) \end{aligned} \tag{E4-3.17}$$

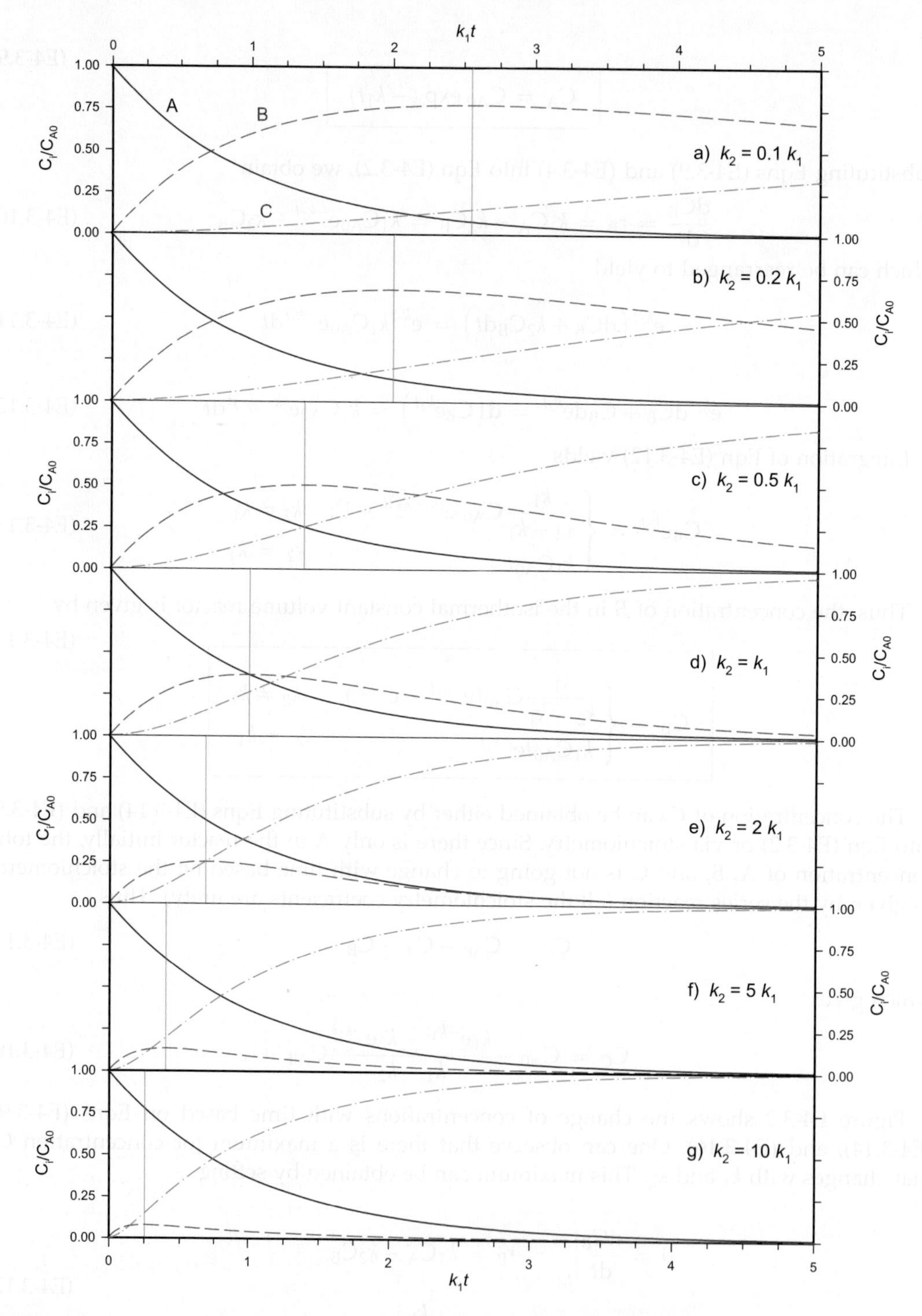

FIGURE E4-3.2 Variation of concentrations with reaction time for series reactions.

TABLE 4.2 Reaction Residence Time Requirement and Concentration Profile for Single Reactions in an Isothermal Constant Volume Batch Reactor for Some Simple Kinetic Models

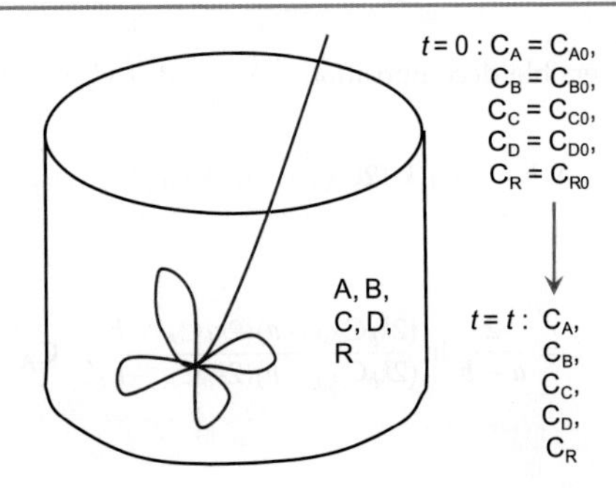

1. Zeroth order: A → products, $r = k$

$t = (C_{A0} - C_A)/k;\ C_A = C_{A0} - k\,t$

2. First order: A → products, $r = k\,C_A$

$t = \ln(C_{A0} - C_A)/k;\ C_A = C_{A0}\exp(-k\,t)$

3. Power-law kinetics: A → products, $r = kC_A^n$

$$t = \frac{C_{A0}^{1-n} - C_A^{1-n}}{(1-n)k};\ C_A = \left[C_{A0}^{1-n} - (1-n)kt\right]^{\frac{1}{1-n}}$$

4. Bimolecular: A + B → products, $r = kC_AC_B$

$$t = \frac{1}{k}\left(\frac{1}{C_A} - \frac{1}{C_{A0}}\right);\ C_A = C_B = \frac{C_{A0}}{1 + kC_{A0}t},\quad \text{if } C_{A0} = C_{B0}$$

$$t = \frac{1}{k(C_{B0} - C_{A0})}\ln\frac{C_{A0}(C_A + C_{B0} - C_{A0})}{C_AC_{B0}};\ C_A = \frac{C_{A0}(C_{B0} - C_{A0})}{C_{B0}\exp[k(C_{B0} - C_{A0})t] - C_{A0}};\ C_B = C_{B0} - C_{A0} + C_A$$

5. Autocatalytic: A + R → 2 R + products, $r = k\,C_AC_R$

$$t = \frac{1}{k(C_{A0} + C_{R0})}\ln\frac{C_{A0}(C_{A0} + C_{R0} - C_A)}{C_AC_{R0}};\ C_A = \frac{C_{A0}(C_{A0} + C_{R0})}{C_{A0} + C_{R0}\exp[k(C_{A0} + C_{R0})t]};\ C_R = C_{A0} + C_{R0} - C_A$$

6. Unimolecular catalytic: A → products, $r = \dfrac{kC_A}{K_A + C_A}$

$$t = \frac{1}{k}\left(K_A\ln\frac{C_{A0}}{C_A} + C_{A0} - C_A\right)$$

7. Unimolecular catalytic: A → products, $r = \dfrac{kC_A^2}{K_A + C_A}$

$$t = \frac{1}{k}\left(\ln\frac{C_{A0}}{C_A} + \frac{K_A}{C_A} - \frac{K_A}{C_{A0}}\right)$$

8. First-order reversible: A ⇄ B, $r = k_f\,C_A - k_bC_B$

$$t = \frac{1}{k_f + k_b}\ln\frac{k_fC_{A0} - k_bC_{B0}}{(k_f + k_b)C_A - k_b(C_{A0} + C_{B0})};\ C_A = \frac{(k_fC_{A0} - k_bC_{B0})\exp\left[-(k_f + k_b)t\right] + k_b(C_{A0} + C_{B0})}{k_f + k_b}$$

$C_B = C_{A0} + C_{B0} - C_A$

9. Catalytic first-order reversible: A ⇄ B, $r = \dfrac{k(C_A - C_B/K_C)}{1 + K_AC_A + K_BC_B}$

$$t = \frac{K_C}{k(1 + K_C)}\left\{(K_A - K_B)(C_{A0} - C_A) + \left[1 + (C_{A0} + C_{B0})\left(K_B + \frac{K_A - K_B}{K_C}\right)\right]\ln\frac{(1 + K_C)C_{A0} - (C_{A0} + C_{B0})}{(1 + K_C)C_A - (C_{A0} + C_{B0})}\right\}$$

$C_B = C_{A0} + C_{B0} - C_A$

(Continued)

TABLE 4.2 Reaction Residence Time Requirement and Concentration Profile for Single Reactions in an Isothermal Constant Volume Batch Reactor for Some Simple Kinetic Models—*Cont'd*

10. Reversible decomposition: $A \rightleftarrows B + C,\ r = k_f C_A - k_b C_B C_C$

$$A, b = k_f + k_b(2C_{A0} + C_{B0} + C_{C0}) \pm \sqrt{[k_f + k_b(2C_{A0} + C_{B0} + C_{C0})]^2 - 4k_b^2(C_{A0} + C_{B0})(C_{A0} + C_{C0})}$$

$$t = \frac{2}{a-b}\ln\frac{(2k_bC_{A0} - a)(2k_bC_A - b)}{(2k_bC_{A0} - b)(2k_bC_A - a)};\quad C_A = \frac{1}{2k_b}\frac{a(2k_bC_{A0} - b)\exp\left(\frac{a-b}{2}t\right) - b(2k_bC_{A0} - a)}{(2k_bC_{A0} - b)\exp\left(\frac{a-b}{2}t\right) - (2k_bC_{A0} - a)}$$

$$C_B = C_{A0} + C_{B0} - C_A;\quad C_C = C_{A0} + C_{C0} - C_A$$

11. Reversible codimerization: $A + B \rightleftarrows C,\ r = k_f C_A C_B - k_b C_C$

$$A, b = k_f(C_{A0} - C_{B0}) - k_b \pm \sqrt{\left[k_f\left(C_{A0} - C_{B0}\right) - k_b\right]^2 + 4k_f k_b(C_{A0} + C_{C0})}$$

$$t = \frac{2}{b-a}\ln\frac{(2k_fC_{A0} - a)(2k_fC_A - b)}{(2k_fC_{A0} - b)(2k_fC_A - a)};\quad C_A = \frac{1}{2k_f}\frac{A(2k_fC_{A0} - b)\exp\left(-\frac{a-b}{2}t\right) - b(2k_fC_{A0} - a)}{(2k_fC_{A0} - b)\exp\left(-\frac{a-b}{2}t\right) - (2k_fC_{A0} - a)}$$

$$C_B = C_{B0} - C_{A0} + C_A;\quad C_C = C_{A0} + C_{C0} - C_A$$

12. Reversible bimolecular: $A + B \rightleftarrows C + D,\ r = k(C_A C_B - C_C C_D / K_C)$

$$\alpha = K_C(C_{A0} - C_{B0}) - 2C_{A0} - C_{C0} - C_{D0};\quad A, b = \alpha \pm \sqrt{\alpha^2 + 4(K_C - 1)(C_{A0} + C_{C0})(C_{A0} + C_{D0})}$$

$$t = \frac{2K_C}{k(b-a)}\ln\frac{[2(K_C - 1)C_{A0} - a][2(K_C - 1)C_A - b]}{[2(K_C - 1)C_{A0} - b][2(K_C - 1)C_A - a]};$$

$$C_A = \frac{1}{2(K_C - 1)}\frac{A[2(K_C - 1)C_{A0} - b]\exp\left(-\frac{a-b}{2K_C}kt\right) - b[2(K_C - 1)C_{A0} - a]}{[2(K_C - 1)C_{A0} - b]\exp\left(-\frac{a-b}{2K_C}kt\right) - [2(K_C - 1)C_{A0} - a]}$$

$$C_B = C_{B0} - C_{A0} + C_A;\quad C_C = C_{A0} + C_{C0} - C_A;\quad C_D = C_{A0} + C_{D0} - C_A$$

which can be rendered to

$$k_1 \frac{k_1}{k_2 - k_1} C_{A0}\, e^{-k_1 t_m} = k_2 \frac{k_1}{k_2 - k_1} C_{A0}\, e^{-k_2 t_m} \tag{E4-3.18}$$

or

$$\boxed{t_m = \frac{\ln(k_2/k_1)}{k_2 - k_1}} \tag{E4-3.19}$$

and the corresponding concentration of B is given by

$$\boxed{C_{B\max} = C_{A0}\left(\frac{k_2}{k_1}\right)^{\frac{-k_2}{k_2 - k_1}}} \tag{E4-3.20}$$

One can observe that at short times, the formation of intermediate product is noticeable. The time at which maximal concentration of B occurs decreases with increasing k_2. However, at long timescale, only the formation of the final product C is important and the series reaction may be simplified to a first-order reaction from reactant A to product C if timescale is long. The reaction rate constant can be approximated by the smaller of the two for the approximate reaction.

When simple kinetics is combined with constant volume or constant density for single reactions in a batch reactor, closed form analytic solutions are usually easy to achieve. A list of some of these cases is shown in Table 4.2.

While simple problems can be solved by hand, this last example showed how tedious for even a simple problem could be. At this point, one can appreciate that an automatic integrator is helpful in solving batch reactor problems. There are many software programs one can use for integration: Maple, Mathcad, Matlab, to name a few. We have also supplied a visual basic code that can run in Microsoft Excel. This is a good option as Microsoft Excel can be applied to solve most of the programs a process engineer encounter when an automatic integrator is added. The excel visual basic program provided is ODExLims. We shall discuss the solution in Numerical Solutions of Batch Reactor Problems.

4.2. BATCH REACTOR SIZING

We have learned now how to compute the required reaction time for a given reaction kinetics to proceed onto a desired reaction extent (or conversion). How big a reactor do we need to carry out the bioprocess? To do this, let us look at Fig. 4.2 to find the answer.

Mass balance of the raw materials leads to

$$Q = \frac{V}{t_B} = \frac{V}{t_P + t_f + t_U} \tag{4.21}$$

where Q is the rate of raw materials coming into the facility, V is the volume of the raw materials can be loaded for each batch, which is the effective reactor volume, and t_B is the batch time or the total time required to complete one batch operation. The batch time required includes the preparation time, t_P, for loading the reactor with reaction mixture and raising the temperature to reaction temperature; the reaction time, t_f, to achieve the desired

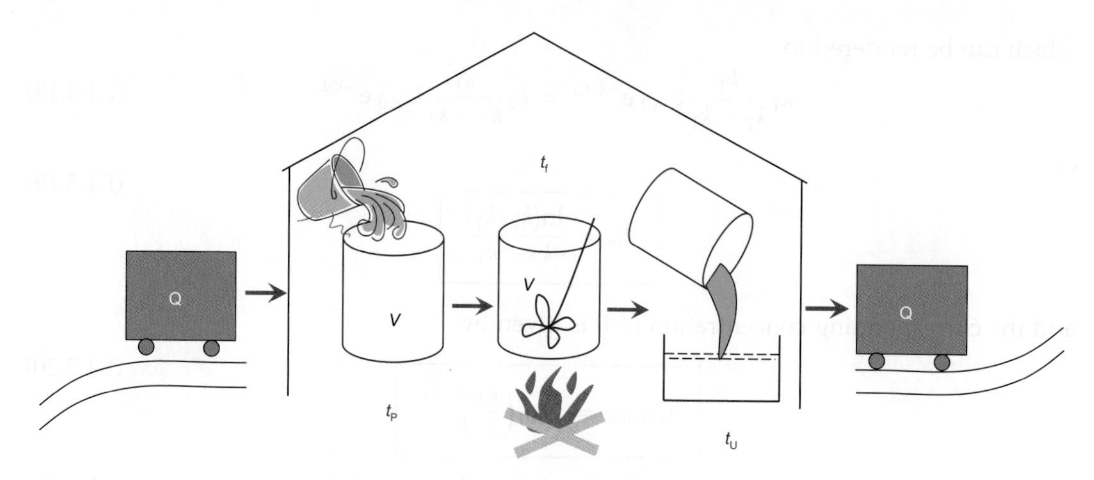

FIGURE 4.2 An illustration of material flow in a bioprocess plant.

conversion f_{Af}; and the unloading time, t_U, for unloading the reaction mixture and returning the reactor to working conditions.

The reactor volume can be obtained from Eqn (4.21) as

$$V = t_B\ Q = \left(t_P + t_f + t_U\right)Q \tag{4.22}$$

Example 4-4. Our winery takes grain in and put the wine on the market. The bottleneck of the operation is the fermenter operation. The fermenter is loaded with 10% sugar (assuming a density of 1000 kg/m^3) and yeast before fermentation. This leads to a 5-h delay before fermentation starts. The fermentation takes 5 days to complete to obtain a 4% alcohol mixture. Finally, to unload the fermenter contents and clean the fermenter requires another 3 h. Assume that the final product wine (4% alcohol) also has a density of 1000 kg/m^3. Determine the fermenter size needed if a daily production of 240 L of wine is needed.

Solution. $t_P = 5$ h; $t_f = 5$ days $= 120$ h; $t_U = 3$ h. Thus, the total time for each batch of fermentation will take $t_B = 5 + 120 + 3$ h $= 128$ h.

The fermenter size can be determined as $V = (240/24) \times 128$ L $= 1280$ L.

Example 4-5. Consider the reaction:

$$\text{A} \longrightarrow \text{B}, \quad k = 0.15\ \text{min}^{-1}$$

in a batch reactor. The loading, preparation, unloading, and cleaning of the reactor requires 10 h for each batch of production. A costs \$2/mole, and B sells for \$5/mole. The cost of operating the reactor (including the preparation time) is \$0.03 per liter per hour. We need to produce 100 moles of B per hour using $C_{A0} = 2$ mol/L. Assume no value or cost of disposal of unreacted A (i.e. separation or recovery cost to A is identical to the fresh A cost).

a. Perform a mole balance on the reactor to relate the conversion with reactor size.
b. What is the optimum conversion and reactor size?
c. What is the cash flow (or profit per mole of *A* feed to the reactor) from the process?
d. At what operating cost do we break even? What is the corresponding conversion?

Solution. Let the reaction time be t and the total preparation time (reactor loading, preparation, unloading, and cleaning) be t_L. The total time required for each batch is then $t_B = t + t_L$.

a. Mole balance of A in the reactor leads to

$$0 - 0 + r_A V = \frac{dn_A}{dt} \tag{E4-5.1}$$

The rate law gives

$$r_A = \nu_A r = -kC_A \tag{E4-5.2}$$

It is understood that the reaction mixture density is not changing. We have

$$C_A = \frac{n_A}{V} = \frac{n_{A0}(1-f_A)}{V} = C_{A0}(1-f_A) \tag{E4-5.3}$$

Substituting Eqns (E4-5.2) and (E4-5.3) into Eqn (E4-5.1) and integrating with the initial point of $f_A = 0$ at $t = 0$, we obtain

$$t = -\frac{\ln(1-f_A)}{k} \tag{E4-5.4}$$

We know the production rate of B, $F_{B0} = 100$ mol/h. From stoichiometry,

$$F_{A0} = \frac{F_B}{f_A} \tag{E4-5.5}$$

Therefore, the reactor volume can be obtained from Eqn (4.22) as

$$V = t_B Q = (t_L + t)\frac{F_B}{C_{A0}f_A} = \left[t_L - \frac{\ln(1-f_A)}{k}\right]\frac{F_B}{C_{A0}f_A} \tag{E4-5.6}$$

b. Based on the economic information at hand, we can estimate the gross profit for the reaction process as

$$GP\$ = \$_B F_B - \$_A F_{A0} - \$_V V \tag{E4-5.7}$$

where $\$_B$, $\$_A$, and $\$_V$ are the molar value of product B, molar cost of reactant A, and the unit operating cost of reactor based on the reactor volume and time, respectively. Substituting Eqns (E4-5.5) and (E4-5.6) into Eqn (E5-4.7), we obtain

$$GP\$ = \$_B F_B - \$_A \frac{F_B}{f_A} - \$_V\left[t_L - \frac{\ln(1-f_A)}{k}\right]\frac{F_B}{C_{A0}f_A} \tag{E4-5.8}$$

To find the optimum conversion, we maximize the gross profit. That is starting by setting

$$\frac{dGP\$}{df_A} = 0 \tag{E4-5.9}$$

Since the flow rate of product B is fixed, not a function of the conversion f_A, we have

$$0 = \frac{dGP\$}{df_A} = 0 + \$_A \frac{F_B}{f_A^2} - \frac{\$_V F_B}{kC_{A0} f_A (1 - f_A)} + \$_V \left[t_L - \frac{\ln(1 - f_A)}{k} \right] \frac{F_B}{C_{A0} f_A^2} \quad \text{(E4-5.10)}$$

which can be reduced to,

$$0 = \frac{\$_A k C_{A0}}{\$_V} - \frac{f_A}{1 - f_A} + kt_L - \ln(1 - f_A) \quad \text{(E4-5.11)}$$

Since

$$\frac{\$_A k C_{A0}}{\$_V} + kt_L = \frac{2(\$/\text{mol}) \times 0.15/\text{min} \times 2(\text{mol/l})}{0.03\$/(\text{L}\cdot\text{h})} + 0.15/\text{min} \times 10\ \text{h}$$

$$= 1290$$

Equation (E-5.11) is reduced to

$$1290 = \frac{f_A}{1 - f_A} + \ln(1 - f_A) \quad \text{(E4-5.12)}$$

This nonlinear equation can be solved to give

$$f_A = 0.9992297$$

Thus, the optimum conversion is $f_A = 0.9992297$. The reactor size can be computed from Eqn (E4-5.6)

$$V = \left[t_L - \frac{\ln(1 - f_A)}{k} \right] \frac{F_B}{C_{A0} f_A} = \left[10 - \frac{\ln(1 - 0.9992297)}{0.15 \times 60} \right] \frac{100}{2 \times 0.9992297}\ \text{L}$$

$$= 540.24\ \text{L}$$

c. The cash flow based on the optimum conversion:

$$\frac{GP\$}{F_{A0}} = \frac{\$_B F_B}{F_{A0}} - \$_A \frac{F_B}{F_{A0} f_A} - \$_V \left[t_L - \frac{\ln(1 - f_A)}{k} \right] \frac{F_B}{F_{A0} C_{A0} f_A}$$

$$= \$_B f_A - \$_A - \left[t_L - \frac{\ln(1 - f_A)}{k} \right] \frac{\$_V}{C_{A0}}$$

$$= 5 \times 0.9992297 - 2 - \left[10 - \frac{\ln(1 - 0.99922297)}{0.15 \times 60} \right] \frac{0.03}{2} \$/\text{mol} - \text{A}$$

$$= \$2.8342\ /\text{mol} - \text{A}$$

d. At breaking even point, the net profit (or in this case the gross profit) is zero. Therefore, at the break-even point, operating cost and the value of product are equal.
The value of product is,

$$\$_B F_B = 5 \times 100\ \$/\text{h} = 500\ \$/\text{h}$$

which is also the operating cost at break even.

The operating conditions for the break-even point can be obtained by setting the gross profit to zero.

$$0 = \mathrm{GP\$} = \$_B F_B - \$_A \frac{F_B}{f_A} - \$_V \left[t_L - \frac{\ln(1-f_A)}{k} \right] \frac{F_B}{C_{A0} f_A} \tag{E4-5.13}$$

which can be rearranged to

$$f_A - \frac{\$_A}{\$_B} - \frac{\$_V}{\$_B} \left[t_L - \frac{\ln(1-f_A)}{k} \right] \frac{1}{C_{A0}} = 0 \tag{E4-5.14}$$

or

$$f_A - 0.43 + \frac{0.001}{3} \ln(1-f_A) = 0 \tag{E4-5.15}$$

Solving Eqn (E4-5.15), we obtain

$$f_A = 0.430187$$

4.3. NON-ISOTHERMAL BATCH REACTORS

The solution of a batch reactor problem involves the solution of sets of ordinary differential equations from the species mole balance in the reactor as we have noted above. Mole balance leads to,

$$r_j V = \frac{dn_j}{dt} \tag{4.2}$$

or

$$\frac{dn_j}{dt} = r_j V \tag{4.23}$$

with initial conditions set in the reactor as $t = 0$, $n_j = n_{j0}$, or $C_j = C_{j0}$. If the reactor is not operated isothermally, an energy balance equation is needed as well, Eqn (3.134), or

$$\sum_{j=1}^{N_S} C_{Pj} n_j \frac{dT}{dt} - \frac{d(pV)}{dt} = \dot{Q} - \dot{W}_s - V \sum_{i=1}^{N_R} r_i \Delta H_{Ri} \tag{4.24}$$

with $t = 0$, $T = T_0$. For liquids, $\frac{d(pV)}{dt} \approx 0$, which further simplifies Eqn (4.24).

The reaction rates r_j's given as functions of the concentrations (and temperature):

$$\frac{dn_j}{dt} = r_j V = V \sum_{i=1}^{N_R} \nu_{ij} r_i \tag{4.25}$$

$$r_i = f(C_k, T) \quad i = 1, 2, 3, \ldots, N_R \tag{4.26}$$

In some cases (for example elementary reactions), the power-law rates can be applied, that is

$$r_i = k_{i0} e^{-\frac{E_i}{RT}} \prod_{j=1}^{N_S} C_j^{O_{R_j}} \tag{4.27}$$

as discussed in Chapter 3. In other cases, the reaction rates are more complicated functions of the concentration and temperature. The concentration and number of moles are related by definition:

$$C_j = \frac{n_j}{V} \tag{4.28}$$

For liquid phase reactions,

$$V = \frac{\rho_0}{\rho} V_0 \tag{4.29}$$

And for gas phase reactions, the ideal gas law may be used to approximate the volume change:

$$V = \frac{RT}{P} \sum_{j=1}^{N_S} n_j \tag{4.30}$$

Therefore, the solution to a non-isothermal batch reactor problem is similar to that to an isothermal batch reactor problem. However, the temperature in the reactor needs to be solved (considered) simultaneously with the reacting species.

The temperature is normally controlled via a heat jacket where thermal energy can be supplied to the reactor or removed from the reactor (Fig. 4.3). When the reactor is insulated, the reactor becomes adiabatic where temperature rise (for exothermic reaction) or decrease (endothermic reaction) depending on the nature of the reaction taking place in the reactor.

$$\dot{Q} = UA_H(T - T_c) \tag{4.31}$$

where U is the overall heat transfer coefficient, A_H is the total heat transfer area, and T_c is the temperature of the fluid in the heat-exchanging jacket. In case of noninsulated

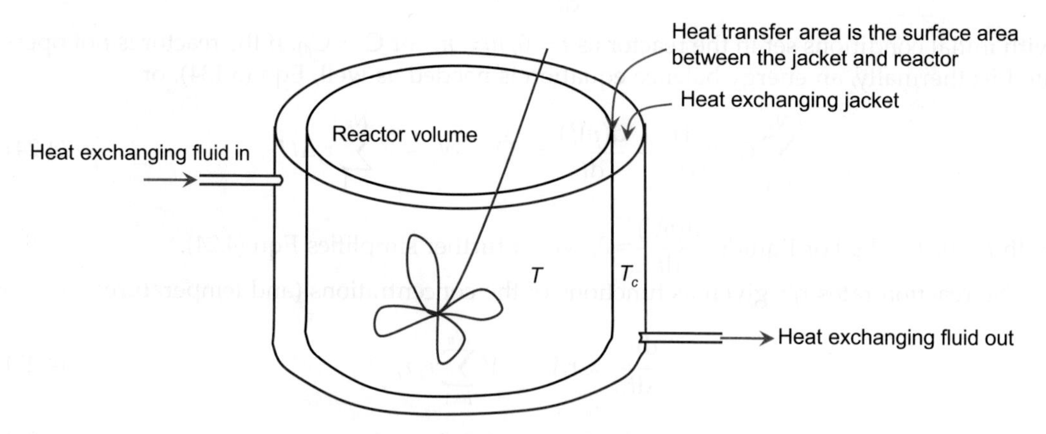

FIGURE 4.3 Schematic diagram of a batch reactor with a heat exchanger jacket.

reactor, T_c is the temperature of the environment (surroundings). For an adiabatic reactor, $\dot{Q} = 0$.

Example 4-6 H-Factor. A reaction with one single temperature-dependent reaction rate constant,

$$-\upsilon_A A + (-\upsilon_B)\, B \longrightarrow \text{products} \qquad r = k(T) C_A^{O_{RA}} C_B^{O_{RB}} \tag{E4-6.1}$$

is carried out in a constant volume batch reactor. Each time when the reactor is loaded and discharged, the temperature profile, i.e. temperature change with time during the intended reaction period

$$T = f(t) \tag{E4-6.2}$$

is different. For comparison purposes, we would like to develop a method to quantify the effect so that operators can control the reaction effectively. A concept of H-factor was developed, which is the effective reaction time equivalent to that at a constant temperature T_R. Figure E4-6.1 illustrates this concept. Derive a formula for the H-factor.

Solution. For reaction occurring in a batch reactor, mole balance of reactant A leads to

$$\overset{0}{\text{In}} - \overset{0}{\text{Out}} + \text{Generation} = \text{Accumulation}$$

$$\nu_A r V = \frac{dn_A}{dt} \tag{E4-6.3}$$

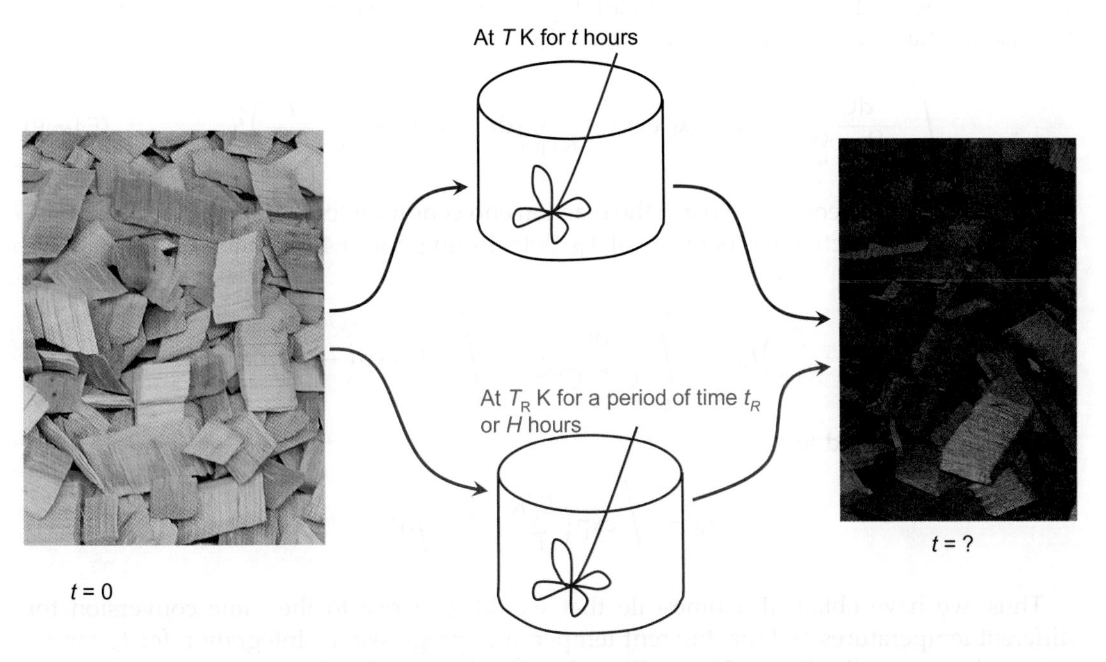

FIGURE E4-6.1 The concept of H-factors as applied to pulping and reactions involving woodchips.

Since the volume is constant (constant volume batch reactor), we further obtain

$$\nu_A k C_A^{O_{RA}} C_B^{O_{RB}} = \frac{dC_A}{dt} \tag{E4-6.4}$$

Based on stoichiometry, we have

$$\frac{n_A - n_{A,0}}{\nu_A} = \frac{n_B - n_{B,0}}{\nu_B} \tag{E4-6.5}$$

For constant volume reactor, Eqn (E4-6.5) is reduced to

$$C_B = C_{B0} + \frac{\nu_B}{\nu_A}(C_A - C_{A0}) \tag{E4-6.6}$$

Therefore, C_B and C_A are related. As the rate constant k is only a function of temperature (Arrhenius relationship), separation of variables for Eqn (E4.3-4) leads to

$$\frac{dC_A}{C_A^{O_{RA}} C_B^{O_{RB}}} = \nu_A k dt = \nu_A k_0 \exp\left(-\frac{E}{RT}\right) dt \tag{E4-6.7}$$

For a desired reaction end condition or conversion, the reaction time can be obtained by integrating Eqn (E4-6.7).

$$\int_{C_{A0}}^{C_A} \frac{dC_A}{C_A^{O_{RA}} C_B^{O_{RB}}} = \int_0^t \nu_A k_0 \exp\left(-\frac{E}{RT}\right) dt \tag{E4-6.8}$$

where C_B is related to C_A via Eqn (E4-6.6). Equation (E4.3-8) is applicable to reaction occurring isothermally at a constant temperature, T_R as well:

$$\int_{C_{A0}}^{C_A} \frac{dC_A}{C_A^{O_{RA}} C_B^{O_{RB}}} = \int_0^{t_R} \nu_A k_0 \exp\left(-\frac{E}{RT_R}\right) dt = \nu_A k_0 \exp\left(-\frac{E}{RT_R}\right) t_R \tag{E4-6.9}$$

where t_R is the time required to reach the reaction end condition (concentration C_A from C_{A0}) isothermally at a reaction temperature of T_R. Substituting Eqn (E4-6.9) into Eqn (E4-6.8), we obtain

$$\nu_A k_0 \exp\left(-\frac{E}{RT_R}\right) t_R = \int_{C_{A0}}^{C_A} \frac{dC_A}{C_A^{O_{RA}} C_B^{O_{RB}}} = \int_0^t \nu_A k_0 \exp\left(-\frac{E}{RT}\right) dt \tag{E4-6.10}$$

which can be reduced to

$$t_R = \int_0^t \exp\left(\frac{E/R}{T_R} - \frac{E/R}{T}\right) dt \tag{E4-6.11}$$

Thus, we have obtained a timescale that would give rise to the same conversion for different temperatures and/or different temperature progressions. Integration for t_R can be achieved numerically (Liu, S. 2010, J. Biotech. Adv., 28: 563–582.)

In chemical pulping, this temperature T_R is usually taken as 100 °C (or 373.15 K) and the resulting t_R is called H-factor. Once the activation energy is known, the effect of temperature and time can be easily lumped together with this single parameter, t_R, or H-factor. This turned out to be smart idea as operators can control the reaction effectively even the temperature varied during the process. Frequently quoted values of the constants are of those of Vroom (1957) for kraft pulping of woodchips as shown below.

$$HF = \int_0^t \exp\left(43.2 - \frac{16115\ \text{K}}{T}\right) dt \tag{E4-6.12}$$

As temperature rises, more solvent evaporates to the vapor phase. As pressure increases, more solvent returns to the liquid phase. Therefore for liquid or liquid–solid reactions at high temperature, the effective reaction volume V changes with temperature and pressure if not with concentration or composition. The constant volume assumption is only approximate. The complexity further arises as the reaction kinetics is not the same when temperature is increased causing different components in the plant biomass to be susceptible to reaction. Thus, the H-factor treatment is only an approximation of the reaction system. One variant of the H-factor is the severity factor. Equation (E4-6.11) can also be written as

$$t_R = \int_0^t \exp\left(\frac{T - T_R}{RT_R T/E}\right) dt \tag{E4-6.13}$$

If one approximates

$$\frac{RT_R T}{E} \approx T_E \tag{E4-6.14}$$

as a constant, then Eqn (E4-2.13) can be written as

$$t_R \approx \int_0^t \exp\frac{T - T_R}{T_E} dt = t \exp\frac{T - T_R}{T_E} \tag{E4-6.15}$$

The severity factor is defined as the log of t_R, that is

$$SF = \log\left(t \exp\frac{T - T_R}{T_E}\right) = \log t + \frac{T - T_R}{T_E \ln 10} \tag{E4-6.16}$$

For hot water extraction of woody biomass, the frequently used T_E is 14.75 °C or 14.75 K to be precise (Overend & Chornet 1987; Montane et al. 1994; Kabel et al. 2006). This is equivalent to $\frac{E}{R} = 10800$ K for hot water extraction of woody biomass or hemicellulose reaction.

Example 4-7. Hot water extraction of woodchips. Hot water extraction is an excellent technique to remove hemicelluloses from wood. Hemicellulose extracted this way can be converted to valuable products at low cost. Kate carefully prepared a batch of woodchips to conduct hot water extraction experiment. She loaded 500 g of sugar maple chips and

2 L water into an M/K digester, quickly ramped up the temperature to 160 °C. After 2 h at 160 °C, she then quenched the reaction mixture down to room temperature. After thoroughly washing the woodchips that were collected from the hot water extraction experiments, Kate found that the woodchips are weighing 385 g.

a. How much mass loss (in %) for the woodchips occurred in the hot water extraction experiment?

b. If Kate were to carry out the experiment at 180 °C, what is the extraction time she should keep in order to obtain roughly the same level of extraction?

Solution

a. Initially, the woodchips weigh 500 g and after extraction they weigh 385 g. Therefore, 500 – 385 g = 115 g of wood was extracted or removed to the liquid phase. The mass loss is thus 115/500 = 23%.

b. Let us assume that the extraction reaction can be approximated by a single temperature varying reaction rate constant. That is the rate of mass removal may be approximated by

$$r = k(T)f(C) \tag{E4-7.1}$$

where C is the concentration of components inside the wood.

For reaction occurring in a batch reactor, mole balance of reactant A leads to

$$\overset{0}{\text{In}} - \overset{0}{\text{Out}} + \text{Generation} = \text{Accumulation}$$

$$\nu_A r V = \frac{dn_A}{dt} \tag{E4-7.2}$$

Since the volume is constant (constant volume batch reactor), we further obtain

$$\nu_A k f(C) = \frac{dC_A}{dt} \tag{E4-7.3}$$

Since the rate constant k is only a function of temperature, separation of variables for Eqn (E4.4-6) leads to

$$\frac{dC_A}{f(C)} = \nu_A k dt = \nu_A k_0 \exp\left(-\frac{E}{RT}\right) dt \tag{E4-7.4}$$

For a desired reaction end condition or conversion, the reaction time can be obtained by integrating Eqn (E4-7.4).

$$\int_{C_{A0}}^{C_A} \frac{dC_A}{f(C)} = \int_0^t \nu_A k_0 \exp\left(-\frac{E}{RT}\right) dt = \nu_A k_0 \exp\left(-\frac{E}{RT}\right) t \tag{E4-7.5}$$

if the temperature is constant. For the reaction to take place at two different temperatures to have the same conversion (or concentration change), we obtain from Eqn (E4-7.5)

$$\nu_A k_0 \exp\left(-\frac{E}{RT_1}\right) t_1 = \nu_A k_0 \exp\left(-\frac{E}{RT_2}\right) t_2 \tag{E4-7.6}$$

which can be reduced to

$$t_2 = \exp\left(\frac{E/R}{T_2} - \frac{E/R}{T_1}\right) t_1 \tag{E4-7.7}$$

We can now estimate the time needed at a different temperature. Let us assume that $\frac{E}{R} = 10800$ K, substitute into Eqn (E4-7.7) to yield

$$\begin{aligned} t_2 &= \exp\left(\frac{10800\text{ K}}{T_2} - \frac{10800\text{ K}}{T_1}\right) t_1 \\ &= \exp\left[\frac{10800\text{ K}}{(180 + 273.15)} - \frac{10800\text{ K}}{(160 + 273.15)\text{K}}\right] \times 2\text{ h} = 0.6654\text{ h} = 39.93\text{ min} \end{aligned} \tag{E4-7.8}$$

That is, at 180 °C, an extraction time of 39.93 min is expected to yield the same level of extraction as 2 h at 160 °C.

4.4. NUMERICAL SOLUTIONS OF BATCH REACTOR PROBLEMS

In summary, a batch reactor problem as described by Eqns (4.2) and (4.23)–(4.31), can be generalized mathematically as

$$\frac{dy_j}{dt} = f_j(t, \mathbf{y}) \tag{4.32}$$

with $t = 0$, $y_j = y_{j0}$. Here $\mathbf{y} = \{y_1, y_2, \ldots\}$.

When you open the ODExLims visual basic code, you will see

```
Option Base 1
Option Explicit

'The following subroutine defines the ordinary differential equations y' = f(x,y,c)
'You may change the lines within Sub Func and Sub Jacobian
'Report bugs to Dr. Shijie Liu

Sub Func(f, ByVal x As Double, ByVal y, Optional c)

f(1) = c(1) * y(1)
f(2) = c(2) * x + c(3) * y(2) ^ c(4) - 0.1 * y(1)

End Sub
```

by default, you only need to change the lines between
"Sub Func(f, ByVal x As Double, ByVal y, Optional c)" and "End Sub."

In between these lines, you are to input the differential equations. You will need to write each equation separately on a different line. In the example shown in the code, there are two differential equations:

f(1) = c(1) * y(1)	$\Rightarrow$	$\frac{dy_1}{dx} = f_1 = c_1 y_1$
f(2) = c(2) * x +c(3) * y(2) ^ c(4) – 0.1 * y(1)	$\Rightarrow$	$\frac{dy_2}{dx} = f_2 = c_2 x + c_3 y_2^{c_4} - 0.1 y_1$

where c_j's are reserved as parameters (i.e. true constants) that one can pass from excel worksheet to the visual basic program at run time. This gives us freedom to make each code to be more general and thus capable of solving a class of problems. When you change the values of c_j's, the solution to the set of equations changes. You will not need to change the visual basic code just for the different values of c_j's.

Example 4-8. Concentration profile for a series reaction with feedback regulation. A liquid reaction system is carried out in a batch reactor:

$$\text{A} \longrightarrow \text{B} \longrightarrow \text{C} \tag{E4-8.1}$$

with

$$r_1 = \frac{k_1 C_A}{K_1 + C_A + K_C C_C} \tag{E4-8.2}$$

$$r_2 = \frac{k_2 C_B}{K_2 + C_B} \tag{E4-8.3}$$

where $k_1 = 1\ \text{mol}\cdot\text{L}^{-1}\cdot\text{h}^{-1}$, $k_2 = 0.5\ \text{mol}\cdot\text{L}^{-1}\cdot\text{h}^{-1}$, $K_1 = 0.1\ \text{mol}\cdot\text{L}^{-1}$, $K_2 = 0.2\ \text{mol}\cdot\text{L}^{-1}$, and $K_C = 100$.

Find the change of concentrations of A, B, and C as a function of time between 0 and 100 h in a constant volume isothermal batch reactor starting with

a. pure A initially at $C_{A0} = 10\ \text{mol}\cdot\text{L}^{-1}$; $C_{B0} = C_{C0} = 0\ \text{mol}\cdot\text{L}^{-1}$
b. $C_{A0} = 10\ \text{mol}\cdot\text{L}^{-1}$, $C_{B0} = 0\ \text{mol}\cdot\text{L}^{-1}$, $C_{C0} = 10\ \text{mol}\cdot\text{L}^{-1}$

Solution. This is a set of two reactions occurring in series. Mole balance for species j leads to

$$\frac{dn_j}{dt} = r_j V \tag{E4-8.4}$$

Since the volume is constant, we have

$$\frac{dC_j}{dt} = r_j \tag{E4-8.5}$$

We next find the rates of reaction (Fig. E4.8-1). Applying Eqn (3.66), we obtain

$$\begin{aligned} r_A &= \nu_{1A} r_1 + \nu_{2A} r_2 \\ &= -r_1 = -\frac{k_1 C_A}{K_1 + C_A + K_C C_C} \end{aligned} \tag{E4-8.6}$$

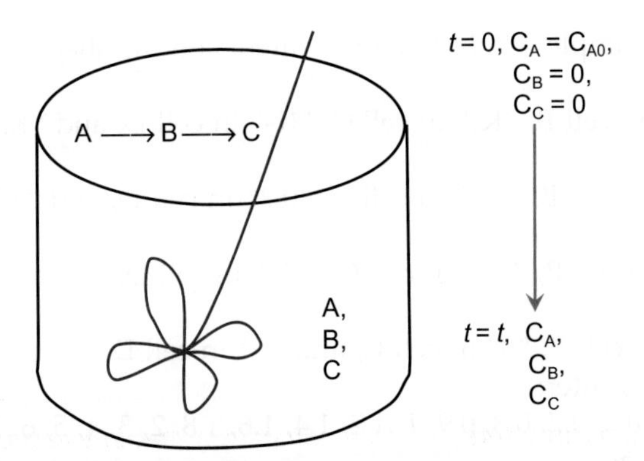

FIGURE E4-8.1 A schematic diagram of the batch reactor.

$$r_B = \nu_{1B} r_1 + \nu_{2B} r_2 = r_1 - r_2 = \frac{k_1 C_A}{K_1 + C_A + K_C C_C} - \frac{k_2 C_B}{K_2 + C_B} \tag{E4-8.7}$$

$$r_C = \nu_{1C} r_1 + \nu_{2C} r_2 = r_2 = \frac{k_2 C_B}{K_2 + C_B} \tag{E4-8.8}$$

Substituting Eqn (E4-8.6) through (E4-8.8) into Eqn (E4-8.5), we obtain the differential equations for the system:

$$\frac{dC_A}{dt} = r_A = -\frac{k_1 C_A}{K_1 + C_A + K_C C_C} \tag{E4-8.9}$$

$$\frac{dC_B}{dt} = r_B = \frac{k_1 C_A}{K_1 + C_A + K_C C_C} - \frac{k_2 C_B}{K_2 + C_B} \tag{E4-8.10}$$

$$\frac{dC_C}{dt} = r_C = \frac{k_2 C_B}{K_2 + C_B} \tag{E4-8.11}$$

Now we are ready to solve the problem with an automatic integrator.

Open the excel file: *odexlims.xls*. If prompted, enable the macro. If not prompted, make sure the macros are allowed to run from this file. You will see

Microsoft Excel - odexlims.xls

File Edit View Insert Format Tools Data Window Help Adobe PDF

E1

	A	B	C	D	G
1	c(1)	c(2)	c(3)	c(4)	
2	-0.5	4	-0.3	1	
3	x	y(1)	y(2)	This example has two equations:	y(1)' =f(1)=c(1)*y(1) and y(2)' =f(2)=c(2)*x+c(3)*y(2)^c(4)-0.1*y(1)
4	0	4	6	<= The initial conditions	The equations can be changed by editing the program
5	0.5	3.11520313	5.14871476		Select Tools -> Macro -> Visual Basic Editor
6	1	2.42612264	5.4533271		and then Change the routine Func as desired
7	1.5	1.88946631	6.7287839	Select the output region, use function (ODExLIMS), and then hold down Ctrl and Shift while pressing Enter	
8	2	1.47151784	8.82112718		
9	2.5	1.14601925	11.6019867		
10	3	0.89252069	14.9640992		

Now save the file as Example 4-7. Delete the contents on the sheet shown.

On row 1, enter:

"k_1" in cell A, "k_2" in cell B, "K_1" in cell C, "K_2" in cell D, and "K_c" in cell E.

On row 2, enter:

"1" in cell A, "0.5" in cell B, "0.1" in cell C, "0.2" in cell D, and "100" in cell E.

On row 3, enter:

"t" in cell A, "C_A" in cell B, "C_B" in cell C, "C_C" in cell D.

On row 4, enter:

"0" in cell A, "10" in cell B, "0" in cell C, and "0" in cell D.

In column 1 after row 4, enter:

0.1, 0.2, 0.3, 0.4, 0.5, 0.6, 0.7, 0.8, 0.9, 1, 1.2, 1.4, 1.6, 1.8, 2, 3, 4, 5, 6, 7, 8, 9, 10, …

It reads on screen now as

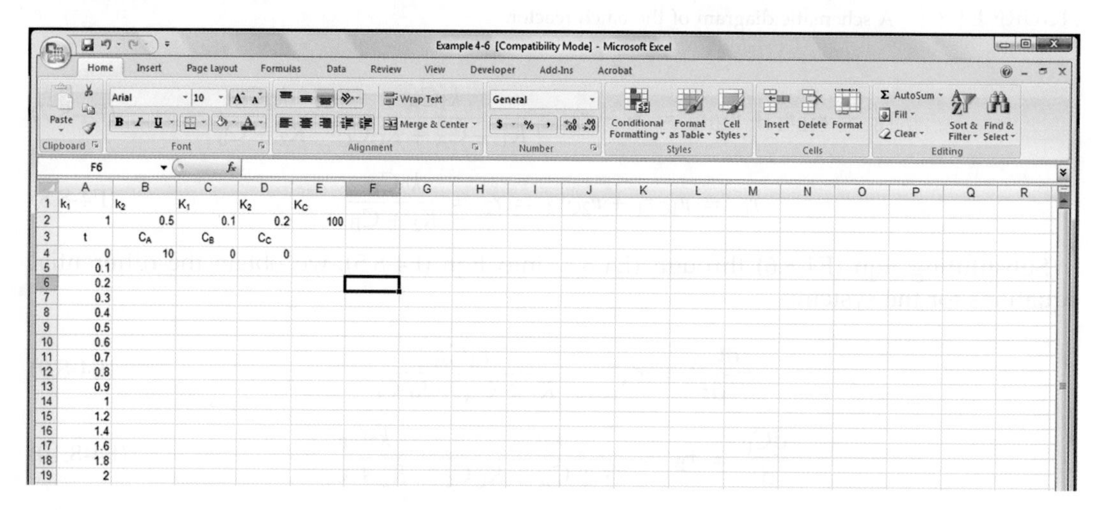

We next open the visual basic editor (from macro). Replace the two equations ["f(1) = …" and "f(2) = …"] with those of Eqns (E4.5-9) through (E4.5-11). In our case, we have three equations, so another line needs to be inserted. Noting from the sequence of parameters we had input on the Excel worksheet earlier: k_1, k_2, K_1, K_2, K_C, which are now available as c(1), c(2), c(3), c(4), and c(5). After entering the equations in the visual basic code, it reads on the screen:

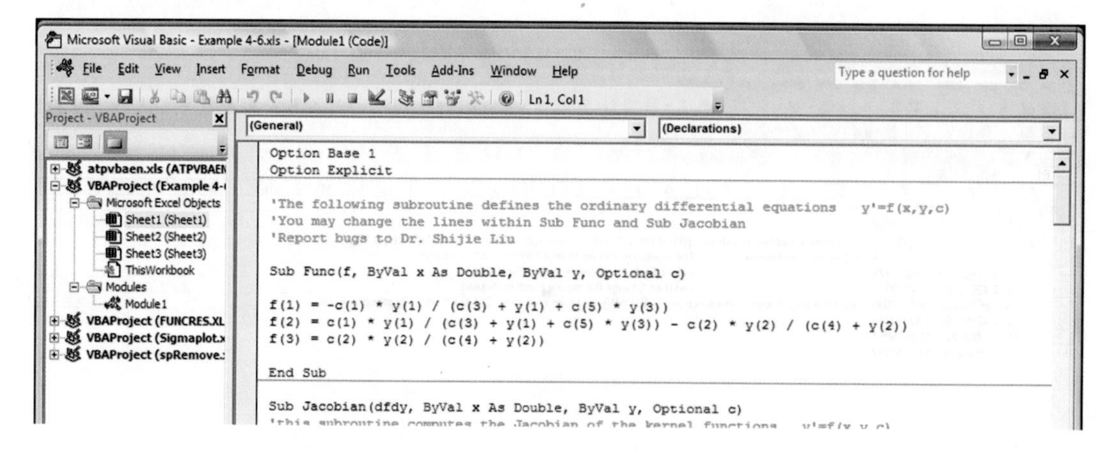

Make sure the equations you entered are correct (as you desired). We next go to the excel worksheet. Select the region below the row of initial values ("0," "10," "0," "0") until the last row you have time entered, between columns for C_A and C_C. Insert function, from "User Defined", find "ODExLIMS." Here is how it reads

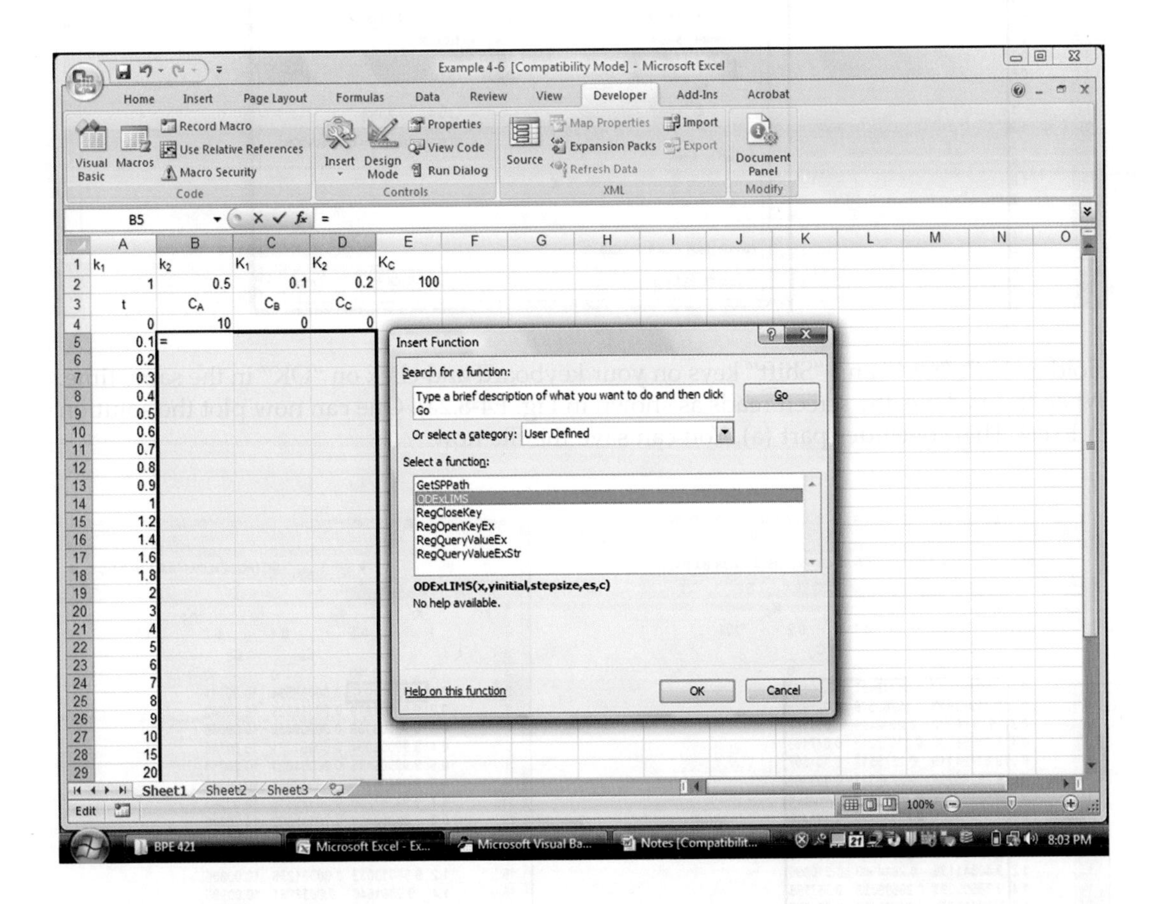

Click on "OK" and the dialog for the ODExLIMs shows up. On the row of "X," enter the locations of the values of t to be solved including the starting point (from $t = 0$ to the last t value you have entered). On the row of "Yintial," enter the location of the initial values (C_{A0}, C_{B0}, C_{C0}), and on the row of "C," enter the location of the parameters needed to be passed into the program, which are the k's values. Make sure the sequence of the "C" values is correct. When this is done, the screen reads,

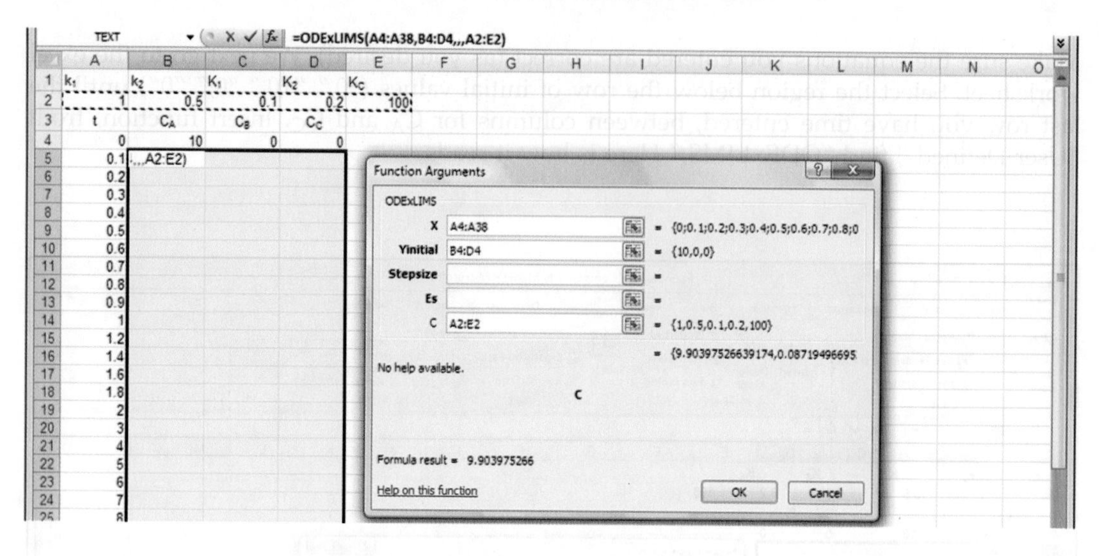

Hold on both "Ctrl" and "Shift" keys on your keyboard and click on "OK" in the same time. When this is done, the screen reads as shown in Fig. E4-8.2a). One can now plot the solution in Excel. This concludes part (a). You can save the file now.

B5 {=ODExLIMS(A4:A38,B4:D4,,,A2:

	A	B	C	D	E
1	k_1	k_2	K_1	K_2	K_C
2	1	0.5	0.1	0.2	100
3	t	C_A	C_B	C_C	
4	0	10	0	0	
5	0.1	9.90397527	0.08719497	0.00883	
6	0.2	9.81973813	0.15263675	0.027625	
7	0.3	9.7486372	0.2002459	0.051117	
8	0.4	9.68858536	0.23422211	0.077193	
9	0.5	9.63724119	0.2579517	0.104807	
10	0.6	9.59269998	0.2739311	0.133369	
11	0.7	9.55352177	0.28397016	0.162508	
12	0.8	9.51863221	0.28939293	0.191975	
13	0.9	9.4872245	0.29118564	0.22159	
14	1	9.45868452	0.29009821	0.251217	
15	1.2	9.40841136	0.2814903	0.310098	
16	1.4	9.36509093	0.26695398	0.367955	
17	1.6	9.32695881	0.24875199	0.424289	
18	1.8	9.292814	0.22849022	0.478696	
19	2	9.26180507	0.20736124	0.530834	
20	3	9.13646561	0.11387618	0.749658	
21	4	9.03757725	0.06407878	0.898344	
22	5	8.95135864	0.04544731	1.003194	
23	6	8.87295	0.0382104	1.08884	
24	7	8.80031839	0.03434443	1.165337	
25	8	8.73233307	0.03164362	1.236023	
26	9	8.66822928	0.02951155	1.302259	
27	10	8.6074413	0.02774281	1.364816	
28	15	8.34061992	0.02187373	1.637506	
29	20	8.11644649	0.01844959	1.865104	

(a)

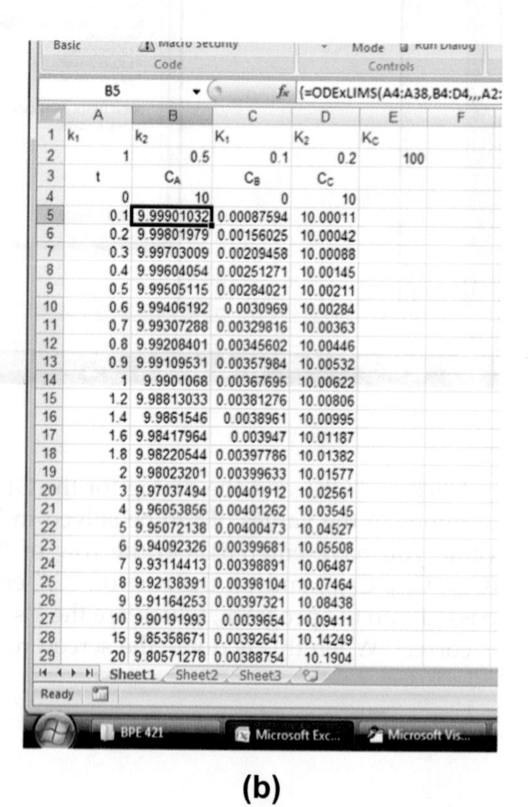

B5 {=ODExLIMS(A4:A38,B4:D4,,,A2:

	A	B	C	D	E
1	k_1	k_2	K_1	K_2	K_C
2	1	0.5	0.1	0.2	100
3	t	C_A	C_B	C_C	
4	0	10	0	10	
5	0.1	9.99901032	0.00087594	10.00011	
6	0.2	9.99801979	0.00156025	10.00042	
7	0.3	9.99703009	0.00209458	10.00088	
8	0.4	9.99604054	0.00251271	10.00145	
9	0.5	9.99505115	0.00284021	10.00211	
10	0.6	9.99406192	0.0030969	10.00284	
11	0.7	9.99307288	0.00329816	10.00363	
12	0.8	9.99208401	0.00345602	10.00446	
13	0.9	9.99109531	0.00357984	10.00532	
14	1	9.9901068	0.00367695	10.00622	
15	1.2	9.98813033	0.00381276	10.00806	
16	1.4	9.9861546	0.0038961	10.00995	
17	1.6	9.98417964	0.003947	10.01187	
18	1.8	9.98220544	0.00397786	10.01382	
19	2	9.98023201	0.00399633	10.01577	
20	3	9.97037494	0.00401912	10.02561	
21	4	9.96053856	0.00401262	10.03545	
22	5	9.95072138	0.00400473	10.04527	
23	6	9.94092326	0.00399681	10.05508	
24	7	9.93114413	0.00398891	10.06487	
25	8	9.92138391	0.00398104	10.07464	
26	9	9.91164253	0.00397321	10.08438	
27	10	9.90191993	0.0039654	10.09411	
28	15	9.85358671	0.00392641	10.14249	
29	20	9.80571278	0.00388754	10.1904	

(b)

FIGURE E4-8.2 The excel solution.

To perform part (b), you will only need to type 10 into the cell for C_{C0}, which is currently 0. The numbers (solution) should change automatically. If not, press "F9" key. You will see the difference immediately. The screen is shown above on the right (Fig. E4-8.2b). Comparing the solutions for part (a) and for part (b), one can observe that an increase in concentration C decreases the rate of conversion for A significantly.

Figure E4-8.3 shows the final solutions as plotted out for the concentrations of A and C (Fig. E4-8.3a) and B (Fig. E4-8.3b) as functions of time. One can observe that as the final

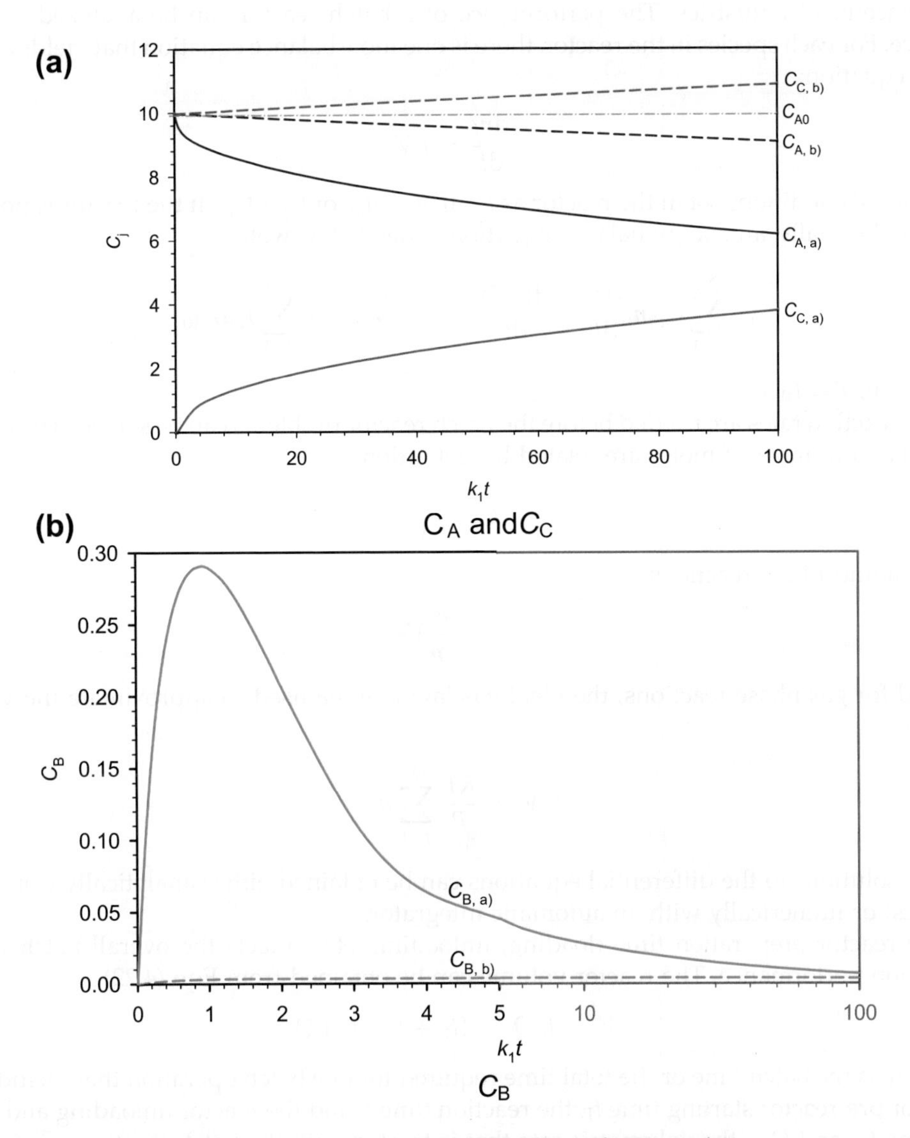

FIGURE E4-8.3 The concentrations of A, B, and C in the reactor as functions of time.

product concentration is high in the reaction mixture, the reaction is slowed significantly due to the feedback regulation. The intermediate product B formed is very low when the final product concentration is high in the reactor.

4.5. SUMMARY

Batch reactor is widely used in industry and is the preferred reactor in laboratories and in pharmaceutical industries. The performance of a batch reactor can be analyzed via mole balance. For each species in the reactor, there is one mole balance equation that yields a differential equation:

$$\frac{dn_j}{dt} = r_j V \tag{4.23}$$

with initial conditions set in the reactor as $t=0$, $n_j = n_{j0}$, or $C_j = C_{j0}$. If the reactor is not operated isothermally, an energy balance equation is needed as well,

$$\sum_{j=1}^{N_S} C_{Pj} n_j \frac{dT}{dt} - \frac{d(pV)}{dt} = \dot{Q} - \dot{W}_s - V \sum_{i=1}^{N_R} r_i \Delta H_{Ri} \tag{4.24}$$

with $t=0$, $T=T_0$.

The reaction rates are needed before the batch reactor problems can be solved. The concentration and number of moles are related by definition:

$$C_j = \frac{n_j}{V} \tag{4.28}$$

For liquid phase reactions,

$$V = \frac{\rho_0}{\rho} V_0 \tag{4.29}$$

And for gas phase reactions, the ideal gas law may be used to approximate the volume change:

$$V = \frac{RT}{P} \sum_{j=1}^{N_S} n_j \tag{4.30}$$

The solutions to the differential equations can be obtained either analytically (for simple kinetics) or numerically with an automatic integrator.

The reactor preparation time (loading, unloading, etc.) affects the overall batch reactor operation performance. The reactor volume can be obtained from Eqn (4.22)

$$V = t_B Q = (t_P + t_f + t_U) Q \tag{4.22}$$

where t_B is the batch time or the total time required for one batch operation that includes the time for pre-reactor starting time t_P, the reaction time t_f and the reactor unloading and cleaning time t_U, and Q is the volumetric rate that is treated with the batch reactor.

Further Reading

Kabel, M.A., Bos, G., Zeevalking, J., Voragen, A.G.J., Schols, H.A., 2006. Effect of pretreatment severity on xylan solubility and enzymatic breakdown of the remaining cellulose from wheat straw. *Bioresource Technology*, 98, 2034–2042.

Liu, S., 2010. Woody biomass: Niche position as a source of sustainable renewable chemicals and energy and kinetics of hot-water extraction/hydrolysis. *J. Biotech. Adv.* 28, 563–582.

Montané, D., Salvadó, J., Farriol, X., Jollez, P., Chornet, E., 1994. Phenomenological kinetics of wood delignification: application of a time-dependent rate constant and a generalized severity parameter to pulping and correlation of pulp properties. *Wood Science and Technology*, 28, 387–402.

Overend, R., Chornet, E., 1986. Fractionation of lignocellulosics by steam-aqueous pretreatment. *The Philosophical Transactions of the Royal Society London*, 321, 523–536.

Vroom, K.E., 1957. The "H" factor: a means of expressing cooking times and temperatures as a single variable. *Pulp Paper Mag. Can.* **58**(3), 228–231.

PROBLEMS

4.1. Our winery has discovered that all of last year's crop now being stored for aging contained 200 ppm of a chemical that gives it garlic flavor. However, we find that the concentration of this chemical is 50 ppm 1 year after it was put in storage. Taste tests in which this chemical was added to good wine shows that it can be detected only if its concentration is greater than 10 ppm. How long will we have to age this wine before we can sell it?

4.2. Our winery chemist has just found that the reaction by which the garlic-flavored compound of the previous problem disappears is by a reaction that produces a tasteless dimer of the chemical.

(a) With this mechanism, how long must we age our wine before we can sell it?

(b) Since we do not entirely trust his judgment (why would a competent chemist work for a winery?), we decide to test his results by analyzing the wine after the second year of aging. What percentages should we find if the reaction is first or second order?

4.3. The carton of milk in your refrigerator contains 20 cells per glass of a strain of *Escherichia coli* which makes people sick. This strain doubles every 2 days, and your immune system can destroy up to 1000 cells per glass without noticeable effects.

(a) When should the carton of milk be poured down the drain?

(b) At room temperature, this strain doubles every 8 h. For how long is the milk drinkable if left on the counter?

4.4. Your neighbor just sneezed on your desk, and the drop contains 200 virus particles. Half of the virus particles are destroyed every 10 min by air oxidation. Can the person who sits at your desk next hour catch his cold?

4.5. Yogurt is produced by adding a small amount of finished yogurt to fresh milk in a process whose kinetics can be described approximately as

$$A \longrightarrow 2A, \quad r = kC_A$$

It is found that with a certain culture, the concentration of product in fresh milk doubles in 8 h. If the process is started by adding 5% of finished yogurt to milk, how long is required to prepare a batch of yogurt?

4.6. A certain drug is metabolized such that its concentration in the bloodstream halves every 4 h. If the drug loses its effectiveness when the concentration falls to 10% of its initial concentration, how frequently should the drug be taken?

4.7. An aqueous ester hydrolysis reaction $A \rightarrow B + C$ has $k = 0.02/\text{min}$ and an equilibrium constant of 10 with all concentrations in mol/L.

(a) Starting with $C_{A0} = 1$ mol/L, and $C_{B0} = C_{C0} = 0$, what is the equilibrium composition?

(b) What is the reverse rate constant in the above reaction?

(c) Find $C_A(t)$, $C_B(t)$, and $C_C(t)$ in a batch reactor for these initial conditions.

4.8. A gaseous reaction

$$A \longrightarrow B + C \quad r = kC_A^2, \text{ with } k = 0.1 \text{ mol}\cdot\text{L}^{-1}\cdot\text{s}^{-1}$$

is occurring in an isothermal constant pressure batch reactor. The reactor is at 373 K charged initially with 1 bar of A and 0.2 bar of N_2 (not A, B, or C), that is not reacting. Determine the time required for the reaction volume to expand by 50%, i.e. $V/V_0 = 1.5$.

4.9. Sterilization is a batch process by which bacteria and molds in food are killed by heat treatment. A can of vegetables that originally contained 10,000 viable spores has 100 spores remaining after heating for 10 min at 250 °F. Assuming first-order kinetics, how long must this can be heated at this temperature to reduce the probability of having a single spore to an average of 1 in 1 million cans?

4.10. In ethanol production by fermentation of corn, hydrolyzed ground corn in a water suspension containing 50% corn by weight is mixed with sufficient enzyme to produce ethanol by the approximate reaction

$$C_6H_{12}O_6 \longrightarrow 2C_2H_5OH + 2CO_2$$

When the solution reaches 12% ethanol, the yeast dies and the reaction stops.

(a) How many bushels of corn are required to produce 500 tons of pure ethanol per day? Assume 1 bushel of corn weighs 56 lb.

(b) The process requires 72 h to go to completion. What size batch reactor tank or tanks are required for this process?

4.11. Consider the reaction

$$A \longrightarrow B, \ r = 0.15/\text{min}\, C_A$$

in a batch reactor. The total preparation time for each batch operation is 8 h. A costs \$2/mole, and B sells for \$4/mole. The cost for operating the reactor is \$0.04 per liter hour. We need to produce 100 moles of B per hour using $C_{A0} = 2$ mol/L. Assume no value or cost of disposal of unreacted A.

(a) What is the optimum conversion and reactor size?

(b) What is the cash flow from the process?

(c) What is the cash flow ignoring operating cost?

(d) At what operating cost do we break even?

4.12. One hundred moles of A per hour are available in concentration of 0.1 mol/L by a previous process. This stream is to be reacted with B to produce C and D. The reaction proceeds by the aqueous-phase reaction,

$$A + B \longrightarrow C + D, \quad k = 5 \text{ mol}^{-1}\cdot\text{L}\cdot\text{h}^{-1}$$

The amount of C required is 95 mol/h. In extracting C from the reacted mixture, A and B are destroyed; hence, recycling of unused reactants is not possible. Calculate the optimum reactor size as well as feed composition for this process if the total preparation time for each batch operation is 10 h.

Data: B costs \$1.25/mol in crystalline form. It is highly soluble in the aqueous solution and even when present in large amounts does not change the concentration of A in solution. Capital and operating costs are \$0.015 $h^{-1}\cdot L^{-1}$.

4.13. One hundred fifty moles of B are to be produced hourly from a feed consisting of a saturated solution of A ($C_{A0} = 0.1$ mol/L) in a batch reactor. The reaction is

$$A \longrightarrow B, \; r = 0.2/hC_A$$

The cost of reactant at $C_{A0} = 0.1$ mol/l is \$A = \$0.50/mol A. The cost of reactor including installation, auxiliary equipment, instrumentation, overhead, labor, depreciation, etc., is $\$m = \$0.01\ h^{-1}\cdot L^{-1}$. The total preparation time for each batch of operation is 9 h.

What reactor size, reactant rate, and conversion should be used for optimum operations? What is the unit cost of B for these conditions if unreacted A is discarded?

4.14. You wish to design a plant to produce 100 tons/day of ethylene glycol from ethane, air, and water. The plant has three reactor stages, ethane dehydrogenation, ethylene oxidation, and ethylene oxide hydration.

(a) What are the reactions?

(b) Both dehydrogenation and hydration have nearly 100% selectivity (with recycle of unreacted reactants), but ethylene to ethylene oxide has only 70% selectivity with an old catalyst and 90% selectivity with a new and expensive catalyst. How many tons/day of ethane do we need to supply to this plant with each of these catalysts?

4.15. We want to hydrolyze 500 lb/day of an ester at an initial concentration of 5 molar (the ester has a molecular weight of 120) in aqueous basic solution in a batch process, and we need product that is 99% hydrolyzed. In bench top experiments in a flask, we find that 50% of the ester hydrolyzes in 15 min for initial ester concentrations of either 1 or 5 molar. We also find that, when we react for 8 h, all the ester has hydrolyzed. It takes 1 h to empty the reactor and refill and heat it to start another batch.

(a) What size reactor will we need?

(b) What size reactor will we need if we can tolerate 90% conversion?

(c) This process was found to have an activation energy of 12 kcal/mol, and we had been operating at 40 °C. What reactor volumes would we need if we can operate at 80 °C?

(d) This hydrolysis reaction is exothermic with $\Delta H_R = -8$ kcal/mol. What must be the average rate of cooling (in watts) during the reaction to maintain the reaction isothermal?

(e) If we started the batch reactor at 40 °C but forgot to turn on the cooling, what would be the final temperature if the reactor were adiabatic (and the vessel would withstand the pressure)? Assume the heat capacity of the solution to be that of water, 1 cal/(cm^3 K).

(f) What cautions do you recommend regarding operation at 80 °C?

4.16. A pulp mill utilizing the saw dust from nearby lumber mills to produce a market pulp for paper production. A recent development had the company thinking of increasing the pulp production by 50% for entering the nonwoven market. A close examination at the pulp mill has the engineers to conclude that the digesters were the bottleneck. Currently, the woodchips were steamed, mixed with a pulping liquor, and underwent delignification at 150 °C for 3 h. For each load of woodchips, a minimum of 2 h is needed for loading, heating the digester up, explosive decompression unloading, and cleaning up the digester for the next load. Your task is to find a way to ease the bottleneck quickly at a low cost. State your assumptions clearly and your solution to the problem as stated.

CHAPTER

5

Ideal Flow Reactors

OUTLINE

In this chapter, we deal with the fundamentals of reaction in continuous flow reactors. For simplicity, we shall focus on the ideal isothermal reactors. Most industrial reactors are operated in a continuous mode instead of batch because continuous reactors produce more products with smaller equipment, require less labor and maintenance, and frequently produce better quality control. Continuous processes are more difficult to start and stop than batch reactors, but they make product without stopping to change batches and they require minimum labor.

Batch processes can be tailored to produce small amounts of product when needed. Batch processes are also ideal to measure rates and kinetics in order to design continuous processes: Here one only wants to obtain *information* rapidly without generating too much product that must be disposed of. In pharmaceuticals, batch processes are sometimes desired to assure

Bioprocess Engineering
http://dx.doi.org/10.1016/B978-0-444-59525-6.00005-6

quality control: Each batch can be analyzed and certified (or discarded), while contamination in a continuous process will invariably lead to a lot of worthless product before certifiable purity is restored. Food and beverages are still made in batch processes in many situations because biological reactions are never exactly reproducible, and a batch process is easier to "tune" slightly to optimize each batch. Besides, it is more romantic to produce beer by "beechwood aging," wine by stamping on grapes with bare feet, steaks by charcoal grilling, and similar batch processes.

We will develop mass and energy balances in flow reactors. In one limit, the reactor is stirred sufficiently to mix the fluid completely (continuous stirred-tank reactor [CSTR] or chemostat), and in the other limit, the fluid is completely unmixed (plug flow reactor [PFR]). In any other situation, the fluid is partially mixed and one cannot specify the composition without a detailed description of the fluid mechanics. However, we will assume the reactors to be either completely mixed or completely unmixed in this chapter. As to any flow equipment, there is a need of mechanical force to push the fluid mixture through. Thus, pressure drop or mechanic energy balance is also needed in addition to the mass and energy balances.

5.1. FLOW RATE, RESIDENCE TIME, SPACE TIME, SPACE VELOCITY, DILUTION RATE

Figure 5.1 shows a schematic of a flow reactor with an inlet and an outlet. In the inlet, we feed in a reaction mixture containing reactants and solvents, with a concentration of C_{j0} for species j. The temperature and pressure of the inlet stream are measured at T_0 and P_0. The volumetric flow rate is Q_0. When the reaction mixture passing through the flow reactor of total effective volume V, chemical or biological reaction(s) occur and the flows are controlled. It outflows the reaction mixture containing unreacted reactants, products, and solvents. For any given species j, its concentration is a concentration of C_{je}. The temperature and pressure of the outlet stream are measured at T_e and P_e, and the volumetric flow rate is Q_e.

The reactor residence time is defined as the average time any fluid particle spent in the reactor, from inlet to outlet. As such, it can be shown that

$$d\bar{t} = \frac{dV}{Q} \tag{5.1}$$

Where $\bar{t}$ is the residence time. Since the volumetric flow rate can vary inside the reactor, the residence time calculation is not straightforward. For constant-volumetric flow reactors, Eqn (5.1) is reduced to

$$\bar{t} = \int_0^V \frac{dV}{Q} = \frac{V}{Q_e} = \frac{V}{Q_0} \tag{5.2}$$

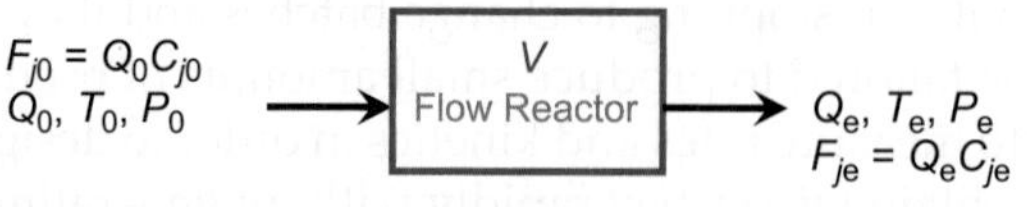

$F_{j0} = Q_0 C_{j0}$
Q_0, T_0, P_0 → V Flow Reactor → Q_e, T_e, P_e
$F_{je} = Q_e C_{je}$

FIGURE 5.1 Schematic diagram of a flow reactor showing the inlet and outlet.

The residence time varies with temperature and pressure, besides the feed flow rate. Therefore, the residence time is not an easy parameter to use when designing and/or operating a reactor.

To simplify the calculation of a time scale, a space time τ is defined. The space time is the time needed to feed a reactor full of reaction mixture through the reactor. It is thus defined as the total volume of the reactor divided by the inlet volumetric flow rate. That is,

$$\tau = \frac{V}{Q_0} \tag{5.3}$$

The space time is especially useful for liquid reactors. Since the density of liquids is relatively constant, we can assume that the flow rate remains nearly constant. In this case, the space time is nearly the same as the residence time.

Figure 5.2 shows the space time scale for a variety of important industrial reactions. One can observe that the required space time is nearly inversely exponentially related to the reaction temperature. Higher temperature requires significantly shorter reaction time.

Alternatively, one can define the frequency of reaction mixture being treated based on the reactor. This is commonly called space velocity. In bioreactions, the biocatalysts are kept in

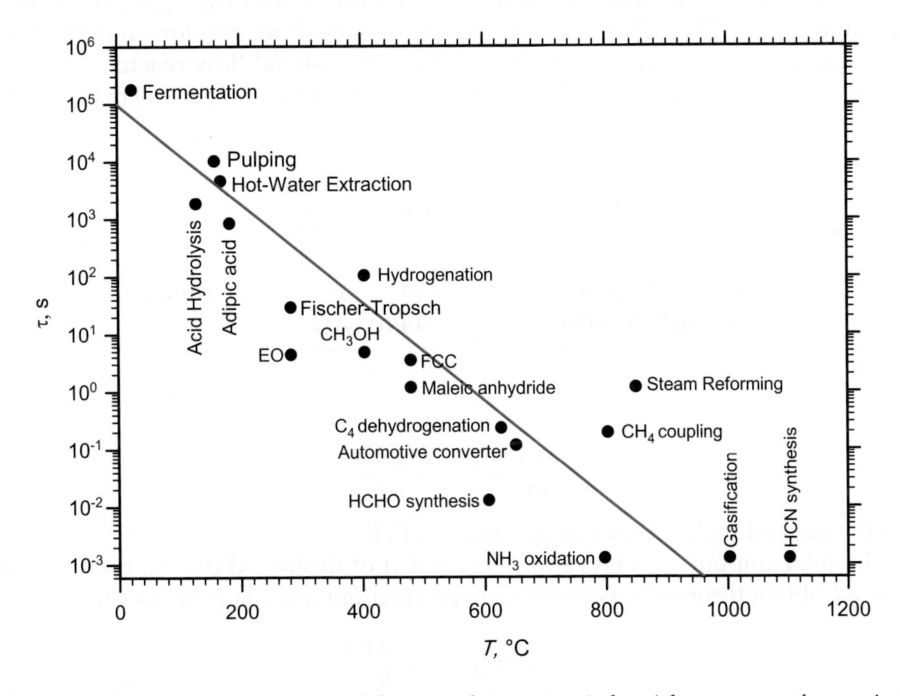

FIGURE 5.2 Nominal space time required for several important industrial reactors vs the nominal reactor operating temperatures. Time scale goes from days (fermentation or bioreactions) down to milliseconds (for ammonia oxidation to form nitric acid). The low-temperature ($T < 200$ °C) long-time ($\tau > 10$ min) processes involve liquids and/or solids as substrates, while the high-temperature short-time processes involve gases, usually at high pressures.

the reactor. Our interest is in maintaining the same level of catalyst. Therefore, the rate of reactor contents being replaced by the feed stream is defined as the dilution rate. Therefore, dilution rate and space velocity are two identical quantities. In this text, we shall not differentiate dilution rate from space velocity.

The space velocity or dilution rate is simply defined as the inlet flow rate divided by the reactor volume. That is

$$D = \frac{Q_0}{V} \tag{5.4}$$

where D stands for *dilution rate* that is commonly used associated with chemostats. For chemical reactors, the quantity defined in Eqn (5.4) is commonly referred to as the *space velocity*.

5.2. PLUG FLOW REACTOR

PFR is an idealized flow reactor such that along the direction of the flow all the reaction mixture are moving along with the same speed, there is no mixing or back flow. The contents in the PFR flow like plugs, from inlet to outlet. On the other hand, the reaction mixture is well mixed, just like that in a batch reactor, within each plug or on the cross-section plane of the PFR. This idealization makes the flow reactor analysis simplified extremely as now one can treat the PFR as a one-dimensional flow reactor.

Figure 5.1 shows a schematic of PFR. Mole balance for a given species j over a differential volume between V and $V + \mathrm{d}V$ leads to

$$F_j\big|_V - F_j\big|_{V+\mathrm{d}V} + r_j \mathrm{d}V = \frac{\partial (C_j \mathrm{d}V)}{\partial t} \tag{5.5}$$

which leads to

$$-\mathrm{d}F_j + r_j \mathrm{d}V = \frac{\partial (C_j \mathrm{d}V)}{\partial t} \tag{5.6}$$

or

$$\frac{\partial C_j}{\partial t} = r_j - \frac{\partial (QC_j)}{\partial V} \tag{5.7}$$

which is the general mole balance equation for a PFR.

Since the total amount of mass cannot be created or destroyed during chemical and bio-reactions, we obtain through mass balance over the differential volume as shown in Fig. 5.3,

$$-\Delta(\rho Q) = \frac{\partial (\rho \Delta V)}{\partial t} \tag{5.8}$$

which is reduced to

$$\frac{\partial \rho}{\partial t} = -\frac{\partial (\rho Q)}{\partial V} \tag{5.9}$$

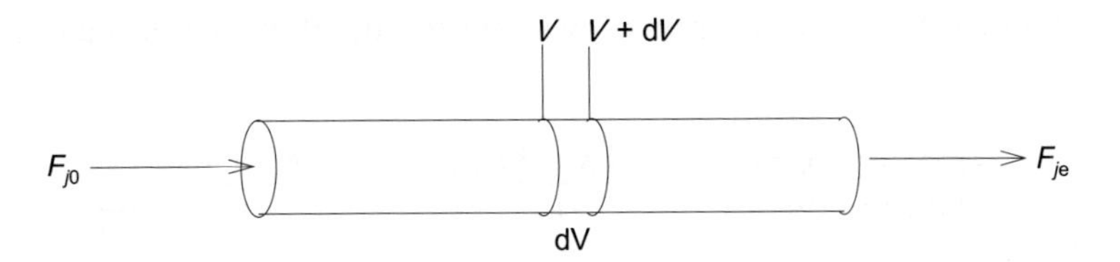

FIGURE 5.3 A schematic diagram of the PFR showing a differential control volume (V, $V + \mathrm{d}V$).

In general,

$$\rho = \sum_{j=1}^{N_S} C_j M_j \tag{5.10}$$

In a general case, Eqn (5.7) needs to be written each for every component (species) except one involved. Thus, we would have N_s partial differential equations to solve even for an isothermal isobaric reactor. If temperature changes, the energy balance equation must be solved simultaneously as well. Pressure drop or momentum balance makes another addition to the equations.

In industrial operations, we would prefer to run the reactor at maximum capacity all the time to maximize the throughput and minimize the unit cost to produce the product. Therefore, often times steady-state operations are desired. When steady state is reached, every quantified measure in the reactor is independent on time, i.e. time derivatives are zero. Equation (5.7) is reduced to

$$r_j = \frac{\mathrm{d}F_j}{\mathrm{d}V} \tag{5.11}$$

For a single reaction that is carried out in a steady PFR, there is only one independent concentration or reaction mixture content variable and all other concentrations can be related through stoichiometry as shown in Chapter 3. Without lose of generosity, let us use component A as the key component of consideration. Equation (5.11) applied to species A gives

$$r_A = \frac{\mathrm{d}F_A}{\mathrm{d}V} \tag{5.12}$$

an ordinary differential equation.

In general, the rate of reaction is a function of concentration and temperature. From Chapter 3, we learned that the stoichiometry can be applied to relate the amount of every species in the reaction mixture. The amount change of a component participating in the reaction divided by its stoichiometric coefficient is the universal extent of reaction for a single reaction. The stoichiometry can be written in a flow reactor as

$$\frac{\mathrm{d}F_j}{\nu_j} = \frac{\mathrm{d}F_A}{\nu_A} = r\mathrm{d}V \tag{5.13}$$

When there is no side feed or outlet stream, Eqn (5.13) can be integrated to give

$$\frac{F_j - F_{j0}}{\nu_j} = \frac{F_A - F_{A0}}{\nu_A} = \frac{F_{A0}}{-\nu_A} f_A \tag{5.14}$$

The total molar flow rate can be computed by summing up all the component (species) flow rates. That is

$$F = \sum_{j=1}^{N_S} F_j = \sum_{j=1}^{N_S} \left(F_{j0} + \nu_j \frac{F_A - F_{A0}}{\nu_A} \right) = F_0 + \frac{F_A - F_{A0}}{\nu_A} \sum_{j=1}^{N_S} \nu_j \tag{5.15}$$

Letting ν_Σ be the total stoichiometric coefficients, i.e.,

$$\nu_\Sigma = \sum_{j=1}^{N_S} \nu_j \tag{5.16}$$

We obtain

$$F = F_0 + \frac{\nu_\Sigma}{\nu_A}(F_A - F_{A0}) = F_0 - \frac{\nu_\Sigma}{\nu_A} F_{A0} f_A \tag{5.17}$$

While the above derivation is concise, we often tabularize the stoichiometry to gain a thorough understanding of the stoichiometry for every species, either be those involved in the reaction or those that are not participating in the actual reaction. The stoichiometry is shown in Table 5.1.

The concentration can be related to the molar flow rate through

$$C_j = \frac{F_j}{Q} = \frac{F_{j0} + \frac{\nu_j}{\nu_A}(F_A - F_{A0})}{Q} = \frac{F_{j0} - \frac{\nu_j}{\nu_A} F_{A0} f_A}{Q} \tag{5.18}$$

The volumetric flow rate Q can be a function of temperature and pressure (density change). Since the mass flow rate does not change if no side inlets or outlets, we have

$$C_j = \frac{\rho}{\rho_0} \frac{F_{j0} + \frac{\nu_j}{\nu_A}(F_A - F_{A0})}{Q_0} = \frac{\rho}{\rho_0} \frac{F_{j0} - \frac{\nu_j}{\nu_A} F_{A0} f_A}{Q_0} \tag{5.19}$$

For isothermal operations, Q is constant for reactions involving condensed matter (liquid or solid) only. For ideal gas, the volumetric flow rate can be related to the molar flow rate through ideal gas law

$$PQ = FRT \tag{5.20}$$

TABLE 5.1 Stoichiometry of a Reaction System with Side Inlets or Outlets

Species	Initial	Change	At V
A	F_{A0}	$F_A - F_{A0}$	F_A
j	F_{j0}	$F_j - F_{j0} = \nu_j \frac{F_A - F_{A0}}{\nu_A}$	$F_j = F_{j0} + \nu_j \frac{F_A - F_{A0}}{\nu_A}$
…	…	…	…
Total	F_0	$\sum_{j=1}^{N} (F_j - F_{j0}) = \nu_\Sigma \frac{F_A - F_{A0}}{\nu_A}$	$\sum_{j=1}^{N} F_j = F_0 + \nu_\Sigma \frac{F_A - F_{A0}}{\nu_A}$

which leads to

$$Q = \frac{P_0 T}{P T_0} \frac{F}{F_0} Q_0 = \frac{P_0 T}{P T_0}\left[1 + \frac{\nu_\Sigma}{\nu_A}\frac{F_A - F_{A0}}{F_0}\right] Q_0 = \frac{P_0 T}{P T_0}\left[1 - \frac{\nu_\Sigma}{\nu_A}\frac{F_{A0}}{F_0} f_A\right] Q_0 \tag{5.21}$$

and

$$C_j = \frac{F_j}{Q} = \frac{P T_0}{P_0 T} \frac{C_{j0} - \frac{\nu_j}{\nu_A} C_{A0} f_A}{1 - \frac{\nu_\Sigma}{\nu_A}\frac{F_{A0}}{F_0} f_A} \tag{5.22}$$

Using the fractional conversion f_A, Eqn (5.12) is reduced to

$$\mathrm{d}V = F_{A0} \frac{\mathrm{d}f_A}{-r_A} \tag{5.23}$$

Integrating Eqn (5.23) gives the required volume of the steady PFR for the desired fractional conversion of f_{Ae},

$$V = F_{A0} \int_0^{f_{Ae}} \frac{\mathrm{d}f_A}{-r_A} \tag{5.24}$$

Correspondingly, the space time (no side inlets or outlets) for a PFR is given by

$$\tau = \frac{V}{Q_0} = C_{A0} \int_0^{f_{Ae}} \frac{\mathrm{d}f_A}{-r_A} \tag{5.25}$$

Comparing Eqn (5.25) with Eqn (4.8), we can observe that the behavior for a PFR is very similar to that of a Batch reactor. In fact, one can show that the time t for a batch reactor and the residence time $\bar{t}$ for a steady PFR are "interchangeable." Table 5.2 shows a list of solutions for some single reactions with simple kinetics.

Example 5-1. An elementary first-order reaction:

$$A \rightarrow B$$

is to be carried out in a PFR. If the rate constant $k = 0.02\ \mathrm{s}^{-1}$ and the volumetric flow rate is constant at 10 L/s, calculate the reactor volume required for 50% conversion.

Solution. Figure E5-1 shows a schematic diagram of the constant density PFR.

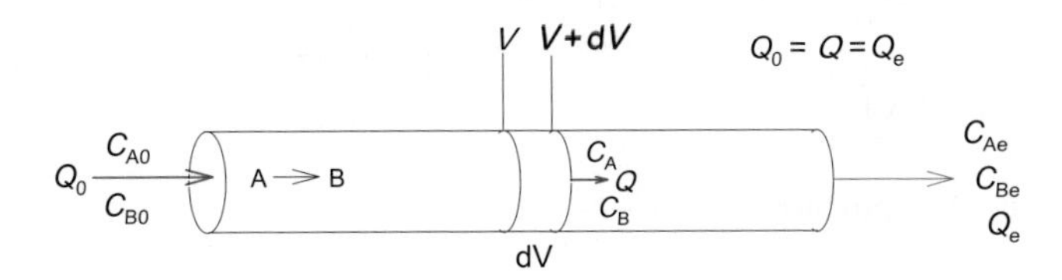

FIGURE E5-1 A schematic diagram of a constant density PFR showing a differential control volume (V, $V + \mathrm{d}V$).

TABLE 5.2 Reaction Space Time Requirement and Concentration Profile for Single Reactions in an Isothermal Constant Density Plug Flow Reactor (PFR) with Simple Kinetic Models

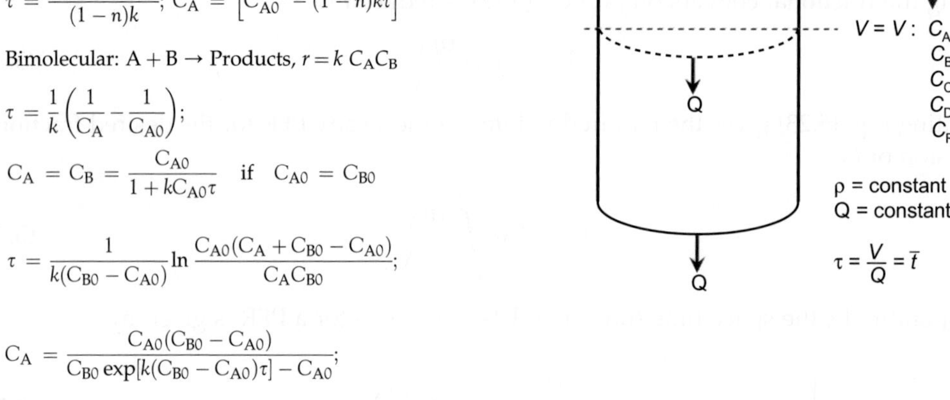

1. Zeroth-order: A → Products, $r = k$

$$\tau = (C_{A0} - C_A)/k;\ C_A = C_{A0} - k\,\tau$$

2. First-order: A → Products, $r = k\,C_A$

$$\tau = \ln(C_{A0}/C_A)/k;\ C_A = C_{A0}\exp(-k\,\tau)$$

3. Power-law kinetics: A → Products, $r = k\,C_A^n$

$$\tau = \frac{C_{A0}^{1-n} - C_A^{1-n}}{(1-n)k};\ C_A = \left[C_{A0}^{1-n} - (1-n)k\tau\right]^{\frac{1}{1-n}}$$

4. Bimolecular: A + B → Products, $r = k\,C_A C_B$

$$\tau = \frac{1}{k}\left(\frac{1}{C_A} - \frac{1}{C_{A0}}\right);$$

$$C_A = C_B = \frac{C_{A0}}{1 + kC_{A0}\tau} \quad \text{if} \quad C_{A0} = C_{B0}$$

$$\tau = \frac{1}{k(C_{B0} - C_{A0})}\ln\frac{C_{A0}(C_A + C_{B0} - C_{A0})}{C_A C_{B0}};$$

$$C_A = \frac{C_{A0}(C_{B0} - C_{A0})}{C_{B0}\exp[k(C_{B0} - C_{A0})\tau] - C_{A0}};$$

$$C_B = C_{B0} - C_{A0} + C_A$$

5. Autocatalytic: A + R → 2R + products, $r = k\,C_A C_R$

$$\tau = \frac{1}{k(C_{A0} + C_{R0})}\ln\frac{C_{A0}(C_{A0} + C_{R0} - C_A)}{C_A C_{R0}};$$

$$C_A = \frac{C_{A0}(C_{A0} + C_{R0})}{C_{A0} + C_{R0}\exp[k(C_{A0} + C_{R0})\tau]};$$

$$C_R = C_{A0} + C_{R0} - C_A$$

6. Unimolecular catalytic: A → products, $r = \frac{kC_A}{K_A + C_A}$

$$\tau = \frac{1}{k}\left(K_A \ln\frac{C_{A0}}{C_A} + C_{A0} - C_A\right)$$

7. Unimolecular catalytic: A → products, $r = \frac{kC_A^2}{K_A + C_A}$

$$\tau = \frac{1}{k}\left(\ln\frac{C_{A0}}{C_A} + \frac{K_A}{C_A} - \frac{K_A}{C_{A0}}\right)$$

(Continued)

TABLE 5.2 Reaction Space Time Requirement and Concentration Profile for Single Reactions in an Isothermal Constant Density Plug Flow Reactor (PFR) with Simple Kinetic Models—*Cont'd*

8. First-order reversible: $A \rightleftarrows B, r = k_f C_A - k_b C_B$

$$\tau = \frac{1}{k_f + k_b} \ln \frac{k_f C_{A0} - k_b C_{B0}}{(k_f + k_b) C_A - k_b (C_{A0} + C_{B0})};$$

$$C_A = \frac{(k_f C_{A0} - k_b C_{B0}) \exp[-(k_f + k_b)\tau] + k_b (C_{A0} + C_{B0})}{k_f + k_b}$$

$$C_B = C_{A0} + C_{B0} - C_A$$

9. Catalytic first-order reversible: $A \rightleftarrows B, r = \dfrac{k(C_A - C_B/K_C)}{1 + K_A C_A + K_B C_B}$

$$\tau = \frac{K_C}{k(1+K_C)} \left\{ (K_A - K_B)(C_{A0} - C_A) + \left[1 + (C_{A0} + C_{B0})\left(K_B + \frac{K_A - K_B}{K_C}\right)\right] \ln \frac{(1+K_C)C_{A0} - (C_{A0} + C_{B0})}{(1+K_C)C_A - (C_{A0} + C_{B0})} \right\}$$

$$C_B = C_{A0} + C_{B0} - C_A$$

10. Reversible decomposition: $A \rightleftarrows B + C, r = k_f C_A - k_b C_B C_C$

$$a, b = k_f + k_b(2C_{A0} + C_{B0} + C_{C0}) \pm \sqrt{[k_f + k_b(2C_{A0} + C_{B0} + C_{C0})]^2 - 4k_b^2 (C_{A0} + C_{B0})(C_{A0} + C_{C0})}$$

$$\tau = \frac{2}{a-b} \ln \frac{(2k_b C_{A0} - a)(2k_b C_A - b)}{(2k_b C_{A0} - b)(2k_b C_A - a)}; \quad C_A = \frac{1}{2k_b} \frac{a(2k_b C_{A0} - b)\exp\left(\frac{a-b}{2}\tau\right) - b(2k_b C_{A0} - a)}{(2k_b C_{A0} - b)\exp\left(\frac{a-b}{2}\tau\right) - (2k_b C_{A0} - a)}$$

$$C_B = C_{A0} + C_{B0} - C_A; \quad C_C = C_{A0} + C_{C0} - C_A$$

11. Reversible codimerization: $A + B \rightleftarrows C, r = k_f C_A C_B - k_b C_C$

$$a, b = k_f (C_{A0} - C_{B0}) - k_b \pm \sqrt{[k_f (C_{A0} - C_{B0}) - k_b]^2 + 4 k_f k_b (C_{A0} + C_{C0})}$$

$$\tau = \frac{2}{b-a} \ln \frac{(2k_f C_{A0} - a)(2k_f C_A - b)}{(2k_f C_{A0} - b)(2k_f C_A - a)}; \quad C_A = \frac{1}{2k_f} \frac{a(2k_f C_{A0} - b)\exp\left(-\frac{a-b}{2}\tau\right) - b(2k_f C_{A0} - a)}{(2k_f C_{A0} - b)\exp\left(-\frac{a-b}{2}\tau\right) - (2k_f C_{A0} - a)}$$

$$C_B = C_{B0} - C_{A0} + C_A; \quad C_C = C_{A0} + C_{C0} - C_A$$

12. Reversible bimolecular: $A + B \rightleftarrows C + D, r = k(C_A C_B - C_C C_D / K_C)$

$$\alpha = K_C (C_{A0} - C_{B0}) - 2C_{A0} - C_{C0} - C_{D0}; \quad a, b = \alpha \pm \sqrt{\alpha^2 + 4(K_C - 1)(C_{A0} + C_{C0})(C_{A0} + C_{D0})}$$

$$\tau = \frac{2K_C}{k(b-a)} \ln \frac{[2(K_C - 1)C_{A0} - a][2(K_C - 1)C_A - b]}{[2(K_C - 1)C_{A0} - b][2(K_C - 1)C_A - a]};$$

$$C_A = \frac{1}{2(K_C - 1)} \frac{a[2(K_C - 1)C_{A0} - b]\exp\left(-\frac{a-b}{2K_C}k\tau\right) - b[2(K_C - 1)C_{A0} - a]}{[2(K_C - 1)C_{A0} - b]\exp\left(-\frac{a-b}{2K_C}k\tau\right) - [2(K_C - 1)C_{A0} - a]}$$

$$C_B = C_{B0} - C_{A0} + C_A; \quad C_C = C_{A0} + C_{C0} - C_A; \quad C_D = C_{A0} + C_{D0} - C_A$$

Mole balance for species A over the differential volume between V and $V + dV$ at steady state leads to

$$-d(QC_A) + r_A dV = 0 \tag{E5-1.1}$$

which leads to

$$Q_0 C_{A0} \frac{df_A}{-r_A} = dV = QC_{A0} \frac{df_A}{kC_A} = QC_{A0} \frac{df_A}{kC_{A0}(1 - f_A)} \tag{E5-1.2}$$

Therefore

$$dV = \frac{Q}{k} \frac{df_A}{1 - f_A} \tag{E5-1.3}$$

Integration of Eqn (E5-1.3) leads to

$$V = -\frac{Q}{k} \ln(1 - f_A) \tag{E5-1.4}$$

Substituting in the volumetric flow rate, rate constant, and conversion, we obtain

$$\boxed{V = -\frac{10\ \text{L/s}}{0.02/\text{s}} \ln(1 - 0.5) = 346.57\ \text{L}}$$

Example 5-2. Calculate (a) the reactor volume, V, (b) the residence time, $\bar{t}$, and (c) the space time, τ, and (d) explain any difference between the two time scales, for the gas-phase production of C_2H_4 from C_2H_6 in a cylindrical PFR of constant diameter, based on the following data and assumptions:

$$C_2H_6(A) \rightarrow C_2H_4(B) + H_2(C) \quad r = kC_A$$

1. The feed is pure C_2H_6 at 1 kg/s, 1000 K and 2 bar.
2. $k = 0.254$/min at 1000 K.
3. The reactor operates isothermally with negligible pressure drop.
4. $f_A = 0.20$ at the outlet.
5. Side reactions are negligible.
6. Ideal gas law can be used.

Solution. Figure E5-2 shows a schematic diagram of the PFR.

Mole balance for species A over a differential volume between V and $V + dV$ at steady state leads to

$$-dF_A + r_A dV = 0 \tag{E5-2.1}$$

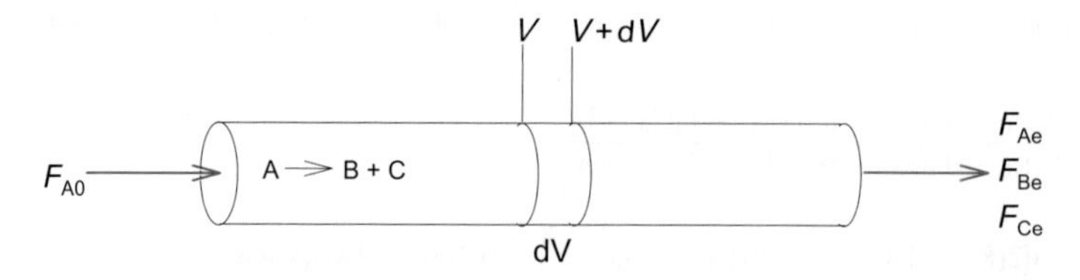

FIGURE E5-2 A schematic diagram of the PFR showing a differential control volume (V, $V + dV$).

which leads to

$$F_{A0}\frac{df_A}{-r_A} = dV = F_{A0}\frac{df_A}{kC_A} \tag{E5-2.2}$$

The concentration of A at any where in the reactor can be calculated through

$$C_A = \frac{F_A}{Q} = F_{A0}\frac{1-f_A}{Q} \tag{E5-2.3}$$

The volumetric flow rate changes in the reactor as the number of moles of the reaction mixture changes. The volumetric flow rate is proportional to the total molar flow rate change. Stoichiometry is needed to find the total molar flow rate. Table E5-2 shows a summary of stoichiometry.

TABLE E5-2 Stoichiometry of the Reaction System

Species	Initial	Change	At V
A	F_{A0}	$-F_{A0}f_A$	$F_{A0}(1-f_A)$
B	0	$F_{A0}f_A$	$F_{A0}f_A$
C	0	$F_{A0}f_A$	$F_{A0}f_A$
Total	F_{A0}	$F_{A0}f_A$	$F_{A0}(1+f_A)$

Based on ideal gas

$$PQ = FRT \tag{E5-2.4}$$

Since the pressure is constant, we have

$$\frac{Q}{Q_0} = \frac{F}{F_0} = 1 + f_A \tag{E5-2.5}$$

Substituting Eqn (E5-2.5) into Eqn (E5-2.3), we obtain

$$C_A = \frac{F_{A0}}{Q_0}\frac{1-f_A}{1+f_A} = C_{A0}\frac{1-f_A}{1+f_A} \tag{E5-2.6}$$

Substituting Eqn (E5-2.6) into Eqn (E5-2.2), we obtain

$$dV = \frac{F_{A0}}{kC_A}df_A = \frac{F_{A0}}{kC_{A0}}\frac{1+f_A}{1-f_A}df_A = \frac{Q_0}{k}\frac{1+f_A}{1-f_A}df_A \tag{E5-2.7}$$

Thus, the volume of the reactor by integration.

$$V = \frac{Q_0}{k}\int_0^{f_{Ae}} \frac{1+f_A}{1-f_A} df_A = \frac{Q_0}{k}\int_0^{f_{Ae}} \frac{2-(1-f_A)}{1-f_A} df_A$$

$$= \frac{Q_0}{k}\int_0^{f_{Ae}} \left[\frac{2}{1-f_A} - 1\right] df_A \qquad \text{(E5-2.8)}$$

$$= \frac{Q_0}{k}\left[-2\ln(1-f_{Ae}) - f_{Ae}\right]$$

Where the volumetric flow rate can be computed from the reactor inlet conditions based on ideal gas law,

$$Q_0 = \frac{F_{A0}RT_0}{p_0} = \frac{\dot{m}_0 RT_0}{p_0 M_A} \qquad \text{(E5-2.9)}$$

1. The required volume of the PFR can thus be computed using Eqn (E5-2.8). First, we need to find the volumetric flow rate at the reactor inlet. Since the mass flow rate is given, as well as the pressure and temperature. Using Eqn (E5-2.9)

$$Q_0 = \frac{\dot{m}_0 RT_0}{p_0 M_A} = \frac{1\text{kg/s} \times 8314\,\text{J/(kmol·K)} \times 1000\,\text{K}}{2 \times 10^5\text{Pa} \times (2 \times 12.011 + 6 \times 1.00794)\,\text{kg/kmol}}$$

$$= 1.38246\,\text{m}^3/s$$

Using Eqn (E5-2.8), we obtain

$$V = \frac{Q_0}{k}\left[-2\ln(1-f_{Ae}) - f_{Ae}\right] = \frac{1.38246\,\text{m}^3/s}{0.254\,\text{min}^{-1}/60(\text{s/min})}\left[-2\ln(1-0.2) - 0.2\right]$$

$$= 80.43\,\text{m}^3$$

2. Residence time for the reaction mixture passing through the differential volume as shown in Fig. E5-2 can be determined by

$$d\bar{t} = \frac{dV}{Q} \qquad \text{(E5-2.10)}$$

Substituting Eqns (E5-2.2) and (E5-2.3) into Eqn (E5-2.10), we obtain

$$d\bar{t} = \frac{dV}{Q} = F_{A0}\frac{df_A}{kC_A} \times \frac{1}{Q} = F_{A0}\frac{df_A}{kQC_A} = F_{A0}\frac{df_A}{kF_A}$$

which leads to

$$d\bar{t} = \frac{1}{k}\frac{df_A}{1-f_A} \qquad \text{(E5-2.11)}$$

Thus,

$$\bar{t} = \frac{1}{k}\int_0^{f_{Ae}} \frac{df_A}{1-f_A} = \frac{-\ln(1-f_{Ae})}{k} \tag{E5-2.12}$$

Plug in the numbers,

$$\bar{t} = \frac{-\ln(1-f_{Ae})}{k} = \frac{-\ln(1-0.2)}{0.254/\text{min}} = 0.8785 \text{ min}$$

3. The space time is defined as the reactor volume divided by the inlet volumetric flow rate,

$$\tau = \frac{V}{Q_0} \tag{E5-2.13}$$

In part (a), we have obtained the values for V and Q_0. Substituting V and Q_0 into the above equation, we obtain

$$\tau = \frac{V}{Q_0} = \frac{80.429 \text{ m}^3}{1.38246 \text{ m}^3/\text{s}} = 58.18 \text{ s} = 0.9696 \text{ min}$$

4. One can observe that $\tau \neq \bar{t}$. This is due to the change of flow rate or density of the reaction mixture in the reactor. As the reaction mixture density decreases in the reactor, the volumetric flow rate (or flow velocity) increases and the residence time decreases. The space time, however, is defined based on the inlet flow rate.

5.3. GASIFICATION AND FISCHER–TROPSCH TECHNOLOGY

Before leaving the tubular reactor discussions, let us examine the promising gasification and synthesis reactions and their reactors. This is a process in which the carbon and hydrogen raw material sources were first converted to basic building block chemicals: CO and H_2 and polymerize together to produce desired products.

$$n\text{CO} + 2n\text{H}_2 \rightarrow (\text{CH}_2)_n + n\text{H}_2\text{O} \tag{5.26}$$

This process was discovered and developed primarily in Germany during World Wars I and II to provide synthetic liquid fuels to compensate for the Allies blockade of crude oil shipment. [The argument can be made that both world wars were essentially fought over access to petroleum in the Caucasus region of Russia and the Middle East. The U.S. blockade of Japanese access to Far East crude oil was a major factor in Japan declaring war on the United States with the bombing of Pearl Harbor. These arguments are summarized in the book *The Prize* by Daniel Yergin.]

Fischer–Tropsch (FT) technology has been practiced on a large scale in South Africa because of the need for an independent source of liquid fuels during their political isolation, and they had abundant coal to make syngas. However, these processes are potentially an exceedingly important replacement for liquid fuels to use when crude oil supplies are

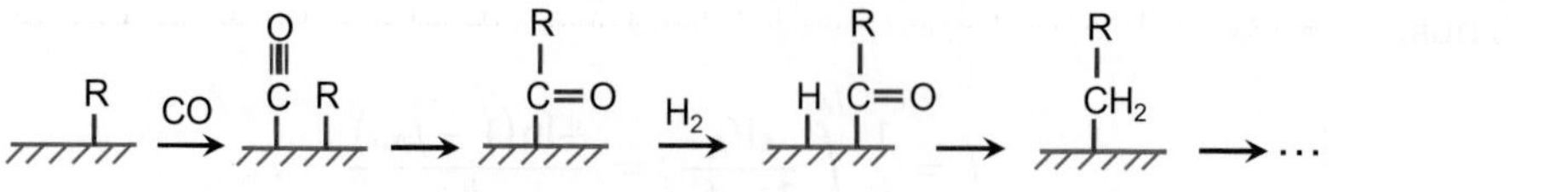

FIGURE 5.4 Proposed mechanism for Fischer–Tropsch polymerization of CO and H_2 to form alkane polymer.

depleted. Using coal (several hundred years supply in the United States alone) and natural gas (more proven reserves than petroleum), we can be assured of sources of liquid fuels for transportation through this technology long after supplies of crude oil and even natural gas have been used up. The more prominent use of Fischer–Tropsch technology is the renewable biomass feedstock, as petroleum, natural gas, and coal will eventually be depleted. Biomass as we know it is renewable and will not be depleted as long as the Sun is sending out rays.

Fischer and Tropsch found that when a mixture of CO and H_2 was heated to about 250 °C at high pressures over an iron catalyst, polymer would form, and under suitable conditions this had the appropriate molecular weight for gasoline and diesel fuel. Different metal catalysts give different molecular weights (Ni produces CH_4) and different amounts of alkanes (Fe and Re), olefins (Ru), and alcohols (Rh); so catalysts and process conditions can be altered to produce a desired molecular weight and distribution.

The products are essentially all linear molecules, which for olefins and alcohols have the double bond or the OH group on the end carbon (α-olefins and α-alcohols). The mechanism of this polymerization process is thought to be similar to (but also very different from) Ziegler Natta (ZN) polymerization of ethylene and propylene on Ti. It is thought that CO adsorbs and hydrogenates (perhaps to form the CH_2 group) on an adsorption site adjacent to an adsorbed alkyl R, as shown in Fig. 5.4. If the CH_2 inserts between the metal and the adsorbed R, one obtains and adsorbed RCH_2-, which can add another CH_2 to form RCH_2CH_2-, and the chain repeats itself indefinitely until the adsorbed alkyl dehydrogenates to olefin, hydrogenates to paraffin, or hydrates to α-alcohol.

The CO and H_2 (syngas) for FT synthesis were initially made by the gasification of coal, which was plentiful in Germany. Coal contains various amounts of H depending on the sources (CH_x, with $0 < x < 1$), but hydrogen content is usually very low. For simplicity, let us consider the gasification of carbon

$$C + H_2O \rightarrow CO + H_2 \tag{5.27}$$

Starting from a stoichiometric feed of carbon and water, the gas-phase equilibrium mixture is dependent on the temperature. In the gas phase, various compounds can form. The most common ones are CO, H_2, CO_2, and CH_4, and other larger molecules. For simplicity, let us consider the four most abundant compounds only. The reactions involved are

$$CO + H_2O \rightarrow CO_2 + 2H_2 \tag{5.28}$$

$$2CO + 2H_2 \rightarrow CO_2 + CH_4 \tag{5.29}$$

Figure 5.5 shows the equilibrium compositions for the gasification of carbon as a function of temperature. One can observe that the gas mixture consists of mostly CO and H_2 at 1:1 at high temperatures (greater than 900 °C). At lower temperatures, equilibrium favors the formation of CO_2 and CH_4 in the gas mixture instead of H_2O.

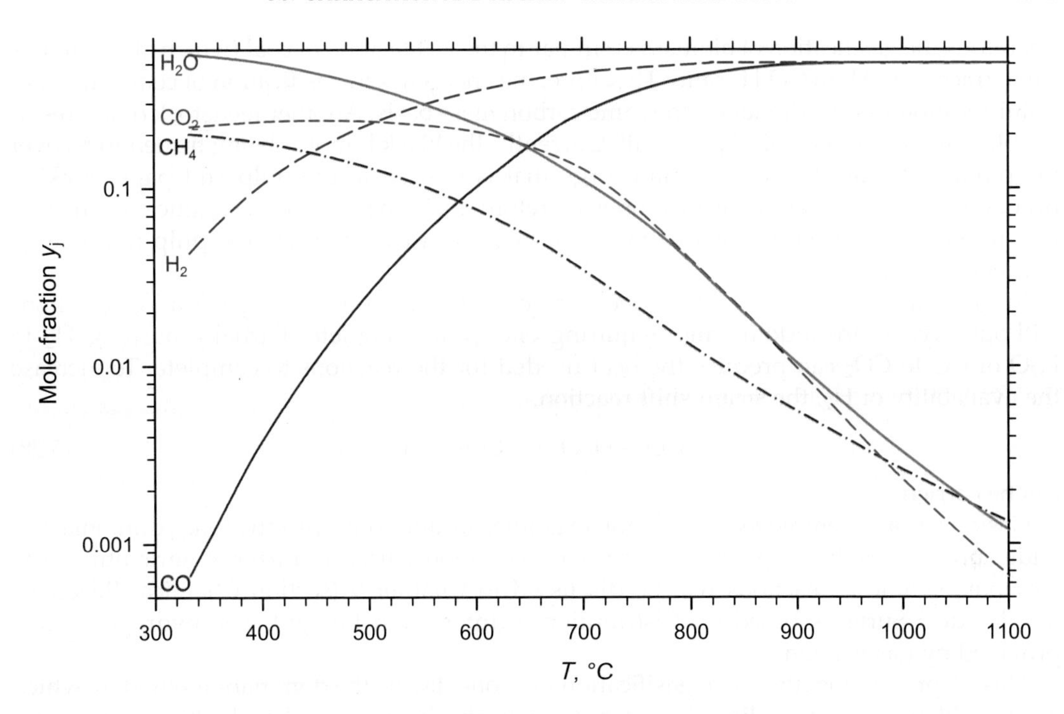

FIGURE 5.5 Equilibrium mole fractions for the carbon-steam reaction as a function of temperature.

Syngas can also be made using naphtha or other hydrocarbon feedstocks, such as the methane from natural gas,

$$CH_4 + H_2O \rightarrow CO + 3H_2 \tag{5.30}$$

Note that coal produces CO and H_2 in a 1:1 ratio, naphtha in a 1:2 ratio, and methane in a 1:3 ratio. Because of the need in thermal energy to shift the reactions forward, oxygen (or air) is usually supplied to partially oxidize the carbon (and hydrogen) to maintain energy balance. An excess of H_2 is thus usually desired; so alkanes are the preferred feedstock.

Existing syngas plants operate by direct oxidation of natural gas

$$CH_4 + {}^1/_2O_2 \rightarrow CO + 2H_2 \tag{5.31}$$

using pure O_2 from a liquid air plant. This process, called autothermal reforming, uses this exothermic reaction in an adiabatic reactor and produces the 1:2 ratio of CO:H_2 that is ideal for methanol or FT processes.

Today, more attention is paid to the gasification of renewable biomass. Lignocellulosic biomass holds the most promising position in a sustainably renewable world. Dry lignocellulosic biomass can be approximated by $CH_{1.47}O_{0.57}$. Gasification of lignocellulosic biomass leads to

$$CH_{1.43}O_{0.57} + (0.43 + 2\nu_{O_2})H_2O - \nu_{O_2}\,O_2 \rightarrow CO + (1.145 + 2\nu_{O_2})H_2 \tag{5.32}$$

Therefore, the gasification of biomass is similar to the gasification of coal (which also contains small fraction of H) in $CO:H_2$ ratio. Therefore, the energetics in gasification of coal and lignocellulosic biomass are similar on the same carbon mass basis. Another feedstock of interest is the black liquor in a chemical pulp mill. Currently, the black liquor is being turned to recover the pulping chemicals and thermal energy that is needed in the pulp and paper making processes. The black liquor gasification is therefore not going to make a significant contribution to our needs in liquid fuel or hydrocarbon, but it can improve the pulp mill energy efficiency.

In gasification, O_2 is usually added for energetics reasons. The gasification reactions without oxygen are indothermic, requiring energy to complete. Partially burning H_2 to H_2O or CO to CO_2 can produce the heat needed for the reactions to complete. To increase the availability of H_2, the steam shift reaction,

$$CO + H_2O \rightarrow CO_2 + H_2 \tag{5.28}$$

can be carried out.

Gasidfication is employed today, for example, in ammonia production. Ammonia has wide applications. It is a precursor for urea, a commonly used fertilizer in agriculture. The ammonia synthesis reactions will be discussed in Chapter 9 (section Chemical Reactions on Nonideal Surfaces Based on Distribution of Interaction Energy). The hydrogen gas is provided by gasification.

This FT process together with gasification may one day be the dominant method by which we will obtain some of our liquid fuels from renewable biomass, and coal. This technology is capable of supplying at least 200 years of liquid hydrocarbons at current consumption rates from known proven reserves of coal. The biomass as renewable resources, on the other hand, can supply our needs for liquid fuel "indefinitely."

Two types of reactors will be discussed, a *straight-through transport reactor,* which is also referred to as a *riser* or *circulating fluidized bed,* and a PBR, which is also referred to as *a fixed-bed reactor.*

Riser. Because the catalyst used in the process decays rapidly at high temperatures (e.g. 350 °C), a *straight-through transport reactor* is ideal. This type of reactor is also called a *riser* and/or a circulating bed. A schematic diagram is shown in Fig. 5.6. Here the catalyst particles are fed to the bottom of the reactor and are shot up through the reactor together with the entering reactant gas mixture and then separated from the gas in a settling hopper. The volumetric gas feed rate is high in order to suspend and transport the particles upward against the gravity. In Sasol plant, South Africa, the gas feed rate is 3×10^5 m^3/h.

A schematic of an industrial *straight-through transport reactor* used at Sasol are shown in Fig. 5.7 together with the composition of the feed and product streams. The products that are condensed out of the product stream before the stream is recycled include Synoil (a synthetic crude), water, methyl ethyl ketone, alcohols, acids, and aldehydes. The reactor is operated at 25 atm and 350 °C and at anyone time contains 150 tons of catalyst. The catalyst feed rate is 6–9.5 tons/s, and the gas recycle ratio is 2:1.

Packed-Bed. Transport of solid particles upward requires high fluid velocity and thus energy consumption. To reduce the energy consumption in the reactor, the solid catalyst can be fixed in the reactor. The packed-bed reactor used at the Sasol plant, South Africa to

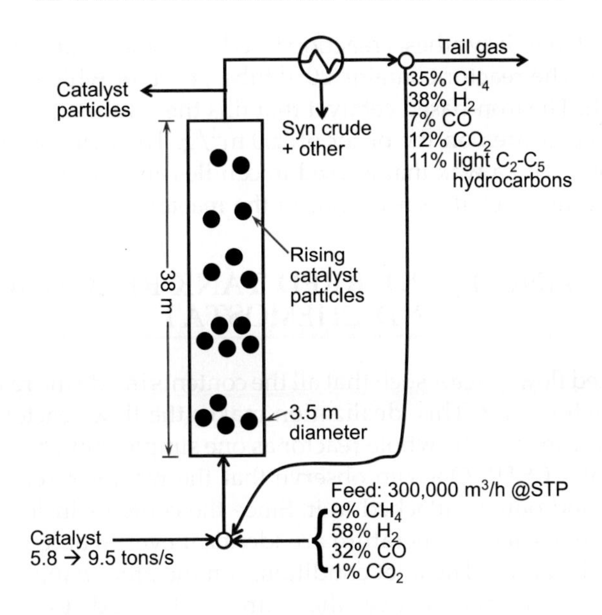

FIGURE 5.6 Schematic of Sasol Fischer–Tropsch process.

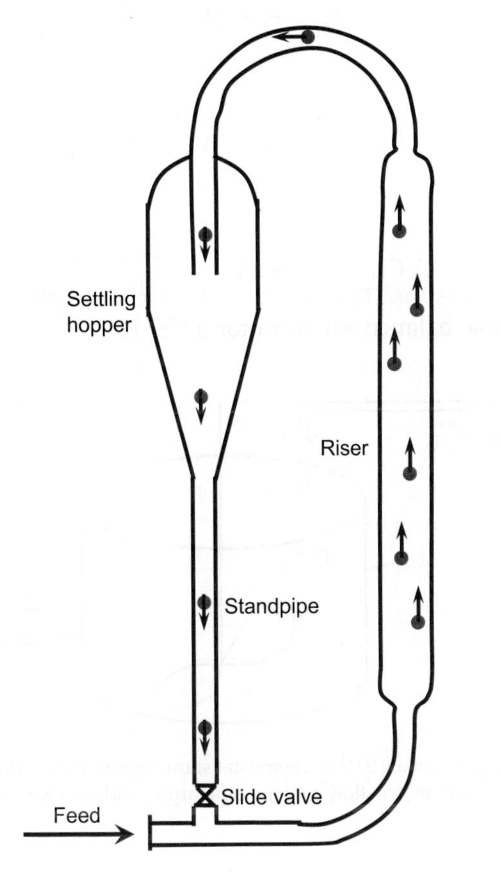

FIGURE 5.7 A schematic of reactor system, where the detailed flow of the riser is shown in Fig. 5.6.

carry out Fischer–Tropsch synthesis reaction is fed at a syngas rate of 30,000 m^3/h (STP) at 240 °C and 27 atm. The reactor contains 2050 tubes, each of which is 5.0 cm in diameter and 12 m in length. The iron-based catalyst that fills these tubes usually contains K_2O and SiO_2 and has a specific area on the order of 200 m^2/g. The reaction products are light hydrocarbons along with a wax that is used in candles and printing inks. Approximately, 50% conversion of the reactant is achieved in the reactor.

5.4. CONTINUOUS STIRRED TANK REACTOR (CSTR) AND CHEMOSTAT

CSTR is an idealized flow reactor such that all the contents inside the reactor are well mixed, just like that in a batch reactor. This idealization makes the flow reactor analysis simplified extremely as now one can treat the whole reactor as one simple unit or "black box." Figure 5.8 shows a schematic of a CSTR. One can observe that the reactor resembles a batch reactor, however with inlets and outlets attached to it. Since the contents inside the reactor are well mixed, the concentrations and temperature are identical everywhere inside the reactor and are equal to those at the outlet. The inlet conditions, on the other hand, can be different.

Mole balance for a given species j over the entire reactor leads to

$$F_{j0} - F_j + r_j V = \frac{dn_j}{dt} \tag{5.33}$$

which leads to

$$F_{j0} - F_j + r_j V = V\frac{dC_j}{dt} + C_j\frac{dV}{dt} \tag{5.34}$$

or

$$Q_0 C_{j0} - QC_j + r_j V = V\frac{dC_j}{dt} + C_j\frac{dV}{dt} \tag{5.35}$$

which is the general mole balance equation for a CSTR.

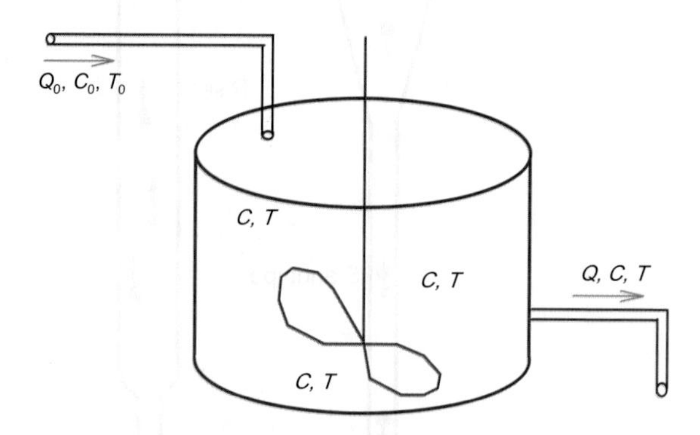

FIGURE 5.8 Schematic diagram of a CSTR or chemostat showing one stream flowing in and one stream flowing out of the reactor, with proper volumetric flow rates, temperature, and concentrations.

Since the total amount of mass cannot be created or destroyed during chemical and bioreactions, we obtain through mass balance over the entire reactor as shown in Fig. 5.6,

$$\rho_0 Q_0 - \rho Q = \frac{\mathrm{d}(\rho V)}{\mathrm{d}t} = \rho \frac{\mathrm{d}V}{\mathrm{d}t} + V \frac{\mathrm{d}\rho}{\mathrm{d}t} \tag{5.36}$$

For condensed matters, density is only a function of temperature. In general,

$$\rho = \sum_{j=1}^{N_S} C_j M_j \tag{5.37}$$

Equations (5.33) through (5.37) are equally applicable to batch reactors. Therefore, these equations are more general mole balance equations for any well-mixed reactors. In a general case, Eqn (5.35) needs to be written each for every component (species) except one involved. Like the plug flow reactions, momentum balance equation is needed to close the problem. Thus, we would have N_S differential equations to solve even for an isothermal reactor. If temperature changes, the energy balance equation must be solved simultaneously as well. In addition, we need to know how Q would vary with time.

We next consider more simplified case, where steady-state condition has reached. In fact, most times when we say CSTR or Chemostat, we mean CSTR at steady state. At steady state, nothing changes with time. Therefore, Eqns (5.33) and (5.35) are reduced to

$$F_{j0} - F_j + r_j V = 0 \tag{5.38}$$

or

$$Q_0 C_{j0} - Q C_j + r_j V = 0 \tag{5.39}$$

which are algebraic equations.

For a single reaction that is carried out in a steady CSTR, there is only one independent concentration or reaction mixture content variable and all other concentrations can be related through stoichiometry as shown in Chapter 3. Without loss of generosity, let us use component A as the key component of consideration. Equation (5.38) applied to species A gives

$$F_{A0} - F_A + r_A V = 0 \tag{5.40}$$

or

$$Q_0 C_{A0} - Q C_A + r_A V = 0 \tag{5.41}$$

These algebraic equations can be solved easily.

$$V = \frac{F_{A0} - F_A}{-r_A} = \frac{F_{A0} f_A}{-r_A} \tag{5.42}$$

or

$$V = \frac{Q_0 C_{A0} - Q C_A}{-r_A} \tag{5.43}$$

Note that the rate of reaction is evaluated at the reactor outlet conditions.

In general, the rate of reaction is a function of concentration and temperature. From Chapter 3, we learned that the stoichiometry can be applied to relate the amount of every species in the reaction mixture. The amount change of a component participating in the reaction divided by its stoichiometric coefficient is the universal extent of reaction for a single reaction. The stoichiometry can be written in a flow reactor as

$$\frac{F_{j0} - F_j}{\nu_j} = \frac{F_{A0} - F_A}{\nu_A} = rV \tag{5.44}$$

The total molar flow rate can be computed by adding all the component (species) flow rates up. That is

$$F = \sum_{j=1}^{N_S} F_j = \sum_{j=1}^{N_S}\left(F_{j0} + \nu_j \frac{F_A - F_{A0}}{\nu_A}\right) = F_0 + \frac{F_A - F_{A0}}{\nu_A}\sum_{j=1}^{N_S}\nu_j \tag{5.45}$$

Letting ν_Σ be the total stoichiometric coefficients, i.e.,

$$\nu_\Sigma = \sum_{j=1}^{N_S}\nu_j \tag{5.46}$$

We obtain

$$F = F_0 + \frac{\nu_\Sigma}{\nu_A}(F_A - F_{A0}) = F_0 - \frac{\nu_\Sigma}{\nu_A}F_{A0}f_A \tag{5.47}$$

While the above derivation is concise, we often tabularize the stoichiometry to gain a thorough understanding of the stoichiometry for every species, either be those involved in the reaction or those that are not participating in the actual reaction. The stoichiometry is shown in Table 5.3.

The concentration can be related to the molar flow rate through

$$C_j = \frac{F_j}{Q} = \frac{F_{j0} - \dfrac{\nu_j}{\nu_A}F_{A0}f_A}{Q} \tag{5.48}$$

The volumetric flow rate Q can be a function of temperature and pressure (density change). Since the mass flow rate does not change if no side inlets or outlets, we have

$$Q = \frac{\rho_0}{\rho}Q_0 \tag{5.49}$$

TABLE 5.3 Stoichiometry of a Reaction System with Side Inlets or Outlets

Species	At inlet	Change	At outlet
A	F_{A0}	$F_A - F_{A0}$	F_A
j	F_{j0}	$F_j - F_{j0} = \nu_j \frac{F_A - F_{A0}}{\nu_A}$	$F_j = F_{j0} + \nu_j \frac{F_A - F_{A0}}{\nu_A}$
...	...	...	...
Total	F_0	$\sum_{j=1}^{N_s}(F_j - F_{j0}) = \nu_\Sigma \frac{F_A - F_{A0}}{\nu_A}$	$\sum_{j=1}^{N_s}F_j = F_0 + \nu_\Sigma \frac{F_A - F_{A0}}{\nu_A}$

$$C_j = \frac{\rho}{\rho_0}\frac{F_{j0} + \dfrac{\nu_j}{\nu_A}(F_A - F_{A0})}{Q_0} = \frac{\rho}{\rho_0}\frac{F_{j0} - \dfrac{\nu_j}{\nu_A}F_{A0}f_A}{Q_0} \tag{5.50}$$

For isothermal operations, Q is constant for reactions involving condensed matter (liquid or solid) only. For ideal gas, the volumetric flow rate can be related to the molar flow rate through ideal gas law

$$PQ = FRT \tag{5.51}$$

which leads to

$$Q = \frac{P_0 T}{P T_0}\frac{F}{F_0}Q_0 = \frac{P_0 T}{P T_0}\left[1 + \frac{\nu_\Sigma}{\nu_A}\frac{F_A - F_{A0}}{F_0}\right]Q_0 = \frac{P_0 T}{P T_0}\left[1 - \frac{\nu_\Sigma}{\nu_A}\frac{F_{A0}}{F_0}f_A\right]Q_0 \tag{5.52}$$

Example 5-3. Rework example 5-1 for a CSTR. An elementary first-order reaction:

$$A \rightarrow B$$

is to be carried out in a CSTR. If the rate constant $k = 0.02/\text{s}$ and the volumetric flow rate is constant at 10 L/s, calculate the reactor volume required for 50% conversion.

Solution. Figure E5-3 shows a schematic diagram of the constant density CSTR.

Mole balance for species A over the entire CSTR volume at steady state leads to

$$(QC_A)_0 - (QC_A) + r_A V = 0 \tag{E5-3.1}$$

which leads to

$$QC_{A0}\frac{f_A}{-r_A} = V = QC_{A0}\frac{f_A}{kC_A} = QC_{A0}\frac{f_A}{kC_{A0}(1 - f_A)} \tag{E5-3.2}$$

Therefore

$$V = \frac{Q}{k}\frac{f_A}{1 - f_A} \tag{E5-3.3}$$

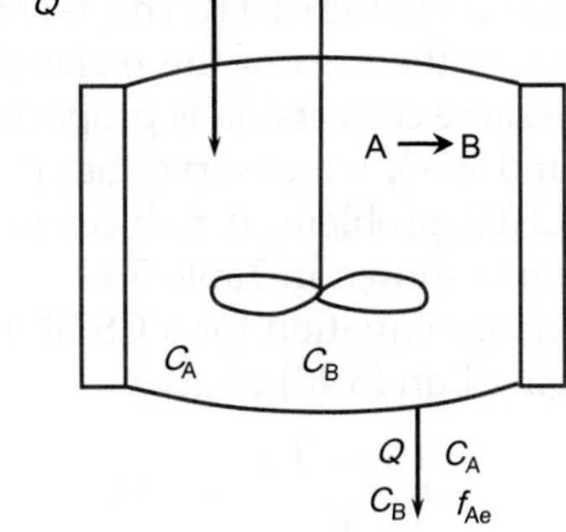

FIGURE E5-3 A schematic diagram of a constant density CSTR.

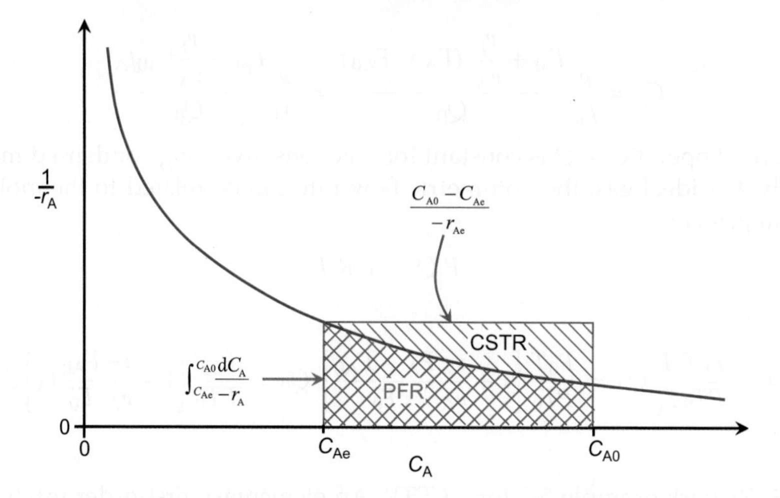

FIGURE 5.9 Schematic diagram of the different reactor volume requirement for a CSTR and a PFR. The volume of CSTR required is proportional to the whole rectangular area, whereas the volume of a PFR required is proportional to the area underneath the curve only.

Substituting in the volumetric flow rate, rate constant, and conversion, we obtain

$$V = \frac{10\ \text{L/s}}{0.02\ \text{s}^{-1}} \times \frac{0.5}{1 - 0.5} = 500\ \text{L}$$

Compared with the 346.57 L required for a PFR at the same reaction conditions, CSTR is much bigger.

Example 5-3 shows that the required reactor volume for a CSTR is bigger than a PFR (Example 5-1) for the same reaction conditions and reactor throughput. The difference is due to the level of concentration inside the reactor. For a PFR, the concentration changes from inlet to outlet with reactant concentration being highest at the inlet, thus faster reaction near inlet when the reactor is run under isothermal conditions. However, for a CSTR, the concentrations are uniform in the reactor and are identical to those in the outlet. Therefore, the reactant concentration is at lowest in the CSTR. This is shown in Fig. 5.9. The CSTR reactor volume required is proportional to the area of the rectangle, whereas the required reactor volume for a PFR to achieve the same conversion is proportional to the area under the curve.

Comparing examples E5-1 and E5-3, we observe that the solution to a CSTR is easier to achieve than to a PFR. For a CSTR problem, it reduces to a (set of) algebraic equation(s). For simple kinetics, this solution is shown in Table 5.4.

The solution to the molar balance equation for a CSTR at steady state, Eqn (5.40), can be visually illustrated by rearranging Eqn (5.40) to give

$$\frac{F_{A0} - F_A}{V} = -r_A \tag{5.53}$$

which is the molar change rate of A in a CSTR per reactor volume. One can observe that the left-hand side is the molar rate of A fed subtracted the molar rate of A letting out of the

TABLE 5.4 Steady-State Solutions of Reactions in a Constant Density CSTR with Simple Rate Law Expressions

1. Zero order: A → Products, $r = k$

$$C_A = \max[C_{A0} - k\tau,\ 0];\ \tau = \frac{C_{A0} - C_A}{k}$$

2. Half-order: A → Products, $r = k\,C_A^{1/2}$

$$C_A = \frac{k^2\tau^2 + 2C_{A0} - k\tau\sqrt{k^2\tau^2 + 4C_{A0}}}{2};\ \tau = \frac{C_{A0} - C_A}{kC_A^{1/2}}$$

3. First-order: A → Products, $r = k\,C_A$

$$C_A = \frac{C_{A0}}{1 + k\tau};\ \tau = \frac{C_{A0} - C_A}{kC_A};$$

4. Second-order: A → Products, $r = k\,C_A^2$

$$C_A = \frac{\sqrt{1 + 4k\tau C_{A0}} - 1}{2k\tau};\ \tau = \frac{C_{A0} - C_A}{kC_A^2};$$

5. Second-order: A + B → Products, $r = k\,C_A C_B$

$$C_A = \frac{\sqrt{[1 - k\tau(C_{A0} - C_{B0})]^2 + 4k\tau C_{A0}} - 1 + k\tau(C_{A0} - C_{B0})}{2k\tau};\ C_B = C_{B0} - C_{A0} + C_A$$

$$\tau = \frac{C_{A0} - C_A}{kC_A(C_{B0} - C_{A0} + C_A)};$$

6. Autocatalytic: A + R → 2R + Products, $r = k\,C_A C_R$

$$C_A = \frac{1 + k\tau(C_{A0} + C_{R0}) - \sqrt{[1 + k\tau(C_{A0} + C_{R0})]^2 - 4k\tau C_{A0}}}{2k\tau};\ C_R = C_{R0} + C_{A0} - C_A$$

$$\tau = \frac{C_{A0} - C_A}{kC_A(C_{A0} + C_{R0} - C_A)};$$

(Continued)

TABLE 5.4 Steady-State Solutions of Reactions in a Constant Density CSTR with Simple Rate Law Expressions—*Cont'd*

7. Unimolecular catalytic: $A \rightarrow$ Products, $r = \dfrac{kC_A}{K_A + C_A}$

$$C_A = \frac{\sqrt{(K_A - C_{A0} + k\tau)^2 + 4K_A C_{A0}} - K_A + C_{A0} - k\tau}{2}; \quad \tau = \frac{C_{A0} - C_A}{kC_A}(K_A + C_A);$$

8. Unimolecular: $A \rightarrow$ Products, $r = \dfrac{kC_A^2}{K_A + C_A}$

$$C_A = \frac{\sqrt{K_A^2 + 4(1 + k\tau)C_{A0}} - K_A}{2(1 + k\tau)}; \quad \tau = \frac{C_{A0} - C_A}{kC_A^2}(K_A + C_A)$$

9. First-order reversible: $A \rightleftarrows B$, $r = k_f C_A - k_b C_B$

$$C_A = \frac{C_{A0} + k_b\tau(C_{A0} + C_{B0})}{1 + (k_f + k_b)\tau}; \quad \tau = \frac{C_{A0} - C_A}{k_f C_A - k_b(C_{A0} + C_{B0} - C_A)};$$

10. First-order reversible catalytic: $A \rightleftarrows B$, $r = \dfrac{k(C_A - C_B/K_C)}{1 + K_A C_A + K_B C_B}$

$$C_A = \frac{\sqrt{[1 + K_B(2C_{A0} + C_{B0}) + k\tau(1 + 1/K_C) - K_A C_{A0}]^2 - 4(K_A - K_B)[C_{A0} + (C_{A0} + C_{B0})(K_B C_{A0} + k\tau/K_C)]} - 1 - K_B(2C_{A0} + C_{B0}) - k\tau(1 + 1/K_C) + K_A C_{A0}}{2(K_A - K_B)};$$

$$C_A = \frac{C_{A0} + (C_{A0} + C_{B0})(K_B C_{A0} + k\tau/K_C)}{1 + K_B(2C_{A0} + C_{B0}) + k\tau(1 + 1/K_C) - K_A C_{A0}} \quad \text{if } K_A = K_B$$

$$\tau = \frac{C_{A0} - C_A}{k[C_A - (C_{A0} + C_{B0} - C_A)/K_C]}[1 + K_A C_A + K_B(C_{A0} + C_{B0} - C_A)]$$

11. Second-order reversible: $A \rightleftarrows B + C$, $r = k_f C_A - k_b C_B C_C$

$$C_A = \frac{1 + k_f\tau + k_b\tau(C_{B0} + C_{C0} + 2C_{A0}) - \sqrt{[1 + k_f\tau + k_b\tau(C_{B0} + C_{C0} + 2C_{A0})]^2 - 4k_b\tau[C_{A0} + k_b\tau(C_{B0} + C_{A0})(C_{C0} + C_{A0})]}}{2k_b\tau};$$

$$\tau = \frac{C_{A0} - C_A}{k_f C_A - k_b(C_{A0} + C_{B0} - C_A)(C_{A0} + C_{C0} - C_A)}$$

12. Second-order reversible: $A + B \rightleftarrows R$, $r = k_f C_A C_B - k_b C_R$

$$C_A = \frac{\sqrt{[1 - k_f\tau(C_{A0} - C_{B0}) + k_b\tau]^2 + 4k_f\tau[C_{A0} + k_b\tau(C_{A0} + C_{R0})]} - 1 + k_f\tau(C_{A0} - C_{B0}) - k_b\tau}{2k_f\tau}$$

$$\tau = \frac{C_{A0} - C_A}{k_f C_A(C_{B0} - C_{A0} + C_A) - k_b(C_{A0} + C_{R0} - C_A)}$$

13. Second-order reversible: $A + B \rightleftarrows C + D$, $r = k_f C_A C_B - k_b C_C C_D$

$$C_A = \frac{\sqrt{[1 - k_f\tau(C_{A0} - C_{B0}) + k_b\tau(C_{C0} + C_{D0} + 2C_{A0})]^2 + 4(k_f - k_b)\tau[C_{A0} + k_b\tau(C_{A0} + C_{C0})(C_{A0} + C_{D0})]} - 1 + k_f\tau(C_{A0} - C_{B0}) + k_b\tau(C_{C0} + C_{D0} + 2C_{A0})}{2(k_f - k_b)\tau}$$

$$C_A = \frac{C_{A0} + k_b\tau(C_{A0} + C_{D0})(C_{A0} + C_{D0})}{1 - k_f\tau(C_{A0} - C_{B0}) + k_b\tau(C_{C0} + C_{D0} + 2C_{A0})} \quad \text{if } k_f = b_b$$

$$\tau = \frac{C_{A0} - C_A}{k_f C_A(C_{B0} - C_{A0} + C_A) - k_b(C_{A0} + C_{C0} - C_A)(C_{A0} + C_{D0} - C_A)}$$

reactor, divided by the reactor volume. Thus, one can refer the left-hand side as the molar supply rate per reactor volume or simply molar supply rate. That is

$$MS_A = \frac{F_{A0} - F_A}{V} \tag{5.54}$$

which can be rearranged to give

$$MS_A = F_{A0}\frac{f_A}{V} = Q_0 C_{A0}\frac{f_A}{V} = \frac{C_{A0} f_A}{\tau} \tag{5.55a}$$

or

$$MS_A = \frac{Q_0 C_{A0} - Q C_A}{V} = \frac{C_{A0} - \frac{\rho}{\rho_0} C_A}{\tau} \tag{5.55b}$$

Therefore, the molar rate supply of A to a CSTR is linearly related to the conversion, Eqn (5.55a). If the density remains constant, $\rho = \rho_0$, then the molar supply rate of A to a CSTR is also linearly related to the concentration of A. In other words, when density is constant, the molar supply rate of A to the CSTR is a straight on the supply rate vs concentration plane.

Let us now look at the right-hand side in the context of molar balance. It is the molar consumption rate (or negative molar generation rate) of A. That is,

$$MC_A = -r_A \tag{5.56}$$

The molar balance equation can thus be expressed as the molar supply rate of A to the reactor (MS_A) equals to the molar consumption rate of A (MC_A) in the reactor. The solution to a CSTR problem is thus visually illustrated in Fig. 5.10: on the two-dimensional graph of "molar

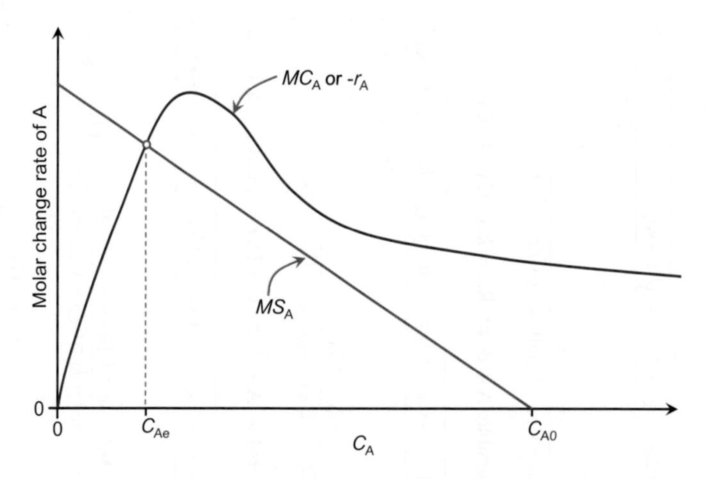

FIGURE 5.10 Realizing mole balances in a CSTR. The molar consumption rate of A, MC_A, is same as the rate of reaction of A, $-r_A$, in the CSTR operating conditions, whereas the molar supply rate of A (molar feed rate of A subtract the molar rate of A letting out of the CSTR), MS_A, changes linearly with the concentration for a constant density reactor.

change rate of A" vs "concentration of A" (or "fractional conversion of A"), the steady-state solution is the intercept between the "molar supply rate" and the "molar consumption rate". That is,

$$MC_A = MS_A \tag{5.57}$$

Example 5-4. Consider the reaction:

$$A \rightarrow B,\ k = 0.15/\text{min}$$

in a CSTR. A costs \$2/mol, and B sells for \$5/mol. The cost of operating the reactor is \$0.03/L/h. We need to produce 100 mol of B/h using $C_{A0} = 2$ mol/L. Assume no value or cost of disposal of unreacted A (i.e. separation or recovery cost to A is identical to the fresh A cost).

1. Perform a mole balance on the reactor to relate the conversion with reactor size.
2. What is the optimum conversion and reactor size?
3. What is the cash flow (or profit per mole of A feed to the reactor) from the process?
4. At what operating cost do we break-even?

Solution. A sketch of the reactor system is shown in Fig. E5-4.

1. It is understood that the CSTR is operating under constant temperature (isothermal) and steady-state conditions, i.e. no accumulation of any sort of materials inside the reactor. Mole balance around the reactor for B yields

$$0 - F_B + r_B V = 0 \tag{E5-4.1}$$

The rate law gives

$$r_B = \nu_B r = kC_A \tag{E5-4.2}$$

It is understood that the reaction mixture density is not changing, i.e. the volumetric flow rates at the reactor inlet and the outlet are nearly unchanged. We have

$$C_A = \frac{F_A}{Q} = \frac{F_{A0}(1 - f_A)}{Q} = C_{A0}(1 - f_A) \tag{E5-4.3}$$

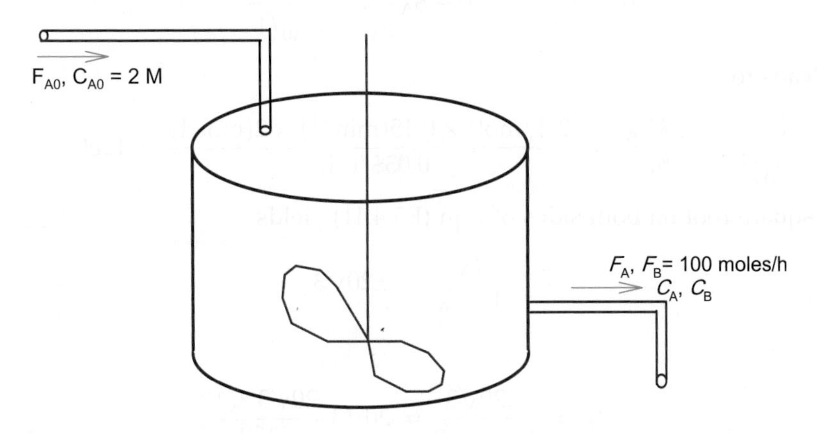

FIGURE E5-4 Well-mixed reaction vessel.

Substituting Eqns (E5-4.2) and (E5-4.3) into Eqn (E5-4.1), we obtain

$$V = \frac{F_B}{r_B} = \frac{F_B}{kC_{A0}(1-f_A)} \tag{E5-4.4}$$

2. Based on the economic information at hand, we can estimate the gross profit for the reaction process as

$$GP\$ = \$_B F_B - \$_A F_{A0} - \$_V V \tag{E5-4.5}$$

where $\$_B$, $\$_A$, and $\$_V$ are the molar value of product B, molar cost of reactant A, and the unit operating cost of reactor based on the reactor volume and time; respectively. Based on the stoichiometry, we have

$$F_B = F_{A0} - F_A = F_{A0} f_A \tag{E5-4.6}$$

which leads to

$$F_{A0} = \frac{F_B}{f_A} \tag{E5-4.7}$$

Substituting Eqns (E5-4.7) and (E5-4.4) into Eqn (E5-4.5), we obtain

$$GP\$ = \$_B F_B - \$_A \frac{F_B}{f_A} - \$_V \frac{F_B}{kC_{A0}(1-f_A)} \tag{E5-4.8}$$

To find the optimum conversion, we maximize the gross profit. That is starting by setting

$$\frac{dGP\$}{df_A} = 0 \tag{E5-4.9}$$

Since the flow rate of product B is fixed, not a function of the conversion f_A, we have,

$$0 = \frac{dGP\$}{df_A} = 0 + \$_A \frac{F_B}{f_A^2} - \frac{\$_V F_B}{kC_{A0}(1-f_A)^2} \tag{E5-4.10}$$

which leads to

$$\frac{f_A^2}{(1-f_A)^2} = \frac{\$_A k C_{A0}}{\$_V} = \frac{2(\$/\text{mol}) \times 0.15(\text{min}^{-1}) \times 2(\text{mol/l})}{0.03\$/(\text{l h})} = 1200 \tag{E5-4.11}$$

Taking square root on both sides of Eqn (E5-4.11) yields

$$\frac{f_A}{1-f_A} = \pm 20\sqrt{3} \tag{E5-4.12}$$

Thus,

$$f_A = \frac{\pm 20\sqrt{3}}{1 \pm 20\sqrt{3}} = 20\sqrt{3}\,\frac{20\sqrt{3} \pm 1}{1199} \tag{E5-4.13}$$

Since the conversion of A must be between 0 (no conversion) and 1 (100% conversion) in order for it to be physically possible, we discard the value that is greater than unit and obtain

$$f_A = 20\sqrt{3}\,\frac{20\sqrt{3}-1}{1199} = 0.97194 \tag{E5-4.14}$$

Next, we check if indeed this conversion gives the maximum gross profit. We can either plot out the variation of GP$ vs f_A to see if we indeed having a maximum GP$ at this f_A value or checking the second derivative of GP$,

$$\frac{d^2GP\$}{df_A^2} = -\frac{2\$_A F_B}{f_A^3} - \frac{2\$_V F_B}{kC_{A0}(1-f_A)^3} \tag{E5-4.15}$$

Plug in the values we know up until this step, we obtain

$$\frac{d^2GP\$}{df_A^2} = -\frac{2\times 2(\$/\text{mol})\times 100(\text{mol/h})}{0.97194^3}$$

$$-\frac{2\times 0.03[\$/(1\,\text{h})]\times 100(\text{mol/h})}{0.15(\text{min}^{-1})\times 60(\text{min/h})\times 2(\text{mol/l})\times(1-0.97194)^3}$$

$$= -15527(\$/\text{h}) < 0$$

A negative second-order derivative means that the value of GP$ is lower for either higher or lower f_A. Thus, we indeed have obtained a maximum value of the gross profit at the conversion of $f_A = 0.97194$. This confirms that the optimum conversion is $f_A = 0.97194$. The reactor size can be computed from Eqn (E5-4.4)

$$V = \frac{F_B}{kC_{A0}(1-f_A)} = \frac{100}{0.15\times 60\times 2\times(1-0.97194)}\,1 = 197.99\,1$$

3. The cash flow based on the optimum conversion:

$$\frac{GP\$}{F_{A0}} = \frac{\$_B F_B}{F_{A0}} - \$_A\frac{F_B}{f_A F_{A0}} - \$_V\frac{F_B}{kC_{A0}(1-f_A)F_{A0}}$$

$$= \$_B f_A - \$_A - \frac{\$_V f_A}{kC_{A0}(1-f_A)}$$

$$= 5\times 0.97194 - 2 - \frac{0.03\times 0.97194}{0.15\times 60\times 2\times(1-0.97194)}\$/\text{mol}-\text{A}$$

$$= \$2.802/\text{mol}-\text{A}$$

4. At breaking even point, the net profit (or in this case the gross profit) is zero. Therefore, at the break-even point, operating cost and the value of product are equal.
The value of product is,

$$\$_B F_B = 5\times 100\,\$/\text{h} = 500\,\$/\text{h}$$

which is also the operating cost at break-even.

The operating conditions for the break-even point can be obtained by setting the gross profit to zero. This was not asked here.

$$0 = \text{GP\$} = \$_B F_B - \$_A \frac{F_B}{f_A} - \$_V \frac{F_B}{kC_{A0}(1-f_A)} \tag{E5-4.16}$$

which can be rearranged to

$$f_A^2 - \left(1 + \frac{\$_A}{\$_B} - \frac{\$_V}{\$_B kC_{A0}}\right) f_A + \frac{\$_A}{\$_B} = 0 \tag{E5-4.17}$$

or

$$f_A^2 - \frac{4199}{3000} f_A + \frac{2}{5} = 0 \tag{E5-4.18}$$

Solving Eqn (E5-4.18), we obtain

$$f_A = 0.99944424 \text{ or } 0.400222$$

This concludes the solution to Example 5-4.

5.5. MULTIPLE REACTORS

Multiple reactors are frequently employed in industry, either because of efficiency or the space/size limitations. Reactors can be connected in parallel or in series. Figures 5.11–5.14 show some examples of the multiple reactor systems.

When performing analysis on multiple reactors, the easiest way is to number the reactors in sequence as illustrated in Fig. 5.11. It is then convenient to work with concentrations and flow rates that are identified for exiting each reactor. Reactors in parallel are analyzed in a manner identical to that for single reactors except that the flow rate is split (only a portion of the total inlet flow to the reactor system enters a particular reactor). For reactors connected in series, the total flow rates are the same as the flow rate entering the reactor system. However, the compositions in each reactor are different. The inlet conditions are identical

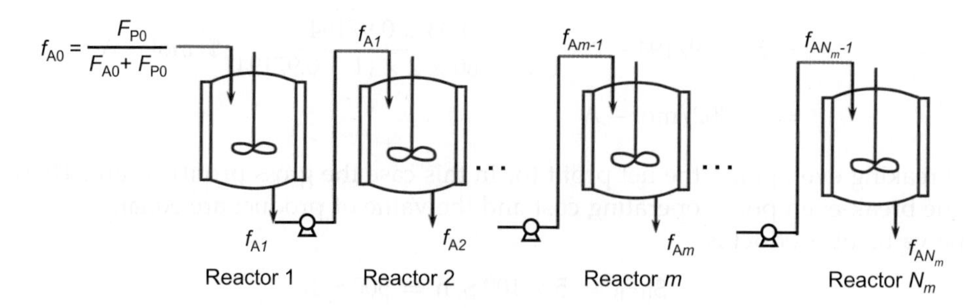

FIGURE 5.11 A CSTR train: multiple CSTR's connected in series.

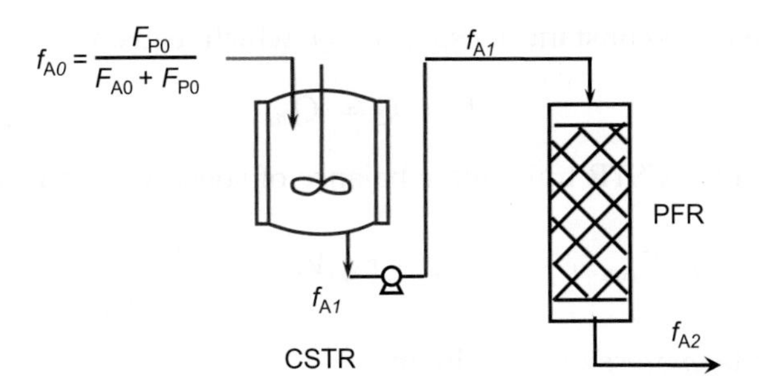

FIGURE 5.12 A CSTR is placed in front of a PFR.

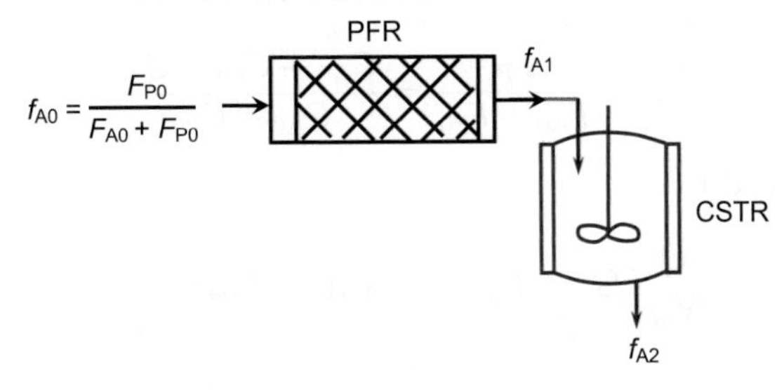

FIGURE 5.13 A PFR is placed in front of a CSTR.

to those exiting the one reactor placed ahead when no heat exchanger (cause temperature change) or separation devices (cause composition and/or flow rate to change) were placed in between the reactors.

If you work with fractional conversion, it is then convenient to define the conversion based on the total "unreacted reactant" in the feed, that is, converting the products back to the reactants. In this way, the fractional conversion is not set to zero at any reactor inlet and thus the fractional conversion becomes a continuous variable that can be used for all the reactors in series.

We use a simple reaction to illustrate the steps of solution

$$A \rightarrow P, \; r = kC_A \tag{5.58}$$

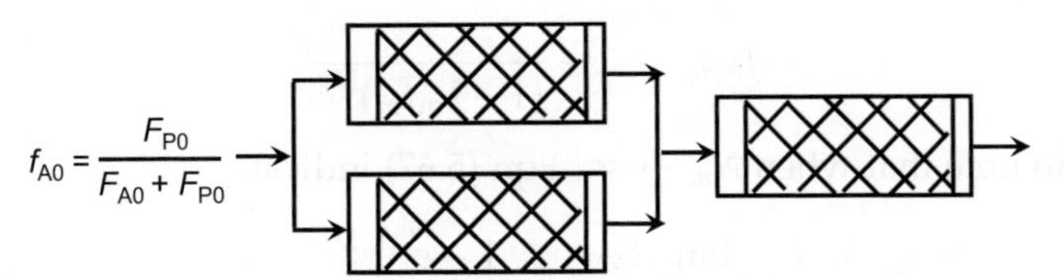

FIGURE 5.14 A schematic of a multiple reactors with two PFR's connected in parallel before connected with another PFR in series.

The reaction mixture has a constant density, $\rho_0 = \rho$, which leads to

$$Q_0 = Q = Q_m \tag{5.59}$$

For the mth reactor in the CSTR train, mole balance of species A leads to

$$Q_{m-1}C_{Am-1} - Q_m C_{Am} + r_{Am} V_m = \left[\frac{dn_A}{dt}\right]_{V_m} = 0 \tag{5.60}$$

Substituting in the rate expression, we obtain

$$\frac{Q}{V_m}(C_{Am-1} - C_{Am}) - k_m C_{Am} = 0 \tag{5.61}$$

Using fractional conversion based on the total unreacted feed:

$$f_A = \frac{F_P}{F_{A0} + F_{P0}} = \frac{C_{A0} + C_{P0} - C_A}{C_{A0} + C_{P0}} \tag{5.62}$$

Equation (5.56) is reduced to

$$\frac{Q}{V_m}(f_{Am} - f_{Am-1}) - k_m(1 - f_{Am}) = 0 \tag{5.63}$$

Letting

$$\bar{t}_m = \frac{V_m}{Q} \tag{5.64}$$

Equation (5.63) can be rearranged to yield

$$f_{Am} = \frac{f_{Am-1} + k_m \bar{t}_m}{1 + k_m \bar{t}_m} \tag{5.65}$$

which can be solved to yield

$$f_{AN_m} = 1 - \frac{1}{\prod_{m=1}^{N_m}(1 + k_m \bar{t}_m)} \tag{5.66}$$

If the reactors are operated at the same temperature, no change in catalyst, and all the reactors are of the same size, Eqn (5.66) can be further reduced to

$$f_{AN_m} = 1 - \frac{1}{(1 + k_m \bar{t}_m)^{N_m}} \tag{5.67}$$

It is interesting to note that when $N_m \to \infty$, Eqn (5.67) indicates

$$\lim_{N_m \to \infty} f_{AN_m} = 1 - e^{k_m \bar{t}_m N_m} \tag{5.68}$$

since the total residence time, $N_m \bar{t}_m$ is finite. The solution for a PFR is recovered.

Example 5-5. The elementary reaction

$$A + R \rightarrow 2R$$

with a rate constant $k = 0.02$ L/mol/s is to be carried out isothermally in flow reactors. We wish to process 120 L/min of a feed containing 5 mol/L of A to the highest conversion possible in the reactor system consisting of one 100-L PFR and one 100-L CSTR, connected as you wish and any feed arrangement.

1. Sketch your recommended design and feed arrangement;
2. Determine the final conversion.

Solution. To begin with the solution, let us first examine the reaction stoichiometry and kinetics. The reaction system can be considered as constant density: isothermal, no molar change. Stoichiometry leads to

$$C_A + C_R = C_{A0} + C_{R0} = C_{A0} \tag{E5-5.1}$$

The reaction rate is given by

$$r_A = \nu_A r = -kC_A C_R = -kC_A(C_{A0} - C_A) \tag{E5-5.2}$$

1. Equation (E5-5.2) shows that when $C_R = 0$, the reaction rate is zero. That is, a PFR with a fresh feed would not convert any reactant to the product. The CSTR is thus placed in the front, followed by the PFR. Figure E5-5.1 shows a sketch of the reactor system.
2. Mole balance of A around the first reactor, CSTR, as shown in Fig. E5-5.1 leads to

$$QC_{A0} - QC_{A1} + r_{A1}V_1 = 0 \tag{E5-5.3}$$

Substituting Eqn (E5-5.2) into (E5-5.3), we obtain

$$QC_{A0} - QC_{A1} - kC_{A1}(C_{A0} - C_{A1})V_1 = 0 \tag{E5-5.3}$$

which is a quadratic equation on C_{A1} that can be solved to give

$$C_{A1} = \frac{Q + kC_{A0}V_1 \pm \sqrt{(Q + kC_{A0}V_1)^2 - 4QkC_{A0}V_1}}{2kV_1} = \frac{Q + kC_{A0}V_1 \pm (Q - kC_{A0}V_1)}{2kV_1} \tag{E5-5.4}$$

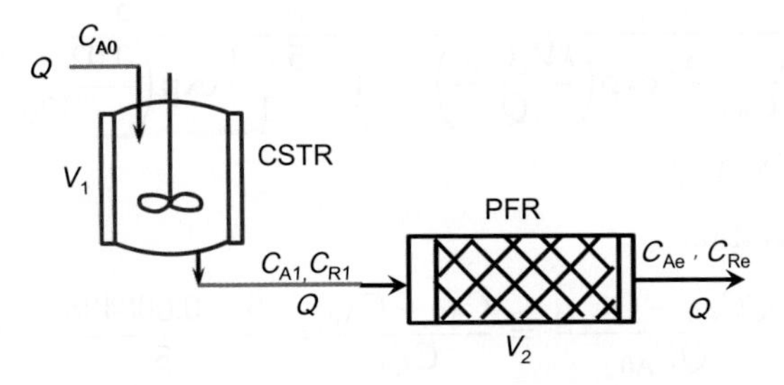

FIGURE E5-5.1 A sketch of the reactor system with one CSTR in front, followed by one PFR, in series.

There are two solutions: $C_{A1} = C_{A0}$ and

$$C_{A1} = \frac{Q}{kV_1} \tag{E5-5.5}$$

Clearly, this second solution is the one desired. The first solution is the trivial solution where no product was present prior to the reactor start-up. Substitute the numbers into Eqn (E5-5.5), we obtain

$$C_{A1} = \frac{Q}{kV_1} = \frac{120/60}{0.02 \times 100}\,\text{mol/L} = 1\ \text{mol/L}$$

Mole balance of A in a differential volume along the axis of the PFR (V, $V + dV$) leads to

$$-d(QC_A) + r_A dV = 0 \tag{E5-5.6}$$

Since Q is constant, substituting Eqn (E5-5.2) into Eqn (E5-5.6) and rearranging, we obtain

$$kdV = -\frac{QdC_A}{C_A(C_{A0} - C_A)} = -\left(\frac{1}{C_A} + \frac{1}{C_{A0} - C_A}\right)\frac{QdC_A}{C_{A0}} \tag{E5-5.7}$$

Integrating Eqn (E5-5.7) around the PFR (or the second reactor in Fig. E5-5.1),

$$\int_0^{V_2} kdV = \int_{C_{A1}}^{C_{Ae}} -\left(\frac{1}{C_A} + \frac{1}{C_{A0} - C_A}\right)\frac{QdC_A}{C_{A0}} \tag{E5-5.8}$$

we obtain

$$kV_2 = \frac{Q}{C_{A0}} \ln \frac{C_{A1}(C_{A0} - C_{Ae})}{C_{Ae}(C_{A0} - C_{A1})} \tag{E5-5.9}$$

Equation (E5-5.9) can be rearranged to give

$$C_{Ae} = \frac{C_{A0}}{1 + \dfrac{C_{A0} - C_{A1}}{C_{A1}} \exp\left(\dfrac{kV_2 C_{A0}}{Q}\right)} \tag{E5-5.10}$$

Substituting in the numbers, we have

$$C_{Ae} = \frac{C_{A0}}{1 + \dfrac{C_{A0} - C_{A1}}{C_{A1}} \exp\left(\dfrac{kV_2 C_{A0}}{Q}\right)} = \frac{5}{1 + \dfrac{5-1}{1} \exp\left(\dfrac{0.02 \times 100 \times 5}{120/60}\right)}\,\text{mol/L}$$
$$= 0.008408\ \text{mol/L}$$

The final conversion is thus

$$f_{Ae} = \frac{QC_{A0} - QC_{Ae}}{QC_{A0}} = \frac{C_{A0} - C_{Ae}}{C_{A0}} = \frac{5 - 0.008408}{5} = 0.9983$$

The conversion is at 99.83%.

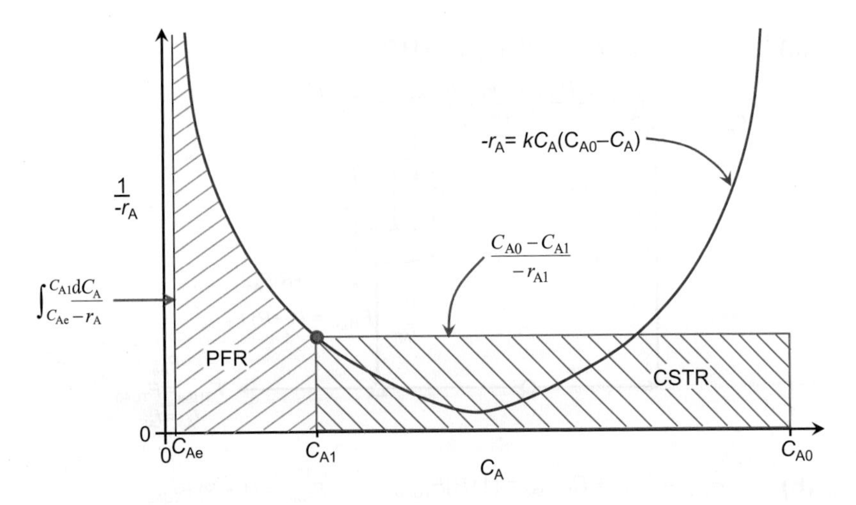

FIGURE E5-5.2 A sketch of the equal-volume CSTR and PFR reactor in series system for an autocatalytic reaction.

Figure E5-5.2 illustrates the solution of this example on the $(-r_A)^{-1}$ vs C_A plot. This figure helps us understand the volume of the CSTR is proportional to the rectangular area with the top line corresponding to the reactor exit condition. Lower $(-r_{Ae})^{-1}$ or higher reaction rate at the reactor outlet reduces the reactor volume requirement. The volume of the PFR, on the other hand, is proportional to the area under the rate curve.

5.6. RECYCLE REACTORS

Recycle reactors represent cases where part of the reactor effluent is returned to the reactor inlet. In particular, this setup is useful for recycling the unreacted reactants, and/or catalysts. To simplify the derivations, we introduced a new (fictitious) flow rate: flow rate of total unreacted A (TUA). TUA means that all the products are reacted (reversely) back to reactant A.

Figure 5.15 shows illustrations of how CSTR and PFR can be setup in general. The feed is consisted of A (F_{A0}) and some products (F_{TUA0} may not be equivalent to F_{A0}). The required effluent from the reactor system consisted of F_{Ae} and overall conversion f_{Ae}. If we use conversion to work through the problem, we have the fractional conversion at the inlet to the reactor system:

$$f_{A0} = \frac{F_{TUA0} - F_{A0}}{F_{TUA0}} \tag{5.69}$$

The fractional conversion of A leaving the reactor system is given by

$$f_{Ae} = \frac{F_{TUAe} - F_{Ae}}{F_{TUAe}} \tag{5.70}$$

Let us assume that the ratio of flow that is recycled is R (recycle ratio) times the flow rate leaving the reactor system. Since there are no other outlets leaving the reactor system, the total molar flow rate at the only inlet (to the reactor system) and the outlet are identical.

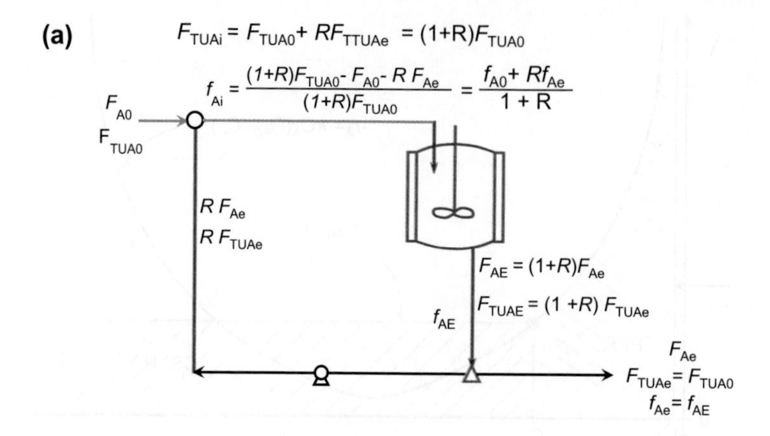

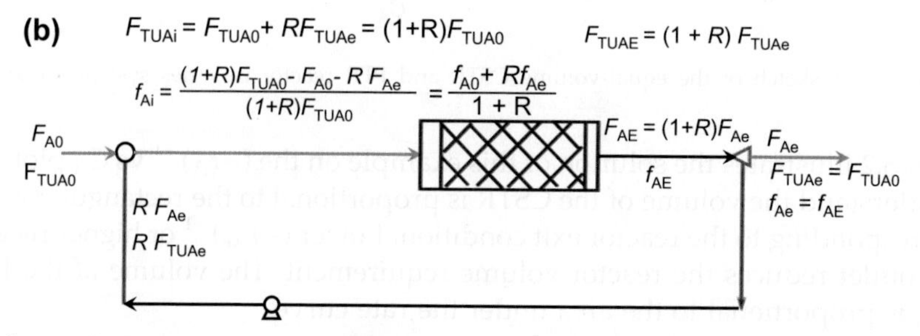

FIGURE 5.15 A schematic of a recycle reactor system. The reactor outlet is split into two fractions, with one fraction returned to the reactor inlet. (a) Recycle CSTR; (b) Recycle PFR.

Because the splitter does not alter the compositions of the streams in this case, the fractional conversion at the reactor outlet is the same as that at the reactor system outlet.

$$f_{AE} = f_{Ae} \tag{5.71}$$

and the total molar flow rate at the reactor outlet is given by

$$F_{TUAE} = (1+R)F_{TUAe} = (1+R)F_{TUA0} \tag{5.72}$$

$$F_{AE} = (1+R)F_{Ae} \tag{5.73}$$

The reactor inlet stream is a combined stream of two, one from the reactor system inlet and the other is the recycle stream. Thus, molar balance leads to

$$F_{TUAi} = F_{TUA0} + RF_{TUAe} = (1+R)F_{TUA0} \tag{5.74}$$

$$F_{Ai} = F_{A0} + RF_{Ae} \tag{5.75}$$

and the fractional conversion of A at the reactor inlet is given by

$$f_{Ai} = \frac{F_{TUAi} - F_{Ai}}{F_{TUAi}} = \frac{(1+R)F_{TUA0} - F_{A0} - RF_{Ae}}{(1+R)F_{TUA0}} = 1 - \frac{1-f_{A0}}{1+R} - R\frac{1-f_{Ae}}{1+R} = \frac{f_{A0} + Rf_{Ae}}{1+R} \tag{5.76}$$

Once we figured out the flow rates passing through the reactor, and the compositions (in this case, we have used the fractional conversion) at the inlet and outlet of the reactor, we can then just focus on the reactor. We perform the reactor analysis the same way as would do for an ideal flow reactor. For example, for a recycle PFR, we have

$$V = \frac{F_{TUAi}}{-\nu_A}\int_{f_{Ai}}^{f_{AE}} \frac{df_A}{r} = \frac{F_{A0}}{-\nu_A}\frac{1+R}{1-f_{A0}}\int_{\frac{f_{A0}+Rf_{Ae}}{1+R}}^{f_{Ae}} \frac{df_A}{r} \tag{5.77}$$

Recycle reactors are useful for autocatalytic reactions as the product is required for the reaction to take place. The key to simplification of recycle reactors, like multiple reactors, is to use the same basis for conversion.

Example 5-6. The elementary reaction

$$A + R \rightarrow 2R$$

with a rate constant $k = 0.02\,\text{L} \cdot \text{mol}^{-1} \cdot \text{s}^{-1}$ is to be carried out isothermally in a plug flow reactor having a working volume of 200 L. We wish to process 120 L/min of a feed containing 5 mol/L of A to the highest conversion possible in the reactor with any feed arrangement. Find the optimum conversion achievable.

Solution. As discussed in Example 5-5, this is an autocatalytic reaction that requires the product in the reactor to proceed. Stoichiometry leads to

$$C_A + C_R = C_{A0} + C_{R0} = C_{A0} \tag{E5-6.1}$$

The reaction rate is given by

$$r_A = \nu_A r = -kC_A C_R = -kC_A(C_{A0} - C_A) \tag{E5-6.2}$$

When PFR is used, one must recycle the final product stream back to the feed in order for the reaction to proceed in the reactor. Figure E5-6.1 shows a sketch of the reactor system.

A simple split at ② is employed for recycle the effluent stream to the feed point ①. Mass balance around point ① (mixing for feed into the reactor) leads to

$$Q_{\text{PFR Feed}} = (S1 + R)Q \tag{E5-6.3}$$

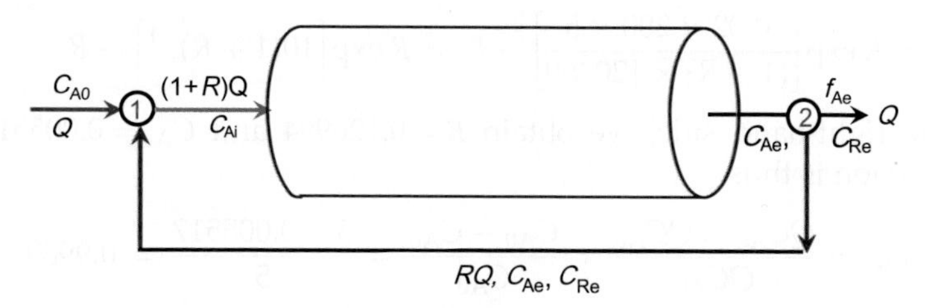

FIGURE E5-6.1 A sketch of a simple recycle PFR system.

and the concentration of A in the feed into PFR is given by

$$C_{Ai} = \frac{QC_{A0} + RQC_{Ae}}{(1+R)Q} = \frac{C_{A0} + RC_{Ae}}{1+R} \tag{E5-6.4}$$

Mole balance of A in a differential volume within the PFR (V, $V + \mathrm{d}V$) leads to

$$-\mathrm{d}[(1+\mathrm{R})QC_A] + r_A\,\mathrm{d}V = 0 \tag{E5-6.5}$$

Since Q is constant, substituting Eqn (E5-6.2) into Eqn (E5-6.5) and rearranging, we obtain

$$k\mathrm{d}V = -\frac{(1+R)Q\mathrm{d}C_A}{C_A(C_{A0} - C_A)} = -\left(\frac{1}{C_A} + \frac{1}{C_{A0} - C_A}\right)\frac{(1+R)Q\mathrm{d}C_A}{C_{A0}} \tag{E5-6.6}$$

Integrating Eqn (E5-6.6) around the PFR,

$$\int_0^V k\mathrm{d}V = \int_{C_{Ai}}^{C_{Ae}} -\left(\frac{1}{C_A} + \frac{1}{C_{A0} - C_A}\right)\frac{(1+R)Q\mathrm{d}C_A}{C_{A0}} \tag{E5-6.7}$$

we obtain

$$kV = \frac{(1+R)Q}{C_{A0}}\ln\frac{C_{Ai}(C_{A0} - C_{Ae})}{C_{Ae}(C_{A0} - C_{Ai})} \tag{E5-6.8}$$

Substituting Eqn (E5-6.4) into Eqn (E5-6.8), we obtain

$$kV = \frac{(1+R)Q}{C_{A0}}\ln\frac{C_{A0} + RC_{Ae}}{RC_{Ae}} \tag{E5-6.9}$$

Equation (E5-6.9) can be rearranged to give

$$C_{Ae} = \frac{C_{A0}}{R\exp\left[\frac{kVC_{A0}}{(1+R)Q}\right] - R} \tag{E5-6.10}$$

or

$$\frac{C_{A0}}{C_{Ae}} = R\exp\left[\frac{kVC_{A0}}{(1+R)Q}\right] - R \tag{E5-6.11}$$

The optimum recycle ratio is one that minimizes C_{Ae} or maximizes C_{A0}/C_{Ae}. Substituting in the numbers in Eqn (E5-6.11), we have

$$\frac{C_{A0}}{C_{Ae}} = R\exp\left[\frac{0.02 \times 200 \times 5}{(1+R) \times 120/60}\right] - R = R\exp\left[10(1+R)^{-1}\right] - R \tag{E5-6.12}$$

Maximizing the right-hand side, we obtain $R = 0.126994$ and $C_{Ae} = 0.005517$ mol/L. The optimum conversion is thus

$$f_{Ae} = \frac{QC_{A0} - QC_{Ae}}{QC_{A0}} = \frac{C_{A0} - C_{Ae}}{C_{A0}} = \frac{5 - 0.005517}{5} = 0.9989$$

The conversion is at 99.89%.

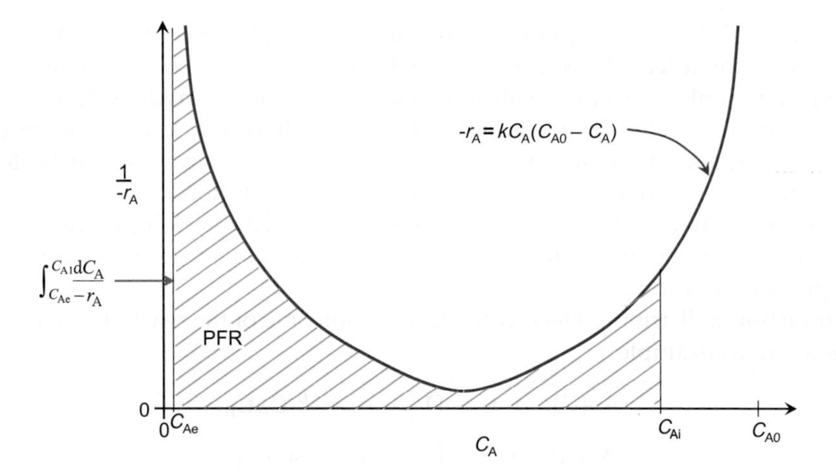

FIGURE E5-6.2 A sketch of one single recycle plug flow reactor on the reciprocal of reaction rate vs concentration plane.

Figure E5-6.2 illustrate the recycle plug flow reactor on the $(-r_A)^{-1}$ vs C_A plot. The recycle of the effluent stream into the reactor caused the concentration of A entering the reactor to be lower than C_{A0} and thus ensures a finite value of $(-r_A)^{-1}$. Since the volume of the PFR is proportional to the area under the rate curve, the finite value of $(-r_A)^{-1}$ ensures a finite reactor volume requirement. For the fixed volume reactor, this ensures the concentration of the effluent to be lower than the feed concentration.

5.7. DISTRIBUTED FEED AND WITHDRAW

Chemical and biological reactions normally involve multiple components and multiple reactions occurring simultaneously. In some cases, the desired products are formed from an equilibrium limiting step whereby the efficiency is restricted due to the maximum amount of desired products can be formed at a given feed composition. In some cases, the desired product is an intermediate product along the overall reaction pathway. Still, in other cases, the reaction that forms the desired product has a different concentration dependence on rate. All these cases would benefit if one could either feed some of the reactants gradually or remove the some of products from reaction mixture.

5.7.1. Distributed Feed

For parallel reactions, multiple products form the same set of reactants at the same reaction conditions. There are several ways to optimize the bioprocess system for desired product production (and thus efficiency) or selectivity $s_{P/A}$ or $S_{P/A}$: 1) selection of pressure (if gas phase reaction), temperature, and different solvents; 2) catalyst selection or development; 3) changing type of reactor; and 3) changing the way the reactants are being added to the reactor. In this section, we are interested in how the selectivity can be altered by changing the way the reactants are fed to the reactor.

One example of interest is pulping or conversion of plant biomass into fibers via chemical processes. There are at least three groups of substances in the woody biomass: hemicelluloses, lignin, and cellulose. All these substances react with sodium hydroxide at high temperatures, with different rates. The concentration of alkali is the key factor in cellulose/hemicellulose degradation, which occurs while lignin is reacting with caustic to degrade into small molecules and become soluble in aqueous solution. Modern kraft pulping digesters are built with distributed white liquor feed as well as black liquor removal capabilities. The aim is to maintain constant alkali concentration (a key reactant for pulping) and degraded product concentration.

To illustrate how a distributed feed can affect the outcome of the reaction, we use a parallel reaction network as example:

$$\mathrm{A} + \mathrm{B} \rightarrow \mathrm{C} + \mathrm{D} \qquad r_1 = k_1 C_\mathrm{A} C_\mathrm{B} \tag{5.78}$$

$$\mathrm{A} + \mathrm{B} \rightarrow \mathrm{E} + \mathrm{F} \qquad r_2 = k_2 C_\mathrm{A} C_\mathrm{B}^m \tag{5.79}$$

If product E is the desired product, we can write the differential selectivity of E as

$$s_{\mathrm{E/A}} = \frac{\mathrm{d}F_\mathrm{A}|_{\text{due to the formation of E}}}{\mathrm{d}F_\mathrm{A}|_{\text{total}}} = \frac{r_{2\mathrm{A}}}{r_{1\mathrm{A}} + r_{2\mathrm{A}}} = \frac{-k_2 C_\mathrm{A} C_\mathrm{B}^m}{-k_1 C_\mathrm{A} C_\mathrm{B} - k_2 C_\mathrm{A} C_\mathrm{B}^m} = \frac{k_2 C_\mathrm{B}^{m-1}}{k_1 + k_2 C_\mathrm{B}^{m-1}} \tag{5.80}$$

Therefore, the level of concentration of B in the reactor affects the selectivity to the formation of product E. Either high or low concentration of B will change the product mix if m is not exactly unity. Figure 5.16 shows three possible selected reactor feeding schemes. Figure 5.16a will give the highest possible concentrations of both A and B in the reactor. Figure 5.16b is a case where the concentration of B is maximum in the reactor, while the concentration A is maintained at minimum (the same as when the reaction is complete, i.e. the outlet). Figure 5.16c is a case where the concentration of A is maximum in the reactor, while the concentration B is maintained at minimum (the same as when the reaction is complete, i.e. the outlet). If a CSTR was chosen, we would have the lowest concentrations of both A and B in the reactor, which would be equivalent to those in the reactor outlet.

Example 5-7. Product distribution for parallel reactions.

We wish to produce R in the following reaction:

$$\mathrm{A} + \mathrm{B} \rightarrow \mathrm{R}, \qquad r_1 = \frac{k_1 C_\mathrm{A} C_\mathrm{B}^{1/2}}{1 + K_\mathrm{A} C_\mathrm{A} + K_\mathrm{B} C_\mathrm{B}^{1/2}} \tag{E5-7.1}$$

Unfortunately a side reaction occurs, where product P is formed

$$\mathrm{A} + \mathrm{B} \rightarrow \mathrm{P}, \qquad r_2 = \frac{k_2 C_\mathrm{B}}{1 + K_\mathrm{A} C_\mathrm{A} + K_\mathrm{B} C_\mathrm{B}^{1/2}} \tag{E5-7.2}$$

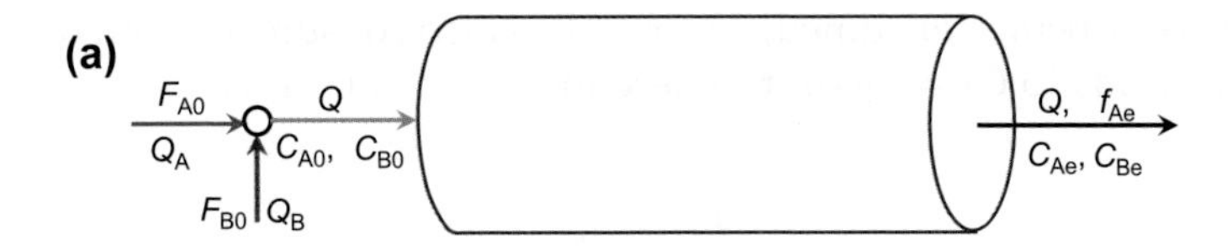

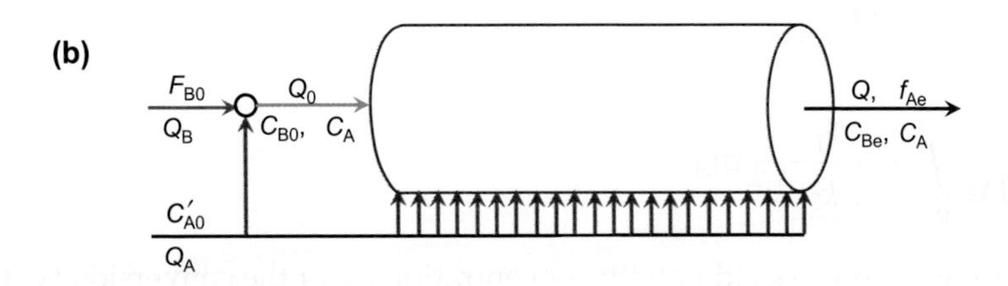

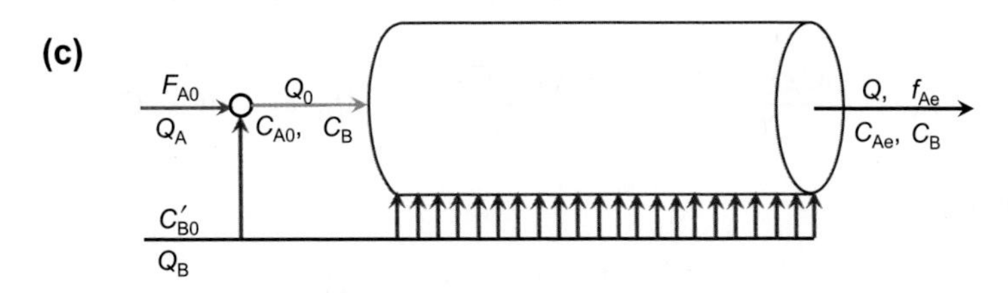

FIGURE 5.16 Selected feed schemes for a two reactant systems in PFR. (a) Feeding both A and B at the beginning. (b) Feeding B at the beginning, while maintaining C_A constant by adjusting the feed distributed along the reactor. (c) Feeding A at the beginning, while maintaining C_B constant by adjusting the feed distributed along the reactor.

For 90% conversion of A, find the concentration of R in the product stream as a function of the reaction rate constants. Equal volumetric flow rates of the A and of the B streams are fed to the reactor, and each stream has a concentration of 20 mol/L of the said reactant. The rate parameters are: $k_1 = 0.1\ \text{mol}^{-1/2} \cdot \text{L}^{1/2} \cdot \text{min}^{-1}$; $k_2 = 0.2\ \text{min}^{-1}$; $K_A = 10\ \text{mol}^{-1} \cdot \text{L}$; and $K_B = 5\ \text{mol}^{-1/2} \cdot \text{L}^{1/2}$. The flow in the reactor follows:

1. PFR;
2. CSTR;
3. The best of the three PFR contacting (feeding) schemes in Fig. 5.16.

Solution. As a warning, be careful to get the concentrations and flow rates right when you mix the streams. To begin with, we find the differential selectivity of the desired product

$$s_{R/A} = \frac{dF_A|_{\text{due to the formation of R}}}{dF_A|_{\text{total}}} = \frac{r_{1A}}{r_{1A} + r_{2A}} = \frac{k_1 C_A}{k_1 C_A + k_2 C_B^{1/2}} \tag{E5-7.3}$$

One can solve the problem by performing mole balances on each species and solve the differential equations using an automatic integrator. We can also do it more illustrative by using the differential selectivity as defined by Eqn (E5-7.3). This is the approach we will be taking here.

1. PFR. Referring to Fig. 5.16a, noting that the starting concentration of each reactant in the combined feed is $C_{A0} = C_{B0} = 20\ \text{mol/L} \div 2 = 10\ \text{mol/L}$. Based on the stoichiometry,

for every mole of A being consumed, 1 mol of B is also consumed (both desired and side reactions). This leads to $C_A = C_B$ everywhere in the reactor. Thus,

$$S_{R/A} = \frac{\Delta F_A|_{\text{due to the formation of R}}}{\Delta F_A|_{\text{total}}} = \frac{\int_0^{f_{Ae}} S_{R/A} df_A}{f_{Ae} - 0} = \frac{1}{f_{Ae}} \int_0^{f_{Ae}} \frac{k_1 C_A}{k_1 C_A + k_2 C_B^{1/2}} df_A \tag{E5-7.4}$$

$$= \frac{1}{f_{Ae}} \int_0^{f_{Ae}} \frac{k_1}{k_1 + k_2 C_A^{1/2}} df_A$$

At this point, we can work either with concentration C_A or the conversion f_A. The flow rate Q remains constant in the reactor. Let us use the concentration for this case:

$$f_A = \frac{QC_{A0} - QC_A}{QC_{A0}} = \frac{C_{A0} - C_A}{C_{A0}} \Rightarrow df_A = -dC_A/C_{A0} \tag{E5-7.5}$$

which leads to

$$S_{R/A} = \frac{-1}{C_{A0} f_{Ae}} \int_{C_{A0}}^{C_{Ae}} \frac{k_1}{k_1 + k_2 C_A^{1/2}} dC_A = \frac{-1}{C_{A0} f_{Ae}} \int_{C_{A0}^{1/2}}^{C_{Ae}^{1/2}} \frac{k_1}{k_1 + k_2 x} dx^2$$

$$= \frac{-1}{C_{A0} f_{Ae}} \int_{C_{A0}^{1/2}}^{C_{Ae}^{1/2}} \frac{2k_1 x}{k_1 + k_2 x} dx = \frac{-2k_1}{k_2 C_{A0} f_{Ae}} \int_{C_{A0}^{1/2}}^{C_{Ae}^{1/2}} \left(1 - \frac{k_1}{k_1 + k_2 x}\right) dx \tag{E5-7.6}$$

$$= \frac{-2k_1}{k_2 C_{A0} f_{Ae}} \left[x - \frac{k_1}{k_2} \ln(k_1 + k_2 x) \right]_{C_{A0}^{1/2}}^{C_{Ae}^{1/2}}$$

$$= \frac{2k_1}{k_2 C_{A0} f_{Ae}} \left[C_{A0}^{1/2} - C_{Ae}^{1/2} - \frac{k_1}{k_2} \ln \frac{k_1 + k_2 C_{A0}^{1/2}}{k_1 + k_2 C_{Ae}^{1/2}} \right]$$

Substituting $f_{Ae} = 0.9$, $C_{A0} = 10$ mol/L, $C_{Ae} = (1 - 0.9) \times 10$ mol/L $= 1$ mol/L, $k_1 = 0.1$ mol$^{-1/2} \cdot$ L$^{1/2} \cdot$ min^{-1} and $k_2 = 0.2$/min into above, we obtain

$$S_{R/A} = \frac{2k_1}{k_2 C_{A0} f_{Ae}} \left[C_{A0}^{1/2} - C_{Ae}^{1/2} - \frac{k_1}{k_2} \ln \frac{k_1 + k_2 C_{A0}^{1/2}}{k_1 + k_2 C_{Ae}^{1/2}} \right] \tag{E5-7.7}$$

$$= \frac{1}{9}(3.162278 - 1 - 0.44631) = 0.19066$$

The final concentrations for the products are:

$$C_{Re} = S_{R/A}\frac{\nu_{1R}}{-\nu_{1A}}(C_{A0} - C_{Ae}) = 1.716 \text{ mol/L}$$

and

$$C_{Qe} = (1 - S_{R/A})\frac{\nu_{2Q}}{-\nu_{2A}}(C_{A0} - C_{Ae}) = 7.284 \text{ mol/L}$$

2. CSTR

Figure E5-7.1 shows a sketch of the CSTR. One can find the parameters already known as $f_A = 0.9$, $C_{A0} = C_{B0} = 10$ mol/L, $C_A = C_B = (1 - 0.9) \times 10$ mol/L $= 1$ mol/L. The selectivity of product R is given by

$$S_{R/A} = s_{R/A} = \frac{k_1 C_A}{k_1 C_A + k_2 C_B^{1/2}} = \frac{1}{3} \tag{E5-7.8}$$

The product stream concentration can be computed as

$$C_{Re} = S_{R/A}\frac{\nu_{1R}}{-\nu_{1A}}(C_{A0} - C_{Ae}) = 3 \text{ mol/L}$$

$$C_{Qe} = (1 - S_{R/A})\frac{\nu_{2Q}}{-\nu_{2A}}(C_{A0} - C_{Ae}) = 6 \text{ mol/L}$$

3. From Eqn (E5-7.3), we infer that the higher the concentration of A and the lower the concentration of B in the reactor will give the highest selectivity to the desired product R. In this case, feeding A from the beginning will render the highest concentration of A available to participate in the reaction. The lowest concentration of B achievable is the concentration at the end of the reactor. Therefore, Fig. E5-7.1c will give the highest selectivity to R.

In this case, the volumetric flow rate Q and the concentration of A are changing in the reactor, while the concentration of B is desired to be constant that equals to the concentration

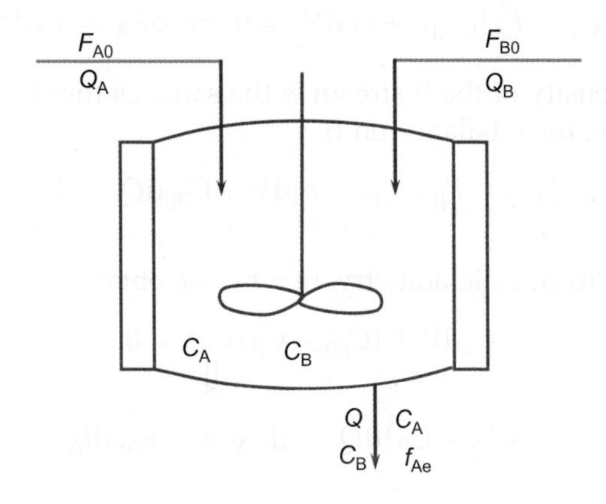

FIGURE E5-7.1 A schematic of a CSTR with two feed streams.

of B at the end of the reaction (90% conversion), $C_B = (1 - 0.9) \times C'_{B0}/2 = 1$ mol/L. We can either solve the problem by direct mole balance and integration (with an automatic integrator) or find out how the concentration is to vary with conversion before we can follow the same steps as we did in part 1.

To aid the solution of the problem, we resketched the PFR feeding scheme diagram as shown in Fig. E5-7.2 and a blowout of the differential section between V and $V + dV$ in Fig. E5-7.3. Both concentration of A and volumetric rate Q are changing in the reactor but not independently from each other. We thus need to figure out how these two are related.

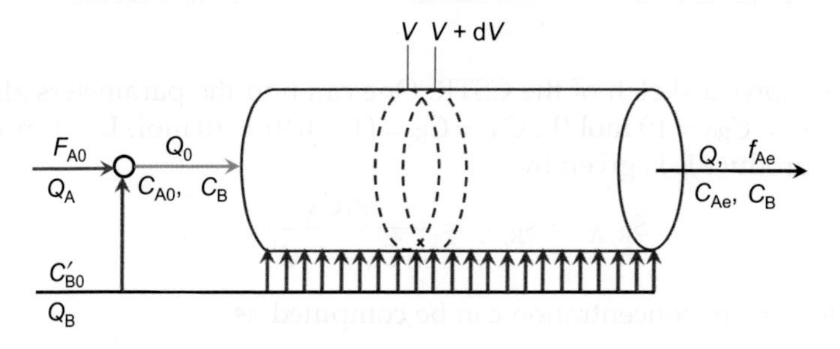

FIGURE E5-7.2 A sketch of the distributed feed PFR.

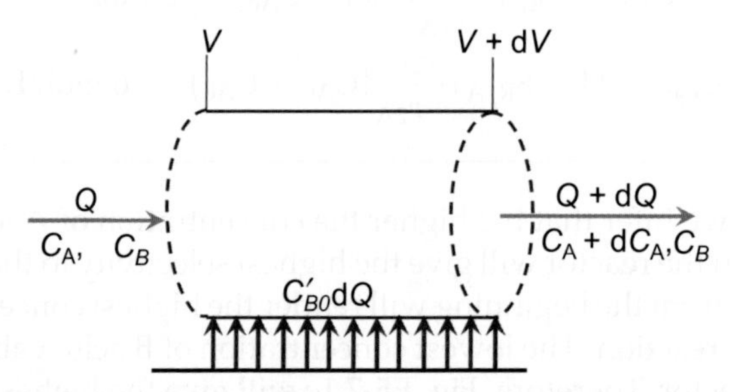

FIGURE E5-7.3 A sketch of a differential volume (section) in the middle of the distributed PFR.

1. Mole balance on A:

$$F_A|_V - F_A|_{V+dV} + r_A dV = 0 \Rightarrow dF_A = r_A dV \tag{E5-7.9}$$

2. Assuming that the density of the B stream is the same as the density of the A stream, as well as to the mixture, mole balance on B:

$$F_B|_V - F_B|_{V+dV} + r_B dV + C'_{B0} dQ = 0 \tag{E5-7.10}$$

Since C_B = constant and from stoichiometry, $r_B = r_A$, we obtain

$$r_A dV + (C'_{B0} - C_B)\, dQ = 0 \tag{E5-7.11}$$

$$\Downarrow$$

$$-(C'_{B0} - C_B) dQ = dF_A = -F_{A0} df_A \tag{E5-7.12}$$

which yields

$$(C'_{B0} - C_B)(Q - Q_0) = F_{A0}f_A \tag{E5-7.13}$$

To find Q_0, we refer to Fig. E5-7.2 for clarity. Mass balance of B for the feed stream to the PFR lead to:

$$(Q_0 - Q_A)C'_{B0} = Q_0\, C_B \tag{E5-7.14}$$

$$\Downarrow$$

$$Q_0 = Q_A + \frac{Q_A C_B}{C'_{B0} - C_B} \tag{E5-7.15}$$

Thus,

$$Q = Q_0 + \frac{F_{A0}}{C'_{B0} - C_B} f_A = \frac{F_{A0}}{C'_{B0} - C_B}(1 + f_A) \tag{E5-7.16}$$

or

$$C_A = \frac{F_A}{Q} = \frac{F_{A0}(1 - f_A)}{\dfrac{F_{A0}}{C'_{B0} - C_B}(1 + f_A)} = (C'_{B0} - C_B)\frac{1 - f_A}{1 + f_A} \tag{E5-7.17}$$

Having established how the concentration changes with the conversion, we can then employ the selectivity to solve the problem.

$$s_{R/A} = \frac{k_1 C_A}{k_1 C_A + k_2 C_B^{1/2}} = \frac{k_1(C'_{B0} - C_B)\dfrac{1 - f_A}{1 + f_A}}{k_1(C'_{B0} - C_B)\dfrac{1 - f_A}{1 + f_A} + k_2 C_B^{1/2}}$$

$$= \frac{k_1(C'_{B0} - C_B)(1 - f_A)}{k_1(C'_{B0} - C_B) + k_2 C_B^{1/2} - \left[k_1(C'_{B0} - C_B) - k_2 C_B^{1/2}\right] f_A} \tag{E5-7.18}$$

$$= \frac{19(1 - f_A)}{21 - 17 f_A}$$

which can be integrated to yield the overall selectivity:

$$S_{R/A} = \frac{\Delta F_A\big|_{\text{due to the formation of R}}}{\Delta F_A\big|_{\text{total}}} = \frac{\int_0^{f_{Ae}} s_{R/A}\,\mathrm{d}f_A}{f_{Ae} - 0} = \frac{1}{f_{Ae}}\int_0^{f_{Ae}} \frac{19(1 - f_A)}{21 - 17 f_A}\,\mathrm{d}f_A$$

$$= \frac{19}{17 f_{Ae}}\int_0^{f_{Ae}} \left[1 - \frac{4}{21 - 17 f_A}\right] \mathrm{d}f_A$$

$$S_{R/A} = \frac{19}{17f_{Ae}}\left\{f_{Ae} + \frac{4}{17}\ln\left[\frac{21 - 17f_{Ae}}{21}\right]\right\} = \frac{19}{0.9 \times 17}\left\{0.9 + \frac{4}{17}\ln\left[\frac{21 - 0.9 \times 17}{21}\right]\right\} = 0.73661$$

The product stream concentration can be computed as.

$$C_{Re} = S_{R/A}\frac{\nu_{1R}}{-\nu_{1A}}(C_{A0} - C_{Ae}) = 6.6295 \text{ mol/L}$$

$$C_{Qe} = (1 - S_{R/A})\frac{\nu_{2Q}}{-\nu_{2A}}(C_{A0} - C_{Ae}) = 2.3705 \text{ mol/L}$$

As a comparison, here is how the three types of reactor arrangement will do to the final product mixture for the particular problem:

PFR	$S_{R/A} = 0.19066$,	$C_{Re} = 1.716$ mol/L
CSTR	$S_{R/A} = 0.33333$,	$C_{Re} = 3$ mol/L
PFR with optimum feed	$S_{R/A} = 0.73661$,	$C_{Re} = 6.6295$ mol/L

The reactor feed strategy greatly affects the product mixture. PFR with optimum (distributed) feed yields significantly more desired product.

5.7.2. Reactive Distillation

Separation of one or more products from the reaction stream via a different phase is an effective way of increasing the process efficiency. Figure 5.17 shows a sketch of a conceptual reactive distillation tower, which looks identical to a tray tower when idealized.

Figure 5.17a shows the overall flow schematic with the liquid reaction mixture being fed from the tower top. The liquid is flowing down the column with a number of stopping stages where catalysts present. While each particular case could have slightly different arrangement, this conceptual column is general enough to describe most of the systems.

Performance analysis of the reactive distillation tower can be done in a manner similar to what we have learned so far for reactor analysis. This is made clear by examining an individual stage i as isolated in Fig. 5.17b and c. This illustration shows that each stage may be treated as a CSTR that is coupled with mass transfer to remove one or more volatile components. Therefore, this idealization of the reactive distillation tower renders it to a CSTR train.

Mole balance of A in the liquid (or reactive) stream in the i-th stage yields:

$$Q_{Li-1}C_{Ai-1} - Q_{Li}C_{Ai} + r_{Ai}V_i - J_{Ai}V_ia_i = 0 \tag{5.81}$$

where a_i is the specific liquid–vapor contacting area (area divided by total liquid volume) at stage i, Q_{Li-1} is the volumetric flow rate of liquid stream flowing into the i-th stage, Q_{Li} is the volumetric flow rate of liquid stream flowing out of the i-th stage, C_{Ai} is the concentration of A in liquid phase at stage i, r_{Ai} is the rate of formation of A in stage i, V_i is the total volume of liquid in stage i, and J_{Ai} is the mass transfer flux of A out of liquid phase in stage i. Mole balance of A in the vapor stream leads to

$$F_{Vi+1}y_{Ai+1} - F_{Vi}y_{Ai} + J_{Ai}V_ia_i = 0 \tag{5.82}$$

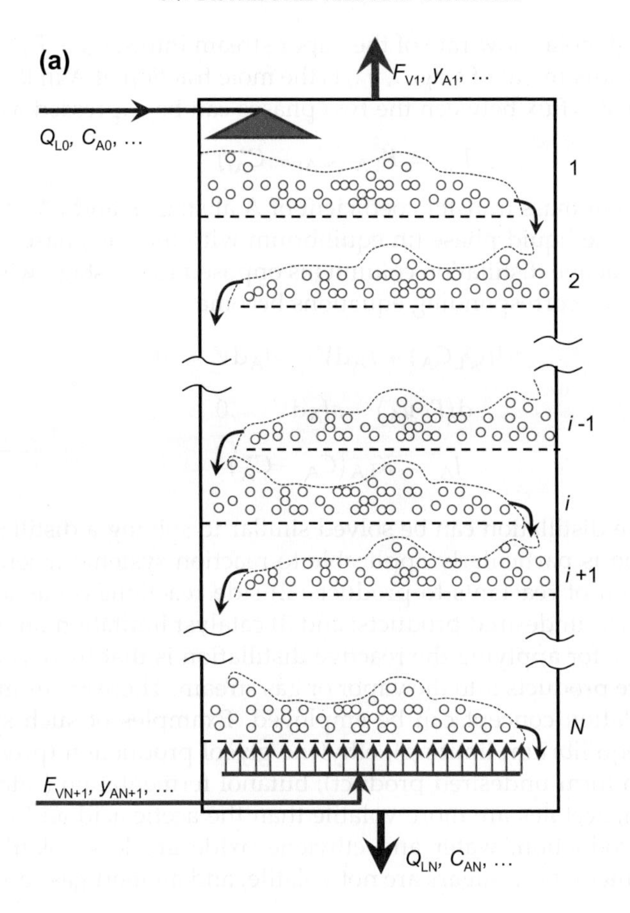

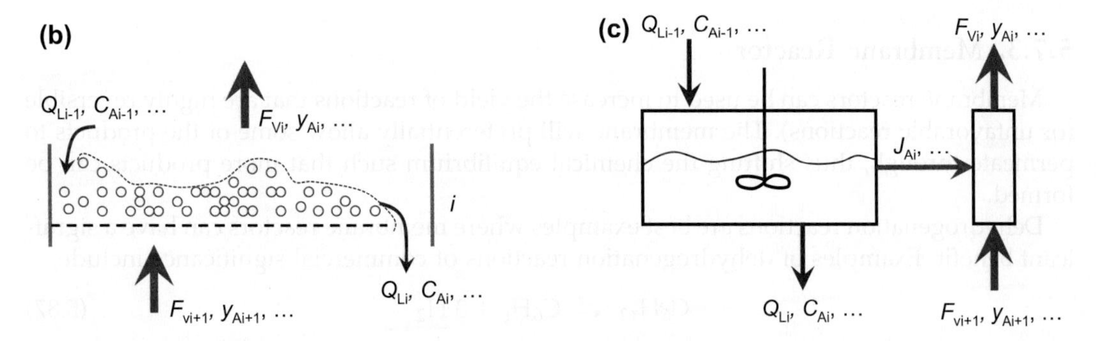

FIGURE 5.17 A schematic diagram and idealization of reactive distillation column. (a) An illustration of a reactive distillation tower. (b) A sketch of the ith stage. (c) An idealization of stage i.

where F_{Vi+1} is the total molar flow rate of the vapor stream into stage i, F_{Vi} is the total molar flow rate of the vapor stream out of stage i, y_{Ai} is the mole fraction of A in the vapor stream at stage i. The mass transfer flux between the two phases can be expressed as

$$J_{Ai} = K_{LAi}(C_{Ai} - C^*_{Ai}) \tag{5.83}$$

where K_{LAi} is the overall mass transfer coefficient of A at stage i, and C^*_{Ai} is the equilibrium concentration of A in the liquid phase (in equilibrium with the gas phase y_{Ai}).

For a continuous reactive distillation column (as opposed to the stage-wise reactive distillation column), the three corresponding equations become

$$-\mathrm{d}(Q_L C_A) + r_A \mathrm{d}V - aJ_A \mathrm{d}V = 0 \tag{5.84}$$

$$\mathrm{d}(F_V y_A) + aJ_A \mathrm{d}V = 0 \tag{5.85}$$

$$J_A = K_{LA}(C_A - C^*_A) \tag{5.86}$$

Therefore, the reactive distillation can be solved similar to solving a distillation column.

Reactive distillation is particularly applicable to reaction systems where 1) equilibrium limiting the conversion of reactants to products; 2) side reactions occur to further render one or more products to undesired products; and 3) catalyst limitation on the final product concentration. The key for applying the reactive distillation is that there is a preferential to evaporate one of more products into the vapor or gas stream. There are numerous examples where reactive distillation concept can be employed. Examples of such systems include: acetate production (equilibrium limiting); ethylene glycol production (product can further react with reactant to form undesired product); butanol fermentation (catalyst inhibition). In acetate production, acetates are more volatile than the acetic acid and the alcohol used. In ethylene glycol production, water and ethylene oxide are less volatile than ethylene glycol. In butanol fermentation, sugars are not volatile, and an inert gas can be used to strip butanol out.

5.7.3. Membrane Reactor

Membrane reactors can be used to increase the yield of reactions that are highly reversible (or unfavorable reactions). The membrane will preferentially allow some of the products to permeate through, thus shifting the chemical equilibrium such that more products can be formed.

Dehydrogenation reactions are best examples where membrane reactors can have a significant benefit. Examples of dehydrogenation reactions of commercial significance include,

$$C_6H_{12} \rightleftarrows C_6H_6 + 3\,H_2 \tag{5.87}$$

Benzene production;

$$C_6H_5CH_2{-}CH_3 \rightleftarrows C_6H_5CH{=}CH_2 + H_2 \tag{5.88}$$

Styrene production (monomer for polymer production);

$$C_4H_{10} \rightleftarrows C_4H_8 + H_2 \tag{5.89}$$

Butene production (monomer for polymer production);

$$C_3H_8 \rightleftarrows C_3H_6 + H_2 \tag{5.90}$$

Propylene production (monomer for polymer production).

These gas phase reactions can also be simplified to

$$A \rightleftarrows B + C \tag{5.91}$$

with one of the product that is significantly smaller in size. The small molecules can permeate through membranes that larger molecules could not. Although these reactions are thermodynamically unfavorable, the removal of H_2 from the reaction mixture can shift the thermodynamic equilibrium that favors the production of alkenes, which are valuable as they are monomers for polymer production.

Figure 5.18 shows an idealization of membrane reactors. From Fig. 5.18, one can conclude that membrane reactor problem can easily be solved just as other reactors. In most situations though, an automatic integrator is needed.

Mole balance of species B in the reactive stream yields:

$$-dF_B + r_B dV - aJ_B dV = 0 \tag{5.92}$$

where a is the specific mass transfer area (surface area of the membrane divided by reaction mixture volume), F_B is the molar flow rate of species B in the reactive stream, r_B is the rate of

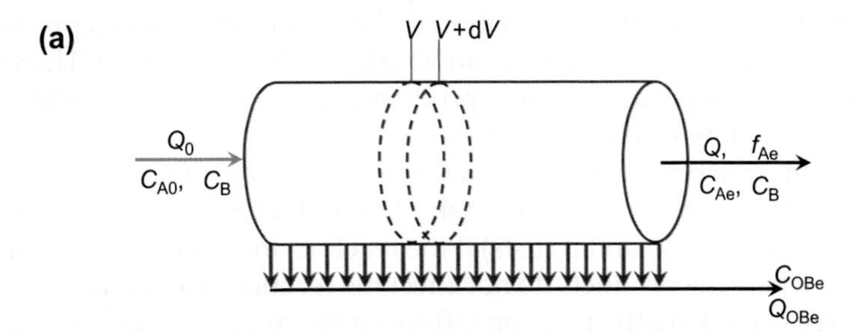

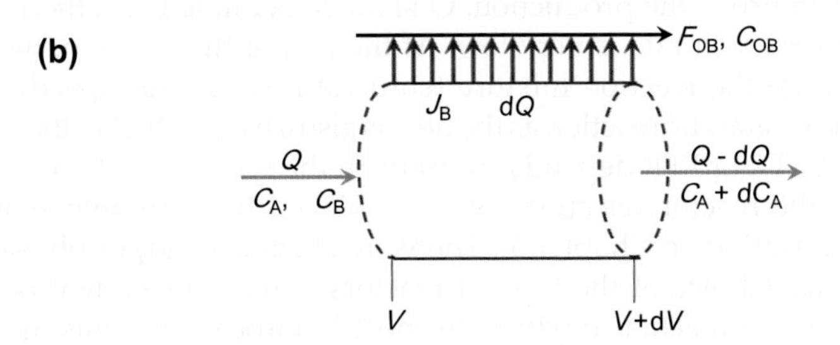

FIGURE 5.18 A schematic of membrane reactor. (a) Some components are allowed to permeate through the membrane and removed from the reaction mixture. (b) Blowout of a differential volume (section) of the membrane reactor.

formation of B, V is the volume of reactive mixture volume, and J_B is the mass transfer flux of B out of reactive stream. Mole balance of species B in the stream over the other side of the membrane (nonreactive stream) leads to

$$-dF_{OB} + aJ_B dV = 0 \tag{5.93}$$

where F_{OB} is the molar flow rate of species B in the nonreactive stream. The mass transfer flux between the two streams can be expressed as

$$J_B = k_{cB}(p_B - p_{OB}) \tag{5.94}$$

where k_{cB} is the permeability of species B through the membrane, p_B is the partial pressure of species B in the reactive stream and p_{OB} is the partial of species B in the nonreactive stream.

Therefore, a membrane reactor problem can be solved in a similar fashion as one would for a plug flow reactor. However, there is an added term for mass transfer.

5.8. PFR OR CSTR?

In this chapter, we have discussed how to solve flow reactor problems. It helps up in designing and/or performing performance evaluations for a reactor. Before we get into the whether a PFR or a CSTR should be chosen, we should look at why we use a flow reactor in the first place. Flow reactors can produce products continuously at a specified quality with a consistent feed. The continuous nature makes it qualify for mass production. It comes also with it less labor cost as automation can be effectively put in place. Therefore, flow reactors are used when mass production of a product is desired and a consistent feed stream is guaranteed for the quality of the product.

We next examining whether a PFR or a CSTR should be chosen. Examples 5-1 and 5-3 showed that a PFR can achieve the same task as that of a CSTR with a smaller volume (and thus less operating as well as capital costs) if the reactors are run under isothermal conditions and for reactions where the products do not affect the reaction rate. What will happen if one or more products are catalyzing the reaction (affecting the reaction rate)? For example, autocatalytic reaction will only occur if there is the product in the reaction mixture. In this case, a CSTR might be preferred as the product is being recirculated inside the reactor. If a PFR is chosen, a recycle stream will improve the production. One other example is exothermic reaction. At low-temperature, the reaction rate is very low. At the end of the reaction, the heat released by the reaction can raise the reaction mixture temperature and thus speedup the reaction. This is similar to an autocatalytic reaction as the heat is also a by-product in the reaction. Therefore, the selection of CSTR or PFR depends strongly on the type of reactions.

While in general, the reactor selection can be achieved by economic analysis (see Bioprocess System Optimization, in Chapter 3). There are chemical and/or physical restrictions for bioprocess systems. Choice of the type of reactors is then dependent on physical and chemical properties of the reaction mixture. In most bioprocess systems, multiple phases: solid, liquid, and/gases are involved as reactants and/or products. For example, a soluble solid is to react with a liquid stream, it might be better off to choose a CSTR as stirring action is need to mix the reaction mixture.

Common analogy to CSTR includes stirred-tank reactor and fluidized bed reactors (solid–liquid, solid–gas, solid–liquid–gas), while tubular reactor and packed-bed reactors are more close to a PFR. There are other types of reactors that taking into mass transfer effects. For example, counter-current flow reactor is a good choice for gas–solid and liquid–solid systems where the aim is to reacting away part of the contents in the solid. This is commonly seen in ore leaching, pulp, and paper, etc. The counter-current flow is achieved by flowing gas (or liquid) up in a vertical reactor, while letting the solid moving down by gravity.

Example 5-8. Consider a simple elementary series reaction system

$$A \overset{k_1}{\to} B \overset{k_2}{\to} C$$

with a feed stream containing C_{A0} mol/L of A. If the intermediate product B is the desired product, determine the optimum type of ideal isothermal flow reactor and contact time required.

Solution. There are two types of ideal flow reactors applicable to this example: 1. PFR and 2. CSTR.

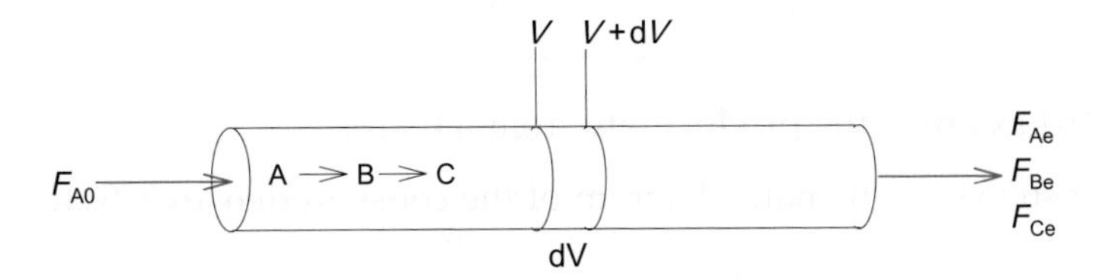

FIGURE E5-8.1 A schematic diagram of the PFR showing a differential control volume (V, $V + dV$).

1. PFR. Figure E5-8.1 shows a sketch of the PFR system. Mole balances for species A and B lead to

$$-dF_A + r_A dV = 0 \tag{E5-8.1}$$

$$-dF_B + r_B dV = 0 \tag{E5-8.2}$$

Since $F_A = C_A Q$, $F_B = C_B Q$, $\tau = V/Q$ and the reaction mixture is of constant density, Eqns (E5-8.1) and (E5-8.2) are rearranged to give

$$\frac{dC_A}{d\tau} = r_A = -r_1 = -k_1 C_A \tag{E5-8.3}$$

$$\frac{dC_B}{d\tau} = r_B = r_1 - r_2 = k_1 C_A - k_2 C_B \tag{E5-8.4}$$

Equations (E5-8.3) and (E5-8.4) can be solved together with the initial conditions $C_A(\tau = 0) = C_{A0}$ and $C_B(\tau = 0) = 0$ (see example 4-3) to give

$$C_A = C_{A0} \exp(-k_1 \tau) \tag{E5-8.5}$$

$$C_B = \frac{k_1}{k_2 - k_1} C_{A0} [e^{-k_1 \tau} - e^{-k_2 \tau}] \tag{E5-8.6}$$

and

$$C_C = C_{A0} - C_A - C_B = C_{A0} - \frac{k_1 e^{-k_2 t} - k_2 e^{-k_1 t}}{k_1 - k_2} C_{A0} \tag{E5-8.7}$$

This maximum concentration of B (or the production rate of B) can be obtained by setting

$$0 = \left.\frac{dC_B}{d\tau}\right|_{\tau_m} = r_B = k_1 C_{A0} e^{-k_1 \tau_m} - k_2 \frac{k_1}{k_2 - k_1} C_{A0} (e^{-k_1 \tau_m} - e^{-k_2 \tau_m}) \tag{E5-8.8}$$

which gives the contact time required for maximum production of B

$$\tau_m = \frac{\ln(k_2/k_1)}{k_2 - k_1} \tag{E5-8.9}$$

and the corresponding concentration of B is given by

$$C_{Bmax} = C_{A0} \left(\frac{k_2}{k_1}\right)^{\frac{-k_2}{k_2 - k_1}} \tag{E5-8.10}$$

2. CSTR. We next examine the productivity from a CSTR.

Figure E5-8.2 shows a schematic diagram of the constant density CSTR.

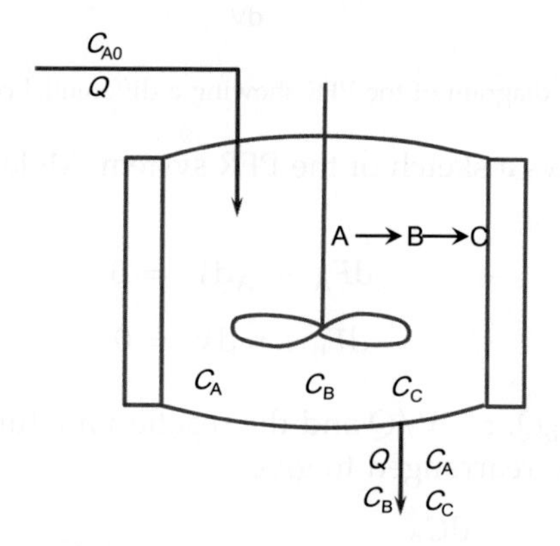

FIGURE E5-8.2 A schematic diagram of a constant density CSTR.

Mole balance for species A and B in the CSTR volume at steady state leads to

$$(QC_A)_0 - (QC_A) + r_A V = 0 \tag{E5-8.11}$$

$$0 - (QC_B) + r_B V = 0 \tag{E5-8.12}$$

Noting also $\tau = V/Q$, we arrive from Eqns (E5-8.11) and (E5-8.12)

$$C_A = \frac{C_{A0}}{1 + k_1 \tau} \tag{E5-8.13}$$

$$C_B = \frac{k_1 \tau C_{A0}}{(1+k_1\tau)(1+k_2\tau)} \tag{E5-8.14}$$

This maximum concentration of B (or the production rate of B) can be obtained by setting

$$0 = \left.\frac{dC_B}{d\tau}\right|_{\tau_m} = \frac{(1+k_1\tau_m)(1+k_2\tau_m) - \tau_m[k_1(1+k_2\tau_m)+k_1(1+k_2\tau_m)]}{(1+k_1\tau_m)^2(1+k_2\tau_m)^2} k_1 C_{A0} \tag{E5-8.15}$$

which gives the contact time required for maximum production of B in a CSTR

$$\tau_m = \frac{1}{\sqrt{k_2 k_1}} \tag{E5-8.16}$$

and the corresponding concentration of B is given by

$$\boxed{C_{Bmax} = C_{A0}\left(1+\sqrt{\frac{k_2}{k_1}}\right)^{-2}} \tag{E5-8.17}$$

Figure E5-8.3 shows the ratio of the maximum concentration B in a PFR, Eqn (E5-8.10) to that in a CSTR, Eqn (E5-8.17), as a function of the kinetic rate constant k_2/k_1. One can observe that the productivity to B is higher in a PFR than in a CSTR, as the ratio is always greater than unity.

Therefore, the optimum reactor type is PFR, with a contact time given by Eqn (E5-8.9) if the desired product is the intermediate product B.

Example 5-8 shows that PFR is better suited for intermediate product production. This can be easily interpreted from the concentration distributions. In a CSTR, the reactant concentration is

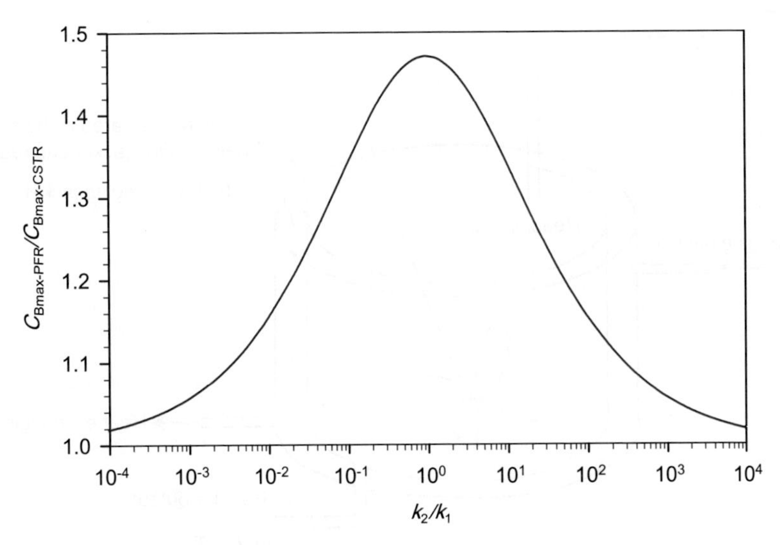

FIGURE E5-8.3 The ratio of the maximum intermediate product B in a PFR to that in a CSTR as a function of the kinetic rate constant ratio.

at its minimal while the product concentration is at its maximal. This situation is not ideal if the product is an intermediate product as the product concentration is high in the reactor and consequently its further reaction to decomposition products is enhanced. On the other hand, in a PFR, the reactant concentration is at its highest and the products are at their lowest in the reactor. This situation favors the product that is the immediate from the reactants. At intermediate contact times, the productivity of the intermediate products reaches maximum.

5.9. STEADY NONISOTHERMAL FLOW REACTORS

We have been focused on the ideal flow reactors so far without considering the change of temperatures. If temperature is not constant, the rate of reaction will not be constant and in turn it will affect the reactor performance. For steady nonisothermal flow reactors, the temperature change in the reactor is governed by the energy balance equation:

$$\sum_{j=1}^{N_S} F_{j0}\left(H_j - H_{j0}\right) + V\sum_{i=1}^{N_R} r_i \Delta H_{Ri} + \sum_{j=1}^{N_S} C_{Pj} n_j \frac{dT}{dt} - \frac{d(pV)}{dt} = \dot{Q} - \dot{W}_s \tag{3.134}$$

by setting $\frac{d}{dt} = 0$. Thus, for a steady nonisothermal CSTR as shown in Fig. 5.19, Eqn (3.134) is reduced to

$$\sum_{j=1}^{N_S} F_{j0}\left(H_j - H_{j0}\right) + V\sum_{i=1}^{N_R} r_i \Delta H_{Ri} = \dot{Q} - \dot{W}_s \tag{5.95}$$

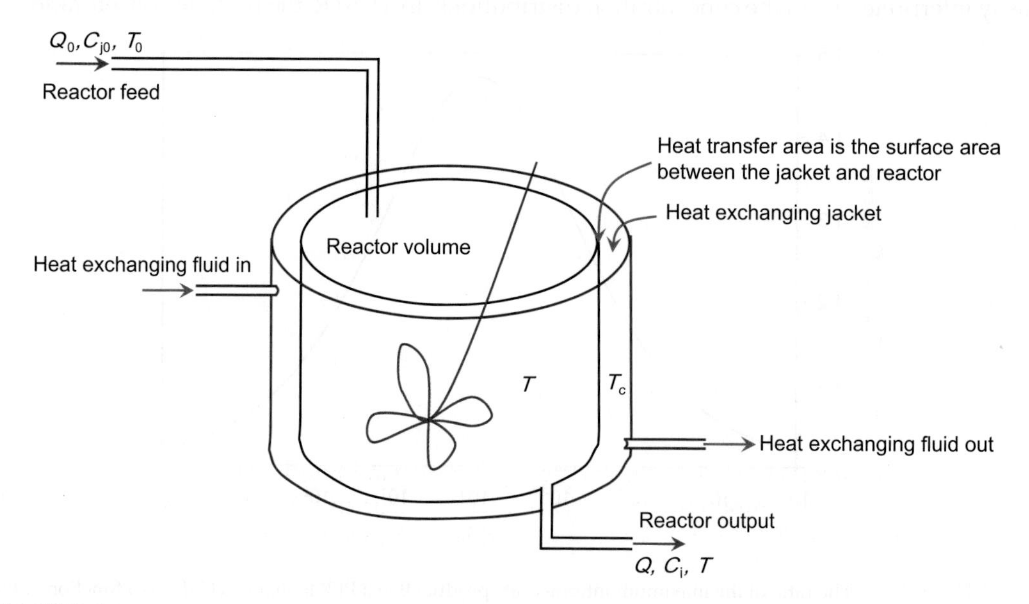

FIGURE 5.19 A schematic of a nonisothermal CSTR with a heat-transfer jacket.

where $\dot{W}_s$ is the shaft work exported out of the reaction mixture, which is the negative of the stirrer output, and $\dot{Q}$ is the heat transfer into the reaction mixture. That is,

$$\dot{Q} = UA_{\mathrm{H}}(T_{\mathrm{c}} - T) \tag{5.96}$$

where U is the overall heat-transfer coefficient and A_{H} is the total heat transfer area. Substituting into Eqn (5.95), we obtain

$$\sum_{j=1}^{N_S} F_{j0}\left(H_j - H_{j0}\right) + V\sum_{i=1}^{N_R} r_i \Delta H_{\mathrm{R}i} = UA_{\mathrm{H}}(T_{\mathrm{c}} - T) - \dot{W}_s \tag{5.97}$$

Thus, the energy balance equation can be solved simultaneously with the mole balance equation to determine the reactor output or reactor volume requirement.

For a steady PFR, Eqn (3.134) is reduced to

$$\sum_{j=1}^{N_S} F_{j0}\mathrm{d}H_j + \sum_{i=1}^{N_R} r_i \Delta H_{\mathrm{R}i}\mathrm{d}V = \mathrm{d}\dot{Q} - \mathrm{d}\dot{W}_s \tag{5.98}$$

Usually, the shaft work is not present or negligible in a PFR, $\dot{W}_s = 0$. The heat transferred into the reactor can be written in the same manner as for a CSTR:

$$\mathrm{d}\dot{Q} = Ua(T_{\mathrm{c}} - T)\mathrm{d}V \tag{5.99}$$

where a is the specific heat transfer area, which equals the heat transfer area divided by the reactor volume. Thus, the energy balance equation for a steady PFR is given by

$$\sum_{j=1}^{N_S} F_{j0}C_{Pj}\mathrm{d}T + \sum_{i=1}^{N_R} r_i \Delta H_{\mathrm{R}i}\mathrm{d}V = Ua(T_{\mathrm{c}} - T)\mathrm{d}V \tag{5.100}$$

which is a differential equation, just like the mole balance equation for PFR.

Example 5-9. The exothermic gas phase reaction:

$$\mathrm{A} \underset{k_{\mathrm{b}}}{\overset{k_{\mathrm{f}}}{\rightleftarrows}} \mathrm{B} + \mathrm{C} \qquad r = k_{\mathrm{f}}p_{\mathrm{A}} - k_{\mathrm{b}}p_{\mathrm{B}}p_{\mathrm{C}}$$

is carried out in a CSTR operating at 50 bar. Calculate the maximum rate if the reactor operates at a 22% conversion of A with a pure A in the feed. Additional data are given below

$$k_{\mathrm{f}} = 0.435\exp\left(-\frac{E_{\mathrm{f}}}{RT}\right)\ \mathrm{mol\,s^{-1}\cdot m^{-3}\cdot bar^{-1}}, \qquad E_{\mathrm{f}} = 20\ \mathrm{kJ/mol}$$

$$k_{\mathrm{b}} = 147\exp\left(-\frac{E_{\mathrm{b}}}{RT}\right)\ \mathrm{mol\,s^{-1}\cdot m^{-3}\cdot bar^{-2}}, \qquad E_{\mathrm{b}} = 60\ \mathrm{kJ/mol}$$

Solution: For nonisothermal reactors, temperature plays an important role in reactor performance. In a CSTR, the temperature is uniform in the reactor and thus is the same as the final (output) temperature. To find the maximum reaction rate, we perform:

$$0 = \frac{\mathrm{d}r}{\mathrm{d}T} = p_{\mathrm{A}}\frac{\mathrm{d}k_{\mathrm{f}}}{\mathrm{d}T} - p_{\mathrm{B}}p_{\mathrm{C}}\frac{\mathrm{d}k_{\mathrm{b}}}{\mathrm{d}T} \tag{E5-9.1}$$

Since the final pressures are not functions of temperature for the required conversion of A. Since based on the rate law,

$$\frac{dk_f}{dT} = k_f \frac{E_f}{RT^2} \qquad \frac{dk_b}{dT} = k_b \frac{E_b}{RT^2} \tag{E5-9.2}$$

We obtain by substituting Eqn (E5-9.2) into Eqn (E5-9.1),

$$0 = p_A k_f \frac{E_f}{RT^2} - p_B p_C k_b \frac{E_b}{RT^2} \tag{E5-9.3}$$

Therefore,

$$\frac{k_f}{k_b} = \frac{p_B p_C}{p_A} \frac{E_b}{E_f} \tag{E5-9.4}$$

For a given conversion f_A, the flow rates of the reaction mixture are given by

$$F_A = F_{A0}(1 - f_A);\ F_B = F_{A0} f_A = F_C;\ \text{and}\ F_T = F_A + F_B + F_C = F_{A0}(1 + f_A).$$

Therefore, the partial pressures in the final reaction mixture are given by

$$p_A = \frac{F_A}{F_T} P = \frac{1 - f_A}{1 + f_A} P \tag{E5-9.5a}$$

$$p_B = \frac{F_B}{F_T} P = \frac{f_A}{1 + f_A} P = p_C \tag{E5-9.5b}$$

Substitute Eqn (E5-9.5) into Eqn (E5-9.4), we obtain

$$\frac{k_f}{k_b} = \frac{f_A^2}{(1 + f_A)(1 - f_A)} \frac{E_b}{E_f} P = \frac{0.22^2}{(1 + 0.22)(1 - 0.22)} \times \frac{60}{20} \times 50\ \text{bar} = 7.63\ \text{bar}$$

Also

$$\frac{k_f}{k_b} = \frac{0.435 \exp\left(-\dfrac{E_f}{RT}\right)}{147 \exp\left(-\dfrac{E_b}{RT}\right)} \text{bar} = \frac{0.435}{147} \exp\left(\frac{E_b - E_f}{RT}\right) \text{bar}$$

Therefore,

$$T = \frac{E_b - E_f}{R \ln\left(\dfrac{k_f}{k_b} \times \dfrac{147}{0.435} \text{bar}^{-1}\right)} = \frac{60000 - 20000}{8.314 \times \ln\left(\dfrac{147}{0.435} \times 7.63\right)} \text{K} = 614.8\ \text{K}$$

Now we have obtained the optimum temperature (for maximum reaction rate). Substitute the temperature and partial pressures into the rate expression, we obtain the maximum reaction rate

$$r = 0.183\ \text{mol} / (\text{m}^3 .\ \text{s})$$

Example 5-10. Nonisothermal PFR. The exothermic gas phase reaction:

$$A \underset{k_b}{\overset{k_f}{\rightleftarrows}} B + C \qquad r = k_f p_A - k_b p_B p_C$$

is carried out in a PFR operating at 50 bar with negligible pressure drop. The feed consists of pure A and the required conversion is 70%. The rate data is given by

$$k_f = 0.435 \exp\left(-\frac{E_f}{RT}\right) \text{ mol s}^{-1}\cdot\text{m}^{-3}\cdot\text{bar}^{-1}, \qquad E_f = 20 \text{ kJ/mol}$$

$$k_b = 147 \exp\left(-\frac{E_b}{RT}\right) \text{ mol s}^{-1}\cdot\text{m}^{-3}\cdot\text{bar}^{-2}, \qquad E_b = 60 \text{ kJ/mol}$$

1. Find the optimum temperature progression in the reactor with the maximum allowed temperature of 350 °C.
2. What is the reactor space time required if the optimum temperature progression is taken?
3. What is the heat to be removed if $C_P \approx 0$?

Solution. The stoichiometry:

	A	$\rightleftarrows$	B	+	C	
$V = 0$	F_{A0}		0		0	
$V = V$	F_A		F_B		F_C	$+) = F_T$
	$F_{A0}(1-f_A)$		$F_{A0}f_A$		$F_{A0}f_A$	$+) = F_{A0}(1+f_A)$

The partial pressures in the reaction mixture are given by

$$p_A = \frac{F_A}{F_T}P = \frac{1-f_A}{1+f_A}P \tag{E5-10.1a}$$

$$p_B = \frac{F_B}{F_T}P = \frac{f_A}{1+f_A}P = p_C \tag{E5-10.1b}$$

Thus, the reaction rate is given by

$$r = k_f P\frac{1-f_A}{1+f_A} - k_b P^2 \frac{f_A^2}{(1+f_A)^2} \tag{E5-10.2}$$

1. The optimum temperature is the temperature that gives rise to the maximum reaction rate, that is,

$$0 = \frac{dr}{dT} = P\frac{1-f_A}{1+f_A}\frac{dk_f}{dT} - P^2\frac{f_A^2}{(1+f_A)^2}\frac{dk_b}{dT} \tag{E5-10.3}$$

Since the final pressures are not functions of temperature for the required conversion of A. Since based on the rate law,

$$\frac{dk_f}{dT} = k_f\frac{E_f}{RT^2} \qquad \frac{dk_b}{dT} = k_b\frac{E_b}{RT^2} \tag{E5-10.4}$$

We obtain by substituting Eqn (E5-10.4) into Eqn (E5-10.3),

$$0 = Pk_f \frac{1-f_A}{1+f_A}\frac{E_f}{RT^2} - P^2 k_b \frac{f_A^2}{(1+f_A)^2}\frac{E_b}{RT^2} \tag{E5-10.5}$$

Therefore,

$$\frac{k_f}{k_b} = P\frac{f_A^2}{(1+f_A)(1-f_A)}\frac{E_b}{E_f} \tag{E5-10.6}$$

Also

$$\frac{k_f}{k_b} = \frac{k_{f0}\exp\left(-\frac{E_f}{RT}\right)}{k_{b0}\exp\left(-\frac{E_b}{RT}\right)} = \frac{k_{f0}}{k_{b0}}\exp\left(\frac{E_b-E_f}{RT}\right) \tag{E5-10.7}$$

Therefore, the optimum temperature in the PFR is given by

$$T = \frac{E_b - E_f}{R\ln\left(\frac{k_f}{k_b}\times\frac{k_{b0}}{k_{f0}}\right)} = \frac{E_b - E_f}{R\ln\left(\frac{f_A^2 P}{1-f_A^2}\times\frac{E_b}{E_f}\times\frac{k_{b0}}{k_{f0}}\right)} \tag{E5-10.8}$$

Substituting in the known numbers, we obtain

$$T = \frac{4811.16\ \text{K}}{\ln\left(\frac{f_A^2}{1-f_A^2}\right)+10.833477} \tag{E5-10.9}$$

From the above equation, we observe that as the conversion (f_A) is increased, the required optimum temperature decreases. Therefore, at low conversions, the optimum temperature calculated could exceed the maximum allowed temperature. At the maximum temperature $T = 350\ ^\circ\text{C} = 623.15$ K, its corresponding conversion can be determined from Eqn (E5-10.9) to be $f_A = 0.206357793$. Therefore, the optimum temperature progression in the PFR is given by

$$T = \begin{cases} 623.15\ \text{K} & f_A \le 0.20636 \\ \dfrac{4811.16\ \text{K}}{\ln\left(\frac{f_A^2}{1-f_A^2}\right)+10.833477} & f_A > 0.20636 \end{cases} \tag{E5-10.10}$$

The temperature progression is plotted in Fig. E5-10. One can observe that temperature decreases along the length of the reactor (or space time). The maximum temperature (at which the reaction stops) is also shown as it progresses through the reactor.

2. To determine the space time (reactor size) requirement, we must perform a mole balance to the PFR. At steady state, the mole balance of A in the differential volume is given by

$$-\text{d}F_A + r_A\text{d}V = 0 \tag{E5-10.11}$$

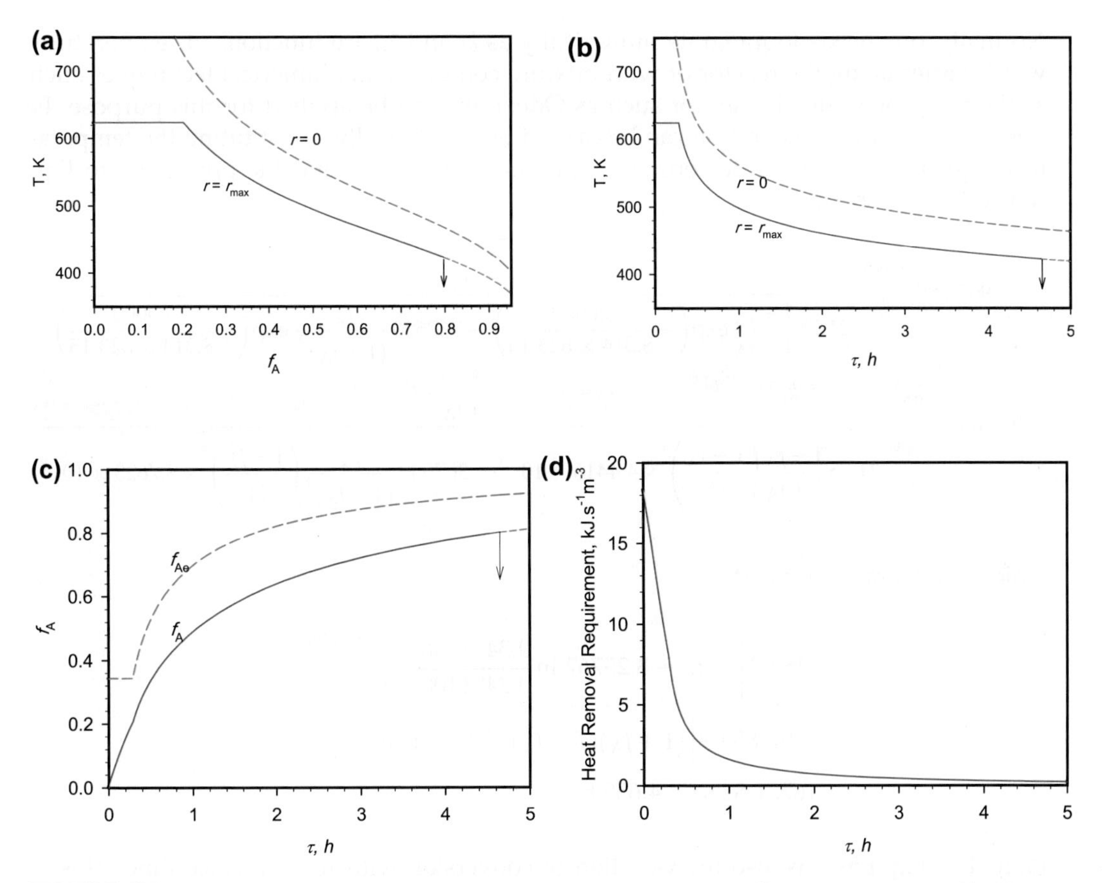

FIGURE E5-10 Optimum temperature progression in a PFR and its effect on conversion. (a) Optimum temperature progression as a function of conversion in the PFR. (b) Optimum temperature progression along the PFR. (c) Conversion at optimum reactor temperature as a function of PFR size. (d) Heat generation of removal needed along the PFR.

Noting that $F_A = F_{A0}(1 - f_A) = Q_0 C_{A0}(1 - f_A)$, Eqn (E5-10.11) can be rendered to give

$$r d\tau = C_{A0} df_A = 0 \tag{E5-10.12}$$

At reactor inlet, $f_A = 0$, $T = T_0 = 523.15$ K:

$$C_{A0} = \frac{P}{RT_0} = \frac{50 \times 10^5}{8.314 \times 623.15} \text{mol/m}^3 = 965.089 \text{ mol/m}^3$$

Integrating Eqn (5-10.12) yield,

$$\tau = C_{A0} \int_0^{f_{Ae}} \frac{df_A}{r} = C_{A0} \int_0^{f_{Ae}} \frac{df_A}{k_f P \frac{1 - f_A}{1 + f_A} - k_b P^2 \frac{f_A^2}{(1 + f_A)^2}} \tag{E5-10.13}$$

Normally, one needs to integrate numerically as k_f and k_b are functions of temperature, which varies along the reactor or with mixture composition. Numerical techniques such as the Simpson's rule, integrator such as OdexLims can be applied for this purpose. In this particular case, integration can be carried out analytically. Substituting the temperature Eqn (E5-10.10), the rate constants, initial concentration, and the pressure into Eqn (E5-10.13), we obtain

$$\tau = 965.089 \int_0^{0.20636} \frac{df_A}{21.75\dfrac{1-f_A}{1+f_A}\exp\left(-\dfrac{20000}{8.314\times 623.15}\right) - 367500\dfrac{f_A^2}{(1+f_A)^2}\exp\left(-\dfrac{60000}{8.314\times 623.15}\right)}$$

$$+965.089 \int_{0.20636}^{0.8} \frac{df_A}{21.75\dfrac{1-f_A}{1+f_A}\left(\dfrac{1-f_A^2}{f_A^2}\right)^{\frac{1}{2}} \times 4.4416\times 10^{-3} - 367500\dfrac{f_A^2}{(1+f_A)^2}\left(\dfrac{1-f_A^2}{f_A^2}\right)^{\frac{3}{2}} \times 8.7623\times 10^{-8}}$$

which is integrated to yield

$$\begin{aligned}\tau &= 248.03\left[-f_A + 3.25762\ln\frac{0.3431108+f_A}{0.3431108-f_A}\right]_0^{0.20636} \\ &\quad + 14985.09\left[(1+f_A)(1-f_A^2)^{-1/2} - \arcsin f_A\right]_{0.20636}^{0.8} \text{ s} \\ &= 16771.86 \text{ s} = 4.659 \text{ h}\end{aligned}$$

Plotted in Fig. E5-10 is also the variation of conversion with reactor space time. This is achieved by integrating for the space time as a function of conversion.

3. Since the heat capacity is negligible, temperature change can be achieved with negligible thermal energy. Therefore, the heat generated during reaction must be removed. Energy balance gives

$$\sum_{j=1}^{N_S} F_{j0}dH_j + r\Delta H_R dV = d\dot{Q} - d\dot{W}_s$$

There is no work input or output. When heat capacity is negligible, the energy balance equation reduces to

$$\frac{d\dot{Q}}{dV} = r\Delta H_R = r(E_f - E_b)$$

which gives the heat required for the reactor. It is the negative of what needs to be removed.

Figure E5-10d shows the heat generated (or removal requirement) along the PFR. One can observe that more heat is being generated at the front end of the reactor.

5.10. REACTIVE EXTRACTION

In renewable resources industries, woody biomass is commonly used as raw materials to produce chemicals and materials. In this section, we devote some effort in learning how a special type of continuous flow reactor with two contacting streams can be analyzed.

Woody biomass is solid and often reacts with a liquid stream to decompose woody biomass to desired products. For example, hot water extraction of woody biomass employs a water stream to extract hemicelluloses from woody biomass. Kraft pulping employs a white liquor (aqueous sodium hydroxide and sodium sulfide solution) to degrade and extracting lignin and other components from woody biomass. In both cases, the woody biomass remains at the end of the reaction. Another example of such a reactive extraction process is the ore leaching: a liquid stream is employed to extract desired element (or compound) from "rocky" materials.

The reactive extraction process can be idealized as reaction occurring in two separate streams with different flow rates (even opposing flowing directions). Without loss of generality, Fig. 5.20 shows a sketch of a conceptual reactive extraction tower. There are three streams: a heavy reacting phase (for example woody biomass and its carrying liquid), a light reacting phase (supplies active reacting agents to the heavy reacting phase), and a heat exchange fluid phase. While the heat exchanging fluid phase is physically separated

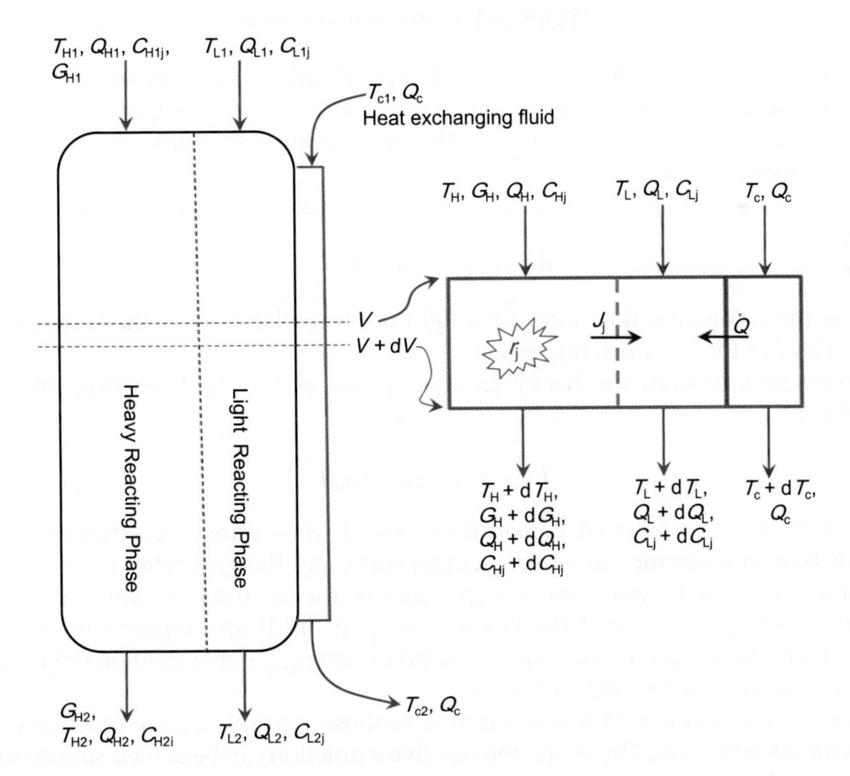

FIGURE 5.20 A schematic diagram and idealization of reactive extraction tower.

from the light reacting phase (and so from the heavy reacting phase), it provides heat to the light reacting phase via heat transfer through the reactor wall surface (or internal tubular insertion wall surfaces). The heavy reacting phase and the light reacting phase are in direct contact, and thus mass transfer of active reacting agents in the fluid (liquid) phase occurs. Each stream is specified by its (liquid or fluid) flow rate, temperature, and compositions. There is an additional flow rate needed to specify for the heavy reacting phase: the solid mass flow rate. Other than the solid mass flow (and the light reacting phase is similar to the heavy reacting phase), the reactive extraction process is identical to a reactive distillation process. Therefore, the analysis for the reactive extraction can be applied to reactive distillation as well.

At steady state, mass balance of the solid materials leads to

$$dG_H = -\sum_{j=1}^{N_S} r_j dV \tag{5.101}$$

where r_j is the (mass) rate of formation of species j in the fluid phase associated with the solid phase. For reactive extraction, there is a net loss in solid mass as components are being dissolved into the fluid phase.

In the heavy reacting phase, mass balance of species j at steady state leads

$$-d\left(Q_H C_{Hj}\right) + r_j dV - aJ_j dV = 0 \tag{5.102}$$

where Q_H is the volumetric flow rate of the heavy (fluid) reacting phase, C_{Hj} is the (mass) concentration of species j in the heavy reacting phase, J_j is the mass transfer flux of species j from the heavy reacting phase, and a is the specific area of contact between the heavy and light reacting phases.

In the light reacting phase, mass balance of species j at steady state leads

$$-d\left(Q_L C_{Lj}\right) + aJ_j dV = 0 \tag{5.103}$$

where Q_L is the volumetric flow rate of the light reacting phase, C_{Lj} is the (mass) concentration of species j in the light reacting phase.

Mass transfer flux from the heavy reacting phase to the light reacting phase can be computed via

$$J_j = K_{Cj}\left(C_{Hj} - C_{Lj}\right) \tag{5.104}$$

where K_{Cj} is the mass transfer coefficient for species j. Mass transfer coefficients are dependent on the type of molecule, flow rates, temperature, and the properties of the solid phase.

In addition to the mass balances, energy balances for the three streams (heavy reacting phase, light reacting phase, and the heat-exchanging fluid) are required to complete the set of the governing equations. The rate of reaction is strongly dependent on the temperature for reactions involved with solid materials.

Equations (5.101) through (5.104) are similar to those governing the extraction processes, with an extra reacting term. Therefore, the reactive extraction can be solved similar to solving an extraction column.

5.11. GRAPHIC SOLUTIONS USING BATCH CONCENTRATION DATA

We have learned so far how to perform reactor analysis for flow reactors based on known reaction rate. The reaction rate is usually experimentally determined via examining the concentration changes in a batch reactor, which will be discussed in Chapter 7. In this section, we shall examine how to design or analyze a flow reactor based on the concentration profile obtained in batch experiments at the same (feed) conditions.

Figure 5.21 shows a typical (reactant) concentration profile obtained in a batch reactor. Initially, the reactor is charged with the raw material with the key reactant concentration of C_{A0}. As the reaction progresses, the concentration of A decreases with time until the reaction is complete. If we look at a key product, the concentration would be increased with increase duration of the reaction, just opposite to the reactant concentration. For ease of discussion, we shall restrict ourself to constant density reactions, for example, condensed phase (liquid and/or solid) reactions.

5.11.1. Solution of a PFR using Batch Concentration Data

For a reaction carried out in a steady PFR, we have learned that mole balance in a differential volume of the PFR leads to

$$r_j = \frac{dF_j}{dV} \tag{5.11}$$

where

$$F_j = Q\,C_j \tag{5.105}$$

For constant density reactions, the volumetric flow rate Q is constant throughout the reactor. Therefore, Eqns (5.11) and (5.105) lead to

$$\frac{dV}{Q} = \frac{dC_j}{r_j} \tag{5.106}$$

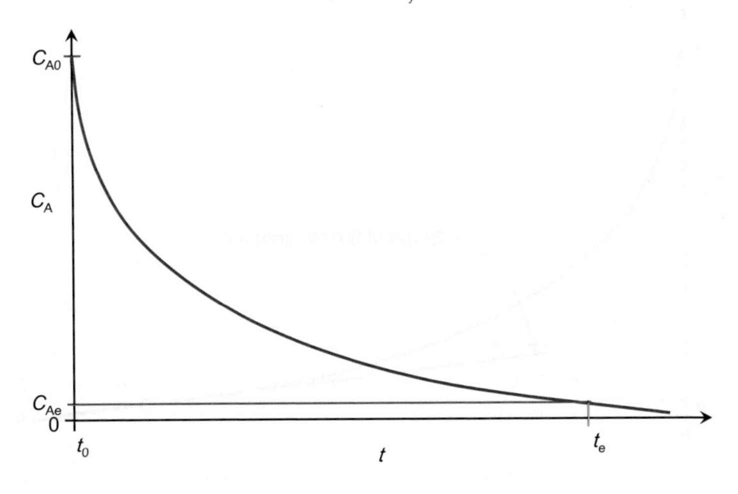

FIGURE 5.21 Variation of concentration with reaction time in a batch reactor.

or

$$\frac{V}{Q} = \int_{C_{j0}}^{C_{je}} \frac{dC_j}{r_j} \tag{5.107}$$

for constant density reactions. To make use of the batch concentration data as shown in Fig. 5.22, we need to know how the reaction rate is related to the concentration change. In a batch reactor, mole balance leads to Eqn (4.2), or

$$r_j V_{\text{Batch}} = \frac{dn_j}{dt} \tag{5.108}$$

Again for constant density reactions ($\rho = \text{constant} \Rightarrow V_{\text{batch}} = \text{constant}$), Eqn (5.108) is reduced to

$$r_j = \frac{dC_j}{dt} \tag{5.109}$$

Thus, the integration of Eqn (5.107) may be taken on the batch concentration data via Eqn (5.109).

$$\frac{V}{Q} = \int_{C_{j0}}^{C_{je}} \frac{dC_j}{r_j} = \int_{C_{j0}}^{C_{je}} \frac{dC_j}{dC_j/dt} = \int_{t@C_{j0}}^{t\,@C_{je}} dt = t_e - t_0 \tag{5.110}$$

Therefore, the integration rates can be read off directly from the batch concentration profile (data). Referring to Fig. 5.22 and Eqn (5.110), if the conversion is known (or specified), we can

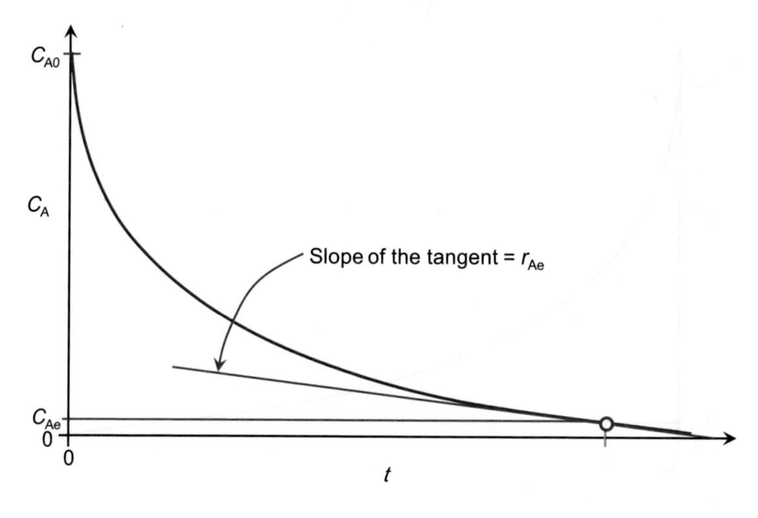

FIGURE 5.22 Finding the rate of reaction from the batch concentration data.

read the time from the batch data at which the desired effluent concentration is obtained, t_e, and the starting time, t_0. The required PFR volume is calculated by

$$V = Q(t_e - t_0) \tag{5.111}$$

On the other hand, if the reactor is given for a given throughput, Fig. 5.22 can be employed to read off the effluent concentration corresponding to the time t_e,

$$t_e = t_0 + \frac{V}{Q} \tag{5.112}$$

The similarity between PFR and batch reactor mathematically makes the solution of a PFR problem rather simple if batch concentration profile is known for the same reaction conditions.

5.11.2. Solution of a CSTR using Batch Concentration Data

Solution of a CSTR has been relatively simple when the reaction rate data is known. Mole balance around a steady CSTR leads to

$$Q_0 C_{j0} - QC_j + r_j V = 0 \tag{5.39}$$

where the flow rate, concentration, and reaction rate are all evaluated at effluent conditions if subscript 0 is not shown. For a constant density reaction, Eqn (5.39) is reduced to

$$Q\frac{C_{je} - C_{j0}}{V} = r_{je} \tag{5.113}$$

If the reactor effluent conditions are known (or specified), the required reaction rate for Eqn (5.113) via Eqn (5.109) from the batch concentration data. Figure 5.23 illustrates how

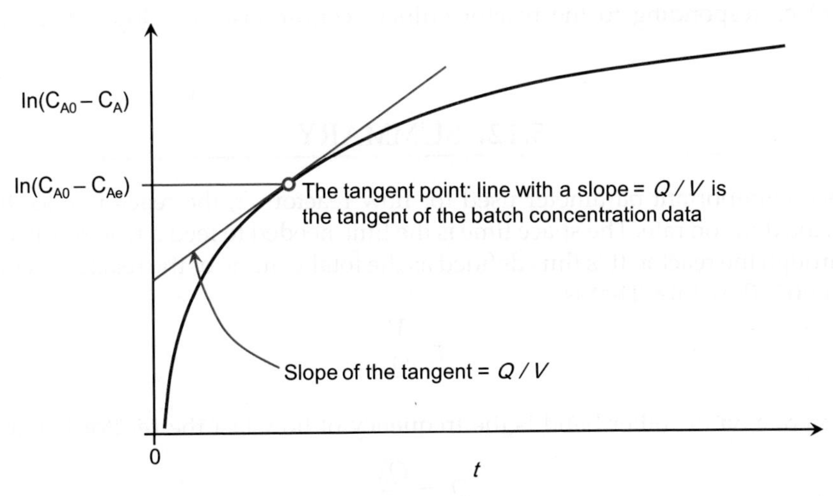

FIGURE 5.23 Finding the space velocity or dilution rate from the batch reactant concentration data.

this reaction rate is determined. The reaction rate to be used in Eqn (5.113) is the slope of the tangent of the batch concentration curve at the reactor effluent concentration. Once the reaction rate is determined, the reactor volume can be obtained by rearranging Eqn (5.113),

$$V = Q\frac{C_{je} - C_{j0}}{r_{je}} \tag{5.114}$$

If on the other hand, the reactor and throughput are known, the reactor effluent concentration can be determined by combining Eqns (5.109) and (5.113). Substituting Eqn (5.109) into Eqn (5.113), we obtain

$$Q\frac{C_{je} - C_{j0}}{V} = \frac{dC_{je}}{dt} \tag{5.115}$$

It is not convenient to use Eqn (5.115) to compute the concentration C_{je} by inspecting the batch concentration data as shown in Fig. 5.21 or Fig. 5.22. Rearranging Eqn (5.115), we can obtain

$$\frac{Q}{V} = \frac{d\ln|C_{je} - C_{j0}|}{dt} \tag{5.116}$$

Equation (5.116) indicates that the solution can be obtained by plotting the batch concentration data (or rather the difference of batch concentration data) on a semilog scale plot. The right-hand side of Eqn (5.116) is the slope of (the tangent to) the batch concentration (difference) data on a semilog plot, which must be equivalent to the dilution rate or space time, Q/V.

Figure 5.23 illustrates how to find the CSTR effluent concentration from the semilog plot of the batch concentration difference data. The line with a slope of Q/V pinches the semilog batch concentration difference data at exactly the effluent conditions. Therefore, the reactor effluent concentration can be read (or computed) from the tangent point as indicated in Fig. 5.23.

Figure 5.23 can also be employed to find the reactor volume if the reactor effluent conditions are known. In this case, draws the tangent to the batch concentration difference data at the point corresponding to the reactor effluent conditions. The slope of the tangent is then Q/V.

5.12. SUMMARY

There is one important parameter used for flow reactors, τ, the reactor space time or its inverse, D, the dilution rate. The space time is the time needed to feed a reactor full of reaction mixture through the reactor. It is thus defined as the total volume of the reactor divided by the inlet volumetric flow rate. That is,

$$\tau = \frac{V}{Q_0} \tag{5.3}$$

The dilution rate on the other hand is the frequency of how fast the reactor is filled:

$$D = \frac{Q_0}{V} \tag{5.4}$$

There are two basic types of ideal flow reactors: PFR and CSTR. PFR represents a one-dimensional flow reactor, like a piston. At steady state, the concentration of reactants as well as products changes along the direction of flow in a PFR. The concentrations of the reactants are the highest in a PFR presented to reaction. The analysis to a PFR is similar to that for a batch reactor, the only difference being the independent variable: rather than time t, it is the volume of reactor V. For PFR, it is the residence time or distance along the reactor flow direction, whereas time is the independent variable for a batch reactor.

Since the reaction mixture changes along the reactor, mole balance for PFR leads to

$$\frac{\partial C_j}{\partial t} = r_j - \frac{\partial (QC_j)}{\partial V} \tag{5.7}$$

When steady state is reached, nothing in the reactor changes with time. Equation (5.7) is then reduced to

$$r_j = \frac{\mathrm{d}F_j}{\mathrm{d}V} \tag{5.11}$$

The reactor volume can be solved for a desired fractional conversion of f_{Ae},

$$V = F_{\mathrm{A0}} \int_0^{f_{\mathrm{Ae}}} \frac{\mathrm{d}f_{\mathrm{A}}}{-r_{\mathrm{A}}} \tag{5.24}$$

Correspondingly, the space time (no side inlets or outlets) for a PFR is given by

$$\tau = \frac{V}{Q_0} = C_{\mathrm{A0}} \int_0^{f_{\mathrm{Ae}}} \frac{\mathrm{d}f_{\mathrm{A}}}{-r_{\mathrm{A}}} \tag{5.25}$$

Table 5.2 shows a list of solutions for some single reactions with simple kinetics. For steady nonisothermal PFR, one more equation needs to solved simultaneously with Eqn (5.11),

$$\sum_{j=1}^{N_S} F_{j0} C_{Pj} \mathrm{d}T + \sum_{i=1}^{N_R} r_i \Delta H_{Ri} \mathrm{d}V = Ua(T_c - T)\mathrm{d}V \tag{5.100}$$

CSTR represents a reactor that is well mixed such that no concentration gradient exits. CSTR is also termed chemostat. Mole balance for a given species j over the entire reactor leads to

$$F_{j0} - F_j + r_j V = \frac{\mathrm{d}n_j}{\mathrm{d}t} \tag{5.33}$$

At steady state, only algebraic equations are resulted in CSTR analysis as the sole derivative in the mole balance Eqn (5.33) is the rate change of moles with time t in the reactor. At steady state, all the time derivatives are zero. Thus, for example, for species A, Eqn (5.33) is reduced to

$$\frac{F_{A0} - F_A}{V} = -r_A \tag{5.53}$$

One can observe that the left-hand side is the molar rate of A fed subtracted the molar rate of A letting out of the reactor, divided by the reactor volume. Thus, one can refer the left-hand side as the molar supply rate per reactor volume or simply molar supply rate. That is,

$$MS_A = \frac{F_{A0} - F_A}{V} \tag{5.54}$$

And the right-hand side is the molar consumption rate (or negative molar generation rate) of A. That is,

$$MC_A = -r_A \tag{5.56}$$

Therefore, the molar balance equation can be expressed as the molar supply rate of A to the reactor (MS_A) equals to the molar consumption rate of A (MC_A) in the reactor. The solution of a CSTR problem is thus visually illustrated in Fig. 5.11. That is,

$$MC_A = MS_A \tag{5.57}$$

For a steady nonisothermal CSTR, there is one more equation needed to be solved together,

$$\sum_{j=1}^{N_S} F_{j0}(H_j - H_{j0}) + V\sum_{i=1}^{N_R} r_i \Delta H_{Ri} = UA_H(T_c - T) - \dot{W}_s \tag{5.97}$$

The concentrations of reactants in a CSTR are at their lowest level in a CSTR and thus least available to reaction. In flow reactor design, our interest is not only on the reactor volume but type of reactors. Usually, a whole bioprocess system optimization (economic analysis) is applied to determine whether CSTR or PFR is employed. In some cases, one can save time by knowingly selecting the right type of reactors. Selection of PFR or CSTR depends on the nature of the reaction mixture and type of reaction (kinetics). One important clue is that CSTR has the highest product concentrations and lowest reactant concentrations in the reactor, which is the opposite for PFR. The reactor feed strategy greatly affects the product mixture. A reactor with optimum feed distribution and/or product separation can yield significantly more desired product.

Further Reading

Fogler, H.S. 1999. *Elements of Chemical Reaction Engineering*, (4th ed.). Prentice-Hall.

Hill, C.G. 1977. *An Introduction to Chemical Engineering Kinetics and Reactor Design*, Wiley & Sons, New York.

Levenspiel, O. 1999. *Chemical Reaction Engineering*, (3rd Ed.). John Wiley & Sons, New York.

Schmidt, L.D. 2005. *The Engineering of Chemical Reactions*, (2nd ed.). Oxford University Press, New York.

PROBLEMS

5.1. Ethylene is the monomer for polyethylene production. Polyethylene is an important commodity plastics widely used today. As a replacement for petroleum products, ethanol is being developed to manufacture ethylene as ethanol can be produced from biomass. The following reaction:

$$C_2H_5OH(A) \rightarrow C_2H_4(B) + H_2O(C)$$

is being considered to be carried out in a PFR. 1) The feed is pure ethanol at 1 kg/s, 500 K, and 2 bar; 2) the kinetics is given by $r = \frac{kC_A}{1 + C_A/K_A}$, $k = 0.1\ \text{min}^{-1}$ and $K_A = 1$ mol/L; 3) the reactor operates isothermally with negligible pressure drop; 4) the final conversion at the outlet of the reactor $f_{Ae} = 0.4$. Compute

(a) The reactor volume V;
(b) The space time τ;
(c) And the dilution rate, D.

5.2. At your favorite fast food joint, the french fries are made by filling a basket with potatoes and dipping them in hot animal or vegetable fat for 4 min and then draining them for 4 min. Every hour the small pieces that fell out of the basket are scooped out because they burn and give a bad taste. At the end of the 16 h day, the fat is drained and sent out for disposal because at longer times the oil has decomposed sufficiently to give a bad taste. Approximately 2 pounds of potatoes are used in 10 gal of oil.

(a) Why is a batch process usually preferred in a restaurant?
(b) Design a continuous process to make 1 ton/day of french fries, keeping exactly the same conditions as above so they will taste the same. Describe the residence times and desired flow patterns in solid and liquid phases. Include the oil recycling loop.
(c) How might you modify the process to double the production rate from that specified for the same apparatus? What experiments would you have to do to test its feasibility?
(d) How would you design this continuous process to handle varying load demands?

5.3. An irreversible first-order reaction gave 95% conversion in a batch reactor in 20 min.

(a) What would be the conversion of this reaction in a CSTR with a 20 min residence time?
(b) What residence time would be required for 95% conversion in a CSTR?
(c) What residence time would be required for 99% conversion in a CSTR?
(d) What residence time would be required for 95% conversion in a PFR?
(e) What residence time would be required for 99% conversion in a PFR?

5.4. Calculate the ratio of residence times in CSTR and PFR for the nth-order irreversible reaction for conversions of 50, 90, 99, and 99.9% for $n = 0$, 1/2, 1, 2, and -1 for $C_{A0} = 1.0$ mol/L.

5.5. Calculate the reactor volumes required to process 100 L/min of 3 mol A in the aqueous reaction $A \rightarrow 2B$ for PFR and CSTR reactors.

(a) 90% conversion, $k = 2\ \text{min}^{-1}$
(b) 99% conversion, $k = 2\ \text{mol} \cdot \text{L}^{-1} \cdot \text{min}^{-1}$
(c) 99.9% conversion, $k = 2\ \text{mol} \cdot \text{L}^{-1} \cdot \text{min}^{-1}$
(d) 90% conversion, $k = 2\ \text{min}^{-1} \cdot \text{L} \cdot \text{mol}^{-1}$
(e) 99.9% conversion, $k = 2\ \text{min}^{-1} \cdot \text{L} \cdot \text{mol}^{-1}$

5.6. Set up the above problems if the feed is pure A, A and B are ideal gases, and the reactors operate at 100 atm.

5.7. An aqueous feed containing reactant A (1 mol/L) enters a 2-L plug flow reactor and reacts with the reaction $2A \rightarrow B$, r (mol/L/min) $= 0.2\ C_A$.
(a) What feed rate (L/min) will give an outlet concentration of $C_A = 0.1$ mol/L?
(b) Find the outlet concentration of A (mol/L) for a feed rate of 0.1 L/min.
(c) Repeat this problem for a stirred-tank reactor.

5.8. An aqueous feed containing reactant A at $C_{A0} = 2$ mol/L at a feed rate $F_{A0} = 100$ mol/min decomposes in a CSTR to give a variety of products. The kinetics of the conversion are represented by

$$A \rightarrow 2.5\ B,\ r = 10\ C_A\ (\text{mol} \cdot \text{L}^{-1} \cdot \text{min}^{-1})$$

(a) Find the volume CSTR needed for 80% decomposition of reactant A.
(b) Find the conversion in a 30 L CSTR.
(c) What flow rate will be required to produce 100 mol/min of B at 80% conversion?

5.9. An ester in aqueous solution is to be saponified in a continuous reactor system. Batch experiments showed that the reaction is first order and irreversible, and 50% reaction occurred in 8 min at the temperature required. We need to process 100 mol/h of 4 mol/L feed to 95% conversion. Calculate the reactor volumes required for this process in
(a) a PFR,
(b) a CSTR,
(c) two equal-volume CSTRs,
(d) four equal-volume CSTRs.

5.10. The aqueous reaction A → products has a rate $r = 2C_A/(1 + C_A)^2$ (rate in $\text{mol} \cdot \text{L}^{-1} \cdot \text{min}^{-1}$) and is to be carried out in a continuous reactor system. We need to process 100 mol/h of 2 mol/L feed to 90% conversion. Calculate the reactor volumes required in
(a) a PFR,
(b) a CSTR,
(c) two equal-volume CSTRs.
(d) Use plots of $1/r$ vs conversion to show these results.
(e) What is the ideal combination of reactors for total minimum volume for this reaction?
(f) Show how you would solve problem (e) analytically. Set up equations and indicate the method of solution.

5.11. We have a 100-gal tank of a product that now contains small particles that must be removed before it can be sold. The product now has 10^4 particles/cm^3, and it is only acceptable for sale if the particle concentration is less than 10^2 particles/cm^3. We have a filter that will effectively remove all particles.

(a) At what rate must the product be pumped through the filter to make the product acceptable within 2 days if the tank is mixed and the filtered product is continuously fed back into the tank?

(b) At the pumping rate of part (a) how long will be required if the filtered product is placed in a separate tank?

(c) Repeat parts (a) and (b) assuming the filter only removes 90% of the particles on each pass.

5.12. **(a)** Find $C_A(\tau)$ and $C_B(\tau)$ for the liquid reaction $A \rightarrow B$ with $r = kC_AC_B$ in a PFR and a CSTR with a feed of $C_{A0} = 2$ mol/L and $C_{B0} = 0$ with $k = 0.2$ L mol^{-1} · min^{-1}.

(b) Why cannot this reaction be carried out in a PFR with this composition?

(c) What modification would be required in a PFR to give finite conversion?

5.13. Sketch $1/r$ vs $C_{A0} - C_A$ or f_A for $A \rightarrow$ products for the reactions $r = kC_A/(1 + K\,C_A)$ for $C_{A0} = 2$ mol/L, $k = 0.1$ min^{-1}, and $K = 1$ L/mol. From this graph, find τ for 90% conversion for

(a) a PFR,

(b) a CSTR,

(c) two equal-volume CSTRs,

(d) the optimal combination of reactors in series.

5.14. An irreversible first-order reaction gave 80% conversion in a batch reactor in 20 min.

(a) Calculate the total residence time for this conversion for CSTRs in series for 1, 2, 3, and 4 equal-volume reactors.

(b) What residence time will be required for a very large number of equal-volume CSTRs? What is the limit of $(1 + k\tau)^{-n}$ in the limit $n \rightarrow \infty$?

5.15. **(a)** What is the optimum combination of ideal reactors for the reaction $A \rightarrow B$ if it is autocatalytic with $r = kC_AC_B$ and $C_A = C_{A0}$, $C_{B0} = 0$? What is the intermediate concentration between reactors?

(b) Solve for 90% conversion if $C_{A0} = 1$ mol/L and $k = 0.25$ L · mol^{-1} · min^{-1}.

5.16. In fermentation processes sugar (A) is converted to ethanol (C) as a by-product of yeast (B) reproduction. In a simple model, we can represent this process as

$$A \rightarrow B + 3C, \quad r = kC_AC_B$$

Starting with 10 weight percent sucrose ($C_{12}H_{22}O_{11}$) in water and assuming that half of the carbon atoms in the sucrose are converted into ethanol (the above stoichiometry), find the times required to produce 3.5 weight percent alcohol (1% sucrose remaining) for initial concentrations of yeast of 0.00001, 0.0001, 0.001, and 0.01 M. It is found that 2 h are required for this conversion if the initial yeast concentration is maintained at 1 M. Assume that the density is that of water.

5.17. The gas-phase reaction $A \rightarrow 3B$ obeys zeroth-order kinetics with $r = 0.25$ mol/L/h at 200 °C. Starting with pure A at 1 atm, calculate the time for 95% conversion of A in

(a) a constant-volume batch reactor,

(b) a constant-pressure batch reactor.

Calculate the reactor volume to process 10 mol/h of A to this conversion in

(c) a constant-pressure PFR,

(d) a constant-pressure CSTR.
(e) Calculate the residence times and space times in these reactors.

5.18. One hundred moles of A per hour are available in concentration of 0.1 mol/L by a previous process. This stream is to be reacted with B to produce C and D. The reaction proceeds by the aqueous-phase reaction,

$$A + B \rightarrow C + D,\ k = 5\,L \cdot mol^{-1} \cdot h^{-1}$$

The amount of C required is 95 mol/h. In extracting C from the reacted mixture A and B are destroyed; hence recycling of unused reactants is not possible. Calculate the optimum reactor size and type as well as feed composition for this process.

Data: B costs \$1.25/mol in crystalline form. It is highly soluble in the aqueous solution and even when present in large amounts does not change the concentration of A in solution. Capital and operating costs are \$0.015/h/L for mixed-flow reactors.

5.19. One-hundred and fifty moles of B are to be produced hourly from a feed consisting of a saturated solution of A ($C_{A0} = 0.1$ mol/L) in a mixed-flow reactor. The reaction is

$$A \rightarrow B,\ r = 0.2(h^{-1})C_A$$

The cost of reactant at $C_{A0} = 0.1$ mol/L is \$A = \$0.50/mol A. The cost of reactor including installation, auxiliary equipment, instrumentation, overhead, labor, depreciation, etc., is $\$m = \$0.01\ h^{-1} \cdot liter^{-1}$.

What reactor size, feed rate, and conversion should be used for optimum operations? What is the unit cost of B for these conditions if unreacted A is discarded?

5.20. Suppose all unreacted A of the product stream of the previous problem can be reclaimed and brought up to the initial concentration $C_{A0} = 0.1$ mol/L at a total cost of \$0. A (125/mol) processed. With this reclaimed A as a recycle stream, find the new optimum operating conditions and unit cost of producing B.

5.21. Consider the reaction

$$A \rightarrow B,\ r = 0.15(min^{-1})\ C_A$$

in a CSTR. A costs \$2/mol, and B sells for \$4/mol. The cost of operating the reactor is \$0.03 per liter per hour. We need to produce 100 mol of B/h using $C_{A0} = 2$ mol/L. Assume no value or cost of disposal of unreacted A.
(a) What is the optimum conversion and reactor size?
(b) What is the cash flow from the process?
(c) What is the cash flow ignoring operating cost?
(d) At what operating cost do we break-even?

5.22. Find an expression for the conversion in a dimerization reaction

$$2A \rightarrow B,\ r = kC_A^2$$

with A and B ideal gases starting with pure A at 1 atm in
(a) a CSTR,
(b) a PFR.

5.23. Find an expression for the conversion in a dimerization reaction

$$2A \rightarrow B,\ r = kC_A^2$$

in a CSTR with A and B ideal gases starting with A at 1 atm for
(a) no diluent in the feed,
(b) 1 atm of inert diluent,
(c) 9 atm of diluent,
(d) 99 atm of diluent.
(e) Compare the volumes required for 90% conversion in these situations with those predicted using the constant-density approximation.

5.24. The aqueous reversible reaction

$$A \leftrightharpoons B, \; r = kC_A - k'C_B$$

is to be carried out in a series of reactors with separation of unreacted B between stages. At each stage, the reaction goes to 50% of the equilibrium composition. How many stages are required for 90% conversion of the initial A for $k = 0.2 \text{ min}^{-1}$, $K_{eq} = 1$ if
(a) all B is extracted between stages,
(b) 50% of B is extracted between stages.
(c) Find τ with complete extraction if the reactors are CSTRs.
(d) Find τ if the reactors are PFRs.

5.25. A reaction A → products is known to obey the rate expression $r = kC_A^n$. Using two 50-L CSTRs in series, it is found that with a feed of 2.0 mol/L, after the first reactor $C_A = 1.0$ mol/L and after the second $C_A = 0.3$ mol/L.
(a) Find n.
(b) What volume PFR will be required to obtain 90% conversion for this reaction at the same feed rate?

5.26. A certain equipment catalog lists CSTRs as costing

$$\text{CSTR} = 1000 + 100V^{1/2}$$

and PFRs as

$$\$\text{PFR} = 500 + 100V$$

where $ is in dollars and V is in liters.
(a) Why might the cost of a chemical reactor be roughly proportional to its surface area? For what reactor geometries might the costs of chemical reactors have these dependences on their volumes? How should the cost of a spherical CSTR depend on its volume?
(b) At what volume will the costs of a CSTR and PFR be equal in this catalog?
(c) We find that a 1000-L PFR will process 500 mol/h of a reactant in a first-order reaction to 90% conversion. How does the cost of this reactor compare with a CSTR for the same conversion?
(d) Repeat this calculation for processing 1000 mol/h to 90% conversion.

5.27. A 10,000-galion holding tank receives an aqueous by-product effluent stream from a continuous chemical process. The tank is well mixed and drains into a river. The tank receives 2400 gal/day of a certain by-product that decomposes in the tank with a rate coefficient of 0.2 h^{-1}.

(a) What fraction of the by-product from the process enters the river?
(b) At this flow rate what size tank would be required to react 99% of the by-product before entering the river?

5.28. A 10,000-gal-holding tank receives an aqueous by-product effluent stream from a batch chemical process. The constant-volume tank is well mixed and drains into a river. A batch process is recycled every 8 h, and in the cleanup of the reactor 1000 gal are rapidly drained into the tank at the end of each batch run. The by-product decomposes in the tank with a rate coefficient of 0.2 h^{-1}.
(a) What fraction of the by-product from the process enters the river?
(b) At this discharge rate what size tank would be required to react 99% of the by-product before entering the river?

5.29. We wish to treat a stream 1 m^3/h containing 2 mol/L A to produce 90% conversion in the reaction

$$A \rightarrow B, \quad r = kC_AC_B$$

with $k = 1/4$ (units of minutes, moles, and liters).
(a) Find τ in the best single reactor.
(b) Find τ in two equal-volume CSTRs.
(c) Find the reactor volumes for minimum τ in two reactors in series.

5.30. We wish to treat 10 L/min of liquid feed containing 1 mol-A/L to 99% conversion. The reaction is given by

$$2A \rightarrow R + U, \; r = \frac{k_1C_A}{1 + k_2C_A}$$

where $k_1 = 2.5\ \text{min}^{-1}$ and $k_2 = 5$ L/mol. Suggest a good arrangement for doing this using two CSTR's. Find the sizes of the two units needed.

5.31. We wish to explore various reactor setups for the transformation of A into R. The feed contains 99% A, 1% R; the desired product is to consist of 10% A, 90% R. The transformation takes place by means of the elementary reaction

$$A + R \rightarrow R + R$$

That is, the rate of reaction is given by $r = k\ C_AC_R$. Here the rate constant $k = 1\ \text{L} \cdot \text{mol}^{-1} \cdot \text{min}^{-1}$. The concentration of active materials is

$$C_{A0} + C_{R0} = C_A + C_R = C_0 = 1\ \text{mol/L}$$

throughout. What reactor holding time (i.e. mean residence time) will yield a product in which $C_R = 0.9$ mol/L?
(a) In a plug flow reactor without recycle?
(b) In a plug flow reactor with optimum recycle?
(c) In a CSTR?
(d) In a minimum size setup without recycle by a combination of one PFR and one CSTR?

5.32. A three-stage CSTR is used for the reaction A → products. The reaction occurs in aqueous solution and is second order with respect to A, with $k_A = 0.040\ \text{L} \cdot \text{mol}^{-1} \cdot \text{min}^{-1}$. The inlet concentration of A and the inlet volumetric flow rate are 1.5 mol · L^{-1} and 2.5 L · min^{-1}, respectively. Determine the maximum fractional conversion (f_A) obtained at the outlet and order of reactors if the three CSTR's available of volume: 10 L, 20 L, and 50 L.

5.33. When B is mixed A, the liquid phase reaction

$$A + B \rightarrow C \qquad r = kC_A$$

Has a rate constant $k = 0.2\ \text{min}^{-1}$. This reaction is to be carried out isothermally in a CSTR at steady state. The reactant A costs \$2/mol and reactant B costs \$0.10/mol. The product C sells for \$6/mol. The cost of operating the reactor is \$0.05 per liter per hour. We wish to produce 360,000 mol of C per day to meet the market demands. The available reactants: A and B, are from different sources: the solution for A has a concentration of 1 mol/L and the solution for B has a concentration of 4 mol per liter. Assume no cost or value to dispose off unreacted A and B.

(a) What is the overall feed stream concentration of A if a stoichiometric feed is chosen? Is this the best choice and why?

(b) Perform a mole balance on the reactor to relate the conversion of A with the reactor size.

(c) Express the profit per mole of A feed to the reactor as a function of the conversion.

(d) What is the optimum conversion of A (for a stoichiometric feed) and what is the corresponding reactor size?

(e) What is the cash flow (or profit per mole of A feed to the reactor) from the process?

5.34. The reaction between ammonia and formaldehyde to give hexamine is

$$4NH_3 + 6HCHO \rightarrow (CH_2)_6N_4 + 6H_2O$$

A 0.5-L CSTR is used for the reaction. Each reactant is fed to the reactor in a separate stream, at the rate of 1.5×10^{-3} L/s each with ammonia concentration 4.0 mol/L and formaldehyde 6.4 mol/L. The reactor temperature is 36 °C. Calculate the concentration of ammonia and formaldehyde in the effluent stream. The reaction rate is

$$-r_A = kC_A C_B^2 \frac{\text{mol-A}}{\text{L} \times \text{s}}$$

where A is ammonia and B is formaldehyde

$$k = 1.42 \times 10^3 \exp\left(\frac{-3090\,K}{T}\right)$$

5.35. The reaction $A + B \rightleftharpoons C + D$ is carried out in an adiabatic plug flow reactor. The following data are available

$$\Delta H_R = -120{,}000\ \text{J/mol}; \qquad C_{p_A} = C_{p_B} = C_{p_C} = C_{p_D} = 100\ \text{J/(mol K)}$$
$$K_e\ (\text{equilibrium constant}) = 500{,}000\ \text{at}\ 50\ ^\circ\text{C}$$
$$F_{A_0} = F_{B_0} = 10\ \text{mol/min}$$

Calculate the maximum conversion that may be achieved if the feed enters at 27 °C and only A and B are in the feed.

5.36. An ideal gas reaction is carried out in a CSTR

$$A \rightarrow 2C$$

The feed to the reactor is 50% A and 50% inert (by volume) at 1 atm and 100 °C. The reaction rate is given by:

$$-r_A = kC_A, k = 1\ s^{-1}$$

The inlet volumetric flow rate is 1 m^3/s. Determine the reactor volume required for 80% conversion of *A*.

5.37. The liquid phase reaction $A + B \rightarrow C + D$ is carried out in a PFR of volume 1 m^3. The inlet volumetric flow rate is 0.5 m^3. The rate expression is

$$-r_A = kC_AC_B, \quad k = 1 \times 10^{-4} \frac{m^3}{mol \times s}$$

The inlet concentrations of *A* and *B* are 1×10^3 mol/m^3. Calculate the outlet fractional conversion.

5.38. Reactant A reacts according to second-order kinetics (assume constant density, isothermal operation), i.e. $-r_A = kC_A^2$. The reaction is carried out in a flow reactor and the outlet conversion is 95%. Suppose that a second reactor is added of identical volume to the first and the overall conversion is 95%. By what factor do we increase the plant throughput under the following scenarios? In each case you must justify your answer using appropriate equations or logic.

(a) The original reactor is a PFR. The added unit is a PFR and the units are operated in parallel.

(b) The original unit is a PFR. The added unit is a PFR and the units are operated in series.

(c) The original unit is a CSTR. The added unit is a CSTR and the reactors are operated in parallel.

(d) The original unit is a CSTR. The added unit is a CSTR and the units are operated in series.

(e) The original unit is a CSTR. The added unit is a PFR which is run in series with the PFR first.

5.39. Consider a liquid phase reaction occurring in two CSTR connected in series. The volume of each reactor is 100 L. The reaction is $A + B \xrightarrow{k} C$, $-r_A = kC_AC_B$ with $k = 1\ L \cdot mol^{-1} \cdot s^{-1}$ to give the rate in $mol \cdot L^{-1} \cdot s^{-1}$.

The feed to the first reactor consists of 1 L/s of a solution of 1 mol/L of A and 0.2 mol/L of B. The feed to the second reactor is the effluent from the first reactor plus another feed stream consisting of 1 L/s of a solution containing 0.8 mol/L of B (no A in this stream).

(a) Calculate the molar flow rate of C from the first reactor.

(b) Calculate the molar flow rate of C from the second reactor.

5.40. Consider the ideal gas reaction

$$A + B \xrightarrow{k} C + D$$

which is conducted in a plug flow reactor. The feed is 50% A, 30% *BB*, and 20% inert on a molar basis. The total inlet molar flow rate 10 mol/s which gives a total volumetric flow rate of 0.1 m^3/s.

(a) determine the reactor volume required to achieve 50% conversion of A.

(b) determine the reactor volume required to achieve 80% conversion of A.

The rate equation is $-r_A = k\, C_A C_B$ with $k = 5 \times 10^{-4}\ m^3 \cdot mol^{-1} \cdot s^{-1}$.

5.41. The intermediate R is to be produced in a steady isothermal liquid CSTR:

$$A \rightarrow R, \qquad r_1 = k_1\, C_A$$

$$R \rightarrow S, \qquad r_2 = k_2\, C_R$$

with $k_1 = 2\ s^{-1}$ and $k_2 = 0.5\ s^{-1}$. Calculate the value of residence time for maximum yield of R, τ_{maxR}. What is the conversion of A, yields of R and S if the residence time in the reactor is τ_{maxR}.

5.42. The reaction system:

$$A \rightarrow R, \qquad r_1 = k_1 C_A$$

$$A \rightarrow S, \qquad r_2 = k_2 C_B$$

Have activation energies of 8 and 10 kcal/mol, respectively. In a 1-L batch reactor at 100 °C, the fractional yield of R is 50% and the conversion is 50% in a reaction time of 10 min with $C_{A0} = 1$ mol/L. The solvent is water and the reactor can be pressurized as needed to maintain liquids at any given temperature.

(a) What temperature and reactor volume are required to produce 90% fractional yield of R at 90% conversion in a CSTR using a feed of 2 mol/L A at a flow rate of 10 L/min?

(b) Repeat a. if a PFR is used instead.

5.43. We wish to produce ethylene by the oxidative dehydrogenation of ethane. Over a suitable catalyst the reactions and rates are found to be

$$C_2H_6 + 0.5\, O_2 \rightarrow C_2H_4 + H_2O, \qquad r_1 = k_1 C_{C_2H_6} C_{O_2}$$

$$C_2H_6 + 3.5\, O_2 \rightarrow 2CO_2 + 3H_2O, \qquad r_2 = k_2 C_{C_2H_6} C_{O_2}^2$$

The reaction is to be run at 1000 K, where it is found that $k_1 = 9$ L/(mol·s) and $k_2 = 1670\ L^2/(mol^2 \cdot s)$. The feed pressures are $p_{C_2H_6} = 2$ atm, $p_{O_2} = 1$ atm, and $p_{N_2} = 4$ atm. Neglect the pressure drop in the reactor and the reaction is to have a residence time such that the product contains 0.05 atm of O_2. Assume that there is sufficient diluent that the density remains constant.

(a) Will a PFR or a CSTR give a higher ethylene fractional yield?

(b) Will a PFR or a CSTR require the longer residence time?

(c) Calculate the fractional yield to ethylene on a carbon atom basis in PFR and CSTR for this O_2 conversion.

(d) Set up the problem to calculate the residence times required in PFR and CSTR. (This illustrates how complex multiple reaction systems can become and why the fractional yield concept is useful. When numerical methods are used, the complexity would not however deter a solution with today's computers.)

5.44. Under ultraviolet radiation, reactant A of $C_{A0} = 10$ kmol/m^3 in a liquid process stream ($Q = 1$ m^3/min) decomposes as follows:

$$A \rightarrow R \quad r_1 = 16C_A^{0.5} \quad \text{kmol}/(\text{m}^3 \cdot \text{min})$$

$$A \rightarrow S \quad r_2 = 12C_A \quad \text{kmol}/(\text{m}^3 \cdot \text{min})$$

$$2A \rightarrow T \quad r_3 = 0.5\,C_A^2 \quad \text{kmol}/(\text{m}^3 \cdot \text{min})$$

We wish to design a reactor setup to maximize the production R.

(a) What type of reactor or reactor scheme is to be selected?

(b) Calculate the fraction of feed transformed into the desired product R as well as the volume of the reactor needed.

(c) Repeat a. and b. if the desired product is S instead.

5.45. The gas-phase decomposing reaction

$$A \rightarrow B + C, \qquad r = k\,C_A$$

is to be carried out adiabatically in a flow reactor. The feed consists of pure A at a temperature of 298 K and a pressure of 1 bar. The feed rate is 0.1 mol/s. Neglect the pressure drop in the reactor.

(a) Calculate the operating temperature and conversion from a CSTR of volume 2 m^3.

(b) Calculate the volume of a PFR for a conversion of 0.99. Comment on your findings.

(c) Recalculate the volume of the PFR for a conversion of 0.99, but the feed to the reactor is preheated to 500 K.

The additional data are: $k = 10^{11}\exp\left(-\dfrac{E}{RT}\right)$ s^{-1}; $\dfrac{E}{R} = 18000$ K; $\Delta H_R = -60$ kJ/mol-A; $\overline{C}_{PA} = 120$ J/(mol·K); $\overline{C}_{PB} = 80$J/(mol·K); $\overline{C}_{PC} = 40$J/(mol·K)

5.46. Consider the elementary reaction: $A + R \rightarrow 2\,R$ with a rate constant equal 0.001 L · mol^{-1} · s^{-1}. We wish to process 1.5 L/s of a feed containing 10 mol/L A to the highest conversion possible in the reactor system consisting of four 150-L CSTR's connected as you wish and any feed arrangement.

(a) Sketch your recommended design and feed arrangement.

(b) Determine the final conversion.

(c) Comment on the reactor start-up conditions.

5.47. We wish to convert A to R in a plug flow reactor by the aqueous decomposition reaction:

$$A \rightarrow R + U, \qquad r_1 = k_1\,C_A$$

where $k_1 = 1.2$ m^3/(mol·min). We realized that A can also be dimerized to S:

$$A + A \rightarrow S, \qquad r_2 = k_2\,C_A^2$$

with $k_2 = 0.8$/min. The aqueous feed contains A by $C_{A0} = 40$ mol/m^3.

(a) Which type of ideal isothermal flow reactors (CSTR or PFR) is preferred? Briefly state why?
(b) What is the yield of R and reactor holding time if the fractional conversion of A is 90% for the reactor chosen in part a.?

5.48. Propylene (P) and chlorine (C) react in gas phase to produce allyl chloride (A)

$$C_3H_6 + Cl_2 \rightarrow H_2C{=}CHCH_2Cl + HCl \qquad r_1 = k_1 p_P p_C$$

and 1,2-dichloropropane (D),

$$C_3H_6 + Cl_2 \rightarrow H_2CClCHClCH_3 \qquad r_2 = k_2 p_P p_C$$

The kinetic experiments show that $k_1 = 206000 \exp\left(-\frac{7610\ K}{T}\right)$ mol/(m^3·s·bar^2) and $k_2 = 11.7 \exp\left(-\frac{1920\ K}{T}\right)$ mol/(m^3·s·bar^2). Allyl chloride is the desired product. Either CSTR or PFR can be used to carry out the reaction. Neglect the pressure drop in the reactor and the reactors can be operated at isothermal conditions between 25 and 450 °C. The feed to the reactor will be 1 bar propylene and 1 bar chlorine.
(a) What is the optimum operating temperature in a CSTR? In a PFR?
(b) Find the local selectivity $s_{A/P}$.
(c) What is the overall selectivity to allyl chloride in a CSTR for a 90% conversion?
(d) What is the overall selectivity to allyl chloride in a PFR for a 90% conversion?

5.49. The liquid phase reaction

$$A \rightleftarrows B \quad r = k_1 C_A - k_b C_B$$

is to be carried out in a flow reactor. The rate constants are: $k_f = \exp\left(13.18 - \frac{39800}{RT}\right)$ min^{-1} and $k_b = \exp\left(24.78 - \frac{82600}{RT}\right)$ min^{-1}. The heat capacities are: $\bar{C}_{PA} = \bar{C}_{PB} = 124$ J/(mol K). The reactor can be operated between 290 and 500 K. The feed will be pure A.
(a) What is the optimum operating temperature or temperature progression if a PFR is used?
(b) What is the maximum possible fractional conversion?
(c) For a CSTR capable of delivering a holding time of 1 min, what is the heat exchanger capability (UA_H) required for a conversion of 0.62 if the feed and heat exchanging fluid are both at 290 K?

5.50. Enzyme E catalyzes the aqueous decomposition of reactant A to products R and B as follows:

$$A \xrightarrow{\text{enzyme}} R + B, \qquad r = \frac{200 C_A C_{E0}}{2 + C_A}$$

where r is in mol/L/min, C_A and C_{E0} are in mol/L. The reaction is to carry out in a plug flow reactor. In the feed stream, the concentrations of the enzyme and reactant A are 0.001 mol/L and 10 mol/L, respectively. How does density change in the reactor? Find the space time and mean residence time required to drop the reactant concentration to 0.025 mol/L.

5.51. A gaseous mixture of A and B at $T_0 = 400$ K, $P_0 = 4$ atm, $C_{A0} = 100$ mol/L and $C_{B0} = 200$ mol/L is fed to a flow reactor where the reaction

$$A + B \rightarrow 2R$$

takes place. In the effluent stream, $T_e = 300$ K, $P_e = 3$ atm and $C_{Ae} = 20$ mol/L. Find f_{Ae}, f_{Be}, and C_{Be}.

5.52. We wish to convert A to R in a CSTR by the aqueous decomposition reaction:

$$A \rightarrow R + U \qquad r_1 = k_1 C_A^2$$

Where $k_1 = 0.9$ m^3/(mol·min). We realized that A can also turn to S through another reaction:

$$A + A \rightarrow S \quad r_2 = k_2 C_A$$

With $k_2 = 1.2$ min^{-1}. The aqueous feed contains A by $C_{A0} = 40$ mol/m^3. Find the optimum operating conditions (f_A, τ, and concentrations) if the cost of separation and recycle of the reactant is too high.

5.53. A fast aqueous reaction network:

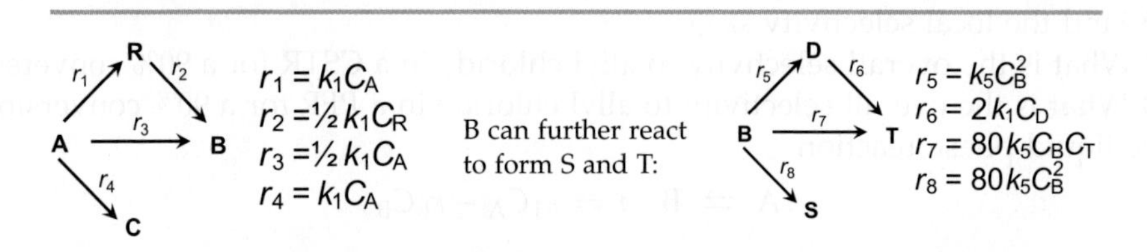

The feed contains 20 mol/L A and there are no other active reactants in the feed. In a batch experiment, when A is properly mixed with catalyst, the conversion of A is found to be 99.9% in 1 s. However, the concentration of B varies with time slowly after.

(a) If the desired product is S, what type and size (small, intermediate, or large) of flow reactor would you choose?

(b) What type and size (small, intermediate, or large) of flow reactor would you choose if the desired product is T instead?

(c) What are the final concentrations (A, B, C, D, and R) after the batch reactor was left alone for a long-time together with its contents? Roughly estimate the final concentrations of S and T.

CHAPTER

6

Kinetic Theory and Reaction Kinetics

OUTLINE

We learned that the reaction rate plays a key role in bioprocess analysis. The reaction rate is the main interest of bioprocess kinetics. In Chapter 3, we learned that the rate of reaction is observed as functions of temperature and concentrations. Based on equilibrium analysis, we further showed that the reaction rate variation with temperature is due to the reaction energy requirement. We also learned that the most commonly used experimental reaction rate law form is power-law form in concentrations. In particular, when nonequilibrium arguments were applied to an elementary reaction,

$$\sum_{j=1}^{N_S} \nu_j A_j = 0 \tag{6.1}$$

The rate of reaction may be written as Eqn (3.52) or

$$r = k^*\left(e^{-\Delta G_f/RT} - e^{-\Delta G_b/RT}\right) \tag{6.2}$$

If the heat capacity is independent on temperature and activity coefficients are independent on the concentrations, the rate expression can be reduced to Eqn (3.101) or

Bioprocess Engineering
http://dx.doi.org/10.1016/B978-0-444-59525-6.00006-8

$$r = k_{f0}e^{-E_f/RT}\prod_{j=1}^{\text{Reactant}} C_j^{-\nu_j} - k_{b0}e^{-E_b/RT}\prod_{j=1}^{\text{Product}} C_j^{\nu_j} \tag{6.3}$$

which is the mathematical basis for transitional state theory of chemical kinetics. Equations (6.2) and (6.3) are highly empirical, in line with nonequilibrium thermodynamics.

In this chapter, we provide this justification of power-law reaction rate relationship in terms of molecular kinetic theory.

6.1. ELEMENTARY KINETIC THEORY

The simplest way in which to visualize a reaction between two chemical species is in terms of a collision between the two. Physical proximity is obviously a necessary condition for reaction, for there can be no interaction between two molecules that are well-separated from each other. In fact, though, collisions are rather difficult to define as discrete events, since the interaction between two molecules extends over a distance that depends on their individual potential energy fields. Fortunately, many useful results can be obtained by using simplified models; for gases, the two most useful are the ideal gas (point-particle) model and the hard-sphere model. In the *ideal gas model*, a molecule is pictured as a point-particle (i.e. dimensionless) of mass equal to the molecular weight with given position and velocity coordinates. For the *hard-sphere model*, the normal analogy is to a billiard ball, a rigid sphere of given diameter and mass equal to the molecular weight. The potential energy curves for intermolecular interactions according to the two models are shown in Fig. 6.la and for a representative real system in Fig. 6.1b. A number of more detailed models have been devised to approximate the potentials corresponding to the interaction of real molecules; however, we shall be able to attain our major objectives here with the use of point-particle or hard-sphere models. It can be seen from Fig. 6.1 that the major deficiency of the models is in ignoring the attractive forces (energy < 0 on the diagrams) which exist in a certain range of intermolecular separation. However, the point-particle model will form the basis for our first try to produce a simple theory of reaction. Before doing this, though, let us take a look at the origin of the distribution laws that are so important in eventual application.

6.1.1. Distribution Laws

The properties of temperature, pressure, and composition which have been used in Chapter 3 to define rate laws refer to the averages of these quantities for the system under consideration. To develop the idea of reaction as a result of intermolecular collision, it is necessary to look at individual molecular events and then assemble them into the overall, observable result. In this task, we must be concerned with what average property arises from a distribution of individual properties. In the case of a gas, for example, the individual molecules are in constant motion as a result of their kinetic energy and consequently are constantly colliding with one another. The velocities of individual molecules thus change continually, and the result is a distribution of velocities about an average value. How can we convince ourselves more quantitatively of the existence of such a distribution? Picture

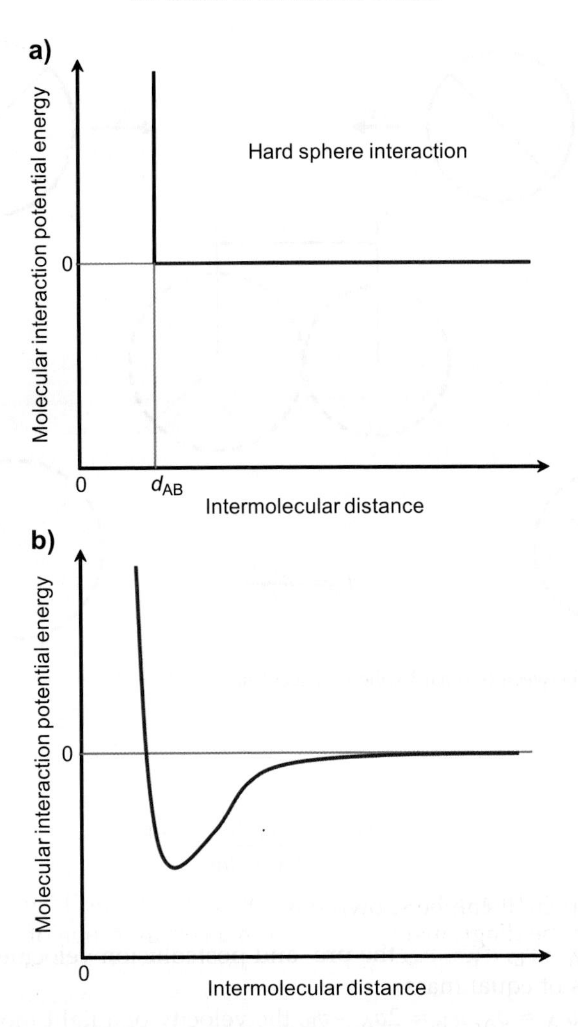

FIGURE 6.1 Mutual potential energy diagrams for model and real systems. (a) Hard-sphere interaction potential as a function of center-to-center intermolecular distance. (b) Molecular interaction potential energy as a function of intermolecular distance.

the collision between two hard-sphere molecules as shown in Fig. 6.2. Before collision, we have molecule A, with mass m_A, diameter σ_A, and velocity v_A, and molecule B, with mass m_B, diameter σ_B, and velocity v_B. If there are no tangential forces acting in the collision, which we shall assume, the velocities involved in energy transfer during collision are those parallel to the line of centers, as indicated on the Fig. 6.2. From momentum and energy conservation balances, one obtains the postcollision velocities in terms of the precollision values:

$$v'_A = \frac{2m_B v_B - v_A(m_B - m_A)}{m_A + m_B} \tag{6.4}$$

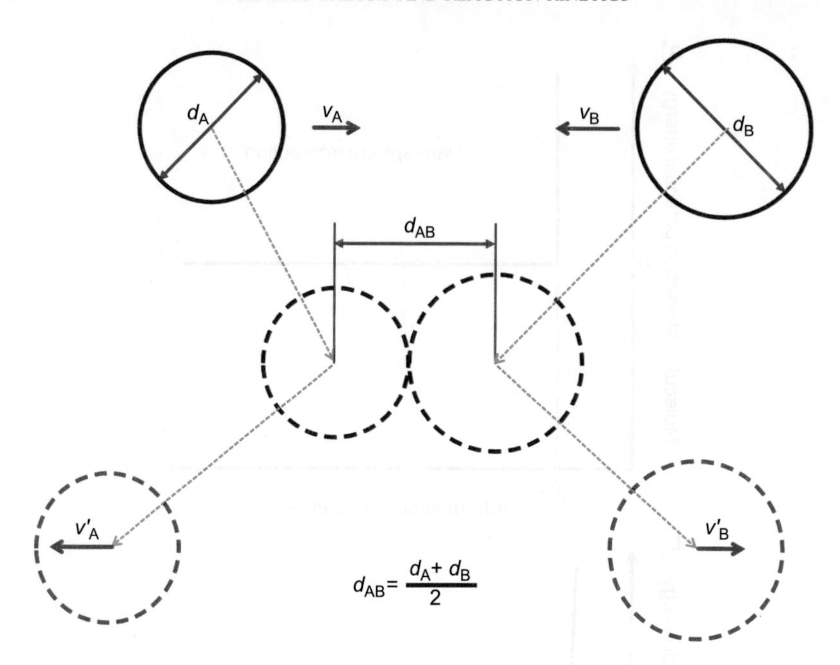

FIGURE 6.2 Collision between two hard-sphere molecules.

$$v'_B = \frac{2m_A v_A - v_B(m_A - m_B)}{m_A + m_B} \tag{6.5}$$

From Eqns (6.4) and (6.5), it can be shown that:

1. When $m_A = m_B$, $v'_A = v_B$, $v'_B = v_A$, the pre- and postcollision velocities are exchanged between molecules of equal mass.
2. When $m_A >> m_B$, $v'_A \approx v_A$, $v'_B \approx 2v_A - v_B$, the velocity of a light molecule is profoundly affected by collision with a heavy molecule, while the velocity of the heavy molecule remains essentially constant.

The exchange of kinetic energy, and thus velocity, as illustrated will ensure the existence of a distribution of velocities: energy is conserved in collisions where velocity is not conserved.

By making some rather general postulates concerning the nature of this distribution, we can derive its specific mathematical form. We shall suppose an isotropic medium at equilibrium such that the number of molecules in any region is the same and the velocities in any direction are "equal," which requires that the components of velocity along any system of the coordinate directions are "equal" and independent of coordinate system. Also, we suppose that the velocities along any three coordinate axes are independent of each other and that the change of a velocity lying between certain limits is a function only of the velocity and the limits considered. The details of the derivation are beyond the scope of our present discussion, but the important result is not. Boltzmann distribution for energies is given by

$$\frac{n_i}{n_T} = \frac{\exp\left(-\frac{E_{mi}}{k_B T}\right)}{\sum_j \exp\left(-\frac{E_{mj}}{k_B T}\right)} \tag{6.6}$$

where n_i is the number of molecules at equilibrium temperature T, with an energy E_{mi}, n_T is the total number of molecules in the system, and k_B is the Boltzmann constant. Because velocity and speed are related to energy, Eqn (6.6) can be used to derive relationships between temperature and the speed of molecules. The denominator in this equation is known as the canonical partition function.

For the case of an "ideal gas" consisting of noninteracting atoms (hard spheres) in the ground state, all energy is in the form of kinetic energy. That is,

$$E_m = m_m \frac{v_x^2 + v_y^2 + v_z^2}{2} \tag{6.7}$$

where m_m is the mass of a molecule, and (v_x, v_y, v_z) are the velocity components in the Cartesian coordinates (x, y, z). We can then rewrite Eqn (6.6) as

$$\frac{n_i}{n_T} = \frac{1}{\hat{g}}\exp\left(-m_m \frac{v_x^2 + v_y^2 + v_z^2}{2k_B T}\right) = \frac{1}{\hat{g}}\exp\left(-M\frac{v_x^2 + v_y^2 + v_z^2}{2RT}\right) \tag{6.8}$$

where $\hat{g}$ is the partition function, corresponding to the denominator in Eqn (6.6). M is the molecular mass and R is the ideal gas constant. This distribution of n_i/n_T is proportional to the probability density function $P(\,)$ for finding a molecule with these values of velocity components. Thus,

$$P(v_x, v_y, v_z) = \frac{c}{\hat{g}}\exp\left(-M\frac{v_x^2 + v_y^2 + v_z^2}{2RT}\right) \tag{6.9}$$

where c is the normalizing constant, which can be determined by recognizing that the probability of a molecule having *any* velocity must be 1. Therefore, the integral of Eqn (6.9) over all v_x, v_y, and v_z must be 1.

$$\int_{-\infty}^{\infty}\int_{-\infty}^{\infty}\int_{-\infty}^{\infty} P(v_x, v_y, v_z)\,dv_x dv_y dv_z = 1 \tag{6.10}$$

It can be shown that

$$\frac{c}{\hat{g}} = \left(\frac{M}{2\pi RT}\right)^{3/2} \tag{6.11}$$

Substituting Eqn (6.11) into Eqn (6.9), we obtain

$$P(v_x, v_y, v_z) = \left(\frac{M}{2\pi RT}\right)^{3/2} \exp\left(-M\frac{v_x^2 + v_y^2 + v_z^2}{2RT}\right) \tag{6.12}$$

where $P(v_x, v_y, v_z)\,dv_x dv_y dv_z$ is the fraction of all molecules having velocities in the range of (v_x, v_y, v_z) to $(v_x + dv_x, v_y + dv_y, v_z + dv_z)$ in the Cartesian (rectangular) coordinate axes of x, y, and z. For an isotropic medium, i.e. the mixture (locally) is uniform, there is directional preference for any changes. Let us do a change of variables by setting

$$\begin{aligned} v &= \sqrt{v_x^2 + v_y^2 + v_z^2} \\ v_x &= v \cos\theta \sin\phi \\ v_y &= v \sin\theta \sin\phi \\ v_z &= v \cos\phi \end{aligned} \tag{6.13}$$

which corresponding to a transformation from Cartesian space of (v_x, v_y, v_z) to spherical space of (v, θ, ϕ). As such, $0 \le \phi \le \pi$, $0 \le \theta \le 2\pi$. This change of variables applies to Eqn (6.12), we have

$$P(v, \theta, \phi)\,dv d\phi d\theta = \frac{v^2 \sin\phi}{(2\pi RT/M)^{3/2}} e^{-Mv^2/(2RT)} dv d\phi d\theta \tag{6.14}$$

where $P(v, \phi, \theta)\,dv d\phi d\theta$ is the fraction of all molecules having velocities in the range v to $v + dv$, with the directions setting between (ϕ, θ) to $(\phi + d\phi, \theta + d\theta)$. Integrating the whole range of $0 \le \phi \le \pi$ and $0 \le \theta \le 2\pi$, we obtain

$$P(v)dv = \frac{4v^2}{(2RT/M)^{3/2}\pi^{1/2}} e^{-Mv^2/(2RT)} dv \tag{6.15}$$

where $P(v)dv$ is the fraction of all molecules having velocities in the range v to $v + dv$. This is the Maxwell–Boltzmann distribution. From this Maxwell–Boltzmann distribution, we obtain other quantities of interest, such as the average velocity and the root-mean-square velocity. These are listed in Table 6.1.

TABLE 6.1 Properties Derived from the Maxwell–Boltzmann Distribution Law

Property	Description	Relation	Value
$\overline{v}$	Average velocity	$\overline{v} = \int_0^\infty vP(v)dv$	$2\sqrt{\frac{2RT}{\pi M}}$
v_m	Median velocity	$\frac{1}{2} = \int_0^{v_m} P(v)dv$	$1.0877\sqrt{\frac{2RT}{M}}$
$\overline{v^2}$	Second momentum of distribution	$\overline{v^2} = \int_0^\infty v^2 P(v)dv$	$\frac{3RT}{M}$
$\sqrt{\overline{v^2}}$	Root-mean-square velocity		$\sqrt{\frac{3RT}{M}}$

6.1.2. Collision Rate

With the distribution laws established, we can now attack the problem that is central to a collision theory of reaction: the number of collisions experienced per molecule per second in the Maxwellian gas. Clearly the magnitude of this collision number is a function of temperature (through the constant α), and if we define a total collision number, collisions of all molecules per second per volume, it will also depend on molecular density (i.e. concentration). Thus, the two independent variables of concentration and temperature used in power-law rate equations will appear in the total collision number.

Consider the simple situation illustrated in Fig. 6.3. Here a single, hard-sphere molecule of A is moving through a gas composed of identical, stationary, hard-sphere B molecules. The speed of A is v_A, and in its path through the matrix of B molecules, A will follow a randomly directed course determined by collisions with B. Collisions are defined to occur when the distance between centers is smaller than:

$$d_{AB} = \frac{d_A + d_B}{2} \tag{6.16}$$

If the matrix of B molecules is not too dense, we can approximate the volume in which collisions occur as that of a cylinder of radius d_{AB}, developing a length of v_A per second. The number of collisions per second for the A molecule, Z(A, B), will then be the volume of this cylinder times the number of B molecules per unit volume, C_B:

$$Z(A, B) = C_B \pi d_{AB}^2 v_A \tag{6.17}$$

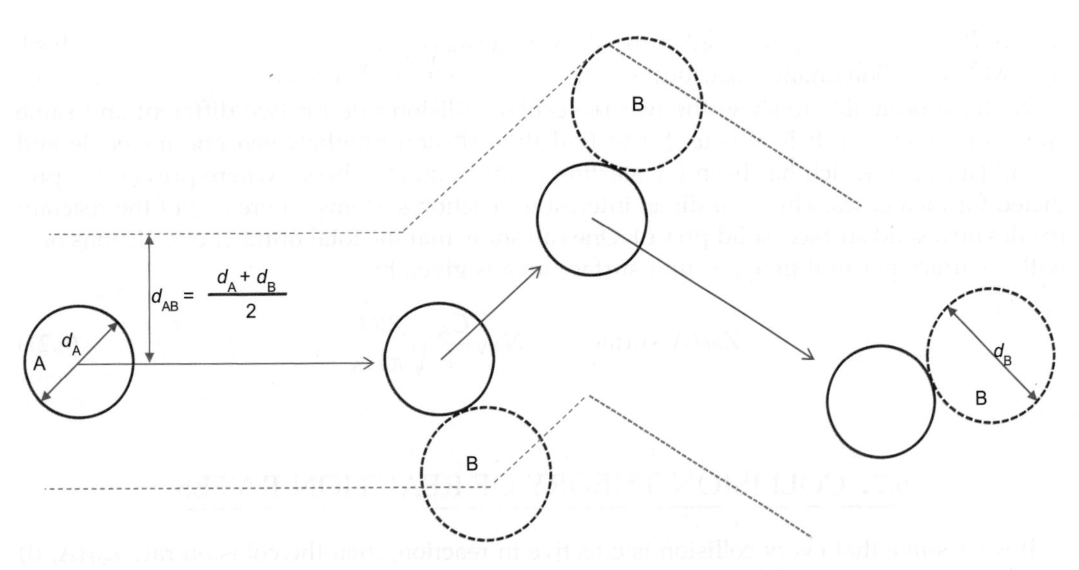

FIGURE 6.3 Trajectory of single molecule A through a stationary matrix of B.

This probably represents the first stop on the way to a collision theory of reaction rates. If, indeed, we have the passage of a single molecule through a dilute, fixed matrix of other molecules (sometimes called a "dusty gas") with a known speed v_A, and with every collision resulting in reaction, then the reaction rate would in fact be given by Eqn (6.17). Yet, we know that we do *not* have a single molecule, we do *not* have a fixed speed, and we do *not* have a dusty gas; so this simple theory needs some cosmetics at this point.

One of the things we need to know is the collision number between molecule A, which is representative of a Maxwellian distribution of speed of A molecules and B molecules themselves possessing a Maxwellian distribution of speed. This can be done by defining a collision volume determined not by v_A but by a mean relative speed, v_r between the Maxwellian populations of A and B. This approach has been discussed by Benson [S.W. Benson, *The Foundations of Chemical Kinetics*, McGraw-Hill Book Co., New York, NY (1960)]. The result, for identifiable molecular species A and B, is simply that

$$v_r = \sqrt{\frac{8RT}{\pi}\left(\frac{1}{M_A}+\frac{1}{M_B}\right)} \tag{6.18}$$

The collision rate we are seeking may now be obtained by direct substitution into Eqn (6.17) using v_r instead of v_A. For the total number of collisions between Maxwellian molecules A and B per unit time, the collision rate, Z_{cT}(A, B), is determined by substitution of v_r from Eqn (6.18) and multiplication by the concentration of A molecules, C_A:

$$Z_{cT}(A,B) = N_{AV}^2 C_A C_B \pi d_{AB}^2 \sqrt{\frac{8RT}{\pi}\left(\frac{1}{M_A}+\frac{1}{M_B}\right)} \tag{6.19}$$

where N_{AV} is the Avogadro's number. A corresponding substitution for like molecules (A = B) into Eqn (6.19) gives

$$Z_{cT}(A,A) = N_{AV}^2 C_A^2 \pi d_A^2 \sqrt{\frac{8RT}{\pi M_A}} \tag{6.20}$$

We have been able to show the two-molecular collision rate for two different and same species in a system. It is also useful to find the collision rate between one molecule and a wall (surface), which has been the starting point of kinetic theory where pressure is predicted for idea gases. This is of direct interest to reaction systems where one of the reactant resides on a solid surface (solid phase). One can show that the total number of collisions of A with a surface per unit time per unit surface area is given by

$$Z_{cT}(A,\text{surface}) = N_{AV}\frac{C_A}{4}\sqrt{\frac{8RT}{\pi M_A}} \tag{6.21}$$

6.2. COLLISION THEORY OF REACTION RATES

If we assume that every collision is effective in reaction, then the collision rate Z_{cT}(A, B) from Eqn (6.19) gives us the rate of the reaction A + B → products directly. However, based on the discussions we have earlier, we know that in order for the reaction to occur, the "molecular bundle" must overcome an energy barrier. That is, there is a switch for the reaction to occur, unless it is the spontaneous decaying reaction like that of nuclear reaction. Therefore, it is expected that not every collision would lead to a successful reaction.

In the new visualization, consider a collision between hard-sphere molecules A and B with relative velocity v_r and b as an impact parameter which can be related to, but is generally not equal to, d_{AB}. The general view corresponds to Fig. 6.4. Here $v_{||}$ and $v_{\perp}$ are velocity components in the parallel and perpendicular directions to the line of motion. We can also write an energy expression in terms of these velocity components

$$E_r = \frac{1}{2}\left(\frac{1}{M_A} + \frac{1}{M_B}\right)^{-1}(v_{||}^2 + v_{\perp}^2) \tag{6.22}$$

The second term of this expression is the energy directed along the line of centers and, in the hard-sphere model, we assume that this is the component of energy involved in the reaction. Let us call this energy along the line of centers E_c. E_c is a function of the distance between two colliding (or interacting) spheres. From Fig. 6.4 we have

$$\begin{aligned} \frac{E_c}{E_r} &= \frac{v_{\perp}^2}{v_{||}^2 + v_{\perp}^2} = 0; \qquad b > d_{AB} \\ \frac{E_c}{E_r} &= \frac{v_{\perp}^2}{v_{||}^2 + v_{\perp}^2} = 1 - \frac{b^2}{d_{AB}^2}; \quad b \le d_{AB} \end{aligned} \tag{6.23}$$

Now, we will further assume that there is an energy-dependent reaction probability and, in the most simple approach, that this is just an "on–off" switch such that the probability of reaction is zero if $E_c < E_a$ and is unity if $E_c > E_a$, where E_a is the minimum energy for reaction. If we write this out formally,

$$\begin{aligned} \delta(E_c) &= 0; \quad E_c < E_a \\ \delta(E_c) &= 1; \quad E_c \ge E_a \end{aligned} \tag{6.24}$$

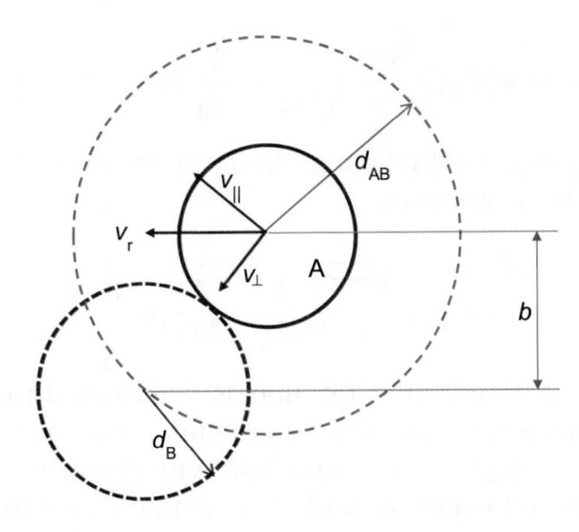

FIGURE 6.4 The reactive hard-sphere model.

The picture to this point then is the collision of hard spheres given in Fig. 6.4, with energies as defined in Eqn (6.23) and probabilities as given in Eqn (6.24). How do we turn this into a reaction rate expression that is compatible with all the work done previously to get to Eqn (6.19)? This can be achieved by defining yet a new quantity: the *reactive cross-section*. We define a reactive cross-sectional area as

$$
\begin{aligned}
S_R(E_r) &= \int_0^\infty \delta[E_c(b)]2\pi b db \\
&= 0; \qquad E_r < E_a \\
&= \pi d_{AB}^2\left(1 - \frac{E_a}{E_r}\right); \quad E_r \geq E_a
\end{aligned}
\tag{6.25}
$$

The energy dependence of S_R is essentially the collision area that the interacting molecules see as a function of the relative energy. Now in order to determine a reaction rate (or rate constant) from the result of Eqn (6.25), we need to integrate over the distribution of E_r and over the range of possible values of $b < b_{max}$ associated with each E_r. After some rather complex geometry, one comes up with a collision rate as a function of the relative energy that says:

$$
Z(E_r) = \frac{2C_A C_B}{(RT)^{3/2}}\sqrt{\frac{2}{\pi}\left(\frac{1}{M_A} + \frac{1}{M_B}\right)}\int_{E_a}^\infty e^{-E_r/(RT)} S_R(E_r) E_r dE_r \tag{6.26}
$$

which yields

$$
Z(E_r) = \pi d_{AB}^2 \sqrt{\frac{8RT}{\pi}\left(\frac{1}{M_A} + \frac{1}{M_B}\right)} e^{-E_a/(RT)} C_A C_B \tag{6.27}
$$

Thus, we have obtained the reactive collision rate.

Often a steric factor, ξ, is introduced to account for all additional factors affecting the collision–reaction probability except for those directly associated with energy. Thus

$$
ZE_r = \pi \xi d_{AB}^2 \sqrt{\frac{8RT}{\pi}\left(\frac{1}{M_A} + \frac{1}{M_B}\right)} e^{-E_a/(RT)} C_A C_B \tag{6.28}
$$

We may now compare Eqn (6.28) with the bimolecular rate law to find what a corresponding rate constant would be. This is given by

$$
k = \pi \xi d_{AB}^2 \sqrt{\frac{8RT}{\pi}\left(\frac{1}{M_A} + \frac{1}{M_B}\right)} e^{-E_a/(RT)} \tag{6.29}
$$

and is the rate constant of a bimolecular reaction as determined from collision theory. It is essentially of the Arrhenius form, since the weak temperature dependence of the preexponential factor is generally negligible in comparison with the activation energy term. Thus, the reaction rate law observed experimentally is explained, and this is the foundation for the discussion of kinetics.

To simplify the collision theory outlined above, we devise a more illustrative simplistic elementary kinetic description for the steps taken as

$$A + B \rightleftharpoons AB^* \tag{6.30}$$

$$AB^* \rightarrow C \tag{6.31}$$

To illustrate the reaction kinetics for a bimolecular reaction

$$A + B \rightarrow C \tag{6.32}$$

In the reaction kinetic steps, AB* is regarded as the active reaction complex, which can be regarded as a transitional state (to achieve required active energy) or as the collision occurrence. Therefore, we regard the transitional state theory, active complex theory, and the more fundamental collision theory to be compatible. It is thus expected that the transitional state theory, active complex theory, and the collision theory would all produce similar rate expressions. No effort will be made to distinguish these three "theories." This discussion will also lead to us to treat the kinetics in simplistic form like Eqns (6.30) and (6.31), whereby no direct reference to the more fundamental representation with collision theory is needed.

It is interesting to note from the collision theory that an elementary reaction should not have more than three reactant molecules involved as the collision of three or more molecules at one location is increasingly rare.

6.3. REACTION RATE ANALYSIS/APPROXIMATION

Collision theory provides a vivid conceptual description of chemicals: contacting of reacting species, activating the reaction, and spontaneous reaction. It offers the form of reaction rates for elementary reactions: frequency of collision depends on the product of reacting species concentrations. In most practical reactions, the process does occur in such a simple fashion. It naturally leads to more steps to complete the reaction path. To illustrate how to deal with reaction rates from multiple-reaction steps or pathways, we use a simplistic example as given by reactions (6.30) and (6.31):

$$A + B \rightleftharpoons AB^* \tag{6.30}$$

$$AB^* \rightarrow C \tag{6.31}$$

where the overall reaction is given by (6.32)

$$A + B \rightarrow C \tag{6.32}$$

There are two steps in this reaction. One can treat the reactions as multiple reactions and thus deal with each reaction equally. At this stage, we have learned how to do so (Chapter 3). The reaction rate for any given species in a multiple reaction can be computed by Eqn (3.66) or

$$r_j = \sum_{i=1}^{N_R} \nu_{ij} r_i \tag{6.33}$$

where r_j is the rate of reaction for species j; r_i is the reaction rate for reaction i as written; N_R is the total number of reactions; and ν_{ij} is the stoichiometric coefficient of species j in reaction i. For example, elementary reaction system described by (6.30) and (6.31) yield

$$r_1 = k_1 C_A C_B - k_{-1} C_{AB*} \tag{6.34}$$

$$r_2 = k_2 C_{AB*} \tag{6.35}$$

$$r_A = -r_1 \tag{6.36}$$

$$r_B = -r_1 \tag{6.37}$$

$$r_C = r_2 \tag{6.38}$$

$$r_{AB*} = r_1 - r_2 \tag{6.39}$$

There are no assumptions or approximations involved in these equations.

While Eqns (6.34)–(6.39) are convenient to use due to the simplistic nature of the reaction system, in other cases, one wish to simplify the reaction as there could be hundreds or even thousands of reaction steps in some practical cases. Usually, we simplify the reactions by considering the relative magnitude of the reaction rates as not all the reactions are preceded at equation rates. Some reaction species in the mixture are of low level, even difficult to detect with conventional techniques. All these information would allow us to simplify the reaction system. This is the subject of discussion in the following subsections.

6.3.1. Fast-Equilibrium Step Approximation

Some reactions or steps are faster than others in a reaction system. In the simplistic example, we have two reactions. Suppose one reaction is much slower than the other one, then the slower reaction would be the one controlling the overall reaction rate. For example, if reaction (6.31) is the rate-limiting step or reaction (6.30) proceeds much faster than reaction (6.30), we would have reaction (6.30) to be in equilibrium while deriving a suitable rate expression. Since reaction (6.31) is slow, reaction (6.30) would be completed while (6.31) is still proceeding slowly. That is to say

$$0 = r_1 = k_1 C_A C_B - k_{-1} C_{AB*} \tag{6.40}$$

Solving Eqn (6.40), we obtain

$$C_{AB*} = \frac{k_1}{k_{-1}} C_A C_B = K_1 C_A C_B \tag{6.41}$$

Thus, the concentration of AB* can be expressed as a function of C_A and C_B, eliminating the need for us to deal with the species AB*. Furthermore, if we assume that K_1 is small, i.e. the concentration C_{AB*} is negligible when compared with C_A and C_B, then we do not need to look at the difference, for example, between C_A and the total concentration A that is not converted to C[1]. Using Eqn (6.41), we arrive at the reaction rate expression for the overall reaction (6.32) as

$$r = r_C = r_2 = k_2 C_{AB*} = k_2 K_1 C_A C_B \tag{6.42}$$

Therefore, we have shown that if the second step is rate liming, the overall reaction rate is of second order and the rate constant is the product of the rate constant of the second reaction and the equilibrium constant of the first step.

What happens if step 1, or reaction (6.30), is really the rate-limiting step? That the reaction (6.31) is fast is equivalent to say that any AB* formed in the reaction system is immediately converted to C and thus the concentration of AB* is zero. Thus, the overall reaction rate is then

$$r = -r_A = r_1 = k_1 C_A C_B \tag{6.43}$$

The reaction rate is equivalent to the forward rate of reaction step 1.

We are now comfortable in approximate the reaction rates if one or more reaction steps are rate-limiting while others are fast.

6.3.2. Pseudosteady-State Hypothesis

In a reaction system, there are species that are of particular interest to us, while there are also species that are of less interest from a practical point of view. For example, in the simplistic reaction system we use, reactions (6.30) and (6.31), reactants A and B are to be supplied, while C is the product of interest, based on the overall reaction (6.32). We are not interested in the value of AB* from a practical standpoint. One can also look at this from a different standpoint. There are species formed in the reaction system that have very low level of concentration and upon completion of the reaction system there is no trace of, or only negligible amount of, them. We call these species intermediates. In most reaction systems, the intermediates formed can hardly be detected with even sophisticated measuring tools available today. Because the concentrations of the intermediates are very low, one can assume that their net rates of formation are zero. This is the essence of pseudosteady-state hypothesis (PSSH).

In reaction system (6.30) and (6.31), species AB* is an intermediate, that is

$$0 = r_{AB*} = r_1 - r_2 = k_1 C_A C_B - k_{-1} C_{AB*} - k_2 C_{AB*} \tag{6.44}$$

[1]If the assumption K_1 is not invoked, one needs to find the concentrations of "free" A and B to be used in Eqn (6.38). The measurable concentrations of A and B are given by (via mass balance).

$$C_{AT} = C_A + C_{AB^*}$$
$$C_{BT} = C_B + C_{AB^*}$$

These two equations must be solved together with Eqn (6.38) to express the concentration of C_{AB*} as a function of the overall concentrations of A and B. This may be more important at the beginning of the reaction (measurable concentration of A and B change "sharply" while very little product C is formed) and toward the completion of the reaction.

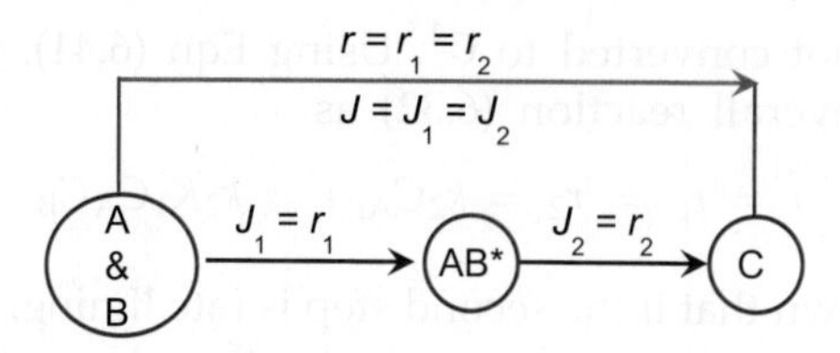

FIGURE 6.5 Analogy of chemical reaction pathway and electric circuit: reaction rates (r's) are interpreted the same as fluxes (J's) moving from one node to the next.

which can be solved to give

$$C_{AB*} = \frac{k_1}{k_{-1} + k_2} C_A C_B \tag{6.45}$$

By virtue, we assume the concentration C_{AB*} is negligibly small as compared with C_A and C_B. If this is not the case, one needs to examine its effect on the concentrations of A and B (see footnote from the previous section). Thus, the overall reaction rate, for reaction (6.32), is given by

$$r = r_C = r_2 = k_2 C_{AB*} = \frac{k_1 k_2}{k_{-1} + k_2} C_A C_B \tag{6.46}$$

Therefore, we have derived at the rate expression using PSSH. This reaction rate expression is quite similar to that obtained from fast-equilibrium step (FES) approximation. However, the reaction rate constant is different. When experiments are conducted to determine the rate expression, one can hardly distinguish Eqn (6.46) from (6.43) or (6.42). Therefore, both FES and PSSH are useful tools for kinetic or reaction rate analyses.

One advantage of PSSH is that if one draws the reaction system in analog with an electric circuit as shown in Fig. 6.5, the reaction rate is like the electric current or flux. The flux is equal throughout the electric circuit, passing any given nodes (or intermediates). There is no loss of mass along the reaction pathway. This assumption is applicable and useful after the reaction starts (some product has already been formed) and before the reaction ends (there are still reactants available). This assumption is also less harsh than the FES approximation. Therefore, PSSH is widely used in kinetic analyses.

6.4. UNIMOLECULAR REACTIONS

In this section, we are dealing with reactions:

$$A \rightarrow \text{products} \tag{6.47}$$

which can be found in isomerization and decomposition reactions. In the stoichiometry, only one molecule or one species (to be more precise) is acting as the reactant.

At first glance, it seems paradoxical to treat unimolecular reactions, in which a single molecule is apparently involved in reaction, in terms of a collision theory based on pairwise interactions. Indeed, we have developed a rather specific picture of a chemical reaction from the hard-sphere collision model, in which the energetics of reaction is represented in terms of relative kinetic energy.

The key phrase in the proceeding paragraph is "apparently involved in reaction." While one may find true first-order reactions, such as nuclear decay reactions, past experience has shown that most apparent first-order reactions can behave differently at different concentrations. The main reason lies here that molecules need to be activated for reaction to occur. Lindemann (1922) was the first to treat the apparent unimolecular reactions through the collisional activation concept. In order for the reaction to occur, one A molecule needs to be activated by colliding with another molecule, i.e.

$$\mathrm{A} + \mathrm{U} \rightarrow \mathrm{A}^* + \mathrm{U} \qquad r_1 = k_1 C_\mathrm{A} C_\mathrm{U} \tag{6.48}$$

$$\mathrm{A}^* + \mathrm{W} \rightarrow \mathrm{A} + \mathrm{W} \qquad r_2 = k_2 C_{\mathrm{A}^*} C_\mathrm{W} \tag{6.49}$$

$$\mathrm{A}^* \rightarrow \text{products} \qquad r_3 = k_3 C_{\mathrm{A}^*} \tag{6.50}$$

The first step involves the activation of the A molecule by collision with another molecule U, in the system to give A*. A second step involves the deactivation of A* by collision with a third molecule W. One can postulate that the activated A* is unstable as it possesses higher energy than normal A molecule. Therefore, a PSS can be applied to A*, i.e. the net formation rate of A* is zero. This gives

$$0 = r_{\mathrm{A}^*} = 1 \times r_1 + (-1) \times r_2 + (-1) \times r_3 = k_1 C_\mathrm{A} C_\mathrm{U} - k_2 C_{\mathrm{A}^*} C_\mathrm{W} - k_3 C_{\mathrm{A}^*} \tag{6.51}$$

from which we obtain,

$$C_{\mathrm{A}^*} = \frac{k_1 C_\mathrm{A} C_\mathrm{U}}{k_2 C_\mathrm{W} + k_3} \tag{6.52}$$

Thus, for the overall reaction

$$\mathrm{A} \rightarrow \text{products} \tag{6.53}$$

The reaction rate is given by

$$r = r_3 = k_3 C_{\mathrm{A}^*} = \frac{k_1 k_3 C_\mathrm{U}}{k_2 C_\mathrm{W} + k_3} C_\mathrm{A} \tag{6.54}$$

which is the general rate law for simple unimolecular reactions. Let us now examine the apparent order of reaction. This would involve the knowledge of U, W, and the concentration ranges.

Case 1. U = W = A. The collisional activation and deactivation can be achieved by colliding with another molecule of A only. This is the widely discussed case in the literature. Equation (6.54) is reduced to

$$r = \frac{k_1 k_3 C_\mathrm{A}^2}{k_2 C_\mathrm{A} + k_3} \tag{6.55}$$

One can infer from Eqn (6.55) that

$$\begin{aligned} r &\approx k_1 C_\mathrm{A}^2; \quad \text{when } C_\mathrm{A} << \frac{k_3}{k_2} \\ &\approx \frac{k_1 k_3}{k_2} C_\mathrm{A}; \quad \text{when } C_\mathrm{A} >> \frac{k_3}{k_2} \end{aligned} \tag{6.56}$$

Therefore, the apparent order of reaction can be first order when the concentration is high, while second order when the concentration is low.

Case 2. U = any molecule in the system and W = A. The collisional activation is achieved by collision of A with any molecule in the system, whereas the deactivation is achieved by collision with another A molecule only. In this case, $C_U = C_T$ and Eqn (6.54) is reduced to

$$r = \frac{k_1 k_3 C_T C_A}{k_2 C_A + k_3} \tag{6.57}$$

One can infer that

$$r = \frac{k_1 k_3 C_T C_A}{k_2 C_A + k_3} \begin{cases} \approx \dfrac{k_1 k_3 C_A^2}{k_2 C_A + k_3}; & \text{when } C_A \approx C_T \\ (k_1 C_T) C_A; & \text{when } C_T = \text{constant and } C_A \ll \dfrac{k_3}{k_2} \\ \dfrac{k_1 k_3 C_T}{k_2}; & \text{when } \dfrac{k_3}{k_2} \ll C_A \text{ and } C_T = \text{constant} \end{cases} \tag{6.58}$$

When A is of small fraction in an inert mixture, the total concentration C_T does not change noticeably with the change of C_A. If there $\nu_\Sigma = 0$, C_T = constant. The last two scenarios indicate that when $C_T \approx$ constant, the apparent order of reaction can be either first order (at low concentrations) or zeroth order (at high concentrations).

6.5. FREE RADICALS

We next look into the active complexes as appeared in the unimolecular kinetic discussions. As we noted earlier, the active complex may or may not be a stable molecule, which is the reason it is active. To start with this discussion, we look into the thermal decomposition of acetaldehyde

$$CH_3CHO \rightarrow CH_4 + CO \tag{6.59}$$

occurs in gas phase at about 500 °C. The rate of this reaction is empirically found to be 3/2 order in acetaldehyde in a wide range of concentrations. That is

$$r = k[CH_3CHO]^{3/2} \tag{6.60}$$

This reaction is of the form A → B + C, but it is clearly not an elementary reaction as the order of reaction is not first order in the only reactant. It does not fit directly to the simplistic collision theory based unimolecular mechanism as described in the preceding section.

This reaction is actually a multiple-reaction system that involves the major steps

$$CH_3CHO \rightarrow \cdot CH_3 + \cdot CHO \quad r_1 \tag{6.61}$$

$$\cdot CH_3 + CH_3CHO \rightarrow CH_4 + CH_3CO\cdot \quad r_2 \tag{6.62}$$

$$CH_3CO\cdot \rightarrow \cdot CH_3 + CO \quad r_3 \tag{6.63}$$

$$\cdot CH_3 + \cdot CH_3 \rightarrow C_2H_6 \quad r_4 \tag{6.64}$$

$$\cdot CHO + \cdot CHO \rightarrow HCHO + CO \quad r_5 \tag{6.65}$$

In words, we describe the process as initiated by the decomposition of acetaldehyde to form the methyl radical $\cdot CH_3$ and the formyl radical $\cdot CHO$. Then methyl attacks the parent molecule acetaldehyde and abstracts an H atom to form methane and leave the acetyl radical $\cdot CH_3CO$, which dissociates to form another methyl radical and CO. Finally, two methyl radicals combine to form the stable molecule ethane. Two formyl radicals react to form HCHO and CO.

Reaction (6.61) is the initiation step, where free radicals are generated as a start. Reactions (6.62) and (6.63) are propagation steps, where new free radicals are generated from the "old:" ones. Reactions (6.64) and (6.65) are termination steps, where free radicals are consumed.

This is a set of four elementary reactions. Examination of these four steps shows that they do involve the reaction of acetaldehyde and that methane is formed by step 2 and CO by step 3. If we add steps 2 and 3, we get

$$CH_3CHO \rightarrow CH_4 + CO \tag{6.59}$$

but this occurs by a sequence of two steps.

Note also that stable products C_2H_6 and HCHO are formed, alongside the free radicals. Ethane C_2H_6 and formaldehyde HCHO are not among the products we said were formed. These species are minor products (no more than 1% of the amount of CH_4 and CO), which can be ignored and perhaps not even measured. When you are uncovering the kinetics though, the detection of trace products, especially the stable products, is paramount.

This reaction system is an example of a chain reaction. The only reactant is acetaldehyde, and there are seven products listed: CH_4, CO, $\cdot CH_3$, $\cdot CHO$, $CH_3CO\cdot$, C_2H_6, and HCHO. The first two, CH_4 and CO, are the major products, and the last two, C_2H_6 and HCHO, are the minor products. The other species, $\cdot CH_3$, $\cdot CHO$, $CH_3CO\cdot$, are free radicals that are very active and never build up to high concentrations.

To show that the above kinetics or mechanism can yield this empirical rate expression of 3/2 order, let us apply the PSS approximation on all the free radicals:

$$0 = r_{\cdot CH_3} = r_1 - r_2 + r_3 - 2r_4$$

$$0 = k_1[CH_3CHO] - k_2[\cdot CH_3][CH_3CHO] + k_3[CH_3CO\cdot] - 2k_4[\cdot CH_3]^2 \tag{6.66}$$

$$0 = r_{\cdot CHO} = r_1 - 2r_5$$

$$0 = k_1[CH_3CHO] - 2k_5[\cdot CHO]^2 \tag{6.67}$$

$$0 = r_{\cdot CH_3CO} = r_2 - r_3$$

$$0 = k_2[\cdot CH_3][CH_3CHO] - k_3[CH_3CO\cdot] \tag{6.68}$$

And the overall rate of reaction,

$$r = r_{CH_4} = r_2 = k_3[\cdot CH_3][CH_3CHO] \tag{6.69}$$

We need only to determine $[\cdot CH_3]$ before the rate expression is determined. We observe that addition of Eqns (6.66) + (6.68) leads to

$$0 = k_1[CH_3CHO] - 2k_4[\cdot CH_3]^2 \tag{6.70}$$

Solving for $[\cdot CH_3]$, we obtain

$$[\cdot CH_3] = \left(\frac{k_1}{2k_4}\right)^{1/2}[CH_3CHO]^{1/2} \tag{6.71}$$

Substituting Eqn (6.71) into Eqn (6.69), we obtain the rate for the overall reaction

$$r = k_3[\cdot CH_3][CH_3CHO] = k_3\left(\frac{k_1}{2k_4}\right)^{1/2}[CH_3CHO]^{3/2} \tag{6.72}$$

Therefore, we predict 3/2 order kinetics with an effective rate coefficient $k = k_3(k_1/2k_4)^{1/2}$.

6.6. KINETICS OF ACID HYDROLYSIS

We have learned the derivation of kinetic equations based on a given mechanism. Next, we apply this technique to a slightly more complex situation: acid hydrolysis of polymers in an aqueous medium. Acid hydrolysis can be described as

$$H_2O \rightleftarrows H_2O^* \tag{6.73}$$

$$HX_nOH\ (aq) + H_2O^* \rightarrow HX_mOH\ (aq) + HX_sOH\ (aq) \tag{6.74}$$

$$HX_nOH\ (aq) + H^+(aq) \rightleftarrows HX_nOH\cdot H^+(aq) \tag{6.75}$$

$$HX_nOH\cdot H^+(aq) + H_2O(aq) \rightarrow HX_mOH\cdot H^+(aq) + HX_sOH\ (aq) \tag{6.76}$$

$$H^+ + H_2O^* \rightleftarrows H_3O^+ \tag{6.77}$$

$$HX_nOH\ (aq) + H_3O^+(aq) \rightleftarrows HX_nOH\cdot H_3O^+(aq) \tag{6.78}$$

$$HX_nOH\cdot H_3O^+(aq) \rightarrow HX_mOH\cdot H^+(aq) + HX_sOH(aq) \tag{6.79}$$

where $m + s = n$; H_2O^* is activated water molecule; H_3O^+ and H^+ are considered to have the same catalytic effect; HX_nOH represents an n-unit oligomer, i.e. for example, xylan: $H(-O-C_5H_8O_3-)_nOH$, $X = OC_5H_8O_3$.

The monomers can further decompose into other products. For example, sugars can dehydrate in the presence of protons to dehydrated products such as furfural, humic acid, levulinic acid, etc.

$$HX_1OH\cdot H^+(aq) \rightarrow H^+ + \text{other dehydration products} \tag{6.80}$$

The reaction (6.74) shows that the breaking of intermonomer bonds is random. If all the intermonomer bonds are equally active, the rate of formation of one particular m-oligomer from an n-oligomer is given by

$$r_{m,\ n\rightarrow m(6.74)} = k_{(2)}C_n[H_2O^*] \tag{6.81}$$

and the decomposition rate of the n-oligomer (with $n-1$ intermonomer bonds) is

$$-r_{n,\ n\rightarrow\forall 1\leq i\leq n-1(6.74)} = (n-1)k_{(2)}C_n[\mathrm{H_2O^*}] \tag{6.82}$$

where C_n is the mole concentration of n-oligomer, $[H_2O^*]$ is the concentration of "free" activated water molecules, and is $k_{(2)}$ the reaction rate constant.

For reaction (6.76), we apply the same assumption that all the $n-1$ intermonomer bonds are equally reactive,

$$-r_{n,\ n\rightarrow\forall 1\leq i\leq n-1(6.76)} = (n-1)k_{(4)}[\mathrm{HX}_n\mathrm{OH\cdot H^+}] \tag{6.83}$$

Combing the fast-equilibrium step, reaction (6.75), Eqn (6.83) is reduced to

$$-r_{n,\ n\rightarrow\forall 1\leq i\leq n-1(6.76)} = (n-1)k_{(4)}K_{(3)}C_n[\mathrm{H^+}] \tag{6.84}$$

where $K_{(3)}$ is the equilibrium constant of reaction (6.75). Similarly, reactions (6.77)–(6.79) give

$$-r_{n,\ n\rightarrow\forall 1\leq i\leq n-1(6.76)} = (n-1)k_{(7)}k_{(6)}C_n[\mathrm{H_3O^+}] = (n-1)k_{(7)}K_{(6)}K_{(5)}C_n[\mathrm{H^+}][\mathrm{H_2O^*}] \tag{6.85}$$

Combing the reaction rates from reactions (6.74), (6.76), and (6.79), one can obtain the following rate law based on Eqns (6.81), (6.82), and (6.85),

$$r_{m,n\rightarrow m} = 2k_{\mathrm{H}}C_n \tag{6.86}$$

$$r_{n,n\rightarrow\forall 1\leq i\leq n-1} = -(n-1)k_{\mathrm{H}}C_n \tag{6.87}$$

where k_H is the rate constant of breaking one single intermonomeric unit bond. The overall rate constant for the intermonomeric unit bond breaking is given by

$$k_{\mathrm{H}} = k_{(4)}K_{(3)}[\mathrm{H^+}] + k_{(7)}K_{(6)}[\mathrm{H_3O^+}] + k_{(2)}[\mathrm{H_2O*}] \tag{6.88}$$

Thus, the net formation rate of m-oligomer is given by

$$r_m = \sum_{i=m+1}^{N} r_{m,i\rightarrow m} + r_{m,m\rightarrow\forall 1\leq i\leq m-1} = \sum_{i=m+1}^{N} 2k_{\mathrm{H}}C_i - (m-1)k_{\mathrm{H}}C_m \tag{6.89}$$

which is valid for all oligomers (excluding monosaccharides). For monosaccharides, one additional reaction (6.80) occurs. Combining Eqn (6.89) and the rate from reaction (6.80), the rate of formation of monomeric unit is

$$r_1 = 2\sum_{i=2}^{N} k_{\mathrm{H}}C_i - k_{\mathrm{D}}C_1 \tag{6.90}$$

where k_D is the rate constant for the degradation of monomeric sugar. For different sugars, this constant can have different values.

For the formation of monomeric sugars, Eqn (6.90) can be reduced to

$$r_1 = 2k_{\mathrm{H}}C_{\Sigma 0} - (2k_{\mathrm{H}} + k_{\mathrm{D}})C_1 \tag{6.91}$$

where $C_{\Sigma 0}$ is the total molar concentration of monomers and oligomers.

$$C_{\Sigma 0} = \sum_{i=1}^{N} C_i \tag{6.92}$$

Equation (6.90) describes the rate for individual oligomer units. However, this is not convenient in most cases as the number of molecular species is not easy to determine. Lumped kinetics can be derived based on Eqn (6.90). Summing up all the oligomers, we obtain

$$r_{\Sigma 1} = \sum_{n=1}^{N} n r_n = \sum_{n=1}^{N} n\left[\sum_{i=n+1}^{N} 2k_H C_i - (n-1)k_H C_n\right] - k_D C_1 = -k_D C_1 \tag{6.93}$$

$$\begin{aligned} r_{\Sigma 0} &= \sum_{n=1}^{N} r_n = \sum_{n=1}^{N} 2 \sum_{i=n+1}^{N} k_H C_i - \sum_{n=2}^{N} (n-1)k_H C_n - k_D C_1 = k_H \sum_{n=1}^{N} (n-1)C_n - k_D C_1 \\ &= k_H(C_{\Sigma 1} - C_{\Sigma 0}) - k_D C_1 \end{aligned} \tag{6.94}$$

where the subscript $\Sigma 1$ denotes the mixture measured based on total number of monomeric units, and subscript $\Sigma 0$ denotes the mixture measured based on total number of molecules.

$$C_{\Sigma 1} = \sum_{i=1}^{N} iC_i \tag{6.95}$$

Equations (6.93) and (6.94) indicate that the reaction mixture in the hydrolyzate solution can be characterized based on the total number of moles and the total number of monomeric units. Effectively, all the oligomers are lumped into two "pseudo-oligomer species: $\Sigma 0$ and $\Sigma 1$."

Since H_3O^+ and H^+ are of the same effect, we have

$$[H_3O^+] + [H^+] = 10^{-pH} \tag{6.96}$$

where pH is the pH value of the aqueous solution. Reactions (6.73) and (6.77) lead to

$$[H_2O^*] = \frac{[H_2O^*]_0}{1 + K_* \times 10^{-pH}} \tag{6.97}$$

where $[H_2O^*]$ is the concentration of "free" activated water and $[H_2O^*]_0$ is the total concentration of activated water. Thus, the rate constant for the hydrolysis is given by

$$k_H = k_1 \times 10^{-pH} + \frac{k_2}{1 + k_3 \times 10^{-pH}} \tag{6.98}$$

This section shows that simple kinetic expressions can be obtained for otherwise a complicated problem when proper assumptions can be made. For acid hydrolysis of polymers, the reaction kinetics may be approximated by three "first-order reaction rate" relationships of lumped component concentrations: 1) moles of monomers in the reaction mixture, 2) total moles of the reaction mixture including monomer and oligomers, and 3) total number of the monomer units in the reaction mixture.

6.7. SUMMARY

While reaction rates are empirical in nature, collision theory does provide a means to estimate the reaction rate. Collision theory gives rise to the correct reaction rate dependence on concentrations and temperature. Based on collision theory, most viable reactions are bimolecular. Reactions with more than three molecules are unfavorable. Therefore, an elementary reaction usually involves three or less molecules on either side of the reaction.

Nonelementary reactions can be decoupled into elementary reaction steps or reaction pathways. The reaction system that forms a nonelementary reaction can be analyzed as if one were dealing with a multiple-reaction system. In many occasions, we find simplification of the nonelementary reaction is necessary. Some reaction steps are fast than others, or some or all the reaction intermediates are present in the reaction system in only trace amount. This observations lead to two methods of simplifying reaction rate expressions: FES and PSSH. FES stands for FES approximation, while PSSH stands for pseudosteady-state hypothesis. FES assumes one or more steps are rate-limiting, and the rest steps are in thermodynamic equilibrium. PSSH assumes that the net rates of formation for the intermediates are zero.

Active reaction intermediates are common as they are means to overcome the activation energies. Active intermediates can be active complex, transitional state (or activated molecules), and free radicals. Nonelementary reactions usually have complicated reaction rate expressions than the simple power-law form. Fractional order (1/2, 3/2, ...) can be observed for free-radical reactions. Transitional state theory is based solely on the activated state approach.

Simple kinetic expressions can be obtained for otherwise a complicated problem when proper assumptions are made. For acid hydrolysis of polymers, the reaction kinetics may be approximated by three "first-order reaction rate" relationships of lumped components, Eqns (6.91), (6.93), and (6.94), despite a complicated composition of the reaction mixture.

Reading Materials

Anslyn, E.V., Dougherty, D.A., 2006. *Modern Physical Organic Chemistry.* Sausalito, CA: University Science Books.

Frost, A.A., Pearson, R.G., 1961. *Kinetics and Mechanism* (2nd ed.). New York: John Wiley & Sons, Inc.

Isaacs, N.S., 1996. *Physical Organic Chemistry* (2nd ed.). NY: Prentice Hall.

Lindemann, F.A. 1922. The radiation theory of chemical reaction. *Trans. Faraday Soc.*, **17**, 588–589.

Moore, J.W., Pearson, R.G., 1981. *Kinetics and Mechanism*. New York: Wiley.

Steinfeld, J.I., Fransico, J.S., Hase, W.L., 1999. *Chemical Kinetics and Dynamics* (2nd ed.). Englewood Cliffs, NJ: Prentice-Hall.

PROBLEMS

6.1. The gas-phase decomposition of azomethane (AZO) to give ethane and nitrogen:

$$(CH_3)_2N_2 \rightarrow C_2H_6 + N_2$$

is believed to progress in the following fashion:

$$2\,(CH_3)_2N_2 \rightleftarrows (CH_3)_2N_2 + [(CH_3)_2N_2]^*$$
$$[(CH_3)_2N_2]^* \rightarrow C_2H_6 + N_2$$

Derive the rate of formation of ethane (C_2H_6) that is consistent with this mechanism. Clearly define the symbols you use and state your assumptions.

6.2. The reaction to form NO: $N_2 + O_2 \rightarrow 2\,NO$, in high-temperature combustion processes, is thought to proceed by the following elementary steps:

$$O_2 \underset{k_{-1}}{\overset{k_1}{\rightleftarrows}} 2O$$

$$N_2 + O \overset{k_2}{\rightarrow} NO + N$$

$$O_2 + N \overset{k_3}{\rightarrow} NO + O$$

Find a reasonable reaction rate for the overall reaction.

6.3. The gas-phase dehydrogenation of ethane to ethylene

$$C_2H_6 \rightarrow C_2H_4 + H_2$$

Proceeds through the elementary reaction steps

$$C_2H_6 + H\cdot \overset{k_1}{\rightarrow} C_2H_5\cdot + H_2$$

$$C_2H_6 \underset{k_{-2}}{\overset{k_1}{\rightleftarrows}} C_2H_5\cdot + H\cdot$$

$$C_2H_5\cdot \overset{k_3}{\rightarrow} C_2H_4 + H\cdot$$

(a) Identify the initiation, propagation, and termination steps.
(b) Find a reasonable expression for the overall reaction rate.
(c) The bond energy of ethane is 104 kcal/mol, and the propagation steps have very low activation energies. What is the approximate activation energy of this reaction?

6.4. The Goldschmidt mechanism (Smith, 1939) for the esterification of methyl alcohol (M) with acetic acid (A) catalyzed by a strong acid (e.g. HCl) involves the following steps:

$$M + H^+ \rightarrow CH_3OH_2^+\ (C);\ \text{rapid} \quad (1)$$

$$A + C \rightarrow CH_3COOCH_3\ (E) + H_3O^+;\ \text{slow} \quad (2)$$

$$M + H_3O^+ \overset{K}{\rightleftarrows} C + H_2O\ (W);\ \text{rapid} \tag{3}$$

(a) Show that the rate law for this mechanism, with M present in great excess, is

$$r_E = kLc_Ac_{HCl}/(L + c_W), \tag{4}$$

where

$$L = c_MK = c_Cc_W/c_{H_3O^+} \tag{5}$$

Assume all H^+ is present in C and in H_3O^+.

(b) Show that the integrated form of Eqn (4) for a constant-volume batch reactor operating isothermally with a fixed catalyst concentration is

$$k = [(L + c_{A0})\ \ln\ (c_{A0}/c_A) - (c_{A0} - c_A)]/c_{HCl}L\,t.$$

This is the form used by Smith (1939) to calculate k and L.

(c) Smith found that L depends on temperature and obtained the following values (what are the units of L?):

T, °C	0	20	30	40	50
L:	0.11	0.20	0.25	0.32	0.42

Does L follow an Arrhenius relationship?

6.5. Consider the following reversible reaction:

$$CO + Cl_2 \rightleftarrows COCl_2$$

The rate of formation of $COCl_2$ has been observed to follow the rate expression:

$$r_{COCl_2} = k_f[Cl_2]^{3/2}[CO] - k_r[Cl_2]^{1/2}[COCl_2]$$

A proposed mechanism is:

$Cl_2 \rightleftarrows 2Cl^*$	Equilibrium
$CO + Cl^* \rightleftarrows COCl^*$	Equilibrium
$COCl^* + Cl_2 \rightleftarrows COCl_2 + Cl^*$	Rate determining

Use the rate-determining step/equilibrium assumption to determine if the proposed mechanism is consistent with the observed rate expression.

6.6. Under the influence of oxidizing agents, hypophosphorous acid is transformed into phosphorous acid: $H_3PO_2 \xrightarrow{\text{oxidizing agent}} H_3PO_3$. The kinetics of this transformation present the following features. At a low concentration of oxidizing agent,

$$r_{H_3PO_3} = k[\text{oxidizing agent}]\ [H_3PO_2]$$

At high concentration of oxidizing agent,

$$r_{H_3PO_3} = k'[H^+]\,[H_3PO_2]$$

To explain the observed kinetics, it has been postulated that, with hydrogen ions as catalyst, normal unreacted H_3PO_2 is transformed reversibly into an active form, the nature of which is unknown. This intermediate then reacts with the oxidizing agent to give H_3PO_3. Show that this scheme does explain the observed kinetics.

6.7. For the decomposition of ozone in an inert gas M, the rate expression is

$$-r_{O_3} = \frac{k[O_3]^2[M]}{[O_2][M] + k'[O_3]}$$

Suggest a mechanism that is consistent with the above rate law.

6.8. Suggest a mechanism that is consistent with the experimentally observed rate expression for the following:

$$2A + B \rightarrow A_2B, \; r = kC_AC_B$$

6.9. Show that the following scheme:

$$N_2O_5 \underset{k_{-1}}{\overset{k_1}{\rightleftarrows}} NO_2 + NO_3\cdot$$

$$NO_3\cdot \xrightarrow{k_2} O_2 + NO\cdot$$

$$NO_3\cdot + NO\cdot \xrightarrow{k_3} 2NO_2$$

Proposed by R. Ogg, J. Chem. Phys., 15, 337 (1947) is consistent with the observed firs-order decomposition of N_2O_5.

6.10. Describe the differences between FES and PSSH.

CHAPTER

7

Parametric Estimation

OUTLINE

In many engineering problems, two or more variables are inherently related. Ideally, if one who is attempting to model the problem also knows the problem well, the relationship between the variables can be established using biological, engineering, physical, and/or chemical principles. To avoid complexity and/or uncertainties, one usually starts with heuristic arguments based on engineering and/or physical principles to derive at a mathematical model to relate these variables qualitatively. Undetermined parameters or coefficients are left in the mathematical model/relationship to guard against any uncertainty and/or unaccounted complexity. The kinetic modeling as discussed in Chapter 6 is a means to achieve the fundamental understanding and accurate models. Field (or experimental) data must be collected to estimate these unknown parameters before any actual use of this model. This leads to the classic problem of *parametric estimation*. While the model is known to be correct (if the parameters are determined accurately), the data contain error due to observation and instrumentation limitations. This situation is in contrary to functional approximation where the data are error-free while the model is not exact. Parametric estimation is commonly

Bioprocess Engineering
http://dx.doi.org/10.1016/B978-0-444-59525-6.00007-X

encountered in bioprocess engineering. For example, finding the kinetic constants of a chemical reaction with known mechanism, finding the exact relationship between flow rate and pressure drop for laminar flow of a liquid through complex network, etc. Parametric estimation is the main topic of this chapter.

In other occasions, one may have no access to the fundamental knowledge locking the underlying problem to be modeled. Sets of data are collected or available for the relations of the variables in question. Although no sound physical or engineering background is required, a mathematical model is needed for process optimization, prediction of outcome at some untested input, or process control. In this case, one must first determine if the variables are related. If they are related, then determine how they are related. This leads to the classic problem of *correlation* or *correlation analysis*. Still, if we know for sure that the variables are related, a mathematical model must be determined from the data set. This latter case is a subset of the former: *correlation analysis*. We call the latter problem *regression analysis* or *curve-fitting*. Correlation and/or regression analysis is a classic subject area in applied mathematics and has been an active subject of discussion for centuries.

The three formal problems or analyses: *parametric estimation*, *regression*, and *correlation* are interrelated. *Regression* or *curve-fitting* consists of selecting a mathematical model, usually of polynomials and then applying *parametric estimation* to determine the unknown coefficients. The mathematical model is thus frequently called regression model. *Correlation* is the most general terminology among these three terminologies. It consists of determining whether the variables are related (or correlated) and then regression/curve-fitting is applied to find a best relationship relating the variables. Because of the close relation among the three terminologies, it is often unclear what the differences are among these three terminologies. Very often, one uses the term correlation or curve-fitting without qualification to substitute all the three terminologies. Because a set of data can be fitted with many different functions with similar quality in the representation of the data, one is not to confuse the correlation with a physically correct mathematical model. As the data contain error, the best-fit model does not necessarily mean the true relationship. Nevertheless, correlation can be applied as the best aid to engineering research and process design and/or modeling.

7.1. REGRESSION MODELS

Regression analysis is a statistical/numerical technique for investigating and/or modeling the relationship between two or more variables. For example, in a bioprocess, suppose that the yield of the product is related to the process-operating temperature. Thermodynamics and chemical/bioprocess engineering principles (including heat transfer, mass transfer, and reaction engineering) can be applied to relate the yield to the operating temperature. However, because of the complexity and uncertainty involved, we often attempt to approach the problem in a heuristic manner. The derived model expression is thus a simplified version of the true underlying relationship. There are model parameters in the derived expression that can only be determined by experimentation. The evaluation of the unknown parameters is thus called parametric estimation. In other occasions, we may not know how the variables are related and model expressions are selected simply based on simplicity. In any case, the experimental data need to be generated for the underlying problem. Regression analysis can then be used to "build" a model or fine-tune the model parameters to predict yield at a given temperature level. This model can also be used for process optimization, such as finding the level of temperature that maximizes yield, or for process control purposes.

As an illustration, consider the data in Table 7.1 generated in our lab. In this table, y is the flow rate of water through a tube, and x is the percentage reading from a rotameter mounted on the tube. Figure 7.1 presents a scatter diagram of the data in Table 7.1. This is just a graph on which each (x_i, y_i) pair is represented as a point plotted in a two-dimensional coordinate system. We know for the fact that the rotameters are scaled linearly to reflect the flow rate for a given fluid passing through it. Inspection of this scatter diagram confirms our knowledge that, although no simple curve will pass exactly through all the points, there is a strong indication that the points lie scattered randomly around a straight line. Therefore, it is reasonable to assume that the mean of the random variable Y is related to x by the following straight-line relationship:

$$E(Y|x) = y = a_0 + a_1 x \tag{7.1}$$

TABLE 7.1 Water Flow Rates and Rotameter Readings

Observation number	Rotameter reading, %	Flow rates, g/s
1	5	0.3261
2	10	0.5912
3	15	0.8908
4	20	1.206
5	25	1.544
6	30	1.844
7	35	2.148
8	40	2.434
9	45	2.753
10	50	3.032
11	55	3.326
12	60	3.573
13	65	3.908
14	70	4.143
15	75	4.471
16	80	4.704
17	85	5.015
18	90	5.263
19	95	5.582

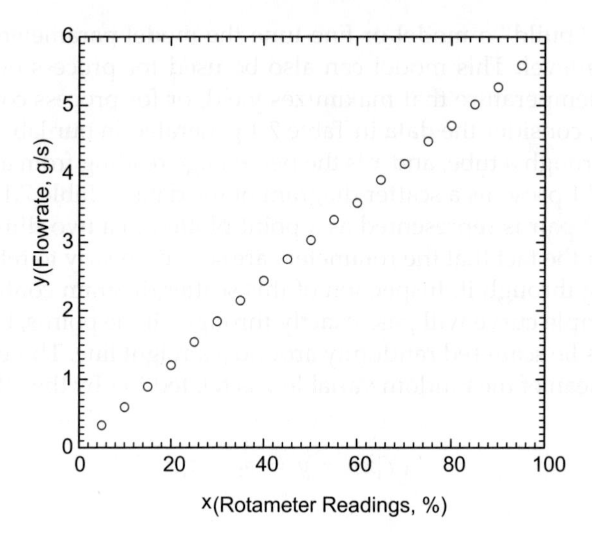

FIGURE 7.1 Scatter diagram of flow rate values versus rotameter reading from Table 7.1.

where the slope and intercept of the line are called model parameters regression coefficients. While the mean of Y or the model for y is a linear function of x, the actual observed value y_i does not fall exactly on a straight line. The deviation of the data from a straight line is due to the error in experimental observation. The appropriate way to generalize this trend indicated by the experimental data to a linear model is to assume that the expected value of Y is a linear function of x, but that for a fixed value of x the actual value of Y is determined by the mean value function (the linear model) plus a random error term, say,

$$Y = y + \varepsilon = a_0 + a_1 x + \varepsilon \tag{7.2}$$

where ε is the random error term. We will call this model the simple linear regression model, because it has only one independent variable or regressor, Y. While we have reasonable confidence that Eqn (7.1) is correct qualitatively, we also know for fact that the experimental data contain error.[1]

To gain more insight into this model, suppose that we can fix the value of x (assuming x is error-free) and observe the value of the random variable Y. Now if x is fixed, the random component ε on the right-hand side of the model in Eqn (7.2) determines the properties of Y. Suppose that the mean and variance of ε are 0 and σ^2, respectively. Then

$$E(Y|x) = E(a_0 + a_1 x + \varepsilon) = a_0 + a_1 x + E(\varepsilon) = a_0 + a_1 x \tag{7.3}$$

[1]Well, the rotameter readings are set visually by manually adjusting the control valve that controls the flow rate each time. In practice, one often generate a calibration curve based on the experimental data. Assuming the same person will be performing the flow rate control, one can therefore "effectively" ignore the error for the rotameter readings. The flow rates were measured by collecting and weighing the out flow water from the tube using a beaker, and the collection time is measured by a stopwatch.

Notice that this is the same relationship that we initially wrote down empirically from the inspection of the scatter diagram in Fig. 7.1. The variance of Y for a given x is

$$V(Y|x) = V(a_0 + a_1 x + \varepsilon) = V(a_0 + a_1 x) + V(\varepsilon) = \sigma^2 \tag{7.4}$$

Thus, the true (regression) model $E(Y|x) = a_0 + a_1 x$ is a line of mean values for the experimental data; that is, the height of the regression line at any value of x is just the expected value of Y for that x. The slope, a_1, can be interpreted as the change in the mean of Y for a unit change in x. Furthermore, the variability of Y at a particular value of x is determined by the error variance σ^2. This implies that there is a distribution of Y-values at each x and that the variance of this distribution is the same at each x.

For example, suppose that the true regression model relating water flow rate to rotameter reading is $y = 0.0661 + 0.05842x$ and suppose that the variance is $\sigma^2 = 0.001554$. Figure 7.2 illustrates this situation. The solid line represents the mean value of Y (or the value of y) and the dashed curves represent the probability (the horizontal distance to the base dashed line: $x = x_1$ or $x = x_2$) at which Y is observed. Notice that we have used a normal distribution to describe the random variation in ε. Since Y is the sum of a constant $a_0 + a_1 x$ (the mean) and a normally distributed random variable, Y is a normally distributed random variable. The variance σ^2 determines the variability in the observations Y on water flow rate. Thus, when σ^2 is small, the observed values of Y will fall close to the line, and when σ^2 is large, the observed values of Y may deviate considerably from the line. Because σ^2 is constant, the variability in Y at any value of x is the same.

The regression model describes the relationship between water flow rate Y and rotameter reading x. Thus, for any value of rotameter reading, water flow rate has a normal distribution

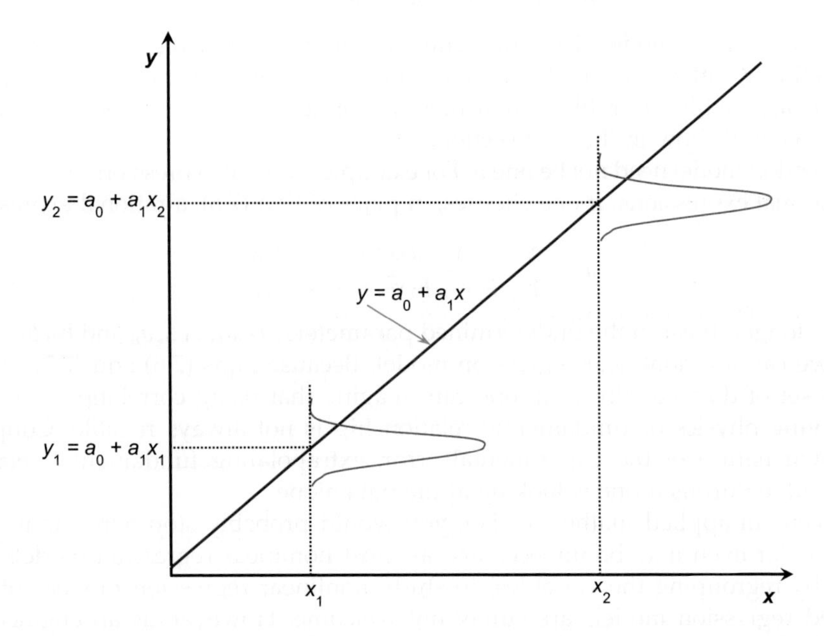

FIGURE 7.2 The distribution of Y for a given value of x.

with mean $0.0661 + 0.05842x$ and variance $\sigma^2 = 0.001554$. For example, if $x = 22$, then Y has a mean value $E(Y|x) = 0.0661 + 0.05842(22) = 1.351$ and variance 0.001554.

In most real-world problems, the values of the intercept and slope (a_0, a_1) and the error variance σ^2 will not be known, and they must be estimated from sample data. Regression analysis is a collection of statistical and numerical tools for finding estimates of the parameters in the regression model. Then this fitted regression equation or model is typically used in prediction of future observations of Y or for estimating the mean response at a particular level of x. To illustrate, a lab technician might be interested in estimating the mean water flow rate when the rotameter reading is $x = 33\%$. This chapter discusses such procedures and applications from simple linear to differential regression models.

7.2. CLASSIFICATION OF REGRESSION MODELS

The water flow rate is linearly related to the rotameter readings. This is the simplest regression model in that only two variables are involved: one independent variable (the rotameter reading) and one dependent variable (the water flow rate). The fundamental mathematical model is algebraically linear in the parameters to be determined:

$$y = a_0 + a_1 x \tag{7.5}$$

In this case, we have enough background to know the exact qualitative functional form. If one is to correlate or regress the data set without any prior knowledge, one may try a more general form:

$$y = a_0 + a_1 x + a_2 x^2 + \cdots + a_n x^n \tag{7.6}$$

which is a polynomial model. The polynomial model is a linear regression model because Eqn (7.6) is linear with respect to the undetermined parameters: $a_0, a_1, \ldots, a_n$. Linear regression models are highly desirable in that there is abundance of literature on it and easy to perform as we will show in the next section.

The regression model need not be linear. For example, rational expressions may be preferred over polynomial expressions. If one chooses, in place of Eqn (7.6), a rational expression,

$$y = \frac{a_0 + a_1 x + a_2 x^2 + \cdots + a_n x^n}{1 + b_1 x + b_2 x^2 + \cdots + b_m x^m} \tag{7.7}$$

then it is no longer linear in the undetermined parameters: $a_0, a_1, \ldots, a_n$ and $b_0, b_1, \ldots, b_m$. In this case, we call it a nonlinear regression model. Because Eqns (7.6) and (7.7) can usually correlate a set of data equally well, one can imagine that using correlation to extrapolate the underlying physics or fundamental relationship is not always reliable. Coupled with the unknown nature of the experimental error, extrapolating fundamental relations are even more adventurous if one is looking at the data alone.

If you were an applied mathematician, you would probably stop here. As it is already cumbersome (or even may be unnecessary, as most nonlinear regression models could be linearized by regrouping the variables) to study nonlinear regression models, other more complicated regression models are surely not welcome. However, as an engineer, we do not have the luxury to ignore other more complicated regression models. In engineering, we often need to interpret experimental or field data in terms of a given known physical model. For example, the concentration of the reactant C can be measured at different times t for the liquid reactant decomposing to liquid products in a well-mixed batch reactor. It might be a perfect example to apply the linear regression model, Eqn (7.6), to correlate the data. However, for process engineers, the simplest regression model for the particular problem is

$$\frac{dC}{dt} = -a_0 C^{a_1} \tag{7.8a}$$

and for bioprocesses:

$$\frac{dC}{dt} = -\frac{a_0 C^{a_1}}{a_2 + C^{a_3}} \tag{7.8b}$$

which are not only nonlinear, but is no longer an algebraic equation. Therefore, the regression model (7.8) does not fit into the same category as we have discussed earlier. We can call this model an ordinary differential regression model. This opens up a whole new class of regression models. Similarly, one may have partial differential regression models, differential-algebraic regression models, and integral regression models as well. In bioprocess engineering, we normally encounter algebraic regression models and (ordinary or partial) differential regression models.

7.3. CRITERIA FOR "BEST" FIT AND SIMPLE LINEAR REGRESSIONS

The case of simple linear regression considers a single regressor or predictor x and a dependent or response variable Y. Suppose that the true relationship between Y and x is a straight line and that the observation Y at each level of x is a random variable. As noted previously, the expected value of Y for each value of x is

$$E(Y|x) = y = a_0 + a_1 x \tag{7.9}$$

where the intercept a_0 and the slope a_1 are unknown regression coefficients. We assume that each observation, Y, can be described by the model

$$Y = a_0 + a_1 x + \varepsilon \tag{7.10}$$

where e is a random error with mean zero and variance σ^2. The random errors corresponding to different observations are also assumed to be uncorrelated random variables.

Suppose that we have n pairs of observations $(x_1, y_1), (x_2, y_2)\ldots (x_n, y_n)$. Figure 7.3 shows a typical scatter plot of observed data and a candidate for the estimated regression line. The estimates of a_0 and a_1 should result in a line that is (in some sense) a "best fit" to the data.

There are several choices for "best" fit by minimizing the norm of the error, $\|\varepsilon\|$. Three of such choices are shown in Fig. 7.4. In Fig. 7.4a, the dashed lines are produced by minimizing the sum of the residuals directly, i.e.,

$$\text{minimizing} \sum_{i=1}^{n} \varepsilon_i = \text{minimizing} \sum_{i=1}^{n} (y_i - a_0 - a_1 x_i)$$

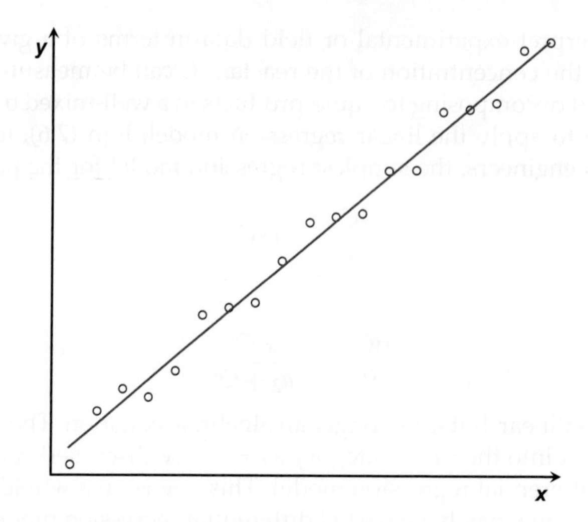

FIGURE 7.3 Deviations of the data from the estimated regression model.

As shown in Fig. 7.4a, this is an inadequate criterion. The "fit" is not unique as all the lines, not only the short-dashed or long-dashed lines but the solid line as well, all satisfy the condition of minimizing the sum of the errors. Obviously, the "best" fit is the solid line. However, any straight line passing through the midpoint (except a perfect vertical line) results in a minimum value for the sum of the residual because the errors cancel.

The second choice might seem to be logical, minimizing the sum of the absolute values of the residuals:

$$\text{minimizing} \sum_{i=1}^{n} |\varepsilon_i| = \text{minimizing} \sum_{i=1}^{n} |y_i - a_0 - a_1 x_i|$$

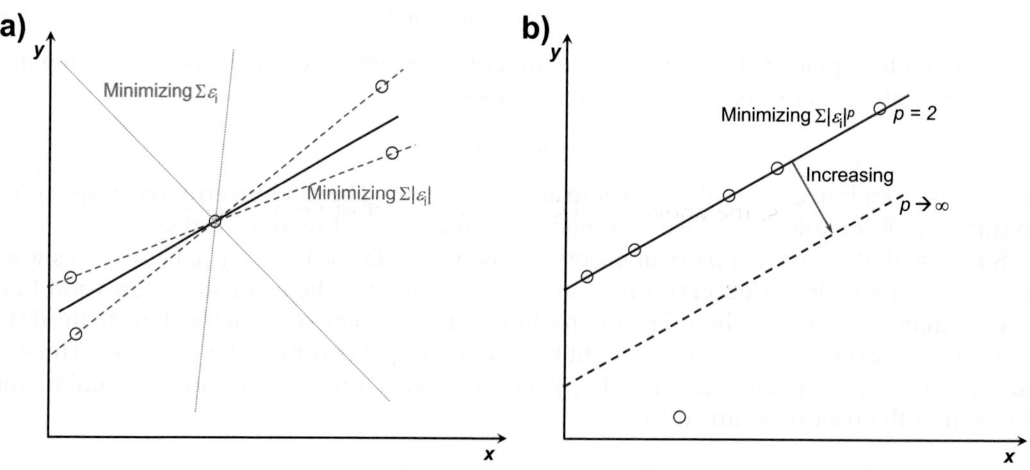

FIGURE 7.4 Examples of "best" fit criteria for regression analysis. (a) Minimizing the sum of errors or the sum of the absolute errors. (b) Minimizing the l_p-norm of the errors.

With this approach, one can avoid the errors being canceled as in the first choice where the sum of the residuals is being minimized. Figure 7.4a illustrates the inadequacy of this criterion: any line lies between the two long-dashed lines will minimize the sum of the absolute values. Therefore, this criterion does not yield a unique fit either.

Alternatively, one can minimize the l_p-norm of the residual for an arbitrary p. This strategy is equivalent to

$$\text{minimizing} \sum_{i=1}^{n} |\varepsilon_i|^p = \text{minimizing} \sum_{i=1}^{n} |y_i - a_0 - a_1 x_i|^p$$

As p is increased, as shown in Fig. 7.4b, it gives undue influence to an outlier, that is, a single point with a large error. This is especially true for $p \to \infty$. Therefore, one cannot just choose any p.

German scientist Karl Gauss (1777–1855) proposed estimating the parameters a_0 and a_1 in Eqn (7.10) in order to minimize the sum of the squares of the vertical deviations in Fig. 7.3. This strategy corresponds to the last choice whereby setting $p = 2$. To be in general, we shall restate the approach as the unknown parameters in the model being determined by minimizing the estimated variance of the data around the model.

We call this criterion for estimating the regression coefficients the method of least squares. Using Eqn (7.10), we may express the n observations in the sample as

$$y_i = a_0 + a_1 x_i + \varepsilon_i, \quad i = 1, 2, \ldots, n \tag{7.11}$$

and the estimated variance of the experimental data around the model is given by

$$\sigma^2 = \frac{1}{n-1} \sum_{i=1}^{n} \varepsilon_i^2 = \frac{1}{n-1} \sum_{i=1}^{n} (y_i - a_0 - a_1 x_i)^2 \tag{7.12}$$

The least squares estimators of a_0 and a_1 must satisfy

$$\frac{\partial \sigma^2}{\partial a_0} = -\frac{2}{n-1} \sum_{i=1}^{n} (y_i - a_0 - a_1 x_i) = 0 \tag{7.13}$$

$$\frac{\partial \sigma^2}{\partial a_1} = -\frac{2}{n-1} \sum_{i=1}^{n} (y_i - a_0 - a_1 x_i) x_i = 0 \tag{7.14}$$

For linear regressions, the above process results in a set of linear algebraic equations in general. Simplifying these two equations, (7.13) and (7.14), yields

$$n a_0 + a_1 \sum_{i=1}^{n} x_i = \sum_{i=1}^{n} y_i \tag{7.15}$$

$$a_0 \sum_{i=1}^{n} x_i + a_1 \sum_{i=1}^{n} x_i^2 = \sum_{i=1}^{n} x_i y_i \tag{7.16}$$

Equations (7.15) and (7.16) are called the least squares normal equations. The solution to the normal equations results in the least squares estimators for a_0 and a_1.

The fitted or estimated regression line is therefore

$$y = a_0 + a_1 x \tag{7.17}$$

Note that each pair of observations satisfies the relationship

$$y_i = a_0 + a_1 x_i + \varepsilon_i, \quad i = 1, 2, \ldots, n \tag{7.18}$$

DEFINITION

The least squares estimates of the intercept and slope in the simple linear regression model are

$$a_0 = \overline{y} - a_1 \overline{x} \tag{7.19}$$

$$a_1 = \frac{\sum_{i=1}^{n} x_i y_i - \frac{1}{n}\left(\sum_{i=1}^{n} y_i\right)\left(\sum_{i=1}^{n} x_i\right)}{\sum_{i=1}^{n} x_i^2 - \frac{1}{n}\left(\sum_{i=1}^{n} x_i\right)^2} \tag{7.20}$$

where $\overline{y} = \frac{1}{n}\sum_{i=1}^{n} y_i$ and $\overline{x} = \frac{1}{n}\sum_{i=1}^{n} x_i$.

where $\varepsilon_i = y_i - y(x_i)$ is called the residual. The residual describes the error in the fit of the model to the ith observation y_i. In the next section, we will use the residuals to provide information about the adequacy of the fitted model.

We have so far discussed the regression by assuming that the data contain error in y_i's and the error is of absolute nature as characterized by Eqn (7.20). For a simple linear regression model, as long as only one variable (either x_i's or y_i's) contains an error of absolute nature, the above procedure is strictly valid. For any other regression models, if the variable x is in experimental error, one will need to minimize the residual square of x. Simply rename x as the regressor in the regression process should suffice. There can be occasions where more than one variable in the same regression model is in experimental error, one should deal with these types of regression with care. If at all possible, experimental technique should be improved to eliminate the errors in the controlling variables (e.g. x). When experimental technique fails, one needs to determine the magnitudes of the errors among different variables. There is no general rule or simple technique to treat these types of regression problems. If the magnitudes of the errors are consistently related with the regression model, then there is no special attention needed and one can apply the regression technique as if only one variable contains measurement error. Otherwise, the usual approach is to minimize the residual square of the variable that has the largest magnitude in error.

Apart from the complicated error structures, there are cases where the regressor contains experimental error of relative nature. That is, for the simple linear regression model as an example,

$$y_i = (a_0 + a_1 x_i) + (1 + d_i), \quad i = 1, 2, \ldots, n \tag{7.21}$$

where d_i is the relative error or relative residual at point (x_i, y_i). The relative residual or error d can be assumed to be distributed normally, rather than the residual or absolute error $e = y \cdot d$.

For example, in obtaining the data of Table 7.1, we have measured the flow rates such that we always have four significant digits irrespective of the magnitude of the flow rates. The number of significant digits can be achieved by using a large enough beaker to collect water. When the flow rate is very small, we collect enough water such that the amount of water can be measured correctly with four digits. When the flow rate is high, we make sure the time lap is long enough such that the accuracy in time has four significant digits. By generating the data in this fashion, we know for sure that the data is accurate to within four digits.

When the relative error in measured y is normally distributed, the regression should be carried out by minimizing the sum of d squared. That is,

$$\text{minimizing} \sum_{i=1}^{n} |d_i|^2 = \text{minimizing} \sum_{i=1}^{n} \left[\frac{y_i}{y(x_i)} - 1 \right]^2$$

or minimizing d^2 with

$$d^2 = \frac{1}{n-1} \sum_{i=1}^{n} d_i^2 = \frac{1}{n-1} \sum_{i=1}^{n} \left[\frac{y_i}{y(x_i)} - 1 \right]^2 \tag{7.22}$$

In general, this approach will lead to nonlinear regression. Even for a simple linear regression model, the above regression approach will require nonlinear analysis.

In bioprocess engineering applications, the regression problems we usually encounter are nonlinear. The minimization of the (relative or absolute) residual square sum can be achieved by applying the optimization techniques. Therefore, there are no special discussions devoted here in this chapter.

7.4. CORRELATION COEFFICIENT

From the perspective of the data set, y_i varies with x_i. The total variation of y_i (a measure of the difference of y_i from the average value of y_i) can be computed from the data set as

$$\text{TV} = \frac{1}{n-1} \sum_{i=1}^{n} (y_i - \bar{y})^2 \tag{7.23}$$

Using the regression model, we can explain part of the total variation. The unexplained portion of the variation is the estimated variance of the data around the model and is given by

$$\text{UV} = \sigma^2 = \frac{1}{n-1} \sum_{i=1}^{n} [y(x_i) - y_i]^2 \tag{7.24}$$

If there is no correlation between the variables, the two variations defined above, Eqns (7.23) and (7.24), are identical. On the other hand, if the regression line passes through all the data points, then the unexplained portion of variation UV or σ^2 is zero. The regression is thus perfect. In practice, because of the error in data, one is not to expect a perfect match between the data and the model. The ratio of the unexplained variation to the total variation is called *random factor*:

$$F_R = \frac{\text{UV}}{\text{TV}} = \frac{(n-1)\sigma^2}{\sum_{i=1}^{n}(y_i - \bar{y})^2} \tag{7.25}$$

The complementary of the *random factor* is usually called the *coefficient of determination* and is defined by

$$R^2 = 1 - F_R = 1 - \frac{(n-1)\sigma^2}{\sum_{i=1}^{n}(y_i - \bar{y})^2} \tag{7.26}$$

The square root of the coefficient of determination, R, is called the *correlation coefficient*, which is sometimes called as *correlation* in short. Therefore, from parametric estimation point of view, the higher the value of R, the more reliable are the model parameters. If R is close to 0 or if F_R is close to unity, we say that x_i and y_i are not correlated (randomly related). If R is close to unity or random factor is close to zero, we say that x_i and y_i are strongly correlated by the model.

From Eqn (7.26), the correlation coefficient can be obtained in general as

$$R = \sqrt{1 - F_R} = \sqrt{1 - \frac{(n-1)\sigma^2}{\sum_{i=1}^{n} y_i^2 - \frac{1}{n}\left(\sum_{i=1}^{n} y_i\right)^2}} \tag{7.27}$$

If the regression is carried out by minimizing σ^2, the computation of the minimum σ^2 or the unexplained variations at final correlation conditions is readily available. Therefore, computation of R will not require extensive computational effort. The value of R is frequently used as an indicator to the quality of fit.

For the flow rate versus rotameter reading data in Table 7.1, the regression model is linear. Minimizing the variance of the data around the model yield the final model as given by

$$y = 0.0661 + 0.05842x \tag{7.28}$$

and the variance of the data in Table 7.1 around the model, Eqn (7.28), is given by

$$\sigma^2 = 0.001554$$

From the data in Table 7.1, we can also compute

$$\sum_{i=1}^{n} y_i^2 = 218.1895, \quad \sum_{i=1}^{n} y_i = 56.75405$$

Therefore,

$$R = \sqrt{1 - \frac{(n-1)\sigma^2}{\sum_{i=1}^{n} y_i^2 - \frac{1}{n}\left(\sum_{i=1}^{n} y_i\right)^2}} = \sqrt{1 - \frac{(19-1)\times 0.001554}{218.1895 - \frac{1}{19}\times 56.75405^2}} = 0.999712$$

In this case, the correlation coefficient is very close to unity. Since the regression model is fundamentally sound, we shall say that the experimental data is very good.

If the regression is carried out by minimizing d^2 instead, the definition of R is not as straightforward. Using Eqn (7.27) hides the fact that the data contain a relative error. One is not to replace σ^2 with d^2 in Eqn (7.27) either. An alternative definition can be used is to normalize the total variation with the mean value of y_i's. That is,

$$R' = \sqrt{1 - \frac{\frac{n-1}{n} d^2}{\frac{n \sum_{i=1}^{n} y_i^2}{\left(\sum_{i=1}^{n} y_i\right)^2} - 1}} \tag{7.29}$$

The correlation coefficient defined by Eqn (7.29) should give a better estimate of the quality of the fit for the data containing relative error.

7.5. COMMON ABUSES OF REGRESSION

Correlation/regression analysis is widely used and frequently misused; several common abuses of regression are briefly mentioned here. The most unforgiving misuse is the sloppiness in selecting variables for correlation. Care should be taken in selecting variables with which to construct regression equations and in determining the form of the model. It is possible to develop statistical relationships among variables that are completely unrelated in practical sense. For example, we might attempt to relate the room temperature with number of boxes of computer paper used in a lab. A straight line may even appear to provide a good fit to the data, but the relationship is an unreasonable one on which to rely. A strong observed association between variables does not necessarily imply that a causal relationship exists between those variables. Designed experiments are the only way to determine causal relationships. Whenever possible, fundamentally sound relationships are to be sought and only parametric estimation is applied. Because of the unknown nature of the experimental error, a slightly smaller variance cannot be used as a criterion either to endorse or to reject a regression model.

The most common misuse of parametric estimation/regression is not minimizing the error variance of data around the model that is generic to the data. It is common not to enquire whether the experimental data is obtained with either an absolute certainty (an absolute error is present, or the data is accurate to within $\pm\varepsilon$) or a relative certainty (relative error is present, or the data is accurate to with $\pm d'\%$). Linearization of regression model is commonly applied irrespective of the error structure. Most common excuse for knowingly taking the incorrect step is only when liner regression was applied that the accompanying numerical problem could be solved in a reasonable time frame. While this was a problem in the computer stone age, one can no longer use it as an excuse today. In engineering, on the other hand, we often consider the linear regression model because a straight line is visually pleasing when data are scattered around it.

Regression relationships are valid only for values of the regressor variable within the range of the original data. This is especially true for correlations. The mathematical relationship that we have tentatively assumed may be valid over the original range of x, but it may be unlikely to remain so as we extrapolate—that is, if we use values of x beyond that range. In other words, as we move beyond the range of values of x for which data were collected, we become less certain about the validity of the assumed model. Regression models are not always valid for extrapolation purposes.

7.6. GENERAL REGRESSION ANALYSIS

It is evident from previous discussion that when the regression model is algebraically linear, the associated least squares problem reduces to solving a set of linear equations. Therefore, linear regression is popular in textbooks as well as in practice. It was often for one to resort to variable transformations to reduce a nonlinear algebraic regression model to a linear regression model. While it was mathematically genius in performing such a transformation at a time when there is virtually no computing power, it is not acceptable conceptually today as computing power is vast available.

Modeling of a physical system with mathematical expressions is an important part of research in science and engineering. When mathematical modeling is involved, there are commonly free parameters left in model equations. Experimental data are utilized to offer a closure to the system or problem under consideration. In order to determine the free parameters, one often seeks a simple equation that directly or indirectly relates to the experimental data. For example, linear algebraic functions or equations (with respect to the free parameters) are highly desired because linear regression can then be easily applied to determine the free parameters. Because of the popularity in linear regression, experimental data are usually converted to suit the needs for simplicity in regression. There are errors involved in the experimental data. Conversion of the experimental data normally causes the error to magnify. In most cases, the errors in the new derived quantities are not linearly related to the errors in the original experimental data. To partially counter the indirect link in error, data treatment would normally be applied by performing data smoothing prior to parameter estimation. However, this exercise puts a high weight on data smoothing. The regression performed based on the converted experimental data is not reliable because the error that is minimized is not linearly related to the error in the original experimental data. Therefore, the parameters obtained in such a fashion are not reliable. To increase the reliability of such a parametric estimation, one normally turns to design or redesign a better experiment. When the experimental error is "eliminated" or "much reduced," the quality of the converted (or derived) data bears less error. Therefore, the parameters estimated in this fashion can be reliable. However, there is a limit in redesigning an experiment. The cost associated with such an exercise is also high. Alternatively, to rectify the discrepancy in errors in the course of regression, one may regress the experimental data directly rather than through some derived quantities other than the original experimental data.

Regression by minimizing the variance of the experimental data around the regression model prediction is the correct approach one should adopt. This approach in general renders a nonlinear regression problem. Fortunately, we now know how to solve an optimization problem. The regression problem is essentially an optimization problem: minimizing the variance of data around the regression model by changing the regression parameters! In this sense, we will not need any other special techniques to perform regression analysis.

7.7. QUALITY OF FIT AND ACCURACY OF DATA

When dealing with regression, we need to address the issues of *accuracy, precision*, and *bias*. The term accuracy is commonly used, for example, as in reference to the accuracy of the weather forecasting or to the accuracy of an opinion poll taken just before a national election. Of interest here is the meaning of the term as it appears to the data as compared to what they should be. It is directly applicable to the quality of fit.

Consider the four targets of Fig. 7.5. Assuming that those shooting at the targets were aiming at the center, the person shooting target A was successful. While not every bullet went through the exact center, the distance between the holes and the center is small. The holes in target B are similarly clustered as in target A, but they show large deviation from the center. The large deviations or errors between the holes and the center of the target suggest a lack of exactness or correctness. While all the holes deviate significantly from the center, there is, however, a measure of consistency in the holes. In summary, the holes in B show two important characteristics: they tend to agree with each other but they deviate considerably from where the shooter was aiming.

The holes in target C are very different in characteristics from the holes in either target A or target B. For one, most holes are not near the center, and two, they are not near to each other. Thus, they lack both correctness and consistency. Because most of them are not near the center of the target, the shooter is not exact. Because of the wide scatter, there is a lack of consistency. In comparing the holes on targets B and C, they both lack exactness, but there is a measure of consistency for the holes in target B that is missing in target C.

The fourth distribution of holes is shown as case D. Like case B, all of the holes are to the lower left of the center; but unlike case B, the holes lack consistency. Both cases C and D show considerable scatter, but with case D, the scatter is concentrated to one side of the target.

A comparison of the four targets indicates that there are three important characteristics of data. The holes in targets A and B show a measure of consistency. In data analysis, this consistency is more formally referred to as precision. Precision is defined as the ability to give multiple estimates that are near to each other. In terms of cases A and B, the shooters were precise. The shooters of cases C and D were imprecise since the holes show a lot of scatter.

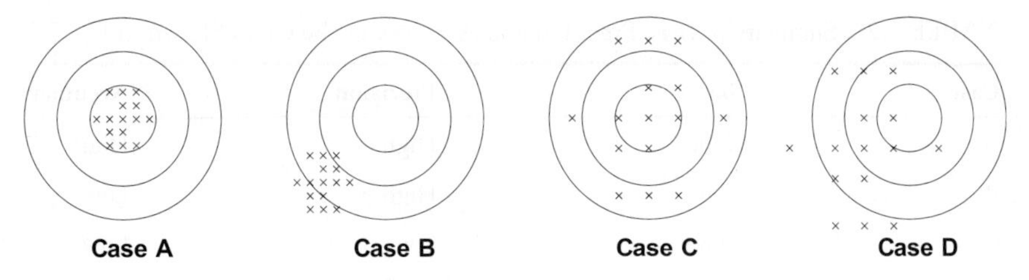

FIGURE 7.5 A schematic of accuracy, precision, and bias.

Bias is a second important characteristic of data. The holes in targets B and D are consistently to the lower left of the center; that is, there is a systematic distribution of the wholes with respect to the center of the target. If we found a point that could represent the center of the holes in any target, then the difference between the center of the holes and the center of the target would be a measure of the shooter's bias. More formally, bias is a systematic deviation of values from the true value. The holes in cases B and D show a systematic deviation to the lower left, while cases A and C are considered to be unbiased because there is no systematic deviation.

Precision and bias are elements of accuracy. Specifically, bias is a measure of systematic deviation and precision is a measure of random deviations. Inaccuracy can result from either a bias or a lack of precision. In referring to the targets, the terms correctness and exactness were used. More formally, accuracy is the degree to which the data deviate from the true value. If the deviations are small, then the method or process that led to the measurement is accurate.

Table 7.2 shows a summary of the concepts of accuracy, precision, and bias as they characterize the holes in the targets of Fig. 7.5. Of course, terms like high, moderate, and low are somewhat objective.

Approximation of one single value of point can be illustrated as neatly as Fig. 7.5. One can observe the precision and bias. For the approximation of a continuous line, one cannot show as clear as for one single point. For the case where the continuous line is not known for sure and the data contain error, the accuracy becomes more difficult to define. For regression or parametric estimation analysis, this is exactly the case.

Similar to Fig. 7.5 for the approximation of a true value by experimentation or shooting a target, Fig. 7.6 shows the regressions of a set of data. In this case, the data contain error but with a true value manifests in the mean. Regression analysis can be applied to reveal the relationship or continuous line. Case A shows a perfect fit to the data: the line represents the mean of the data. The data scatter around the line and there is no systematic bias in appearance. One can therefore observe the error distribution in the data.

In case B, the continuous line shows the same trend as the data qualitatively. However, the data are consistently off the line: the mean of the data is shifted away from the continuous line. There is a systematic error in the parameters of the line. This is similar to case B of Fig. 7.5. Corrections to the parameters are needed.

In case C, the line represents the overall mean of the data. However, the line lacks the detailed agreement with the data: a hump in the middle of the range cannot be explained as simply the experimental error. Therefore, the regression model is biased and unable to reveal the detail of the data. In case D, the regression model has the same problem as

TABLE 7.2 Summary of Bias, Precision and Accuracy of the Cases Shown in Fig. 7.5

Case	Bias	Precision	Accuracy
A	None	High	High
B	High	High	Low
C	None	Low	Low
D	Moderate	Low	Low

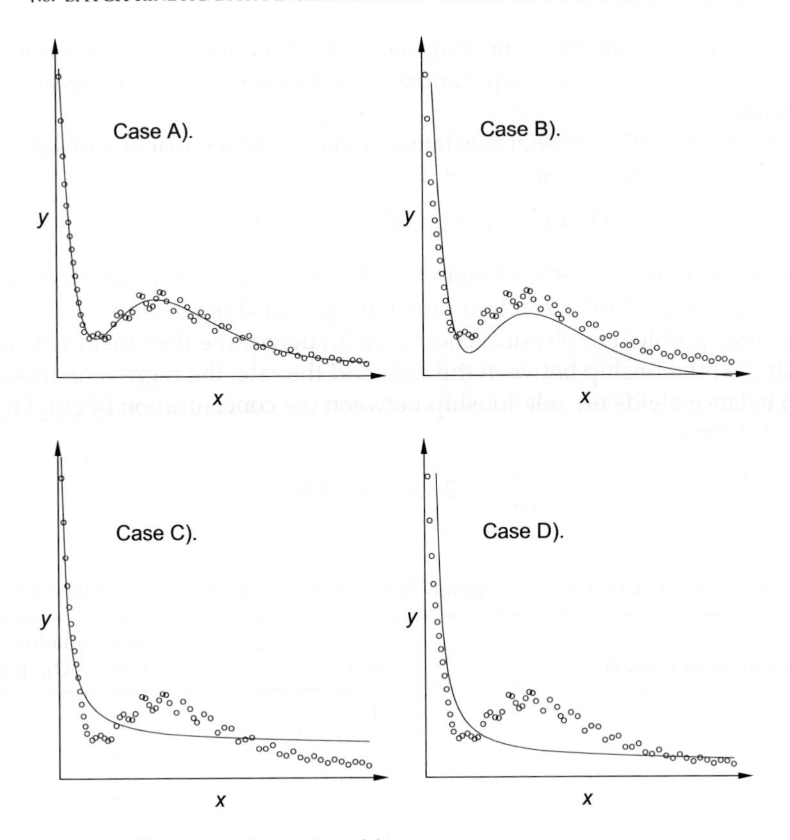

FIGURE 7.6 Schematics illustrating the quality of fits.

case C. In addition, the data are consistently higher the regression line. It becomes obvious that the regression model missed the hump in data in the middle range.

In regression analysis, we know that the data contain error. However, we shall assume that the data do not have systematic error. Therefore, we must require the regression line to be lie in the center of the data—bias of the data in relative to the regression line means either the parameters are not correctly estimated or the model needs to be improved. Whether the data and regression show any bias, graphic illustrations are the best means to detect. Bias and/or imprecision is not easy to define and detect mathematically. One must visually assess the quality of the fit. If there is a bias in the fit, one can improve the regression by adjusting the initial guess (as there might be more solutions to the nonlinear optimization problem) and/or improving the regression model.

7.8. BATCH KINETIC DATA INTERPRETATION: DIFFERENTIAL REGRESSION MODEL

In this section, we shall discuss the parametric estimation for one particular class of regression model: differential model. This type of problem is commonly encountered in Physical

Chemistry, Reaction Engineering, and Bioprocess Engineering, where reaction kinetic relationships are obtained by batch experimentation. Further to our discussions, let us use a real-life example:

Hellin and Jungers (1957) present the data in Table 7.3 on the reaction of sulfuric acid with diethylsulfate in aqueous solution at 22.9 °C:

$$H_2SO_4 + (C_2H_5)_2SO_4 \rightleftarrows 2C_2H_5HSO_4 \quad (7.30)$$

Initial concentrations of H_2SO_4 (denoted as A) and $(C_2H_5)_2SO_4$ (denoted as B) are each 5.5 mol/L ($=C_{A0}=C_{B0}$). Find a reaction rate equation for this reaction.

This is a classic problem in physical chemistry. To determine the rate of reaction, we must first establish the relationship between the data and the rate: the regression model. A simple mass (mole) balance yields the relationship between the concentration of ethyl hydrosulfate, $C_2H_5HSO_4$, and time

$$\frac{dC_C}{dt} = 2r = f(C_A, C_B, C_C) \quad (7.31)$$

TABLE 7.3 Kinetic Data for Aqueous Reaction of Sulfuric Acid with Diethylsulfate

Measurement number	t, min	Concentration of $C_2H_5HSO_4$, mol/L
	0	0
1	41	1.18
2	48	1.38
3	55	1.63
4	75	2.24
5	96	2.75
6	127	3.31
7	146	3.76
8	162	3.81
9	180	4.11
10	194	4.31
11	212	4.45
12	267	4.86
13	318	5.15
14	368	5.32
15	379	5.35
16	410	5.42
	∞	5.80

where r is the rate of reaction. From stoichiometry, the concentration of A, B, and C are related through

$$C_A = C_{A0} - \frac{1}{2}C_C = C_B \tag{7.32}$$

Applying the simplest form (power-law rate expression) of kinetics to this homogeneous reaction leads to

$$\frac{dC_C}{dt} = k_f(C_A C_B)^{\frac{n}{2}} - k_b C_C^n = k_f\left(C_{A0} - \frac{1}{2}C_C\right)^n - k_b C_C^n \tag{7.33}$$

Here, k_f, k_b, and n are termed kinetic constants. We also know that the chemical equilibrium is established at infinite time or the rate of change of C_C is zero at infinite time, and k_f, k_b, and n are related by

$$k_b = \left[\left(\frac{C_{A0} - 0.5C_C}{C_C}\right)^n\right]_{t\to\infty} k_f = \left(\frac{13}{29}\right)^n k_f \tag{7.34}$$

Thus, two parameters can be varied and the experimental data can be used to estimate these parameters. To this point, we have the regression model:

$$\frac{dC_C}{dt} = k_f\left(C_{A0} - \frac{1}{2}C_C\right)^n - k_f\left(\frac{13}{29}C_C\right)^n \tag{7.35}$$

which is a nonlinear ordinary differential regression model.

Determining the parameters: k_f and n of Eqn (7.35) from the data in Table 7.3 is not an easy task. This problem is tackled traditionally through linear regressions. Because straight lines are visually pleasing and easy to spot the scattering of experimental data around the line, the regression is normally done by transforming the model to a linear model. There are two general methods used in the literature: the integral methods and the differential methods, all of which attempts to reduce the differential model, such as Eqn (7.35), to a linear (algebraic) model. The linearization of the kinetic model in terms of regression needs is not unique in some cases. For example, the well-known two parameters (r_{max} and K_m) Michaelis–Menten equation

$$r = \frac{r_{max}S}{K_m + S} \tag{7.36}$$

can be linearized in multiple ways. They include

(1) the Lineweaver–Burk plot (the double reciprocal plot $1/r \sim 1/S$)

$$\frac{1}{r} = \frac{1}{r_{max}} + \frac{K_m}{r_{max}}\frac{1}{S} \tag{7.37}$$

In terms of two new parameters ($a_0 = 1/r_{max}$ and $a_1 = K_m/r_{max}$), the regression model is linear: $y = a_0 + a_1 x$. Here, $y = 1/r$ and $x = 1/S$.

(2) the Eadie–Hofstee plot ($r \sim r/S$)

$$r = r_{\max} - K_m \frac{r}{S} \tag{7.38}$$

The regression model is linear: $y = r_{\max} + K_m x$. Here, $y = r$ and $x = r/S$. And

(3) the Hanes–Woolf plot ($S/r \sim S$)

$$\frac{S}{r} = \frac{1}{r_{\max}} S + \frac{K_m}{r_{\max}} \tag{7.39}$$

In terms of two new parameters ($a_1 = 1/r_{\max}$ and $a_0 = K_m/r_{\max}$), the regression model is linear: $y = a_0 + a_1 x$. Here, $y = S/r$ and $x = S$.

These classic approaches have contributed to the early successes in the "slide rule" age when computing power is nonexistent. We will examine the validity of such approaches in the following.

7.8.1. Integral Methods

In the integral method approach, Eqn (7.35) is first integrated to obtain an algebraic equation. In this case, one can assume an order before starting the process. For example, we assume $n = 2$, Eqn (7.35) can be integrated to obtain

$$\ln\left(\frac{C_{A0} - \frac{3}{58}C_C}{C_{A0} - \frac{55}{58}C_C}\right) = \frac{26}{29} k_f C_{A0} t \tag{7.40}$$

Letting

$$y = \ln\left(\frac{C_{A0} - \frac{3}{58}C_C}{C_{A0} - \frac{55}{58}C_C}\right) \tag{7.41}$$

Equation (7.40) is reduced to

$$y = \frac{26}{29} k_f C_{A0} t \tag{7.42}$$

or

$$y = at \tag{7.43}$$

By converting the data of C_C in Table 7.3 to y using Eqn (7.41), one can transform the initial differential model to a linear model using Eqn (7.43). If this procedure fails, a different n can be selected to repeat the process.

Table 7.4 shows the transformed data set from Table 7.3 using Eqn (7.41). With this approach, the regression becomes very simple and visually favorable. There might be some trial-and-error involved, still, given the complexity of the problem it is welcomed among the Physical Chemistry and Reaction Engineering communities. Figure 7.7 shows the straight-line plot generated from the integral method. One can observe a pleasing straight line passing through the data points on the (t, y) plane. The straight line is the best fit (from the procedure discussed earlier):

$$y = 0.006607\,t \tag{7.44}$$

with a correlation coefficient of

$$R = 0.99912 \tag{7.45}$$

Since the regression is very good with the correlation coefficient close to unity and the data scattering is minimal in Fig. 7.7, one has confidence that Eqn (7.44) can represent the transformed data (Table 7.4). Therefore, the kinetic parameters are given by $n = 2$ and $k_f = 0.006607 \times \dfrac{29}{26C_{A0}} = 0.001340.$

TABLE 7.4 Transformed Data from Table 7.3 for Integral Method of Kinetic Data Interpretation, $n = 2$

t, min	$y = \ln\left(\dfrac{C_{A0} - \frac{3}{58}C_C}{C_{A0} - \frac{55}{58}C_C}\right)$
0	0
41	0.2163
48	0.2587
55	0.3145
75	0.4668
96	0.6165
127	0.8140
146	1.009
162	1.033
180	1.194
194	1.318
212	1.415
267	1.773
318	2.139
368	2.441
379	2.505
410	2.673

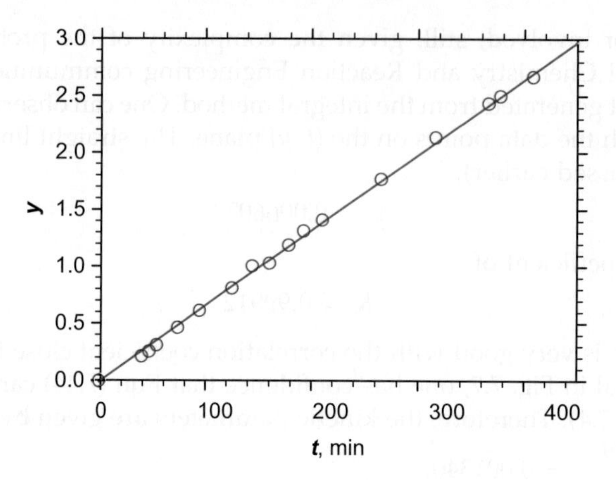

FIGURE 7.7 Kinetic parametric estimation using an integral method.

7.8.2. Differential Methods

With the integral methods of approaches, one often has to assume a value for the order of reaction. Trial-and-error may not be everyone's favorite. To avoid the trial-and-error nature of the integral method, the experimental data in Table 3 can be differentiated to obtain

$$z = \frac{dC_C}{dt} = k_f\left(C_{A0} - \frac{1}{2}C_C\right)^n - k_f\left(\frac{13}{29}C_C\right)^n \tag{7.46}$$

The values of z at selected values of C_C's can be obtained either through direct numerical differentiation of the data (C_C, t) series or by first regressing the data series according to a polynomial form

$$C_C = a_0 + a_1 t + a_2 t + a_2 t^2 + a_3 t^3 \ldots \tag{7.47}$$

and then differentiating to obtain the derivative or z.

By so doing, one effectively reduces the differential model to an algebraic regression model. However, Eqn (7.46) is still nonlinear. One will need to use a nonlinear regression program to perform the parametric estimation. Therefore, this is still not favorable in the Physical Chemistry and Reaction Engineering texts. Steps are often taken during the planning of experiments to avoid this situation. For this problem, one can notice that if C_C is small, Eqn (7.46) may be approximated by

$$z \approx k_f\left(C_{A0} - \frac{1}{2}C_C\right)^n \tag{7.48}$$

Equation (7.48) can be rearranged to give

$$\ln z \approx \ln k_f + n \ln\left(C_{A0} - \frac{1}{2}C_C\right) \tag{7.49}$$

Letting,

$$y = \ln z = \ln \frac{dC_C}{dt} \tag{7.50}$$

and

$$x = \ln\left(C_{A0} - \frac{1}{2}C_C\right) \tag{7.51}$$

one can transform the initial differential regression model to a linear regression model:

$$y = ax + b \tag{7.52}$$

Therefore, the final regression is very easy to perform and visually pleasing. Here, the discrepancy between the linear model, Eqn (7.52), and the initial differential model, Eqn (7.35), can be reduced by good practice in experimental design.

However, because of the range of data in Table 7.3, the simplified approach outlined above is not suitable as new experimentation is not feasible. To illustrate the linear regression from a differential method, we let

$$x_n = \left(C_{A0} - \frac{1}{2}C_C\right)^n - \left(\frac{13}{29}C_C\right)^n \tag{7.53}$$

the Eqn (7.46) becomes

$$z = k_f x_n \tag{7.54}$$

Table 7.5 shows the experimental data (Table 7.3) as converted to the new coordinates (x_n, z) for $n = 1.5$ and 2. The derivatives, z, is evaluated by a central difference scheme, i.e.

$$x_{n,i} = \frac{\left(C_{A0} - \frac{1}{2}C_{C,i}\right)^n - \left(\frac{13}{29}C_{C,i}\right)^n + \left(C_{A0} - \frac{1}{2}C_{C,i+1}\right)^n - \left(\frac{13}{29}C_{C,i+1}\right)^n}{2} \tag{7.55}$$

and

$$z_i = \frac{C_{C,i+1} - C_{C,i}}{t_{i+1} - t_i} \tag{7.56}$$

where i is the index for the data points, in incremental time.

Figure 7.8 shows the correlation on the (x_n, z) plane. The correlation for $n = 1.5$ is shown in Fig. 7.8a, whereas the correlation using $n = 2$ is shown in Fig. 7.8b. The best-fit lines are given by

$$z = 0.003024x_{1.5} \tag{7.57}$$

and

$$z = 0.001344x_2 \tag{7.58}$$

The corresponding correlation coefficients are given by 0.9165 and 0.9124, respectively.

TABLE 7.5 Transformed Data from Table 7.3 Based on the Differential Method

C_C, mol/L	$x_{1.5}=\left(C_{A0}-\frac{1}{2}C_C\right)^{1.5}-\left(\frac{13}{29}C_C\right)^{1.5}$	$x_2=\left(C_{A0}-\frac{1}{2}C_C\right)^2-\left(\frac{13}{29}C_C\right)^2$	$z=\frac{dC_C}{dt}$
0.59	11.74	27.02	0.02878
1.28	10.28	23.29	0.02857
1.505	9.79	22.08	0.03571
1.935	8.84	19.79	0.03050
2.495	7.59	16.83	0.02429
3.03	6.38	14.04	0.01807
3.535	5.22	11.42	0.02368
3.785	4.64	10.14	0.003125
3.96	4.239	9.24	0.01667
4.21	3.663	7.96	0.01429
4.38	3.271	7.10	0.007778
4.655	2.636	5.71	0.007455
5.005	1.829	3.95	0.005686
5.235	1.299	2.802	0.00340
5.335	1.069	2.304	0.002727
5.385	0.954	2.055	0.002258

The correlation as shown in Fig. 7.8 is not strongly supportive of the straight line (either in Fig. 7.8a or Fig. 7.8b). The data points might have been suggesting that a curve should have been drawn rather than a straight line. Nevertheless, others may be content with the regression as the correlation coefficient is at 0.91. Let us take the value of $n=2$, then the kinetic parameters determined from the differential method are given by $n=2$ and $k_f=0.001344$.

7.8.3. Which Methods to Use: Differential or Integral?

Traditionally, kinetic parameters have been determined through linear regression. One can observe the physical simplicity a straight-line plot, such as Fig. 7.7 or Fig. 7.8, implied. In some cases, the regression model is not easily rearranged into a linear form, nonlinear regression has been used as well. However, the two methods are still held as the only means of obtaining the kinetic parameters: integral method and differential method. Here an integral method refers to any procedure of regression that involves converting a differential model to an algebraic model through analytic integration. In other words, the differential equation is solved analytically before regression. On the other hand, a differential method refers to any

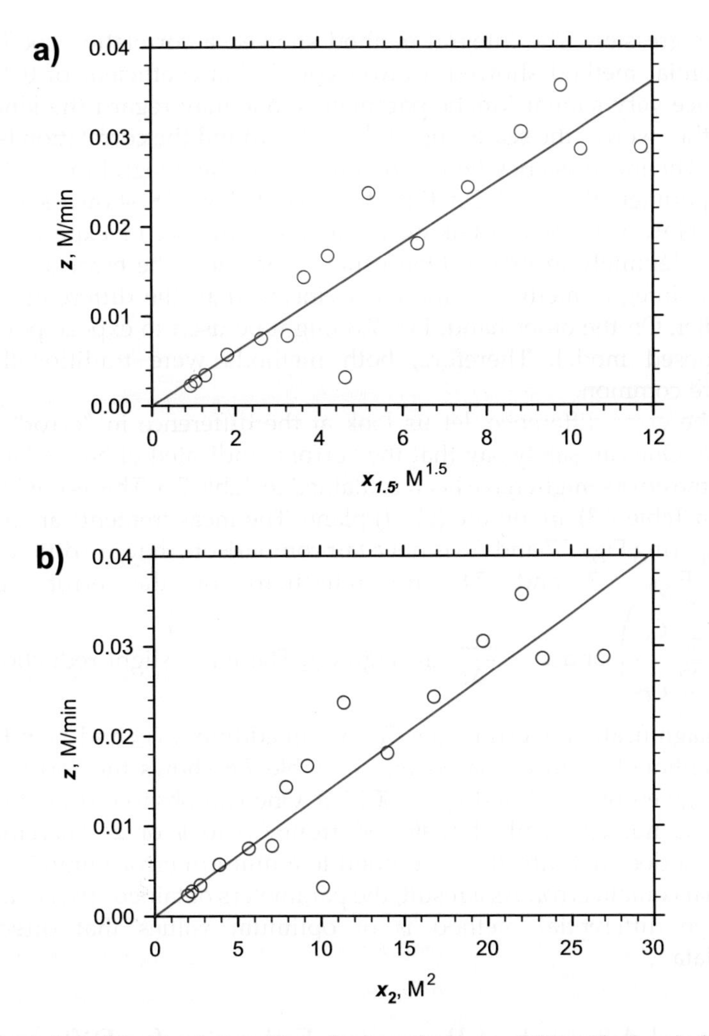

FIGURE 7.8 Correlation of the kinetic data (a) on the ($x_{1.5}$, z) plane and (b) on the (x_2, z) plane.

procedure that involves numerically differentiating the (experimental) data to obtain the derivative or derivatives in the differential model. In so doing, one can rename the derivative to a new variable. Thus, there are no derivatives to deal with directly at regression.

For the same kinetic data, sections Integral Methods and Differential Methods showed different correlations. When the same kinetic equation is imposed:

$$\frac{dC_C}{dt} = k_f\left(C_{A0} - \frac{1}{2}C_C\right)^2 - k_f\left(\frac{13}{29}C_C\right)^2 \tag{7.59}$$

One can infer that slightly different values of k_f are obtained. While one can argue that the difference in the values of k_f is small, there is a marked difference in the perception of the quality of the regression. The integral method showed a correlation coefficient of 0.9991 and the differential method showed a lower correlation coefficient of 0.9124. Since both methods produce very similar kinetic parameters, one may regard the kinetic parameters as correct. In other words, the scattering of the data around the correlation is due to "experimental error." The inconsistency here is that based on the integral method, Fig. 7.7 shows very little "experimental error." On the other hand, Fig. 7.8 shows significant "experimental error." However, we are talking about the same set of experimental data. This "conclusion" is definitely incorrect. One usually considers the error as correlation error. In this case, the integral method is more convincing than the differential method as the "error" is smaller. On the other hand, Fig. 7.8 might be used to expose potential problems with the proposed model. Therefore, both methods were traditionally used before computers were common.

To resolve the error difference, let us look at the difference in "error" represented by Figs 7.7 and 7.8. One can safely say that the "errors" indicated either in Fig. 7.7 or Fig. 7.8 directly reflect the errors might have been contained in Table 7.3. This is obvious as the experimental data (in Table 7.3) are on the (C_C, t) plane. The measurements are in C_C, not y or z. Therefore, comparing Figs 7.7 and 7.8 is not a fair comparison: they are different. The "errors" indicated in Figs 7.7 and 7.8 are reflections of the errors propagated to $y = \ln\left(\dfrac{C_{A0} - \frac{3}{58}C_C}{C_{A0} - \frac{55}{58}C_C}\right)$ and $z = \dfrac{\Delta C_C}{\Delta t}$ through C_C. There is a slight reduction of error from C_C to y, but a magnification of error from C_C to z. In addition, $x_{1.5}$ and x_2 in Fig. 7.8 contains error as well, although reduced based on C_C. Table 7.6 shows the "errors" if the kinetic parameters are given by $n = 2$ and $k_f = 0.001340$. One can observe from Table 7.6 that the error structure is not uniformly transferred from C_C to y or z. Therefore, minimizing the error in y or z does not directly correspond to a uniform error minimization for C_C, the original data that contain error. As a result, the parameters obtained from neither the integral method nor the differential method is of optimum values that directly reflect the experimental data.

7.8.4. A General Approach of Parametric Estimation for Differential Models

One can conclude from the previous discussions that since the experimental data is given as a time series in C_C, we will need to minimize the variance of the experimental data C_C around the regression model predictions. To this end, the integral method (Integral Methods) may be redesigned to achieve this task by not looking for a linear regression model, but explicit in the dependent variable. However, the regression model is, in general, a nonlinear differential equation of C_C with respect to time t. Therefore, we will need to solve the regression model numerically for C_C.

A viable approach is to use a general differential equation solver (or integrator) to compute the value of C_C for a given time series and then minimize the variance associated with predicted and experimental values of C_C. There are many integrators available both commercially and on the web (for example, adaptive Runge–Kutta methods based and extrapolation methods based integrators of particular utility). We shall introduce one that

TABLE 7.6 "Errors" of the Data and Various Transformations in Figs 7.7 and 7.8

t_i	$C_{C,i}$	C_C	ε_C	y_i	ε_y	Fig. 7.8						
0	0	0	0	0	0	t_i	$x_{2,i}$	x_2	ε_{x_2}	z_i	Z	ε_z
41	1.18	1.436068	**−0.256***	0.2163	**−0.0546**	20.5	27.02	26.0362	**0.99**	0.02878	0.034885	**−0.00610**
48	1.38	1.641458	**−0.261**	0.2587	**−0.0585**	44.5	23.29	21.8960	**1.39**	0.02857	0.029338	**−0.00077**
55	1.63	1.836816	**−0.207**	0.3145	**−0.0489**	51.5	22.08	20.8266	**1.26**	0.03571	0.027905	**0.00781**
75	2.24	2.344248	**−0.104**	0.4668	**−0.0287**	65.0	19.79	18.9188	**0.87**	0.03050	0.025349	**0.00515**
96	2.75	2.805283	**−0.055**	0.6165	**−0.0178**	85.5	16.83	16.3693	**0.46**	0.02429	0.021933	**0.00235**
127	3.31	3.373303	**−0.063**	0.8140	**−0.0251**	111.5	14.04	13.6474	**0.39**	0.01807	0.018286	**−0.00022**
146	3.76	3.665667	**0.094**	1.009	**0.0443**	136.5	11.42	11.4757	**−0.06**	0.02368	0.015376	**0.00831**
162	3.81	3.883856	**−0.074**	1.033	**−0.0371**	154.0	10.14	10.1723	**−0.04**	0.00313	0.013630	**−0.01050**
180	4.11	4.102335	**0.008**	1.194	**0.0045**	171.0	9.239	9.05287	**0.19**	0.01667	0.012130	**0.00454**
194	4.31	4.254627	**0.055**	1.318	**0.0359**	187.0	7.964	8.11548	**−0.15**	0.01429	0.010874	**0.00341**
212	4.45	4.430265	**0.020**	1.415	**0.0143**	203.0	7.101	7.27782	**−0.18**	0.00778	0.009751	**−0.00197**
267	4.86	4.851535	**0.008**	1.773	**0.0089**	239.5	5.710	5.68303	**0.03**	0.00746	0.007615	**−0.00016**
318	5.15	5.124676	**0.025**	2.139	**0.0380**	292.5	3.951	3.97739	**−0.03**	0.00569	0.005329	**0.00036**
368	5.32	5.315579	**0.004**	2.441	**0.0091**	343.0	2.802	2.83619	**−0.04**	0.00340	0.003800	**−0.00040**
379	5.35	5.349688	**0.000**	2.505	**0.0007**	373.5	2.304	2.31376	**−0.01**	0.00273	0.003100	**−0.00037**
410	5.42	5.433392	**−0.014**	2.673	-0.0357	394.5	2.055	2.01158	**0.04**	0.00226	0.002695	**−0.00044**

* *The bold numbers are errors (of model compared with the data).*

is based on extrapolation and the symmetric two-step midpoint method with stiffness removal, the GBS approach (Hairer et al. 1987).

The easiest way is to perform the regression analysis on a spreadsheet such as Excel® and Quattro Pro®. As these spreadsheet programs have built-in optimization routines, allow the interface of user-defined visual basic routines and have the graphical capabilities to bring the regression analysis visually at every step of the way. We will show the use of the Excel® to solve the same kinetic parametric estimation problem dealt in the previous sections. We have developed a general-purpose visual basic routine for solving a set of ordinary differential equations named ODExLIMS to be served as an integrator to the differential regression model (interested reader can e-mail sliu@esf.edu for a copy of the visual basic routine).

Figure 7.9 shows the setup of the problem initially on an Excel® worksheet. We first load the ODExLIMS.xls on to Excel®. Delete the contents on the worksheet. We input the measured data, time, initial guess of k_f and n; input the formulas for calculating the residual squared and the variance of the experimental data around the model predictions, and saved the file as kinetic.xls. We also generate a graph of C_C versus t with the experimental data shown as circles and the predictions as a continuous line. Presently, we have not computed

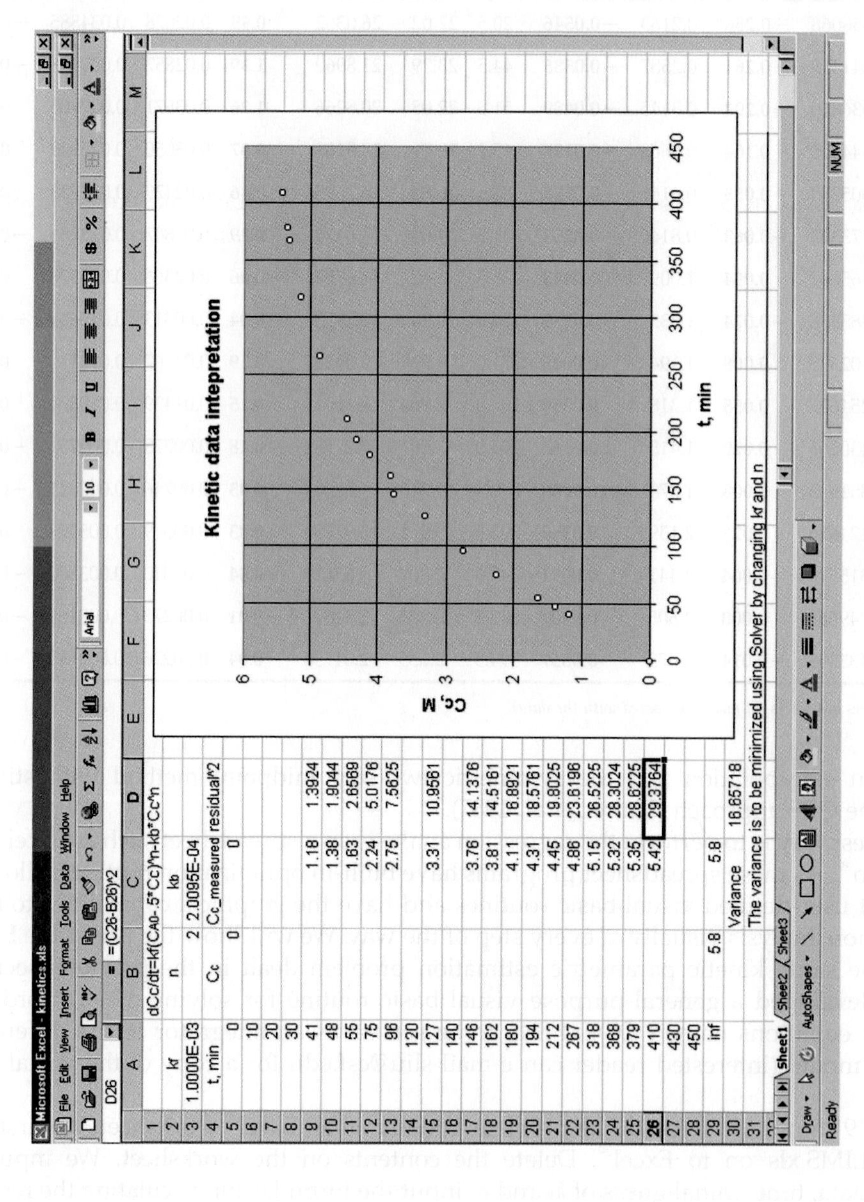

FIGURE 7.9 Setting up the Excel® worksheet to perform the regression analysis.

any predicted values of C_C yet and that column is empty. To ensure the prediction shown as a smooth line, we added a few point in the time series. After setting up the worksheet, we then open the visual basic editor to change the differential equation (*Sub FUNC* of the ODExLIMS program) to our differential regression model: Eqn (7.33). There is only one single differential equation. Let y(1) denotes C_C, x denotes t, c(1) denotes k_f, c(2) denotes n, and c(3) denotes k_b. In our case, k_b is directly related to k_f and n through Eqn (7.34). Figure 7.10 shows the differential equation in the visual basic module. Therefore, only two parameters can be varied: k_f and n, corresponding to c(1) and c(2).

After the regression model has been entered to the visual basic routine, we then go back to the Excel® worksheet. As solution of an ordinary differential equation requires an initial condition, enter the zero for time $t = 0$ for the prediction column (column 2). Select the rest of the cells in column 2 for the times we need solutions for C_C and press the function button (f_x) to bring up the function dialog. Select *ODExLIMS* from *user-defined* category. Then the dialog box shows up for the integrator. Figure 7.11 shows the dialog of the ODExLIMS program. After filling the required items, hold on the *cntrl* and the *Shift* keys while press the *Enter* keys at the same time, you will immediately notice a line showing up on the chart generated and the numbers in the prediction column are filled.

Now we are ready to perform the regression analysis. As there is an optimization routine in Excel®, we can use the Solver® to minimize the variance by changing the two "free parameters": k_f and n. The solver can be located from the *Tools* button on the worksheet menu. When you choose Solver®, a dialog (Fig. 7.12) will show up. After filling the required items, we press *Solve* button on the solver dialog to see the numbers in the prediction column and graph change. If the numbers become # signs, adjust the initial guesses for k_f and n and retry the Solver® program. When the parameters are out of range, either the solution overflows or become nonexistent. This can be avoided by a better initial guess. One can also restrict k_f such that it will not go to a negative number as we know that the forward reaction can only proceed forward. By setting up constraints, one can make sure that the solution makes sense physically and also makes the optimization routine narrowing the searching range so that the solution is easier to find. Figure 7.12 shows the Solver® dialog. We want to minimize the variance, setting the target cell as *D30*, where we entered the formula to calculate the variance. Choose *Equal to* Min and By Changing Cells: *A3:B3*, where the initial guess of k_f and n are entered.

Figure 7.13 shows the solution obtained by minimizing the variance of the data C_C around the regression model with Solver® by changing k_f and n. The minimum variance is obtained as $\sigma^2 = 0.01109$, with $k_f = 3.657 \times 10^{-3}$ $(\text{mol/L})^{-0.373}$ s^{-1}, $n = 1.373$, and $k_b = 1.215 \times 10^{-3}$ $(\text{mol/L})^{-0.373}$ s^{-1}. For someone who is only interested in representing the data, it is satisfactory to accept the solution by now. Further checking at the quality of the solution obtained is necessary now to ensure that our effort is not wasted.

The quality of the regression analysis can be judged by examining the correlation coefficient and by examining the visual appearance of the model prediction in relation to the data. Therefore, it is very important to plot the solutions while the regression analysis is being performed. One can interfere if the regression model misses the general trend of the experimental data. One can compute the correlation coefficient R for the solution obtained.

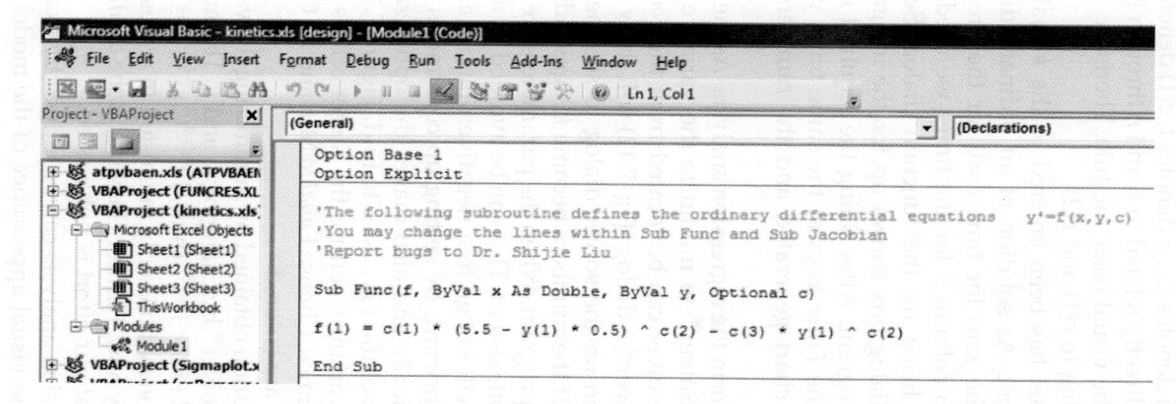

FIGURE 7.10 Differential equation, Eqn (7.33), in visual basic code in ODExLIMS routine.

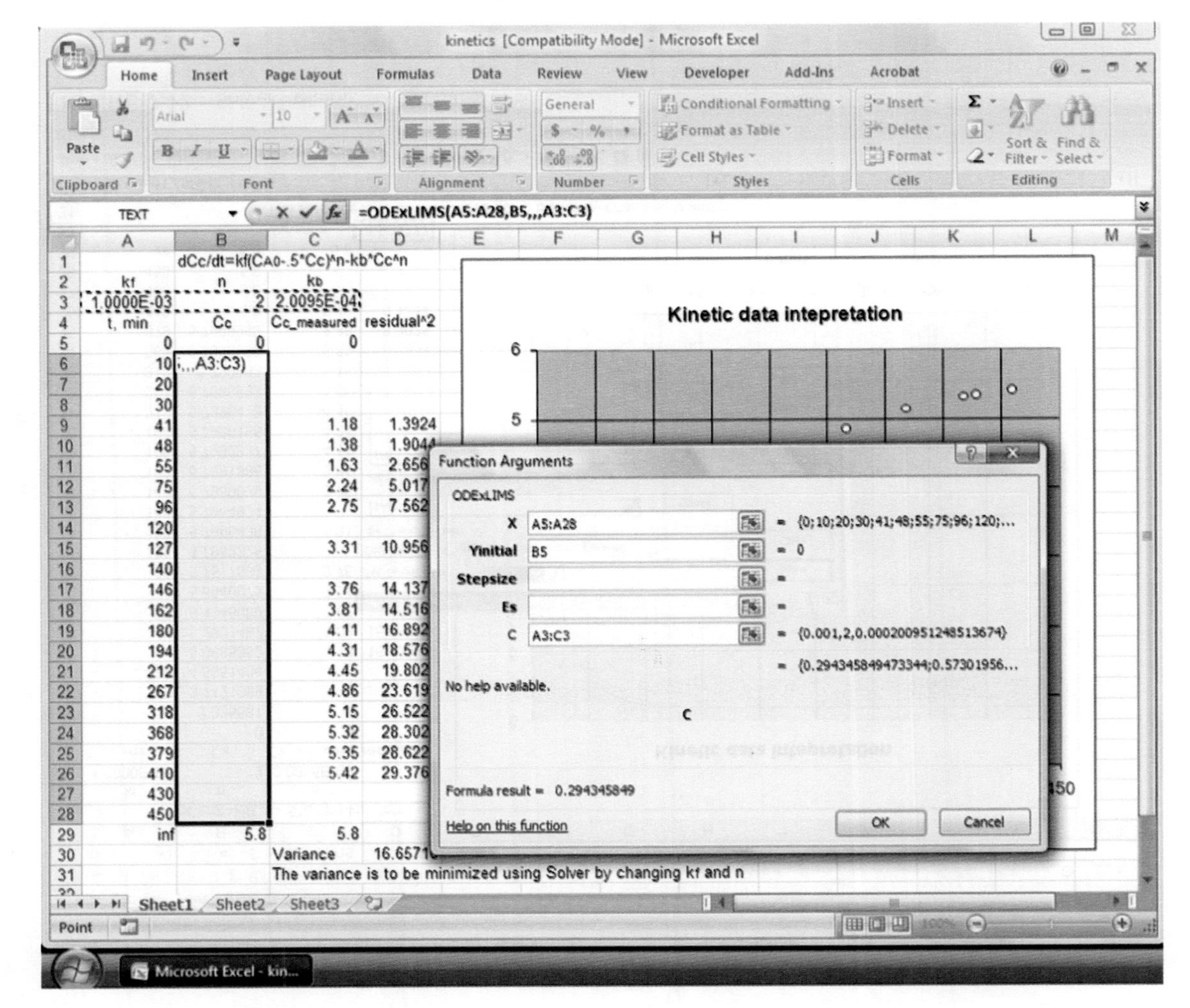

FIGURE 7.11 Dialog for the ODExLIMS routine.

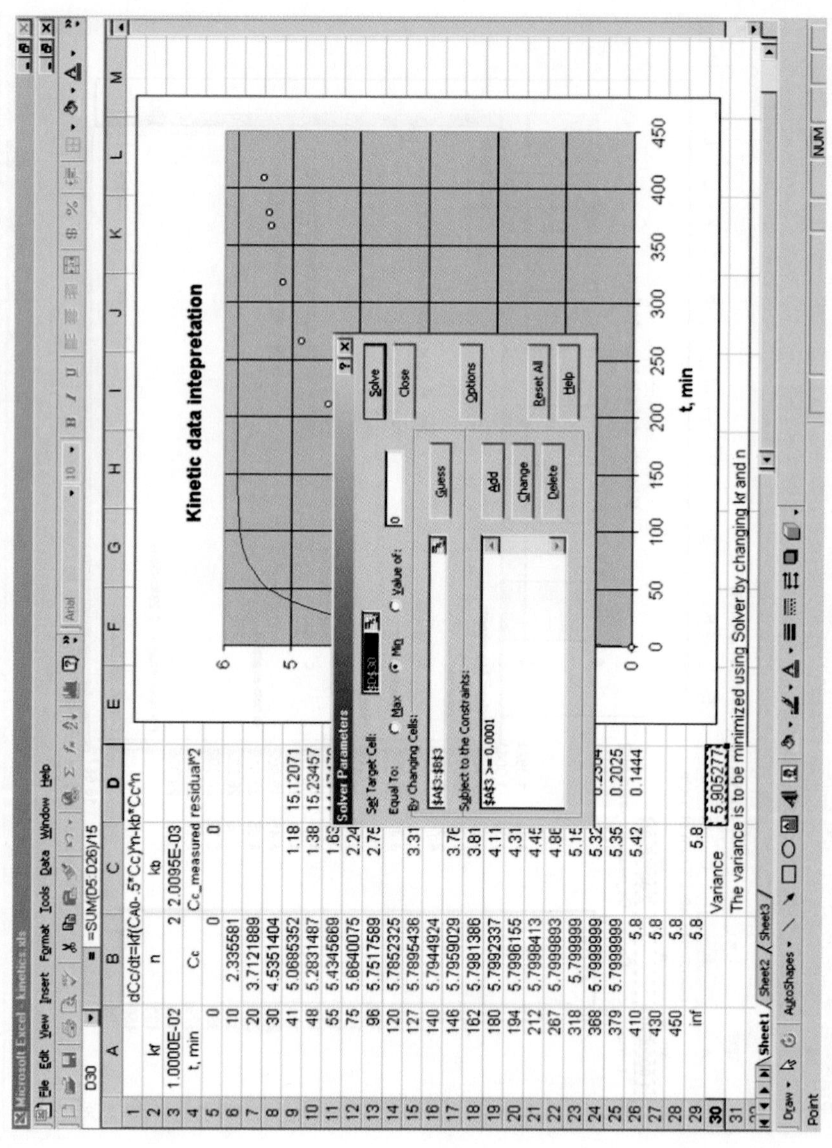

FIGURE 7.12 Solver® dialog.

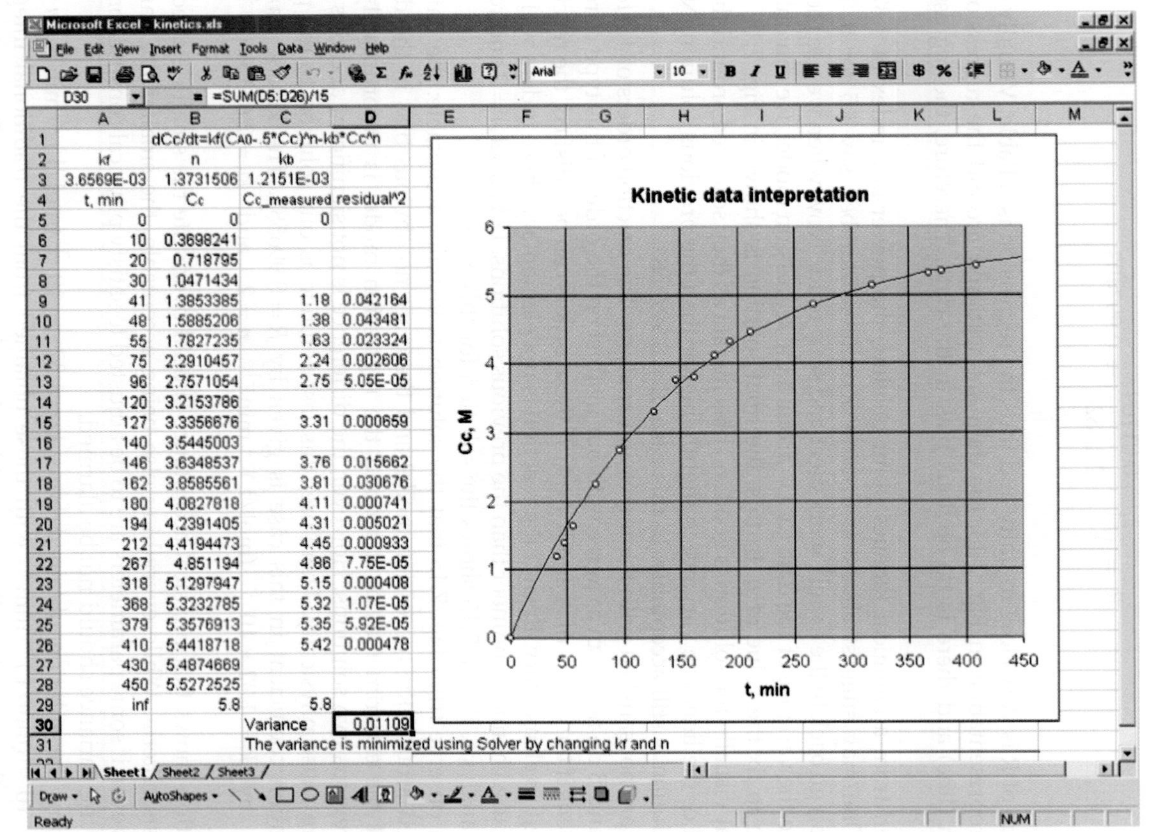

	A	B	C	D
1		dCc/dt=kf(CA0-.5*Cc)^n-kb*Cc^n		
2	kf	n	kb	
3	3.6569E-03	1.3731506	1.2151E-03	
4	t, min	Cc	Cc_measured	residual^2
5	0	0	0	
6	10	0.3698241		
7	20	0.718795		
8	30	1.0471434		
9	41	1.3853385	1.18	0.042164
10	48	1.5885206	1.38	0.043481
11	55	1.7827235	1.63	0.023324
12	75	2.2910457	2.24	0.002606
13	96	2.7571054	2.75	5.05E-05
14	120	3.2153786		
15	127	3.3356676	3.31	0.000659
16	140	3.5445003		
17	146	3.6348537	3.76	0.015662
18	162	3.8585561	3.81	0.030676
19	180	4.0827818	4.11	0.000741
20	194	4.2391405	4.31	0.005021
21	212	4.4194473	4.45	0.000933
22	267	4.851194	4.86	7.75E-05
23	318	5.1297947	5.15	0.000408
24	368	5.3232785	5.32	1.07E-05
25	379	5.3576913	5.35	5.92E-05
26	410	5.4418718	5.42	0.000478
27	430	5.4874669		
28	450	5.5272525		
29	inf	5.8	5.8	
30			Variance	0.01109
31			The variance is minimized using Solver by changing kf and n	

FIGURE 7.13 Solution of the kinetic parametric estimation problem by varying k_f and n in the Excel® environment.

$$\sum_{i=1}^{16} C_{Ci} = 59.03 \quad \sum_{i=1}^{16} C_{Ci}^2 = 249.8577 \quad \frac{\sum_{i=1}^{16} C_{Ci}^2 - \frac{1}{16}\sum_{i=1}^{16} C_{Ci}}{16-1} = 2.13826$$

$$R = \sqrt{1 - \frac{0.01109}{2.13826}} = 0.997403$$

The value of R is very close to unity and thus the regression is reliable. Visually from the graphical representation in Fig. 7.13, the data are scattered around the regression model predication (line) and there is no obvious bias in the data. Therefore, the regression is a success.

However, from a chemical kinetics point of view, the power-law index of 1.373 is not pleasing. One may suggest choosing a more acceptable number, say 1.5 for n. If this is done, we can go back to the Excel® worksheet and set n to 1.5. Now when we use the Solver® to minimize the variance of the data for C_C around the regression model, we can only vary k_f as we wish to fix the value of n. In this, the final solution is shown in Fig. 7.14. One can observe that visually the solution is good: no bias in data as they scattered around the regression model or the line. The variance is slightly higher than the previous solution. Nevertheless, the solution is still acceptable. In this case, $R = 0.997368$.

Still, we are not satisfied with the regression analysis. The reaction orders of 1.5 for C and 0.75 for A and B do not seem to agree with our instinct on the order of this type of reactions. What happens if the orders of A and B are 1? If these orders can be satisfied, the reaction may be explained as elementary. Even if the reaction is not elementary, these orders will be more convincing to a chemical engineer than the previous solutions. Let us set $n = 2$ and repeat the regression analysis. Figure 7.15 shows the solution for this case.

One can observe from Fig. 7.15 that the solution is visually acceptable: the data points are scattered around the regression model and there are no obvious bias in the data. The variance of the experimental data around the regression model is unfortunately higher than the previous two solutions. However, the difference is not significant and this solution makes more sense physically. Therefore, this last solution is our solution to the problem. The correlation coefficient in this case is given by $R = 0.996588$. The kinetic parameters are given by $k_f = 1.32 \times 10^{-3}$ $(\text{mol/L})^{-1}\,\text{min}^{-1}$, $n = 2$, and $k_b = 2.653 \times 10^{-4}$ $(\text{mol/L})^{-1}\,\text{min}^{-1}$.

This section shows that physical acceptance should overwrite the small detailed regression analysis criteria. While everything else being acceptable, the smaller the variance is better. However, if some parameters are to be adjusted to satisfy physical constrictions, slight increase in the variance should not be alarmed.

Comparing the solution obtained here: $k_f = 1.32 \times 10^{-3}$ $(\text{mol/L})^{-1}\,\text{min}^{-1}$, $n = 2$ and $k_b = 2.653 \times 10^{-4}$ $(\text{mol/L})^{-1}\,\text{min}^{-1}$ with those obtained from the traditional integral and differential methods, sections Regression Models and Classification of Regression Models, we notice a slight difference in k_f. As the error being minimized is the experimental data compared with the model prediction in this general approach, we can trust the solution obtained here. In terms of complexity in solution, the general approach requires more

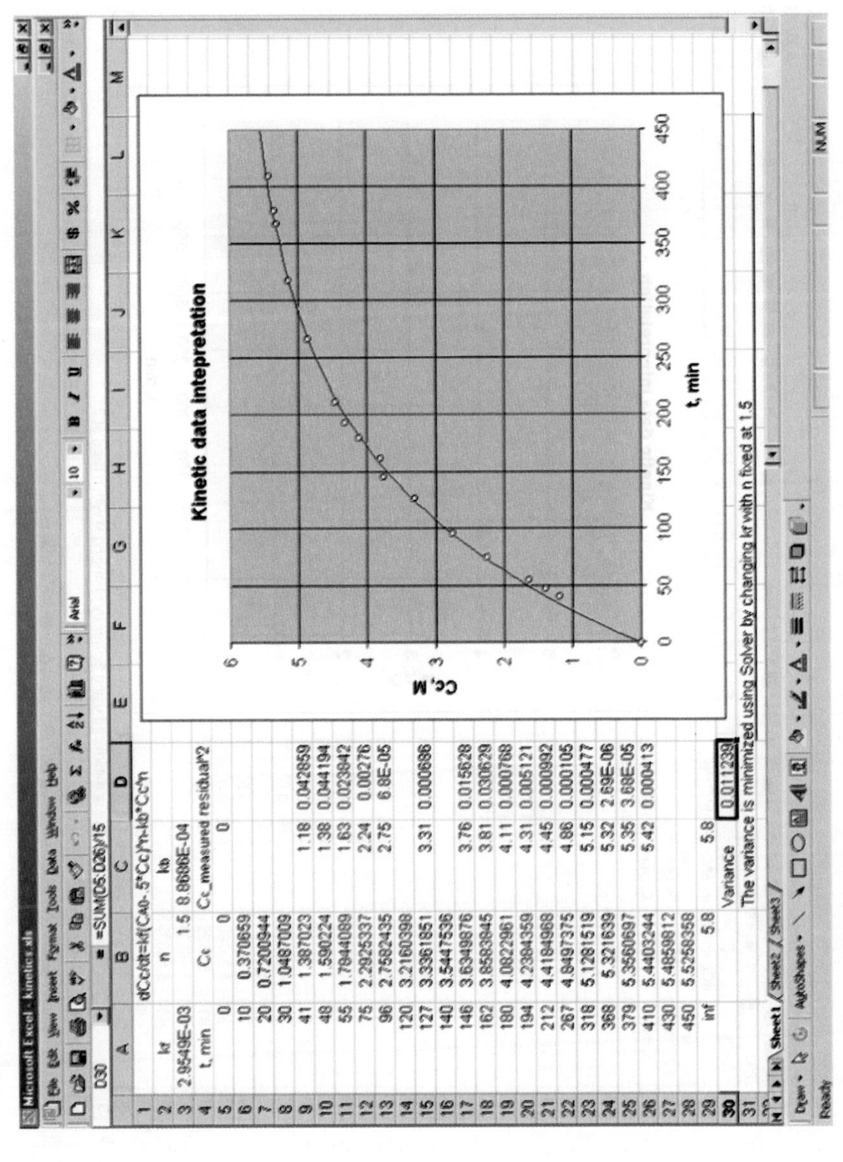

FIGURE 7.14 Minimizing the variance by setting $n = 1.5$ and varying k_f.

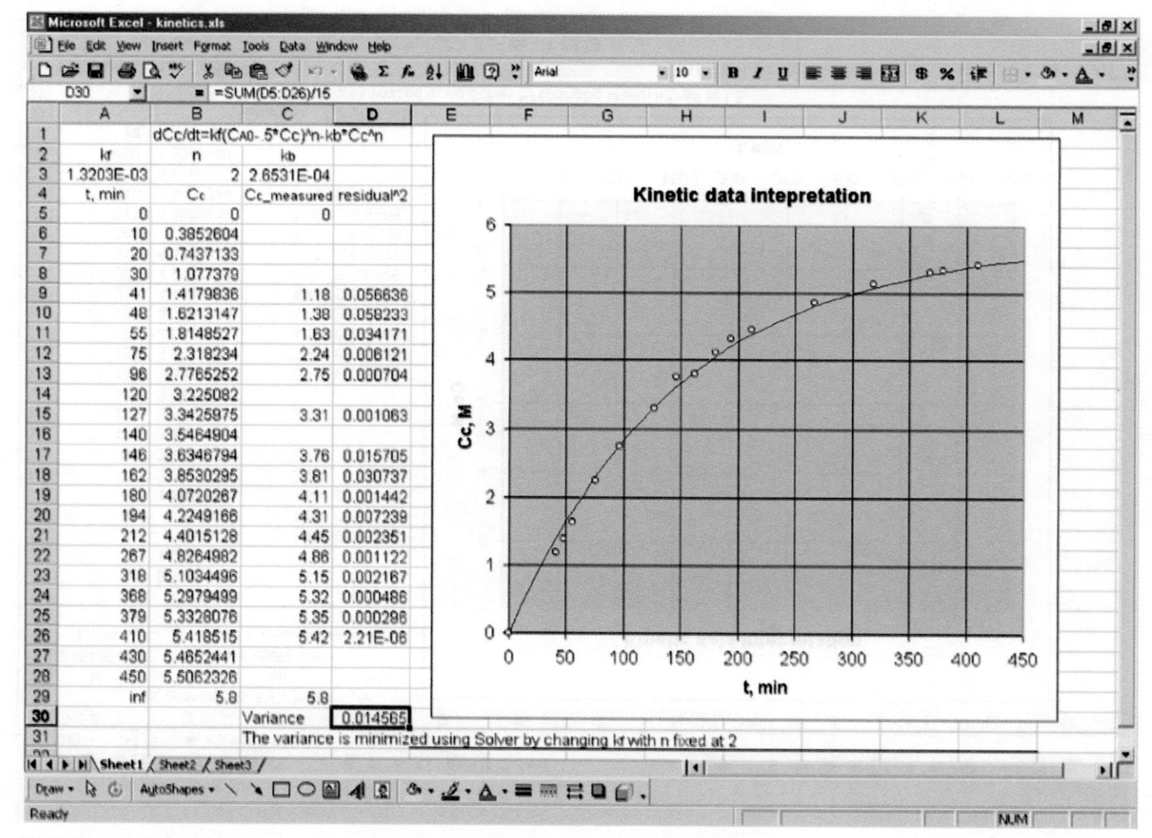

	A	B	C	D
1		dCc/dt=kf(CA0-.5*Cc)^n-kb*Cc^n		
2	kf	n	kb	
3	1.3203E-03	2	2.6531E-04	
4	t, min	Cc	Cc_measured	residual^2
5	0	0	0	
6	10	0.3852604		
7	20	0.7437133		
8	30	1.077379		
9	41	1.4179836	1.18	0.056636
10	48	1.6213147	1.38	0.058233
11	55	1.8148527	1.63	0.034171
12	75	2.318234	2.24	0.006121
13	96	2.7765252	2.75	0.000704
14	120	3.225082		
15	127	3.3425975	3.31	0.001063
16	140	3.5464904		
17	146	3.6346794	3.76	0.015705
18	162	3.8530295	3.81	0.030737
19	180	4.0720267	4.11	0.001442
20	194	4.2249166	4.31	0.007239
21	212	4.4015128	4.45	0.002351
22	267	4.8264982	4.86	0.001122
23	318	5.1034496	5.15	0.002167
24	368	5.2979499	5.32	0.000486
25	379	5.3328076	5.35	0.000296
26	410	5.418515	5.42	2.21E-06
27	430	5.4652441		
28	450	5.5062326		
29	inf	5.8	5.8	
30			Variance	0.014565
31			The variance is minimized using Solver by changing kf with n fixed at 2	

FIGURE 7.15 Minimizing the variance by setting $n = 2$ and varying k_f.

effort if one need to write the integrator routine as well. However, if one takes the integrator routine developed here in this paper, the general approach becomes easier to apply than the traditional integral and differential methods.

7.9. SUMMARY

In this chapter, the basic regression approaches have been discussed. Regression model is a mathematical equation intended to be applied to describe a given set of experimental or observed data. To perform parametric analysis, one must first understand the error and error structure of the data. One should not cater to a linear regression model just because straight lines are easy to deal with and visually pleasing. More fundamental regression models do however bring complexity into the parametric estimation. In particular, one common type of regression mode: differential regression model is discussed in detail and an example has used for further discussions. In the Physical Chemistry and Reaction Engineering literature, the integral methods and the differential methods have been standardized for solving the differential regression model problems. Irrespective of the error structure in data, it had been a common practice to transform the regression models into linear ones. The integral method is marked by its trial-and-error nature and the differential method generally shows higher degrees of uncertainty. Discussions with these two frequently used methods especially for computer illiterates are made with the real batch kinetic estimation problem. The basis for not trusting the kinetic parameters obtained using these two methods is the ignorance of the error structure of data during regression. To this end, a viable approach to parametric estimation for the differential regression model problem is preferred. However, one does need to use computer to carry out the analysis. The viable method is combining a general numerical integrator such as ODExLIMS and the utilization of the solver program in Excel®. As such, the trial-and-error nature and the tedious calculations of the traditional (precomputer age) methods can be eliminated. Above all, the parameters estimated directly reflect the quality of the data series and thus can be trusted over those obtained from the traditional methods.

Further Reading

Adamson, A.W., 1986. *A Textbook of Physical Chemistry* (3rd ed.). Orlando: Academic Press College Division.

Alberty, R.A., Silbery, R.J., 1992. *Physical Chemistry.* Wiley: New York, NY. p. 635.

Butt, J.B., 1999. *Reaction Kinetics and Reactor Design* (2nd ed.). New York: Marcel Dekker, Inc.

Chapra, S.C., Canale, R.P., 1998. *Numerical Methods for Engineers* (3rd ed.). Toronto: McGraw-Hill.

Fogler, H.S., 1999. *Elements of Chemical Reaction Engineering* (3rd ed.). Upper Saddle River, New Jersey: Prentice Hall.

Hairer, E., Nørsett, S.P., Wanner, G. 1987. *Solving Ordinary Differential Equations: 2 Stiff and Differential-algebraic Problems.* New York: Springer-Verlag.

Hellin, M., Jungers, J.C., 1957. *Bull. Soc. Chim. France*, 386.

Hinshelwood, C.N., Hutchison, W.K., 1926. A Comparison between Unimolecular and Bimolecular Gaseous Reactions. The Thermal Decomposition of Gaseous Acetaldehyde. *Proc. R. Soc. Lond. A*, 111: 380–385.

Kremenic, G., Nieto, J.M.L., Weller, S.W., Tascon, J.M.D., Tejuca, L.G. 1987. Selective oxidation of propene on a molybdenum-prasedodymium-bismuth catalyst. *Ind. Eng. Chem. Res.*, **26**(7), 1419–1424.

Levenspiel, O., 1999. *Chemical Reaction Engineering* (3rd ed.). Toronto: John Wiley & Sons.

Rodriguez, Tijero. 1989. *Can. J. Chem. Eng.*, **67**(6), 963–968.

PROBLEMS

7.1. At 518 °C, acetaldehyde vapor decomposes into methane and carbon monoxide according to $CH_3CHO \rightarrow CH_4 + CO$. In a particular experiment carried out in a constant-volume BR (Hinshelwood and Hutchison, 1926), the initial pressure of acetaldehyde was 48.4 kPa, and the following increases of pressure (ΔP) were noted (in part) with increasing time:

t, s	42	105	242	480	840	1440
ΔP, kPa	4.5	9.9	17.9	25.9	32.5	37.9

From these results, determine the order of reaction and calculate the value of the rate constant in pressure units (kPa) and in concentration units (mol L^{-1}).

7.2. Rate constants for the first-order decomposition of nitrogen pentoxide (N_2O_5) at various temperatures are as follows (Alberty and Silbey, 1992, p. 635):

T, K	273	298	308	318	328	338
k, 10^{-5} s^{-1}	0.0787	3.46	13.5	49.8	150	487

Show that the data obey the Arrhenius relationship and determine the values of the Arrhenius parameters.

7.3. The oxidation of propene to acrolein was carried out over a Mo-Pr-Bi Catalyst [*Ind. Eng. Chem. Res.*, 26, 1419(1987)].

$$CH_3CH = CH_2 + O_2 \rightarrow CH_2 = CHCHO + H_2O$$

It has been proposed to correlate the data using the power-law model for the rate law.

$$r_{\text{acrolein}} = k\, p_P^{\alpha}\, p_{O_2}^{\beta}$$

The reaction was carried out in a differential reactor with 0.5 g catalyst at 623 K. From the data below, determine the reaction orders with respect to propene and oxygen and the specific reaction rate.

F_A, mmol/h	0.21	0.48	0.09	0.39	0.60	0.14	1.44
p_P, atm	0.1	0.2	0.05	0.3	0.4	0.05	0.5
p_{O_2}, atm	0.1	0.2	0.05	0.01	0.02	0.4	0.5

where F_A = exiting molar flow rate of acrolein, p_P = entering partial pressure of propene, and p_{O_2} = entering partial pressure of oxygen.

7.4. Brown and Stock (H.C. Brown and L.M. Stock, *J. Am. Chem. Soc.*, 79, 5175, 1957) reported some data on the chlorination of toluene in 99.8% acetic acid at 25 °C:

Time, s	Toluene, mol/L	Chlorine, mol/L
0	0.1908	0.0313
2790	0.1833	0.0238
7690	0.1745	0.0150
9690	0.1719	0.0123
14,000	0.1682	0.0086
19,100	0.1650	0.0055

Determine a reasonable kinetic sequence (reaction pathways) to explain these data and the values of the appropriate rate constants.

7.5. In pulp and paper processing, anthraquinone (AQ) accelerates the delignification of wood and improves liquor selectivity. The kinetics of the liquid-phase oxidation of anthracene (AN) to AQ with NO_2 in acetic acid as solvent has been studied by Rodriguez and Tijero (1989) in a semibatch reactor (batch with respect to the liquid phase), under conditions such that the kinetics of the overall gas–liquid process is controlled by the rate of the liquid-phase reaction. This reaction proceeds through the formation of the intermediate compound anthrone (ANT):

$$C_{14}H_{10}(AN) \xrightarrow[k_1]{NO_2} C_{14}H_9O(ANT) \xrightarrow[k_2]{NO_2} C_{14}H_8O_2(AQ)$$

The following results (as read from a graph) were obtained for an experiment at 95 °C, in which $C_{AN,0} = 0.0337$ mol L^{-1}:

t, min	C_{AN} (mol L^{-1})	C_{ANT} (mol L^{-1})	C_{AQ} (mol L^{-1})
0	0.0337	0	0
10	0.0229	0.0104	0.0008
20	0.0144	0.0157	0.0039
30	0.0092	0.0181	0.0066
40	0.0058	0.0169	0.0114
50	0.0040	0.0155	0.0144
60	0.0030	0.0130	0.0178
70	0.0015	0.0114	0.0209
80	0.0008	0.0088	0.0240
90	0.0006	0.0060	0.0270

Determine the orders of reactions and the values of the rate constants k_1 and k_2.

7.6. A wastewater stream is treated biologically with a reactor containing immobilized cells in porous particles. Table P7.6 shows the rate data obtained for a particular particle size when the external mass transfer effects are negligible. Internal mass transfer effects are known to be present. Determine if Michaelis–Menten equation, i.e.

$$r = \frac{r_{\mathrm{max}} S}{K_{\mathrm{m}} + S}$$

even mass transfer effects are not negligible. Determine the apparent kinetic parameters.

S_0, g/L	0.00	0.10	0.25	0.50	1.00	2.00
r, g/(L·h)	0.000	0.085	0.200	0.360	0.630	1.000

7.7. An understanding of bacteria transport in porous media is vital to the efficient operation of the water flooding of petroleum reservoirs. Bacteria can have both beneficial and harmful effects on the performance of the reservoir. In enhanced microbial oil recovery, EMOR, bacteria are injected to secrete surfactants to reduce the interfacial tension at the oil–water interface so that the oil will flow out more easily. However, under some circumstances the bacteria can be harmful, by plugging the pore space (due to excessive growth and wall attachment) and thereby block the flow of water and oil. One bacteria that has been studied, *Leuconostoc mesenteroides*, has the unusual behavior that when it is injected into a porous medium and fed sucrose, it greatly reduces the flow (i.e. damages the formation and reduces permeability). When the bacteria are fed fructose or glucose, there is no damage to the porous medium (Lappan R. and Fogler H.S. *SPE Prod. Eng.*, 7: 167–171, 1992). The cell concentration, X, is given in Table P8.13 as a function of time for different initial sucrose concentrations.

(a) From Table P7.7, determine the time to reach the stationary phase, the saturation constant, K_S, and the maximum specific growth rate, μ_{max}. $r = \mu_G X$ and $\mu_G = \frac{\mu_{\mathrm{max}} S}{K_S + S}$.

S is the substrate concentration, while X is the cell concentration.

(b) Will an inhibition model of the form

$$\mu_G = \mu_{\mathrm{max}} \left(1 - \frac{X - X_0}{X_\infty}\right)^n$$

where n and X_∞ are parameters, fit the data?

7.8. Yogurt is produced by a mixed culture of *Lactobacillus bulgaricus* and *Streptococcus thermophilus* to pasteurize milk. At a temperature of 110 °F, the bacteria grow and produce lactic acid. The acid contributes flavor and causes the proteins to coagulate, giving the characteristic properties of yogurt. When sufficient acid has been produced (about 0.90%), the yogurt is cooled and stored until eaten by consumers. A lactic acid level of 1.10% is the limit of acceptability. One limit on the shelf life of yogurt is "postacidification" or continued production of acid by the yogurt cultures during

TABLE P7.7 Cell Concentration, 10^{10} cells/L, as Functions of Time and Sucrose Concentration

	Sucrose			
Time, h	**10 g/L**	**50 g/L**	**100 g/L**	**150 g/L**
0.00	3.00	2.00	2.00	1.33
1.00	4.16	3.78	6.71	5.27
2.00	5.34	5.79	1.11	0.30
3.00	7.35		5.72	3.78
4.00	6.01	9.36	3.71	7.65
5.00	8.61	6.68	8.32	10.3
6.00	10.1	17.6	21.1	17.0
7.00	18.8	35.5	37.6	38.4
8.00	28.9	66.1	74.2	70.8
9.00	36.2	143	180	194
10.0	42.4	160	269	283
11.0	44.4	170	237	279
12.0	46.9	165	256	306
13.0	46.9	163	249	289

storage. Table P7.8 shows acid production (% lactic acid) in yogurt versus time at four different temperatures.

For the purpose of this problem, assume that the saturation constant is large (very rarely in reality) and thus the acid production follows first-order kinetics with respect to the consumption of lactose in the yogurt to produce lactic acid. At the start of acid production, the lactose concentration is about 1.5%, the bacteria concentration is 10^{11} cells/L, and the acid concentration at which all metabolic activity ceases is 1.4% lactic acid.

Time, days	35 °F	40 °F	45 °F	50 °F
1	1.02	1.02	1.02	1.02
14	1.03	1.05	1.14	1.19
28	1.05	1.06	1.15	1.24
35	1.09	1.10	1.22	1.26
42	1.09	1.12	1.22	1.31
49	1.10	1.12	1.22	1.32
56	1.09	1.13	1.24	1.32
63	1.10	1.14	1.25	1.32
70	1.10	1.16	1.26	1.34

(a) Determine the activation energy for the reaction.
(b) How long would it take to reach 1.10% acid at 38 °F?
(c) If you left yogurt out at room temperature, 77 °F, how long would it take to reach 1.10% lactic acid?

7.9. Table P7.9 shows data on bakers' yeast in a particular medium at 23.4 °C and various oxygen partial pressures were obtained:

p_{O_2}, mmHg	0	0.5	1	1.5	2.5	3.5	5
$-\mu_{O_2}$, mmHg, no sulfanilamide	0	23.5	33	37.5	42	43	43
$-\mu_{O_2}$, mmHg, with 20 g/L sulfanilamide	0	17.4	25.6	30.8	36.4	39.6	40

(a) Calculate the maximum oxygen uptake rate $-\mu_{O_2\max}$ and the Monod saturation constant K_S when no sulfanilamide is present. Monod equation is given by

$$-\mu_{O_2} = \frac{\mu_{O_2\max} S}{K_S + S}$$

where S is the concentration of oxygen. In this case, oxygen pressure could be used.

(b) Determine whether sulfanilamide is a competitive or noncompetitive inhibitor to the O_2 uptake. For competitive inhibition

$$-\mu_{O_2} = \frac{\mu_{O_2\max} S}{K_S + S + K_I I}$$

and for noncompetitive inhibition

$$-\mu_{O_2} = \frac{\mu_{O_2\max} S}{(K_S + S)(1 + I/K_I)}$$

where I is the concentration of the inhibitor.

7.10. Diene 110 is synthesized in benzene via:

$$2\,\text{A} \xrightarrow{[(CH_3)_2CHO]_3Al} \text{B}$$

A: CHO, CH_3; B: $C(O)OCH_2$, CH_3, CH_3

At 28 °C, the concentration of A was measured as given in Table P7.10.

t, h	0	3	6	9	12
C_A, mol/L	2	1.08	0.74	0.56	0.46

Determine the reaction rate expression.

CHAPTER

8

Enzymes

OUTLINE

Bioprocess Engineering
http://dx.doi.org/10.1016/B978-0-444-59525-6.00008-1

Enzymes are usually proteins of high molecular weight (15,000 < M < several million daltons) that act as catalysts. Recently, it has been shown that some RNA molecules are also catalytic, but the vast majority of cellular reactions are mediated by protein catalysts. RNA molecules that have catalytic properties are called *ribozymes.* Enzymes are specific, versatile, and very effective biological catalysts, resulting in much higher reaction rates as compared to chemically catalyzed reactions under ambient conditions. More than 2000 enzymes are known. Enzymes are named by adding the suffix *-ase* to the end of the substrate, such as urease, or the reaction catalyzed, such as alcohol dehydrogenase. Some enzymes have a simple structure, such as a folded polypeptide chain (typical of most hydrolytic enzymes). Many enzymes have more than one subunit. Some protein enzymes require a nonprotein group for their activity. This group is either a cofactor, such as metal ions, Mg, Zn, Mn, Fe, or a coenzyme, such as a complex organic molecule, NAD, FAD, CoA, or some vitamins. An enzyme containing a nonprotein group is called a *holoenzyme.* The protein part of this enzyme is the *apoenzyme* (holoenzyme = apoenzyme + cofactor). Enzymes that occur in several different molecular forms, but catalyze the same reaction, are called *isozymes.* Some enzymes are grouped together to form enzyme complexes. Enzymes are substrate specific and are classified according to the reaction they catalyze. Major classes of enzymes and their functions are listed in Table 8.1.

Enzymes have been classified into six main types, depending on the nature of the reaction catalyzed. A four-digit coding (numbering scheme) for enzymes has been developed, in which the classes are distinguished by the first of four digits. The second and third digits describe the type of reaction catalyzed, and the fourth digit is employed to distinguish between the types of the same function on the basis of the actual substrate in the reaction catalyzed. This scheme has proven useful in clearly delineating many enzymes that have similarities. It was developed by the Nomenclature Commission of the International Union of Biochemistry and Molecular Biology, and the prefix EC (stands for Enzyme Code, or Enzyme Commission as it was originally initiated) is generally employed with the numerical scheme. This classification scheme is useful as it unambiguously identifies the enzyme in question. Earlier nomenclature often resulted in one enzyme being identified by several names if its activity was broad.

Example: Alcoholdehydrogenase (trivial name)
Systematic name: alcohol: NAD^+ oxidoreductase (an alcohol is the electron donor and NAD^+ is the electron acceptor)

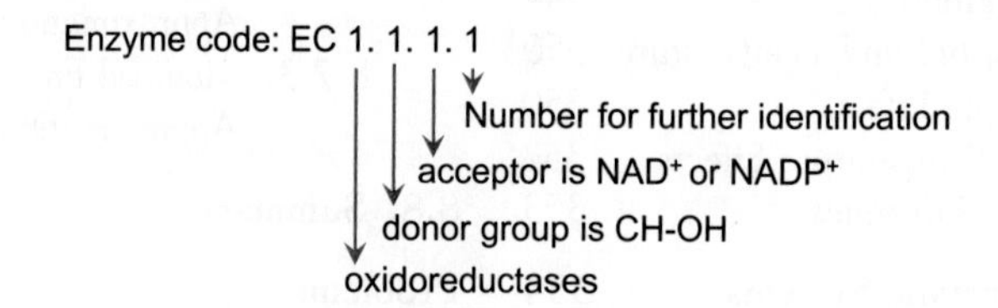

Figure 8.1 shows the structure and active sites of one alcoholdehydrogenase. While enzymes are specific in function, the degree of specificity varies. Some may act on closely related substrates (eg. based on a functional group) and are said to exhibit *group specificity;*

TABLE 8.1 International Classification of Enzymes: Code Numbers (EC 1st Digit, 2nd Digit, 3rd Digit, 4th Digit) and Types of Reactions Catalyzed

1st Digit (Class)	2nd Digit	3rd Digit	4th
1. Oxidoreductases	Donor of hydrogen or electron	Acceptor of hydrogen	
Transfer of hydrogen or oxygen	1 Alcohol	or electron	
atoms or electrons from one	2 Aldehyde or ketone	1 NAD^+ or $NADP^+$ or	
substrate to another: oxidases or	3 Alkene, –CH=CH–	peroxidase	
dehydrogenases	4 Primary amine: $CH-NH_2$	2 Cytochrome or heme	
	5 Secondary amine: CH–NH–	protein	
	6 NADH or NADPH	3 O_2	
	7 Nitrogenous compound	4 S–S	
	8 Sulfur group	5 Quinone or similar	
	9 Heme group	6 Nitrogenous group	
	10 Diphenols or related	7 Iron–sulfur–protein	
	11 Peroxide	8 Flavin	
	12 Hydrogen	11 Incorporating two O	
	13 Single donor with O_2	12 Incorporating one O	
	14 Paired donors, with O_2	98 Other, known	
	15 Acting on superoxide	99 Other	
	16 Oxidizing metal ion		
	17 Acting on CH or CH_2 groups		
	18 Iron–sulfur–protein		
	19 Reduced flavodoxin		
	20 Phosphorous or arsenic		
	21 on XH and YH to form XY		
	97 Oxidoreductases		
	98 Other, using H_2 as reductant		
	99 Other, using O_2 as oxidant		
2. Transferases	General type of group	Nature of group	
Group transfer excluding hydrogen	1 1-Carbon group	transferred	
or oxygen:	2 Aldehyde or ketone		
$AX + B \rightarrow BX + A$	3 Acyl group–COR		
	4 Glycosyl group		
	5 Alkyl or aryl, other than methyl		
	6 Nitrogenous groups		
	7 Phosphate group		
	8 Sulfur-containing groups		
	9 Selenium-containing groups		
3. Hydrolases	Type of bond hydrolyzed		
Catalyzes hydrolysis:	1 Ester		
$A{-}X + H_2O \rightarrow X{-}OH + HA$	2 Glycosylases		
	3 Ether		
	4 Peptide		
	5 C–N bonds other than peptides		
	6 Acid anhydrides		
	7 C–C		
	8 Halide		
	9 Phosphorus–nitrogen		
	10 S–N		
	11 C–phosphorus		
	12 S–S		
	13 S–S		

(*Continued*)

TABLE 8.1 International Classification of Enzymes: Code Numbers (EC 1st Digit, 2nd Digit, 3rd Digit, 4th Digit) and Types of Reactions Catalyzed—*Cont'd*

1st Digit (Class)	2nd Digit	3rd Digit	4th
4. Lyases Nonhydrolytic removal of groups with product usually contains double bond	Type of bond broken 1 C–C 2 C–O 3 C–N 4 C–S 5 C-halide 6 P–O 99 Other	Group removed 1 Carboxyl 2 Aldehyde 3 Ketoacid	
5. Isomerases	Type of reaction 1 Racemizationor epimerization 2 *cis–trans* isomerizations 3 Intramolecular oxidoreductases 4 Intramolecular transfer reactions 5 Intramolecular lyases 99 Other	Type of molecule 1 Amino acids 2 Hydroxyacids 3 Carbohydrates	
6. Ligases Synthesis of bonds with breaking down of ATP or nucleoside triphosphates	Type of bond formed 1 C–O 2 C–S 3 C–N 4 C–C 5 Phosphoric ester 6 N-metal		

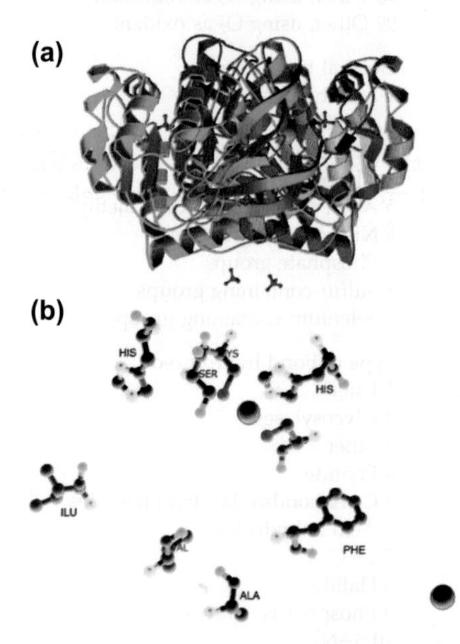

FIGURE 8.1 Alcoholdehydrogenase: structure and active sites. (a) Crystallographic structure of human ADH 5. (b) The active site consists of a zinc atom, His-67, Cys-174, Cys-46, Ser-48, His-51, Ile-269, Val-292, Ala-317, and Phe-319. The zinc coordinates the substrate (alcohol). The zinc is coordinated by Cys-146, Cys-174, and His-67, Phe-319, Ala-317, His-51, Ile-269, and Val-292 stabilize NAD^+ by forming hydrogen bonds. His-51 and Ile-269 form hydrogen bonds with the alcohols on nicotinamide ribose. Phe-319, Ala-317, and Val-292 form hydrogen bonds with the amide on NAD^+.

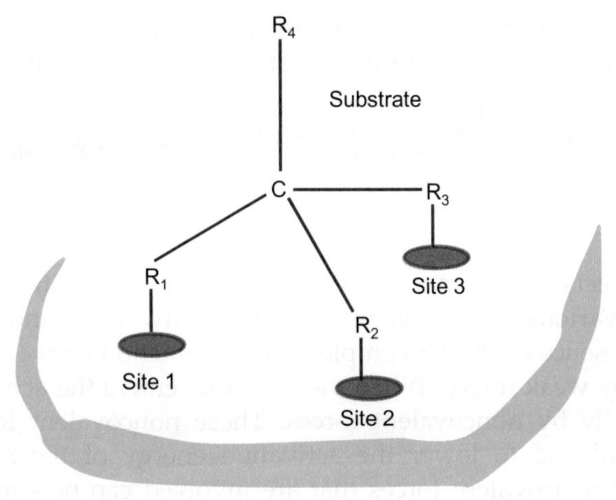

FIGURE 8.2 Representation of the three-point interaction of substrate with enzyme.

others are more exacting in their substrate requirements and are said to be *absolutely specific.* The product formed from a particular enzyme and substrate is also unique. Enzymes are able to distinguish between stereochemical forms and only one isomer of a particular substrate may be catalyzed to react. Surprisingly, enzyme reactions may yield stereospecific products from substrates that possess no asymmetric carbon atoms, as long as one carbon is *prochiral*. This chirality is a result of at least three-point interaction between substrate and enzyme in the active site of the enzyme. In Fig. 8.2, sites 1, 2, and 3 are binding sites on the enzyme. When two of the R groups on the substrate are identical, the molecule has a *prochiral* center and a chiral center can result from the enzymatic reaction, as the substrate can only "fit" into the active site in one configuration if the site has binding selectivity for three of the R-group substituents. If the substrate has four different R groups, then chirality can be preserved in the reaction as a result of the multipoint attachment.

8.1. HOW ENZYMES WORK

Enzymes lower the activation energy of the reaction catalyzed by binding the substrate and forming an enzyme-substrate complex. Enzymes do not affect the free-energy change or the equilibrium constant. Figure 8.3 illustrates the action of an enzyme from the activation-energy point of view. For example, the activation energy for the decomposition of hydrogen peroxide varies depending on the type of catalysis. The activation energy E of the uncatalyzed reaction at 20 °C is 75 kJ per mole (kJ/mol), whereas the E values for chemically catalyzed (by colloidal platinum) and enzymatically catalyzed (catalase) decomposition are 54 and 29 kJ/mol, respectively. That is, catalase accelerates the rate of reaction by a factor of about 10. One should note that this large change in rate for a relatively small change in activation energy is due to the exponential dependence of rate on activation energy. In this case,

the ratio of the rates is $\dfrac{e^{-\frac{29,000}{8.314\times293}}}{e^{-\frac{75,000}{1.987\times293}}} = e^{\frac{75,000-29,000}{8.314\times293}} = 1.59\times10^{8}$ if the preexponent factor remains the same.

The molecular aspects of enzyme–substrate (ES) interaction differ for different enzyme and substrate pairs. Various studies using crystallography, X-ray, and Raman spectroscopy have revealed the presence of the ES complex. The interaction between the enzyme and its substrate is usually by weak forces. When the substrate enters the active site of an enzyme, it will be held initially by noncovalent forces. These noncovalent forces responsible for binding may be employed to lower the activation energy of the reaction as shown in Fig. 8.3. The types of noncovalent forces that are involved can be summarized as follows: a) *Electrostatic interactions* include charge–charge ($1/d_{\text{S-enz}}$, i.e. inversely proportional to the distance between the charged enzyme active site to the charged substrate), dipole–dipole ($d_{\text{S-enz}}^{-6}$), charge-induced dipole ($d_{\text{S-enz}}^{-4}$), and dipole-induced dipole ($d_{\text{S-enz}}^{-6}$) interactions. The magnitude of these forces depends on the distance between molecules, varying with the distance ($d_{\text{S-enz}}$) in the manner indicated above. All depend inversely on the dielectric constant of the solvent between the ions or dipoles. b) *van der Waals forces* are comprised of electron cloud repulsion ($d_{\text{S-enz}}^{-12}$) and attractive dispersion forces (London forces) ($d_{\text{S-enz}}^{-6}$). The sum of these is described by the Lennard–Jones 6–12 potential. Dispersion forces are not large, but in an enzyme, the sum of all such forces between substrate and enzyme may be quite significant. c) *Hydrogen bonds* are important in biological systems and occur when two electronegative atoms are bound to a common proton. Often oxygen *is* one of the atoms. d) *Hydrophobic forces* reflect the tendency of apolar molecules to partition from an aqueous

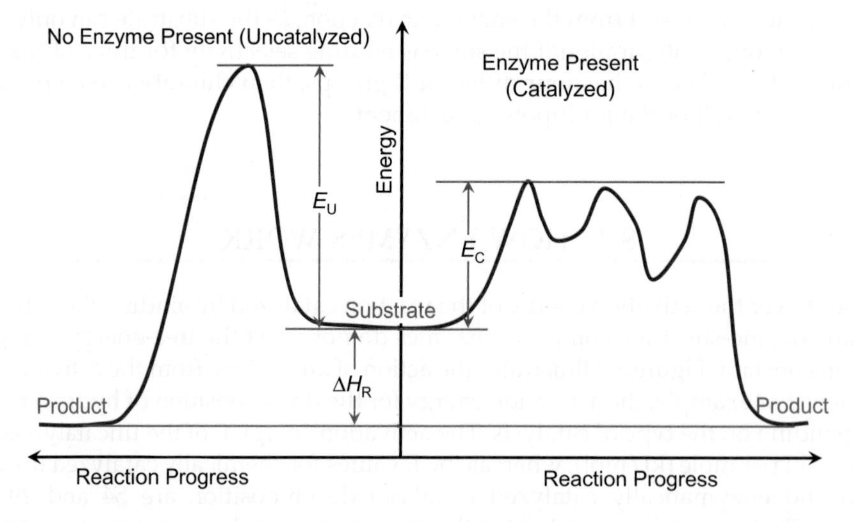

FIGURE 8.3 Activation energies of enzymatically catalyzed and uncatalyzed reactions. Note that $E_U < E_C$.

environment to a hydrophobic one. The driving force for such movement can be thought of as a result of the entropy gain when water molecules, which must be structured around an apolar molecule, are able to assume a more random arrangement when the molecule is transferred. The magnitude of this force *is* found experimentally to depend on the surface area of the molecule.

When the substrate moves from the external aqueous environment to the active site of the enzyme, *its* salvation shell is lost and one or more of the above forces are important in determining the strength of its binding. Hydrogen bonding and electrostatic interactions are generally most important. The difference in energies between the solvated state and that of the ES complex determines the strength of substrate binding. The substrate binds to a specific site on the enzyme known as the *active site.* The substrate is a relatively small molecule and fits into a certain region on the enzyme molecule, which is a much larger molecule. The simplest model describing this interaction is the lock-and-key model, in which the enzyme represents the lock and the substrate represents the key, as described in Fig. 8.4.

In multisubstrate enzyme-catalyzed reactions, enzymes can hold substrates such that reactive regions of substrates are close to each other and to the enzyme's active site, which is known as the *proximity effect.* This is the simplest mechanism by which an enzyme may enhance the rate of a reaction. The reactants were brought at the active sites and would then be present at local concentrations that are much higher than those present in solution. How large a rate enhancement might we expect from such approximation? Some insight into this can be obtained by examining *intramolecular* catalysis. Here one group adjacent to a reacting group provides catalytic assistance in the reaction.

An example of intramolecular catalysis is provided by the hydrolysis of tetramethyl succinanilic acid. This reaction is illustrated as

$$\mathrm{HO{-}C({=}O){-}C(CH_3)_2{-}C(CH_3)_2{-}C({=}O){-}NH{-}C_6H_5} + \mathrm{H_2O} \longrightarrow \mathrm{HO{-}C({=}O){-}C(CH_3)_2{-}C(CH_3)_2{-}C({=}O){-}OH} + \mathrm{NH_2{-}C_6H_5} \qquad (8.1)$$

The carboxylic acid moiety provides intramolecular assistance in the hydrolysis of the amide bond. At pH 5, the reaction occurs with a half-life of 30 min, whereas the corresponding hydrolysis of the unsubstituted acetanilide is some 300 years! This difference in rates corresponds to a rate enhancement of 1.6×10^8. Unsubstituted succinanilic acid is hydrolyzed 1200 times more slowly than the tetramethyl substituted compound; the methyl groups are important in bringing the catalytic group close to the reacting amide bond.

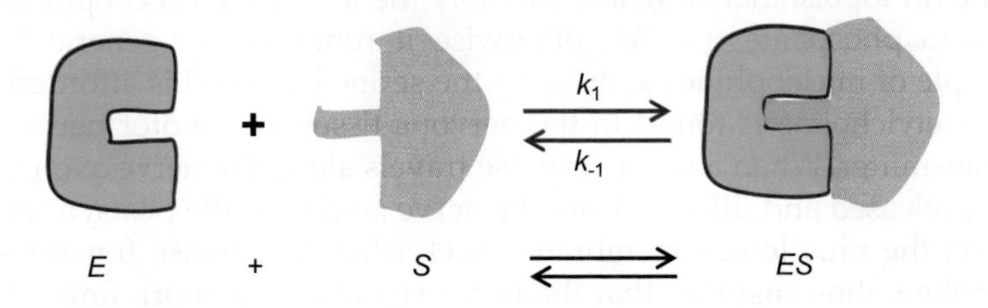

FIGURE 8.4 Schematic of the lock-and-key model of enzyme catalysis.

The differences in rates between intramolecular catalysis and the corresponding intermolecular catalysis can be employed to define an apparent concentration of reactant at the reaction site in intramolecular catalysis. In intermolecular catalysis, reactants A and B may react at a rate which is first order in both A and B, the overall rate can be expressed as $k_2[A][B]$, where k_2 is a second-order rate constant ($1\ mol^{-1} \cdot s^{-1}$). In the case of intramolecular catalysis, both A and B are present in the same compound, and the rate will now be $k_1[A{-}B]$, with k_1 (s^{-1}) being a first-order rate constant. Thus, the ratio k_1/k_2, which has units of molarity, represents the effective concentration of reactant A which would need to be present at the catalytic site to cause a smaller concentration of B to react at a pseudo-first-order rate equivalent to that of the intramolecularly catalyzed rate. Hence k_1/k_2 can then be thought of as an "effective" concentration of catalyst A at the reaction site. Such concentrations can be extremely high. When the effective molarities exceed attainable values, then other factors influencing catalysis, in addition to approximation, must be important.

In enzyme-catalyzed reactions, this enhanced local concentration effect can account for some of the rate enhancement but is generally not sufficiently large. It does provide a lower limit to the rate acceleration that might be expected however. We must turn to other mechanisms to provide an explanation for the catalytic abilities of enzymes.

Covalent Catalysis: Electrophilic and Nucleophilic Catalysis is another main route an enzyme may employ to enhance the reaction rate. An enzyme can *form* a covalent bond with one or more reactants and so alter the reaction path from that observed in the uncatalyzed case. The discovery that enzymes may indeed *form* covalent intermediates relied on early kinetic observations, including "burst" kinetics and the observation of constant rates of product release from substrates with varying substituents. Today, the crystallographic structures of many enzymes and their substrate-containing intermediates are well-known, providing further evidence for the formation of such covalent intermediate compounds.

Covalent catalysis is divided into two types: electrophilic and nucleophilic catalysis. In nucleophilic catalysis, the nucleophilic groups on the enzyme are more electron donating than the normal attacking groups, and a reactive intermediate is *formed* which breaks down rapidly to *form* the products. Electrophilic catalysis on the other hand involves catalysts that withdraw electrons from the reaction center of the intermediate. We will first consider nucleophilic catalysis.

The most common nucleophiles in enzymes are the serine hydroxyl (found in serine proteases, esterases, lipases, and phosphatases), the cysteine thiol (thiol proteases), the carboxylic group of aspartic acid, the amino group of lysine (aldolase, transaldolase, DNA ligase), the -OH of tyrosine (in topoisomerases), and possibly the imidazole (in conjunction with phosphoryl groups in phosphate transfer, otherwise it functions by general base catalysis). A simple example of nucleophilic catalysis by the serine hydroxyl is afforded by acetylcholine esterase. Acetylcholine is found in the nervous tissue and motor nerve tracts; it is an active neurotransmitter. When a nerve impulse travels along the nerve axon to the synapse, acetylcholine is released and diffuses from the nerve ending to the postsynaptic receptor for acetylcholine on the muscle cell membrane. Acetylcholine esterase functions by breaking down acetylcholine, thus ensuring that the nerve signal is of a short, finite duration. If the enzyme is inhibited, tetanic shock and muscle paralysis follow. The enzyme is thus the target for nerve gases and some insecticides. The enzyme has two subsites; one contains the nucleophilic serine which is involved in the formation of an acetyl–enzyme intermediate (called the esteratic site), and the other is negatively charged and provides a salt bridge to enhance recognition and binding of the trimethylammonium region of acetylcholine. The serine acts a nucleophile and attacks the ester linkage, presumably via the formation of a tetrahedral intermediate. Then the choline is released, and an acyl enzyme intermediate is formed. Water (OH) then releases the acetate from the acyl intermediate. The reaction mechanism is shown in Fig. 8.5.

The enzyme is remarkably efficient; it has a turnover number (k_{cat}, or the first-order reaction rate constant) of 25,000 and thus cleaves one substrate molecule every 40 μs. This rapid rate of cleavage is crucial as nerve impulses can be carried at a rate of 1000 impulses/s, necessitating the rapid removal of acetylcholine from the postsynaptic receptor.

Electrophilic catalysts, in contrast to nucleophilic catalysis, act by withdrawing electrons from the reaction center of the intermediate and are thus *electron sinks.* They stabilize a negative charge. Examples of this mechanism involve coenzymes thiamine pyrophosphate and pyridoxal phosphate. In many cases, including these coenzymes, electrophilic catalysis involves the formation of Schiff bases. For example, acetoacetate decarboxylase catalyzes the decarboxylation of acetoacetate to acetone and CO_2. The mechanism involves the formation of a Schiff base involving a lysine residue. Acetoacetate decarboxylase participates in the production of acetone by fermentation of sugars by anaerobic bacteria, such as *Clostridium acetobutylicum.* This fermentation process was an important route to acetone in World War I, when acetone was employed in the production of the explosive cordite and chemical routes were not available. Other important Schiff base reactions include aldolase and transaldolase reactions.

Acids and bases can catalyze reactions by either donating or accepting a proton which is transferred in the transition state. When such a charged group develops in the transition

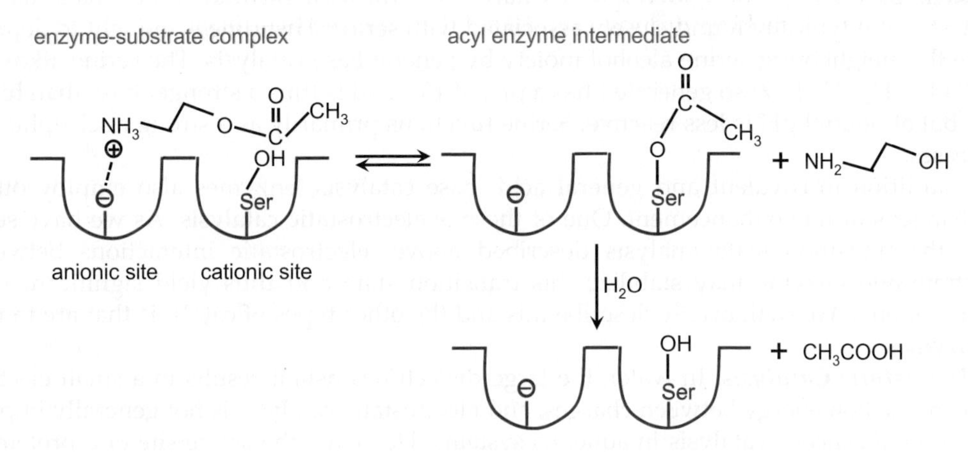

FIGURE 8.5 The mechanism of action of acetylcholine esterase.

state, the resulting positive or negative charge makes the transition state unfavorable. The presence of acids or bases results in a stabilization of such a transition state. By providing acid or base groups at the active site, an enzyme is thus able to stabilize the charged transition state. This mechanism is employed by a wide variety of enzymes.

Two types of acid or base catalysis can be distinguished: *general* and *specific*. The distinction between specific and general acids and bases can be best understood by examining experimental observations of catalytic reaction rates. Consider, for example, the hydrolysis of an ester in buffered solutions. The hydrolysis rate can be determined at a constant pH (by maintaining the ratio of acid and base forms of the buffer at a constant value), at several different total concentrations of buffer. If the rate of reaction increases with increasing buffer concentration, then the buffer must be involved in the reaction and act as a catalyst. This is *general* acid or base catalysis. If the rate is unaffected by buffer concentration, then the reaction involves *specific* acid or base catalysis. The reacting species would be only proton (H^+) or hydroxyl anion (OH^-), and the buffer simply serves to maintain these species at constant concentrations.

How does an enzyme obtain the rate enhancements made possible by general acid–base catalysis? The answer lies in the combination of pK_a values for amino acid moieties involved in acid–base catalysis and the typical values of proton dissociation constant K_a, describing proton transfer. An acid with a pK_a of 5 is a better general acid catalyst than one with a pK_a of 7. At pH 7, however, typical of the optimal pH of many enzymes, only 1% of the acid with a pK_a of 5 will be unionized and active in catalysis. The acid with a pK_a of 7 will be 50% unprotonated. The same trend applies to base catalysis. If we consider the amino acids, we see that histidine contains an imidazole moiety which has a pK_a value around 6–7. Therefore, histidine is widely found in enzymes involved in base catalysis as it is 50% ionized at neutral pH. The imidazole moiety may thus be considered as the most effective amino acid base existing at neutral pH. In fact, all enzymatic acyl transfers catalyzed by proteases (e.g. trypsin, chymotrypsin) involve histidine. The imidazole group of histidine can also function as a nucleophile, and we must be careful to determine whether histidine acts a general base catalyst or a nucleophilic catalyst. In proteases, histidine functions as a base catalyst, but it typically found closely associated with serine. Histidine is thought to deprotonate this neighboring serine alcohol moiety by general base catalysis. The serine alkoxide ion ($^-O{-}CH_2CH{-}Enz$) so generated has a pK_a of 13.7 and is thus a stronger base than histidine but at neutral pH is less reactive. Serine functions primarily as a strong nucleophile in proteases.

In addition to covalent and general acid–base catalysis, enzymes also employ other mechanisms of rate enhancement. One of these is electrostatic catalysis. As we have seen from the transition state analysis described above, electrostatic interactions between substrate and enzyme may stabilize this transition state and thus yield significant rate enhancements. We shall briefly describe this and the other types of catalysis that are found in enzymes.

Electrostatic Catalysis. In water, the large dielectric constant results in a small electrostatic interaction energy between charges, and electrostatic catalysis is not generally important in homogeneous catalysis in aqueous systems. However, the active site of a protein is very heterogeneous, and the dielectric constant of the medium between charged groups may be quite different from water. The aromatic and aliphatic amino acid residues present at the active site act to reduce the dielectric constant and charged amino acid residues act as fixed dipoles, thus stabilizing charge quite effectively. The electrostatic interaction energy depends on the charges and is inversely proportional to the dielectric constant and distance between charges.

Lowering the dielectric constant can increase this energy considerably. Proteins may thus use parts of their own structure to solvate transition states and induce electrostatic strain. In fact, enzymes may stabilize charged groups in the transition state better than water, as the amino acids which function as dipoles are rigidly positioned and have a direction in relation to the substrate, whereas in water this directionality is lost.

The overall significance of electrostatic catalysis in enzymes is still not clear, as determination of the local dielectric constant is difficult. Electrostatic stabilization of charged transition states certainly plays some role, however.

Catalysis Involving Metal Ions. In metalloenzymes, a metal ion is present at the active site, and this ion plays an important role in stabilizing negative charges that are formed in electrophilic catalysis. Zinc, copper, and cobalt are commonly involved in coordination of oxyanions involved as reaction intermediates. The enzyme carboxypeptidase-A, which is a carboxyl-terminus exopeptidase (i.e. it acts by hydrolyzing the peptide from the carboxylic acid terminus), contains Zn^{2+} which polarizes the carbonyl oxygen of the terminal peptide bond. The terminal carboxylate is charge paired with the guanidinium cation of Arg 145 leading to polarization of the terminal carboxylic carbonyl group. This polarization increases the electrophilicity of the carbonyl carbon and facilitates nucleophile-mediated hydrolysis of the amide bond. This is illustrated in Fig. 8.6. In addition to stabilizing negative charges, metal ions serve as a source of potent nucleophilic hydroxyl ions. Metal-bound water molecules provide these nucleophilic hydroxyl groups at neutral pH.

An example is the extremely rapid hydration of CO_2 by carbonic anhydrase to produce bicarbonate. The enzyme contains zinc coordinated to the imidazole groups of three histidines, with the fourth ligand being water, which is ionized. The zinc-bound hydroxyl has a pK_a of 8.7, and the reaction mechanism is thought to that shown in Fig. 8.7.

Also, enzymes may hold the substrates at certain positions and angles to improve the reaction rate, which is known as the *orientation effect.* In some enzymes, the formation of an ES

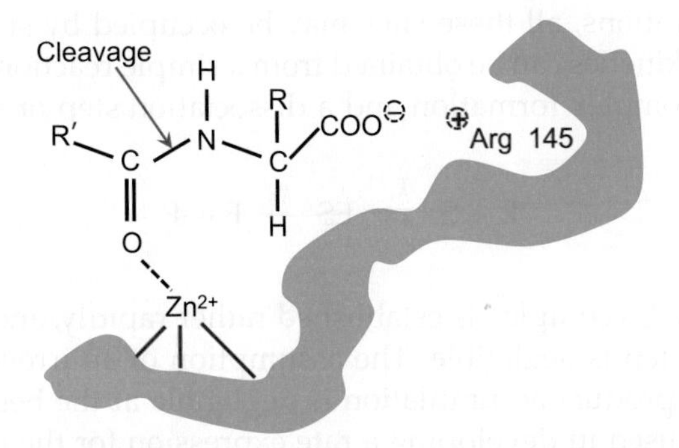

FIGURE 8.6 Metalloenzyme carboxypeptidase-A facilitates nucleophile-mediated hydrolysis of an amide bond.

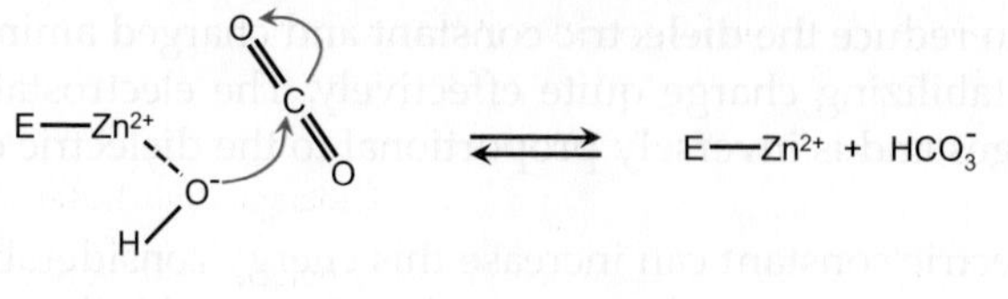

FIGURE 8.7 Metalloenzyme carbonic anhydrase facilitates the hydration of CO_2 to bicarbonate.

complex causes slight changes in the three-dimensional shape of the enzyme. This induced fit of the substrate to the enzyme molecule may contribute to the catalytic activity of the enzyme, too. The enzymes lysozyme and carboxypeptidase-A have been observed to change their three-dimensional structure upon complexing with the substrate. Enzyme catalysis is affected not only by the primary structure of enzymes but also by the secondary, tertiary, and quaternary structures. The properties of the active site of enzymes and the folding characteristics have a profound effect on the catalytic activity of enzymes. Certain enzymes require coenzymes and cofactors for proper functioning.

Table 8.2 lists some enzymes and their cofactors and coenzymes.

8.2. ENZYME KINETICS

8.2.1. Introduction

A mathematical model of the kinetics of single substrate-enzyme-catalyzed reactions was first developed by V. C. R. Henri in 1902 and by L. Michaelis and M. L Menten in 1913. Kinetics of simple enzyme-catalyzed reactions are often referred to as Michaelis–Menten kinetics or *saturation* kinetics. The qualitative features of enzyme kinetics are shown in Fig. 8.8, which is similar to Langmuir–Hinshelwood kinetics (Chapter 9). These models are based on data from batch reactors with constant liquid volume in which the initial substrate, $[S]_0$, and enzyme, $[E]_0$, concentrations are known. More complicated ES interactions such as multisubstrate–multienzyme reactions can take place in biological systems. An enzyme solution has a fixed number of active sites to which substrates can bind. At high substrate concentrations, all these sites may be occupied by substrates or the enzyme is *saturated.* Saturation kinetics can be obtained from a simple reaction scheme that involves a reversible step for ES complex formation and a dissociation step of the ES complex.

$$E + S \underset{k_{-1}}{\overset{k_1}{\rightleftarrows}} ES \overset{k_2}{\rightarrow} E + P \tag{8.2}$$

It is assumed that the ES complex is established rather rapidly, and the rate of the reverse reaction of the second step is negligible. The assumption of an irreversible second reaction often holds only when product accumulation is negligible at the beginning of the reaction. Two major approaches used in developing a rate expression for the enzyme-catalyzed reactions are (1) rapid-equilibrium approach and (2) pseudosteady-state approach.

TABLE 8.2 Cofactors (Metal Ions) and Coenzymes of Some Enzymes

Cofactors	Coenzymes	Entity transferred
Zn^{2+}	Nicotinamide adenine dinucleotide	Hydrogen atoms
Alcohol dehydrogenase	Nicotinamide adenine dinucleotide phosphate	Hydrogen atoms
Carbonic anhydrase		
Carboxypeptidase	Flavin mononucleotide	Hydrogen atoms
Mg^{2+}	Flavin adenine dinucleotide	Hydrogen atoms
Phosphohydrolases		
Phosphotransferases	Coenzyme Q	Hydrogen atoms
Mn^{2+}	Thiamin pyrophosphate	Aldehydes
Arginase		
Phosphotransferases	Coenzyme A	Acyl groups
Fe^{2+} or Fe^{3+}	Lipoamide	Acyl groups
Cytochromes		
Peroxidase	Cobamide coenzyme	Alkyl groups
Catalase	Biocytin	Carbon dioxide
Ferrodoxin	Pyridoxal phosphate	Amino groups
Cu^{2+} or Cu^{+} Tyrosinase Cytochrome oxidase	Tetrahydrofolate coenzyme	Methyl, methylene, formyl, or formino groups
K^{+}		
Pyruvate kinase (also require Mg^{2+})		
Na^{2+}		
Plasma membrane ATPase (also requires K^{+} and Mg^{2+})		

8.2.2. Mechanistic Models for Simple Enzyme Kinetics

Both the pseudosteady-state approximation and the assumption of rapid equilibrium share the same few initial steps in deriving a rate expression for the mechanism in Eqn (8.3), where the rate of product formation

$$r_P = r_2 = K_2[\mathrm{ES}] \tag{8.3}$$

The rate constant k_2 is often denoted as k_{cat} in the biological literature. The rate of formation of the ES complex is

$$r_{ES} = r_1 - r_2 = k_1[\mathrm{E}][\mathrm{S}] - k_{-1}[\mathrm{ES}] - k_2[\mathrm{ES}] \tag{8.4}$$

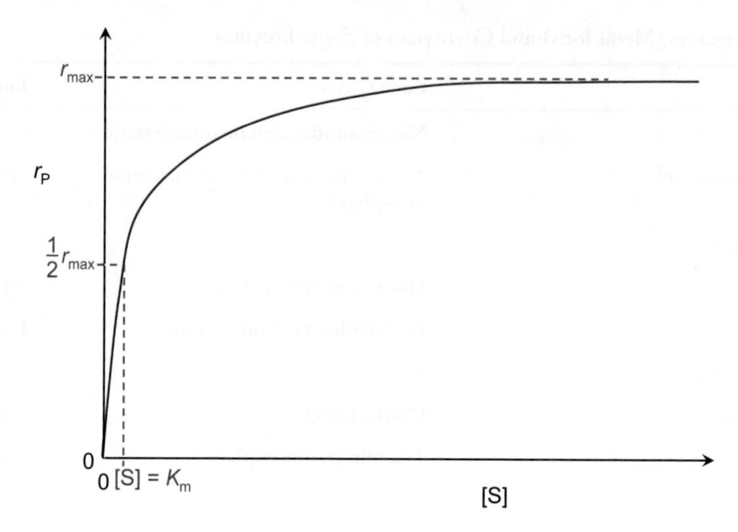

FIGURE 8.8 Effect of substrate concentration on the rate of product formation for an enzyme-catalyzed reaction.

Since the enzyme is not consumed, the conservation equation on the enzyme yields

$$[E] = [E]_0 - [ES] \tag{8.5}$$

At this point, an assumption is required to simplify the rate expression eliminating the requirement of concentrations other than the enzyme loading and substrate and product concentrations.

8.2.2.1. The Fast Equilibrium Step Assumption

Henri and Michaelis and Menten used essentially this approach. Assuming the first step is very fast, and equilibrium is reached when one considers the second step. That is to say

$$0 = r_1 = k_1[E][S] - K_{-1}[ES] \tag{8.6}$$

(Do you see why the rate is zero? This is contrary to what it states that this first step is very fast.) Equation (8.6) yields

$$K_m = \frac{k_{-1}}{k_1} = \frac{[E][S]}{[ES]} \tag{8.7}$$

Apply Eqn (8.5) if enzyme is conserved, then

$$[ES] = \frac{[E]_0[S]}{K_m + [S]} \tag{8.8}$$

Substituting Eqn (8.8) into Eqn (8.3) yields

$$r_P = k_2[ES] = \frac{k_2[E]_0[S]}{K_m + [S]} = \frac{r_{max}[S]}{K_m + [S]} \tag{8.9}$$

where $r_{max} = k_2[E]_0$.

In this case, the maximum forward rate of the reaction is r_{max}. The value of r_{max} changes if more enzyme is added, but the addition of more substrate has no influence on r_{max}. K_m is often called the Michaelis–Menten constant. A low value of K_m suggests that the enzyme has a high affinity for the substrate. Also, K_m corresponds to the substrate concentration at which the reaction rate is half of the maximal reaction rate.

An equation of exactly the same form as Eqn (8.9) can be derived with a different, more general assumption applied to the reaction scheme in Eqn (8.2).

8.2.2.2. The Pseudosteady-State Hypothesis

In many cases, the assumption of rapid equilibrium following mass-action kinetics is not valid, although the ES reaction still shows saturation-type kinetics.

G. E. Briggs and J. B. S. Haldane first proposed using the pseudosteady-state assumption in 1925. In most experimental systems, a closed system (batch reactor) is used in which the initial substrate concentration greatly exceeds the initial enzyme concentration. They suggest that since $[E]_0$ was small, $r_{ES} \approx 0$. (This logic is flawed. Do you see why?) Exact solutions of the actual time course represented by Eqns (8.3), (8.4), and (8.5) have shown that *in a closed system, the pseudosteady-state hypothesis (PSSH) holds* after a brief transient *if* $[S]_0 >> [E]_0$. Figure 8.9 displays one such time course.

By applying PSSH to Eqn (8.4), we find

$$[ES] = \frac{k_1[E][S]}{k_{-1}+k_2} \tag{8.10}$$

Substituting the enzyme conservation Eqn (8.3) in Eqn (8.8) and solve for [ES], we obtain

$$[ES] = \frac{[E]_0[S]}{\frac{k_{-1}+k_2}{k_1}+[S]} \tag{8.11}$$

Substituting Eqn (8.11) into Eqn (8.3) yields

$$r_P = k_2[ES] = \frac{k_2[E]_0[S]}{\frac{k_{-1}+k_2}{k_1}+[S]} \tag{8.12}$$

or

$$r_P = \frac{r_{max}[S]}{K_m+[S]} \tag{8.13}$$

which is identical to Eqn (8.9). However,

$$K_m = \frac{k_{-1}+k_2}{k_1} \tag{8.14}$$

which is not the equilibrium constant as that in Eqn (8.7). Under most circumstances (simple experiments), it is impossible to determine whether Eqn (8.7) or Eqn (8.14) is more suitable. Since K_m results from the more general derivation, we will use it in the rest of our discussions.

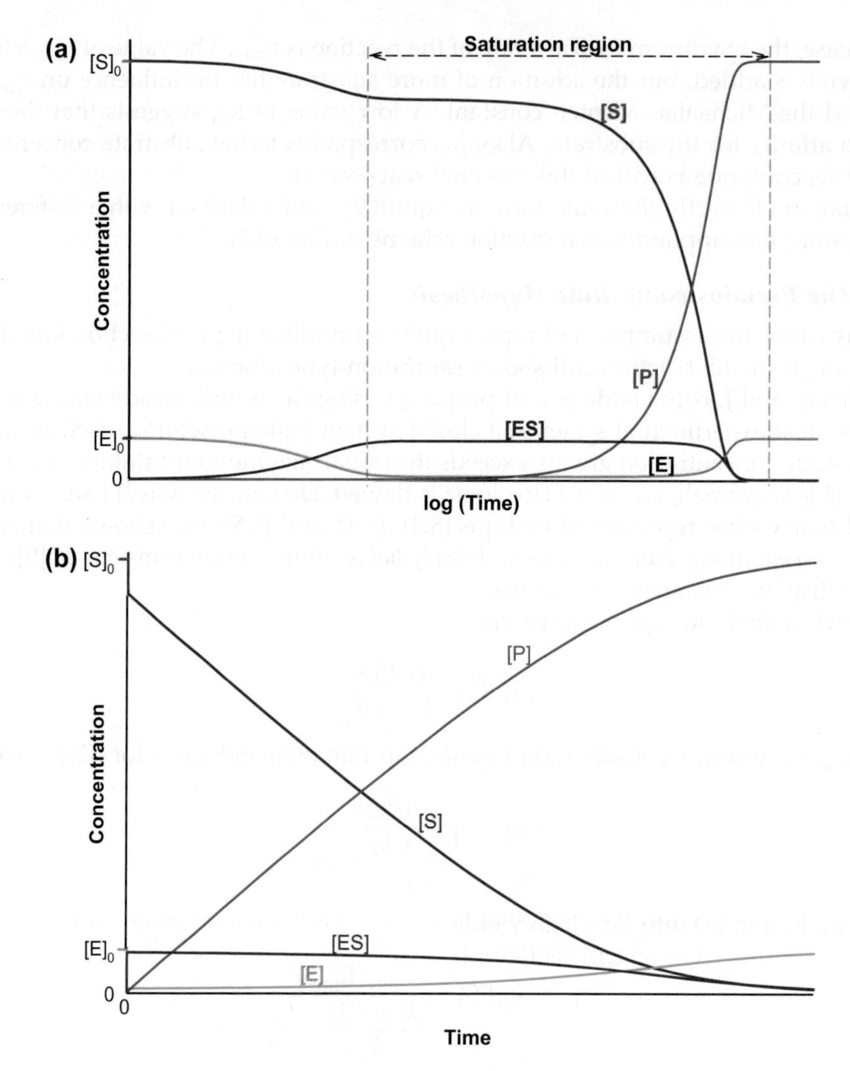

FIGURE 8.9 Time course of the formation of an enzyme/substrate complex and initiation of the pseudosteady state and the completion in a batch reactor, as derived from the two kinetic steps on a typical enzyme, Eqn (8.2) with $k_2 = 0.01\,k_1$, $k_{-1} = 0.8\,k_1$, and $[S]_0 = 10\ [E]_0$. (a) Concentration verse log (time). The pseudosteady state, i.e. when constant concentrations of [ES] and [E] are reached and beyond, is shown clearly in this plot. (b) Concentration verse time plot. The establishment of the pseudosteady state is accomplished in a very short time period, and it nearly shows a step change at time 0 in this linear plot.

8.2.3. Specific Activity

Enzyme concentrations are often given in terms of "units" rather than in mole or mass concentration. We rarely know the exact mass of the enzyme in a sample, since it is generally prepared via isolation of the enzyme from microorganisms or animal or plant tissues and often contains a great deal of non-catalytic protein, the amount of which may vary from sample to sample. Hence a different approach must be adopted, and enzyme concentration is reported in units of *specific activity.* A "unit" is defined as the amount of enzyme (e.g. microgram) which gives a certain amount of catalytic activity under specified conditions (e.g. producing 1.0 μmol of product per minute in a solution containing a substrate concentration sufficiently high to be in the "saturation" region, as shown in Fig. 8.9 where [ES] and [E] are relatively invariant).

Thus different suppliers of enzymes may have preparations with different units of activity, and care must be taken in analyzing kinetic data. Thus, a purified enzyme preparation will have a higher specific activity than a crude preparation; often a protein is considered pure when a constant specific activity is reached during the purification steps.

$$\text{Specific acivity} = \frac{\text{Activity}}{\text{mg-protein}} = \frac{\text{mmol-product}}{\text{mg-protein} \times \text{min} \times \text{ml}} \tag{8.15}$$

The activity is given by the amount of product formed or substrate consumed in the reaction mixture, under the conditions specified (temperature, pH, buffer type, substrate and enzyme concentrations, etc.). If the molecular weight of the enzyme is known, the specific activity can also be defined as:

$$\text{Specific acivity} = \frac{\text{Activity}}{\text{mmol-protein}} = \frac{\text{mmol-product}}{\text{mmol-protein} \times \text{min} \times \text{ml}} \tag{8.16}$$

Example 8-1. To measure the amount of glucoamylase in a crude enzyme preparation, 1 mL of the crude enzyme preparation containing 8-mg protein is added to 9 mL of a 4.44% starch solution. One unit of activity of glucoamylase is defined as the amount of enzyme which produces 1 μmol of glucose/min in a 4% solution of Linter starch at pH 4.5 and at 60 °C. Initial rate experiments show that the reaction produces 0.6 μmol of glucose/(mL · min). What is the specific activity of the crude enzyme preparation?

Solution. The total amount of glucose made is 10 mL × 0.6 μmol glucose/(mL·min) or 6 μmol glucose/min. The specific activity is then:

$$\begin{aligned}\text{Specific activity} &= \frac{6\text{ units}}{1\text{ ml protein solution} \times 8\text{ mg/ml}}\\ &= 0.75\text{ units/mg-protein}\end{aligned}$$

The maximum reaction rate r_{max} must have units such as mol-product/(L min). Since $r_{max} = k_2[E]_0$, the dimensions of k_2 must reflect the definition of units in $[E]_0$. In the above example, we had a concentration of enzyme of 8-mg protein/10-mL solution: 0.75 units/mg-protein or 600 units/L. If, for example, $r_{max} = 1$ mol/(L min), then $k_2 = 1$ mol/(L min) ÷ 600 units/L or $k_2 = 1.67$ μmol/(unit min).

8.2.4. Models for More Complex Enzyme Kinetics

8.2.4.1. Kinetics of Multisubstrate Reactions

The majority of enzymes do not involve just one substrate; they usually involve two. Often the second substrate is a cofactor, such as NAD^+ in oxidoreductases. Many of the concepts we have developed to date can be applied to situations where one of the substrates is held at a constant concentration; the kinetics then follow one of the forms described earlier. Most types of multisubstrate reactions fall into one of two classes, depending on the order of substrate binding and release of products. The description of the reaction in these terms is referred to as the "formal kinetic mechanism." In the first case, when all substrates are added to the enzyme prior to the reaction or conversion, a complex ES intermediate exists. With two-substrate reactions, the mechanism is referred to as a *ternary complex mechanism.* In the second case, when one product is released before the second substrate is bound (for example, when a group is transferred from one reactant to another), the mechanism is referred to as an *enzyme-substituted mechanism.*

In the case of two-substrate enzyme-substituted systems, there is thus a required order of substrate binding (i.e. a *sequential* mechanism). In the case of ternary complex mechanisms, a number of possible binding orders arise. For example, binding of one substrate may not be possible until a particular substrate is first bound, as this may result in a conformational change in enzyme structure which then permits the binding of the second substrate. This is referred to as *compulsory* order. When such order is not important, the mechanism is known as *random* order. This is summarized in Table 8.3 for two-substrate reactions.

We will consider the two main classes of mechanisms described above using the simplest case, that of two-substrate reactions as an example. The reaction to be considered

$$A + B \rightarrow P + Q \tag{8.17}$$

For situations where a ternary complex mechanism is involved, four possibilities can be considered: either a compulsory order or random mechanism with either pseudosteady-state or rapid equilibrium assumptions being used to describe the behavior of the various ES complexes formed. The enzyme-substituted mechanism (also referred to as a double-displacement or ping-pong mechanism) is yet another possibility, distinct from the ternary complex mechanism. In all of these situations, we shall see that the initial rates of reaction can be written in the following form:

$$r_P = \frac{k_2[E]_0[A][B]}{1 + K_{12}[A][B] + K_1[A] + K_2[B]} \tag{8.18}$$

We shall examine the various classes of two substrate reactions to determine detailed rate equations which provide expressions for rate of reaction.

TABLE 8.3 Possible Mechanisms for Single-Site Enzyme with Two Substrates

Ternary complex mechanism: (EAB) formed		**Enzyme-substituted mechanism: A binds and is released; group transferred to B**
Compulsory order	Random order	Compulsory binding order
A binds before B	A or B can bind first	(Sequential mechanism)

Compulsory Order Reactions

Pseudosteady-State Hypothesis

In compulsory order, steady-state systems, one substrate must be added prior to the addition of the second substrate. The reaction pathway can thus be visualized as:

$$\begin{array}{ccccc} & & \text{EAB} \underset{k_{-R}}{\overset{k_R}{\rightleftharpoons}} \text{EPQ} \xrightarrow{k_Q} \text{EP} + \text{Q} \\ & & k_B \uparrow\downarrow k_{-B} \qquad\qquad\qquad \downarrow k_P \\ & & \text{B} \qquad\qquad\qquad\qquad \text{E} + \text{P} \\ & & + \\ \text{E} + \text{A} & \underset{k_{-A}}{\overset{k_A}{\rightleftharpoons}} & \text{EA} \end{array} \tag{8.19}$$

The substrates must be added in the order A and then B, and products are released in compulsory order as well. We can write the equation below for the total amount of enzyme in the system as

$$[E]_0 = [E] + [EA] + [EAB] + [EPQ] + [EP] \tag{8.20}$$

The analysis proceeds by assuming that all ES complexes are at pseudosteady state and that the rate of formation of P is given by

$$r_P = k_P[EP] \tag{8.21}$$

Expressions for each of the ES and enzyme–product complexes can now be written:

$$0 = r_{EA} = k_A[E][A] - k_{-A}[EA] - k_B[EA][B] + k_{-B}[EAB] \tag{8.22}$$

$$0 = r_{EAB} = k_B[EA][B] - k_{-B}[EAB] - k_R[EAB] + k_{-R}[EPQ] \tag{8.23}$$

$$0 = r_{EPQ} = k_R[EAB] - k_{-R}[EPQ] - k_Q[EPQ] \tag{8.24}$$

$$0 = r_{EP} = k_Q[EPQ] - k_P[EP] \tag{8.25}$$

Using these equations, we can eliminate the intermediates starting from Eqn (8.25) to obtain

$$[EP] = \frac{k_Q}{k_P}[EPQ] \tag{8.26}$$

$$[EPQ] = \frac{k_R}{k_{-R} + k_Q}[EAB] \tag{8.27}$$

$$[EAB] = \frac{k_B[B]}{k_{-B} + k_R - \dfrac{k_R k_{-R}}{k_{-R} + k_Q}}[EA] = \frac{k_B[B]}{k_{-B} + \dfrac{k_R k_Q}{k_{-R} + k_Q}}[EA] \tag{8.28}$$

$$[EA] = \frac{k_A[A]}{k_{-A} + k_B[B] - \dfrac{k_{-B} k_B[B]}{k_{-B} + \dfrac{k_R k_Q}{k_{-R} + k_Q}}}[E] = \frac{k_A[A]}{k_{-A} + \dfrac{k_B k_R k_Q}{k_{-B}(k_{-R} + k_Q) + k_R k_Q}[B]}[E] \tag{8.29}$$

Back substitution of [EA] to [EAB], [EPQ], and [EP], we express all the concentrations of complexes to [E], [A], and [B]. Applying the enzyme balance, Eqn (8.20), we then obtain.

$$[\mathrm{E}] = \frac{[\mathrm{E}]_0}{1 + \dfrac{k_\mathrm{A}[\mathrm{A}]}{k_{-\mathrm{A}} + \dfrac{k_\mathrm{B}k_\mathrm{R}k_\mathrm{Q}}{k_{-\mathrm{B}}(k_{-\mathrm{R}} + k_\mathrm{Q}) + k_\mathrm{R}k_\mathrm{Q}}[\mathrm{B}]} \left\{ 1 + \dfrac{k_\mathrm{B}}{k_{-\mathrm{B}} + \dfrac{k_\mathrm{R}k_\mathrm{Q}}{k_{-\mathrm{R}} + k_\mathrm{Q}}} [\mathrm{B}] \left(1 + \dfrac{k_\mathrm{R}}{k_{-\mathrm{R}} + k_\mathrm{Q}} \times \dfrac{k_\mathrm{P} + k_\mathrm{Q}}{k_\mathrm{P}} \right) \right\}} \tag{8.30}$$

The overall rate expression is then

$$r_\mathrm{P} = \frac{[\mathrm{E}]_0[\mathrm{A}][\mathrm{B}]}{\dfrac{k_{-\mathrm{A}}(k_{-\mathrm{B}}k_{-\mathrm{R}} + k_{-\mathrm{B}}k_\mathrm{Q} + k_\mathrm{R}k_\mathrm{Q})}{k_\mathrm{A}k_\mathrm{B}k_\mathrm{R}k_\mathrm{Q}} + \dfrac{[\mathrm{B}]}{k_\mathrm{A}} + \dfrac{k_{-\mathrm{B}}k_{-\mathrm{R}} + k_{-\mathrm{B}}k_\mathrm{Q} + k_\mathrm{R}k_\mathrm{Q}}{k_\mathrm{B}k_\mathrm{R}k_\mathrm{Q}}[\mathrm{A}] + \dfrac{\dfrac{1}{k_\mathrm{P}} + \dfrac{1}{k_\mathrm{Q}} + k_{-\mathrm{R}} + k_\mathrm{Q}}{k_\mathrm{R}k_\mathrm{Q}}[\mathrm{A}][\mathrm{B}]} \tag{8.31}$$

Under conditions where both substrates are present in excess, Eqn (8.31) can be reduced to

$$r_\mathrm{P} = \frac{[\mathrm{E}]_0}{\dfrac{\dfrac{1}{k_\mathrm{P}} + \dfrac{1}{k_\mathrm{Q}} + k_{-\mathrm{R}} + k_\mathrm{Q}}{k_\mathrm{R}k_\mathrm{Q}}} = r_\mathrm{max} \tag{8.32}$$

If only one of the substrates is present in excess, we retain the terms containing the other substrate and obtain the reaction rates as functions of the limiting substrates:

$$r_\mathrm{P} = \frac{[\mathrm{E}]_0[\mathrm{A}]}{\dfrac{1}{k_\mathrm{A}} + \dfrac{\dfrac{1}{k_\mathrm{P}} + \dfrac{1}{k_\mathrm{Q}} + k_{-\mathrm{R}} + k_\mathrm{Q}}{k_\mathrm{R}k_\mathrm{Q}}[\mathrm{A}]} \tag{8.33a}$$

$$r_\mathrm{P} = \frac{[\mathrm{E}]_0[\mathrm{B}]}{\dfrac{k_{-\mathrm{B}}k_{-\mathrm{R}} + k_{-\mathrm{B}}k_\mathrm{Q} + k_\mathrm{R}k_\mathrm{Q}}{k_\mathrm{B}k_\mathrm{R}k_\mathrm{Q}} + \dfrac{\dfrac{1}{k_\mathrm{P}} + \dfrac{1}{k_\mathrm{Q}} + k_{-\mathrm{R}} + k_\mathrm{Q}}{k_\mathrm{R}k_\mathrm{Q}}[\mathrm{B}]} \tag{8.33b}$$

We recover the single (limiting)-substrate rate expression as discussed in the previous section.

Fast Equilibrium Step Analysis

By assuming that the ES complexes are all in equilibrium, the analysis is considerably simplified. Let

$$K_\mathrm{A} = \frac{k_{-\mathrm{A}}}{k_\mathrm{A}}; \; K_\mathrm{B} = \frac{k_{-\mathrm{B}}}{k_\mathrm{B}}; \; K_\mathrm{R} = \frac{k_{-\mathrm{R}}}{k_\mathrm{R}} \tag{8.34}$$

where K's are dissociation constants for the complexes.

By following an analysis similar to that used previously, we eliminate the concentrations of intermediates by using the equilibrium expressions, and write the reaction rate as

$$r_P = \frac{k_Q[E]_0[A][B]}{K_A K_B K_R + K_B K_R[A] + K_R[A][B]} \tag{8.35}$$

Random-Order Reactions

In the case of random-order reactions, we must consider two parallel pathways for the addition of substrates A and B to the enzyme. The resulting EAB complex then undergoes reaction to form EPQ, and these products are then released in any order. The reaction pathway is shown schematically below for the simplest case of rapid equilibrium between all the ES complexes.

$$\begin{array}{l}
E + A \underset{k_{-A}}{\overset{k_A}{\rightleftharpoons}} EA, \quad EA + B \underset{k_{-B}}{\overset{k_B}{\rightleftharpoons}} EAB \\
E + B \underset{k_{-B}}{\overset{k_B}{\rightleftharpoons}} EB, \quad EB + A \underset{k_{-A}}{\overset{k_A}{\rightleftharpoons}} EAB \\
EAB \underset{k_{-R}}{\overset{k_R}{\rightleftharpoons}} EPQ \xrightarrow{k_Q} EP + Q, \quad EP \xrightarrow{k_P} E + P
\end{array} \tag{8.36}$$

Using the same method as before to eliminate the concentrations of the ES complexes apart from EAB in the overall enzyme conservation equation, we can derive the following expression for the rate of reaction.

$$r_P = \frac{k_Q[E]_0[A][B]}{K_A K_B + K_A[A] + K_B[B] + [A][B]} \tag{8.37}$$

The case of steady state existing among the ES complexes rather than equilibrium is considerably more complex to analyze. We must consider the two possible routes for release of products P and Q from the EPQ complex.

Enzyme-Substituted Reactions (the Ping-Pong Mechanism)

In enzyme-substituted or double-displacement mechanisms, both substrates need not be bound together at the active site of the enzyme. No ternary intermediate is formed. This mechanism occurs when, for example, a phosphate-transferring enzyme, such as phosphoglycerate mutase, is phosphorylated. One substrate (A) reacts with the enzyme to give E* (e.g. a phosphorylenzyme) which then transfers the phosphoryl group to the second substrate B.

$$\begin{array}{l}
E + A \underset{k_{-A}}{\overset{k_A}{\rightleftharpoons}} EA \xrightarrow{k_Q} E^* + Q \\
E^* + B \underset{k_{-B}}{\overset{k_B}{\rightleftharpoons}} E^*B \xrightarrow{k_P} E + P
\end{array} \tag{8.38}$$

Kinetics of this type thus provides information about the existence of a covalent intermediate. Often the finding of double-displacement (or "ping-pong") kinetics is used as evidence for the existence of this intermediate, but other confirming information should be sought. The kinetic pattern of this type of mechanism is unique. Following the same technique we used earlier, the rate expression can be derived as

$$r_P = \frac{[E]_0[A][B]}{\left(\frac{1}{k_Q} + \frac{1}{k_P}\right)[A][B] + \frac{k_{-A} + k_Q}{k_A + k_Q}[B] + \frac{k_{-B} + k_P}{k_B + k_P}[A]} \tag{8.39}$$

8.2.4.2. Allosteric Enzymes

Some enzymes have more than one substrate-binding site. The binding of one substrate to the enzyme facilitates binding of other substrate molecules. This behavior is known as *allostery* or *cooperative binding*, and regulatory enzymes show this behavior. The rate expression in this case is

$$r_P = \frac{r_{max}[S]^n}{K'_m + [S]^n} \tag{8.40}$$

where n = cooperativity coefficient and $n > 1$ indicates positive cooperativity. Figure 8.10 compares Michaelis–Menten kinetics with allosteric enzyme kinetics, indicating a sigmoidal shape of $r_P \sim [S]$ plot for allosteric enzymes. The shape of curve is different as the increase in the reaction rate is slower at low substrate concentration due to effectively higher reaction rate as expressed by Eqn (8.16).

8.2.4.3. Inhibited Enzyme kinetics

Certain compounds may bind to enzymes and reduce their activity. These compounds are known to be enzyme inhibitors. Enzyme inhibitions may be irreversible or reversible.

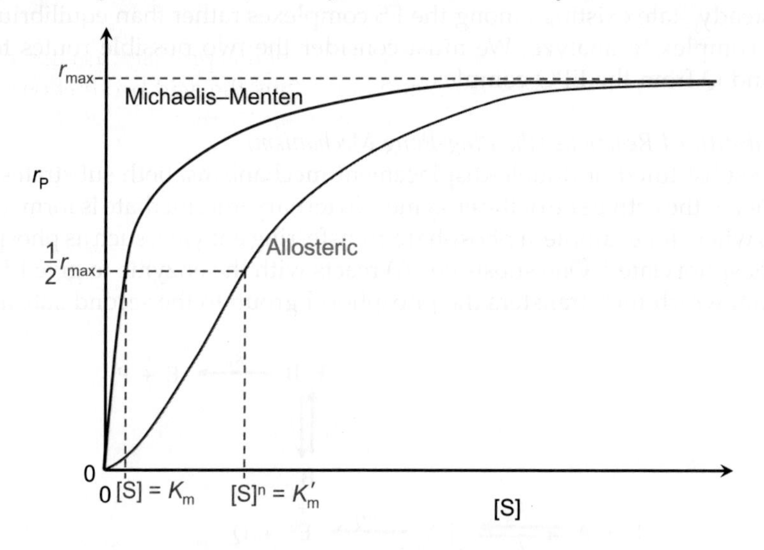

FIGURE 8.10 Comparison of Michaelis–Menten and allosteric enzyme kinetics.

Irreversible inhibitors such as heavy metals (lead, cadium, mercury, and others) form a stable complex with enzyme and reduce enzyme activity. Such enzyme inhibition may be reversed only by using chelating agents such as ethylenediaminetetraacetic acid (EDTA) and citrate. Reversible inhibitors may dissociate more easily from the enzyme after binding. The three major classes of reversible enzyme inhibitions are competitive, noncompetitive, and uncompetitive inhibitions. The substrate may act as an inhibitor in some cases.

Competitive inhibitors are usually substrate analogs and compete with substrate for the active site of the enzyme. The competitive enzyme inhibition scheme can be described as

$$\begin{array}{l} E + S \underset{k_{-1}}{\overset{k_1}{\rightleftharpoons}} ES \xrightarrow{k_2} E + P \\ + \\ I \\ \updownarrow K_I \\ EI \end{array} \tag{8.41}$$

Assuming rapid equilibrium and with the definition of

$$K_m = \frac{k_{-1}}{k_1} = \frac{[E][S]}{[ES]} \tag{8.42}$$

$$K_I = \frac{[E][I]}{[EI]} \tag{8.43}$$

$$[E]_0 = [E] + [ES] + [EI] \tag{8.44}$$

and

$$r_p = k_2[ES] \tag{8.45}$$

we can develop the following equation for the rate of enzymatic conversion:

$$r_P = \frac{r_{max}[S]}{K_m\left(1 + \frac{[I]}{K_I}\right) + [S]} \tag{8.46}$$

or

$$r_P = \frac{r_{max}[S]}{K_{m,app} + [S]} \tag{8.47}$$

where

$$K_{m,app} = K_m\left(1 + \frac{[I]}{K_I}\right) \tag{8.48}$$

The net effect of competitive inhibition is an increased value of $K_{m,app}$ and, therefore, reduced reaction rate. Competitive inhibition can be overcome by high concentrations of substrate.

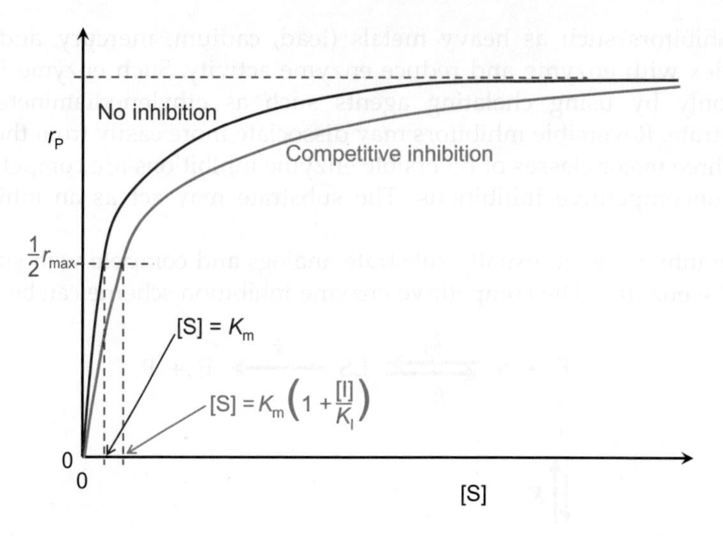

FIGURE 8.11 Comparison of Michaelis–Menten and competitive inhibition enzyme kinetics.

Figure 8.11 shows a comparison between the rate with the competitive enzyme inhibition and that of the Michaelis–Menten kinetics. One can observe that the general shape of the curve is the same, except a stretch of the curve along the substrate concentration axis.

Noncompetitive inhibitors are not substrate analogs. Inhibitors bind on sites other than the active site and reduce enzyme affinity to the substrate. Noncompetitive enzyme inhibition can be described as follows:

$$\begin{array}{ccccc} E + S & \underset{}{\overset{K_m}{\rightleftharpoons}} & ES & \xrightarrow{k_2} & E + P \\ + & & + & & \\ I & & I & & \\ \Big\updownarrow K_I & & \Big\updownarrow K_I & & \\ EI + S & \overset{K_m}{\rightleftharpoons} & EIS & & \end{array} \tag{8.49}$$

$$K_m = \frac{[E][S]}{[ES]} = \frac{[EI][S]}{[EIS]} \tag{8.50}$$

$$K_I = \frac{[E][I]}{[EI]} = \frac{[ES][I]}{[EIS]} \tag{8.51}$$

$$[E]_0 = [E] + [ES] + [EI] + [EIS] \tag{8.52}$$

and

$$r_P = k_2[ES] \tag{8.53}$$

We can develop the following equation for the rate of enzymatic conversion:

$$r_P = \frac{r_{max}[S]}{\left(1 + \frac{[I]}{K_I}\right)(K_m + [S])} \tag{8.54}$$

or

$$r_P = \frac{r'_{max}[S]}{K_m + [S]} \tag{8.55}$$

where

$$r'_{max} = \frac{r_{max}}{1 + \frac{[I]}{K_I}} \tag{8.56}$$

The net effect of noncompetitive inhibition is a reduction in r_{max}. High substrate concentrations would not overcome noncompetitive inhibition. Figure 8.12 illustrates the noncompetitive rate as compared with the Michaelis–Menten kinetics. Other reagents need to be added to block binding of the inhibitor to the enzyme. In some forms of noncompetitive inhibition r_{max} is reduced and K_m is increased. This occurs if the complex ESI can form product.

Uncompetitive inhibitors bind to the ES complex only and have no affinity for the enzyme itself. The scheme for uncompetitive inhibition is

$$\begin{array}{ccc} E + S \overset{K_m}{\rightleftarrows} & ES & \xrightarrow{k_2} E + P \\ & + & \\ & I & \\ & \Big\downarrow\!\Big\uparrow K_I & \\ & ESI & \end{array} \tag{8.57}$$

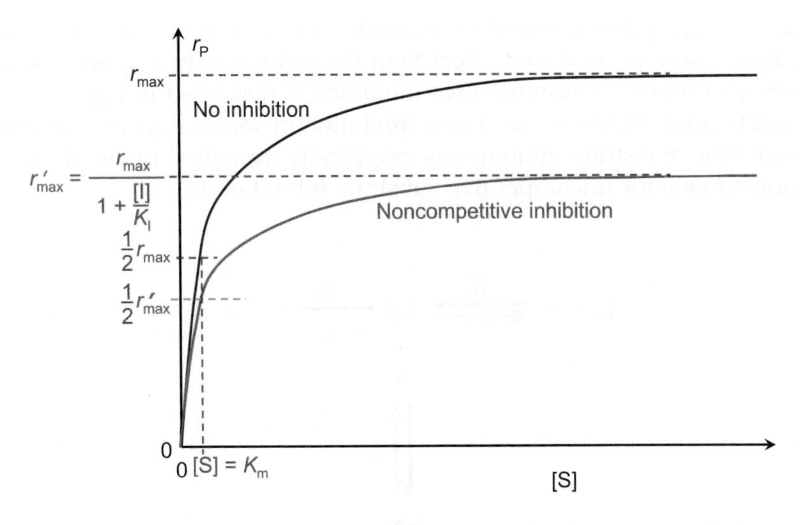

FIGURE 8.12 Comparison of Michaelis–Menten and noncompetitive inhibition enzyme kinetics.

$$K_m = \frac{[E][S]}{[ES]} \tag{8.58}$$

$$K_I = \frac{[ES][I]}{[ESI]} \tag{8.59}$$

$$[E]_0 = [E] + [ES] + [ESI] \tag{8.60}$$

and

$$r_P = k_2[ES] \tag{8.61}$$

we can develop the following equation for the rate of enzymatic conversion:

$$r_P = \frac{r_{max}[S]}{K_m + \left(1 + \frac{[I]}{K_I}\right)[S]} \tag{8.62}$$

or

$$r_P = \frac{r'_{max}[S]}{K'_m + [S]} \tag{8.63}$$

where

$$r'_{max} = \frac{r_{max}}{1 + \frac{[I]}{K_I}} \tag{8.64}$$

$$K'_m = \frac{K_m}{1 + \frac{[I]}{K_I}} \tag{8.65}$$

The net effect of uncompetitive inhibition is a reduction in both r_{max} and K_m values. Reduction in r_{max} has a more pronounced effect than the reduction in K_m, and the net result is a reduction in reaction rate. Uncompetitive inhibition is described in Fig. 8.13.

High substrate concentrations may cause inhibition in some enzymatic reactions, known as *substrate inhibition*. Substrate inhibition is graphically described in Fig. 8.14.

The reaction scheme for uncompetitive substrate inhibition is

$$\begin{array}{ccccc} E + S & \overset{K_m}{\rightleftharpoons} & ES & \xrightarrow{k_2} & E + P \\ & & + & & \\ & & S & & \\ & & \updownarrow K_{S2} & & \\ & & ES_2 & & \end{array} \tag{8.66}$$

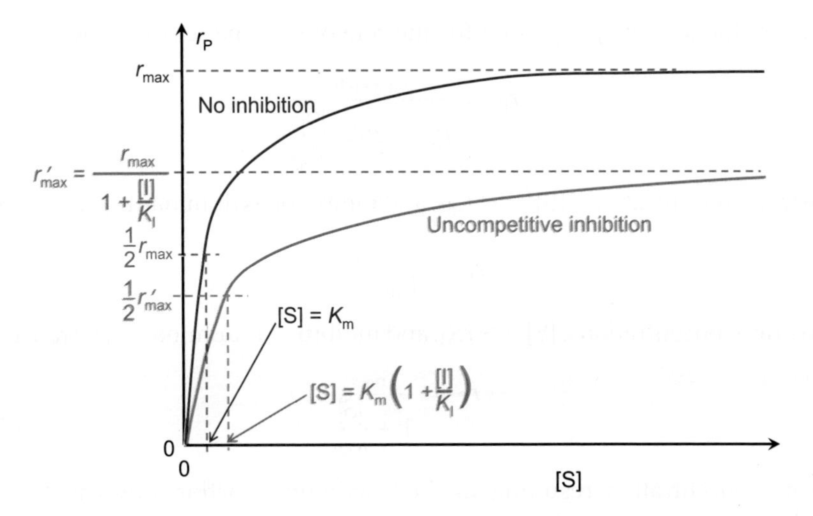

FIGURE 8.13 Comparison of Michaelis–Menten and uncompetitive inhibition enzyme kinetics.

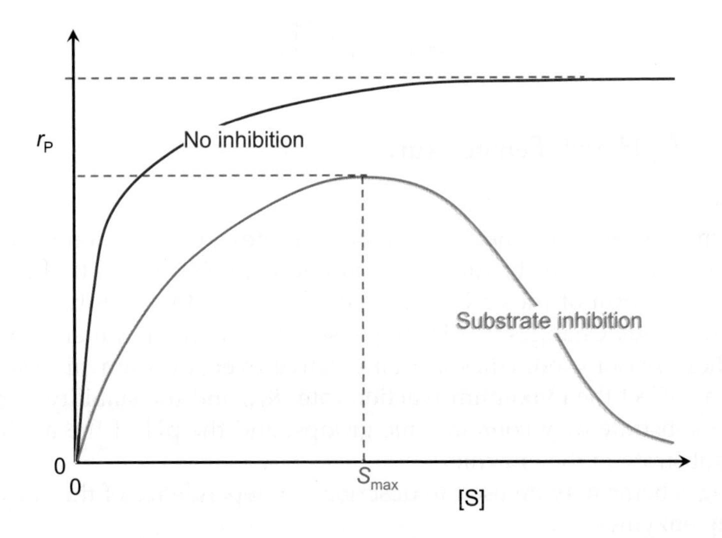

FIGURE 8.14 Comparison of substrate inhibited and uninhibited enzymatic reactions.

$$K_m = \frac{[E][S]}{[ES]} \tag{8.67}$$

$$K_{S2} = \frac{[ES][S]}{[ES_2]} \tag{8.68}$$

$$[E]_0 = [E] + [ES] + [ES_2]$$

and

$$r_P = k_2[ES] \tag{8.70}$$

we can develop the following equation for the rate of enzymatic conversion:

$$r_P = \frac{r_{max}[S]}{K_m + [S] + \frac{[S]^2}{K_{S2}}} \tag{8.71}$$

At low substrate concentrations, $[S]^2 << K_{S2}$, and inhibition is dominant. The rate in this case is

$$r_P = \frac{r_{max}[S]}{K_m + [S]} \tag{8.72}$$

At high substrate concentrations, $[S] >> K_M$, and inhibition is dominant. The rate in this case is

$$r_P = \frac{r_{max}}{1 + \frac{[S]}{K_{S2}}} \tag{8.73}$$

The substrate concentration resulting in the maximum reaction rate can be determined by setting $\frac{dr_P}{d[S]} = 0$. The $[S]_{max}$ is given by

$$S_{max} = \sqrt{K_m K_{S2}} \tag{8.74}$$

8.2.5. Effects of pH and Temperature

8.2.5.1. pH Effects

Certain enzymes have ionic groups on their active sites, and these ionic groups must be in a suitable form (acid or base) to function. Variations in the pH of the medium result in changes in the ionic form of the active site and changes in the activity of the enzyme and hence the reaction rate. Changes in pH may also alter the three-dimensional shape of the enzyme. For these reasons, enzymes are only active over a certain pH range. The pH of the medium may affect the maximum reaction rate, K_m, and the stability of the enzyme. In some cases, the substrate may contain ionic groups, and the pH of the medium affects the affinity of the substrate to the enzyme.

The following scheme may be used to describe pH dependence of the enzymatic reaction rate for ionizing enzymes.

$$\begin{array}{l} E^- + H^+ \\ \quad \Updownarrow K_{a2} \\ EH + S \underset{}{\overset{K_m}{\rightleftharpoons}} EHS \xrightarrow{k_2} EH + P \\ + \\ H^+ \\ \quad \Updownarrow K_{a1} \\ EH_2^+ \end{array} \tag{8.75}$$

With the definition of

$$K_{\mathrm{m}} = \frac{[\mathrm{EH}][\mathrm{S}]}{[\mathrm{EHS}]} \tag{8.76}$$

$$K_{\mathrm{a1}} = \frac{[\mathrm{EH}][\mathrm{H}^+]}{[\mathrm{EH}_2^+]} \tag{8.77}$$

$$K_{\mathrm{a2}} = \frac{[\mathrm{EH}]}{[\mathrm{E}^-][\mathrm{H}^+]} \tag{8.78}$$

$$[\mathrm{E}]_0 = [\mathrm{E}^-] + [\mathrm{EH}] + [\mathrm{EH}_2^+] \tag{8.79}$$

and

$$r_{\mathrm{p}} = k_2[\mathrm{ES}] \tag{8.80}$$

We can derive the following rate expression:

$$r_{\mathrm{P}} = \frac{r_{\max}[\mathrm{S}]}{K_{\mathrm{m}}\left(1 + \frac{K_{\mathrm{a2}}}{[\mathrm{H}^+]} + \frac{[\mathrm{H}^+]}{K_{\mathrm{a1}}}\right) + [\mathrm{S}]} \tag{8.81}$$

or

$$r_{\mathrm{P}} = \frac{r_{\max}[\mathrm{S}]}{K_{\mathrm{m,app}} + [\mathrm{S}]} \tag{8.82}$$

where

$$K_{\mathrm{m,app}} = K_{\mathrm{m}}\left(1 + \frac{K_{\mathrm{a2}}}{[\mathrm{H}^+]} + \frac{[\mathrm{H}^+]}{K_{\mathrm{a1}}}\right) \tag{8.83}$$

As a result of this behavior, the pH optimum of the enzyme is between pK_{a1} and pK_{a2}.

For the case of ionizing substrate, the resulting rate expression is similar to the case of ionizing enzymes. Consider

$$\begin{array}{l} \mathrm{E} + \mathrm{SH} \overset{K_{\mathrm{m}}}{\rightleftharpoons} \mathrm{ESH} \overset{k_2}{\longrightarrow} \mathrm{E} + \mathrm{PH} \\ \quad\ \ \Big\downarrow\!\!\uparrow K_{\mathrm{a1}} \\ \quad\ \ \mathrm{S} + \mathrm{H}^+ \end{array} \tag{8.84}$$

The rate expression can be developed:

$$r_{\mathrm{P}} = \frac{r_{\max}[\mathrm{S}]}{K_{\mathrm{m}}\left(1 + \frac{K_{\mathrm{a1}}}{[\mathrm{H}^+]}\right) + [\mathrm{S}]} \tag{8.85}$$

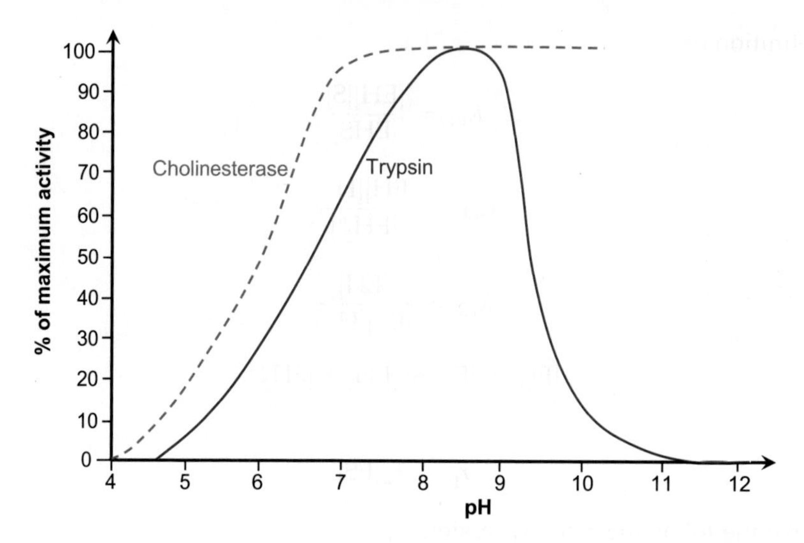

FIGURE 8.15 The pH-activity profiles of two enzymes.

Theoretical prediction of the pH optimum of enzymes requires a knowledge of the active site characteristics of enzymes, which are very difficult to obtain. The pH optimum for an enzyme is usually determined experimentally. Figure 8.15 depicts variation of enzymatic activity with pH for two different enzymes.

8.2.5.2. Temperature Effects

The rate of enzyme-catalyzed reactions increases with temperature up to a certain limit. Above a certain temperature, enzyme activity decreases with temperature because of enzyme denaturation. Figure 8.16 depicts the variation of reaction rate with temperature and the presence of an optimal temperature. The ascending part of Fig. 8.16 is known as *temperature activation*. The rate varies according to the Arrhenius equation in this region.

$$r_{max} = k_2[E] \tag{8.86}$$

$$k_2 = k_{20} \exp\left(-\frac{E_a}{RT}\right) \tag{8.87}$$

where E_a is the activation energy (kJ/mol), and [E] is the active enzyme concentration.

The descending part of Fig. 8.16 is known as *temperature inactivation* or *thermal denaturation*. The kinetics of thermal denaturation can be expressed as.

$$-\frac{d[E]}{dt} = k_d[E] \tag{8.88}$$

$$[E] = [E]_0 e^{-k_d t} \tag{8.89}$$

where $[E]_0$ is the initial enzyme concentration and k_d is the denaturation constant. k_d also varies with temperature according to the Arrhenius equation.

$$k_d = k_{d0} \exp\left(-\frac{E_d}{RT}\right) \tag{8.90}$$

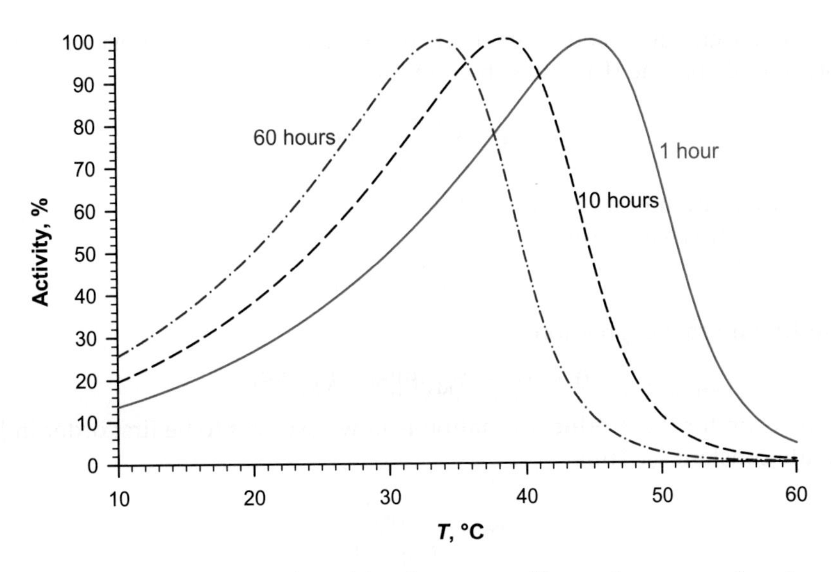

FIGURE 8.16 Effect of temperature on the activity of an enzyme. Here we have assumed a value of $E_a = 46$ kJ/mol, $E_d = 301$ kJ/mol, and $k_{d0} = 1.0 \times 10^{49}$/h. The increase in maximum rate is due to the increase in the activity via Arrhenius law, while the descending of the curve is due to the dominance of the thermal denaturation. The enzyme activity or relative maximum rate is averaged for a total exposure of 1-hour, 10-hour, and 60-hour to the temperature, which is shown in Eqn (8.92).

where E_d is the deactivation energy (kJ/mol). Consequently,

$$r_{max} = k_{20}[E]_0 \exp\left(-\frac{E_a}{RT}\right) e^{-k_d t} \tag{8.91}$$

The activity or average maximum rate for a total exposure time of t is thus given by

$$\bar{r}_{max} = \frac{\int_0^t r_{max} dt}{t} = k_{20}[E]_0 \exp\left(-\frac{E_a}{RT}\right) \frac{1 - e^{-k_d t}}{k_d t} \tag{8.92}$$

The activation energies of enzyme-catalyzed reactions are within the 15–85 kJ/mol range (mostly about 46 kJ/mol). Deactivation energies E_d vary between 170 and 550 kJ/mol (mostly about 300 kJ/mol). That is, enzyme denaturation by temperature is much faster than enzyme activation. A rise in temperature from 30–40 °C results in a 1.8-fold increase in enzyme activity but a 45-fold increase in enzyme denaturation. Variations in temperature may affect both r_{max} and K_m values of enzymes. Figure 8.15 is plotted using Eqn (8.92).

8.2.6. Insoluble Substrates

Enzymes are often used to attack large, insoluble substrates such as woodchips (in biopulping for paper manufacture) or cellulosic residues from agriculture (e.g. cornstalks). In these cases, access to the reaction site on these biopolymers by enzymes is often limited by enzyme diffusion. The number of potential reactive sites exceeds the number of enzyme molecules. This situation is opposite to that of the typical situation with soluble substrates, where access to the enzyme's active site limits reaction. For example, considering the equilibrium adsorption of enzyme (E) onto substrate (S)

$$E + S \underset{k_{des}}{\overset{k_{ads}}{\rightleftarrows}} ES \tag{8.93}$$

If the total concentration of adsorption sites on the substrate surface is $[S]_0$, expressed per liquid volume, then we can write

$$[S]_0 = [S] + [ES] \tag{8.94}$$

and the equilibrium rate expression

$$0 = r_1 = k_{ads}[E][S] - k_{des}[ES] \tag{8.95}$$

The rate of reaction for the product formation is now assumed to be first order in [ES], with a constant rate constant k_2. Thus,

$$r_P = \frac{r_{max}[E]}{K_{eq} + [E]} \tag{8.96}$$

where

$$r_{max} = k_2[S]_0 \tag{8.98}$$

and

$$K_{eq} = \frac{k_{des}}{k_{ads}} \tag{8.99}$$

The previous equation assumes slow binding of enzyme (i.e. $[E] \approx [E]_0$). S_0 is the number of substrate bonds available initially for breakage, and k_{des} and k_{ads} refer to rates of enzyme desorption and adsorption onto the insoluble matrix, respectively.

8.3. IMMOBILIZED ENZYME SYSTEMS

The restriction of enzyme mobility in a fixed space is known as *enzyme immobilization.* In many applications, immobilization of enzymes provides important advantages, such as enzyme reutilization and elimination of enzyme recovery and purification processes, and may provide a better environment for enzyme activity. Since enzymes are expensive, catalyst reuse is critical for many processes. Immobilized enzymes are typically macroscopic catalysts that are retained in the reactor; therefore, continuous replacement of the enzyme is not necessary, and separation of the enzyme from other components in the reaction mixture is simplified. Immobilized enzymes can be employed in a wide range of different reactor configurations and, because high concentrations of catalyst can be obtained, correspondingly high volumetric productivities are possible. Higher reactor productivities lead to lower capital costs. Moreover, immobilized enzymes are often more stable than enzymes in solution. It is also important to note that the properties of the support, for example, its ionic charge, can in some cases be exploited to modify the behavior of the enzyme. Since some

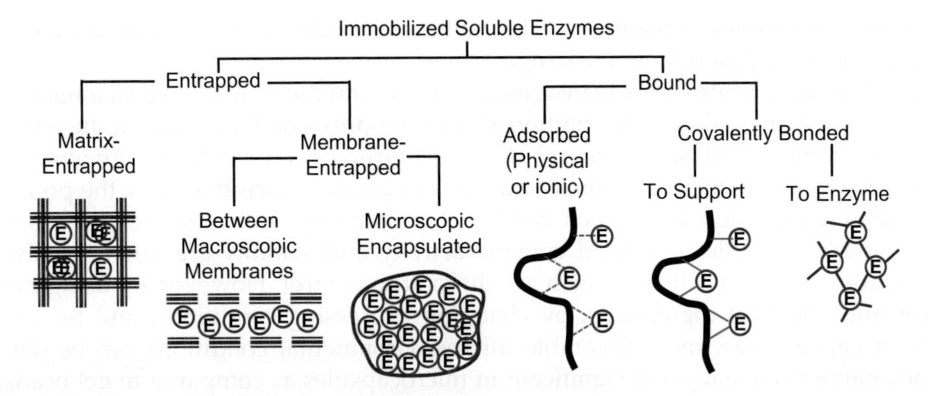

FIGURE 8.17 Major immobilization methods.

of the intracellular enzymes are membrane bound, immobilized enzymes provide a model system to mimic and understand the action of some membrane-bound intracellular enzymes. Product purity is usually improved, and effluent handling problems are minimized by immobilization.

8.3.1. Methods of Immobilization

Major methods of immobilization are summarized in Fig. 8.17. The two major categories are entrapment and surface immobilization.

8.3.1.1. Entrapment

Entrapment is the physical enclosure of enzymes in a small space. Matrix entrapment and membrane entrapment, including microencapsulation, are the two major methods of entrapment.

Matrices used for enzyme immobilization are usually polymeric materials such as Ca-alginate, agar, κ-carrageenin, polyacrylamide, and collagen. However, some solid matrices such as activated carbon, porous ceramic, and diatomaceous earth can also be used for this purpose. The matrix can be a particle, a membrane, or a fiber. When immobilizing in a polymer matrix, enzyme solution is mixed with polymer solution before polymerization takes place. Polymerized gel-containing enzyme is either extruded or a template is used to shape the particles from a liquid polymer–enzyme mixture. Entrapment and surface attachment may be used in combination in some cases.

Membrane entrapment of enzymes is possible; for example, hollow-fiber units have been used to entrap an enzyme solution between thin, semipermeable membranes. Membranes of nylon, cellulose, polysulfone, and polyacrylate are commonly used. Configurations, other than hollow fibers, are possible, but in all cases, a semipermeable membrane is used to retain high molecular weight compounds (enzyme), while allowing small molecular weight compounds (substrate or products) access to the enzyme.

A special form of membrane entrapment is *microencapsulation.* In this technique, microscopic hollow spheres are formed. The spheres contain the enzyme solution, while the sphere is enclosed within a porous membrane. The membrane can be polymeric or an enriched interfacial phase formed around a micro drop.

Despite the aforementioned advantages, enzyme entrapment may have its inherent problems, such as enzyme leakage into solution, significant diffusion limitations, reduced enzyme activity and stability, and lack of control of microenvironmental conditions. Enzyme leakage can be overcome by reducing the molecular weight cutoff of membranes or the pore size of solid matrices. Diffusion limitations can be eliminated by reducing the particle size of matrices and/or capsules. Reduced enzyme activity and stability are due to unfavorable microenvironmental conditions, which are difficult to control. However, by using different matrices and chemical ingredients, by changing processing conditions, and by reducing particle or capsule size, more favorable microenvironmental conditions can be obtained. Diffusion barrier is usually less significant in microcapsules as compared to gel beads.

8.3.1.2. Surface Immobilization

The two major types of immobilization of enzymes on the surfaces of support materials are adsorption and covalent binding.

Adsorption is the attachment of enzymes on the surfaces of support particles by weak physical forces, such as van der Waals or dispersion forces. The active site of the adsorbed enzyme is usually unaffected, and nearly full activity is retained upon adsorption. However, desorption of enzymes is a common problem especially in the presence of strong hydrodynamic forces, since binding forces are weak. Adsorption of enzymes may be stabilized by cross-linking with glutaraldehyde. Glutaraldehyde treatment can denature some proteins. Support materials used for enzyme adsorption can be inorganic materials, such as alumina, silica, porous glass, ceramics, diatomaceous earth, clay, and bentonite, or organic materials, such as cellulose (CMC, DEAE-cellulose), starch, and activated carbon, and ion-exchange resins, such as Amberlite, Sephadex, and Dowex. The surfaces of the support materials may need to be pretreated (chemically or physically) for effective immobilization.

Covalent binding is the retention of enzyme on support surfaces by covalent bond formation. Enzyme molecules bind to support material via certain functional groups, such as amino, carboxyl, hydroxyl, and sulfhydryl groups. These functional groups must not be in the active site. One common trick is to block the active site by flooding the enzyme solution with a competitive inhibitor prior to covalent binding. Functional groups on support material are usually activated by using chemical reagents, such as cyanogen bromide, carbodiimide, and glutaraldehyde. Support materials with various functional groups and the chemical reagents used for the covalent binding of proteins are listed in Table 8.4.

Binding groups on the protein molecule are usually side groups (R) or the amino or carboxyl groups of the polypeptide chain. The cross-linking of enzyme molecules with each other using agents such as glutaraldehyde, bis-diazobenzidine, and 2,2-disulfonic acid is another method of enzyme immobilization. Cross-linking can be achieved in several different ways: enzymes can be cross-linked with glutaraldehyde to form an insoluble aggregate, adsorbed enzymes may be cross-linked, or cross-linking may take place following the impregnation of porous support material with enzyme solution. Cross-linking may cause significant changes in the active site of enzymes, and also severe diffusion limitations may result.

The most suitable support material and immobilization method vary depending on the enzyme and particular application. Two major criteria used in the selection of support

TABLE 8.4 Methods of Covalent Binding of Enzymes to Supports

Supports with –OH end group

a) Using cyanogen bromide

$$\begin{matrix}|\\HC{-}OH\\|\\HC{-}OH\\|\end{matrix} + CNBr \longrightarrow \begin{matrix}|\\HC{-}O\\|\\HC{-}O\\|\end{matrix}\!\!>\!C{=}NH \xrightarrow{+\ H_2N{-}Protein} \begin{matrix}|\\HC{-}O{-}NH{-}Protein\\|\\HC{-}OH\\|\end{matrix}$$

b) Using S-triazine derivatives

$$\vdash OH + Cl{-}(C_3N_3R){-}Cl \longrightarrow \vdash O{-}(C_3N_3R){-}Cl \xrightarrow{+\ H_2N{-}Protein} \vdash O{-}(C_3N_3R){-}NH{-}Protein$$

Supports with $-NH_2$ end group

a) By diazotization

$$\vdash C_6H_4{-}NH_2 \xrightarrow[HCl]{+\ NaNO_2} \vdash C_6H_4{-}N_2^+Cl^- \xrightarrow{+\ Protein} \vdash C_6H_4{-}N{=}N{-}Protein$$

b) Using glutaraldehyde

$$\vdash NH_2 + HCO{-}(CH_2{-})_3CHO \longrightarrow \vdash N{=}CH{-}(CH_2{-})_3CHO \xrightarrow{+\ H_2N{-}Protein} \vdash N{=}CH{-}(CH_2{-})_3CH{=}N{-}Protein$$

Supports with –COOH end group

a) via azide derivative

$$\vdash OCH_2COOH \xrightarrow[H^+]{+\ CH_3OH} \vdash OCH_2COOCH_3 \xrightarrow{+\ H_2NNH_2} \vdash OCH_2CONHNH_2 \xrightarrow[HCl]{+\ NaNO_2} \vdash OCH_2CON_3 \xrightarrow{+\ H_2N{-}Protein} \vdash OCH_2CONH{-}Protein$$

b) Using a carbodiimide

$$\vdash COOH + \begin{matrix}N{-}R_1\\\|\\C\\\|\\N{-}R\end{matrix} \longrightarrow \vdash \overset{O}{\overset{\|}{C}}{-}O{-}\begin{matrix}HN{-}R_1\\|\\C\\\|\\N{-}R\end{matrix} \xrightarrow{+\ H_2N{-}Protein} \vdash \overset{O}{\overset{\|}{C}}{-}NH{-}Protein + \begin{matrix}HNR_1\\|\\O{=}C\\|\\HNR\end{matrix}$$

Supports containing anhydrides

$$\begin{matrix}|\\CH_2\\|\\CH{-}C(=O)\\|\quad\ \ >O\\CH{-}C(=O)\\|\\CH_2\\|\end{matrix} \xrightarrow{+\ H_2N{-}Protein} \begin{matrix}|\\CH_2\\|\\CH{-}C(=O){-}NH{-}Protein\\|\\CH{-}C(=O){-}OH\\|\\CH_2\\|\end{matrix}$$

TABLE 8.5 Effects of Immobilization Methods on the Retention of Enzymatic Activity of Aminoacylase

Support	Method	Observed activity, units	Immobilized enzyme activity, %
Polyacrylamide	Entrapment	526	52.6
Nylon	Encapsulation	360	36.0
DEAE-cellulose	Ionic binding	668	55.2
DEAE-Spephadex A-50	Ionic binding	680	56.2
CM-Sephadex C-50	Ionic binding	0	0
Iodoacetyl cellulose	Covalent binding	472	39.0
CNBr-activated Sephadex	Covalent binding	12	1.0
AE-cellulose	Cross-linked with glutaraldehyde	8	0.6

Source: Chibata I., Tosa T., Sato T., Mori T. and Matuo Y., Proc. of the 4th Int. Fermentation Symp.: Fermentation Technology Today, *1972, p. 383–389.*

material are (1) the binding capacity of the support material, which is a function of charge density, functional groups, porosity, and hydrophobicity of the support surface, and (2) stability and retention of enzymatic activity, which is a function of functional groups on support material and microenvironmental conditions. If immobilization causes some conformational changes on the enzyme, or if reactive groups on the active site of the enzyme are involved in binding, a loss in enzyme activity can take place upon immobilization.

Usually, immobilization results in a loss in enzyme activity and stability. However, in some cases, immobilization may cause an increase in enzyme activity and stability due to more favorable microenvironmental conditions. Because enzymes often have more than one functional site that can bind the surface, an immobilized enzyme preparation may be very heterogeneous. Even when binding does not alter enzyme structure, some enzyme can be bound with the active site oriented away from the substrate solution and toward the support surface, decreasing the access of the substrate to the enzyme. Retention of activity varies with the method used. Table 8.5 summarizes the retention of activity of arninoacylase immobilized by different methods.

8.3.2. Electrostatic and Steric Effects in Immobilized Enzyme Systems

When enzymes are immobilized in a charged matrix as a result of a change in the microenvironment of the enzyme, the apparent bulk pH optimum of the immobilized enzyme will shift from that of soluble enzyme. The charged matrix will repel or attract substrates, product, cofactors, and H^+ depending on the type and quantity of surface charge. For an enzyme immobilized onto a charged support, the shift in the pH-activity profile is given by

$$\Delta pH = pH_i - pH_e = \frac{zN_F\Psi}{RT} \tag{8.100}$$

where pH_i and pH_e are internal and external pH values, respectively; z is the charge (valence) on the substrate; N_F is the Faraday constant (96,500 C/eq. g); Ψ is the electrostatic potential; and R is the gas constant. Expressions similar to Eqn (8.100) apply to other nonreactive-charged medium components. The intrinsic activity of the enzyme is altered by the local changes in pH and ionic constituents. Further alterations in the apparent kinetics are due to the repulsion or attraction of substrates or inhibitors.

The activity of an enzyme toward a high molecular weight substrate is usually reduced upon immobilization to a much greater extent than for a low-molecular-weight substrate. This is mainly because of steric hindrance by the support. Certain substrates, such as starch, have molecular weights comparable to those of enzymes and may therefore not be able to penetrate to the active sites of immobilized enzymes.

Immobilization also affects the thermal stability of enzymes. Thermal stability often increases upon immobilization due to the presence of thermal diffusion barriers and the constraints on protein unfolding. However, decreases in thermal stability have been noted in a few cases. The pH stability of enzymes usually increases upon immobilization, too.

8.4. ANALYSIS OF BIOPROCESS WITH ENZYMATIC REACTIONS

Enzymatic reactions are normally carried out in batch reactors. They can be carried out in flow reactors especially when enzymes are immobilized. Analysis with enzymatic reactions can be performed in the same manner as we have learned in Chapters 4 and 5.

Example 8-2. Urease catalyzed urea decomposition reaction

$$NH_2CONH_2 \rightarrow 2NH_3 + CO_2$$

is to be carried out in a batch reactor. The Michaelis–Menten rate parameters determined from experiment with an enzyme loading of 5 g/L are given by $r_{max} = 1.35 \text{ mol} \times l^{-1} \times s^{-1}$ and $K_m = 0.0265 \text{ mol/L}$. Determine the time needed for 90% conversion of urea to ammonia and carbon dioxide of a solution containing 0.2 mol/L of urea in a 2-l reactor. The enzyme loading is 0.001 g/L.

Solution. The Michaelis–Menten rate law is given by

$$r = \frac{r_{max} S}{K_m + S} \tag{E8-2.1}$$

We know that $K_m = 0.0265 \text{ mol/L}$. Since r_{max} is proportional to the enzyme loading, we have $r_{max} = 1.35 \times 0.001/5 \text{ mol} \times l^{-1} \times s^{-1} = 2.7 \times 10^{-4} \text{ mol} \times l^{-1} \times s^{-1}$.

Mole balance of substrate (urea) in the reactor gives

$$0 - 0 + r_s V = \frac{dn_s}{dt} \tag{E8-2.2}$$

The reactor volume is constant (isothermal liquid/suspended phase reaction). Equation (E8-2.2) is reduced to

$$-\frac{dS}{dt} = \frac{r_{max} S}{K_m + S} \tag{E8-2.3}$$

Separation of variable leads to,

$$\left(\frac{K_m}{S}+1\right)dS = -r_{max}dt \tag{E8-2.4}$$

Integrating Eqn (E8-2.4) from $t=0$ and $S=S_0$, we obtain

$$K_m \ln\frac{S}{S_0}+S-S_0 = -r_{max}t \tag{E8-2.5}$$

The conversion of substrate is defined as

$$f_S = \frac{S_0-S}{S_0} \tag{E8-2.6}$$

Substitute Eqn (E8-2.6) into Eqn (E8-2.5), we obtain

$$t = \frac{S_0 f_S - K_m \ln(1-f_S)}{r_{max}} \tag{E8-2.7}$$

Thus, the time required for 90% conversion is

$$t = \frac{S_0 f_S - K_m \ln(1-f_S)}{r_{max}} = \frac{0.1\times 0.9 - 0.0265\ln(1-0.9)}{2.7\times 10^{-4}}\ \text{s} = 559.3\ \text{s} = 9.322\ \text{min}$$

Example 8-3. Consider the reaction:

$$S \rightarrow P$$

catalyzed by enzyme E. Michaelis–Menten rate parameters are $r_{max}=0.15$/min and $K_m=0.01$ mol/L when the enzyme loading 0.1 g/L. CSTR has been selected to produce 100 mol of P per hour from a stream of substrate containing 1 mol-S/L. S costs \$0.1/mol, P sells for \$1/mol, and the enzyme E cost \$100/g. The cost of operating the reactor is \$0.1/L/h. Assume no value or cost of disposal of unreacted S (i.e. separation or recovery cost to S is identical to the fresh S cost).

(a) What is the relationship between rate of formation of P and enzyme loading?

(b) Perform a mole balance on the reactor to relate the concentration of exiting S with reactor size.

(c) What is the optimum concentration of S at the outlet of the reactor? What is the optimum enzyme loading?

(d) What is the cash flow per mole of product from the process?

Solution. A sketch of the reactor system is shown in Fig. E8-3. Substrate and enzyme are fed to the CSTR. The enzyme is let out unchanged, while some substrate is turned into product P.

(a) The maximum rate is proportional to the enzyme loading, that is,

$$r_{max} = kE_0 \tag{E8-3.1}$$

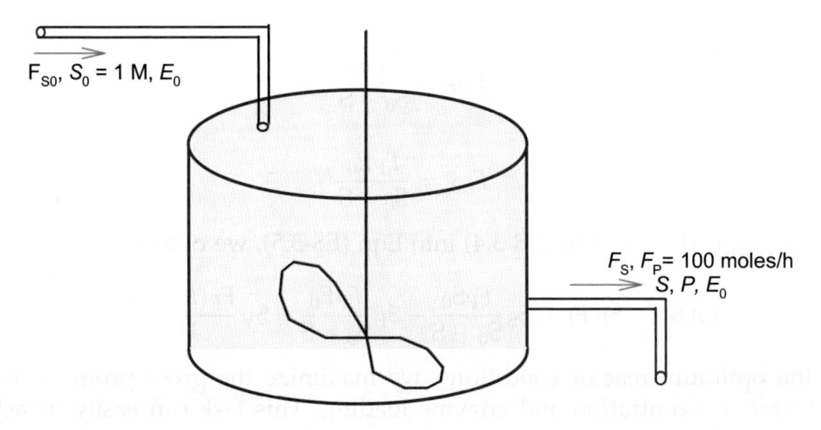

FIGURE E8-3 Well-mixed reaction vessel.

Thus, the rate of formation of P is given by

$$r_P = \frac{kE_0S}{K_m + S} \tag{E8-3.2}$$

$$K_m = 0.01 \text{ mol/L} \quad \text{and} \quad k = 0.15 \text{ min}^{-1}/(0.1 \text{ g/L}) = 1.5 \text{ L} \cdot \text{min}^{-1} \cdot \text{g}^{-1}.$$

(b) It is understood that the CSTR is operating under constant temperature (isothermal) and steady-state conditions, i.e. no accumulation of any sort of materials inside the reactor. Mole balance around the reactor for P yields

$$0 - F_P + r_P V = 0 \tag{E8-3.3}$$

Substituting Eqn (E8-3.2) into Eqn (E8-3.3), we obtain

$$V = \frac{F_P}{r_P} = F_P \frac{K_m + S}{kE_0S} \tag{E8-3.4}$$

(c) Based on the economic information at hand, we can estimate the gross profit for the reaction process as

$$GP\$ = \$_P F_P - \$_S F_{S0} - \$_E F_{E0} - \$_V V \tag{8-3.5}$$

where $\$_P$, $\$_S$, $\$_E$, and $\$_V$ are the molar value of product P, molar cost of substrate S, unit cost of enzyme, and the unit operating cost of reactor based on the reactor volume and time, respectively.

Based on the stoichiometry, we have

$$Q = \frac{F_P}{P} = \frac{F_P}{S_0 - S} \tag{E8-3.6}$$

which leads to

$$F_{S0} = \frac{F_P S_0}{S_0 - S} \tag{E8-3.7a}$$

$$F_{E0} = \frac{F_P E_0}{S_0 - S} \tag{E8-3.7b}$$

Substituting Eqns (E8-3.7) and (E8-3.4) into Eqn (E8-3.5), we obtain

$$\text{GP\$} = \$_P F_P - \$_S \frac{F_P S_0}{S_0 - S} - \$_E \frac{F_P E_0}{S_0 - S} - \$_V \frac{F_P(K_m + S)}{k E_0 S} \tag{E8-3.8}$$

To find the optimum reactor conditions, we maximize the gross profit by varying the effluent substrate concentration and enzyme loading. This task can easily be achieved by an optimizer like the Excel Solver. Substituting the known parameters into Eqn (E8-3.8), we obtain

$$\text{GP\$} = 1 \times 100 - 0.1 \times \frac{100 \times 1}{1 - S} - 100 \frac{100\, E_0}{1 - S} - 0.1 \times \frac{100 \times (0.01 + S)}{1.5 \times 60\, E_0 S} \$/\text{h}$$

which is reduced to

$$\text{GP\$} = 100 - \frac{10}{1 - S} - \frac{10000\, E_0}{1 - S} - \frac{0.01 + S}{9\, E_0 S} \$/\text{h} \tag{E8-3.9}$$

Maximizing the gross profit GP\$, we obtain: $S = 0.075969$ mol/L, $E_0 = 0.0024102$ g/L, and GP\$ = \$10.9256/h.

Therefore, we have found the optimum enzyme loading and the effluent substrate concentration.

(d) The cash flow based on Eqn (E8-3.8),

$$\frac{\text{GP\$}}{F_P} = \$_P - \$_S \frac{S_0}{S_0 - S} - \$_E \frac{E_0}{S_0 - S} - \$_V \frac{(K_m + S)}{k E_0 S} \tag{E8-3.14}$$

Or since we have GP\$ value already,

$$\frac{\text{GP\$}}{F_P} = \frac{10.9256}{100} \$/\text{mol-P} = \$0.109256/\text{mol-P}$$

This concludes the example. One must be careful of the units whenever numbers are inserted into the equation.

Example 8-3 shows that enzyme cost can be significant. Therefore, separate and reuse of enzyme is very important for bioprocess systems.

Example 8-4. It has been observed that substrate inhibition occurs in the following enzymatic reaction:

$$E + S \rightarrow P + E$$

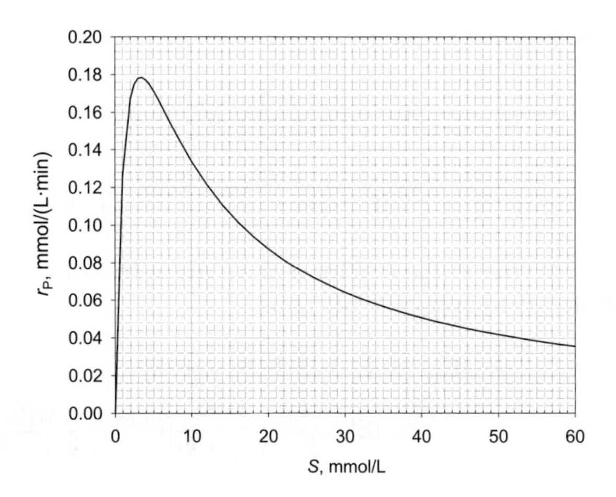

FIGURE E8-4.1

(a) Show that the rate law for substrate inhibition is consistent with the data shown in the Fig. E8-4.1 for r_P versus the substrate concentration of S.

(b) If this reaction is carried out in a fluidized CSTR that has a working volume of 5000 L, to which the volumetric flow rate is 15 L/min and the feed concentration of the substrate is 60 mmol/L, determine the possible conversion of substrate to the desired product. Since the enzyme is immobilized on the solid particle, assume that there is no loss of the enzyme to the effluent.

(c) What would be the effluent substrate concentration if the enzyme loading is 25% lower?

Solution. For substrate inhibition, the mechanism is given by

$$\mathrm{E + S} \underset{k_{-1}}{\overset{k_1}{\rightleftarrows}} \mathrm{E{\cdot}S} \tag{E8-4.1}$$

$$\mathrm{E{\cdot}S} \overset{k_2}{\rightarrow} \mathrm{P + E} \tag{E8-4.2}$$

$$\mathrm{E{\cdot}S + S} \underset{k_{-3}}{\overset{k_3}{\rightleftarrows}} \mathrm{S{\cdot}E{\cdot}S} \tag{E8-4.3}$$

The inhibition step, reaction (E8-4.3), renders the enzyme ineffective and thus slows down the overall reaction rate of utilizing the substrate. The rate of formation for P is given by

$$r_P = k_2[\mathrm{E{\cdot}S}] \tag{E8-4.4}$$

where the intermediate concentration can be obtained through pseudosteady-state hypotheses for the intermediates:

$$0 = r_{\mathrm{E\cdot S}} = k_1[\mathrm{E}][\mathrm{S}] - k_{-1}[\mathrm{E{\cdot}S}] - k_2[\mathrm{E{\cdot}S}] - k_3[\mathrm{E{\cdot}S}] + k_{-3}[\mathrm{S{\cdot}E{\cdot}S}] \tag{E8-4.5}$$

$$0 = r_{\mathrm{S\cdot E\cdot S}} = k_3[\mathrm{E{\cdot}S}][\mathrm{S}] - k_{-3}[\mathrm{S{\cdot}E{\cdot}S}] \tag{E8-4.6}$$

Equations (E8-4.5) and (E8-4.6) lead to

$$[\mathrm{E{\cdot}S}] = \frac{k_1[\mathrm{S}]}{k_{-1}+k_2}[\mathrm{E}] \tag{E8-4.7}$$

$$[\mathrm{S{\cdot}E{\cdot}S}] = \frac{k_3}{k_{-3}}[\mathrm{E{\cdot}S}][\mathrm{S}] = \frac{k_3}{k_{-3}}\frac{k_1[\mathrm{S}]}{k_{-1}+k_2}[\mathrm{E}][\mathrm{S}] \tag{E8-4.8}$$

The total amount of enzyme in the reactor is the sum of free enzyme [E] and those associated with the substrate, [E·S] and [S·E·S]. Thus,

$$\begin{aligned}[\mathrm{E}]_0 &= [\mathrm{E}] + [\mathrm{S{\cdot}E{\cdot}S}] + [\mathrm{E{\cdot}S}] \\ &= [\mathrm{E}] + \frac{k_3}{k_{-3}}\frac{k_1[\mathrm{S}]}{k_{-1}+k_2}[\mathrm{E}][\mathrm{S}] + \frac{k_1[\mathrm{S}]}{k_{-1}+k_2}[\mathrm{E}]\end{aligned} \tag{E8-4.9}$$

which leads to

$$[\mathrm{E}] = \frac{[\mathrm{E}]_0}{1+\dfrac{k_3}{k_{-3}}\dfrac{k_1[\mathrm{S}]}{k_{-1}+k_2}[\mathrm{S}]+\dfrac{k_1[\mathrm{S}]}{k_{-1}+k_2}} \tag{E8-4.10}$$

and

$$[\mathrm{E{\cdot}S}] = \frac{k_1[\mathrm{S}]}{1+\dfrac{k_3}{k_{-3}}\dfrac{k_1[\mathrm{S}]}{k_{-1}+k_2}[\mathrm{S}]+\dfrac{k_1[\mathrm{S}]}{k_{-1}+k_2}}\frac{[\mathrm{E}]_0}{k_{-1}+k_2} \tag{E8-4.11}$$

Substitute Eqns (E8-4.10) and (E8-4.11) into Eqn (E8-4.4), we obtain

$$r_\mathrm{P} = \frac{k_2[\mathrm{E}]_0[\mathrm{S}]}{\dfrac{k_{-1}+k_2}{k_1}+[\mathrm{S}]+\dfrac{k_3}{k_{-3}}[\mathrm{S}]^2} \tag{E8-4.12}$$

(a) Equation (E8-4.12) leads to

(1) When $[\mathrm{S}]=0$, $r_\mathrm{P}=0$;

(2) When [S] is low, r_P increases with S;

(3) When [S] is very high, r_P decreases with increasing [S] because of the $[\mathrm{S}]^2$ term in the denominator;

(4) There is only one maximum (peak) value for r_P as only [S] in the numerator and [S] and $[\mathrm{S}]^2$ in the denominator.

Therefore, the data or curve shown in Fig. E8-4.1 is consistent with Eqn (E8-4.12).

(b) Mole balance on the substrate around the CSTR (Fig. 8-4.2) leads to:

$$QS_0 - QS + r_\mathrm{S}V = 0$$

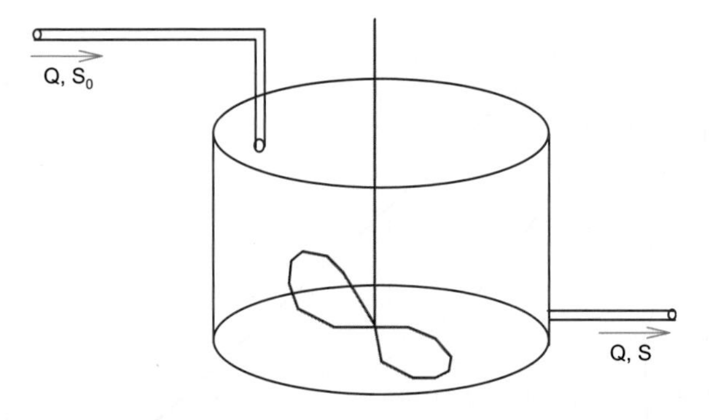

FIGURE 8-4.2 A schematic of a CSTR.

From stoichiometry, $\frac{r_S}{\nu_S} = \frac{r_P}{\nu_P}$. Thus

$$r_P = -r_S = \frac{QS_0 - QS}{V} = D(S_0 - S) \tag{E8-4.13}$$

$$D = Q/V = 15/5000/\text{min} = 3 \times 10^{-3}\ \text{min}^{-1}$$

Therefore, the mole balance Eqn (E8-4.13) is a straight line on the (S, r_P) plane with a negative slope of $-D$ (-3×10^{-3} min^{-1}) and intercept on the S-axis of $S_0 = 60$ mmol/L. Plot the mole balance line (red line) on to the Fig. 8-4.1 yields Fig. 8-4.3.

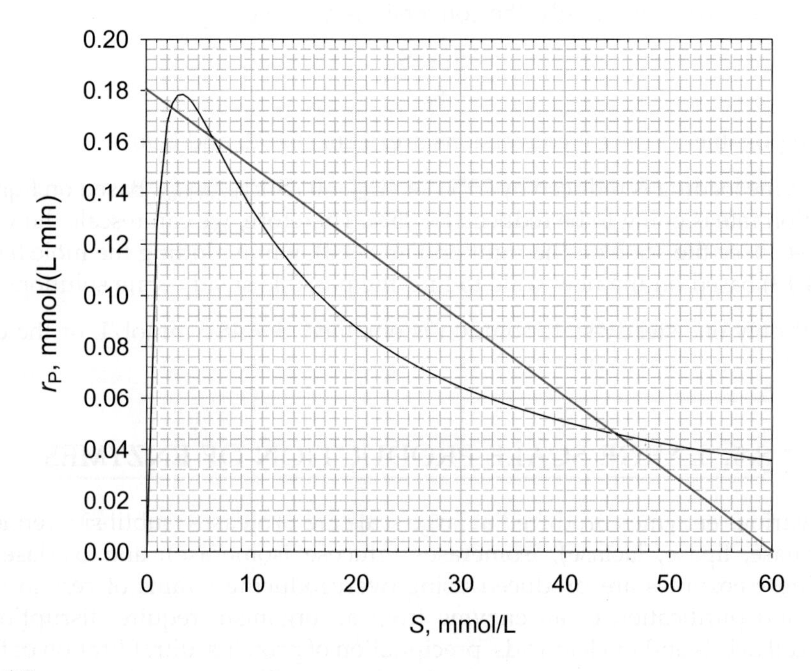

FIGURE 8-4.3

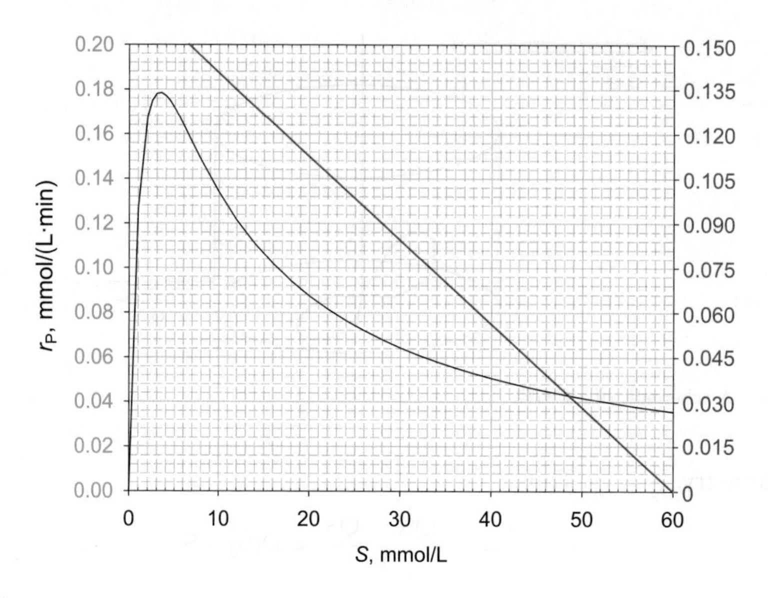

FIGURE 8-4.4

The mole balance line intercepts with the consumption rate of substrate (=generation rate of product) three times. Therefore, there are three possible steady state solutions: $S = 44$, 6.5, and 2.3 mmol/L. Correspondingly, the conversions are given by

$$f_S = \frac{S_0 - S}{S_0} = 1 - \frac{S}{S_0}$$

The three possible fractional conversions are: 0.267, 0.892, and 0.962.

(c) If the enzyme loading is reduced by 25%, i.e. $[E]_0 = 0.75[E]_{0\text{previous}}$. Based on Eqn (E8-4.12), the reaction rate is going to be reduced by 25%. Therefore, we can rescale the vertical axis of Fig. 8-4.1 (see the scale on the right on Fig. 8-4.4), while plotting the mole balance line, Eqn (8-4.13) based on the new scale to find the possible steady-state solutions.

Now that only one steady-state solution is obtained. $S = 48.5$ mmol/L or the conversion $f_S = 0.192$.

8.5. LARGE-SCALE PRODUCTION OF ENZYMES

Among various enzymes produced at large scale are proteases (subtilisin, rennet), hydrolases (pectinase, lipase, lactase), isomerases (glucose isomerase), and oxidases (glucose oxidase). These enzymes are produced using overproducing strains of certain organisms. Separation and purification of an enzyme from an organism require disruption of cells, removal of cell debris and nucleic acids, precipitation of proteins, ultrafiltration of the desired enzyme, chromatographic separations (optional), crystallization, and drying. The process scheme varies depending on whether the enzyme is intracellular or extracellular. In some cases, it may be more advantageous to use inactive (dead or resting) cells with the desired enzyme activity in immobilized form. This approach eliminates costly enzyme separation and purification steps and is therefore economically more feasible. Details of protein separations are covered later in the text.

The first step in the large-scale production of enzymes is to cultivate the organisms producing the desired enzyme. Enzyme production can be regulated and fermentation conditions can be optimized for overproduction of the enzyme. Proteases are produced by using overproducing strains of *Bacillus*, *Aspergillus*, *Rhizopus*, and *Mucor*; pectinases are produced by *Aspergillus niger*; lactases are produced by yeast and *Aspergillus*; lipases are produced by certain strains of yeasts and fungi; and glucose isomerase is produced by *Flavobacterium arborescens* or *Bacillus coagulans*. After the cultivation step, cells are separated from the media usually by filtration or sometimes by centrifugation. Depending on the intracellular or extracellular nature of the enzyme, either the cells or the fermentation broth is further processed to separate and purify the enzyme. The recovery of intracellular enzymes is more complicated and involves the disruption of cells and removal of cell debris and nucleic acids. Figure 8.18 depicts a schematic of an enzyme plant producing extracellular enzymes.

In some cases, enzyme may be both intracellular and extracellular, which requires processing of both broth and cells. Intracellular enzymes may be released by increasing the permeability of cell membrane. Certain salts such as $CaCl_2$ and other chemicals such as

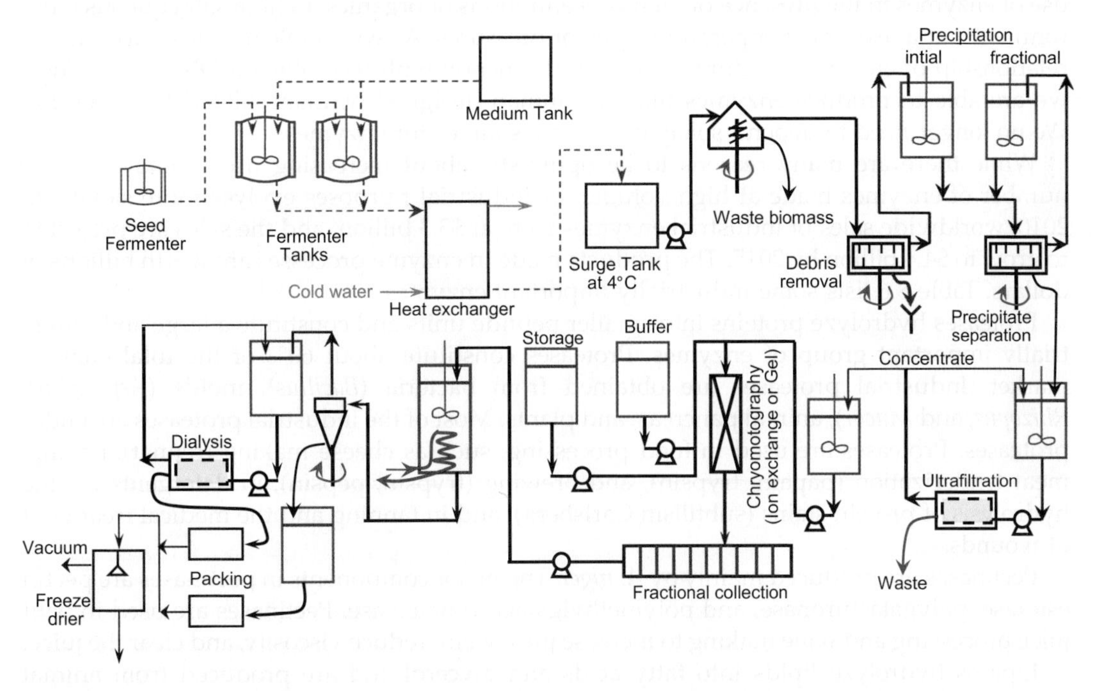

FIGURE 8.18 A flowsheet for the production of an extracellular enzyme.

dimethylsulfoxide and pH shift may be used for this purpose. If enzyme release is not complete, then cell disruption may be essential.

The processes used to produce these industrial enzymes have much in common with our later discussions on processes to make protein from recombinant DNA.

8.6. MEDICAL AND INDUSTRIAL UTILIZATION OF ENZYMES

Enzymes have been significant industrial products for over a century. The range of potential application is still increasing rapidly. With the advent of recombinant DNA technology, it has become possible to make formerly rare enzymes in large quantities and, hence, reduce cost. Also, in pharmaceutical manufacture, the desire to make chirally pure compounds is leading to new opportunities. Chirality is important in a product; in a racemic mixture, one enantiomer is often therapeutically useful while the other may cause side effects and add no therapeutic value. The ability of enzymes to recognize chiral isomers and react with only one of them can be a key component in pharmaceutical synthesis. Processes that depend on a mixture of chemical and enzymatic synthesis are being developed for a new generation of pharmaceuticals.

Technological advances have facilitated the use of enzymes over an increasingly broad range of process conditions. Enzymes from organisms that grow in unusual environments (e.g. deep ocean, salt lakes, hot springs, and industrial waste sites) are increasingly available for study and potential use. New enzymes and better control of reaction conditions allow the use of enzymes in the presence of high concentrations of organics, in high salt aqueous environments, or at extreme temperatures, pH, or pressures. As we couple new insights into the relationship of enzyme structure to biological function with recombinant DNA technology, we are able to produce enzymes that are human designed or manipulated (Chapter 14). We no longer need to depend solely on natural sources for enzymes.

While there are many reasons to be optimistic about increasing use of enzymes, the number of enzymes made at high volume for industrial purposes evolves more slowly. In 2010, worldwide sales of industrial enzymes were at $3.3 billion, and the sales are projected to grow to $4.4 billion by 2015. The products made in enzyme processes are worth billions of dollars. Table 8.6 lists some industrially important enzymes.

Proteases hydrolyze proteins into smaller peptide units and constitute a large and industrially important group of enzymes. Proteases constitute about 60% of the total enzyme market. Industrial proteases are obtained from bacteria (*Bacillus*), molds (*Aspergillus*, *Rhizopus*, and *Mucor*), animal pancreas, and plants. Most of the industrial proteases are endoproteases. Proteases are used in food processing, such as cheese making (rennet), baking, meat tenderization (papain, trypsin), and brewing (trypsin, pepsin); in detergents for the hydrolysis of protein stains (subtilisin Carlsberg); and in tanning and the medical treatment of wounds.

Pectinases are produced mainly by *A. niger.* The major components in pectinases are pectin esterase, polygalacturonase, and polymethylgalacturonatelyase. Pectinases are used in fruit juice processing and wine making to increase juice yield, reduce viscosity, and clear the juice.

Lipases hydrolyze lipids into fatty acids and glycerol and are produced from animal pancreas, some molds, and yeasts. Lipases may be used to hydrolyze oils for soap

TABLE 8.6 Some Industrially Important Enzymes

Name	Example of sources	Application
Amylase	*Bacillus subtilis, Aspergillus niger*	Starch hydrolysis, glucose production
Glucoamylase	*A. niger, Rhizopus niveus, Endomycopsis*	Saccharification of starch, glucose production
Trypsin	Animal pancreas	Meat tenderizer, beer haze removal
Papain	Papaya	Digestive aid, meat tenderizer, medical applications
Pepsin	Animal stomach	Digestive aid, meat tenderizer
Rennet	Calf stomach and/or recombinant *Escherichia coli*	Cheese manufacturing
Glucose isomerase	*Flavobacterium arborescens, Bacillus coagulans, Lactobacillus brevis*	Isomerization of glucose to fructose
Penicillinase	*Bacillus subtilis*	Degradation of penicillin
Glucose oxidase	*A. niger*	Glucose → gluconic acid, dried-egg manufacture
Lignases	Fungal	Biopulping of wood for paper manufacture
Lipases	*Rhizopus*, pancreas	Hydrolysis of lipids, flavoring, and digestive aid
Invertase	*Saccharomyces cerevisiae*	Hydrolysis of sucrose for further fermentation
Pectinase	*Aspergillus oryzae, A. niger, Aspergillus flavus*	Clarification of fruit juices, hydrolysis of pectin
Cellulase	*Trichoderma viride*	Cellulose hydrolysis

manufacture and to hydrolyze the lipid–fat compounds present in waste-water streams; interesterification of oils and fats may be catalyzed by lipase. Lipases may also be used in the cheese and butter industry to impart flavor as a result of the hydrolysis of fats. Lipase-containing detergents are an important application of lipases.

Amylases are used for the hydrolysis of starch and are produced by many different organisms, including *A. niger* and *B. subtilis.* Three major types of amylases are α-amylase, β-amylase, and glucoamylase. α-amylase breaks α-1,4 glycosidic bonds randomly on the amylose chain and solubilizes amylase. For this reason, α-amylase is known as the starch-liquefying enzyme. β-amylase hydrolyzes α-1,4 glycosidic bonds on the nonreducing ends of amylose and produces maltose residues. β-amylase is known as a saccharifying enzyme. α-1,6 Glycosidic linkages in the amylopectin fraction of starch are hydrolyzed by glucoamylase, which is also known as a saccharifying enzyme. In the United States on the average, nearly 5.9×108 kg/year of glucose is produced by the enzymatic hydrolysis of starch. The enzyme pullulase also hydrolyzes α-1,6 glycosidic linkages in starch selectively.

Cellulases are used in the hydrolysis of cellulose and are produced by some *Trichoderma* species, such as *Trichoderma viride* or *Trichoderma reesei*; by some molds, such as *A. niger* and *Thermomonospora*; and by some *Clostridium* species. Cellulase is an enzyme complex and its formation is induced by cellulose. *Trichoderma* cellulose hydrolyzes crystalline cellulose, but *Aspergillus* cellulase does not. Cellulose is first hydrolyzed to cellobiose by cellulase, and cellobiose is further hydrolyzed to glucose by β-glucosidase. Both of these enzymes are inhibited by their end products, cellobiose and glucose. Cellulases are used in cereal processing, alcohol fermentation from biomass, brewing, and waste treatment.

Hemicellulases hydrolyze hemicellulose and are produced by some molds, such as white rot fungi and *A. niger.* Hemicellulases are used in combination with other enzymes in baking doughs, brewing mashes, alcohol fermentation from biomass, and waste treatment.

Lactases are used to hydrolyze lactose in whey to glucose and galactose and are produced by yeast and some *Aspergillus* species. Lactases are used in the fermentation of cheese whey to ethanol.

Other microbial β-1,4 glucanases produced by *Bacillus amyloliquefaciens, A. niger,* and *Penicillium emersonii* are used in brewing mashes containing barley or malt. These enzymes improve filtration efficiency and extract yield.

Penicillin acylase is used by the antibiotic industry to convert penicillin G to 6-aminopenicillanic acid (6-APA), which is a precursor for semi-synthetic penicillin derivatives.

Among other important industrial applications of enzymes are the conversion of fumarate to L-aspartate by aspartase. In industry, this conversion is realized in a packed column of immobilized dead *Escherichia coli* cells with active aspartase enzyme. Fumarate solution is passed through the column, and aspartate is obtained in the effluent stream. Aspartate is further coupled with L-phenylalanine to produce aspartame, which is a low-calorie sweetener known as "Nutrasweet®."

The conversion of glucose to fructose by immobilized glucose isomerase is an important industrial process. Fructose is nearly 1.7 times sweeter than glucose and is used as a sweetener in soft drinks. Glucose isomerase is an intracellular enzyme and is produced by different organisms, such as *F. arborescens, Bacillus licheniformis,* and some *Streptomyces* and *Arthrobacter* species. Immobilized inactive whole cells with glucose isomerase activity are used in a packed column for fructose formation from glucose. Cobalt (Co^{2+}) and magnesium (Mg^{2+}) ions (4×10^{-4} M) enhance enzyme activity. Different immobilization methods are used by different companies. One uses flocculated whole cells of *F. arborescens* treated with glutaraldehyde in the form of dry spherical particles. Entrapment of whole cells in gelatin treated with glutaraldehyde, the use of glutaraldehyde-treated lysed cells in the form of dry particles, and immobilization of the enzyme on inorganic support particles such as silica and alumina are methods used by other companies.

DL-Acylaminoacids are converted to a mixture of L- and D-aminoacids by immobilized aminoacylase. L-Aminoacids are separated from D-acylaminoacid, which is recycled back to the column. L-Aminoacids have important applications in food technology and medicine.

Enzymes are commonly used in medicine for diagnosis, therapy, and treatment purposes. Trypsin can be used as an antiinflammatory agent; lysozyme, which hydrolyzes the cell wall of gram-positive bacteria, is used as an antibacterial agent; streptokinase is used as an antiinflammatory agent; and urokinase is used in dissolving and preventing blood clots. Asparaginase, which catalyzes the conversion of L-asparagineto L-aspartate, is used as an anticancer agent. Cancer cells require L-asparagine and are inhibited by asparaginase. Asparaginase is produced by *E. coli.* Glucose oxidase catalyzes the oxidation of glucose-to-gluconic acid and hydrogen peroxide, which can easily be detected. Glucose oxidase is used for the determination of glucose levels in blood and urine. Penicillinases hydrolyze penicillin and are used to treat allergic reactions against penicillin. Tissue plasminogen activator (TPA) and streptokinase are used in the dissolution of blood clots (particularly following a heart attack or stroke).

The development of biosensors using enzymes as integral components is proceeding rapidly. Two examples of immobilized enzyme electrodes are those used in the determination of glucose and urea by using glucose oxidase and urease immobilized on the electrode membrane, respectively. Scarce enzymes (e.g. TPA) are finding increasing uses, as the techniques of genetic engineering now make it possible to produce usable quantities of such enzymes. The preceding list of enzymes and uses is not exhaustive, but merely illustrative.

8.7. KINETIC APPROXIMATION: WHY MICHAELIS–MENTEN EQUATION WORKS

In Enzyme Kinetics Section, we have discussed the kinetic models of enzyme-catalyzed reactions via two approximations: 1) rapid equilibrium steps and 2) PSSH. Either approach lead to an equation that looks similar and when the parameters are lumped, the two equations become identical. The resulting equation is commonly referred to as Michaelis–Menten equation. The success or usefulness of this equation cannot be underestimated as it has been applied to cases where the simple mechanistic model it implies is not nearly close to the real case. We shall examine why this is the case in this section.

Before we proceed on the discussion, let us consider a simple bioreaction network or pathway that is illustrated in Fig. 8.18 to be carried out in a batch reactor,

$$\mathrm{S + E \rightleftarrows S{\cdot}E} \tag{8.101}$$

$$\mathrm{S{\cdot}E \rightleftarrows P{\cdot}E} \tag{8.102}$$

$$\mathrm{P{\cdot}E \rightleftarrows P + E} \tag{8.103}$$

$$+) = \text{overall} \quad \mathrm{S} \rightleftarrows P \tag{8.104}$$

The uptake of substrate by the enzyme (or substrate–enzyme complexing) is described as a reversible reaction, i.e.

$$r_1 = k_1 C_\mathrm{S} C_\mathrm{E} - k_{-1} C_\mathrm{SE} \tag{8.105}$$

The catalytic reaction occurring or assisted by the enzyme is governed by

$$r_2 = k_\mathrm{C} C_\mathrm{SE} - k_{-\mathrm{C}} C_\mathrm{PE} \tag{8.106}$$

and finally, the discharging of product is governed by

$$r_3 = k_3 C_\mathrm{PE} - k_{-3} C_\mathrm{P} C_\mathrm{E} \tag{8.107}$$

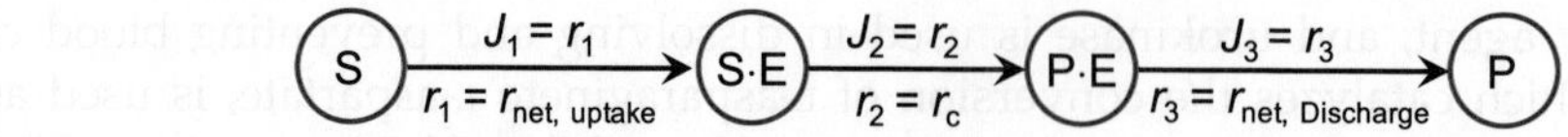

$$\text{S} \xrightarrow[r_1 = r_{\text{net, uptake}}]{J_1 = r_1} \text{S·E} \xrightarrow[r_2 = r_c]{J_2 = r_2} \text{P·E} \xrightarrow[r_3 = r_{\text{net, Discharge}}]{J_3 = r_3} \text{P}$$

FIGURE 8.19 A schematic of reaction pathway showing the rates and fluxes between each adjacent intermediates or substances for the enzymatic isomerization of substrate S to product P.

Since all the steps are already assumed to be reversible and the rates are net rates, the fluxes passing from one "node" to another "node" as shown in Fig. 8.19 are identical to the net reaction rates. As the pathway is still simple enough for attempting on full solution, we shall show how this problem can be solved without further approximation.

Mole balances of all the species in the batch reactor lead to

$$\frac{dC_S}{dt} = -k_1(C_S C_E - C_{SE}/K_S) \tag{8.108}$$

$$\frac{dC_P}{dt} = k_{-3}(C_{PE}/K_P - C_P C_E) \tag{8.109}$$

$$\frac{dC_{SE}}{dt} = k_1(C_S C_E - C_{SE}/K_S) - k_c(C_{SE} - C_{PE} K_S/K_P/K_C) \tag{8.110}$$

$$\frac{dC_{PE}}{dt} = k_c(C_{SE} - C_{PE} K_S/K_P/K_C) - k_{-3}(C_{PE}/K_P - C_P C_E) \tag{8.111}$$

$$C_{E0} = C_E - C_{SE} - C_{PE} \tag{8.112}$$

where K_S and K_P are association (or saturation) constants of S and P with the enzyme; respectively, and K_C is the equilibrium constant of the overall reaction (8.104). That is,

$$K_S = \frac{k_1}{k_{-1}} \tag{8.113}$$

$$K_P = \frac{k_{-3}}{k_3} \tag{8.114}$$

$$K_C = \frac{k_c}{k_{-c}} \times \frac{K_S}{K_P} \tag{8.115}$$

The five Eqns (8.108) through (8.112) can be solved simultaneously together with the initial conditions (in the reactor at time 0)

$$C_S = C_{S0}; C_E = C_{E0}; C_P = 0; C_{SE} = 0; C_{PE} = 0 \quad \text{when } t = 0$$

That is to say, the batch reactor is loaded with the substrate S and the free enzyme E at time 0.

We shall use an integrator to show how this problem can be solved on computer. In this case, we use the ODE × LIMS to integrate Eqns (8.108) through (8.111). Let

$$y_1 = C_S; y_2 = C_p; y_3 = C_{SE}; Y_4 = C_{PE}; \text{and independent variable } x = t$$

$$\text{parameters } c_1 = k_1 C_{E0};\ c_2 = K_S C_{E0};\ c_3 = k_c;\ c_4 = K_C;\ c_5 = K_P C_{E0};\ c_6 = k_{-3} C_{E0}$$

The kernel functions can then be input into the visual basic module as shown in Fig. 8.20. The setup and solution on excel worksheet for one set of parameters is shown in Fig. 8.21. Some of the results for selected values of the parameters are shown in Figs 8.22 through 8.26.

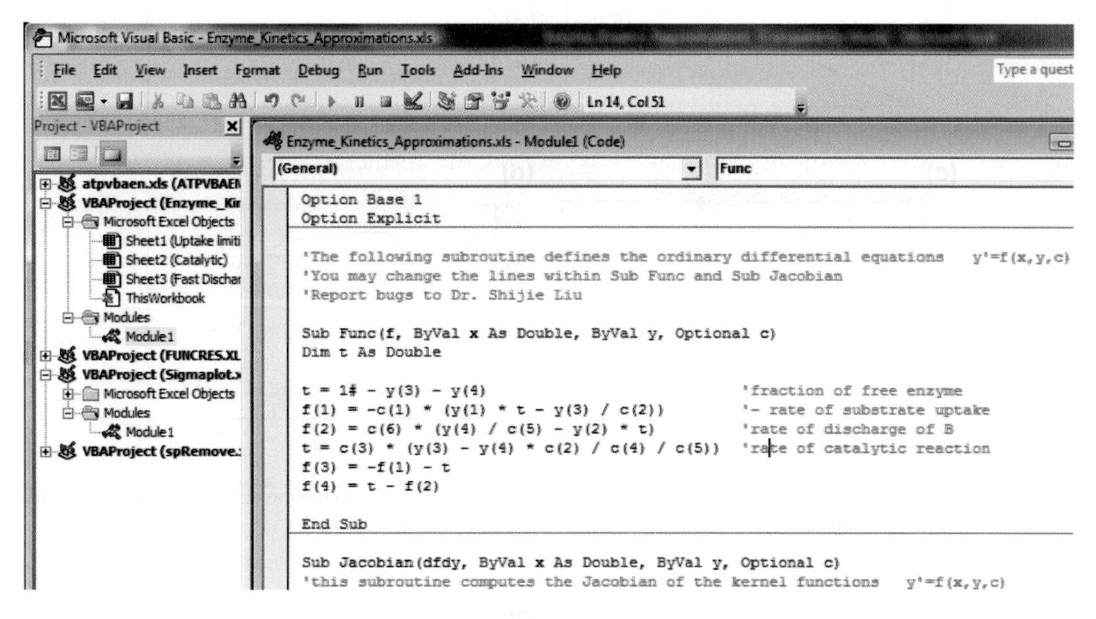

FIGURE 8.20 Visual basic module shown the integral kernels for the enzyme-catalyzed reaction.

B6 {=ODExLIMS(A5:A124,B5:E5,,,A3:F3)}

	A	B	C	D	E	F
1	C(1)	C(2)	C(3)	C(4)	C(5)	C6)
2	k1CE0	Ks = k1/k	kc	Kc=Ksk	KP=k-3/k3	k-3CE0
3	10	1	1	5	0.5	10
4	t	CS/CE0	CP/CE0	CSE	CPE	CE
5	0	10	0	0	0	1
6	0.0001	9.995012	3.66668E-11	0.004988	1.25E-07	0.995012
7	0.0002	9.985132	1.11427E-09	0.014867	1.12E-06	0.985132
8	0.0005	9.956188	2.98657E-08	0.043802	9.91E-06	0.956188
9	0.001	9.910188	2.75845E-07	0.089768	4.32E-05	0.910188
10	0.002	9.825937	2.30029E-06	0.173887	0.000174	0.82594
11	0.003	9.750952	7.6867E-06	0.24866	0.00038	0.75096
12	0.005	9.624454	3.39129E-05	0.37453	0.000982	0.624488
13	0.007	9.523437	8.79144E-05	0.474696	0.001779	0.523525
14	0.008	9.480719	0.000127471	0.516919	0.002235	0.480846
15	0.009	9.442427	0.000176298	0.554675	0.002722	0.442603
16	0.01	9.408075	0.000234943	0.588456	0.003234	0.40831
17	0.015	9.282037	0.000689044	0.711227	0.006048	0.282726
18	0.02	9.207426	0.001430699	0.782103	0.00904	0.208857
19	0.025	9.16265	0.00246618	0.822878	0.012006	0.165116
20	0.03	9.135355	0.003786404	0.846022	0.014837	0.139142
21	0.035	9.11834	0.005374267	0.858804	0.017482	0.123714
22	0.04	9.107363	0.007209013	0.865505	0.019922	0.114572
23	0.05	9.0945	0.011532153	0.869775	0.024194	0.106032
24	0.06	9.086607	0.016589658	0.869075	0.027728	0.103196

FIGURE 8.21 Excel worksheet for the enzyme-catalyzed reaction (8.101) through (8.103).

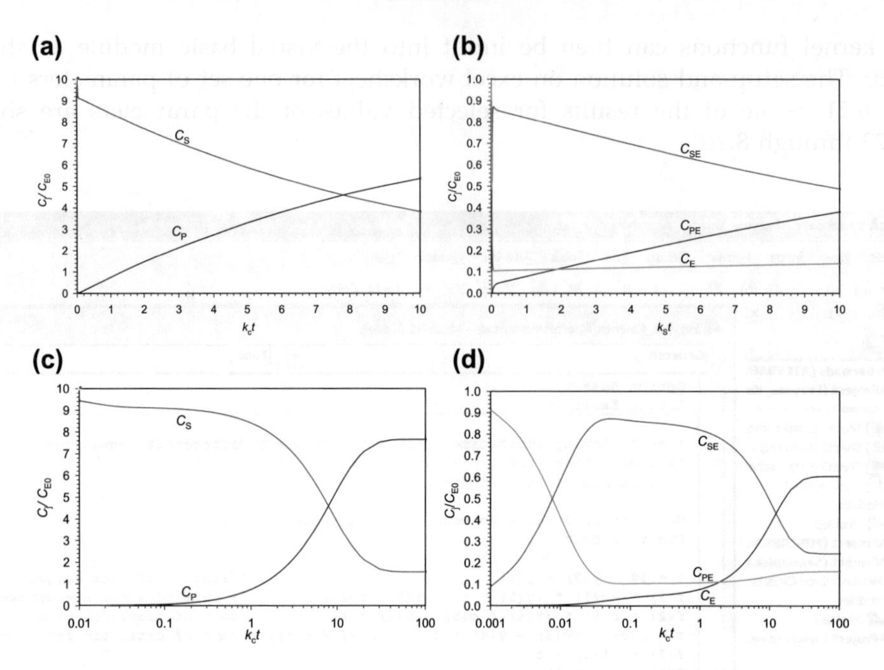

FIGURE 8.22 Variations of free substrate and free product (a) and (c), and enzyme concentrations (b) and (d) with time for $k_1\ C_{E0} = 10\,K_c$; $K_S = 1/C_{E0}$; $K_C = 5$; $K_P = 0.5/C_{E0}$; and $k_{-3}\ C_{E0} = 10\,k_c$.

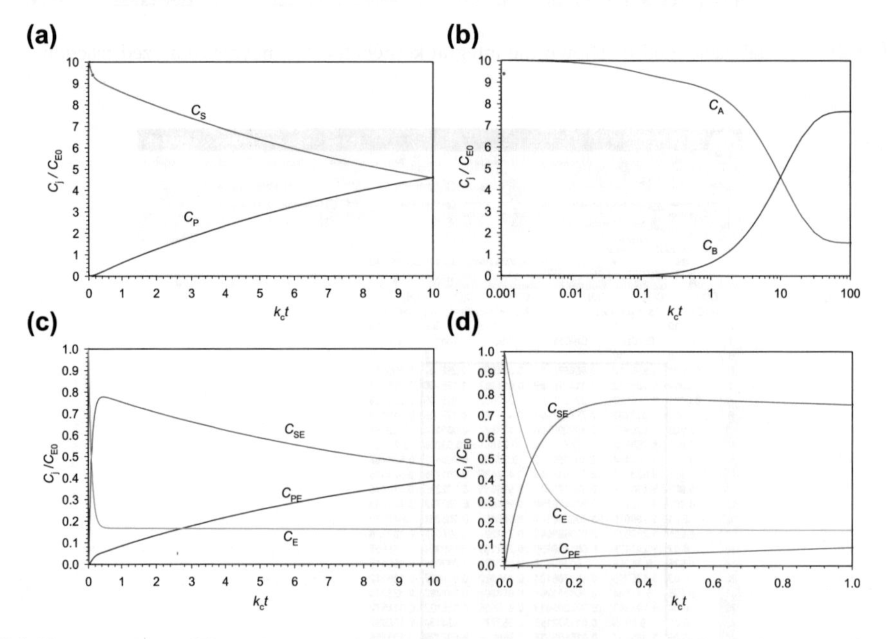

FIGURE 8.23 Variations of free substrate and free product concentrations, (a) and (b), and enzyme distributions, (c) and (d), as function of time for $k_1\ C_{E0} = k_c$; $K_S = 1/C_{E0}$; $K_C = 5$; $K_P = 0.5/C_{E0}$; and $k_{-3}\ C_{E0} = 10\ k_c$.

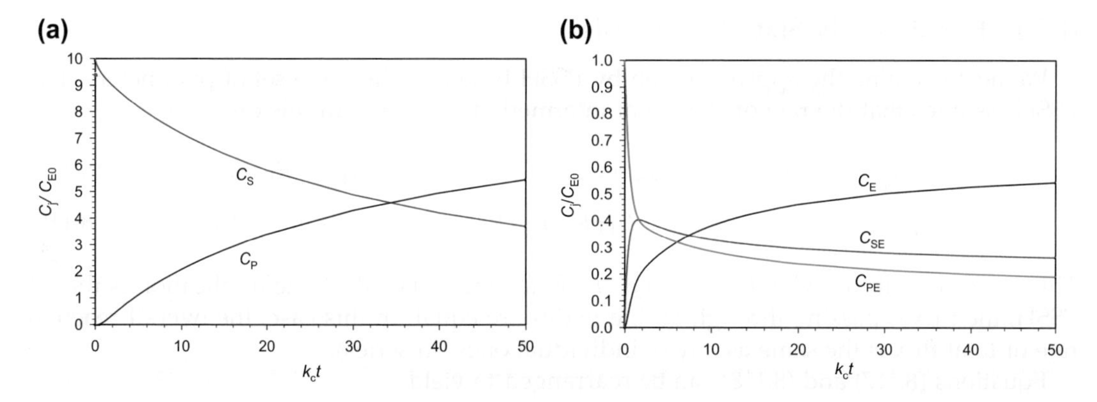

FIGURE 8.24 Variations of free substrate and product concentrations (a) and enzyme distributions (b) with time for $k_1\ C_{E0} = 0.1\,k_c$; $K_S = 1/C_{E0}$; $K_C = 5$; $K_P = 0.5/C_{E0}$; and $k_{-3}\ C_{E0} = k_c$.

We first examine a case where the catalytic reaction rate is limiting. For this case, we scale the time with the catalytic reaction rate constant. The solutions for $C_{S0} = 10\ C_{E0}$; $k_1\ C_{E0} = 10k_c$; $K_S = 1/C_{E0}$; $K_C = 5$; $K_P = 0.5/C_{E0}$; and $k_{-3}\ C_{E0} = 10\,k_c$ are shown in Fig. 8.22. One can observe that in the batch operation, the free substrate concentration (Fig. 8.22a) experiences a quick drop before the free product in the reaction mixture is observed. The decrease is simply due to the complexing of substrate with enzyme and thus is dependent on the amount of enzyme or total enzyme activity. Since the product P is also associated with enzyme, the fraction of enzyme associated with substrate S increases sharply at the start (Fig. 8.22b and d), reaches a maximum, and then decreases, as the product P is being formed. The fraction of enzyme associated with product P increases with time, and as more product P is formed, it also discharged to the reaction mixture and causes the concentration of free product P to increase. The concentration of free product shows almost a delay initially before graduate increase with time (Fig. 8.22a and c).

In the second case, we examine the situation where the uptake of substrate or association of substrate S with enzyme and catalytic reaction are of the similar rates, but the discharge of product from the enzyme is fast. The results are shown in Fig. 8.23. One can observe that there is a drop in the concentration of free substrate S initially, but the drop is gradually at the time scale of reaction (Fig. 8.23a and b). C_{SE} reached maximum gradually and not as obvious as compared Fig. 8.23c with Fig. 8.23b. After C_{SE} reached maximum, and the fraction of free enzyme become "steady" at about $k_ct = 0.25$ (Fig. 8.23d).

We then examine the case when uptake of substrate S is the rate-limiting step as shown in Fig. 8.24. In this case, the decrease in C_S initially is not as apparent in the time scale of reaction (and as the previous two cases). The increase in the concentration of free product P showed almost a "delay." Therefore, the effect of substrate uptake rate is still important.

The effects of the amount of enzyme, substrate, and product saturation constants are important if there are significant amount of enzyme being added to a batch system.

8.7.1. Pseudosteady-State Hypothesis

We next examine the approximation by PSSH based on the same set of parameters. The PSSH assumes that the rate of change of intermediates be zero. In this case,

$$0 = r_{SE} = r_1 - r_2 = k_1(C_E C_S - C_{SE}/K_S) - k_c(C_{SE} - C_{PE}K_S/K_P/K_C) \tag{8.117}$$

$$0 = r_{PE} = r_2 - r_3 = k_c(C_{SE} - C_{PE}K_S/K_P/K_C) - k_{-3}(C_{PE}/K_P - C_E C_B) \tag{8.118}$$

This is equivalent to saying that $r_1 = r_2 = r_3$. Referring to Fig. 8.18, the implication is that at PSSH, the fluxes passing through all the nodes are equal. In this case, the overall reaction rate or total flux is the same as any of individual ones (in series).

Equations (8.117) and (8.118) can be rearranged to yield

$$-C_{SE}(k_1/K_S + k_c) + C_{PE}k_c K_S/K_P/K_C + C_E k_1 C_S = 0 \tag{8.119}$$

$$C_{SE}k_c - C_{PE}(k_c K_S/K_P/K_C + k_{-3}/K_P) + C_E k_{-3} C_P = 0 \tag{8.120}$$

Equations (8.119) and (8.120) can be solved to give

$$C_{SE} = \frac{(K_C^{-1}k_{-3}^{-1} + K_S^{-1}k_c^{-1})C_S + K_C^{-1}k_1^{-1}C_P}{K_C^{-1}k_{-3}^{-1} + K_S^{-1}k_c^{-1} + k_1^{-1}} K_S C_E \tag{8.121}$$

$$C_{PE} = \frac{(k_1^{-1} + K_S^{-1}k_c^{-1})C_P + k_{-3}^{-1}C_S}{K_C^{-1}k_{-3}^{-1} + K_S^{-1}k_c^{-1} + k_1^{-1}} K_P C_E \tag{8.122}$$

Total enzyme balance leads to

$$\begin{aligned} C_{E0} &= C_E + C_{SE} + C_{PE} \\ &= C_E + \frac{(K_C^{-1}k_{-3}^{-1} + K_S^{-1}k_c^{-1})C_S + K_C^{-1}k_1^{-1}C_P}{K_C^{-1}k_{-3}^{-1} + K_S^{-1}k_c^{-1} + k_1^{-1}} K_S C_E \\ &\quad + \frac{(k_1^{-1} + K_S^{-1}k_c^{-1})C_P + k_{-3}^{-1}C_A}{K_C^{-1}k_{-3}^{-1} + K_S^{-1}k_c^{-1} + k_1^{-1}} K_P C_E \end{aligned} \tag{8.123}$$

Thus,

$$C_E = \frac{C_{E0}}{1 + \dfrac{(K_S K_C^{-1}k_{-3}^{-1} + k_c^{-1} + k_{-3}^{-1}K_P)C_S + (K_C^{-1}k_1^{-1}K_S + k_1^{-1}K_P + K_S^{-1}k_c^{-1}K_P)C_P}{K_C^{-1}k_{-3}^{-1} + K_S^{-1}k_c^{-1} + k_1^{-1}}} \tag{8.124}$$

Substituting Eqn (8.124) into Eqns (8.121) and (8.122), we obtain the concentration of enzyme that is associated with substrate or product.

The overall rate of reaction:

$$r = -r_S = r_1 = k_1 C_S C_E - k_{-1} C_{SE} \tag{8.125}$$

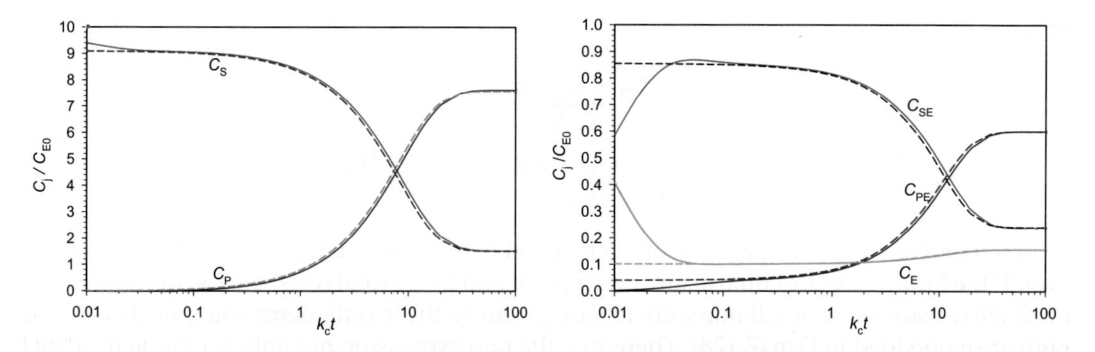

FIGURE 8.25 Variations of free substrate, free product, and enzyme concentrations with time for $k_1\ C_{E0} = 10\,K_c$; $K_S = 1/C_{E0}$; $K_C = 5$; $K_P = 0.5/C_{E0}$; and $k_{-3}\ C_{E0} = 10\,k_c$. The dashed lines are the predictions from PSSH kinetics, whereas the solid lines are from the full solutions.

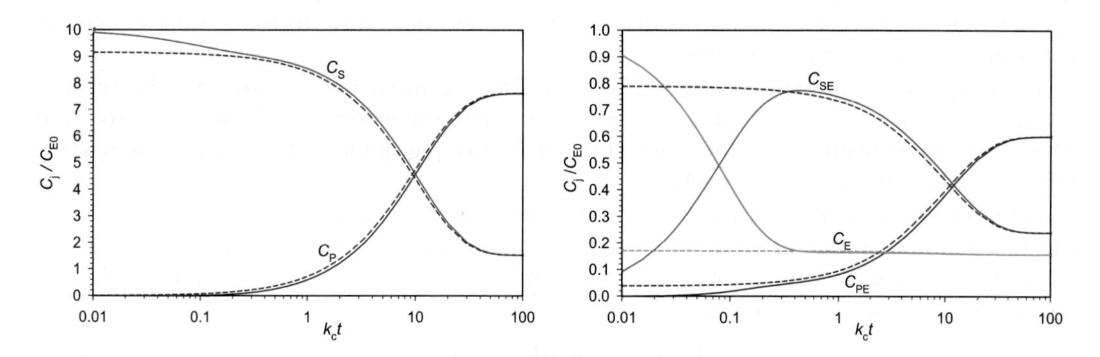

FIGURE 8.26 Variations of free substrate, free product, and enzyme concentrations with time for $k_1\ C_{E0} = k_c$; $K_S = 1/C_{E0}$; $K_C = 5$; $K_P = 0.5/C_{E0}$; and $k_{-3}\ C_{E0} = 10\,k_c$. The dashed lines are the predictions from PSSH kinetics, whereas the solid lines are from the full solutions.

That is

$$r = k_1(C_S C_E - C_{SE}/K_S) \tag{8.126}$$

Substituting the concentration of ES complex A and the concentration of free enzyme in the reaction mixture, Eqn (8.126) renders

$$\begin{aligned} r &= k_1\left[C_S - \frac{(K_C^{-1}k_{-3}^{-1} + K_S^{-1}k_c^{-1})C_S + K_C^{-1}k_1^{-1}C_P}{K_C^{-1}k_{-3}^{-1} + K_S^{-1}k_c^{-1} + k_1^{-1}}\right]C_E \\ &= \frac{C_S - K_C^{-1}C_P}{K_C^{-1}k_{-3}^{-1} + K_S^{-1}k_c^{-1} + k_1^{-1}}C_E \end{aligned} \tag{8.127}$$

or

$$r = \frac{\dfrac{C_S - K_C^{-1}C_P}{K_C^{-1}k_B^{-1} + K_A^{-1}k_S^{-1} + k_A^{-1}}C_{E0}}{1 + \dfrac{(K_S K_C^{-1}k_{-3}^{-1} + k_c^{-1} + k_{-3}^{-1}K_P)C_S + (K_C^{-1}k_1^{-1}K_S + k_1^{-1}K_P + K_S^{-1}k_c^{-1}K_P)C_P}{K_C^{-1}k_{-3}^{-1} + K_S^{-1}k_c^{-1} + k_1^{-1}}} \tag{8.128}$$

Based on Fig. 8.19, one can think of the reaction network in analogy to the electric conduction: 1) the fluxes must be equal at any given point and 2) the total resistance is the summation of all the resistors in series. If one were to look carefully, these statements could be detected as both are embedded in Eqn (8.128). Therefore, the rate expression not only is unique for PSSH but also brings the reaction network to be directly in analog to electric circuit.

At this point, one may look back at the full solutions as illustrated in Figs 8.22 through 8.24, especially with Figs 8.22b and d, 8.23c and d, and 8.25b, that the concentrations of intermediates (in this case, the concentrations of enzyme associated with S and with P) are hardly constant or at "steady state" in any reasonably wide regions where we would like to have the solutions meaningful. Therefore, the assumption is rather strong for the directly involved species that we have eliminated from the rate expression. How do the solutions actually measure up with the full solutions?

To apply the PSSH expression (8.127) or (8.128), we must first ensure that the reaction mixture in already in pseudo-steady state to minimize the error may cause in the solution. This error can be negligible if the amount of catalyst is negligible or for steady flow reactors where steady state is already reached.

Let us consider again the case where no P is present in the reaction mixture at the start of the reaction. The concentrations of S and P charged into the batch reactor are C_{ST0} and $C_{ST0} = 0$. Since there is no P present in the initial reaction mixture, $C_{P0} = 0$. Overall mole balance at the onset of the reaction leads to

$$C_{ST0} = C_{S0} + C_{SE0} + C_{PE0} \tag{8.129}$$

where C_{SE0} and C_{PE0} satisfy Eqns (8.121) and (8.122). Since $C_{P0} = 0$, substituting Eqns (8.121) and (8.122) into Eqn (8.129), we obtain

$$C_{ST0} = C_{S0} + \frac{(K_S K_C^{-1}k_{-3}^{-1} + k_c^{-1} + k_{-3}^{-1}K_P)C_{S0}C_{E0}}{K_C^{-1}k_{-3}^{-1} + K_S^{-1}k_c^{-1} + k_1^{-1} + (K_S K_C^{-1}k_{-3}^{-1} + k_c^{-1} + k_{-3}^{-1}K_P)C_{S0}} \tag{8.130}$$

This quadratic equation can be solved to give

$$C_{S0} = \frac{C_{ST0} - C_{E0} - a + \sqrt{(C_{ST0} - C_{E0} - a)^2 + 4aC_{ST0}}}{2} \tag{8.131}$$

where

$$a = \frac{K_C^{-1}k_{-3}^{-1} + K_S^{-1}k_c^{-1} + k_1^{-1}}{K_S K_C^{-1}k_{-3}^{-1} + k_c^{-1} + k_{-3}^{-1}K_P} \tag{8.132}$$

Figure 8.25 shows the comparison between the full solutions and those from PSSH treatment for the particular case of $k_1 C_{E0} = 10 k_c$ and $k_{-3} C_{E0} = 10 k_c$. One can observe that solutions based on PSSH are surprisingly close to the full solutions. Although we have used the argument that all the intermediates remain at steady state (pseudosteady state) and the solutions do not appear to be the case, the computed enzyme distributions (dashed lines) agree quite well with the full solutions (solid lines) when $k_c t > 0.05$.

To show the reasonable agreement with the solutions from the PSSH approximation to the process, Fig. 8.26 shows a comparison between the full solutions (solid lines) and those from PSSH treatment for the case of $k_1 C_{E0} = k_c$ and $k_{-3} C_{E0} = 10 k_c$ (dashed lines). One can observe that the agreement between the full solutions and the PSSH solutions is rather good at "long" times when $k_c t > 0.3$.

8.7.2. Fast Equilibrium Step Approximation

We next examine how Fast Equilibrium Step (FES) assumption is applied to approximate the enzyme reaction network. If the catalytic reaction is the rate-limiting step (Michaelis–Menten), we have the overall rate for reaction (8.104):

$$r = r_2 = k_c C_{SE} - k_{-c} C_{PE} \tag{8.133}$$

The other two steps (8.103) and (8.105) are in equilibrium,

$$0 = r_1 = k_1 C_S C_E - k_{-1} C_{SE} \tag{8.134}$$

$$0 = r_3 = k_3 C_{PE} - k_{-3} C_P C_E \tag{8.135}$$

which can be rearranged to give

$$C_{SE} = \frac{k_1}{k_{-1}} C_S C_E = K_S C_S C_E \tag{8.136}$$

and

$$C_{PE} = \frac{k_{-3}}{k_3} C_B C_E = K_P C_P C_E \tag{8.137}$$

Total enzyme balance:

$$C_{E0} = C_E + C_{SE} + C_{PE} = C_E + K_S C_S C_E + K_P C_P C_E \tag{8.138}$$

Thus,

$$C_E = \frac{C_{E0}}{1 + K_S C_S + K_P C_P} \tag{8.139}$$

Substituting (8.135) into (8.136), (8.137), and then (8.133), we obtain

$$C_{SE} = \frac{K_S C_S}{1 + K_S C_S + K_P C_P} \tag{8.140}$$

$$C_{PE} = \frac{K_P C_P}{1 + K_S C_S + K_P C_P} \tag{8.141}$$

$$r = k_c C_{E0} K_S \frac{C_S - C_P/K_C}{1 + K_S C_S + K_P C_P} \tag{8.142}$$

Equations (8.128) and (8.142) are quite similar when the rate constants are lumped together. If one were to use Eqn (8.128) to correlate experimental data, one would not be able to distinguish whether it is PSSH model or Michaelis–Menten model. The appeal of the PSSH approach is that it may be able to approximate the reaction rate in general (i.e. all the fluxes are considered), without imposing a particular step as the rate-limiting step as illustrated in Fig. 8.18. This approximation is particular useful when the beginning (reactants) and end (products) are only of concern. Still, Eqn (8.142) looks simpler to use.

At time $t = 0$ in the batch reactor, the reaction is not started yet. However, the rapid equilibrium approximated expression (8.142) requires that the uptake of substrate is already in equilibrium. While this requirement is not of issue for reactions carried out in flow reactors (after the transient period) or when the amount of enzyme is negligible, it becomes important when noticeable amount of enzyme is employed in a batch reactor. For example, the concentration of free substrate S can be obtained via mole balance,

$$C_{ST0} = C_{S0} + C_{SE0} = C_{S0} + \frac{K_S C_{S0}}{1 + K_S C_{S0} + K_P C_{P0}} C_{E0} \tag{8.143}$$

The concentrations of free substrate S and product P charged into the batch reactor are C_{ST0} and $C_{PT0} = 0$, assuming only substrate S was loaded. Since there is no P present in the initial reaction mixture, $C_{P0} = 0$. From Eqn (8.143), we can solved for the free substrate concentration in the batch reactor as

$$C_{S0} = \frac{C_{ST0} - C_{E0} - K_S^{-1} + \sqrt{(C_{ST0} - C_{E0} - K_S^{-1})^2 + 4K_S^{-1} C_{ST0}}}{2} \tag{8.144}$$

Mole balances on substrate S and product P in the reactor lead to

$$\frac{dC_S}{dt} = -r = k_c C_{E0} K_S \frac{C_S - C_P/K_C}{1 + K_S C_S + K_P C_P} \tag{8.145}$$

$$\frac{dC_P}{dt} = r = k_c C_{E0} K_S \frac{C_S - C_P/K_C}{1 + K_S C_S + K_P C_P} \tag{8.146}$$

The solutions from the rapid equilibrium (Michaelis–Menten) model can be obtained by solving Eqns (8.145) and (8.146) with initial conditions given by C_{S0} (Eqn 8.144) and $C_{P0} = 0$ at $t = 0$. Subsequently, the enzyme distributions can be obtained from Eqns (8.140) and (8.141). One should note that the initial conditions set for Michaelis–Menten model must have taken the substrate uptake and product discharge equilibria into consideration.

Instead of having four equations to solve, we now have only two equations to solve. The solutions to one case consistent with the approximation to the first case discussed earlier are

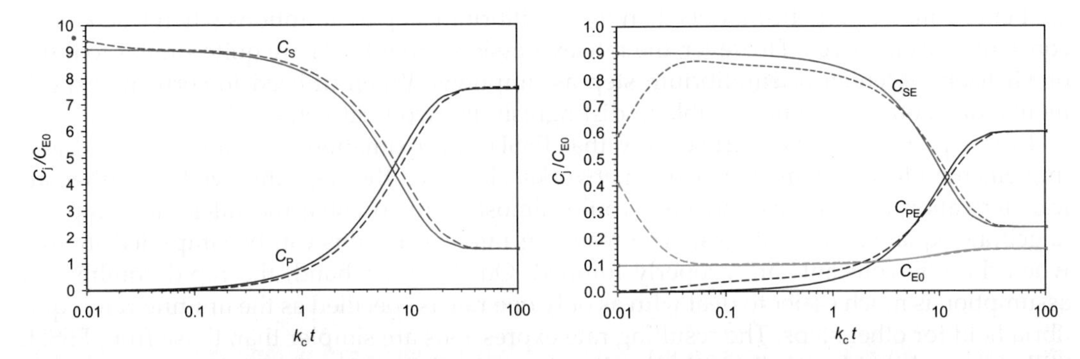

FIGURE. 8.27 Variations of free substrate, free product, and enzyme concentrations with time for $K_S = 1/C_{E0}$; $K_C = 5$; $K_P = 0.5/C_{E0}$. The solid lines are the predictions from Michaelis–Menten kinetics assuming the catalytic reaction is the rate-limiting step, whereas the dashed lines are for $k_1 C_{E0} = 10 k_c$ and $k_{-3} C_{E0} = 10 k_c$, as shown earlier.

shown in Fig. 8.27. For comparison purposes, we have also plotted the full solutions as shown in dashed lines. One can observe that the enzyme distributions as predicted by the Michaelis–Menten approximation are quite similar to the full solutions. Michaelis–Menten approximation becomes suitable once the free enzyme concentration becomes nearly constant.

Figure 8.27 shows the variations of free substrate, free product, and enzyme concentrations with reaction time for a case where the catalytic reaction rate is one tenth of those of the other two steps. The Michaelis–Menten approximation are shown as solid lines, whereas the dashed line are full solutions. One can observe that the Michaelis–Menten approximation agrees reasonably well with the actual system, although there is a noticeable time shift due to the small difference among the rates of the three steps. In deriving at Michaelis–Menten approximation, we have assumed that the rates of the other two steps are very fast. The 10-fold difference in the rate constant is still noticeable.

One can observe from Fig. 8.27 that while the variation of free substrate concentrations for Michaelis–Menten approximation looks similar to the full solutions, there is a shift log t (to the right) that could make the agreement closer. This is due to the fact that the finite rates of uptake of substrate S (or enzyme complexing of S) and discharge of P contribute to the decline of overall rate as used by Michaelis–Menten approximation. As a result, the Michaelis–Menten approximations overpredicted the reaction rate and thus leading to a quicker change in the bulk phase concentrations. Overall, the shape of the curve (or how the concentrations change with time) is remarkably similar. Therefore, if one were to correlate the experimental data, the difference between the quality of full solutions and the quality of fit from Michaelis–Menten approximations would not be noticeable.

8.7.3. Modified Fast Equilibrium Approximation

Comparing Figs 8.25 and 8.27, one can observe that PSSH approximation is closer to the full solutions. Also, PSSH approximation can be applied to a variety of systems, whereas the rapid equilibrium approximation is more specific. Therefore, the PSSH approximations are better suited as kinetic models than the equilibrium step assumptions when true kinetic constants are employed. However, the rate expressions from PSSH are quite similar to those of Michaelis–Menten or equilibrium step assumptions. When utilized to correlate experimental data, one would not be able to distinguish the two treatments.

To this point, we have learned now that PSSH approximation is easily visualized and implemented to approximate reaction networks. However, the steps involved in mathematical derivation are tedious and one would almost want to solve the rates via computer (algebraic equations or matrices). The resulting rate expressions can be simplified though when the rate constants are properly lumped. On the other hand, the rapid equilibrium assumption is much easier to deal with as only one rate is specified as the limiting rate, equilibria hold for other steps. The resulting rate expressions are simpler than those from PSSH. Still, one needs to identify the right rate-limiting step. Comparing the PSSH and rapid equilibrium approximations with the full solutions, one can infer that PSSH approximation is closer to the full solution. When the rates are significantly different, i.e. there is a truly one rate limiting step, one may not find any difference between the three solutions when the initial moments were ignored.

To accommodate the rate difference and making rapid equilibrium approximations more useful, we can make further approximations to recover some of the error incurred due to the assumption of rapid equilibrium steps. This can be accomplished by

$$r = \left(r_1^{-1} + r_2^{-1} + r_3^{-1}\right)^{-1} \approx \frac{r_1|_{r_2=0,r_3=0}}{1 + \dfrac{k_1 C_{E0}}{k_c} + \dfrac{K_P}{k_{-3} K_C} k_1 C_{E0}} \tag{8.147a}$$

$$r = \left(r_1^{-1} + r_2^{-1} + r_3^{-1}\right)^{-1} \approx \frac{r_2|_{r_1=0,r_3=0}}{1 + \dfrac{k_c}{k_1 C_{E0}} + \dfrac{K_P}{k_{-3} K_C} k_c} \tag{8.147b}$$

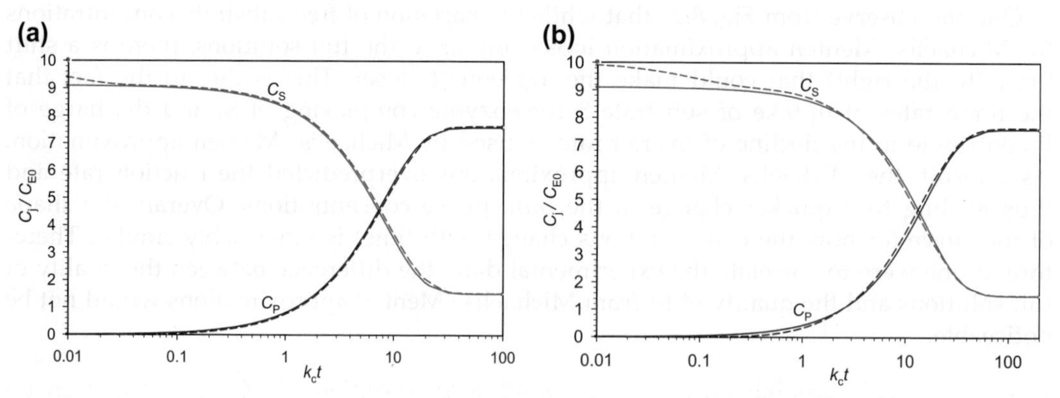

FIGURE. 8.28 Variations of free substrate, free product and enzyme concentrations with time for $K_S = 1/C_{E0}$; $K_C = 5$; $K_P = 0.5/C_{E0}$, $k_1 C_{E0} = 10 k_c$ and $k_{-3} C_{E0} = 10 k_c$. Two cases are shown: (a) $k_1 C_{E0} = 10 k_c$ as shown in Fig. 8.27 and (b) $k_1 C_{E0} = k_c$ which does not qualify for single rate liming step assumption. The solid lines are the predictions from Michaelis–Menten kinetics with the rate coefficient k_c replaced by $(k_c^{-1} + k_1^{-1} C_{E0}^{-1} + K_P k_{-3}^{-1} C_{E0}^{-1})^{-1}$ or the time rescaled.

$$r = \left(r_1^{-1} + r_2^{-1} + r_3^{-1}\right)^{-1} \approx \frac{r_3|_{r_1=0,r_2=0}}{1 + \dfrac{k_{-3}K_C}{k_1 C_{E0} K_P} + \dfrac{k_{-3}K_C}{k_c K_P}} \tag{8.147c}$$

Figure 8.28 shows the variations of free substrate and product concentrations with reaction time comparing the full solutions with the approximate kinetics. One can observe that the rescaled Michaelis–Menten approximation agrees with full solutions reasonably well.

Therefore, one can conclude that Michaelis–Menten equation can be applied to model enzyme reactions after the initial "mixing" period without knowing if there is a rate-limiting step. The rate constants: r_{max} and K_m are functions of the rate constants of all the steps involved.

8.8. SUMMARY

Enzymes are protein, glycoprotein, or RNA molecules that catalyze biologically important reactions. Enzymes are very effective, specific, and versatile biocatalysts. Enzymes bind substrate molecules and reduce the activation energy of the reaction catalyzed, resulting in significant increases in reaction rate. Some protein enzymes require a nonprotein group for their activity as a cofactor.

The kinetics of enzyme-catalyzed reactions is usually modeled after FES: the catalytic reaction step is the rate-limiting step while other steps are in equilibrium or their rates are zero. The resulting rate expression is usually referred to as the Michaelis–Menten equation. The rapid equilibrium assumption produces simplest rate expression and is easy to apply. However, it has the limitation requiring other steps to be much faster. PSSH is more general, and it puts reaction networks in direct analogy with electric circuit. The final rate expression on the other hand, is quite similar to Michaelis–Menten equation when the kinetic parameters are lumped together. Finally, the Michaelis–Menten rate expression can be employed to correlate experimental data, without a true rate-limiting step.

The activity of some enzymes can be altered by inhibitory compounds, which bind the enzyme molecule and reduce its activity. Enzyme inhibition may be competitive, noncompetitive, and uncompetitive. High substrate and product concentrations may be inhibitory, too.

Enzymes require optimal conditions (pH, temperature, ionic strength) for their maximum activity. Enzymes with an ionizing group on their active site show a distinct optimal pH that corresponds to the natural active form of the enzyme. The activation energy of enzyme-catalyzed reactions is within 16–84 kJ/mol. Above the optimal temperature, enzymes lose their activity, and the inactivation energy is on the order of 170–540 kJ/mol.

Enzymes can be used in suspension or in immobilized form. Enzymes can be immobilized by entrapment in a porous matrix, by encapsulation in a semipermeable membrane capsule or between membranes, such as in a hollow-fiber unit, or by adsorption onto a solid support surface. Enzyme immobilization provides enzyme reutilization, eliminates costly enzyme recovery and purification, and may result in increased activity by providing a more suitable microenvironment for the enzyme. Enzyme immobilization may result in diffusion limitations within the matrix. Immobilization may also cause enzyme instability, loss of activity, and shift in optimal conditions (pH, ionic strength). To obtain maximum reaction rates, the particle size of the support material and enzyme loading need to be optimized, and a support material with the correct surface characteristics must be selected.

Enzymes are widely used in industry and have significant medical applications. Among the most widely used enzymes are proteases (papain, trypsin, subtilisin), amylases (starch hydrolysis), rennet (cheese manufacturing), glucose isomerase (glucose-to-fructose conversion), glucose oxidase (glucose-to-gluconic acid conversion), lipases (lipid hydrolysis), and pectinases (pectin hydrolysis). Enzyme production and utilization are a multibillion-dollar business with a great potential for expansion.

Reactor performance for enzymatic reactions can be carried out in the same manner as other chemical reactors. Enzymatic reactions are commonly carried out in batch reactors, while flow reactors can be used when enzymes are immobilized.

Further Reading

Adams, M.W.W., Kelly, R.M., 1995. Enzymes from Microorganisms in Extreme Environments, *Chemical & Engineering News* 32–42. (Dec. 18).

Bailey, J.E., Ollis, D.F., 1986. *Biochemical Engineering Fundamentals,* 2nd ed. McGraw-Hill Book Co., New York.

Blanch, H.W., Clark, D.S., 1996. *Biochemical Engineering,* Marcel Dekker, Inc., New York.

Katchalski-Katzir, E., 1993. Immobilized Enzymes-Learning from Past Successes and Failures, *Trends in Biotechnology* 11, 471–478.

Moran, L.A., Scrimgeourh, K.G., Horton, R., Ochs, R.S., Rawn, J.D., 1994. *Biochemistry,* Prentice-Hall, Inc., Upper Saddle River, NJ.

Nielsen, J., Villadsen, J,. Liden, G., 2003. Bioreaction Engineering Principles, 2nd ed. Kluwer Academic/Plenum Publishers, New York.

Sellek, G.A., Chaudhuri, J.B., 1999. Biocatalysis in Organic Media Using Enzymes from Extremophiles, *Enzyme Microbial Technol.* 25, 471–482.

Stinson, S.C., 1998. Counting on Chiral Drugs, *Chemical & Engineering News* (Sept. 21), 83–104.

Walsh, G., 2002. Proteins – Biochemistry and Biotechnology, John Wiley & Sons: New York.

PROBLEMS

8.1. Chymotrypsin is a serine protease that cleaves the amide linkages in proteins and peptides. It has a binding pocket which is selective for the aromatic residues of amino acids. The reaction occurs by the reversible formation of a Michaelis–Menten complex, followed by acylation of Ser-195 to give a tetrahedral acyl enzyme intermediate. Chymotrypsin will also act as an esterase; we can write the elementary reaction steps in the following form, where RCO-X is an amide or an ester

$$\mathrm{E + RCO{-}X \rightleftarrows RCO{-}X{\cdot}E \rightarrow RCO{-}E' + XH}$$

$$\mathrm{RCO{-}E' + H_2O \rightarrow RCOOH + E}$$

Where $X = \mathrm{NH{-}R'}$ (amide) or $X = \mathrm{O{-}R'}$ (ester) and RCO–E is the acyl enzyme intermediate. This can be written more simply as

$$\mathrm{E + S} \underset{k_{-1}}{\overset{k_1}{\rightleftarrows}} \mathrm{ES_1} \overset{k_2}{\rightarrow} \mathrm{ES_2} \overset{k_3}{\rightarrow} \mathrm{E + P}$$

Derive the rate of formation of P that is consistent with this mechanism.

8.2. Consider the reversible product-formation reaction in an enzyme-catalyzed bioreaction:

$$E+S \underset{k_{-1}}{\overset{k_1}{\rightleftarrows}} ES \underset{k_{-2}}{\overset{k_2}{\rightleftarrows}} E+P$$

Develop a rate expression for product formation using the pseudosteady-state approximation and show that

$$r_P = \frac{r_{max}}{K_m}\frac{[S]-K_C^{-1}[P]}{1+K_m^{-1}[S]+K_P^{-1}[P]}$$

where $K_m = \dfrac{k_{-1}+k_2}{k_1}$, $K_P = \dfrac{k_{-1}+k_2}{k_{-2}}$, $K_C = \dfrac{k_1k_2}{k_{-1}k_{-2}}$, and $r_{max}=k_2[E]_0$

8.3. The enzyme-catalyzed aqueous reaction

$$A \rightarrow \text{products}$$

has a rate $r=1.2\ C_A/(0.01+C_A)$ with rate in moles/(L · min) and concentration in moles/liter. We need to process a stream consisting of 100 mol-A/h at 2 mol/L substrate A to 95% conversion. Batch operations were chosen. For each batch of operations, the total preparation time (loading, raising temperature, unloading after reaction, and cleaning) is 5 h. Calculate the reactor volumes required.

8.4. We wish to treat 10 L/min of liquid feed containing 1 mol-A/L to 99% conversion. The reaction stoichiometry is given by

$$2A \rightarrow R+U, \quad r=\frac{k_1C_A}{K_m+C_A}$$

where $k_1=0.5$ moles · liter^{-1} · min^{-1} and $K_m=0.2$ mol/L. Suggest a good arrangement for doing this using two CSTRs. Find the sizes of the two units needed.

8.5. Enzyme E catalyzes the aqueous decomposition of substrate A to products R and B as follows:

$$A \xrightarrow{\text{enzyme}} R + B, \quad r=\frac{200C_AC_{E0}}{0.1+C_A}$$

where r is in mol · L^{-1} · min^{-1} and C_A and C_{E0} are in mol/L. The reaction is to carry out in a plug flow reactor. In the feed stream, the concentrations of the enzyme and substrate A are 0.001 and 10 mol/L, respectively. How does density change in the reactor? Find the space time and mean residence time required to drop the substrate concentration to 0.025 mol/L.

8.6. The enzyme-catalyzed aqueous reaction

$$A \rightarrow \text{products}$$

has a rate $r=2\ C_A/(0.01+C_A)$ with rate in moles/(L min) and concentration in moles/liter. We need to process 100 mol/h of 2 mol/L feed to 95% conversion. Calculate the reactor volumes required if the reactor system were consisted of

(a) a PFR,

(b) a CSTR,

(c) two equal-volume CSTRs.
(d) an ideal combination of reactors for total minimum volume for two CSTRs.

8.7. It has been observed that substrate inhibition occurs in the following enzymatic reaction:

$$E + S \rightarrow P + E$$

(a) Show that the rate law for substrate inhibition is consistent with the data shown in the Fig. P8.7 below for r_P, mmol/(L · min) versus the substrate concentration of S, mmol/L.
(b) If this reaction is carried out in a fluidized CSTR with an immobilized enzyme system. The reactor has a working volume of 1000 L, to which the volumetric flow rate is 3.2 L/min and the feed concentration of the substrate is 50 mmol/L, determine the possible conversion of substrate to the desired product. Assume that there is no loss of the enzyme to the effluent and the effectiveness factor of the immobilized enzymes is 100%, i.e. no impact of immobilization on the enzyme on catalytic activity.
(c) How many possible solutions have you obtained in part b)? If more than one operation outputs are possible, which one would you like to choose to operate?
(d) What is the dilution rate in part b)? What would be the effluent substrate concentration if the dilution rate is increased by 25%?

8.8. The enzyme-catalyzed reaction:

$$E + S \rightleftarrows P + E$$

The rate of formation P is observed in the lab as shown in Fig. P8.7 with an enzyme loading of $E_0 = 50$ Units/L. In an industrial application, it is decided that enzyme loading can be raised to 75 Units/L. This reaction is to be carried out in a fluidized CSTR with an immobilized enzyme system. The volumetric flow rate is 380 L/h and the feed concentration of the substrate is 60 mmol/L. Assume that there is no loss of the enzyme to the effluent, and the effectiveness factor of the immobilized enzymes

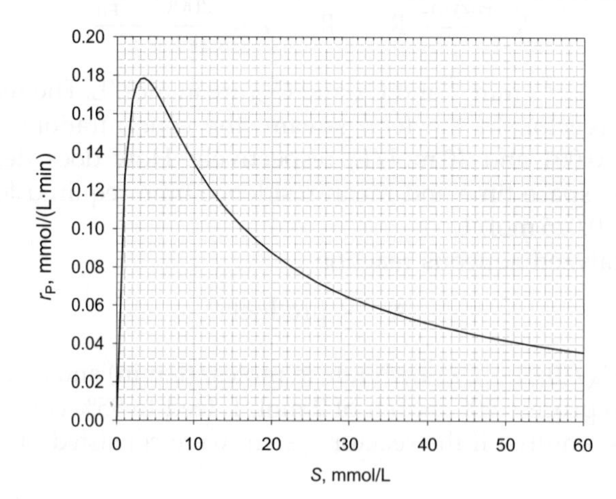

FIGURE P8.7

is 100%, i.e. no impact of immobilization on the enzyme on catalytic activity. Determine the conversion of substrate if the reactor has a working volume of 1000 L.

8.9. In an enzymatic reaction, substrate S is converted irreversibly to produce P. It is suspected that the product inhibits the reaction, and consequently the rate of the reaction is determined for four values of S at each of four levels of the product concentration P. The 16 rate measurements are collected in Table P8.9. Determine the rate constants and type of product inhibition.

TABLE P8.9 Enzymatic Rate Data r_P at Four Levels of S and P

	P, mg/L			
S, g/L	**3**	**9**	**27**	**81**
0.1	0.073	0.058	0.036	0.017
0.4	0.128	0.102	0.064	0.030
1.6	0.158	0.126	0.079	0.037
6.4	0.168	0.134	0.084	0.039

8.10. Decarboxylation of glyoxalate (S) by mitochondria is inhibited by malonate (I). Using data in Table P8.10 obtained in batch experiments, determine the following:

TABLE P8.10

Glyox	Rate of CO_2 evolution, r_{CO_2}, mmol/(L h)		
S, mmol/L	$I = 0$	$I = 1.26$ mmol/L	$I = 1.95$ mmol/L
0.25	1.02	0.73	0.56
0.33	1.39	0.87	0.75
0.40	1.67	1.09	0.85
0.50	1.89	1.30	1.00
0.60	2.08	1.41	1.28
0.75	2.44	1.82	1.39
1.00	2.50	2.17	1.82

(a) What type of inhibition is this?
(b) Determine the constants r_{max}, K_m, and K_I

8.11. We wish to treat 50 L/min of liquid feed containing 1 mol-A/L to 98% conversion with a batch reactor system. The overall reaction stoichiometry is given by

$$2A \rightarrow R + U, \quad r = \frac{k_1 C_A}{K_m + C_A}$$

where $k_1 = 0.8$ moles · liter^{-1} · min^{-1} and $K_m = 0.025$ mol/L. For each batch of operation, 6 h of total preparation time is needed. Determine the reactor size needed to complete the task.

8.12. We wish to treat a stream containing 150 mol-A/min at 1.2 mol-A/L to 99% conversion with a batch reactor system. The overall reaction stoichiometry is given by

$$1.2\text{A} \rightarrow \text{R} + \text{U}, \quad r = \frac{k_1 C_A}{K_m + C_A}$$

where $k_1 = 0.8$ moles · liter^{-1} · min^{-1} and $K_m = 0.012$ mol/L. For each batch of operation, 3 h of total preparation time is needed. Determine the reactor size needed to complete the task.

8.13. We wish to treat a stream containing 250 mol-A/min at 2 mol-A/L to 99.9% conversion with a flow reactor system. The overall reaction stoichiometry is given by

$$\text{A} \rightarrow \text{R} + \text{U}, \quad r = \frac{k_1 C_A}{K_m + C_A}$$

where $k_1 = 0.75$ mol/L/min and $K_m = 0.012$ mol/L. It is decided that one PFR and one CSTR were to be chosen to carry out the task. Determine the optimum arrangement and reactor sizes needed.

8.14. We wish to treat a liquid stream of 360 L/min containing at 1.5 mol-A/L to 98% conversion with a flow reactor system. The overall reaction stoichiometry is given by

$$\text{A} \rightarrow \text{R} + \text{U}, \quad r = \frac{k_1 C_A}{K_m + C_A}$$

where $k_1 = 0.9$ mol/L/min and $K_m = 0.001$ mol/L. It is decided that two CSTRs were to be chosen to carry out the task. Determine the reactor sizes needed.

8.15. The enzymatic hydrolization of fish oil extracted from crude eel oil has been carried out using lipase L. One of the desired products is docosahexaenic acid, which is used as a medicine in China. For 40 mg of enzyme, the Michaelis–Menten saturation constant is 6.2×10^{-2} mmol/L and r_{max} is 5.6 mmol · liter^{-1} · min^{-1}.

(a) Calculate the time necessary to reduce the concentration of fish oil from 1.4% to 0.2 vol %.

(b) Calculate the time necessary to reduce the concentration of fish oil from 1.2% to 0.1 vol % if the enzyme loading is 60 mg.

8.16. Beef catalase has been used to accelerate the decomposition of hydrogen peroxide to yield water and oxygen. The concentration of hydrogen peroxide is given as a function of time for a reaction mixture with a pH of 6.76 maintained at 30 °C as shown in Table P8.16.

TABLE P8.16

t, min	0	10	20	50	100
$C_{H_2O_2}$, mol/L	0.02	0.01775	0.0158	0.0106	0.005

(a) Determine the Michaelis–Menten parameters: r_{max} and K_m.

(b) If the enzyme loading is tripled, what will be the substrate concentration be after 20 min?

8.17. The production of L-malic acid (used in medicines and food additives) was produced over immobilized cells of *Bacillus flavum* MA-3.

$$HOOCCH = CHCOOH + H_2O \xrightarrow{\text{fumarase}} HOOCCH_2CH(OH)COOH$$

The following rate law was obtained for the rate of formation of product:

$$r_P = \frac{r_{max}S}{K_m + S}\left(1 - \frac{P}{P_\infty}\right)$$

where $r_{max} = 76$ Mol/(L · day), $K_m = 0.048$ mol/L, and $P_\infty = 1.69$ mol/L. Design a reactor to process 10 m^3/day of 1.2 mol/L of fumaric acid (S).

(a) A batch reactor is chosen. The required conversion of fumaric acid is 99%. The total preparation time (loading, unloading and cleaning) is 3 h for each batch.

(b) A CSTR is chosen. The required fumaric acid conversion is 99%.

8.18. One-hundred fifty moles of S per hour are available in concentration of 0.5 mol/L by a previous process. This stream is to be reacted with B to produce P and *D*. The reaction proceeds by the aqueous-phase reaction and catalyzed by an enzyme E,

$$S + B \rightleftarrows P + D$$

S is the limiting substrate, and B is in excess. Michaelis–Menten rate parameters are $r_{max} = 2.0$ mol · L^{-1} · min^{-1} and $K_m = 0.02$ mol/L when the enzyme loading 0.001 g/L. CSTR has been selected to carry out the process. S costs $0.1/mol, P sells for $0.8/mol, and the enzyme E costs $50/g. The cost of operating the reactor is $0.1 L^{-1} · h^{-1}. Assume no value or cost of disposal of unreacted S and entrained enzyme E (i.e. separation or recovery cost to S is identical to the fresh S cost).

(a) What is the relationship between rate of formation of P and enzyme loading?

(b) Perform a mole balance on the reactor to relate the concentration of exiting S with reactor size.

(c) What is the optimum concentration of S at the outlet of the reactor? What is the optimum enzyme loading? What is the optimum reactor size?

(d) What is the cash flow per mole of product from the process?

(e) What is the cost of enzyme per unit cost of substrate?

8.19. We have an opportunity to supply 500 mol of P per hour to enter the market. P is to be produced by

$$S \rightarrow P$$

Catalyzed by an enzyme E. Michaelis–Menten rate parameters are $r_{max} = 0.1$ mol · L^{-1} · min^{-1} and $K_m = 0.01$ mol/L when the enzyme loading 0.001 g/L. CSTR has been selected to carry out the process. There is a stream containing S at 2 mol/L is available for use. S costs $0.2/mol, P sells for $1.5/mol, and the enzyme E costs $80/g. The cost of operating the reactor is $0.1 L^{-1} · h^{-1}. Assume no value or cost of disposal of unreacted S and entrained enzyme E (i.e. separation or recovery cost to S is identical to the fresh S cost).

(a) What is the relationship between rate of formation of P and enzyme loading?
(b) Perform a mole balance on the reactor to relate the concentration of exiting S with reactor size.
(c) What is the optimum concentration of S at the outlet of the reactor? What is the optimum enzyme loading? What is the optimum reactor size?
(d) What is the cash flow per mole of product from the process?
(e) What is the cost of enzyme per unit cost of substrate?

CHAPTER

9

Chemical Reactions on Solid Surfaces

OUTLINE

In Chapter 8, we have learned that enzyme can be employed such that a specific product can be produced from a given substrate. In the process, enzyme is not consumed. This is commonly seen in making wine, cheese, and bread: small amount of the previous batch is added to make a new batch (in practice for more than 2000 years).

In 1835, Berzelius realized that the small amounts of a foreign substance could greatly affect the course of chemical reactions. Later in 1894, Ostwald formally states that catalysts

Bioprocess Engineering
http://dx.doi.org/10.1016/B978-0-444-59525-6.00009-3

are substances that accelerate the rate of chemical reactions without being consumed. Catalyst has been employed in industry today to selectively speed up desired reactions. The most common and preferred catalysts are solids as solids can be separated and recovered more easily from reaction mixture.

It is thus rightly so that the single case of reactions most important in bioprocess engineering application are those which occur on solid surfaces when either an heterogeneous catalyst is used to promote the rate of reaction (catalysis) or one main reactant is in solid phase. Solid catalysts are easy to be recovered and reused for carrying out reactions otherwise involving only fluids (gaseous and/or liquid substances). Solid feedstock and/or products are also common in bioprocesses where renewable biomass is being converted. Reactions occurring on surfaces are remarkably similar kinetically. Catalysts for various reactions are found among a wide variety of metals, metal oxides, and metals on various support materials such as carbon and metal oxides. One property of most catalysts is that they provide a large amount of surface per unit volume on which reaction can occur, which normally requires the effective surface to be contained within a porous matrix of some sort. This particular characteristic leads to a number of interesting and important problems arising from the interaction of the rates of transport of mass and energy through such porous matrices, which we shall discuss in detail later.

Common catalytic reactions are

1. Alkylation and dealkylation reactions. Alkylation is the addition of an alkyl group to an organic compound. It is commonly carried out with Friedel–Crafts catalysts, $AlCl_3$ along with trace of HCl. For example,

$$CH_3CH_2CH{=}CH_2 + C_4H_{10} \xrightarrow{AlCl_3} C_8H_{18}$$

SiO_2–Al_2O_3, SiO_2–MgO, and montmorillonite clay are common dealkylation catalysts.

2. Isomerization reactions. Acid-promoted Al_2O_3 is a catalyst used in conversion of normal (straight chain) hydrocarbons to branched hydrocarbons. Acid and base catalysts are both found suited in most isomerization reactions.
3. Hydrogenation and dehydrogenation. The most ingredients involving hydrogen are *d*-orbital containing metals Co, Ni, Rh, Ru, Os, Pd, Ir, Pt, and metal oxides MoO_2 and Cr_2O_3. Dehydrogenation is favored at high temperatures (>600 °C) and hydrogenation is favored at low temperatures. For example,

$$CH_3CH{=}CHCH_3 \rightarrow CH_2{=}CHCH{=}CH_2 + H_2$$

is catalyzed by calcium nickel phosphate, Cr_2O_3, etc.

4. Oxidation reactions. The transition group (IUPAC group 8, 10, 11) elements are commonly used. Ag, Cu, Pt, Fe, Ni, their oxides, and V_2O_5 and MnO_2 are good oxidation catalysts. For example

$$2C_2H_4 + O_2 \xrightarrow{Ag} 2C_2H_4O$$

$$2SO_2 + O_2 \xrightarrow{V_2O_5} 2SO_3$$

$$2C_2H_5OH + O_2 \overset{Cu}{\rightarrow} 2CH_3CHO + 2H_2O$$

$$2CH_3OH + O_2 \overset{Ag}{\rightarrow} 2HCHO + 2H_2O$$

$$4NH_3 + 5O_2 \overset{Pt}{\rightarrow} 4NO + 6H_2O$$

$$2C_2H_6 + 7O_2 \overset{Ni}{\rightarrow} 4CO_2 + 6H_2O$$

5. Hydration and dehydration (or condensation). This type of reactions are catalyzed by substances that have strong affinity to water. Al_2O_3, SiO_2-Al_2O_3 gel, MgO, clay, phosphoric acid, and salts are good catalysts. For example,

$$CH_2{=}CH_2 + H_2O \rightarrow CH_3CH_2OH$$

which is an interesting reaction. It used to be a cheap way to produce ethanol from petroleum-based ethylene. The reverse of the reaction is more important today as ethanol can be produced from renewable resources, and ethylene is a valuable monomer for higher alkenes (jet-fuel) and polymer production.

6. Halogenation and dehalogenation. These reactions are commonly catalyzed with an active ingredient of $CuCl_2$, AgCl, or Pd. Halogenation can occur without catalyst. However, catalyst is used to improve selectivity.

Solid catalysts usually have fine pores such that reactants can be "fixed" or brought tightly together by active centers on the surface for reaction to occur. Fig. 9.1 shows a schematic of typical zeolite catalysts.

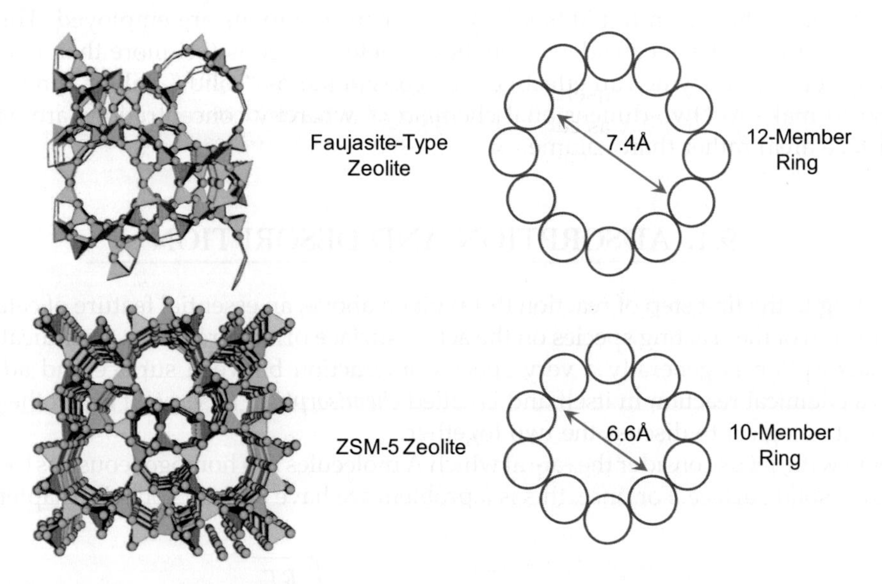

FIGURE 9.1 Typical zeolite (alumina-silica or Al_2O_3-SiO_2) catalyst: 3-D pore formed by 12 oxygen ring and 1-D pore formed by 10 oxygen ring. More zeolite structures can be found at http://www.iza-structure.org/databases/.

Another characteristic of catalytic reactions is that it cannot in general be assumed, once reaction is established at a certain rate under given conditions, that the rate will remain constant with the passage of time. Catalysts normally lose some or all of their specific activity for a desired chemical transformation with time of utilization. This effect, normally referred to as *deactivation*, can come from a number of different sources and is often very important in the analysis and/or design of catalytic processes and reactors.

It is most convenient to consider surface reactions as a series of several steps, in essence a type of chain reaction, which (as we have seen in Chapter 3) employs the active centers of reaction in a closed sequence. Let us again turn to the simple example of an isomerization reaction, $A \rightarrow B$, now taking place on a surface containing one type of active center, σ. The individual reaction steps are:

$$A + \sigma \rightleftarrows A\cdot\sigma \tag{9.1a}$$

$$A\cdot\sigma \rightarrow B\cdot\sigma \tag{9.1b}$$

$$B\cdot\sigma \rightleftarrows B + \sigma \tag{9.1c}$$

The first step in this sequence, which we have written as a chemical reaction, represents the adsorption of A on the surface; the second is the reaction of the surface-adsorbed A species, $A\cdot\sigma$, to the corresponding B species on the surface, $B\cdot\sigma$; and third is the desorption of product B from the surface. We will have to develop our ideas concerning surface reactions by considering each of three steps individually, much as we did in examining the *Lindemann* scheme. The development is based mostly on gas/solid systems, which comprise the most common types of heterogeneous catalytic reactions, however the analysis is also generally valid for liquid/solid systems. Normally for gas/solid systems the expressions for adsorption equilibrium and reaction rate are written in terms of partial pressures of reactant and product species, whereas in liquid/solid systems concentrations are employed. This is not the first time that we have considered kinetics in heterogeneous (i.e. more than one phase) reaction systems, as enzyme can effectively be considered as "solid." Still, it is not an easy transition to make to "two-dimensional chemistry," whereby concentrations are based on area (surface area) rather than volume.

9.1. ADSORPTION AND DESORPTION

According to the first step of reaction (9.1a) given above, an essential feature of catalysis is the adsorption of the reacting species on the active surface prior to reaction. As indicated, this type of adsorption is generally a very specific interaction between surface and adsorbate which is a chemical reaction in itself and is called *chemisorption*. *Desorption* is just the reverse of this, so it is logical to discuss the two together.

To begin with, let us consider the rate at which A molecules in a homogeneous gas (or liquid) will strike a solid surface. For once, this is a problem we have already solved (Chapter 6).

$$Z_{cT}(\mathrm{A, surface}) = N_{AV}C_A\sqrt{\frac{RT}{2\pi M_A}} \tag{6.21}$$

This would give us the maximum possible rate of adsorption (the forward reaction in Eqn (9.1a)) in any system if every molecule striking the surface was adsorbed. This is independent of whether the adsorption is chemisorptions or physisorption, which we will define later. Thus, it is not difficult to imagine the net adsorption–desorption rate is given by

$$r = k_{ad} C_A \theta C_\sigma - k_{des} \theta_A C_\sigma \tag{9.2}$$

where k_{ad} is the adsorption rate constant, C_A is the concentration of the adsorbate in the bulk fluid phase, θ is the fraction of the total possible available positions where A can be adsorbed that are not occupied by any adsorbate molecules, C_σ is the surface concentration of the total possible available positions or sites where A can be adsorbed, θ_A is the fraction of the total possible available positions that are occupied by A. Eqn (9.2) is analogous to the (elementary) reaction rate for a stoichiometry shown in Eqn (9.1a). This is the basis of our discussion on the adsorption and desorption. We still need to figure out what are C_σ and the two rate constants. Before we move further, we shall need to define the surface and type of interactions.

9.1.1. Ideal Surfaces

Molecules we already know something about, so in the present instance we need more detail on the nature of the surface. The simplest model of a surface, the *ideal surface* is one in which each adsorption site, σ, has the same energy of interaction with the adsorbate molecules, which is not affected by the presence or absence of adsorbate molecules on adjacent adsorbent sites and in which each site can accommodate only one adsorbate molecule or atom. We might represent the energy contours of each a surface qualitatively as shown in Fig. 9.2. Adsorption would occur when a molecule or atom of adsorbate with the required energy strikes an unoccupied site, and the energy contours (or energy variation when approaching the adsorbent surface) would be unaffected by the extent of adsorption, as depicted by Fig. 9.3 for ideal enthalpy change.

These requirements for reaction (adsorption) to occur look very similar to those we imposed on the bimolecular collision number in order to derive the reactive collision

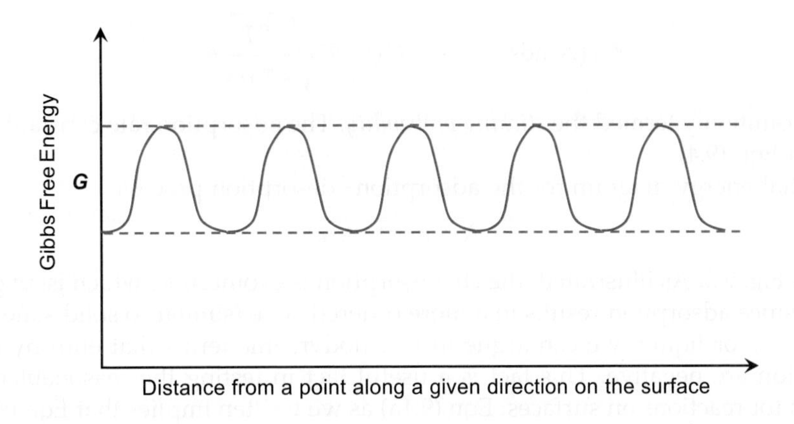

FIGURE 9.2 A schematic of atomic force (interaction energy) on an energetically homogeneous surface.

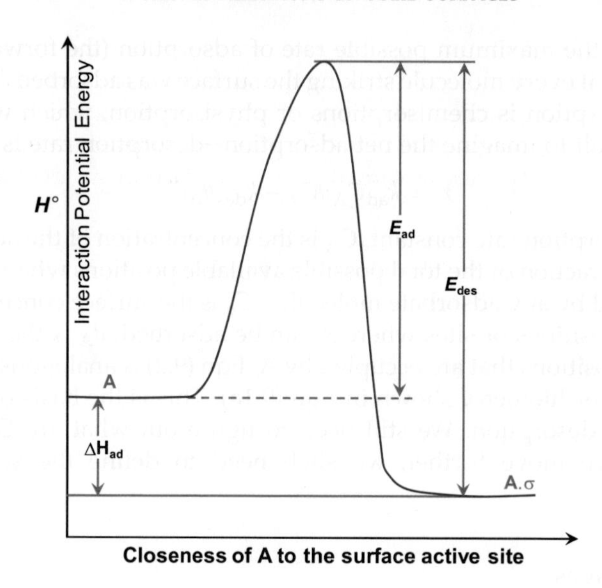

FIGURE 9.3 Interaction potential between molecule A and the active site σ on the surface.

frequency, $Z_{cT}(A, B)$, of Eqn (6.20). If we designate E as the activation energy required for chemisorption, C_σ as the total concentration of sites available for chemisorption, θ the fraction of free sites available for chemisorption, and θ_A the fraction of sites on the surface covered by the adsorbate molecule A, the following analog to Eqn (6.21) may be written as

$$Z_{cT}(\mathrm{A, ads}) = N_{AV}C_A\sqrt{\frac{RT}{2\pi M_A}}C_\sigma\theta e^{-\frac{E_{ad}}{RT}} \tag{9.3}$$

We may also include a term analogous to the steric factor to be used as a measure of the deviation of chemisorption rates from this ideal limit.

$$Z_{cT}(\mathrm{A, ads}) = N_{AV}C_AC_\sigma\theta\xi\sqrt{\frac{RT}{2\pi M_A}}e^{-\frac{E_{ad}}{RT}} \tag{9.4}$$

where ξ is commonly termed the *sticking probability*. The adsorption rate constant is thus predicted from Eqn (9.4).

A potential-energy diagram for the adsorption—desorption process

$$A + \sigma \rightleftarrows A \cdot \sigma \tag{9.1a}$$

is shown in Fig. 9.3. As illustrated, the chemisorption is exothermic, which is, in general, the case. Also, since adsorption results in a more ordered state (similar to solid state) compared to the bulk gas or liquid, we can argue in thermodynamic terms that entropy changes on chemisorption are negative. This fact is a useful fact in testing the reasonableness of rate expressions for reactions on surfaces. Eqn (9.1a) as we written implies that Eqn (9.2) is valid, for which we will call the Langmuir adsorption rate.

An important step in the consideration of surface reactions is the equilibrium level of adsorption on a surface. With Eqn (9.1a), the rate is shown to be reversible and equilibrated at a long enough timescale, so the rate of adsorption equals the rate of desorption. It is convenient to think of this as a process of dynamic equilibrium, where the net rate of change is zero. Assuming A is the only species adsorbed on the surface or at least on the active site of interest, from Eqns (9.2) and (9.4), we have

$$\frac{\theta_A}{\theta C_A} = \frac{k_{ad}}{k_{des}} = \frac{k_{ad0}}{k_{des0}} e^{-\frac{E_{ad}-E_{des}}{RT}} = \frac{k_{ad0}}{k_{des0}} e^{\frac{-\Delta H_{ad}}{RT}} \tag{9.5}$$

This expression is extraordinarily useful, since it permits us to obtain some information concerning the surface coverage factors, θ and θ_A, about which we have been rather vague. The point is that these factors cannot be measured conveniently, while macroscopic quantities such as C_A and the heat of absorption can. Eqn (9.5) provides a link between the two. Solving for the ratio θ_A/θ it can be seen that the surface coverage at equilibrium (or at least some function of it) is determined by the temperature of the system and the partial pressure of adsorbate. Such an equation for fixed temperature and varying partial pressure expresses the *adsorption isotherm* for the adsorbate, or, for fixed partial pressure and varying temperature, the *adsorption isobar.* The heat of adsorption, ΔH_{ad}, appears in Eqn (9.5) since in solving for the ratio of surface coverage functions the difference ($E_{des} - E_{ad}$) appears in the exponential; from Fig. 9.3 we see that this is equal in magnitude to the heat of adsorption.

Eqn (9.5) is termed the Langmuir isotherm, which we may write in more general notation as

$$\frac{\theta_A}{\theta} = K_A C_A = K_A^{\circ} e^{\frac{-\Delta H_{ad}}{RT}} C_A \tag{9.6}$$

where

$$K_A = \frac{k_{ad}}{k_{des}} \tag{9.7}$$

The total number of active sites or centers is fixed for a given amount of surfaces. Therefore, an active site (just the same as the active sites in enzymes) balance leads to

$$\theta_A + \theta = 1 \tag{9.8}$$

if A is the only adsorbate on the particular type of active centers. The site balance is not dependent on temperature or concentration. Combining Eqns (9.6) and (9.8), we obtain

$$\theta_A = \frac{K_A C_A}{1 + K_A C_A} \tag{9.9}$$

which is the Langmuir isotherm equation for the nondissociative adsorption of a single species on a surface (i.e. single molecule on a single-type active site).

In many cases of practical importance, the adsorbate molecule will dissociate on adsorption (e.g. H_2 on many metals) or occupy two adjacent active sites by bonding at two points in the molecule (e.g. ethylene on nickel). In such cases,

$$A_2 + 2\sigma \rightleftarrows 2A\cdot\sigma \tag{9.10}$$

or

$$A + 2\sigma \rightleftarrows \sigma{\cdot}A{\cdot}\sigma \tag{9.11}$$

and the corresponding adsorption equilibrium is

$$r = k_{ad}\theta^2 C_\sigma^2 C_{A_2} - k_{des}\theta_A^2 C_\sigma^2 = 0 \tag{9.12}$$

$$\left(\frac{\theta_A}{\theta}\right)^2 = \frac{k_{ad}}{k_{des}} C_{A_2} \tag{9.13}$$

which leads to the isotherm equation

$$\theta_A = \frac{(K_A C_{A_2})^{1/2}}{1 + (K_A C_{A_2})^{1/2}} \tag{9.14}$$

If the adsorbate molecule is immobile on the surface, the occupancy of nearest-neighbor active sites should be accounted. This is not a large refinement, however, and Eqn (9.12) will be employed without reference to the detailed nature of the adsorbate layer.

A second modification of practical importance is when more than one adsorbate species is present on the surface competing for the same type of active centers (or sites). For example, consider the adsorption equilibrium (no surface reaction)

$$A + \sigma \rightleftarrows A{\cdot}\sigma$$

$$B{\cdot}\sigma \rightleftarrows B + \sigma$$

where A and B are chemisorbed on the same type of surface site, σ; that is, they are competitively adsorbed on the surface. In this case, Eqn (9.6) is applicable to both A and B (with different heats of adsorption) as dictated by the net adsorption rate of zero at equilibrium, i.e. $\frac{\theta_A}{\theta} = K_A C_A$ and $\frac{\theta_B}{\theta} = K_B C_B$. The total number of active site balance is now

$$\theta_A + \theta_B + \theta = 1$$

as the active sites are shared by three parts: active sites occupied by A, active sites occupied by B, and free active sites available for adsorption. Therefore, the corresponding isotherm equations for the surface coverages of A and B are

$$\theta_A = \frac{K_A C_A}{1 + K_A C_A + K_B C_B} \tag{9.15a}$$

$$\theta_B = \frac{K_B C_B}{1 + K_A C_A + K_B C_B} \tag{9.15b}$$

A major property of the Langmuir isotherm is that of saturation. In Eqn (9.9), for example when $K_A C_A >> 1$, $\theta_A \to 1$, and no further adsorption occurs. This is a result of the surface model, in which each adsorption site can accommodate only one adsorbate molecule. Saturation of the surface, then, corresponds to the occupancy of all sites and is called *monolayer coverage.* At low concentrations, $K_A C_A << 1$ and Eqn (9.9) assumes a linear form in C_A corresponding to Henry's law of adsorption. These general features are shown in Fig. 9.4. Experimentally, one measures either the weight or volume of material adsorbed, and the ratio of

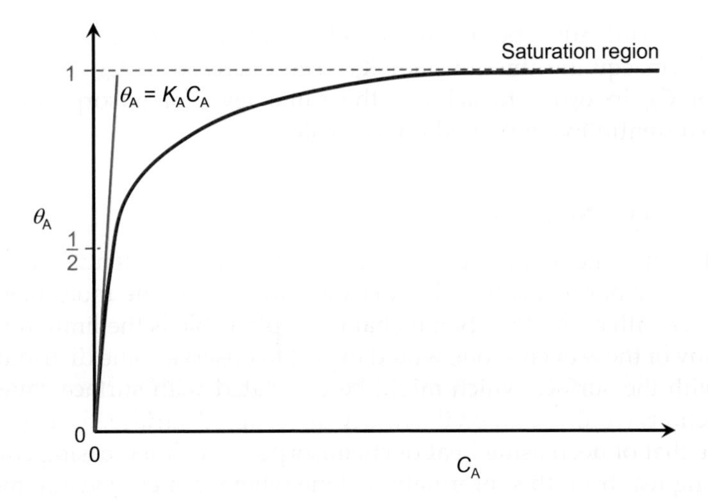

FIGURE 9.4 Monolayer surface coverage, typical Langmuir adsorption isotherm.

this quantity at a given partial pressure (for adsorption from gas phase) or concentration to that at saturation can be taken as a direct measure of surface coverage. Mathematically,

$$\theta_A = \frac{n_{AS}}{n_{max}} \tag{9.16}$$

where n_{AS} is the number of moles of A adsorbed on the surface and n_{max} is the maximum number of moles that can be adsorbed on the surface.

At this point, we observe that the ideal (or Langmuir) adsorption isotherms for a single component and a multicomponent mixture are quite similar. Indeed, in general, the ideal adsorption isotherm or coverage for a particular species j is given by

$$\theta_j = \frac{K_j C_j}{1 + \sum_{m=1}^{N_s} K_m C_m} \tag{9.17}$$

where θ_j is the fraction of sites that are covered by species j. If there are dissociative species in the mixture, modification of Eqn (9.17) needs to be made for the dissociative species in the same fashion as that in Eqn (9.14).

The interpretation of data on adsorption in terms of the Langmuir isotherm is most easily accomplished using the procedure previously described for reaction rate data. As pointed out earlier, the total number of active site is not dependent on the temperature or concentration, the Langmuir isotherm is restricted then by the total amount of adsorbate could be adsorbed on the surface.

Examples of false obedience to the Langmuir isotherm abound. These usually arise when adsorption data have not been obtained over a sufficiently wide range of concentrations or partial pressures (of gas adsorbate); a good test is to see if value of the saturated adsorbate n_{max} evaluated from isotherm data at different temperatures are equal, since within the framework of the Langmuir surface model the saturation capacity should not vary with the temperature. It can be difficult to tell, however, in view of experimental error. It is, on the other hand, very difficult experimentally, as higher temperature usually results in lowers adsorption isotherm equilibrium constant K_A. The decrease in K_A requires much higher concentration of C_A in order to achieve the same level of adsorption as depicted by Fig. 9.5, where concentration is plotted on log scale.

9.1.2. Idealization of Nonideal Surfaces

It is not hard to imagine that no real surface could have the potential-energy distribution as depicted in Fig. 9.2 nor is it reasonable to expect that adsorbate molecules on the surface would not interact with each other. Somewhat more plausible is the limitation of monolayer adsorption. In any of these events, one would expect to observe some distribution of energies of interaction with the surface which might be correlated with surface coverage. Since the strongest interactions would occur on the nearly unoccupied surface, the experimental observation would be that of decreasing heat of chemisorption with increasing coverage. It is not possible to distinguish from this information alone whether energetic inhomogeneity of the surface or adsorbate interactions are the cause, but in most of the practical applications with which we are concerned, this amount of detail is not necessary. In the following discussion, the case of an inhomogeneous surface shall be considered, using the specific example of non-dissociative adsorption of a single species for illustration.

Consider that the surface may be divided into a number of groups of sites, each characterized with a similar heat of chemisorption and so capable of being represented by a Langmuir isotherm. The fractional coverage of each of these for a single adsorbate A is

$$\theta_{Ai} = \frac{K_{Ai}C_A}{1 + K_{Ai}C_A} \tag{9.18}$$

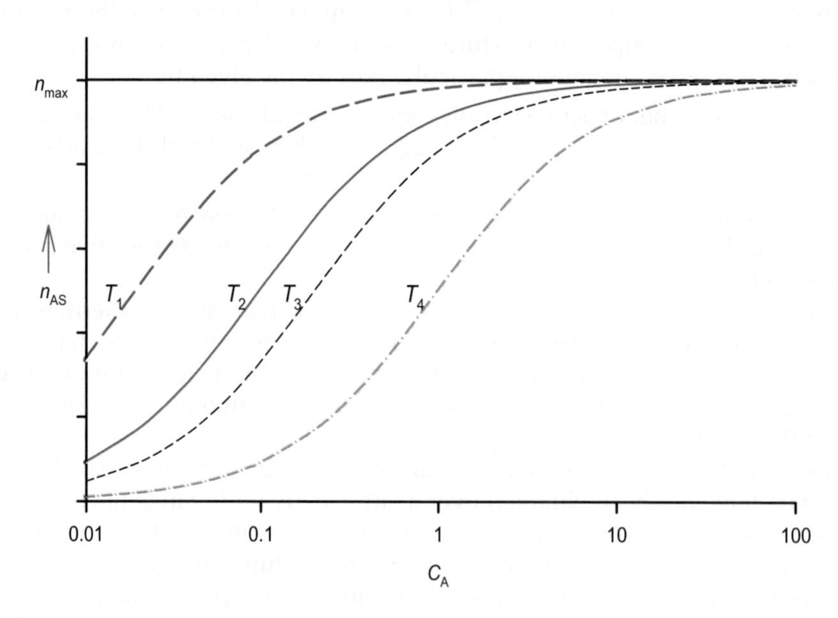

FIGURE 9.5 Variation of adsorption isotherm with temperature following Langmuir adsorption.

and the total coverage is

$$\theta_A n_\sigma = \sum_{i=1}^{n_T} \theta_{Ai} n_{\sigma i} \tag{9.19}$$

where $n_{\sigma i}$ is the number of adsorption sites belonging to group i and can be represented by an appropriate distribution function. It is reasonable to write this distribution function in terms of the heat of chemisorption, ΔH_{ad}, as the interaction between the adsorbate and adsorbent molecules is expected to vary. With different distribution functions, one would expect different adsorption isotherms and deviating differently from the Langmuir adsorption isotherm.

9.1.2.1. ExLan Isotherm

One simplistic distribution function for a nonideal surface the available adsorption sites are exponentially distributed with the excess interaction energy,

$$dn_{\sigma i} = f_{\sigma 0} e^{-\frac{E_s}{RT}} dE_s \tag{9.20}$$

where $E_s = \Delta H^0_{ad} - \Delta H_{ad}$, $f_{\sigma 0}$ is a scaling constant and $dn_{\sigma i}$ the fraction of sites with heats of chemisorption between $-\Delta H^0_{ad} + E_s$ and $-\Delta H^0_{ad} + E_s + dE_s$. If we further assume, as indicated by the form of Eqn (9.20), that the groups of sites do not differ greatly in energy level as one goes from one level to the next, the summation may be replaced by integration with respect to the distribution function.

$$n_\sigma = \int_0^{n_\sigma} dn_{\sigma i} = \int_0^{E_{max}} f_{\sigma 0} e^{-\frac{E_s}{RT}} dE_s = RT f_{\sigma 0}\left(1 - e^{-\frac{E_{max}}{RT}}\right) \tag{9.21}$$

where n_σ is the total number of active (adsorption) sites available, $-\Delta H^0_{ad}$ and $-\Delta H^0_{ad} + E_{max}$ are the maximum adsorption heats required for the adsorbate molecule to be adsorbed on the adsorbent surface, where the minimum merely corresponds to a phase change to the more orderly state on the adsorbent surface. It is expected that the minimum adsorption heat is at least higher than the condensation (from gas to liquid) while could be lower than the solidification (from gas to solid) for gas adsorbate molecules. For liquid adsorbate molecules, this minimum adsorption heat could be lower than the solidification (from liquid to solid) heat. Eqn (9.21) is reduced to

$$f_{\sigma 0} = \frac{n_\sigma}{RT\left(1 - e^{-\frac{E_{max}}{RT}}\right)} \tag{9.22}$$

The fraction of active sites that are occupied by the adsorbate molecules is

$$\theta_A = \frac{1}{n_\sigma} \int_0^{n_\sigma} \theta_{Ai} dn_{\sigma i} = \frac{f_{\sigma 0}}{n_\sigma} \int_0^{E_{max}} e^{-\frac{E_s}{RT}} \frac{K_A^\circ e^{\frac{-\Delta H^0_{ad} + E_s}{RT}} C_A}{1 + K_A^\circ e^{\frac{-\Delta H^0_{ad} + E_s}{RT}} C_A} dE_s \tag{9.23}$$

Integration of Eqn (9.23) leads to

$$\theta_A = -\frac{f_{\sigma 0}}{n_\sigma}RT\int_0^{E_{max}}\frac{\overline{K}_A C_A}{e^{-\frac{E_s}{RT}}+\overline{K}_A C_A}de^{-\frac{E_s}{RT}} = -RT\frac{f_{\sigma 0}}{n_\sigma}\overline{K}_A C_A \ln\left(e^{-\frac{E_s}{RT}}+\overline{K}_A C_A\right)\Big|_0^{E_{max}}$$

$$= RT\frac{f_{\sigma 0}}{n_\sigma}\overline{K}_A C_A \ln\frac{1+\overline{K}_A C_A}{e^{-\frac{E_{max}}{RT}}+\overline{K}_A C_A} \tag{9.24}$$

where

$$\overline{K}_A = K_A^0 e^{-\frac{\Delta H_{ad}^0}{RT}} \tag{9.25}$$

Substituting Eqn (9.22) into Eqn (9.24), we obtain a generalized logarithm coverage.

$$\theta_A = \frac{\overline{K}_A C_A}{1-e^{-\frac{E_{max}}{RT}}}\ln\frac{1+\overline{K}_A C_A}{e^{-\frac{E_{max}}{RT}}+\overline{K}_A C_A}$$

Eqn (9.26) may be referred to as ExLan (*Ex*ponential distribution *Lan*gmuir) model. The higher limit on the adsorption heat is generally at least a few times higher than *RT*. Without loosing much utility, one can assume that $E_{max} \to \infty$ because of the fast decrease in the exponential function. Taking this limit on Eqn (9.26), we obtain an expression that has exactly the same number of parameters as the Langmuir isotherm,

$$\theta_A = \overline{K}_A C_A \ln[1+(\overline{K}_A C_A)^{-1}] \tag{9.27}$$

which is effectively still a one parameter nonideal isotherm expression. There is no increase in the number of parameters as compared with the Langmuir isotherm.

Example 9-1 Adsorption of phenol on activated carbon from aqueous solutions. A comparison of nonideal isotherm and ideal isotherm.

Table E9-1.1 shows the experimental data collected in an undergraduate lab run for the adsorption of phenol on activated carbon. Examine the suitability of Langmuir isotherm and exponential energy distribution nonideal isotherm to describe the experimental data.

TABLE E9-1.1 Equilibrium Concentrations of Phenol in Aqueous Solution and in Activated Carbon

Phenol concentration in aqueous solution C_A, mg/L	Phenol concentration is activated carbon C_{As}, mg/g
0	0
1.5	53.0
2.0	62.4
5.1	82.8
6.6	105.0
22.9	137.0
51.6	172.2
80.2	170.9

Solution. This example is typical of adsorption experiments where the concentrations of adsorbate (phenol in this example) are measured in the bulk fluid phase and in the adsorbent. This is different from the coverage we have been discussed in Langmuir isotherm and the nonideal isotherms. However, it is clear that

$$\theta_A = \frac{C_{As}}{C_{As\infty}} \tag{9.28}$$

where $C_{As\infty}$ is the concentration of adsorbate on the adsorbent surface when the concentration of the adsorbate in the bulk fluid phase is infinitely high, i.e. all the active sites on the adsorbent surface are covered by the adsorbate. This quantity is a property of the adsorbent and adsorbate pair and is not a function of temperature.

Substitute Eqn (9.27) into Eqn (9.9), we obtain the Langmuir model

$$C_{As} = \theta_A C_{As\infty} = C_{As\infty}\frac{K_A C_A}{1 + K_A C_A} \tag{9.29}$$

Therefore, we can fit the experimental data with Eqn (9.29) to check if the model can reasonably describe the experimental data. For this exercise, a spreadsheet program is convenient to use as illustrated in Table E9-1.2.

One can observe from Table E9-1.2 that the Langmuir model fit is consistent with the experimental data: the errors or deviations are consistent with the errors apparent in the experimental data. However, the fit is better at high coverage than the lower coverage (concentrations). Fig. E9-1 shows the visual quality of the fit. Visual inspection of the data shown in Fig. E9-1 agrees with our assessment based on Table E9-1.2. Furthermore, visual inspection shows the data are scattered around the model (solid line). Therefore, the Langmuir model is consistent with experimental data within the experimental accuracy.

TABLE E9-1.2 Least Square Parameter Estimation for the Langmuir Isotherm. The Final Solution Shown Are for $C_{As\infty} = 178.1$ mg-phenol/g-activated carbon and $K_A = 0.21732$ (mg/L)$^{-1}$, Which Were Obtained by Minimizing the Variance between the Langmuir Model and the Experimental Data, σ_L, While Changing $C_{As\infty}$ and K_A

Aqueous solution C_A, mg/L	On activated carbon C'_{As}, mg/g	Eqn (9.29) C_{As}, mg/g	Error^2 $(C_{As} - C'_{As})^2$
0	0	0	0
1.5	53.0	43.78934	84.8362
2.0	62.4	53.96358	71.17314
5.1	82.8	93.63607	117.4205
6.6	105.0	104.9492	0.002578
22.9	137.0	148.3163	128.0591
51.6	172.2	163.5351	75.07994
80.2	170.9	168.4535	5.985588

$$\sigma_L = \sqrt{\frac{\sum_{i=1}^{8}(C_{As,i} - C'_{As,i})^2}{8-1}} = 8.302814$$

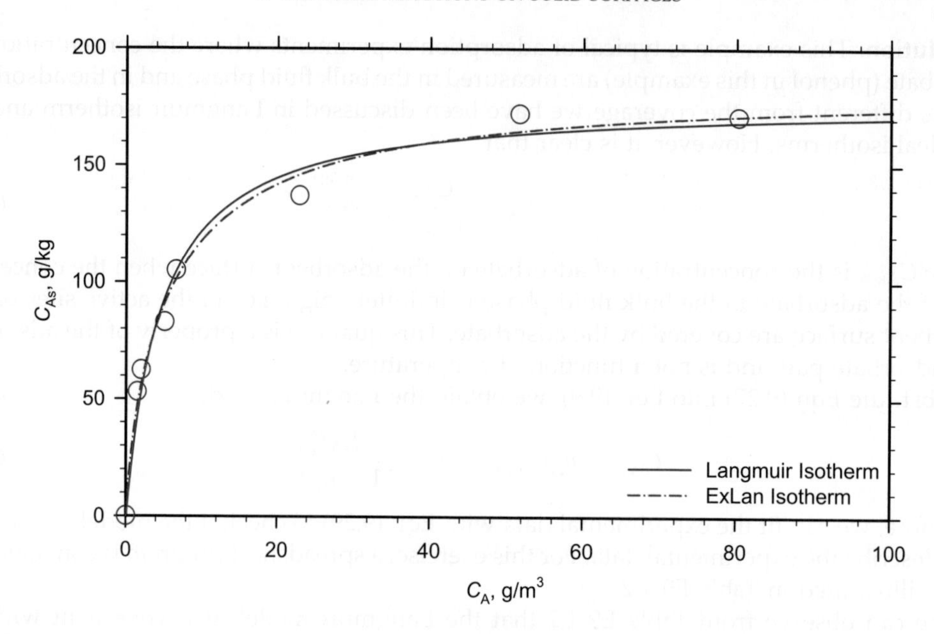

FIGURE E9-1 Langmuir isotherm and ExLan isotherm fits to the experimental data of phenol adsorption on activated carbon.

We next examine the suitability of the exponential adsorption energy distribution nonideal adsorption isotherm, Eqn (9.27). Substitute Eqn (9.28) into Eqn (9.27), we obtain the ExLan model

$$C_{As} = C_{As\infty}\overline{K}_A C_A \ln[1 + (\overline{K}_A C_A)^{-1}] \tag{9.30}$$

The data fit is performed the same way as that for the Langmuir adsorption isotherm model and illustrated in Table E9.1-3 for the ExLan adsorption model. The fitted line is also shown in Fig. E9-1 as the dot-dashed line.

One can observe both from Fig. E9-1 and Table E9-1.3 that one-parameter nonideal adsorption isotherm describes the experimental data well within the apparent experimental error. Comparing with Langmuir model fit (Table E9-1.2), the ExLan adsorption isotherm fit improved the low coverage region, and the overall fit is slightly better using the nonideal adsorption isotherm (lower standard deviation or variance).

One can conclude that despite their simplicity, both Langmuir adsorption isotherm and the nonideal adsorption isotherm describe the experimental data quite well.

One can show that the one-parameter nonideal adsorption isotherm for dissociative adsorption is given by

$$C_{As} = C_{As\infty}\sqrt{\overline{K}_{A_2} C_{A_2}}\ \ln\left[1 + (\overline{K}_{A_2} C_{A_2})^{-1/2}\right] \tag{9.31}$$

So far, we have learned that the nonideal adsorption isotherm has similar qualitative behavior as the ideal (Langmuir) isotherm. The ExLan (nonideal adsorption) isotherm correlates experimental better. We have been dealing with single component adsorption only.

TABLE E9-1.3 Least Square Parameter Estimation for the One-Parameter Nonideal Adsorption Isotherm. The Final Solution Shown Are for $C_{As\infty} = 185.0$ mg-phenol/g-Activated Carbon and $\overline{K}_A = 0.07557\ (\text{mg/L})^{-1}$, Which Were Obtained by Minimizing the Variance between the Nonideal Adsorption Model and the Experimental Data, σ_L, While Changing $C_{As\infty}$ and $\overline{K}_A$

Aqueous solution C_A, mg/L	On activated carbon C'_{As}, mg/g	Eqn (9.30) C_{As}, mg/g	Error^2 $(C_{As} - C'_{As})^2$
0	0	0	0
1.5	53.0	47.91687	25.83822
2.0	62.4	56.77735	31.61424
5.1	82.8	91.23779	71.19638
6.6	105.0	101.5365	11.99601
22.9	137.0	146.0282	81.50787
51.6	172.2	164.7061	56.15872
80.2	170.9	171.2536	0.125006
		$\sigma_L = \sqrt{\dfrac{\sum_{i=1}^{8}(C_{As,i} - C'_{As,i})^2}{8-1}}$	$= 6.306872$

To have the theory useful, we must extend the derivations to multicomponent adsorptions. To do this, we note that the interaction energy between the adsorbate molecule and the adsorption center (or active site) can be divided into two parts: "surface energy" and "adsorbate bonding energy." The "adsorbate bonding energy" is dependent on adsorbate molecule and the adsorbent pair but not dependent on the location of the surface where the adsorption occurs. At this point, we can assume that the "adsorbate bonding energy" is equivalent to the minimum heat of adsorption or adsorption heat under ideal conditions. The "surface energy" is a property of the adsorbent surface only, unrelated to the adsorbate molecules, although it has an effect only when an adsorbate molecule approaches or is bonded on. Thus, the "surface energy" is the nonideal component of the adsorbate–adsorbent interaction energy. Based on this assumption, we can write the adsorption heat in the Langmuir adsorption isotherm as

$$\Delta H_{\text{ad},j} = \Delta H_{\text{ad},j0} - E_s \tag{9.32}$$

where $\Delta H_{\text{ad},j}$ is the adsorption heat for species j adsorbing onto the adsorbent; $\Delta H_{\text{ad},j0}$ is the "bonding energy" of the species j to the adsorbent surface, which can be thought of as the adsorption energy of species j on the adsorbent surface under ideal adsorption conditions; E_s is the "surface energy" and different for different adsorption site.

For each group (i) of sites that has identical "surface energy," the site coverage according to the Langmuir adsorption isotherm is Eqn (9.17), or

$$\theta_{ji} = \frac{K_{ji}C_j}{1 + \sum_{m=1}^{N_s} K_{mi}C_m} \tag{9.17}$$

Noting that

$$K_{ji} = K_j^\circ \mathrm{e}^{-\frac{\Delta H_{\mathrm{ad},ji}}{RT}} \tag{9.33}$$

Substituting Eqn (9.32) into Eqn (9.33), we obtain

$$K_{ji} = K_j^\circ \mathrm{e}^{-\frac{\Delta H_{\mathrm{ad},j0} - E_s}{RT}} = \overline{K}_j \mathrm{e}^{\frac{E_s}{RT}} \tag{9.34}$$

Now applying the exponential surface energy distribution to E_s, similar to the steps in Eqns (9.19) through (9.23), we obtain

$$\theta_j = \frac{1}{n_\sigma}\int_0^{E_{\max}} f_{\sigma 0}\mathrm{e}^{-\frac{E_s}{RT}} \frac{\overline{K}_j C_j \mathrm{e}^{\frac{E_s}{RT}}}{1+\sum_{m=1}^{N_s}\overline{K}_m C_m \mathrm{e}^{\frac{E_s}{RT}}}\mathrm{d}E_s = -RT\frac{f_{\sigma 0}}{n_\sigma}\overline{K}_j C_j \ln\left(\mathrm{e}^{-\frac{E_s}{RT}} + \sum_{m=1}^{N_s}\overline{K}_m C_m\right)\Bigg|_0^{E_{\max}}$$

where $E_{\max}$ is the maximum (upper limit) of the "surface energy" deviation from the minimum. Thus,

$$\theta_j = \frac{\overline{K}_j C_j}{1-\mathrm{e}^{-\frac{E_{\max}}{RT}}}\ln\frac{1+\sum_{m=1}^{N_s}\overline{K}_m C_m}{\mathrm{e}^{-\frac{E_{\max}}{RT}} + \sum_{m=1}^{N_s}\overline{K}_m C_m} \tag{9.35}$$

Assuming whole spectrum of energy distribution, i.e. $E_{\max} \to \infty$, Eqn (9.35) is reduced to

$$\theta_j = \overline{K}_j C_j \ln\left[1+\left(\sum_{m=1}^{N_s}\overline{K}_m C_m\right)^{-1}\right] \tag{9.36}$$

Therefore, the generalization of multiple component and dissociative adsorption to nonideal adsorption would be straightforward.

9.1.2.2. UniLan Isotherm

We have seen how the "surface energy" distribution using an exponential expression can be treated elegantly for adsorption of multiple species mixture based on Langmuir adsorption isotherm. One other simplistic distribution is the uniform distribution, i.e. all the available active centers (sites) are distributed linearly along the surface energy rise:

$$\mathrm{d}n_{\sigma i} = \frac{n_\sigma}{E_{\max}}\mathrm{d}E_s \tag{9.37}$$

where E_s varies between 0 and $E_{\max}$. The fractional coverage by species j is then

$$\theta_j = \frac{1}{n_\sigma}\int_0^{n_\sigma}\theta_{ji}\mathrm{d}n_{\sigma i} = \frac{1}{E_{\max}}\int_0^{E_{\max}}\frac{\overline{K}_j \mathrm{e}^{\frac{E_s}{RT}} C_j}{1+\sum_{m=1}^{N_s}\overline{K}_m C_m \mathrm{e}^{\frac{E_s}{RT}}}\mathrm{d}E_s \tag{9.38}$$

Integration of Eqn (9.38) yields

$$\theta_j = \frac{RT\overline{K}_jC_j}{E_{\max}\sum_{m=1}^{N_s}\overline{K}_mC_m}\ln\frac{1+\sum_{m=1}^{N_s}\overline{K}_mC_m e^{\frac{E_{\max}}{RT}}}{1+\sum_{m=1}^{N_s}\overline{K}_mC_m} \tag{9.39}$$

For single species adsorption, Eqn (9.39) is reduced to

$$\theta_A = \frac{RT}{E_{\max}}\ln\frac{1+\overline{K}_AC_Ae^{\frac{E_{\max}}{RT}}}{1+\overline{K}_AC_A} \tag{9.40}$$

which is also know as the UniLan (*uni*form distribution *Lan*gmuir) model.

Fig. 9.6 shows the change of coverage with bulk phase concentration as predicted by the three models: Langmuir, UniLan, and ExLan. One can observe that the general shape (or qualitative behaviors) of the three models are quite similar. However, compared with the ideal Langmuir isotherm, the nonideality introduced to the isotherms (either UniLan or ExLan models) causes the isotherm to bend upward, i.e. coverage increases quicker at low bulk phase concentration. This is due to the nonideal adsorption models we used: the interaction energy level distributes from the base line of that corresponds to the ideal surfaces (when equating $\overline{K}_j$ and K_j). Therefore, as one would expect, adsorbate molecules prefer to adsorb to high interaction energy sites (with higher $-\Delta H_{ad}$ values) than lower ones (with lower $-\Delta H_{ad}$ values). The level of adsorption increases with nonideality (or introduction of higher interaction energy sites).

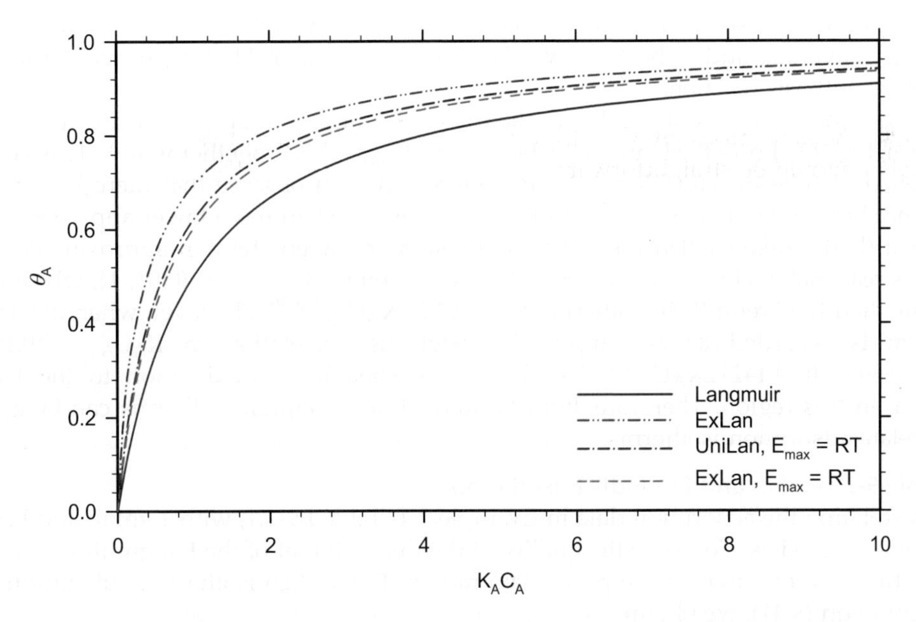

FIGURE 9.6 The adsorption isotherms as predicted by ideal Langmuir adsorption, exponential interaction energy distribution (ExLan) and uniform interaction energy distribution (UniLan).

9.1.3. Common Empirical Isotherms

While our discussions in ideal (Langmuir) and nonideal adsorption isotherms have led to more general adsorption isotherms that could be applicable to a variety of surfaces, we shall make a detour and mention a couple of empirical isotherms. These isotherms were thought of as accounting for nonideality of the adsorbent surfaces. They are approximations to a variety of ideal and nonideal isotherms. As such, their utilities are more restrictive than the above isotherms. The reason we introduce these isotherms is that there are a few classic applications that have utilized these empirical isotherms.

In the low coverage region well before the coverage levels off as the bulk concentration is increased, the Langmuir isotherm (9.9) as well as the generalized logarithm coverage Eqn (9.27) can be approximated by

$$\theta_A = cC_A^m \tag{9.41}$$

In addition, one can note that the dissociative adsorption Eqn (9.14) can be approximated by Eqn (9.37) as well in the low coverage region. This versatile approximation, Eqn (9.41), is called the *Freundlich isotherm*.

In the intermediate coverage region,

$$1 << \overline{K}_A C_A e^{\frac{E_{max}}{RT}} \quad \text{and} \quad 1 >> \overline{K}_A C_A$$

Eqn (9.40) may be approximated by

$$\theta_A \approx \frac{RT}{E_{max}} \ln\left(\overline{K}_A C_A e^{\frac{E_{max}}{RT}}\right) \tag{9.42}$$

which is the Temkin isotherm. Eqn (9.42) correlates experimental data better in the midrange of surface coverage and is best known for the adsorption of Hydrogen and Nitrogen in ammonia synthesis reactions.

To show the closeness of the Freundlich isotherm and Temkin isotherm to the UniLan isotherm, Fig. 9.7 shows the UniLan isotherm with $E_{max} = 5\,RT$ together with ExLan isotherm and Temkin isotherm with identical parameters. One can observe that there is significant difference between ExLan and UniLan isotherms since ExLan has a lower apparent adsorption heat than UniLan when the same parameters are taken. Temkin approximation, Eqn (9.42), is reasonably close to the original UniLan isotherm if $K_A C_A \in (0.01, 1)$, which is less accurate than the Freundlich isotherm, $\theta_A = 0.9128(K_A C_A)^{0.2636}$. However, when the Temkin isotherm is regarded as an empirical model, its correlation in $K_A C_A \in (0.1, 10)$, $\theta_A = 10.804^{-1}\ln(0.14212\overline{K}_A C_A e^{10.804})$, showed reasonable approximation to the UniLan isotherm in this region. Therefore, both Freundlich and Temkin isotherms can be applied to correlate adsorption isotherms.

Example 9-2 Temkin and Freundlich Isotherms.

Recorrelating the adsorption data in Example 9-1, Table E9-1.1, with Temkin and Freundlich isotherm models. Compare the quality of the fits with that of the Langmuir isotherm fit.

Solution. We first look at the power-law model (Freundlich isotherm). Substituting Eqn (9.28) into Eqn (9.41), we obtain

$$C_{As} = c' C_A^m \tag{9.43}$$

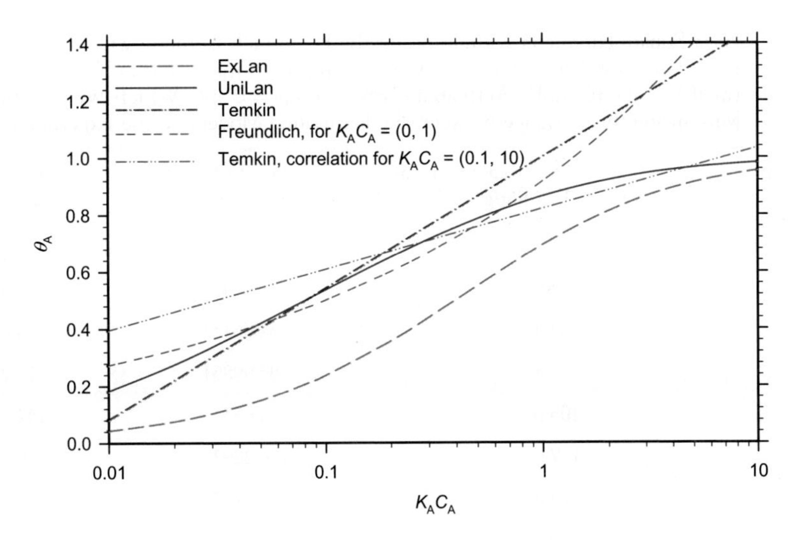

FIGURE 9.7 Approximation of UniLan isotherm by Temkin and Freundlich isotherms, and comparison with ExLan isotherm having the same parameter: $E_{max} = 5\ RT$. Freundlich isotherm were correlated for $K_AC_A \in (0, 1)$: $\theta_A = 0.9128(K_AC_A)^{0.2636}$, and the Temkin isotherm correlation is for $K_AC_A \in (0.1, 10)$: $\theta_A = 10.804^{-1}\ln(0.14212\overline{K}_AC_Ae^{10.804})$.

Therefore, we can fit the experimental data with Eqn (9.43) to check if the model can reasonably describe the experimental data. Since the power-law model is not valid at high coverages, we performed the least square fits on spreadsheet program either with the highest coverage point removed or kept. The solutions are illustrated in Tables E9-2.1 and E9-2.2.

TABLE E9-2.1 Least Square Parameter Estimation for the Freundlich Isotherm. The Final Solution Shown Are for $c' = 55.85$ (mg/L)$^{-m}$·mg-phenol/g-Activated Carbon and $m = 0.271$, Which Were Obtained by Minimizing the Variance between the Freundlich Model and the Experimental Data, σ_L, While Changing c' and m

Aqueous solution C_A, mg/L	On activated carbon C'_{As}, mg/g	Eqn (9.43) C_{As}, mg/g	Error² $(C_{As} - C'_{As})^2$
0	0	0	0
1.5	53.0	62.33299	87.10465
2.0	62.4	67.38618	24.86198
5.1	82.8	86.8411	16.33046
6.6	105.0	93.12478	141.0209
22.9	137.0	130.4549	42.83818
51.6	172.2	162.5764	92.61345
80.2	170.9	183.2113	151.5683

$$\sigma_L = \sqrt{\frac{\sum_{i=1}^{8}(C_{As,i} - C'_{As,i})^2}{8-1}} = 8.914979$$

TABLES E9-2.2 Least Square Parameter Estimation for the Freundlich Isotherm with the Highest Coverage Data Point Not Accounted for in Data-Fitting. The Final Solution Shown Are for $c' = 52.21$ $(\text{mg/L})^{-m}$·mg-phenol/g-Activated Carbon and $m = 0.306$, Which Were Obtained by Minimizing the Variance between the Freundlich Model and the Experimental Data, σ_L

Aqueous solution C_A, mg/L	On activated carbon C'_{As}, mg/g	Eqn (9.43) C_{As}, mg/g	Error² $(C_{As} - C'_{As})^2$
0	0	0	0
1.5	53.0	59.11624	37.40836
2.0	62.4	64.56151	4.672121
5.1	82.8	85.99851	10.23046
6.6	105.0	93.0651	142.4419
22.9	137.0	136.2292	0.594159
51.6	172.2	174.7157	6.328751
80.2	170.9		
		$\sigma_L = \sqrt{\frac{\sum_{i=1}^{7}(C_{As,i} - C'_{As,i})^2}{7-1}} = 5.79764$	

One can observe from Tables E9-2.1 that the Freundlich model fit is not as good as the Langmuir fit as shown in Example 9-1. The deviation of the model with the experimental data is higher at the high coverage region. Fig. E9-2.1 shows the visual quality of the fit. Visual inspection of the data shown in Fig. E9-2.1 reinforces our assessment based on Table E9-2.1.

One can observe from Table E9-2.2 and Fig. E9-2.1 that the Freundlich model fit with the highest coverage data removed has improved quality of fit. Within the region of fit, the Freundlich isotherm fit and the Langmuir isotherm fit are of similar quality, i.e. both within the apparent experimental data error.

We next examine the Temkin isotherm fit to the same data. Substituting Eqn (9.28) into Eqn (9.42), we obtain

$$C_{As} = f_T \ln(K_{AT} C_A) \tag{9.44}$$

where $f_T = \frac{RT}{E_{max}} C_{As\infty}$ and $K_{AT} = \overline{K}_A e^{\frac{E_{max}}{RT}} = K_A^{\circ} e^{\frac{-\Delta H_{ad} + E_{max}}{RT}}$. Since the Temkin isotherm is only valid in the intermediate coverage region, we remove the zero coverage data from consideration. Table E9-2.3 shows the least square fit using Temkin isotherm to the experimental data. Visual representation of the fit as compared with Langmuir isotherm fit is shown in Fig. E9-2.2.

One can observe from Table E9-2.3 and Fig. E9-2.2 that the Temkin model fit is consistent with the experimental data. Within the region of fit, the Temkin isotherm fit and the Langmuir isotherm fit are of similar quality, both within the apparent experimental data error.

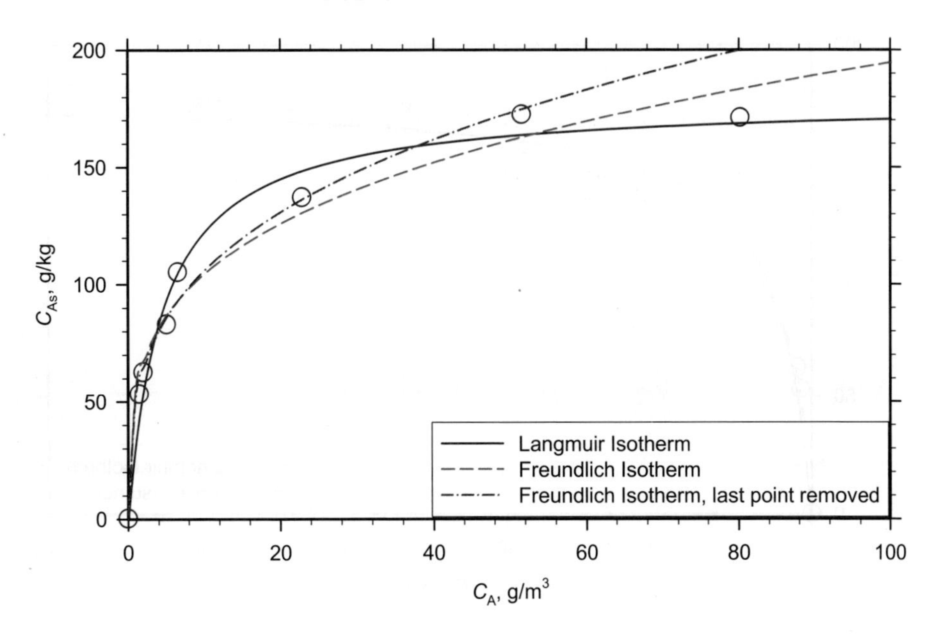

FIGURE E9-2.1 Freundlich isotherm model fit as compared with the Langmuir isotherm fit for the adsorption of phenol on activated carbon.

TABLE E9-2.3 Least Square Parametric Estimation for the Temkin Isotherm. The Final Solution Shown are for $f_T = 31.42$ mg-phenol/g-Activated Carbon and $K_{AT} = 3.545$ L/mg, Obtained by Minimizing the Variance between the Temkin Model and the Experimental Data, σ_L, While Changing f_T and K_{AT}

Aqueous solution C_A, mg/L	On activated carbon C'_{As}, mg/g	Eqn (9.44) C_{As}, mg/g	Error^2 $(C_{As} - C'_{As})^2$
0	0		
1.5	53.0	52.49601	0.254001
2.0	62.4	61.53407	0.749841
5.1	82.8	90.94313	66.31056
6.6	105.0	99.0433	35.48232
22.9	137.0	138.1279	1.272193
51.6	172.2	163.6504	73.09481
80.2	170.9	177.5053	43.63024

$$\sigma_L = \sqrt{\frac{\sum_{i=2}^{8}(C_{As,i} - C'_{As,i})^2}{7-1}} = 6.066217$$

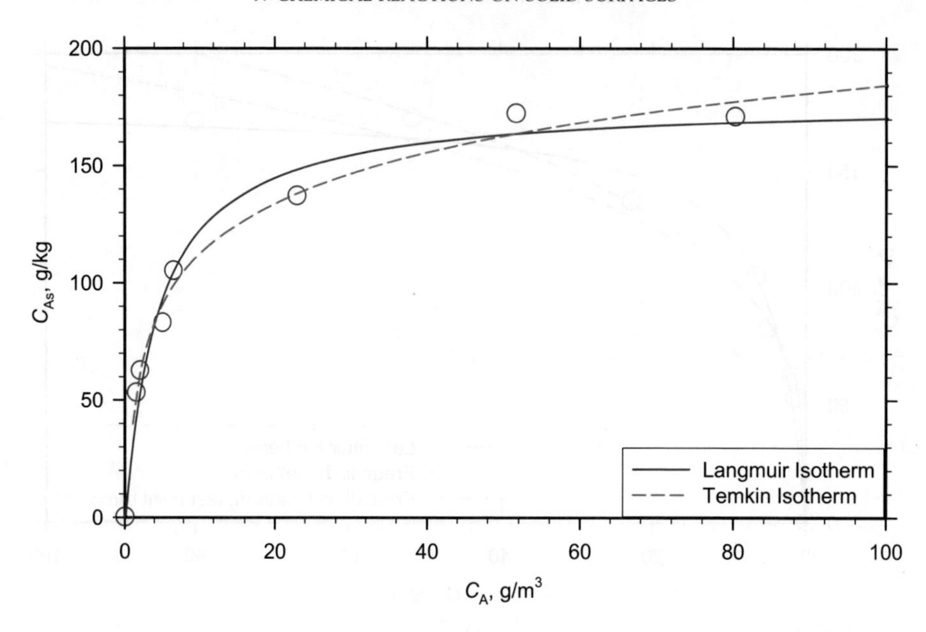

FIGURE E9-2.2 Temkin isotherm model fit as compared with the Langmuir isotherm fit for the adsorption of phenol on activated carbon.

9.1.4. Adsorption at High Surface Coverage

Thus, so far we have examined only the process of ideal (and nonideal) chemisorptions where the adsorbate molecules only interact with the adsorbent surfaces and no interactions with adjacent adsorbate molecules. At high surface coverage, this idealization is no longer valid. It is well known that adsorbate molecules "pack" very closely on the adsorbent surface, which result in significant adsorbate–adsorbate interactions. We next continue our discussion on the nonideal chemisorption to high surface coverages where adsorbate–adsorbate molecule interactions must be accounted for.

To further our consideration, let us once again recall the collision theory of gas molecules (atoms) with surfaces:

$$Z_{cT}(\mathrm{A}, \mathrm{surface}) = N_{AV} C_{\mathrm{A}} \sqrt{\frac{RT}{2\pi M_{\mathrm{A}}}} \tag{6.21}$$

which is equivalent to

$$Z_{cT}(\mathrm{A}, \mathrm{surface}) = \frac{N_{AV} p_{\mathrm{A}}}{\sqrt{2\pi M_{\mathrm{A}} RT}} \tag{9.45}$$

Therefore, adsorption (and reaction in general) can be considered either in concentrations or in partial pressures for gas adsorption. Now let us make up a little picture of the surface (which is two-dimensional) and adsorbed molecules that the collisions are involved with, as in Fig. 9.8.

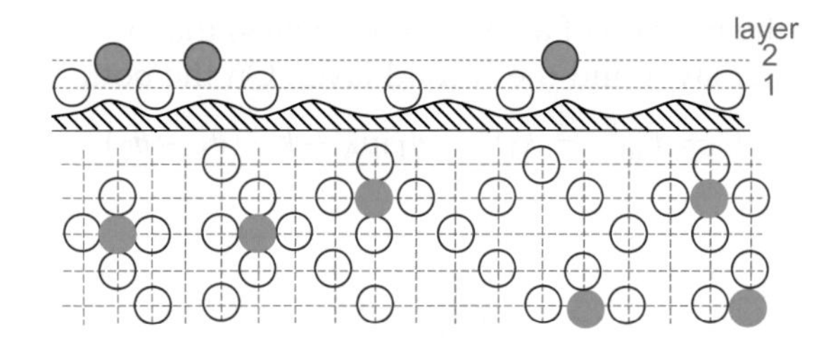

FIGURE 9.8 Two dimensional surface idealization of surface adsorption sites: lower sketch—planar view of a typical idealized adsorbate surface where the active centers are shown; and upper sketch—front view normal to the adsorbate surface. Open circles represent molecules "locked on" as the first layer adsorbate molecules and the filled circles represent molecules "locked on" as the second layer adsorbate molecules.

To start with the discussion, let us consider a typical surface where multiple active centers exist. At each active center, one adsorbate molecule can be adsorbed. However, the centers can be more attractive or less attractive to the adsorbate molecules depending on their locations on the adsorbent surface. One can think of the centers as two layers: the lower layer is more preferred by the adsorbate molecules to "lock" on for its lower energy well (or more attractive to adsorbate molecules), and the upper layer is less attractive to adsorbate molecules but can have adsorbate molecules "locking on" if the adjacent lower layer sites are occupied. Once this upper (or second) layer sites are adsorbed with adsorbate molecules they would serve as steric barriers for the lower layer adsorbed molecules, preventing the adsorbate molecules at the lower layer from leaving the surface.

Fig. 9.8 shows the active centers in two dimensions: on the adsorbate surface plane (bottom sketch) and normal to the surface plane (top sketch). While the two-layer model shown in Fig. 9.8 is straightforward in helping us understand the nature of adsorption, it is not simple to translate it into a mathematical model. To further simplify the adsorption mechanism while without loss of generosity, we further idealize the adsorption by stacking the two layers as shown in Fig. 9.9.

Fig. 9.9 can be translated into mathematical expression more readily. In either layer, there is a dynamic equilibrium with the bulk fluid phase (or in particular gas phase). The adsorption is governed in a manner similar to Eqn (9.1a). On the top layer, the adsorbate molecule can only be adsorbed on to a site if the site below or on the first (or lower) layer is already occupied. This is true because when an adsorbate molecule gets close to the particular site would "slide" to that on the first layer if it is available. Thus, the adsorption–desorption on the top layer is governed by

$$0 = r_{\mathrm{ad},2} = k_2(\theta_1 - \theta_2)p_{\mathrm{A}} - k_{-2}\theta_2 \tag{9.46}$$

where k_2 and k_{-2} are the adsorption and desorption rate constants on the second layer; respectively; θ_1 is the fraction of active centers (sites) that are covered by the adsorbate molecules on

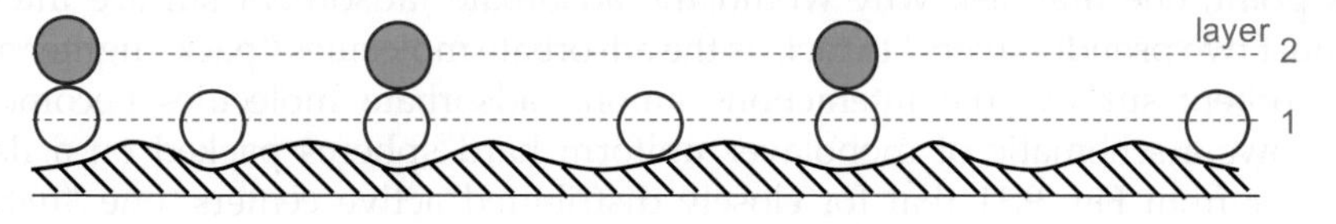

FIGURE 9.9 Bilayer surface adsorption model: two layers are stacked.

the first layer, and θ_2 is the fraction of active centers (sites) that are covered by the adsorbate molecules on both the first layer and the second layer. On the bottom (or first) layer,

$$0 = r_{\mathrm{ad},1} = k_1(1-\theta_1)p_\mathrm{A} - k_{-1}(\theta_1-\theta_2) \tag{9.47}$$

Let,

$$\frac{k_2}{k_{-2}} = \alpha \tag{9.48}$$

be the adsorption isotherm constant for the upper layer. The adsorption isotherm constant for the base (or lower) layer is

$$\frac{k_1}{k_{-1}} = \alpha c \tag{9.49}$$

Eqns (9.46) and (9.47) give

$$\alpha(\theta_1-\theta_2)p_\mathrm{A} = \theta_2 \tag{9.50}$$

$$\alpha c(1-\theta_1)p_\mathrm{A} = \theta_1-\theta_2 \tag{9.51}$$

which can be solved to yield

$$\theta_1 = \frac{\alpha c p_\mathrm{A}(1+\alpha p_\mathrm{A})}{1+\alpha c p_\mathrm{A}(1+\alpha p_\mathrm{A})} \tag{9.52}$$

$$\theta_2 = \frac{\alpha^2 c p_\mathrm{A}^2}{1+\alpha c p_\mathrm{A}(1+\alpha p_\mathrm{A})} \tag{9.53}$$

The number of moles of adsorbate on the adsorbent surface is thus the sum of the molecules on the first layer and the second layer. That is,

$$n_\mathrm{As} = \frac{n_\mathrm{max}}{2}(\theta_1+\theta_2) = \frac{n_\sigma}{2}\frac{\alpha c p_\mathrm{A}(1+2\alpha p_\mathrm{A})}{1+\alpha c p_\mathrm{A}(1+\alpha p_\mathrm{A})} \tag{9.54}$$

where n_σ is the total number of active sites on the adsorbent surface, which is equivalent to the maximum number of adsorbate molecules that could be adsorbed or number of saturation adsorbate molecules. In terms of concentration, the "bi-layer adsorption" can be written as

$$n_\mathrm{As} = \frac{n_\sigma}{2}\frac{cK_\mathrm{A}C_\mathrm{A}(1+2K_\mathrm{A}C_\mathrm{A})}{1+cK_\mathrm{A}C_\mathrm{A}(1+K_\mathrm{A}C_\mathrm{A})}$$

Fig. 9.10 shows a schematic of the isotherm as described by Eqn (9.55). One can observe that the feature differs qualitatively from the Langmuir isotherm (Fig. 9.4) at low coverage ratios where the adsorbate concentration in the adsorbent increases more slowly.

At this point, one may ask why would the adsorbate–adsorbent surface interaction be limited to just two pseudo-layers? In fact, as the adsorbate molecules "pack" tighter and tighter on the adsorbent surface, the interactions among adsorbate molecules become stronger. Fig. 9.11 shows a schematic of monolayer uniform hard spheres packed on a flat surface. One can infer from Fig. 9.11 that for closely distributed active centers, one "hard sphere" can have up to six neighboring "hard spheres" of the same size closely packed on a perfectly

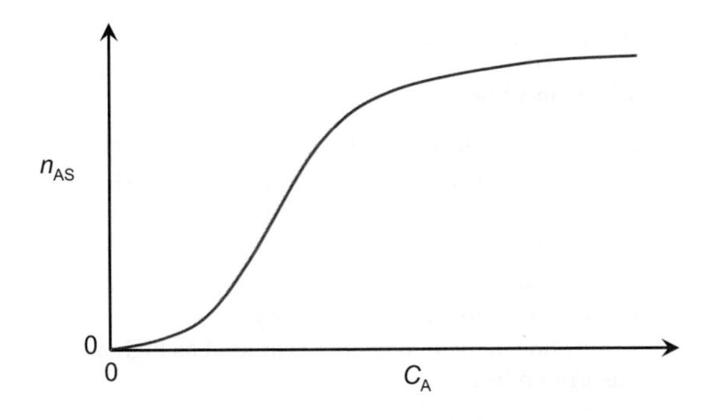

FIGURE 9.10 A schematic of nonideal isotherm with adsorbate–adsorbate interactions.

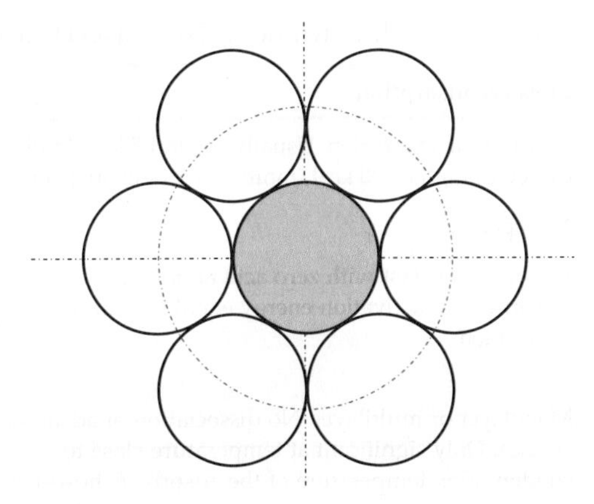

FIGURE 9.11 Uniform hard spheres packed closely on a flat surface.

flat "hard surface". Therefore, there can be up to seven pseudo-layers of adsorption for hard spheres on flat surfaces as there are differences on the number of interacting hard spheres. For real adsorbate and adsorbent surface, the situation can be more completed. Therefore, the apparent layer of adsorption can be more than two. While the adsorbate–adsorbent interaction can be chemical (i.e. chemical bonds formed), the interactions between adsorbate and adsorbate near or at contact is physical. The orderly state of adsorbate molecules on the adsorbent surface is at a lower energy well than that in the bulk fluid phase. While the actual physical orientation of the adsorbate molecules on the adsorbent surface is monolayer, the adsorption mechanism needs not be. Thus, modeling the adsorbate–adsorbent and adsorbate–adsorbent–adsorbate interactions is best to be accomplished with multiple layers. We will deal with this idealization in the proceeding sections.

9.1.4.1. Chemisorption, Physisorption and the BET Theory

We have so far been focused on the interactions between the adsorbent surface and the adsorbate molecules. The difference on the adsorbent surface has led us to a pseudo-two layer adsorption model. The adsorption models so far are applicable to both chemisorptions and physisorption. What happens if more than one layers of adsorbate can truly be adsorbed on the surface? This would lead to pure physical adsorptions, since the interaction between the adsorbate molecules and the adsorbent surfaces become negligible on layers above the adsorbed molecules. If we summarize to this point, chemisorption is a chemical interaction between the adsorbate and the surface. The heats and activation energies of chemisorption are typical of those of a chemical reaction, and that is exactly what it is: a chemical reaction, albeit three-dimensional (in the bulk fluid phase) on one side of the arrow and two-dimensional (on the adsorbent surface) on the other side. The activation energies are such that the species involved have sufficient energy to cross the activation energy barrier at temperature levels that are experimentally accessible and of practical importance.

Now we need to talk about physical adsorption, which, though it is not generally considered to be a crucial factor in surface reactions, is of importance in relation to the topic as

TABLE 9.1 Characteristics of Physical and Chemical Adsorption

Physical adsorption	Chemisorption
Low heat of adsorption. Usually around 5 kcal/mol, but can be as high as 20 kcal/more. Always exothermic.	High heat of adsorption. Usually higher than 20 kcal/mol, but can be less, even endothermic is possible.
Not specific.	Highly specific.
Adsorption is fast with zero activation energy. Desorption is activation energy equal to heat of adsorption.	Adsorption is slow with activation energy, but could be fast with aero activation energy. Desorption activation energy is at least as high as adsorption heat.
Monolayer or multilayer. No dissociation of adsorbed species. Only significant at temperature close to condensation temperature of the adsorbate, however, Kelvin effect can occur for some porous adsorbents.	Monolayer only, but can appear to be multilayer (in isotherms) due to interaction energy distribution nonuniformity. Adsorbate may involve dissociation. Possible over a wide range of temperature.
No effect on the adsorbent electric conductivity.	May have an effect on the adsorbent electric conductivity.
No electron transfer although polarization of adsorbate may occur.	Electron transfer leading to bond formation between adsorbate and surface.

a whole. One might say that physical adsorption does things a bit differently from chemisorption, as is shown in Table 9.1. The analysis of physical adsorption can be complicated, even more so than for chemisorption, because attractive–repulsive interactions are involved that may be more complex than direct chemisorptive interactions. Nevertheless, for adsorption to occur, the adsorbate molecule has to "collide" with the center where adsorption is to take place. Therefore, Eqns (9.1a) and (9.2) apply equally well to physisorptions.

We need to examine a particular model for physical adsorption that has been extremely useful over the years in the characterization of the porous materials that are often employed as catalyst support structures or as catalysts in their own right. The basic question is how to measure the internal (pore) surface area of a material that is perhaps 50% void and has an average pore diameter on the order of 5 nm. We want to know this surface area because it is presumably important in determination of the overall rate of reaction per unit volume of catalyst in a given application.

The analysis of physical adsorption in general and that used to approach this particular problem, derives from a classification later summarized by Brunauer (S. Brunauer, *The Adsorption of Gases and Vapors*, Princeton University Press, Princeton, NJ, 1945). He classified the isotherms for physical adsorption of gases on surfaces into five general types, as shown in Fig. 9.12. Isotherms I and V are already recognizable. Isotherm I is a typical Langmuir isotherm, while isotherm V is a typical bi-layer adsorption isotherm. Isotherms II–IV show the various complexities of physical adsorption. Early work showed that that isotherm II was typical for adsorption of nitrogen (at liquid nitrogen temperatures) on a large number of porous adsorbents. The result of that observation led to the derivation of an appropriate analytical theory to describe this type of adsorption and to use it for physical characterization, in terms of internal surface area of the adsorbent (S. Brunauer, P.H. Emmett and E.J. Teller, J. *Amer. Chem. Soc.*, 60, 309, 1938). From the last initials of the authors comes the name "BET theory."

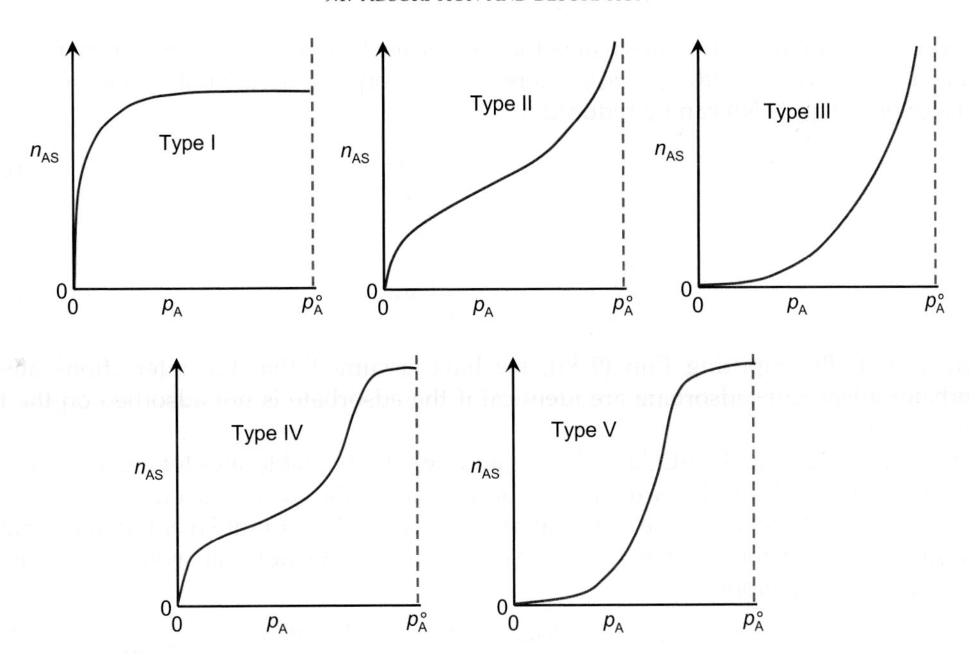

FIGURE 9.12 Classification of adsorption isotherms based on the adsorption of gas on a solid material. The horizontal axes are the partial pressure of the adsorbate gas, and the vertical axes are the amount of gas adsorbed on the surfaces.

At this point, we know that the adsorption can be described using concentrations as we have done so far and equally well with partial pressures as discussed earlier. Whether the adsorption is chemisorptions or physisorption, the adsorption and desorption rates are similar: adsorption requires the adsorbate molecules to get close enough to the adsorption site or active centers and the desorption occurs when the adsorbed molecules leave the adsorbent surface.

9.1.4.2. Multilayer Adsorption of Single Species

Fig. 9.13 shows a schematic of multilayer adsorption, which is a direct extension of Fig. 9.7. The similarity of the model leads us to similar analysis. As we have discussed for bi-layer adsorption, in each layer, there is a dynamic equilibrium with the bulk gas phase. The adsorption is governed in a manner similar to Eqn (9.1a). The adsorbate molecule can only be adsorbed on to a site on a layer if the site on the lower layer is occupied. On the top layer, the adsorption–desorption is governed by

$$0 = r_{ad,N} = k_N(\theta_{N-1} - \theta_N)p_A - k_{-N}\theta_N \tag{9.56}$$

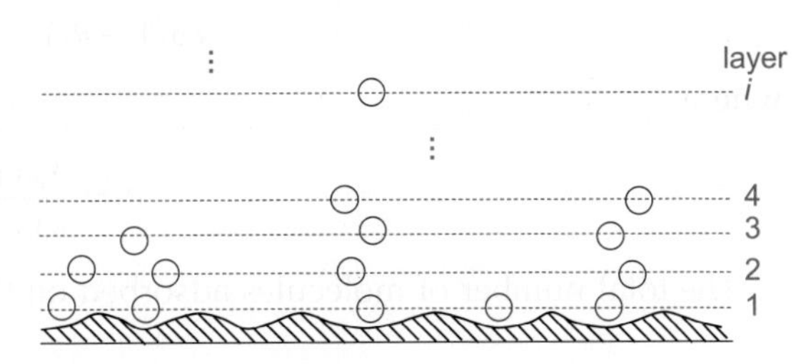

FIGURE 9.13 Multilayer surface adsorption model for the BET isotherm.

The adsorption occurs on the sites where the second last layer is covered (θ_{N-1}) but not occupied by the last layer, i.e. ($\theta_{N-1} - \theta_N$), whereas the desorption occurs only from the covered last layer (θ_N). Eqn (9.50) can be reduced to

$$\beta(\theta_{N-1} - \theta_N) = \theta_N \tag{9.57}$$

where

$$\frac{k_N}{k_{-N}} p_A = \ldots = \frac{k_i}{k_{-i}} p_A = \beta \tag{9.58}$$

where $i \neq 1$. By imposing Eqn (9.58), we have assumed that the interactions among adsorbate–adsorbent–adsorbate are identical if the adsorbate is not adsorbed on the first layer.

For the adsorption in the *i*-th layer (in the middle), the available sites for adsorption is the covered sites by the lower layer (θ_{i-1}) but not covered on the current layer, i.e. $\theta_{i-1} - \theta_i$. The desorption can only occur on the sites that are covered by the current layer but not occupied above. The coverage of the site on top of the current adsorbate molecule would be prevented it from leaving. Therefore,

$$0 = r_{ad,i} = k_i(\theta_{i-1} - \theta_i)p_A - k_{-i}(\theta_i - \theta_{i+1}) \tag{9.59}$$

Since the adsorption and desorption are occurring on top of the adsorbed molecules (like condensation), we have assumed that the adsorption and desorption rate constants are identical from layer to layer by imposing Eqn (9.58). Eqn (9.53) leads to

$$\theta_i - \theta_{i+1} = \beta(\theta_{i-1} - \theta_i) \tag{9.60}$$

and adsorption on the first layer or directly on the adsorbent surface,

$$0 = r_{ad,1} = k_{ad,1}(1 - \theta_1)p_A - k_{des,1}(\theta_1 - \theta_2) \tag{9.61}$$

which is different from the rest of the layers on top of the first layer. The adsorption is on the adsorbent surface, where the interaction between the adsorption site on the adsorbent and the adsorbate molecule is different from the interaction between adsorbed molecule and the adsorbate molecule. Still, the adsorption can only occur on the free sites (not occupied by the adsorbate molecules), whereas the desorption can only occur to the adsorbed molecules which are not covered from the top. Eqn (9.61) can be reduced to

$$c\beta(1 - \theta_1) = \theta_1 - \theta_2 \tag{9.62}$$

where

$$c = \frac{k_{ad,1}}{k_{des,1}} \frac{k_{-i}}{k_i} \tag{9.63}$$

The total number of molecules adsorbed on the adsorbent surface is

$$n_{As,N} = n_{\sigma 1} \sum_{i=1}^{N} \theta_i \tag{9.64}$$

where $n_{\sigma 1}$ is the maximum number of adsorption sites available on each layer. Solving the discrete Eqn (9.60), we obtain,

$$\theta_i = A + B\beta^i \tag{9.65}$$

which is obtained by assuming $\theta_i = \gamma^i$, similar to one would do when solving a homogeneous ordinary differential equation. We have two free parameters in Eqn (9.65). Eqn (9.65) needs to be satisfied also by the first layer, Eqn (9.62) and the topmost layer, Eqn (9.57). Substituting Eqn (9.65) into Eqn (9.57), we obtain

$$A + B\beta^{N+1} = 0 \tag{9.66}$$

Substituting Eqn (9.65) into Eqn (9.62), we obtain

$$c(1 - A - B\beta) = B(1 - \beta) \tag{9.67}$$

Solving Eqns (9.66) and (9.67), we obtain

$$B = \frac{c}{1 - (1 - c)\beta - c\beta^{N+1}} \tag{9.68a}$$

$$A = \frac{-c\beta^{N+1}}{1 - (1 - c)\beta - \beta^{N+1}} \tag{9.68b}$$

Substituting Eqn (9.68) into Eqn (9.65), we obtain the fractional coverage of layer i

$$\theta_i = \frac{c(\beta^i - \beta^{N+1})}{1 - (1 - c)\beta - \beta^{N+1}} \tag{9.69}$$

Therefore, the total number of molecules adsorbed is

$$\begin{aligned} n_{\mathrm{As,N}} &= n_{\sigma 1} \sum_{i=1}^{N} \theta_i = n_{\sigma 1} c \sum_{i=1}^{N} \frac{\beta^i - \beta^{N+1}}{1 - (1 - c)\beta - c\beta^{N+1}} \\ &= n_{\sigma 1} c \frac{\beta \dfrac{1 - \beta^N}{1 - \beta} - N\beta^{N+1}}{1 - (1 - c)\beta - c\beta^{N+1}} = n_{\sigma 1} c\beta \frac{1 - [1 + N(1 - \beta)]\beta^N}{(1 - \beta)[1 - (1 - c)\beta - c\beta^{N+1}]} \end{aligned} \tag{9.70}$$

Since

$$\beta = \frac{k_i}{k_{-i}} p_{\mathrm{A}} = \alpha p_{\mathrm{A}} \tag{9.71}$$

Eqn (9.70) is reduced to

$$n_{\mathrm{As,N}} = n_{\sigma 1} c \alpha p_{\mathrm{A}} \frac{1 - [1 + N(1 - \alpha p_{\mathrm{A}})](\alpha p_{\mathrm{A}})^N}{(1 - \alpha p_{\mathrm{A}})[1 - (1 - c)\alpha p_{\mathrm{A}} - c(\alpha p_{\mathrm{A}})^{N+1}]} \tag{9.72}$$

which is the general multilayer adsorption isotherm. It is applicable to multiadsorption site chemisorptions (strong adsorbent–adsorbate molecular interactions) as well as physisorptions. In general, the multilayer adsorption isotherm is written as

$$n_{\mathrm{As},N} = n_{\sigma 1} c K_{\mathrm{A}} C_{\mathrm{A}} \frac{1-[1+N(1-K_{\mathrm{A}}C_{\mathrm{A}})](K_{\mathrm{A}}C_{\mathrm{A}})^{N}}{(1-K_{\mathrm{A}}C_{\mathrm{A}})[1-(1-c)K_{\mathrm{A}}C_{\mathrm{A}}-c(K_{\mathrm{A}}C_{\mathrm{A}})^{N+1}]} \tag{9.72}$$

Because of interaction with adsorbent surface is the key for the adsorption to occur, the number of layers of adsorption is thus restricted. Most commonly held belief is that chemisorptions has to be monolayer, which stems from this notion. Correctly so, adsorption without adsorbent surface–adsorbate molecule interaction would be meaningless. Molecules can be more compact when adsorbed actually than in their solid state due to the geometric confinement and interactions with the adsorbent surface. Therefore, at this point, Eqn (9.73) is general although only two levels of interactions were allowed in deriving this equation.

9.1.4.3. BET Isotherm and Physisorption

We next turn our attention to physisorption only. At this point, Eqns (9.72) and (9.73) are applicable to both chemisorption and physisorption. Because of the weak adsorbate–adsorbate and adsorbate–adsorbent interactions in physisorption, we can further simplify Eqns (9.72) and (9.73). While chemisorptions can only be modeled with finite number of layers, physisorptions could actually occur on multiple layers where the adsorbate–adsorbent interactions are nearly negligible. Therefore, it is unique to physisorption that 1) an infinite number of layers could take place if the geometric restriction is absent and 2) the adsorbate molecules could not be differentiated with the liquid or solid adsorbate molecules. When the partial pressure of the adsorbate in the bulk gas phase reaches the vapor pressure of the "liquefied" or "solidified" adsorbate, the adsorption reaches maximum as there is no difference between the molecules in the liquid phase and the adsorbed molecules. That is to say, when $p_{\mathrm{A}} = p_{\mathrm{A}}^{\circ}$, $n_{\mathrm{As}} \rightarrow \infty$. Based Eqn (9.72), we have

$$\alpha p_{\mathrm{A}} = \beta = \frac{p_{\mathrm{A}}}{p_{\mathrm{A}}^{\circ}} \tag{9.74}$$

Therefore, Eqn (9.72) is reduced to

$$n_{\mathrm{As},N} = n_{\sigma 1} c \frac{p_{\mathrm{A}}}{p_{\mathrm{A}}^{\circ}} \frac{1-\left[1+N\left(1-\frac{p_{\mathrm{A}}}{p_{\mathrm{A}}^{\circ}}\right)\right]\left(\frac{p_{\mathrm{A}}}{p_{\mathrm{A}}^{\circ}}\right)^{N}}{\left(1-\frac{p_{\mathrm{A}}}{p_{\mathrm{A}}^{\circ}}\right)\left[1-(1-c)\frac{p_{\mathrm{A}}}{p_{\mathrm{A}}^{\circ}}-c\left(\frac{p_{\mathrm{A}}}{p_{\mathrm{A}}^{\circ}}\right)^{N+1}\right]} \tag{9.75}$$

which is applicable only for physisorptions.

Eqns (9.72) and (9.75) can describe all the cases or types of adsorption shown in Fig. 9.11. When $N = 1$, Eqn (9.72) is reduced to

$$n_{\mathrm{As},1} = n_{\sigma 1} \frac{c\frac{p_{\mathrm{A}}}{p_{\mathrm{A}}^{\circ}}}{1+c\frac{p_{\mathrm{A}}}{p_{\mathrm{A}}^{\circ}}} \tag{9.76}$$

for which we have recovered the form of the Langmuir adsorption isotherm. Eqn (9.76) describes the monolayer coverage and is identical to Langmuir isotherm.

Assuming that there is an infinite number of layers of adsorbate possible ($N \to \infty$), Eqn (9.75) is reduced

$$n_{\mathrm{As},\infty} = \frac{n_{\sigma 1} c \dfrac{p_{\mathrm{A}}}{p_{\mathrm{A}}^{\circ}}}{\left(1 - \dfrac{p_{\mathrm{A}}}{p_{\mathrm{A}}^{\circ}}\right)\left[1 - (1-c)\dfrac{p_{\mathrm{A}}}{p_{\mathrm{A}}^{\circ}}\right]} \tag{9.77}$$

which is the well-known BET isotherm. The mole ratio of the total multilayer absorbate molecules to monolayer adsorbate molecules is given by

$$\frac{n_{\mathrm{As},\infty}}{n_{\mathrm{As},1}} = \frac{1 + c \dfrac{p_{\mathrm{A}}}{p_{\mathrm{A}}^{\circ}}}{\left(1 - \dfrac{p_{\mathrm{A}}}{p_{\mathrm{A}}^{\circ}}\right)\left[1 - (1-c)\dfrac{p_{\mathrm{A}}}{p_{\mathrm{A}}^{\circ}}\right]} \tag{9.78}$$

Of the two parameters in Eqn (9.78), the most informative is probably $n_{\mathrm{As},1}$, the capacity at monolayer coverage. We stated earlier that the physical adsorption of nitrogen on many surfaces resembled Type II in the classification of Brunauer (as it turns out, Type III is also seen in a number of instances). Nonetheless, the idea is that if Eqn (9.78) is obeyed we can obtain a value for $n_{\mathrm{As},1}$ and, following some judicious assumptions, a value of the internal surface area. However, one should note that this assumption is flawed since the site on the adsorbent surface could also behave similar to a site on upper layers.

Type IV and Type V adsorptions are recovered when the number of layers is finite, for example, when $N = 2$, Eqn (9.72) gives.

$$\begin{aligned} n_{\mathrm{As},2} &= n_{\sigma 1} c \alpha p_{\mathrm{A}} \frac{1 - (3 - \alpha p_{\mathrm{A}})(\alpha p_{\mathrm{A}})^2}{(1 - \alpha p_{\mathrm{A}})[1 - (1-c)\alpha p_{\mathrm{A}} - c(\alpha p_{\mathrm{A}})^3} \\ &= n_{\sigma 1} c \alpha p_{\mathrm{A}} \frac{(1 - \alpha p_{\mathrm{A}})[1 + \alpha p_{\mathrm{A}} - 2(\alpha p_{\mathrm{A}})^2]}{(1 - \alpha p_{\mathrm{A}})^2[1 + c\alpha p_{\mathrm{A}} + c(\alpha p_{\mathrm{A}})^2]} \end{aligned}$$

which is reduced to

$$n_{\mathrm{As},2} = n_{\sigma 1} \frac{c \alpha p_{\mathrm{A}}(1 + 2\alpha p_{\mathrm{A}})}{1 + c\alpha p_{\mathrm{A}}(1 + \alpha p_{\mathrm{A}})} \tag{9.48}$$

Thus, Eqn (9.72) describes type V isotherms when $N = 2$.

Example 9-3 Adsorption of Water Vapor on Silica Gel.

Experimental adsorption data given by Knaebel (Knaebel, K.S. "14 Adsorption", in Lyle F. Albright ed. *Albright's Chemical Engineering Handbook*, CRC Press, Taylor & Francis Group, Boca Raton, FL, 2009) for water vapor on silica gel at 25 °C is shown in Table E9-3.1. Perform data fit to Langmuir isotherm, bilayer isotherm, and the multilayer isotherm. Comment on your solutions.

Solution. We first examine the quality of fit for the Langmuir model as it is the simplest of all the isotherms with a theoretical basis. Eqn (9.9) can be rearranged to give

$$C_{\mathrm{As}} = C_{\mathrm{As}\infty} \frac{\alpha p_{\mathrm{A}} / p_{\mathrm{A}}^{\circ}}{1 + \alpha p_{\mathrm{A}} / p_{\mathrm{A}}^{\circ}} \tag{E9-3.1}$$

TABLE E9-3.1 Adsorption Isotherm Data for Water Vapor on Silica Gel at 25 °C (taken from Knaebel, K.S. "14 Adsorption", in Lyle F. Albright ed. *Albright's Chemical Engineering Handbook*, CRC Press, Taylor & Francis Group, Boca Raton, FL, 2009)

Relative humidity, p/p°	Loading, mol/L
0.0000	0.00
0.0116	1.73
0.0198	2.23
0.0378	3.53
0.0600	4.84
0.1330	8.68
0.1770	11.20
0.1800	11.82
0.2180	13.67
0.2380	15.26
0.2410	15.59
0.2560	17.08
0.2780	17.40
0.2790	17.94
0.2920	20.03
0.3070	20.43
0.3500	23.45
0.3690	25.28
0.5260	30.97
0.5390	32.04
0.6490	33.03
0.6970	33.32
0.7580	33.87
0.8250	34.11
0.8250	34.15

TABLE E9-3.2 Langmuir Isotherm Fit. The Parameters in Eqn (E9-3.1) were Evaluated by Minimizing the Variance between Calculated Values (Eqn (E9-3.1)) and the Experimental Data. The Parameters Obtained Are: $\alpha = 1.2773$; $C_{As\infty} = 70.52$ mol/L/

Relative humidity, p/p°	**Loading, C'_{As}, mol/L**	**Langmuir, Eqn (E9-3.1) C_{As}, mol/L**	**Error^2 $(C'_{As} - C_{As})^2$**
0	0	0	0
0.0116	1.73	1.029687	0.490439
0.0198	2.23	1.739614	0.240478
0.0378	3.53	3.248241	0.079388
0.0600	4.84	5.020141	0.032451
0.1330	8.68	10.24104	2.436832
0.1770	11.2	13.00431	3.255539
0.1800	11.82	13.18352	1.859187
0.2180	13.67	15.36051	2.857832
0.2380	15.26	16.4412	1.395238
0.2410	15.59	16.59966	1.019421
0.2560	17.08	17.37825	0.088951
0.2780	17.4	18.48034	1.167138
0.2790	17.94	18.52935	0.347336
0.2920	20.03	19.15819	0.76006
0.3070	20.43	19.86512	0.319086
0.3500	23.45	21.78792	2.762496
0.3690	25.28	22.5918	7.226397
0.5260	30.97	28.34119	6.910619
0.5390	32.04	28.75603	10.78443
0.6490	33.03	31.9647	1.13487
0.6970	33.32	33.21535	0.010951
0.7580	33.87	34.6923	0.676181
0.8250	34.11	36.18538	4.307213
0.8250	34.15	36.18538	4.142783

$$\sigma_L = \sqrt{\frac{\sum_{i=1}^{24}(C_{As,i} - C'_{As,i})^2}{24-1}} = 1.536587$$

Table E9-3.2 shows the results of fitting the Langmuir model, Eqn (E9-3.1) to the experimental data. To show the visual appearance of the fit, Fig. E9-3.1 show the experimental data (as circles) and the Langmuir model fit (as solid line). One can observe that the fit is reasonably well. However, there is noticeable deviation at high surface coverage.

We next examine the quality fit for the bilayer isotherm as it was developed to accommodate high coverage cases. Eqn (9.55) can be rearranged to give

$$C_{As} = C_{As1\infty} \frac{c\alpha p_A/p_A^\circ(1+2\alpha p_A/p_A^\circ)}{1+c\alpha p_A/p_A^\circ(1+\alpha p_A/p_A^\circ)} \tag{E9-3.2}$$

Table E9-3.3 shows the results of fitting the Bi-layer isotherm model, Eqn (E9-3.2) to the experimental data. Fig. E9-3.2 shows the experimental data (as circles) and the Bi-layer model fit (as solid line). One can observe that the fit is reasonably well. The quality of fit showed slight improvement over the Langmuir fit as the final variance is smaller and the curve follows the data better. There is clear improvement in the high coverage area over the Langmuir fit as compared with Figs. E9-3.1 and E9-3.2. However, there is a shift in the low surface coverage area.

We now examine the quality fit can be achieved from the more general multilayer isotherm. Eqn (9.72) can be rearranged to give

$$C_{As} = C_{As1\infty} c\alpha' \frac{p_A}{p_A^\circ} \frac{1-\left[1+N(1-\alpha' p_A/p_A^\circ)\right](\alpha' p_A/p_A^\circ)^N}{(1-\alpha' p_A/p_A^\circ)\left[1-(1-c)\alpha' p_A/p_A^\circ - c(\alpha' p_A/p_A^\circ)^{N+1}\right]} \tag{E9-3.3}$$

Table E9-3.4 shows the results of fitting the general multilayer isotherm model, Eqn (E9-3.3) to the experimental data. The parameters obtained are: $N = 6.947093$;

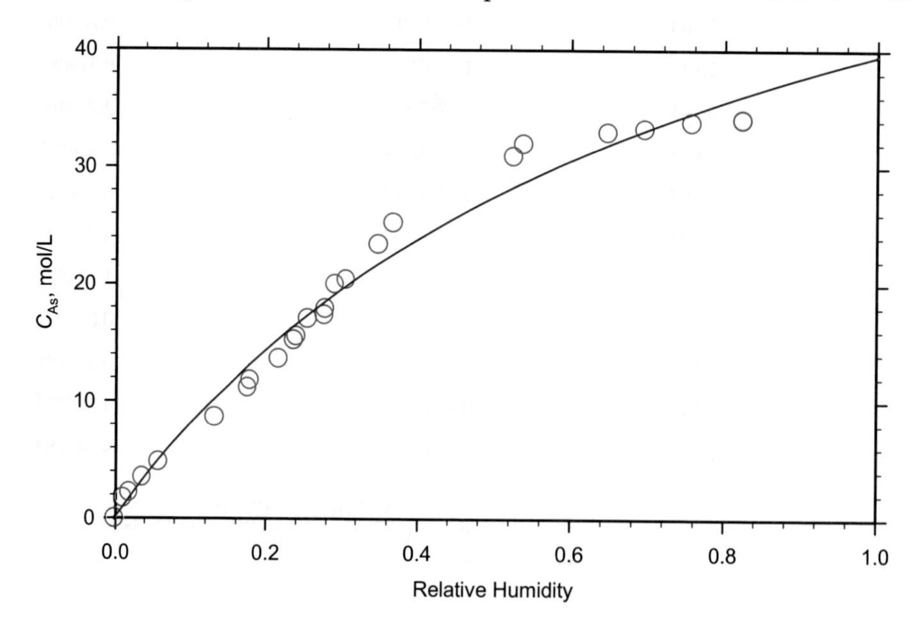

FIGURE E9-3.1 Langmuir isotherm fit to water vapor adsorption on silica gel at 25 °C.

TABLE E9-3.3 Bilayer Isotherm. The Parameters in Eqn (E9-3.2) were Evaluated by Minimizing the Variance between Calculated Values (Eqn 9-3.2) and the Experimental Data: $\alpha = 5.89318$; $c = 0.25734$; $C_{As1\infty} = 21.94268844$

Relative humidity, p/p°	Loading, C'_{As}, mol/L	Bilayer isotherm, Eqn (E9-3.2), C_{As}, mol/L	Error^2$(C'_{As} - C_{As})^2$
0	0	0	
0.0116	1.73	0.430697949	1.688185819
0.0198	2.23	0.786288834	2.08430193
0.0378	3.53	1.699189971	3.351865362
0.0600	4.84	3.034825939	3.25865339
0.1330	8.68	8.357010977	0.104321909
0.1770	11.2	11.73956394	0.291129245
0.1800	11.82	11.96619131	0.021371898
0.2180	13.67	14.75161947	1.16990067
0.2380	15.26	16.14021113	0.774771631
0.2410	15.59	16.34329563	0.567454299
0.2560	17.08	17.33746428	0.066287853
0.2780	17.4	18.72980716	1.768387071
0.2790	17.94	18.79120919	0.724557091
0.2920	20.03	19.57444197	0.207533121
0.3070	20.43	20.443662	0.00018665
0.3500	23.45	22.73512949	0.511039847
0.3690	25.28	23.65695094	2.634288264
0.5260	30.97	29.51002499	2.131527024
0.5390	32.04	29.87921643	4.668985652
0.6490	33.03	32.49447776	0.286784074
0.6970	33.32	33.40233338	0.006778786
0.7580	33.87	34.39831764	0.279119526
0.8250	34.11	35.32549301	1.477423267
0.8250	34.15	35.32549301	1.381783826

$$\sigma_L = \sqrt{\frac{\sum_{i=1}^{24}(C_{As,i} - C'_{As,i})^2}{24-1}} = 1.131690505$$

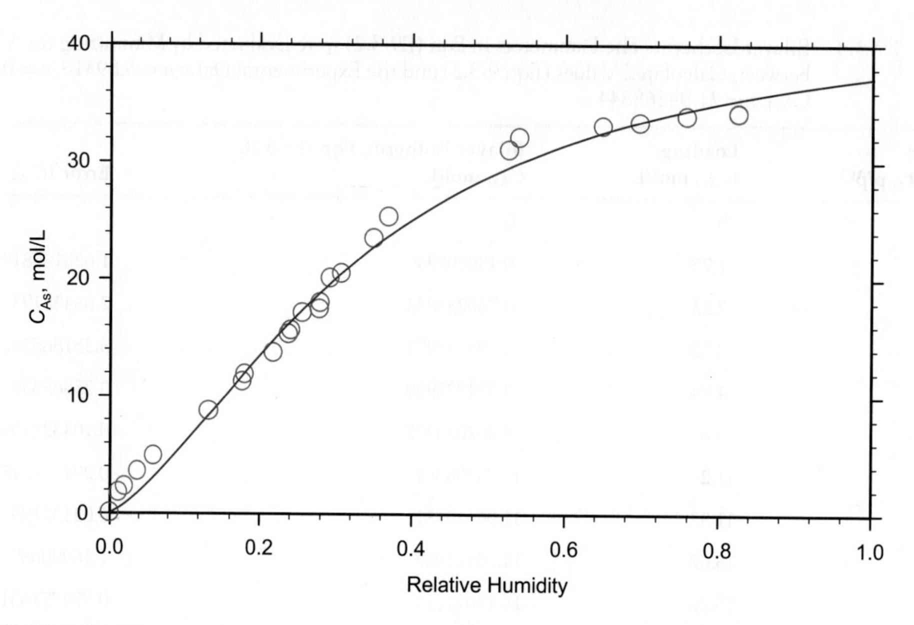

FIGURE E9-3.2 Bilayer isotherm fit to water vapor adsorption on silica gel at 25 °C.

TABLE E9-3.4 General Multilayer Isotherm. The Parameters in Eqn (E9-3.3) Were Evaluated by Minimizing the Variance between Calculated Values (Eqn E9-3.3) and the Experimental Data. The Parameters Obtained Are: $N = 6.947093$; $\alpha' = 3.158229$; $c = 11.119$; $C_{As1\,\infty} = 5.45012$

Relative humidity, $N\ p/p^{\circ}$	Loading, C'_{As}, mol/L	Multilayer isotherm, Eqn (E9-3.3), C_{As}, mol/L	Error² $(C'_{As} - C_{As})^2$
0	0	0	
0.0116	1.73	1.681284	0.002373
0.0198	2.23	2.475732	0.060384
0.0378	3.53	3.720649	0.036347
0.0600	4.84	4.856002	0.000256
0.1330	8.68	8.275699	0.16346
0.1770	11.2	10.89403	0.093618
0.1800	11.82	11.09386	0.527277
0.2180	13.67	13.82702	0.024656
0.2380	15.26	15.37385	0.012961
0.2410	15.59	15.60923	0.00037
0.2560	17.08	16.79091	0.083576

TABLE E9-3.4 General Multilayer Isotherm. The Parameters in Eqn (E9-3.3) Were Evaluated by Minimizing the Variance between Calculated Values (Eqn E9-3.3) and the Experimental Data. The Parameters Obtained Are: $N = 6.947093$; $\alpha' = 3.158229$; $c = 11.119$; $C_{As1\infty} = 5.45012$—*Cont'd*

Relative humidity, $N\ p/p^{\circ}$	**Loading,** C'_{As}, **mol/L**	**Multilayer isotherm, Eqn (E9-3.3),** C_{As}, **mol/L**	**Error**^{2} $(C'_{As} - C_{As})^2$
0.2780	17.4	18.51244	1.237517
0.2790	17.94	18.5897	0.422111
0.2920	20.03	19.58186	0.20083
0.3070	20.43	20.69135	0.068302
0.3500	23.45	23.5883	0.019127
0.3690	25.28	24.71373	0.320664
0.5260	30.97	30.73444	0.055487
0.5390	32.04	31.03673	1.00655
0.6490	33.03	32.92047	0.011997
0.6970	33.32	33.477	0.024648
0.7580	33.87	34.03667	0.027779
0.8250	34.11	34.51437	0.163514
0.8250	34.15	34.51437	0.132765

$$\sigma_L = \sqrt{\frac{\sum_{i=1}^{24}(C_{As,i} - C'_{As,i})^2}{24 - 1}} = 0.451883$$

$\alpha' = 3.158229$; $c = 11.119$; $C_{As1\infty} = 5.45012$ and the variance is small, $\sigma_L = = 0.451883$. Since the number of layers N is close to 7, we next fixed the value of N at 7 and re-evaluated the parameters. Table E9-3.5 shows the final results after fixing the number of layers at 7. The variance change is very minimum and at 0.452307. Therefore, there is no sacrifice with the quality of fit by fixing $N = 7$.

Fig. E9-3.3 shows the experimental data (as circles) and the general multilayer isotherm model fit (as solid line). One can observe that the fit is very well. The quality of fit showed improvement over the bilayer model fit as the final variance is smaller and the curve follows the data right on capturing the details of the change.

9.1.4.4. *Multispecies Multilayer Adsorption Isotherms*

We have so far been focused on the multilayer adsorption of single species. We have seen that they can be treated elegantly and predicting the trends of the adsorption isotherms observed experimentally. In this section, we give the corresponding isotherms for multispecies adsorptions. They can be derived very much the same as for single species.

TABLE E9-3.5 Multilayer Isotherm. The Parameters in Eqn (E9-3.4) Were Reevaluated after Fixing the Number of Layers $N = 7$ by Minimizing the Variance between Calculated Values (Eqn E9-3.3) and the Experimental Data. The Parameters Obtained Are: $\alpha' = 3.166397$; $c = 11.43623$; $C_{As1\infty} = 5.401089$

Relative humidity, p/p°	Loading, C'_{As}, mol/L	Multilayer Isotherm, Eqn (E9-3.3), C_{As}, mol/L	Error^2 $(C'_{As} - C_{As})^2$
0	0	0	
0.0116	1.73	1.702611	0.00075
0.0198	2.23	2.497471	0.071541
0.0378	3.53	3.733997	0.041615
0.0600	4.84	4.856824	0.000283
0.1330	8.68	8.247731	0.186857
0.1770	11.2	10.86153	0.114565
0.1800	11.82	11.06152	0.57529
0.2180	13.67	13.80213	0.017459
0.2380	15.26	15.35626	0.009267
0.2410	15.59	15.59288	8.31E-06
0.2560	17.08	16.78111	0.089337
0.2780	17.4	18.51268	1.238057
0.2790	17.94	18.5904	0.423014
0.2920	20.03	19.58829	0.195106
0.3070	20.43	20.7039	0.075023
0.3500	23.45	23.6139	0.026864
0.3690	25.28	24.74268	0.288709
0.5260	30.97	30.75523	0.046126
0.5390	32.04	31.05566	0.968916
0.6490	33.03	32.92434	0.011165
0.6970	33.32	33.47527	0.02411
0.7580	33.87	34.02885	0.025233
0.8250	34.11	34.501	0.152885
0.8250	34.15	34.501	0.123204

$$\sigma_L = \sqrt{\frac{\sum_{i=1}^{24}(C_{As,i} - C'_{As,i})^2}{24 - 1}} = 0.452307$$

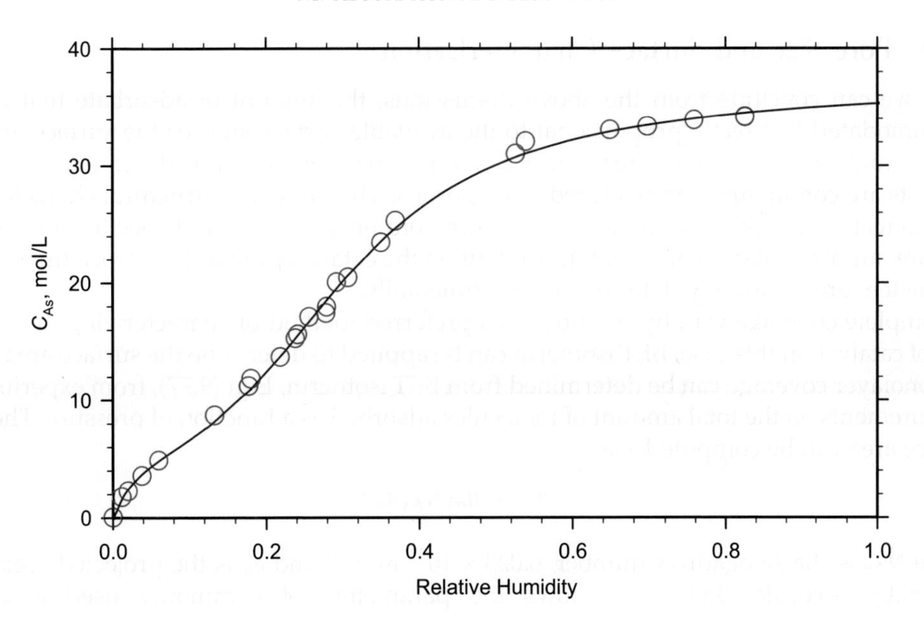

FIGURE E9-3.3 General multilayer isotherm fit to water vapor adsorption on silica gel at 25 °C.

For multispecies adsorption on the same sites nonselectively, the coverage of species j on layer i (among the total of N layers) is given by

$$\theta_{ij} = \frac{c(\beta^{i-1} - \beta^N)}{1 - (1-c)\beta - \beta^{N+1}} K_j C_j \tag{9.79}$$

Where K_j is the adsorption isotherm constant for species j for all layers above the first one layer, c is ratio of the adsorption isotherm constant of the first layer to that of layers above

$$c = \frac{K_{1j}}{K_j}, \tag{9.80}$$

and

$$\beta = \sum_{j=1}^{N_S} K_j C_j \tag{9.81}$$

The total number of species j molecules adsorbed is given by

$$\begin{aligned} n_{js,N} &= n_{\sigma 1} \sum_{i=1}^{N} \theta_{ij} = n_{\sigma 1} c \sum_{i=1}^{N} \frac{\beta^{i-1} - \beta^N}{1 - (1-c)\beta - c\beta^{N+1}} K_j C_j \\ &= n_{\sigma 1} c \frac{\dfrac{1-\beta^N}{1-\beta} - N\beta^N}{1 - (1-c)\beta - c\beta^{N+1}} K_j C_j = n_{\sigma 1} c \frac{1 - [1 + N(1-\beta)]\beta^N}{(1-\beta)[1 - (1-c)\beta - c\beta^{N+1}]} K_j C_j \end{aligned} \tag{9.82}$$

Therefore, we have the general multispecies multilayer adsorption isotherms.

9.1.5. Pore Size and Surface Characterization

As we can conclude from the above discussions, the amount of adsorbate that can be accommodated is directly proportional to the available surface sites or the surface area. To achieve high specific surface area (surface area per mass of solid adsorbent material), solid catalysts are commonly manufactured to be porous. Therefore, the structural characteristics of solid (catalyst) materials are important. Pore volume, pore size, and specific pore surface area are important parameters that dependent on the catalyst preparation procedures. These parameters are commonly determined experimentally.

Complete coverage via physisorption is a preferred method of characterizing the surface area of catalyst. In this case, BET isotherm can be applied to determine the surface area as $n_{\sigma 1}$ or monolayer coverage can be determined from BET isotherm, Eqn (9.77), from experimental measurements on the total amount of molecules adsorbed as a function of pressure. The total surface area can be computed via

$$a_T = n_{\sigma 1} N_{Av} a_\sigma \tag{9.83}$$

where N_{Av} is the Avogadro's number, 6.023×10^{23} mol^{-1}, and a_σ is the projected area of an adsorbate molecule. Table 9.2 shows the parameters of commonly used adsorbate molecules.

Pore volume and pore size are measured by Mercury penetration. Because Mercury is a nonwetting liquid, it is not capable of penetrating pores smaller than 75,000 Å (or 7.5×10^{-7} m) at atmospheric conditions. At high pressure, Mercury can be forced into fine pores as the surface tension is overcome by external pressure. The pore size and the pressure is related by

$$r_P = \frac{7.5 \times 10^{-7}\,\text{m}\cdot\text{bar}}{p} \tag{9.84}$$

By measuring the amount of Mercury penetration as the pressure is increased, we can determine the pore size distributions as well as the pore volume.

TABLE 9.2 Properties of Commonly Used Adsorbates for Catalyst Surface Characterization

Adsorbate	Adsorption temperature, K	Saturation vapor pressure $p°$, MPa	Projected molecular area a_σ, 10^{-20} m^2
N_2	77.4	0.10132	16.2
Kr	77.4	3.456×10^{-4}	19.5
Ar	77.4	0.03333	14.6
C_6H_6	293.2	9.879×10^{-3}	40
CO_2	195.2	0.10132	19.5
CH_3OH	293.2	0.01280	25

9.2. LHHW: SURFACE REACTIONS WITH RATE-CONTROLLING STEPS

At the beginning of this chapter, it was stated that reaction sequences involving surface steps (for example, Eqn 9.1) could be visualized as a type of chain reaction. This is indeed so and it naturally leads to the utility of pseudo-steady state hypothesis (PSSH) derivations for kinetic rate simplifications. However, also associated with the development of the theory of surface reaction kinetics has been the concept of the rate-limiting or rate-controlling step. This presents a rather different view of sequential steps than does pure chain reaction theory, since if a single step controls the rate of reaction then all other steps must be at (rapid) equilibrium. This is a result that is not a consequence of the general PSSH. As we have learned that both PSSH and rapid equilibrium steps lead to similar asymptotic rate expressions, there are no clear advantages gained by using one or the other for a complicated reaction network. Langmuir isotherm is generally applied in surface reaction analyses, which was formalized by Hinshelwood, Hougen, and Watson.

In fact, pursuing the example in Eqn (9.1) a bit further in this regard, if the surface reaction is rate limiting, we can express the net rate of reaction directly in terms of the surface species concentrations, $n_\sigma\theta_A$ and $n_\sigma\theta_B$:

$$r = k_S n_\sigma \theta_A - k_{-S} n_\sigma \theta_B \tag{9.85}$$

where k_S and k_{-S} are rate constants for the forward and reverse surface reaction steps. This represents a considerable simplification from the normal chain reaction analysis, because the first and third steps of (9.1) are at equilibrium and the surface species concentrations are entirely determined by their adsorption/desorption equilibrium on the surface.

Substitution of Eqn (9.15) into Eqn (9.85) gives the rate of reaction in terms of the bulk fluid phase concentrations of the reacting species.

$$r = k_S n_\sigma \frac{K_A(C_A - C_B/K_C)}{1 + K_A C_A + K_B C_B} \tag{9.86}$$

where

$$K_C = \frac{K_A k_s}{K_B k_{-s}} \tag{9.87}$$

is the equilibrium constant. In fact, the value *of* n_σ may be a somewhat elusive quantity, so that in practice this is often absorbed into the rate constant as,

$$r = k\frac{C_A - C_B/K_C}{1 + K_A C_A + K_B C_B} \tag{9.88}$$

The rates of catalytic reactions are usually expressed in terms of unit mass or unit total surface (not external surface) of the catalyst. This is understood because of the active sites are proportional to the total surface area.

As a second example of surface reaction rate control, consider the slightly more complicated bimolecular reaction on one single type of active sites:

$$A + \sigma \rightleftarrows A\cdot\sigma \tag{9.89a}$$

$$B + \sigma \rightleftarrows B \cdot \sigma \tag{9.89b}$$

$$A \cdot \sigma + B \cdot \sigma \rightleftarrows C \cdot \sigma + D \cdot \sigma \tag{9.89c}$$

$$C \cdot \sigma \rightleftarrows C + \sigma \tag{9.89d}$$

$$D \cdot \sigma \rightleftarrows D + \sigma \tag{9.89e}$$

$$+) = \text{overall} \quad A + B \rightarrow C + D \tag{9.89f}$$

Let us assuming that the surface reaction (9.89c) is the rate-limiting step, whereas the adsorption–desorption steps are fast equilibrium steps. The adsorption step (9.89a) is a fast equilibrium step, that is

$$0 = r_{\text{ad-des,A}} = k_A n_\sigma \theta C_A - k_{-A} n_\sigma \theta_A \tag{9.90}$$

which yields after rearrangement

$$\theta_A = K_A \theta C_A \tag{9.91}$$

where

$$K_A = \frac{k_A}{k_{-A}} \tag{9.92}$$

is the Langmuir isotherm constant for species A on the catalyst surface. Similarly, one can write for B, C, and D:

$$\theta_B = K_B \theta C_B \tag{9.93}$$

$$\theta_C = K_C \theta C_C \tag{9.94}$$

$$\theta_D = K_D \theta C_D \tag{9.95}$$

There are four species adsorbed on the same type of active sites. Site balance leads to the summation of the fraction of vacant (i.e. available sites) and the fractions of the sites occupied by A, B, C, and D make unity:

$$\theta + \theta_A + \theta_B + \theta_C + \theta_D = 1 \tag{9.96}$$

Substituting Eqns (9.91) and (9.93) through (9.95) into Eqn (9.96), we obtain after rearrangement

$$\theta = \frac{1}{K_A C_A + K_B C_B + K_C C_C + K_D C_D} \tag{9.97}$$

Since the surface reaction (9.89c) is the rate-limiting step, the overall reaction rate for (9.89f) is identical to that for (9.89c) as the stoichiometric coefficients are the same for A, B, C and D. That is,

$$r = r_S = k_S n_\sigma^2 \theta_A \theta_B \tag{9.98}$$

Substituting Eqns (9.97), (9.91), and (9.93) into Eqn (9.98), we obtain

$$r = \frac{k_S n_\sigma^2 K_A K_B C_A C_B}{(K_A C_A + K_B C_B + K_C C_C + K_D C_D)^2} \tag{9.99}$$

It is clear from Eqn (9.98) that when a surface reaction step is rate controlling, one needs only information concerning adsorption equilibria of reactant and product species in order to write the appropriate rate equation. Table 9.3 shows a collection of the LHHW rate expressions.

As shown in Table 9.3, in each of these reactions, the active centers or sites form a closed sequence in the overall reaction. According to this view, when the stoichiometry between reactants and products is not balanced, the concentration of vacant active centers also enters the rate equation, reaction 2 in Table 9.3.

The bimolecular reaction involving one reactant nonadsorbed is sometimes referred to as a *Rideal* or *Eley-Rideal mechanism.* It is encountered primarily in interpretation of catalytic hydrogenation kinetics. In general, when a reactant or product is no adsorbed on the surface, this particular species is not to appear in the denominator of the rate expression if the surface reaction is the rate-limiting step.

The rate-controlling steps other than surface reaction on ideal surfaces are also shown in Table 9.3. If, for example, the rate of adsorption of a reactant species on the surface is slow compared to other steps, it is no longer correct to suppose that its surface concentration is determined by adsorption equilibrium. Rather, there must be chemical equilibrium among all species on the surface, and the surface concentration of the species involved in the rate-limiting step is determined by this equilibrium. The actual concentration of the rate-limiting adsorbate consequently will not appear in the adsorption terms (denominator) of the rate equation but is replaced by that concentration corresponding to the surface concentration level established by the equilibrium of other steps. Again consider the isomerization example of Eqn (9.1), this time in which the rate of adsorption of A is controlling. From Eqn (9.2), we may write the net rate of reaction as the difference between rates of adsorption and desorption of A:

$$r = k_A C_A \theta C_\sigma - k_{-A} \theta_A C_\sigma \tag{9.100}$$

in which k_A (or k_{ad}), and k_{-A} (or k_{des}) are adsorption and desorption rate constants (i.e. $k_A = k_A^\circ e^{-\frac{E_A}{RT}}$) and θ_A is the fraction of surface coverage by A as determined by the equilibrium of all other steps. Since the surface reaction (9.1b) is a rapid equilibrium step, we have

$$0 = r_s = k_s \theta_A C_\sigma - k_{-s} \theta_B C_\sigma \tag{9.101}$$

which leads to

$$K_s = \frac{k_s}{k_{-s}} = \frac{\theta_B}{\theta_A} \tag{9.102}$$

or

$$\theta_A = \frac{\theta_B}{K_s} \tag{9.103}$$

TABLE 9.3 Some Examples of LHHW Rate Expressions

Overall reaction	Mechanism/ controlling step	Rate expression
1) Isomerization $A \rightleftarrows B$	$A + \sigma \rightleftarrows A\cdot\sigma$	$r = k_A C_\sigma \dfrac{C_A - C_B/K_{eq}}{1 + K_B C_B + K_{eq}^{-1} K_A C_B}$
	$A\cdot\sigma \rightleftarrows B\cdot\sigma$	$r = k_s K_A C_\sigma \dfrac{C_A - C_B/K_{eq}}{1 + K_A C_A + K_B C_B}$
	$B\cdot\sigma \rightleftarrows B + \sigma$	$r = k_B C_\sigma \dfrac{K_{eq} C_A - C_B}{1 + K_A C_A + K_{eq} K_B C_A}$
2) Decomposition (Double site) $A \rightleftarrows B + C$	$A + \sigma \rightleftarrows A\cdot\sigma$	$r = k_A C_\sigma \dfrac{C_A - C_B C_C/K_{eq}}{1 + K_A K_{eq}^{-1} C_B C_C + K_B C_B + K_C C_C}$
	$A\cdot\sigma + \sigma \rightleftarrows B\cdot\sigma + C\cdot\sigma$	$r = k_s K_A C_\sigma^2 \dfrac{C_A - C_B C_C/K_{eq}}{(1 + K_A C_A + K_B C_B + K_C C_C)^2}$
	$B\cdot\sigma \rightleftarrows B + \sigma$	$r = k_B C_\sigma \dfrac{K_{eq} C_A - C_B C_C}{K_B K_{eq} C_A + (1 + K_A C_A + K_C C_C) C_C}$
	$C\cdot\sigma \rightleftarrows C + \sigma$	$r = k_C C_\sigma \dfrac{K_{eq} C_A - C_B C_C}{K_C K_{eq} C_A + (1 + K_A C_A + K_B C_B) C_B}$
3) Bimolecular (single site) $A + B \rightleftarrows C + D$	$A + \sigma \rightleftarrows A\cdot\sigma$	$r = k_A C_\sigma \dfrac{C_A C_B - C_C C_D/K_{eq}}{K_A K_{eq}^{-1} C_C C_D + (1 + K_B C_B + K_C C_C + K_D C_D) C_B}$
	$B + \sigma \rightleftarrows B\cdot\sigma$	$r = k_B C_\sigma \dfrac{C_A C_B - C_C C_D/K_{eq}}{K_B K_{eq}^{-1} C_C C_D + (1 + K_A C_A + K_C C_C + K_D C_D) C_A}$
	$A\cdot\sigma + B\cdot\sigma \rightleftarrows C\cdot\sigma + D\cdot\sigma$	$r = k_s K_A K_B C_\sigma^2 \dfrac{C_A C_B - C_C C_D/K_{eq}}{(1 + K_A C_A + K_B C_B + K_C C_C + K_D C_D)^2}$
	$C\cdot\sigma \rightleftarrows C + \sigma$	$r = k_C C_\sigma \dfrac{K_{eq} C_A C_B - C_C C_D}{K_{eq} K_C C_A C_B + (1 + K_A C_A + K_B C_B + K_D C_D) C_C}$
	$D\cdot\sigma \rightleftarrows D + \sigma$	$r = k_D C_\sigma \dfrac{K_{eq} C_A C_B - C_C C_D}{K_{eq} K_D C_A C_B + (1 + K_A C_A + K_B C_B + K_C C_C) C_D}$
4) Bimolecular (dissociative) $\frac{1}{2}A_2 + B \rightleftarrows C + D$	$A_2 + 2\sigma \rightleftarrows 2A\cdot\sigma$	$r = k_{A_2} C_\sigma^2 \dfrac{C_{A_2} C_B^2 - C_C^2 C_D^2/K_{eq}^2}{[K_{A_2}^{1/2} K_{eq}^{-1} C_C C_D + (1 + K_B C_B + K_C C_C + K_D C_D) C_B]^2}$
	$B + \sigma \rightleftarrows B\cdot\sigma$	$r = k_B C_\sigma \dfrac{C_{A_2}^{1/2} C_B - C_C C_D/K_{eq}}{K_B K_{eq}^{-1} C_C C_D + (1 + \sqrt{K_{A_2} C_{A_2}} + K_C C_C + K_D C_D) C_A}$
	$A\cdot\sigma + B\cdot\sigma \rightleftarrows C\cdot\sigma + D\cdot\sigma$	$r = k_s K_{A_2}^{1/2} K_B C_\sigma^2 \dfrac{C_{A_2}^{1/2} C_B - C_C C_D/K_{eq}}{(1 + \sqrt{K_{A_2} C_{A_2}} + K_B C_B + K_C C_C + K_D C_D)^2}$
	$C\cdot\sigma \rightleftarrows C + \sigma$	$r = k_C C_\sigma \dfrac{K_{eq} C_{A_2}^{1/2} C_B - C_C C_D}{K_{eq} K_C C_{A_2}^{1/2} C_B + (1 + \sqrt{K_{A_2} C_{A_2}} + K_B C_B + K_D C_D) C_C}$
	$D\cdot\sigma \rightleftarrows D + \sigma$	$r = k_D C_\sigma \dfrac{K_{eq} C_{A_2}^{1/2} C_B - C_C C_D}{K_{eq} K_D C_{A_2}^{1/2} C_B + (1 + \sqrt{K_{A_2} C_{A_2}} + K_B C_B + K_C C_C) C_D}$

TABLE 9.3 Some Examples of LHHW Rate Expressions—*Cont'd*

Overall reaction	Mechanism/ controlling step	Rate expression
5) Bimolecular (Dual site) $A + B \rightleftarrows C + D$	$A + \sigma_1 \rightleftarrows A{\cdot}\sigma_1$	$r = k_A C_{\sigma_1} \dfrac{C_A C_B - C_C C_D / K_{eq}}{K_A K_{eq}^{-1} C_C C_D + (1 + K_C C_C) C_B}$
	$B + \sigma_2 \rightleftarrows B{\cdot}\sigma_2$	$r = k_B C_{\sigma_2} \dfrac{C_A C_B - C_C C_D / K_{eq}}{K_B K_{eq}^{-1} C_C C_D + (1 + K_D C_D) C_A}$
	$A{\cdot}\sigma_1 + B{\cdot}\sigma_2 \rightleftarrows C{\cdot}\sigma_1 + D{\cdot}\sigma_2$	$r = k_s K_A K_B C_{\sigma_1} C_{\sigma_2} \dfrac{C_A C_B - C_C C_D / K_{eq}}{(1 + K_A C_A + K_C C_C)(1 + K_B C_B + K_D C_D)}$
	$C{\cdot}\sigma_1 \rightleftarrows C + \sigma_1$	$r = k_C C_{\sigma_1} \dfrac{K_{eq} C_A C_B - C_C C_D}{K_{eq} K_C C_A C_B + (1 + K_A C_A) C_C}$
	$D{\cdot}\sigma_2 \rightleftarrows D + \sigma_2$	$r = k_D C_{\sigma_2} \dfrac{K_{eq} C_A C_B - C_C C_D}{K_{eq} K_D C_A C_B + (1 + K_B C_B) C_D}$
6) Bimolecular (Eley-Rideal) $A + B \rightleftarrows C$	$A + \sigma \rightleftarrows A{\cdot}\sigma$	$r = k_A C_\sigma \dfrac{C_A C_B - C_C / K_{eq}}{K_A K_{eq}^{-1} C_C + (1 + K_C C_C) C_B}$
	$A{\cdot}\sigma + B \rightleftarrows C{\cdot}\sigma$	$r = k_s K_A C_\sigma \dfrac{C_A C_B - C_C / K_{eq}}{1 + K_A C_A + K_C C_C}$
	$C{\cdot}\sigma \rightleftarrows C + \sigma$	$r = k_C C_\sigma \dfrac{K_{eq} C_A C_B - C_C}{1 + K_A C_A + K_{eq} K_C C_A C_B}$

The desorption of B (Eqn 9.1c) is also a rapid equilibrium step,

$$0 = r_{B,\text{des-ad}} = k_{-B} \theta_B C_\sigma - k_B C_B \theta C_\sigma \tag{9.104}$$

which gives

$$\theta_B = \frac{k_B}{k_{-B}} \theta C_B = K_B C_B \theta \tag{9.105}$$

The total active site balance leads to

$$\theta + \theta_A + \theta_B = 1 \tag{9.106}$$

Substituting Eqns (9.103) and (9.105) into Eqn (9.106), we obtain after rearrangement

$$\theta = \frac{1}{1 + K_B C_B + K_S^{-1} K_B C_B} \tag{9.107}$$

and the fraction of sites occupied by A and B are given by

$$\theta_B = K_B C_B \theta = \frac{K_B C_B}{1 + K_B C_B + K_S^{-1} K_B C_B} \tag{9.108}$$

$$\theta_A = K_S^{-1}\theta_B = \frac{K_S^{-1}K_B C_B}{1 + K_B C_B + K_S^{-1}K_B C_B} \tag{9.109}$$

Substituting Eqns (9.107) and (9.109) into (9.100), we obtain

$$r = C_\sigma \frac{k_A C_A - k_{-A}K_S^{-1}K_B C_B}{1 + K_B C_B + K_S^{-1}K_B C_B} = k_A C_\sigma \frac{C_A - k_A^{-1}k_{-A}K_S^{-1}K_B C_B}{1 + K_B C_B + K_S^{-1}K_B C_B} \tag{9.110}$$

At equilibrium, $r = 0$, we have

$$K_{eq} = \frac{C_{B,eq}}{C_{A,eq}} = \frac{1}{k_A^{-1}k_{-A}K_S^{-1}K_B} \tag{9.111}$$

also noting that

$$K_A = \frac{k_A}{k_{-A}} \tag{9.112}$$

we have

$$K_{eq} = \frac{K_S K_A}{K_B} \tag{9.113}$$

Eqn (9.110) can be rewritten as

$$r = k_A C_\sigma \frac{C_A - K_{eq}^{-1}C_B}{1 + K_B C_B + K_{eq}^{-1}K_A C_B} \tag{9.114}$$

Eqn (9.114) can also be written as

$$r = k_A C_\sigma \frac{C_A - K_{eq}^{-1}C_B}{1 + K_B C_B + K_A C_A^*} \tag{9.115}$$

By noting that

$$C_A^* = K_{eq}^{-1}C_B \tag{9.116}$$

as the equilibrium constant is not dependent on the nature of the surfaces. C_A^* is the virtual or equilibrium concentration of A in the bulk fluid phase with the surface overage. This is derivable because the concentration of A on the surface is in equilibrium with other components (or species) in the system as the rest of the steps that govern the overall reaction are fast equilibrium steps. One can observe from Table 9.3 that it holds true for all other cases. Comparing Eqn (9.115) with Eqn (9.110), we note that

$$\theta = \frac{1}{1 + K_B C_B + K_A C_A^*} \tag{9.117}$$

and

$$\theta_A = \frac{K_A C_A^*}{1 + K_B C_B + K_A C_A^*} \tag{9.118}$$

which recovers the Langmuir isotherm includes species A, although the adsorption of A is not in equilibrium. The nonequilibrium of A in the isotherm is accommodated by the replacement of C_A with the virtual concentration of A that is in equilibrium with other species in the system. Therefore, the virtual concentration may be applied to simplify the derivation for adsorption controlled processes or provide a check on the final expression.

Example 9-4 The reaction network of isomerization on a solid catalyst follows the following scheme:

$$\mathrm{A} + \sigma \rightleftarrows \mathrm{A}\cdot\sigma \tag{E9-4.1}$$

$$\mathrm{A}\cdot\sigma \rightleftarrows \mathrm{B}\cdot\sigma \tag{E9-4.2}$$

$$\mathrm{B}\cdot\sigma \rightleftarrows \mathrm{B} + \sigma \tag{E9-4.3}$$

$$+) = \text{overall} \quad \mathrm{A} \rightleftarrows \mathrm{B} \tag{E9-4.4}$$

Discuss the relevance of LHHW kinetics based on the detailed kinetics as the reaction being performed in a batch reactor. Treat the reaction network via a) microkinetics (i.e. full solutions), b) using LHHW approximations, i.e. rate-limiting step assumptions; and c) PSSH on intermediates.

Solution. This is the simplest case of surface catalyzed reaction shown in Table 9.3. As we have discussed in detail the derivation of LHHW kinetic expressions, we now go back to the detailed reaction network analysis before turning to the LHHW simplifications (assumptions).

a) Microkinetics (Full Solutions)

As the reaction rate expression follows stoichiometry for elementary steps, reactions (E9-4.1) through (E9-4.3):

$$r_1 = k_A C_A \theta C\sigma - k_{-A}\theta_A C\sigma \tag{E9-4.5}$$

$$r_2 = k_S \theta_A C\sigma - k_{-S}\theta_B C\sigma \tag{E9-4.6}$$

$$r_3 = k_{-B}\theta_B C\sigma - k_B C_B \theta C\sigma \tag{E9-4.7}$$

Mole balances of all the species in the batch reactor lead to

$$\frac{dC_A}{dt} = -k_A(C_A\theta - \theta_A/K_A)C_\sigma \tag{E9-4.8}$$

$$\frac{dC_B}{dt} = k_B(\theta_B/K_B - \theta C_B)C_\sigma \tag{E9-4.9}$$

$$\frac{d\theta_A}{dt} = k_A(\theta C_A - \theta_A/K_A) - k_S(\theta_A - \theta_B K_A/K_B/K_C) \tag{E9-4.10}$$

$$\frac{d\theta_B}{dt} = k_S(\theta_A - \theta_B K_A/K_B/K_C) - k_B(\theta_B/K_B - \theta C_B) \tag{E9-4.11}$$

$$\theta = 1 - \theta_A - \theta_B \tag{E9-4.12}$$

where

$$K_A = \frac{k_A}{k_{-A}} \tag{E9-4.13}$$

$$K_B = \frac{k_B}{k_{-B}} \tag{E9-4.14}$$

$$K_C = \frac{k_S}{k_{-S}} \times \frac{K_A}{K_B} \tag{E9-4.15}$$

K_A and K_B are adsorption equilibrium constants of A and B, respectively, and K_C is the equilibrium constant.

The five Eqns (E9-4.8) through (E9-4.12) can be solved simultaneously together with the initial conditions (in the reactor at time 0):

$$C_A = C_{A0}; C_\sigma; C_B = 0; \theta = 1; \theta_A = 0; \theta_B = 0 \text{ when } t = 0.$$

We shall use an integrator to show how this problem can be solved on computer. In this case, we use the ODexLims to integrate Eqns (E9-4.8) through (E9-4.11). Let

$$y_1 = C_A; y_2 = C_B; y_3 = \theta_A; y_4 = \theta_B; \text{ and the independent variable } x = t$$

$$\text{Parameters } c_1 = k_A C_\sigma;\ c_2 = K_A C_\sigma;\ c_3 = k_S;\ c_4 = K_C;\ c_5 = K_B C_\sigma;\ c_6 = k_B\, C_\sigma.$$

The kernel functions can then be input into the visual basic module as shown in Fig. E9-4.1. The set-up and solution on excel worksheet for one case (one set of parameters) is shown in Fig. E9-4.2. Some of the results for selected values of the parameters are shown in Figs. E9-4.3 through E9-4.5.

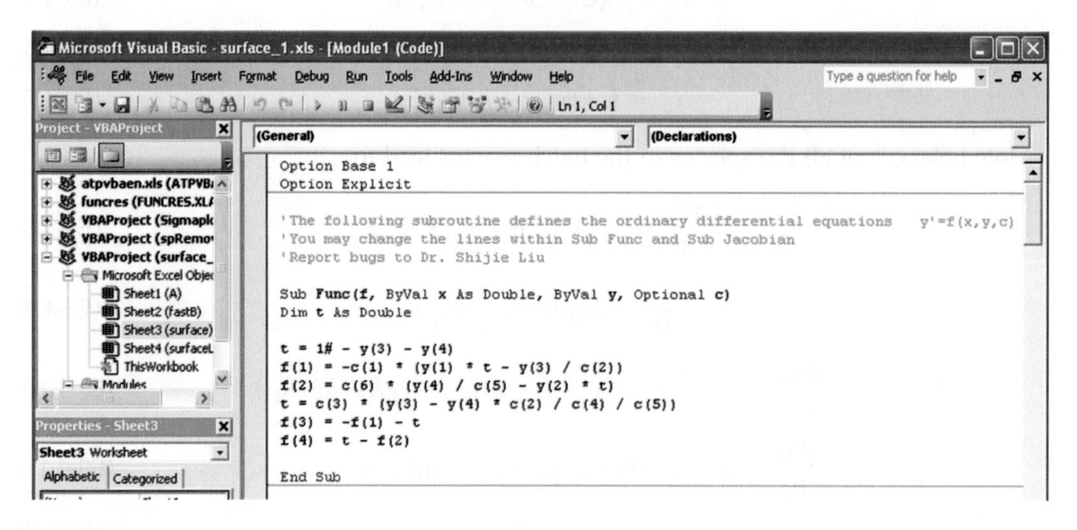

FIGURE E9-4.1 Visual basic module shown the integral kernels for example 9.4.

surface_1 [Compatibility Mode] - Microsoft Exc

B6 f_x {=ODExLIMS(A5:A124,B5:E5,,,A3:F3)}

	A	B	C	D	E	F
1	C(1)	C(2)	C(3)	C(4)	C(5)	C6)
2	kACσ	KA=kA/k-	ks	KC=KAks	KB=kB/k-1	kBCσ
3	10	1	1	4	1	10
4	t	CA/Cσ	CB/Cσ	θA	θB	θ
5	0	10	0	0	0	1
6	0.0001	9.995012	1.58394E-11	0.004988	1.25E-07	0.995012
7	0.0002	9.985132	5.54854E-10	0.014867	1.12E-06	0.985132
8	0.0005	9.956188	1.49472E-08	0.043802	9.93E-06	0.956188
9	0.001	9.910187	1.38253E-07	0.089769	4.33E-05	0.910187
10	0.002	9.825935	1.15589E-06	0.173889	0.000175	0.825937
11	0.003	9.750951	3.87246E-06	0.248661	0.000384	0.750955
12	0.005	9.624454	1.71733E-05	0.37453	0.000999	0.624472
13	0.007	9.523442	4.47512E-05	0.47469	0.001823	0.523487
14	0.008	9.480728	6.50567E-05	0.516908	0.002299	0.480793
15	0.009	9.442442	9.02121E-05	0.554659	0.002809	0.442532
16	0.01	9.408097	0.000120537	0.588432	0.00335	0.408218
17	0.015	9.28213	0.000358217	0.711129	0.006383	0.282488
18	0.02	9.207662	0.000753732	0.781858	0.009726	0.208416
19	0.025	9.163121	0.00131667	0.822393	0.013169	0.164438
20	0.03	9.136158	0.002048511	0.845201	0.016593	0.138206
21	0.035	9.119571	0.002946051	0.85755	0.019933	0.122517

FIGURE E9-4.2 Excel worksheet for Example 9-4.

We first examine a case where the surface reaction rate is limiting. For this case, we scale the time with the surface reaction rate constant. The solutions for $C_{A0} = 10\ C_\sigma$; $k_A\ C_\sigma = 10\ k_S$; $K_A = 1/C_\sigma$; $K_C = 4$; $K_B = 1/C_\sigma$; and $k_B\ C_\sigma = 10\ k_S$ are shown in Fig. E9-4.3. One can observe that in the batch operation, the concentration of the reactant in the bulk fluid phase experiences a quick drop before the product formation is observed (Fig. E9-4.3A and Fig. E9-4.3C). The decrease is simply due to the adsorption of reactants on the catalyst surface and thus is dependent on the amount of catalysts or total amount of adsorption sites. Since the product B is also adsorbed on the surface, the coverage of A increases sharply at the start, reaches a maximum, and then decreases, as the product B is being formed and adsorbed on the surface. The coverage of B increases with time, and as more product B is formed, it also desorbs to the bulk phase and cause the concentration B in the bulk phase to increase.

In the second case, we examine the situation where the adsorption of A and surface reaction are the same, but the desorption rate of B is fast. The results are shown in Fig. E9-4.4. One can observe that there is a drop in the concentration of A initially, but the drop is gradual or at much slower speed that Fig. E9-4.3. θ_A reached maximum more gradually and not as obvious as compared Fig. E9-4.4C with Fig. E9-4.3B. After θ_A reached maximum, and the vacant site fraction become "steady" at about $k_S t = 0.3$ (Fig. E9-4.4D).

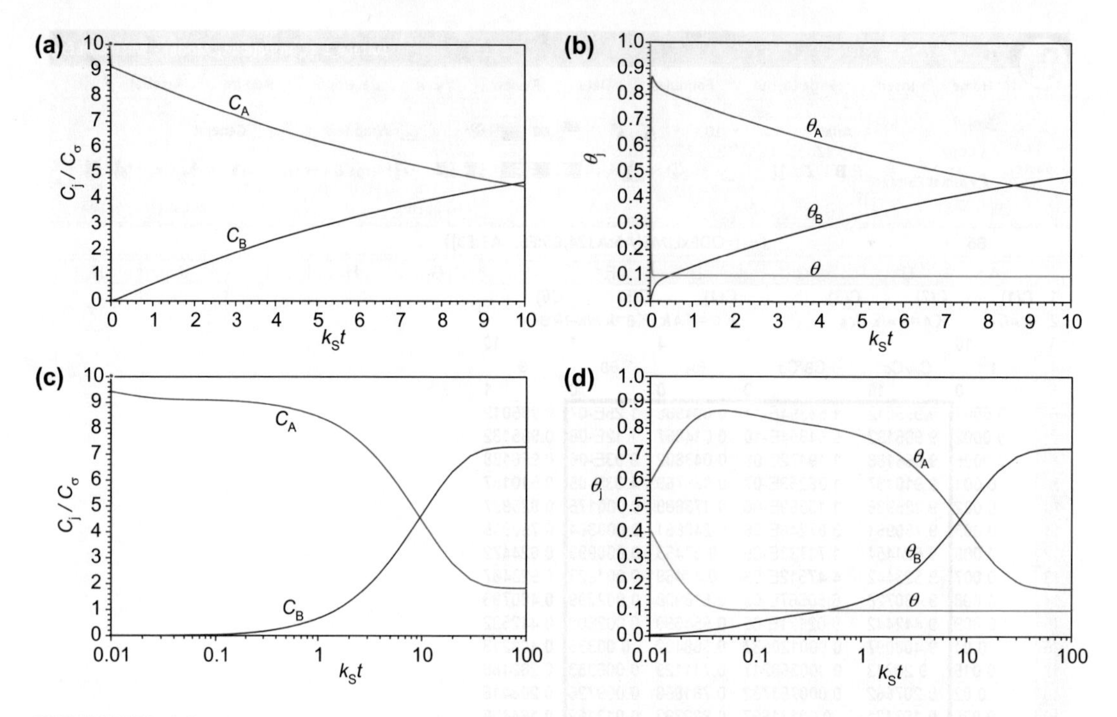

FIGURE E9-4.3 Variations of concentrations in the bulk phase (a, c), and surface coverages (b, d) as functions of time for $k_A C_\sigma = 10\ k_S$; $K_A = 1/C_\sigma$; $K_C = 4$; $K_B = 1/C_\sigma$; and $k_B C_\sigma = 10\ k_S$.

We then examine the case when adsorption of A is the rate-limiting step as shown in Fig. E9-4.5. In this case, the decrease in C_A initially is not as apparent as the previous two cases. The increase in the concentration of B in the bulk phase showed almost a "delay." Therefore, the effect of adsorption is still important.

The effects of catalyst and adsorption on the concentrations of reactants and products are important if there are significant amount of catalysts being added for batch systems. Therefore, once we perform LHHW analysis, we need to take the adsorption into consideration.

b) LHHW approximation

We next use the LHHW assumption to examine one case: the surface rate-limiting case to see how LHHW approximates the first we have discussed in this example. If the surface reaction is the rate-limiting step, we have the overall rate for reaction (E9-4.4):

$$r = r_2 = k_S C_\sigma \theta_A - k_{-S} C_\sigma \theta_B \tag{E9-4.16}$$

The other two steps (E9-4.3) and (E9-4.5) are in equilibrium,

$$0 = r_1 = k_A C_A \theta C_\sigma - k_{-A} \theta_A C_\sigma \tag{E9-4.17}$$

$$0 = r_3 = k_{-B} \theta_B C_\sigma - k_B C_B \theta C_\sigma \tag{E9-4.18}$$

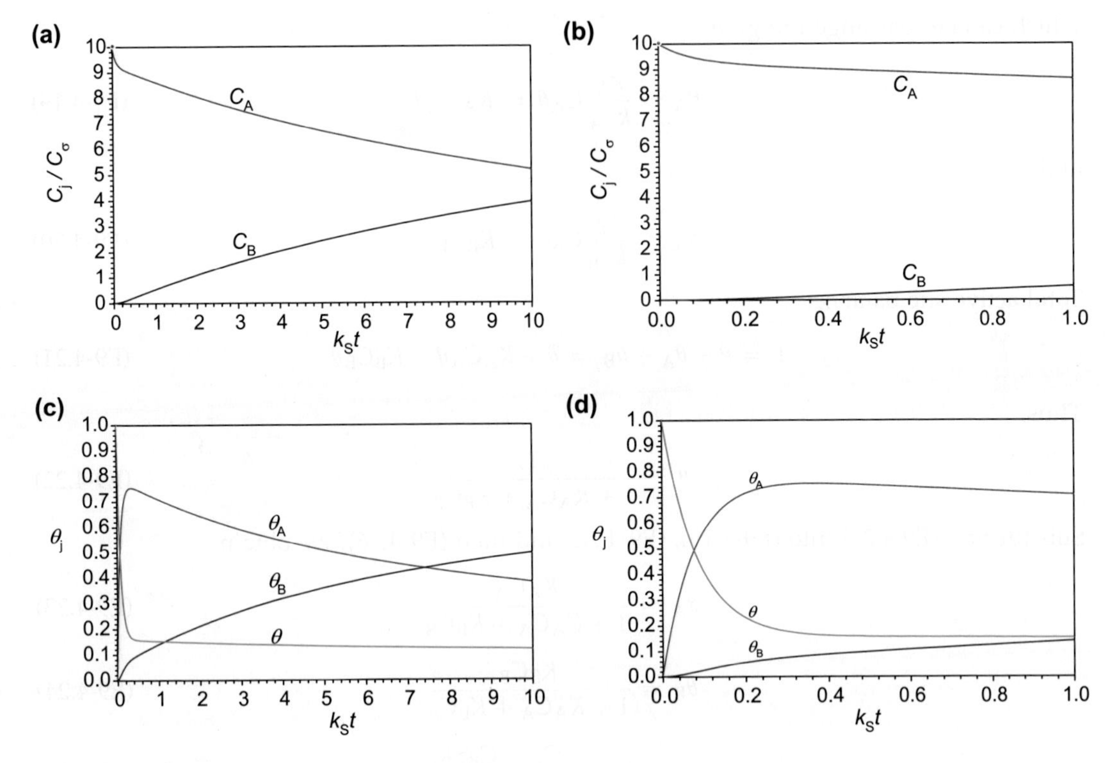

FIGURE E9-4.4 Variations of concentrations in the bulk phase (a, b) and surface coverages (c, d) as functions of time for $k_A C_\sigma = k_S$; $K_A = 1/C_\sigma$; $K_C = 4$; $K_B = 1/C_\sigma$; and $k_B C_\sigma = 10\ k_S$.

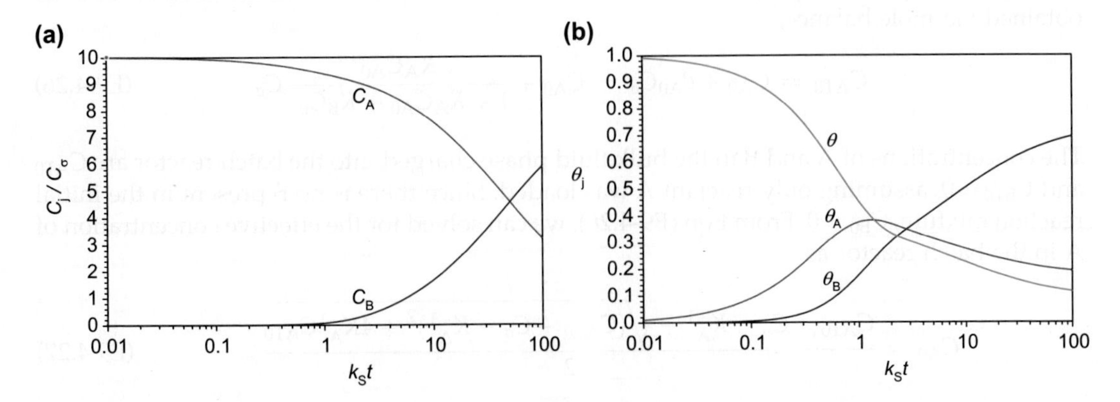

FIGURE E9-4.5 Variations of concentrations in the bulk phase (a) and surface coverages (b) for $k_A C_\sigma = 0.1\ k_S$; $K_A = 1/C_\sigma$; $K_C = 4$; $K_B = 1/C_\sigma$; and $k_B C_\sigma = k_S$.

which can be rearranged to give

$$\theta_A = \frac{k_A}{k_{-A}} C_A \theta = K_A C_A \theta \tag{E9-4.19}$$

and

$$\theta_B = \frac{k_B}{k_{-B}} C_B \theta = K_B C_B \theta \tag{E9-4.20}$$

Total active site balance:

$$1 = \theta + \theta_A + \theta_B = \theta + K_A C_A \theta + K_B C_B \theta \tag{E9-4.21}$$

Thus,

$$\theta = \frac{1}{1 + K_A C_A + K_B C_B} \tag{E9-4.22}$$

Substituting (E9-4.22) into (E9-4.19), (E9-4.20) and then (E9-4.16), we obtain

$$\theta_A = \frac{K_A C_A}{1 + K_A C_A + K_B C_B} \tag{E9-4.23}$$

$$\theta_B = \frac{K_B C_B}{1 + K_A C_A + K_B C_B} \tag{E9-4.24}$$

$$r = k_S C_\sigma K_A \frac{C_A - C_B/K_C}{1 + K_A C_A + K_B C_B} \tag{E9-4.25}$$

At time $t = 0$ in the batch reactor, the reaction is not started yet. However, LHHW expression (E9-4.25) requires that the adsorption and desorption are already in equilibrium. While this requirement is not of issue for reactions carried out in flow reactors (after the transient period) or when the amount of catalyst is negligible, it becomes important when noticeable amount of catalysts is employed in a batch reactor. For example, the concentration of A can be obtained via mole balance,

$$C_{AT0} = C_{A0} + \theta_{A0} C_\sigma = C_{A0} + \frac{K_A C_{A0}}{1 + K_A C_{A0} + K_B C_{B0}} C_\sigma \tag{E9-4.26}$$

The concentrations of A and B in the bulk fluid phase charged into the batch reactor are C_{AT0} and $C_{BT0} = 0$, assuming only reactant A was loaded. Since there is no B present in the initial reaction mixture, $C_{B0} = 0$. From Eqn (E9-4.26), we can solved for the effective concentration of A in the batch reactor as

$$C_{A0} = \frac{C_{AT0} - C_\sigma - K_A^{-1} + \sqrt{(C_{AT0} - C_\sigma - K_A^{-1})^2 + 4K_A^{-1} C_{AT0}}}{2} \tag{E9-4.27}$$

That is to say that the concentration of A in the bulk fluid phase at $t = 0$ is smaller than that in the original bulk fluid phase before contacting with the solid catalyst.

Mole balances on A and B in the reactor leads to

$$\frac{dC_A}{dt} = -r = k_S C_\sigma K_A \frac{C_A - C_B/K_C}{1 + K_A C_A + K_B C_B} \tag{E9-4.28}$$

$$\frac{dC_B}{dt} = r = k_S C_\sigma K_A \frac{C_A - C_B/K_C}{1 + K_A C_A + K_B C_B} \tag{E9-4.29}$$

The solutions from LHHW model can be obtained by solving Eqn (E9-4.28) and Eqn (E9-4.29) with initial conditions given by C_{A0} (Eqn E9-4.27) and $C_{B0} = 0$ at $t = 0$. Subsequently, the fractional coverages can be obtained from Eqn (E9-4.23) and (E9-4.24). One should note that the initial conditions set for surface-rate limiting LHHW model must have taken the adsorption equilibria into consideration.

Instead of having four equations to solve, we now have only two equations to solve. The solutions to one case consistent with the approximation to the first case discussed earlier are shown in Fig. E9-4.6. For comparison purposes, we have plotted the LHHW approximations as dashed lines and the original solutions with individual rates are shown as solid lines.

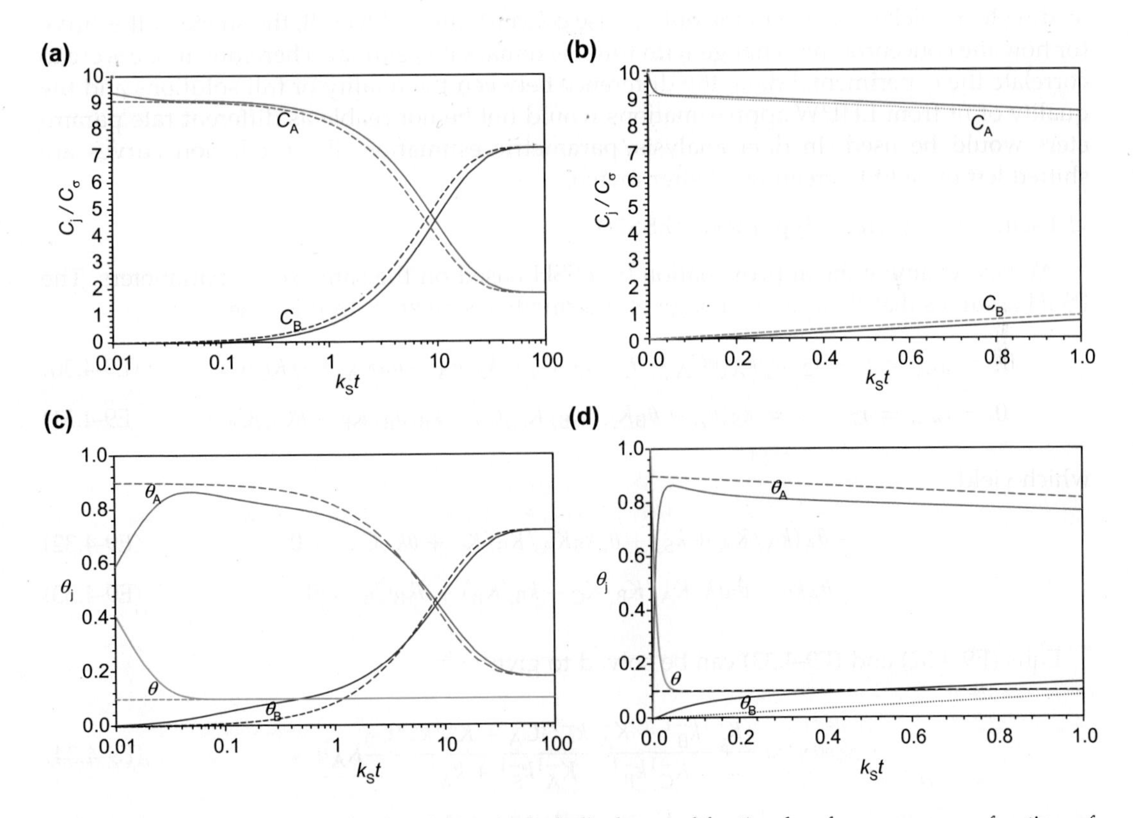

FIGURE E9-4.6 Variations of concentrations in the bulk phase and fractional surface coverages as functions of time for $K_A = 1/C_\sigma$; $K_C = 4$; $K_B = 1/C_\sigma$. The dashed lines are the predictions from LHHW kinetics assuming that the surface reaction is the rate-limiting step, whereas the solid lines are for $k_A\ C_\sigma = 10\ k_S$ and $k_B\ C_\sigma = 10\ k_S$.

Figs. E9-4.6A and B show the change of bulk phase concentrations with reaction time. One can observe that LHHW approximation agrees with the full rate description reasonably well at the shape of curves. In this case, the adsorption of A and desorption of B are one tenth of the rate of surface reaction, the effects of adsorption and desorption are still observable, but the simplification is reasonable. Wider differences in rates would make the approximation less obvious.

The fractional coverages on the catalyst surface are computed via Eqns (E9-4.23) and (E9-4.24) after the bulk phase concentrations were obtained. Figs. E9-4.6C and E9-4.6D show the variations of surface coverage as a function of reaction time. One can observe that the fractional surface coverage as predicted by the LHHW approximation is quite similar to the full rate descriptions. LHHW approximation becomes suitable once the fraction of vacant sites becomes steady (nearly constant).

One can observe from Fig. E9-4.6A that while the variation of bulk concentrations for LHHW approximation looks similar to the full solutions, there is a shift log t (to the right) that could make the agreement closer. This is due to the fact that the finite rates of adsorption of A and desorption of B contributes to the decline of overall rate as used by LHHW approximation. As a result, the LHHW approximations over-predicted the reaction rate and thus leading to a quicker change in the bulk phase concentrations. Overall, the shape of the curve (or how the concentrations change with time) is remarkably similar. Therefore, if one were to correlate the experimental data, the difference between the quality of full solutions and the quality of fit from LHHW approximations would not be noticeable as different rate parameters would be used. In data analysis/parametric estimation, the prediction curves are shifted left or right to creating a better match.

c) Pseudosteady State Hypothesis (PSSH)

We next examine the approximation by PSSH based on the same set of parameters. The PSSH assumes that the rate of change of intermediates be zero. In this case,

$$0 = r_{\sigma\cdot A} = r_1 - r_2 = k_A(\theta C_A - \theta_A/K_A)C_\sigma - k_S(\theta_A - \theta_B K_A/K_B/K_C)C_\sigma \tag{E9-4.30}$$

$$0 = r_{\sigma\cdot B} = r_2 - r_3 = k_S(\theta_A - \theta_B K_A/K_B/K_C)C_\sigma - k_B(\theta_B/K_B - \theta C_B)C_\sigma \tag{E9-4.31}$$

which yield

$$-\theta_A(k_A/K_A + k_S) + \theta_B k_S K_A/K_B/K_C + \theta k_A C_A = 0 \tag{E9-4.32}$$

$$\theta_A k_S - \theta_B(k_S K_A/K_B/K_C + k_B/K_B) + \theta k_B C_B = 0 \tag{E9-4.33}$$

Eqns (E9-4.32) and (E9-4.33) can be solved to give

$$\theta_A = \frac{(K_C^{-1}k_B^{-1} + K_A^{-1}k_S^{-1})C_A + K_C^{-1}k_A^{-1}C_B}{K_C^{-1}k_B^{-1} + K_A^{-1}k_S^{-1} + k_A^{-1}} K_A\theta \tag{E9-4.34}$$

$$\theta_B = \frac{(k_A^{-1} + K_A^{-1}k_S^{-1})C_B + k_B^{-1}C_A}{K_C^{-1}k_B^{-1} + K_A^{-1}k_S^{-1} + k_A^{-1}} K_B\theta \tag{E9-4.35}$$

Total site balance leads to

$$1 = \theta + \theta_A + \theta_B$$
$$= \theta + \frac{(K_C^{-1}k_B^{-1} + K_A^{-1}k_S^{-1})C_A + K_C^{-1}k_A^{-1}C_B}{K_C^{-1}k_B^{-1} + K_A^{-1}k_S^{-1} + k_A^{-1}}K_A\theta + \frac{(k_A^{-1} + K_A^{-1}k_S^{-1})C_B + k_B^{-1}C_A}{K_C^{-1}k_B^{-1} + K_A^{-1}k_S^{-1} + k_A^{-1}}K_B\theta \tag{E9-4.36}$$

Thus,

$$\theta = \frac{1}{1 + \dfrac{(K_AK_C^{-1}k_B^{-1} + k_S^{-1} + k_B^{-1}K_B)C_A + (K_C^{-1}k_A^{-1}K_A + k_A^{-1}K_B + K_A^{-1}k_S^{-1}K_B)C_B}{K_C^{-1}k_B^{-1} + K_A^{-1}k_S^{-1} + k_A^{-1}}} \tag{E9-4.37}$$

Substituting Eqn (E9-4.37) into Eqns (E9-4.34) and (E9-4.35), we obtain the fractional coverages on the catalyst surface.

The overall rate of reaction:

$$r = -r_A = r_1 = k_AC_A\theta C_\sigma - k_{-A}\theta_AC_\sigma \tag{E9-4.38}$$

That is,

$$r = k_A(C_A\theta - \theta_A/K_A)C_\sigma \tag{E9-4.39}$$

Substituting the fractional coverage of A and the fraction of vacant sites, Eqn (E9-4.40) renders

$$r = k_A\left[C_A - \frac{(K_C^{-1}k_B^{-1} + K_A^{-1}k_S^{-1})C_A + K_C^{-1}k_A^{-1}C_B}{K_C^{-1}k_B^{-1} + K_A^{-1}k_S^{-1} + k_A^{-1}}\right]\theta C_\sigma = \frac{C_A - K_C^{-1}C_B}{K_C^{-1}k_B^{-1} + K_A^{-1}k_S^{-1} + k_A^{-1}}\theta C_\sigma \tag{E9-4.40}$$

or

$$r = \frac{\dfrac{C_A - K_C^{-1}C_B}{K_C^{-1}k_B^{-1} + K_A^{-1}k_S^{-1} + k_A^{-1}}C_\sigma}{1 + \dfrac{(K_AK_C^{-1}k_B^{-1} + k_S^{-1} + k_B^{-1}K_B)C_A + (K_C^{-1}k_A^{-1}K_A + k_A^{-1}K_B + K_A^{-1}k_S^{-1}K_B)C_B}{K_C^{-1}k_B^{-1} + K_A^{-1}k_S^{-1} + k_A^{-1}}} \tag{E9-4.41}$$

which is the rate expression for the first case shown in Table 9.3. However, the rate expression is derived from PSSH, not from a rate-limiting step assumption. The expression (E9-4.41) is quite similar to the three rate expressions based on different rate limiting assumptions, although the rate constants are different from any one of them. In fact, one can reduce Eqn (E9-4.41) to the three expressions in Table 9.3 case 1) by assuming $k_S^{-1} = 0$ and $k_B^{-1} = 0$ for adsorption of A being rate limiting; $k_A^{-1} = 0$ and $k_B^{-1} = 0$ for surface reaction being rate limiting; and $k_A^{-1} = 0$ and $k_S^{-1} = 0$ for desorption of B being rate limiting. Therefore, PSSH is more general and carries less degree of approximation/simplifications than the LHHW approximations.

If one were to use Eqn (E9-4.41) to correlate experimental data, one would not be able to distinguish whether it is PSSH model or LHHW with a rate-limiting step as the parameters would need to be lumped together. The appeal of the PSSH approach is that it may be able to approximate the reaction rate in general (i.e. all the fluxes are considered), without imposing a particular step as the rate-limiting step as illustrated in Fig. E9-4.7. This approximation is particularly useful when the beginning (reactants) and end (products) are only of concern.

Based on Fig. E9-4.7, one can think of the reaction network in analogy to the electric conduction: 1) the fluxes must be equal at any given point and 2) the total resistance is the summation of all the resistors in series. If one were to look carefully, these statements could be detected as both are embedded in Eqn (E9-4.41).

At this point, one may look back at the full solutions as illustrated in Figs E9-4.3 through E9-4.5, especially with Figs. E9-4.3B and D, E9-4.4C and D, and E9-4.5B, that the concentrations of intermediates (in this case, the fractional coverage of A and the fractional coverage of B) are hardly constant or at "steady state" in any reasonably wide regions where we would like to have the solutions meaningful. Therefore, the assumption is rather strong. How do the solutions actually measure up with the full solutions?

To apply the PSSH expression (E9-4.40) or (E9-4.41), we must first ensure that the reaction mixture in already in pseudo-steady state to minimize the error may cause in the solution. This error can be negligible if the amount of catalyst is negligible or for steady flow reactors where steady state is already reached.

Let us consider again the case where no B is present in the reaction mixture at the start of the reaction. The concentrations of A and B charged into the batch reactor are C_{AT0} and $C_{BT0} = 0$. Since there is no B present in the initial reaction mixture, $C_{B0} = 0$. Overall mole balance at the onset of the reaction leads to

$$C_{AT0} = C_{A0} + \theta_{A0} C_\sigma + \theta_{B0} C_\sigma \tag{E9-4.42}$$

where θ_{A0} and θ_{B0} satisfy Eqns (E9-4.34) and (E9-4.35). Since $C_{B0} = 0$, substituting Eqns (E9-4.34) and (E9-4.35) into Eqn (9-4.42), we obtain

$$C_{AT0} = C_{A0} + \frac{(K_A K_C^{-1} k_B^{-1} + k_S^{-1} + k_B^{-1} K_B) C_\sigma C_{A0}}{K_C^{-1} k_B^{-1} + K_A^{-1} k_S^{-1} + k_A^{-1} + (K_A K_C^{-1} k_B^{-1} + k_S^{-1} + k_B^{-1} K_B) C_{A0}} \tag{E9-4.43}$$

This quadratic equation can be solved to give

$$C_{A0} = \frac{C_{AT0} - C_\sigma - a + \sqrt{(C_{AT0} - C_\sigma - a)^2 + 4a C_{AT0}}}{2} \tag{E9-4.44}$$

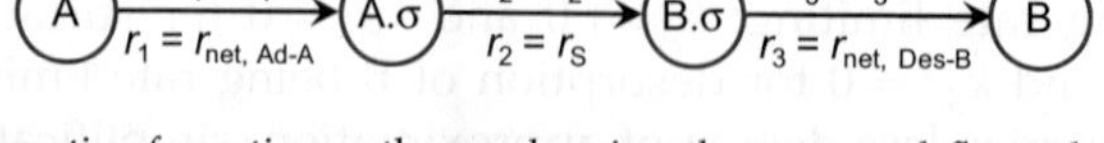

FIGURE E9-4.7 A schematic of reaction pathway showing the rates and fluxes between each adjacent intermediates or substances for isomerization of A to B carried out on a solid catalyst.

where

$$a = \frac{K_C^{-1}k_B^{-1} + K_A^{-1}k_S^{-1} + k_A^{-1}}{K_A K_C^{-1}k_B^{-1} + k_S^{-1} + k_B^{-1}K_B} \tag{E9-4.45}$$

Fig. E9-4.8 shows the comparison between the full solutions and those from PSSH treatment for the particular case of $k_A = 10\ k_S$ and $k_B = 10\ k_S$ where we have also shown the LHHW solutions. One can observe that bulk phase concentration solutions based on PSSH are surprisingly close to the full solutions ($k_St > 0.02$), better than the LHHW solutions as shown in Fig. E9-4.8. Although we have used the argument that all the intermediates remain at steady state (pseudo-steady state) and the solutions (of surface coverages, Fig. E9-4.8B) do not appear to be the case, the computed fractional coverages agree quite well with the full solutions. There is still an apparent shift of the dashed curves to the left but smaller than that in Fig. E9-4.6.

To show the reasonable agreement with the solutions from the PSSH approximation to the process, Fig. E9-4.9 shows the comparison between the full solutions and those from PSSH

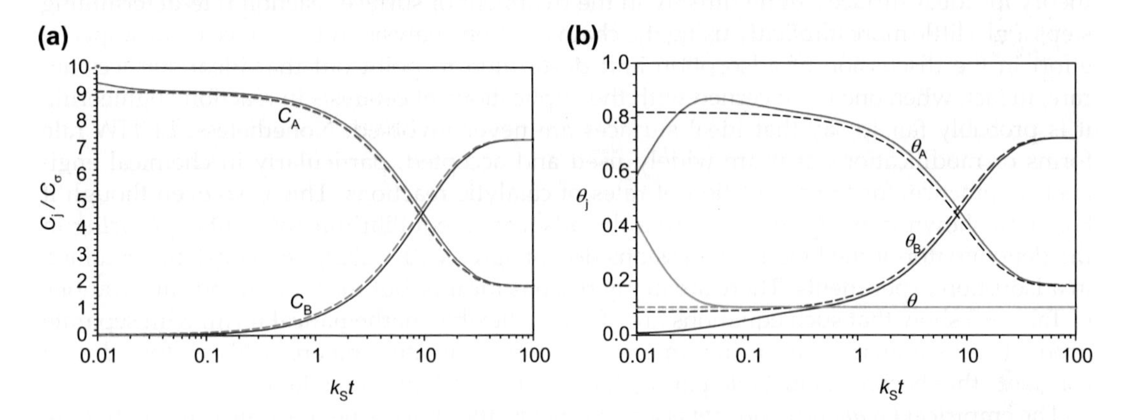

FIGURE E9-4.8 Variations of bulk phase concentrations and fractional surface coverage with time for $k_A C_\sigma = 10\ k_S$; $k_B C_\sigma = 10\ k_S$; $K_A = 1/C_\sigma$; $K_C = 4$; $K_B = 1/C_\sigma$. The dashed lines are the predictions from PSSH kinetics, whereas the solid lines are from the full solutions.

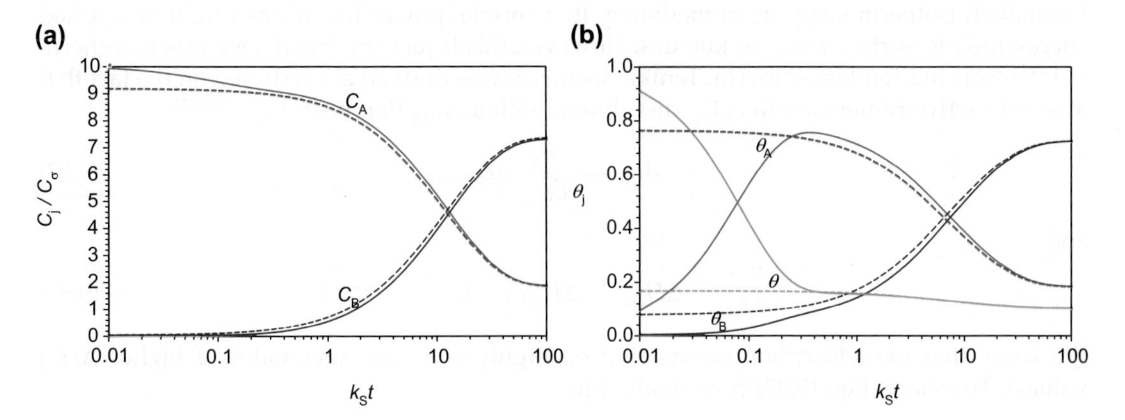

FIGURE E9-4.9 Variations of bulk phase concentrations (a) and fractional coverages (b) with time for $k_A C_\sigma = k_S$; $k_B C_\sigma = 10\ k_S$; $K_A = 1/C_\sigma$; $K_C = 4$; $K_B = 1/C_\sigma$. The dashed lines are the predictions from PSSH kinetics, whereas the solid lines are from the full solutions.

treatment for the case where the rates of reactions are the same for the adsorption and the surface reaction with $k_A = k_S$ and $k_B = 10\ k_S$. This is a case where we did not show any solutions from the equilibrium step assumptions. One can observe that the agreement between the full solutions and the PSSH solutions is rather good for the bulk phase concentrations ($k_S t > 0.1$) despite the fact that two steps together are rate-controlling steps.

Therefore, the PSSH approximations are better suited as kinetic models than the equilibrium step assumptions when true kinetic constants are employed. However, the rate expressions are quite similar to those of LHHW or equilibrium step assumptions. When utilized to correlate experimental data, one would not be able to distinguish the two treatments.

9.3. CHEMICAL REACTIONS ON NONIDEAL SURFACES BASED ON DISTRIBUTION OF INTERACTION ENERGY

The development presented for rates of surface reactions has thus far involved only the theory for ideal surfaces, quite directly in the treatment of surface reaction rate-determining steps and a little more implicitly using the chain reaction analysis. Yet, we have made a special effort in the discussion of adsorption and desorption to point out that ideal surfaces are rare; in fact, when one is concerned with the applications of catalysis in reaction engineering it is probably fair to say that ideal surfaces are never involved. Nonetheless, LHHW rate forms or modifications of it are widely used and accepted, particularly in chemical engineering practice, for the correlation of rates of catalytic reactions. This is so even though it has been shown in many instances that the adsorption equilibrium constants appearing in the denominator of the kinetic expressions do not agree with adsorption constants obtained in adsorption experiments. There are many reasons for this, but the voluminous illustrations of Table 9.3 show that such equations are of a very flexible mathematical form, with separate product and summation terms in numerator and denominator and are richly endowed with constants that become adjustable parameters when correlating rate data.

The empirical *Freundlich isotherm* is a favorable isotherm for kinetic studies although there is no rigorous theoretical basis behind it. Although Freundlich isotherm is not as good as Langmuir and other isotherms that have a theoretical basis, it is accurate enough in low coverage regions as it is an approximation to a variety of isotherms. The success of the Freundlich isotherm suggests immediately that simple, power-law forms might be applied successfully to surface reaction kinetics. However, this is just empirical. One other isotherm of interest is the Temkin isotherm. Temkin isotherm was derived above based on the fact that available active centers are linearly distributed with adsorption heat, Eqn (9.37)

$$\mathrm{d}n_{\sigma i} = \frac{n_\sigma}{E_{\max}}\mathrm{d}E_s \tag{9.37}$$

and

$$\Delta H_{\mathrm{ad}} = \Delta H_{\mathrm{ad},0} - E_s \tag{9.32}$$

We know that the adsorption occurs first on highly energetic sites (sites of higher ΔH_{ad} values). Therefore, Eqn (9.37) is equivalent to

$$d\theta = \frac{1}{E_{max}} dE_s \tag{9.119a}$$

where θ is the available (vacant) active site fraction. Integrating Eqn (9.119a), we obtain

$$E_s = E_{max}\theta \tag{9.119b}$$

which can be rewritten for adsorption of a single species

$$E_s = E_{max}(1 - \theta_A) \tag{9.120}$$

i.e. the adsorbed molecules exhibit an adsorption heat fluctuation (E_s) linearly related to the site coverage. Using Eqn (9.32),

$$\Delta H_{ad}(\theta_A) = \Delta H^0_{ad} - E_s = \Delta H^0_{ad} - E_{max}(1 - \theta_A) \tag{9.121}$$

Therefore, one can imagine that the activation energy of adsorption should be linearly related to the site coverage as well,

$$E_{ad}(\theta_A) = E^0_{ad} + E_\alpha \theta_A \tag{9.122}$$

where $E_{ad}(\theta_A)$ is the activation energy of adsorption for A when the fractional surface coverage of A is θ_A. It is expected that at lower coverage, the activation energy is lower. The activation energy increases as the coverage is increased. E^0_{ad} is the activation energy of adsorption for A when no A has been adsorbed on the surface, and E_α is a positive scaling constant. Since (see Eqn 9.5)

$$\Delta H_{ad} = E_{ad} - E_{des} \tag{9.123}$$

Substitute Eqn (9.122) into Eqn (9.123), we have

$$E_{des}(\theta_A) = E_{ad} - \Delta H_{ad}(\theta_A) = E^0_{ad} - \Delta H^0_{ad} + E_{max} - (E_{max} - E_\alpha)\theta_A \tag{9.124}$$

We now derived at the activation energies for the adsorption and desorption as a function of the surface coverage. Since we expect the desorption activation energy to decrease with increasing coverage, i.e.

$$-(E_{max} - E_\alpha) < 0 \tag{9.125}$$

We have

$$0 < E_\alpha < E_{max} \tag{9.126}$$

This forms the basis for studying the kinetics involving nonideal surfaces.

One example of kinetics involving the application of the nonideal surfaces theory is the ammonia synthesis from Nitrogen and Hydrogen. The synthesis of ammonia has changed the world food production (V. Smil, 2001). The Haber—Bosch process has remained the dominant process in generating ammonia from nitrogen separated from air and hydrogen. Over an Iron catalyst or a promoted Ru/C catalyst:

$$N_2 + 2\sigma \rightleftarrows 2N\cdot\sigma \tag{9.127a}$$

$$H_2 + 2\sigma \rightleftarrows 2H\cdot\sigma \tag{9.127b}$$

$$H\cdot\sigma + N\cdot\sigma \rightleftarrows NH\cdot\sigma + \sigma \tag{9.127c}$$

$$H\cdot\sigma + NH\cdot\sigma \rightleftarrows NH_2\cdot\sigma + \sigma \tag{9.127d}$$

$$H\cdot\sigma + NH_2\cdot\sigma \rightleftarrows NH_3\cdot\sigma + \sigma \tag{9.127e}$$

$$NH_3\cdot\sigma \rightleftarrows NH_3 + \sigma \tag{9.127f}$$

$$+) = \text{overall} \qquad N + 3H_2 \rightleftarrows 2NH_3 \tag{9.127g}$$

The adsorption of Nitrogen was found to be the rate-limiting step and all the other steps are rapid equilibrium steps. As such, the overall rate of reaction is determined by the adsorption of nitrogen or reaction (9.127a). The rate is given by

$$r = -r_{N_2} = k_{N_2} C_\sigma^2 \theta^2 p_{N_2} - k_{-N_2} C_\sigma^2 \theta_N^2 \tag{9.128}$$

Noting that

$$k_{N_2} = k_{N_2}^0 e^{-\frac{E_{ad}}{RT}} = k_{N_2}^0 e^{-\frac{E_{ad}^0 + E_\alpha \theta_N}{RT}} = k_{N_2}^0 e^{-\frac{E_{ad}^0}{RT}} e^{-\frac{E_\alpha \theta_N}{RT}} \tag{9.129}$$

$$k_{-N_2} = k_{-N_2}^0 e^{-\frac{E_{des}}{RT}} = k_{-N_2}^0 e^{\frac{E_{ad}^0 + E_{max} - \Delta H_{ad}^0}{RT}} e^{\frac{(E_{max} - E_\alpha)\theta_N}{RT}} \tag{9.130}$$

Combining the constants together, Eqn (9.130) is reduced to

$$r = \hat{k}_{N_2} \theta^2 p_{N_2} e^{-\frac{E_\alpha \theta_N}{RT}} - \hat{k}_{-N_2} \theta_N^2 e^{\frac{(E_{max} - E_\alpha)\theta_N}{RT}} \tag{9.131}$$

Temkin isotherm, which was derived from the linear distribution of adsorption heat, is given by

$$\theta_N \approx \frac{RT}{E_{max}} \ln\left(\overline{K}_{N_2} p_{N_2}^* e^{\frac{E_{max}}{RT}}\right) \tag{9.132}$$

Since the nitrogen adsorption is the rate-limiting step and the surface coverage of Nitrogen is in equilibrium with hydrogen and ammonia via other surface reaction steps. The pressure in the adsorption isotherm, $p_{N_2}^*$, is thus not the actual partial pressure of nitrogen. This virtual partial pressure of N_2 is evaluated by the partial pressures of hydrogen and ammonia by

$$K_P = \frac{p_{NH_3}^2}{p_{N_2}^* p_{H_2}^3} \tag{9.133}$$

Substituting Eqn (9.133) into Eqn (9.132), we obtain

$$\theta_N = \frac{RT}{E_{max}} \ln\left(\overline{K}_{N_2} \frac{p_{NH_3}^2}{K_P p_{H_2}^3} e^{\frac{E_{max}}{RT}}\right) \tag{9.134}$$

Since the dependence of fractional coverage is dominated by the exponential terms, one can neglect the change in the power-law terms of the fractional coverage in Eqn (9.131) while applying the Temkin approximation of θ_N. Thus, Eqn (9.131) is approximated by

$$r = \hat{k}_{N_2} p_{N_2} \left(\overline{K}_{N_2} \frac{p_{NH_3}^2}{K_P p_{H_2}^3} e^{\frac{E_{max}}{RT}}\right)^{-\frac{E_\alpha}{RT} \times \frac{RT}{E_{max}}} - \hat{k}_{-N_2} \left(\overline{K}_{N_2} \frac{p_{NH_3}^2}{K_P p_{H_2}^3} e^{\frac{E_{max}}{RT}}\right)^{\frac{E_{max} - E_\alpha}{RT} \times \frac{RT}{E_{max}}} \tag{9.135}$$

Noting that at thermodynamic equilibrium the reaction rate becomes zero, we can combine the constant terms together for Eqn (9.135) to give

$$r = kp_{N_2}\left(\frac{p_{H_2}^3}{p_{NH_3}^2}\right)^m - \frac{k}{K_P}\left(\frac{p_{NH_3}^2}{p_{H_2}^3}\right)^{1-m} \tag{9.136}$$

where $m = \dfrac{E_\alpha}{E_{max}}$ and $k = \hat{k}_{N_2}\left(\dfrac{K_P}{\overline{K}_{N_2}}e^{-\frac{E_{max}}{RT}}\right)^m$. Eqn (9.136) is known as the Temkin equation.

This illustrates that the linear energy distribution with Temkin simplification also leads to power-law kinetic expressions. The power-law appearance after Temkin simplification has it attractive as it is analogous to homogenous reactions. Because of the approximation made in the Temkin model that the coverage be in the intermediate region and the variation of the

TABLE 9.4 Comparison of LHHW Rate Expressions with Power-Law Expressions

Reaction and data source	LHHW	Power-law
SO_2 oxidation $SO_2 + \frac{1}{2}O_2 \rightleftarrows SO_3$ W.K. Lewis and E.D. Ries, *Ind. Eng. Chem.*, 19, 830, 1937 O.A. Uyehara and K.M. Watson, *Ind. Eng. Chem.* 35, 541, 1943.	$r = \dfrac{k(p_{SO_2}p_{O_2}^{1/2} - p_{SO_3}/K_P)}{[1 + (K_{O_2}p_{O_2})^{1/2} + K_{SO_2}p_{SO_2}]^2}$ 15.4% deviations over 12 experiments on variation of partial pressures of SO_2 and SO_3.	$r = k(p_{SO_2}p_{SO_3}^{-1/2} - p_{SO_3}^{1/2}p_{O_2}^{-1/2}/K_P)$ 13.3% deviations over 12 experiments on variation of partial pressures of SO_2 and SO_3.
Hydrogenation of codimer (C) $H_2 + C \rightleftarrows P$ J.L. Tschernitz et al. *Trans. Amer. Inst. Chem. Eng.*, 42, 883, 1946	$r = \dfrac{kp_{H_2}p_C}{(1 + K_{H_2}p_{H_2} + K_Cp_C + K_Pp_P)^2}$ 20.9% deviation at 200 °C 19.6% deviation at 275 °C 19.4% deviation at 325 °C	$r = k(p_{H_2}p_C)^{1/2}$ 19.6% deviation at 200 °C 32.9% deviation at 275 °C 21.4% deviation at 325 °C
Phosgene synthesis $CO + Cl_2 \rightleftarrows COCl_2$ C. Potter and S. Baron, *Chem. Eng. Progr.* 47, 473, 1951.	$r = \dfrac{kp_{CO}p_{Cl_2}}{(1 + K_{Cl_2}p_{Cl_2} + K_{COCl_2}p_{COCl_2})^2}$ 3.4% deviation at 30.6 °C 5.6% deviation at 42.7 °C 2.6% deviation at 52.5 °C 7.0% deviation at 64.0 °C	$r = kp_{CO}p_{Cl_2}^{1/2}$ 13.0% deviation at 30.6 °C 9.1% deviation at 42.7 °C 13.9% deviation at 52.5 °C 3.0% deviation at 64.0 °C
Toluene alkylation by methanol $T + M \rightleftarrows X + W$ J.L. Sotelo et al., "Kinetics of Toluene Alkylation with Methanol over Mg-Modified ZSM-5", *Ind. Eng. Chem. Res.* 1993, 32, 2548–2554.	$r = \dfrac{k(P_MP_T - P_Xp_W/K_P)}{P_W + K_Mp_M + K_Xp_X}$ 2.07% deviation Eley–Rideal model (Fraenkel D. "Role of External Surface Sites in Shape Selective Catalysis over Zeolites." *Ind. Eng. Chem. Res.* 1990,29, 1814–1821)	$r = kp_Tp_M$ 4.65% deviation

power-law terms of the coverage function are negligible as compared with the exponential variations, the kinetic expressions derived is not expected to be valid in as wide ranges as one would expect from LHHW expressions. In most cases, the expressions derived from this approach are merely comparable to LHHW expressions. Table 9.4 shows a comparison of some examples where both LHHW and power-law form correlations have been made.

Tables 9.5 and 9.6 show some of the rate expressions based on the ExLand and UniLan adsorption isotherms when surface reaction is limiting. One can observe that when ExLan and UniLan are employed to derive the rate expressions, the reaction rate expressions are quite similar to those of the LHHW expressions.

TABLE 9.5 Some Examples of Rate Expressions with ExLan Adsorption Where Surface Reaction is the Rate-Limiting Step

Overall reaction		Rate expression
1) Isomerization A $\rightleftarrows$ B	$\beta = \overline{K}_A C_A + \overline{K}_B C_B$	$r = k_s \overline{K}_A C_\sigma (C_A - C_B/K_{eq}) \ln(1+\beta^{-1})$
2) Bimolecular A + B $\rightleftarrows$ C + D	$\beta = \overline{K}_A C_A + \overline{K}_B C_B + \overline{K}_C C_C + \overline{K}_D C_D$	$r = k_s \overline{K}_A \overline{K}_B C_\sigma^2 (C_A C_B - C_C C_D/K_{eq}) \ln^2(1+\beta^{-1})$
3) Bimolecular (dissociative) $\frac{1}{2}A_2 + B \rightleftarrows C + D$	$\beta = \overline{K}_{A_2}^{\frac{1}{2}} C_{A_2}^{\frac{1}{2}} + \overline{K}_B C_B + \overline{K}_C C_C + \overline{K}_D C_D$	$r = k_s K_{A_2}^{1/2} K_B C_\sigma^2 (C_{A_2}^{1/2} C_B - C_C C_D/K_{eq}) \ln^2(1+\beta^{-1})$
4) Bimolecular (Eley-Rideal) A + B $\rightleftarrows$ C	$\beta = \overline{K}_A C_A + \overline{K}_C C_C$	$r = k_s \overline{K}_A C_\sigma (C_A C_B - C_C/K_{eq}) \ln(1+\beta^{-1})$

TABLE 9.6 Some Examples of Rate Expressions with UniLan Adsorption Where Surface Reaction Is the Rate-Limiting Step

Overall reaction		Rate expression
1) Isomerization A $\rightleftarrows$ B	$\beta = \overline{K}_A C_A + \overline{K}_B C_B$	$r = k_s \overline{K}_A C_\sigma (C_A - C_B/K_{eq}) \dfrac{RT}{E_{max}\beta} \ln \dfrac{1+\beta\exp\left(\frac{E_{max}}{RT}\right)}{1+\beta}$
2) Bimolecular A + B $\rightleftarrows$ C + D	$\beta = \overline{K}_A C_A + \overline{K}_B C_B + \overline{K}_C C_C + \overline{K}_D C_D$	$r = k_s \overline{K}_A \overline{K}_B C_\sigma^2 \left(C_A C_B - \dfrac{C_C C_D}{K_{eq}}\right) \left(\dfrac{RT}{E_{max}\beta}\right)^2 \ln^2 \dfrac{1+\beta\exp\left(\frac{E_{max}}{RT}\right)}{1+\beta}$
3) Bimolecular (dissociative) $\frac{1}{2}A_2 + B \rightleftarrows C + D$	$\beta = \overline{K}_{A_2}^{\frac{1}{2}} C_{A_2}^{\frac{1}{2}} + \overline{K}_B C_B + \overline{K}_C C_C + \overline{K}_D C_D$	$r = k_s K_{A_2}^{\frac{1}{2}} K_B C_\sigma^2 \left(C_{A_2}^{\frac{1}{2}} C_B - \dfrac{C_C C_D}{K_{eq}}\right) \left(\dfrac{RT}{E_{max}\beta}\right)^2 \ln^2 \dfrac{1+\beta\exp\left(\frac{E_{max}}{RT}\right)}{1+\beta}$
4) Bimolecular (Eley-Rideal) A + B $\rightleftarrows$ C	$\beta = \overline{K}_A C_A + \overline{K}_C C_C$	$r = k_s \overline{K}_A C_\sigma (C_A C_B - C_C/K_{eq}) \dfrac{RT}{E_{max}\beta} \ln \dfrac{1+\beta\exp\left(\frac{E_{max}}{RT}\right)}{1+\beta}$

9.4. CHEMICAL REACTIONS ON NONIDEAL SURFACES WITH MULTILAYER APPROXIMATION

In the previous section, we have learned how Temkin approximation can be applied to perform kinetic analysis to render surface catalyzed reactions with a power-law rate expression. The UniLan and ExLan adsorption isotherms can be applied to derive kinetic models for chemical reactions on nonideal surfaces. Besides the interaction energy distribution modeling, multilayer adsorption can also be applied to model nonideal surfaces. In this section, we apply the multilayer adsorption model to reactions occurring on the surfaces.

When surface reaction is limiting, the overall rate expression is dependent only on the concentrations of the reactants on the surface. For example, the reaction network of isomerization on a solid catalyst follows the following scheme:

$$A + \sigma \rightleftarrows A\cdot\sigma \tag{9.137}$$

$$A\cdot\sigma \rightleftarrows B\cdot\sigma \tag{9.138}$$

$$B\cdot\sigma \rightleftarrows B + \sigma \tag{9.139}$$

$$+) = \text{overall} \qquad A \rightleftarrows B \tag{9.140}$$

Assuming that only step (9.138) is elementary as the adsorption steps are occurring on nonideal surfaces. The reaction rate expression for the overall reaction is then

$$r = k_S C_{AS} - k_{-S} C_{BS} \tag{9.141}$$

The surface coverage of species A and B can be obtained from Eqn (9.82) for nonselective multilayer adsorptions. That is,

$$C_{jS} = C_\sigma c \frac{1 - [1 + N(1-\beta)]\beta^N}{(1-\beta)[1-(1-c)\beta - c\beta^{N+1}]} K_j C_j \tag{9.142}$$

where $j = $ A or B, and β is given by Eqn (9.81) or

$$\beta = K_A C_A + K_B C_B \tag{9.143}$$

Substituting Eqn (9.142) into Eqn (9.141), we obtain the rate expression for reaction of Eqn (9.140) on nonideal surfaces as modeled by nonselective multilayer adsorption:

$$r = k_S C_{AS} - k_{-S} C_{BS} = k_S C_\sigma c K_A \frac{1 - [1 + N(1-\beta)]\beta^N}{(1-\beta)[1-(1-c)\beta - c\beta^{N+1}]} (C_A - C_B / K_{eq}) \tag{9.144}$$

where

$$K_{eq} = \frac{k_S K_A}{k_{-S} K_B} \tag{9.145}$$

is the equilibrium constant for the reaction.

TABLE 9.7 Some Examples of Rate Expressions with Multilayer Adsorption Where Surface Reaction Is the Rate-Limiting Step

Overall reaction	Rate expression	
1) Isomerization $A \rightleftarrows B$	$\beta = K_A C_A + K_B C_B$	$r = k_s c K_A C_\sigma \dfrac{C_A - C_B/K_{eq}}{1-\beta} \times \dfrac{1-[1+N(1-\beta)]\beta^N}{1-(1-c)\beta - c\beta^{N+1}}$
2) Bimolecular $A + B \rightleftarrows C + D$	$\beta = K_A C_A + K_B C_B + K_C C_C + K_D C_D$	$r = k_s c^2 K_A K_B C_\sigma^2 \dfrac{C_A C_B - C_C C_D/K_{eq}}{(1-\beta)^2} \times \left\{\dfrac{1-[1+N(1-\beta)]\beta^N}{1-(1-c)\beta - c\beta^{N+1}}\right\}^2$
3) Bimolecular (dissociative) $\frac{1}{2}A_2 + B \rightleftarrows C + D$	$\beta = K_{A_2}^{\frac{1}{2}} C_{A_2}^{\frac{1}{2}} + K_B C_B + K_C C_C + K_D C_D$	$r = k_s c^2 K_{A_2}^{1/2} K_B C_\sigma^2 \dfrac{C_{A_2}^{1/2} C_B - C_C C_D/K_{eq}}{(1-\beta)^2} \times \left\{\dfrac{1-[1+N(1-\beta)]\beta^N}{1-(1-c)\beta - c\beta^{N+1}}\right\}^2$
4) Bimolecular (Eley Rideal) $A + B \rightleftarrows C$	$\beta = K_A C_A + K_C C_C$	$r = k_s c K_A C_\sigma \dfrac{C_A C_B - C_C/K_{eq}}{1-\beta} \times \dfrac{1-[1+N(1-\beta)]\beta^N}{1-(1-c)\beta - c\beta^{N+1}}$

For chemical reactions with surface reaction as the limiting step, some examples of the reaction rates are listed in Table 9.7 when multilayer adsorption is employed to model the nonideality of the surfaces.

9.5. KINETICS OF REACTIONS ON SURFACES WHERE THE SOLID IS EITHER A PRODUCT OR REACTANT

In the previous section, we have learned that with solid catalysis the surface active centers are not generated or consumed during reaction. When solid phase is one of the reactants, for example, dissolution reactions, combustion reactions, or products, for example vapor deposition, the active centers on the surface changes. The change of surface active centers could lead to changes in the kinetic analysis. In this section, we shall use the reactions on woody biomass to focus our discussions.

Renewable biomass has increasingly become the chemical and energy source for commodity and chemical industry. Reactions involving biomass are usually heterogeneous with the biomass being solid. Pulp and paper are the earliest and remaining application. Based on the surface reaction theory, Liu (e.g. S. Liu "A Kinetic Model on Autocatalytic Reactions in Woody Biomass Hydrolysis", *J. Biobased Materials and Bioenergy,* 2, 135–147, 2008) inserted LWWH type of kinetics into bleaching, pulping, and extraction reactions involving wood and fibers. A series of studies followed resulted in simplestic kinetic relationships. A brief review of the kinetics of "acid-hydrolysis" and hot water extraction is shown here as an example of reactions involving surfaces. There are multitudes of chemical components in wood that participate in the reactions. At high temperatures, water molecule can be activated and directly attack carbohydrates, resulting thermal-hydrodepolymerization. In the case of acid hydrolysis, hydrogen ions act as catalyst to soften the glycosidic bonds and induce their depolymerization. The glycosidic bond breakage is enhanced when the breakaway oligomers are attracted away from the solid surface. High temperature and high electrolyte content favor the oligomers to be dissolved in the liquor phase.

As an example, we shall examine the hot water extraction or hydrolysis of wood in the following. The mechanism for hydrolysis can be very complicated when mass transfer is coupled with the chemistry. However, when viewed on each component, one can deduce that:

1. Transport of hydrogen ion and/or small strong hydrogen bond-forming molecules from the bulk liquor to the surface of the solid particle;
2. Chemisorptions (hydrogen bond formation, for example) occur on the solid surface;
3. Surface reaction between the hydrogen ion (proton) and xylan;
4. Desorption or cleavage of the dissoluble xylooligomer;
5. Diffusion and transport of the dissolved xylooligomer to the bulk liquor.

which is typical of LHHW kinetics. However, the solid phase is not acting as a catalyst. The solid phase contains both the reactant and the desired product.

Under normal conditions, transport steps 1) and 5) are probably unimportant, especially when the effective thickness of the wood chips is less than the critical thickness, i.e. 2–3 mm. *However, the particle size still poses a strong influence on the reaction as only the active components on the surface can be reacted.* These transport steps reach a negligible extent to the overall observed extraction rate. Step 3, the surface reaction step, can be complicated in nature. However, there exists a controlling substep in the chemistry of xylan hydrolysis: breakage of a glycosidic bond. Therefore, step 3 can be simplified to an elementary step representing the glycosidic bond breakage. The chemical reaction involved is said to be the rate-controlling step. In this case, the overall reaction rate is dependent on steps 3–5 directly. In this paper, we are interested in the intrinsic kinetics, i.e. steps (3) through (5), only.

Under autocatalytic conditions, the hydrogen ion concentration is initially very low. However, acetyl groups are present in wood as they are associated with, extractives, lignin as well as hemicellulose. Hydration of the acetyl groups lead to the acidification of the liquor and thus formation of hydrogen ions.

According to these considerations, the extraction-hydrolysis involving solid woodchips can be represented by a simplistic model:

$$\mathrm{H_2O} \rightleftarrows \mathrm{H_2O^*} \tag{9.146}$$

$$\text{R-X}_n\text{OH (s)} + \mathrm{H_2O^*} \rightleftarrows \text{R-X}_n\text{OH}\cdot\mathrm{H_2O^*}\text{(s)} \tag{9.147}$$

$$\text{R-X}_n\text{OH}\cdot\mathrm{H_2O^*}\text{(s)} \rightarrow \text{R-X}_m\text{OH(s)} + \text{HX}_s\text{OH (aq)} \tag{9.148}$$

$$\text{R-POAc (s)} + \mathrm{H_2O^*}\text{(aq)} \rightleftarrows \text{R-POAc}\cdot\mathrm{H_2O}\text{ (s)} \tag{9.149}$$

$$\text{R-POAc}\cdot\mathrm{H_2O}\text{ (s)} \rightleftarrows \text{R-POH(s)} + \text{HOAc (aq)} \tag{9.150}$$

$$\text{R-POAc}\cdot\mathrm{H_2O}\text{ (s)} \rightleftarrows \text{R-OH (s)} + \text{HPOAc (aq)} \tag{9.151}$$

$$\text{HOAc (aq)} \rightleftarrows \mathrm{H^+}\text{(aq)} + \mathrm{OAc^-}\text{(aq)} \tag{9.152}$$

$$\text{R-X}_n\text{OH (s)} + \mathrm{H^+}\text{(aq)} \rightleftarrows \text{R-X}_n\text{OH}\cdot\mathrm{H^+}\text{(s)} \tag{9.153}$$

$$\text{R-X}_n\text{OH}\cdot\mathrm{H^+}\text{(s)} + \mathrm{H_2O}\text{ (aq)} \rightarrow \text{R-X}_m\text{OH}\cdot\mathrm{H^+}\text{(s)} + \text{HX}_s\text{OH (aq)} \tag{9.154}$$

$$HX_nOH\ (aq) + H^+(aq) \rightleftarrows HX_nOH\cdot H^+(aq) \tag{9.155}$$

$$HX_nOH\cdot H^+(aq) + H_2O(aq) \rightarrow HX_mOH\cdot H^+(aq) + HX_sOH\ (aq) \tag{9.156}$$

where $m + s = n$, R- denotes the cellulose and/or lignin bonding connected with the fibers, and P represents a segment/subunit of hemicellulose or lignin. X_n represents an n-xylo-polymer middle group, i.e. $(-O-C_5H_8O_3-)_n$, whereas HX_nOH is an n-xylooligomer. HOAc represents the acetic acid molecule, where $Ac = CH_3CO$.

Eqn (9.153) represents the adsorption of hydrogen ions onto the woody biomass surface, and Eqn (9.154) represents the surface reaction whereby one xylo-oligomer is cleaved from the woody biomass. One should note that the actual entity participating in the extraction reaction/hydrolysis reactions can be either H^+ or H_3O^+. In fact, one may write

$$H^+ + H_2O^* \rightleftarrows H_3O^+ \tag{9.157}$$

and

$$R\text{-}X_nOH\ (s) + H_3O^+ \rightleftarrows R\text{-}X_nOH\cdot H_3O^*(s) \tag{9.158}$$

$$R\text{-}X_nOH\cdot H_3O^+(s) \rightarrow R\text{-}X_mOH\cdot H^+(s) + HX_sOH\ (aq) \tag{9.159}$$

$$R\text{-}POAc\ (s) + H_3O^+(aq) \rightleftarrows R\text{-}POAc\cdot H_3O^+(s) \tag{9.160}$$

$$R\text{-}POAc\cdot H_3O^+(s) \rightleftarrows R\text{-}POH\cdot H^+(s) + HOAc\ (aq) \tag{9.161}$$

$$R\text{-}POAc\cdot H_3O + (s) \rightleftarrows R\text{-}OH\ (s) + HPOAc\cdot H^+\ (aq) \tag{9.162}$$

$$HX_nOH(aq) + H_3O^+(aq) \rightleftarrows HX_nOH\cdot H_3O^+(aq) \tag{9.163}$$

$$HX_nOH\cdot H_3O^+\ (aq) \rightarrow HX_mOH\cdot H^+(aq) + HX_sOH\ (aq) \tag{9.164}$$

Kinetically, the steps as shown in Eqns (9.146) through (9.164) can represent the extraction/hydrolysis reactions.

The monomeric sugar can further dehydrate in the presence of proton to dehydrated products such as furfural, humic acid, Levulinic acid, etc.

$$HX_1OH\cdot H^+(aq) \rightarrow H^+ + H_2O + \text{furfural, and other dehydration products} \tag{9.165}$$

Besides the extraction reaction, the polysaccharides can condense back to the woody biomass:

$$R\text{-}X_nOH\cdot H^+\ (s) + HX_sOH\ (aq) \rightarrow R\text{-}X_{n+s}OH\cdot H^+(s) + H_2O\ (aq) \tag{9.166}$$

or

$$R\text{-}X_nOH\ (s) + HX_sOH\cdot H^+(aq) \rightarrow R\text{-}X_{n+s}OH\cdot H^+(s) + H_2O\ (aq) \tag{9.167}$$

Also, the dehydration polymerization of the xylo-oligomers occurs

$$HX_nOH\cdot H^+(aq) + HX_mOH\ (aq) \rightarrow HX_{n+m}OH\cdot H^+(aq) + H_2O\ (aq) \tag{9.168}$$

The polymerization reactions (9.166) through (9.168) can have a significant effect on the extraction and/or hydrolysis process.

Reactions (9.148), (9.150), (9.151), (9.154), (9.156), (9.159), (9.161), (9.162), and (9.164) through (9.168) are pseudo-elementary steps. There have been numerous studies aimed at revealing the chemistry of these steps. However, for our purposes, we will consider them elementary steps. The reaction rate so defined represents that from the rate-controlling sub-steps based on detailed chemistry.

With the reaction mechanism given by Eqns (9.146) through (9.168), one can write reaction rate expressions for any given component of interest. However, the reaction rate expressions could potentially involve a large number of kinetic parameters due to the number of reactions involved. The kinetic parameters are not easy to determine theoretically based on chemistry and physics of matter. Therefore, further simplification is desirable. The following assumptions are made:

1. The condensation reactions are neglected, i.e. reactions (9.166) through (9.168) are neglected;
2. The breakage of glycosidic bonds has an equal rate or reactivity as long as they are in the same phase;
3. The affinities of glycosidic bonds to hydrogen ions (H^+ and H_3O^+) are the same, as long as they are in the same phase.

The above three assumptions form the basis for the discussions to follow.

It is assumed that the adsorption and desorption reactions occur at much faster rates than those of surface reactions on the woody biomass surface. Therefore, one can assume that the adsorption steps are always in equilibrium. The adsorption process can be represented as the elementary reversible reactions such as that shown by Eqn (9.153). Thus, at the timescale of the surface reactions, the adsorption isotherm for hydrogen ions is given by

$$K_S = \frac{\theta_{n-H^+}}{\theta_{nV} C_{H^+}} \tag{9.169}$$

where K_S is the adsorption equilibrium constant of H^+ onto X_n on the biomass solid surface (or R-X_nOH); $\theta_{n\text{-}H^+}$ is the concentration or fraction of X_n on the biomass solid surface that is associated with H^+. θ_{nV} is the concentration or fraction of X_n on the biomass solid surface that is not associated with H^+; and C_{H^+} is the concentration of H^+ in the extract liquor. The total concentration of xylan on the biomass solid surface is given by

$$\theta_{n-H^+} + \theta_{nV} = \theta_n \tag{9.170}$$

Substituting Eqn (9.169) into Eqn (9.170), we obtain

$$\theta_{n-H^+} = \frac{K_S C_{H^+} \theta_n}{1 + K_S C_{H^+}} \tag{9.171}$$

Ideally, θ_j is the surface concentration of component j on the woody biomass surface. θ_j can be conveniently expressed as moles per g-inert (or water insoluble/undissoluble) biomass. The total surface area can be assumed to be constant during the extraction process.

Intermediate formation in the liquid phase as shown in Eqn (9.155):

$$C_{n-H^+} = K_H C_n C_{H^+} \tag{9.172}$$

where K_H is the equilibrium constant of reaction (9.155) or for H^+ to be chemically associated with HX_nOH in the extract liquor; $C_{n\text{-}H}{}^+$ is the concentration HX_nOH in the extraction liquor that is chemically associated with H^+; and C_n is the concentration of HX_nOH in the extraction liquor.

The dissolution reaction rate, based on reactions (9.148), (9.154), and (9.159), is given by:

$$r_{\theta s,\theta n \to \theta s} = k_{en^*}\theta_{n^*} + k_e\theta_{n-H^+} = \left(\frac{k_{en^*}K_{S^*}[H_2O^*]}{1+K_{S^*}C_{H^+}} + k_{en}\frac{K_S C_{H^+}}{1+K_S C_{H^+}}\right)\theta_n \tag{9.173}$$

where $r_{\theta s,\theta n \to \theta s}$ is the rate of formation of s-oligomer on the solid phase from the n-oligomer on the solid phase. The hydrolysis reaction rate, based on (9.155), (9.156), (9.157), (9.163), and (9.164), can be written as

$$r_{s,n \to s} = 2(k_{h^*}[H_2O^*] + k_h K_H C_{H^+})C_n \tag{9.174}$$

Here, $r_{s,n \to s}$ is the rate of formation of s-oligomer in aqueous phase from the n-oligomer in aqueous phase. The factor 2 is resulted from the fact that either 2 mol of s-oligomers are formed from breaking one bond or breaking of two different bonds in the n-oligomer can each lead to one s-oligomer.

While there are n-bonds can be broken from an n-oligomer on the solid phase, there is only one bond can be broken at any given time. Letting

$$k_E = n\left(\frac{k_{en^*}K_{S^*}[H_2O^*]}{1+K_{S^*}C_{H^+}} + k_{en}\frac{K_S C_{H^+}}{1+K_S C_{H^+}}\right) \tag{9.175}$$

and,

$$k_H = k_{h^*}\frac{K_{H^*}[H_2O^*]}{1+K_{H^*}C_{H^+}} + k_h\frac{K_H C_{H^+}}{1+K_H C_{H^+}} \tag{9.176}$$

we obtain

$$r_{\theta s,\theta n \to \theta s} = \frac{k_E}{n}\theta_n \tag{9.177}$$

$$r_{s,\theta n \to s} = \frac{k_E}{n}\theta_n \tag{9.178}$$

$$r_{s,n \to s} = 2k_H C_n \tag{9.179}$$

Neglecting the condensation reactions, we obtain the formation of s-xylo-oligomers in the liquor as:

$$r_s = \sum_{n=s+1}^{N} r_{s,n\to s} + \sum_{n=s}^{N} r_{s,\theta n\to s} - r_{s,s\to}\ \forall 1 \le i \le s-1 \tag{9.180}$$

where $r_{s,s\rightarrow\forall 1\leq i\leq s\text{-}1}$ is the rate of s-oligomer decomposing into all the lesser oligomers (and monomers). Thus,

$$r_{s,s\rightarrow\forall 1\leq i\leq s-1} = (s-1)k_H C_s \tag{9.181}$$

$$r_s = 2\sum_{n=s+1}^{N} k_H C_n + \sum_{n=s}^{N} \frac{k_E}{n}\theta_n - (s-1)k_H C_s \tag{9.182}$$

for $s > 1$. Comparing with the hydrolysis reaction alone, Eqn (6.85), there is one additional term appeared in Eqn (9.182) due to the production of s-oligomer from the solid material.

Cleavage of xylo-oligomers from the woody biomass when the condensation reactions are neglected is obtained as:

$$\begin{aligned} r_{\theta m} &= -r_{\theta m,\theta m\rightarrow\forall\theta 0\leq\theta i\leq\theta m-1} + \sum_{n=m+1}^{N} r_{\theta m,\theta n\rightarrow\theta m} \\ &= -k_E\theta_m + \sum_{n=m+1}^{N}\frac{k_E}{n}\theta_n \end{aligned} \tag{9.183}$$

The reaction is near the zeroth order with respect to xylan content initially and near the first order near complete dissolution of xylan from woody biomass.

For all the accessible oligomers on the solid surface, the rate of extract can also be expressed in terms of the total number of monomeric units extractable as

$$r_E = \sum_{m=1}^{N} m r_{\theta m} = -k_E\sum_{m=1}^{N} m\theta_m + \sum_{m=1}^{N} m \sum_{n=m+1}^{N}\frac{k_E}{n}\theta_n \tag{9.184}$$

where r_E is the rate of formation of oligomers on the solid phase in terms of the number of monomer units. Eqn (9.184) can be rewritten as

$$r_E = -k_E\sum_{m=1}^{N}\frac{m+1}{2}\theta_m \tag{9.185}$$

Let,

$$P_S = \sum_{m=1}^{N} m\theta_m \tag{9.186}$$

be the concentration of total monomer units in extractable oligomers and the degree of polymerization for the extractable oligomers in the solid phase be given by

$$\mathrm{DP} = \frac{\sum_{m=1}^{N} m\theta_m}{\sum_{m=1}^{N}\theta_m} \tag{9.187}$$

then, the rate of extraction can be written as

$$r_E = -\frac{k_E}{2}\left(1+\frac{1}{\mathrm{DP}}\right)P_S \tag{9.188}$$

Thus, the extraction is of first order with respect to the extractable monomer units. At start, the degree of polymerization is high, resulting in a lower rate constant. Toward the end of extraction, the degree of polymerization is low, resulting in a higher rate constant.

In the liquid phase, the formation rate of monomers is given by

$$r_1 = 2\sum_{n=1}^{N} k_H C_n + \sum_{n=1}^{N} \frac{k_E}{n}\theta_n - (2k_H + k_D)C_1 \tag{9.189}$$

where k_D is the rate constant for the decomposition of monomers, reaction (9.165). As shown in §6.6, the composition in the liquid phase may be described by two pseudo-components to lump all the oligomers. Let

$$C_{\Sigma i} = \sum_{i=1}^{N} iC_i \tag{9.190}$$

$$C_\Sigma = \sum_{i=1}^{N} C_i \tag{9.191}$$

The lumped rates are given by

$$r_{\Sigma i} = \sum_{i=1}^{N} ir_i = \frac{k_E}{2}\sum_{n=1}^{N}(n+1)\theta_n - k_D C_1 \tag{9.192}$$

$$r_\Sigma = \sum_{i=1}^{N} r_i = k_H(C_{\Sigma i} - C_\Sigma) + k_E\sum_{n=1}^{N}\theta_n - k_D C_1 \tag{9.193}$$

where $r_{\Sigma i}$ is the rate of formation of total number of monomer units in the solution ($C_{\Sigma i}$) and r_Σ is the rate of formation of total number of molecules in monomer and oligomer forms in the solution (C_Σ). Substitute Eqns (9.191) into Eqn (9.189), we obtain

$$r_1 = 2k_H C_\Sigma + \sum_{n=1}^{N}\frac{k_E}{n}\theta_n - (2k_H + k_D)C_1 \tag{9.194}$$

9.6. DECLINE OF SURFACE ACTIVITY: CATALYST DEACTIVATION

One particular aspect of solid catalysis that is not encountered in reactions that are not catalytic is a progressive decrease in the activity of the surface with its time of utilization. The reasons for this are numerous, but we will divide them into three general categories.

Poisoning: loss of activity due to strong chemisorption of a chemical impurity on the active sites of the surface, denying their access by reactant molecules. This should not be confused with inhibition as expressed by adsorption terms in the denominator of LHHW rate expressions.

Coking or *fouling:* loss of activity, normally in reactions involving hydrocarbons or carbon-based substrates, due to reactant or product degradation, producing a carbonaceous residue on the surface blocking reactants from accessing the active centers on the catalyst surface.

Sintering: loss of activity due to a decrease in active surface per volume of catalyst, normally the result of excessively high temperatures.

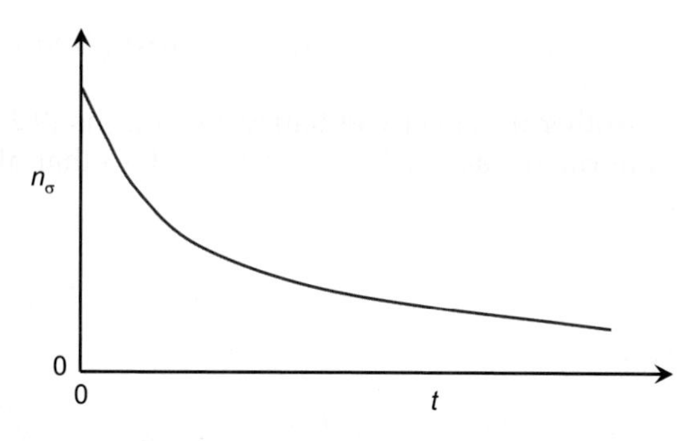

FIGURE 9.14 Variation of number of active centers with the service time of a catalyst.

A vast effort has been expended over the years in investigation of these types of deactivation as they are encountered in catalytic reactions and catalysts of technological importance. The uninitiated are often amazed at the fact that many reaction-system process designs are dictated by the existence of catalyst deactivation, as are process operation and optimization strategies. In some cases, the deactivation behavior is so pronounced as to make detailed studies of intrinsic kinetics of secondary importance.

In the catalytic reaction rate expressions we have seen so far, the number of active centers is the key factor or activity of the catalyst. When viewed in mathematical terms, catalyst deactivation is reduced to the change of the number of active centers. This is illustrated in Fig. 9.14. The loss of active centers can be due to a number of reasons as outlined above. From this point on, the mechanism of catalyst deactivation can be modeled again via reaction kinetics. Therefore, the kinetics we have been discussing so far can be applied to catalyst deactivation as well.

9.7. SUMMARY

Reactions occurring on solid surface start with reactants or catalyst from the fluid phase collide and associate with active centers (or sites) on the surface.

$$\mathrm{A} + \sigma \rightleftarrows \mathrm{A}\cdot\sigma \tag{9.1a}$$

or for dissociative adsorption

$$\mathrm{A_2} + 2\sigma \rightleftarrows 2\mathrm{A}\cdot\sigma \tag{9.10}$$

which is governed by

$$-r_\mathrm{A} = k_\mathrm{A}^0 \mathrm{e}^{-\frac{E_\mathrm{ad}}{RT}} \theta C_\sigma C_\mathrm{A} - k_{-\mathrm{A}}^0 \mathrm{e}^{-\frac{E_\mathrm{des}}{RT}} \theta_\mathrm{A} C_\sigma \tag{9.2a}$$

or in terms of dissociative adsorption

$$-r_{\mathrm{A}_2} = k_{\mathrm{A}_2}^0 \mathrm{e}^{-\frac{E_\mathrm{ad}}{RT}} \theta^2 C_\sigma^2 C_{\mathrm{A}_2} - k_{-\mathrm{A}_2}^0 \mathrm{e}^{-\frac{E_\mathrm{des}}{RT}} \theta_\mathrm{A}^2 C_\sigma^2 \tag{9.12a}$$

These equations form the bases for analyses of the reactive fluid–surface interactions. The adsorption isotherms are derived from Eqn (9.2) and/or Eqn (9.12) together with the total active center balance when the adsorption is at equilibrium, or the net adsorption rate is zero.

Isotherms directly obtained from Eqns (9.2) or(9.12) are termed Langmuir isotherms as uniform surface activity is assumed so that all the rate constants are not functions of the coverage,

$$\theta_A = \frac{K_A C_A}{1 + K_A C_A} \tag{9.9}$$

and

$$\theta_A = \frac{\sqrt{K_{A_2} C_{A_2}}}{1 + \sqrt{K_{A_2} C_{A_2}}} \tag{9.14}$$

Since the dissociative adsorption is a special case of the adsorption where the concentration is replaced by the square root of concentration as noted from Eqns (9.14) and (9.9), we shall now focus on the nondissociative adsorption.

$$K_A = \frac{k_A^0}{k_{-A}^0} e^{-\frac{E_{ad} - E_{des}}{RT}} = K_A^0 e^{-\frac{\Delta H_{ad}}{RT}} \tag{9.5a}$$

For adsorption of multiple component mixture at the same active center, Langmuir adsorption isotherm is given by

$$\theta_j = \frac{K_j C_j}{1 + \sum_{m=1}^{N_s} K_m C_m} \tag{9.17}$$

Nonideal surfaces can be modeled by a distribution of interaction energy (adsorption heat ΔH_{ad}, and/or E_{ad} and E_{des}). An exponential distribution of available sites with an excess adsorption heat between 0 and E_{max} leads to

$$\theta_j = \frac{\overline{K}_j C_j}{1 - e^{-\frac{E_{max}}{RT}}} \ln \frac{1 + \sum_{m=1}^{N_s} \overline{K}_m C_m}{e^{-\frac{E_{max}}{RT}} + \sum_{m=1}^{N_s} \overline{K}_m C_m} \tag{9.35}$$

Eqn (9.35) may be referred to as ExLan (*Ex*ponential energy distribution *Lang*muir) adsorption isotherm. For adsorption of single species,

$$\theta_A = \frac{\overline{K}_A C_A}{1 - e^{-\frac{E_{max}}{RT}}} \ln \frac{1 + \overline{K}_A C_A}{e^{-\frac{E_{max}}{RT}} + \overline{K}_A C_A} \tag{9.26}$$

Assuming whole spectrum of energy distribution, i.e. $E_{max} \to \infty$, Eqn (9.35) is reduced to

$$\theta_j = \overline{K}_j C_j \ln \left[1 + \left(\sum_{m=1}^{N_s} \overline{K}_m C_m \right)^{-1} \right] \tag{9.36}$$

For single species adsorption, Eqn (9.36) is reduced to

$$\theta_A = \overline{K}_A C_A \ln[1 + (\overline{K}_A C_A)^{-1}] \tag{9.27}$$

If the available adsorption sites are linearly distributed about the excess interaction energy between 0 and E_{max}, then the adsorption isotherm becomes

$$\theta_j = \frac{RT\overline{K}_j C_j}{E_{max}\sum_{m=1}^{N_s}\overline{K}_m C_m}\ln\frac{1+\sum_{m=1}^{N_s}\overline{K}_m C_m e^{\frac{E_{max}}{RT}}}{1+\sum_{m=1}^{N_s}\overline{K}_m C_m} \tag{9.39}$$

For single species adsorption, Eqn (9.39) is reduced to

$$\theta_A = \frac{RT}{E_{max}}\ln\frac{1+\overline{K}_A C_A e^{\frac{E_{max}}{RT}}}{1+\overline{K}_A C_A} \tag{9.40}$$

which is also known as the UniLan (*uni*form distribution *Lan*gmuir) model.
In the intermediate coverage region,

$$1 << \overline{K}_A C_A e^{\frac{E_{max}}{RT}} \quad \text{and} \quad 1 >> \overline{K}_A C_A$$

Eqn (9.40) may be approximated by

$$\theta_A \approx \frac{RT}{E_{max}}\ln(\overline{K}_A C_A e^{\frac{E_{max}}{RT}}) \tag{9.42}$$

which is the Temkin isotherm.
Nonideal surfaces can also be modeled with multilayer adsorptions as the adsorbate–adsorbate molecular interactions and steric interactions can be introduced via multilayer adsorption concept. True multilayer adsorption is common in physisorptions. Assuming that 1) on the first layer, the interaction is only between adsorbate and adsorbent surface, and this interaction is uniform; 2) the interactions among adsorbate–adsorbate and adsorbate–adsorbent are uniform and identical for all other layers; we obtain for single species N-layer adsorptions,

$$n_{As,N} = n_{\sigma 1} c K_A C_A \frac{1-[1+N(1-K_A C_A)](K_A C_A)^N}{(1-K_A C_A)[1-(1-c)K_A C_A - c(K_A C_A)^{N+1}]} \tag{9.73}$$

or

$$C_{As,N} = C_{As1\infty} c K_A C_A \frac{1-[1+N(1-K_A C_A)](K_A C_A)^N}{(1-K_A C_A)[1-(1-c)K_A C_A - c(K_A C_A)^{N+1}]} \tag{9.73a}$$

In terms of partial pressure in the bulk phase,

$$n_{As,N} = n_{\sigma 1} c \alpha p_A \frac{1-[1+N(1-\alpha p_A)](\alpha p_A)^N}{(1-\alpha p_A)[1-(1-c)\alpha p_A - c(\alpha p_A)^{N+1}]} \tag{9.72}$$

When $N=1$, the Langmuir adsorption isotherm, Eqn (9.9), is recovered. If $N=2$, Eqn (9.73) is reduced to

$$n_{As,2} = n_{\sigma 1}\frac{cK_A C_A(1+2K_A C_A)}{1+cK_A C_A(1+K_A C_A)} \tag{9.55}$$

which is the bilayer adsorption isotherm.

If the adsorption is truly physisorption, the adsorbed adsorbate may be considered to be equivalent to "liquefied" or "solidified" adsorbate, in which case,

$$\alpha p_A = \beta = \frac{p_A}{p_A^\circ} \tag{9.74}$$

One parameter can be eliminated, and the adsorption isotherm is reduced to

$$n_{As,N} = n_{\sigma 1} c \frac{p_A}{p_A^\circ} \frac{1 - \left[1 + N\left(1 - \frac{p_A}{p_A^\circ}\right)\right]\left(\frac{p_A}{p_A^\circ}\right)^N}{\left(1 - \frac{p_A}{p_A^\circ}\right)\left[1 - (1-c)\frac{p_A}{p_A^\circ} - c\left(\frac{p_A}{p_A^\circ}\right)^{N+1}\right]} \tag{9.75}$$

which is applicable only to physisorptions.

Assuming that there is an infinite number of layers of adsorbate possible ($N \to \infty$), Eqn (9.75) is reduced

$$n_{As,\infty} = \frac{n_\sigma c \frac{p_A}{p_A^\circ}}{\left(1 - \frac{p_A}{p_A^\circ}\right)\left[1 - (1-c)\frac{p_A}{p_A^\circ}\right]} \tag{9.77}$$

Eqns (9.74), (9.75), and (9.77) are not applicable to chemisorptions because the interactions between adsorbate and adsorbent are stronger. Adsorbate molecules can be packed together on the adsorbent surface much tighter than the solid state of the adsorbate, which result in a much smaller p_A° than actual vapor pressure if these equations were used.

In summary, the adsorption isotherms exhibit different dependence on the bulk adsorbate concentration:

Type I isotherm can be either chemisorptions or physisorption. There is a saturation adsorption on the adsorbent surface. The capacity of adsorption is limited by the available active centers on the adsorbent surface. It is the simplest kind and widely seen in solid catalysts.

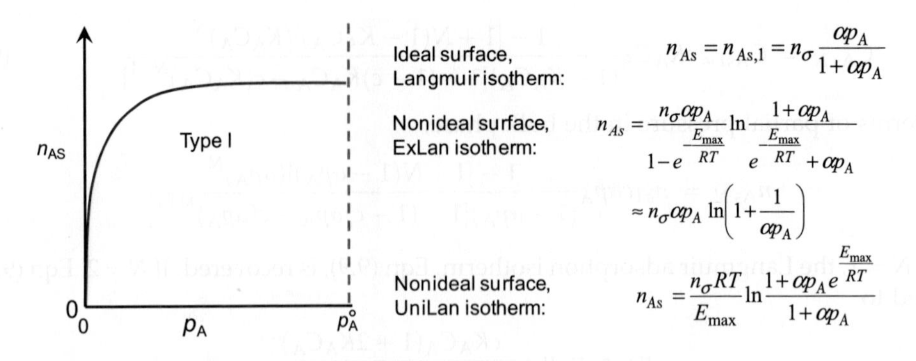

Types II and III, on the other hand, are only seen for physisorptions, where a saturation bulk phase adsorbate concentration exists. There is no limit on the capacity of the adsorption on the adsorbent surface. However, the monolayer coverage deduced from the BET model may not be true monolayer coverage, however it may be used to correlate the surface area.

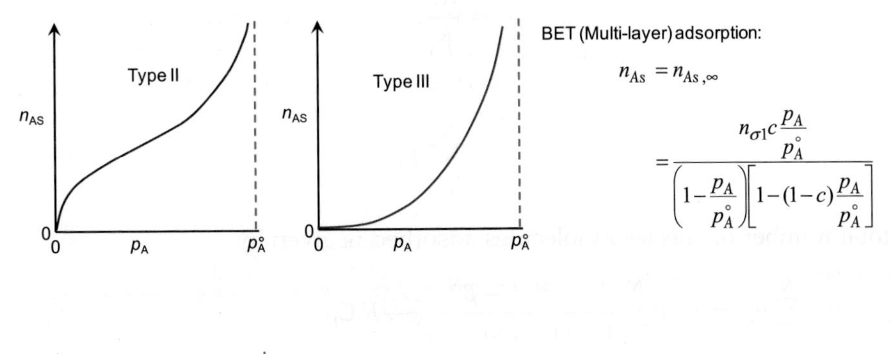

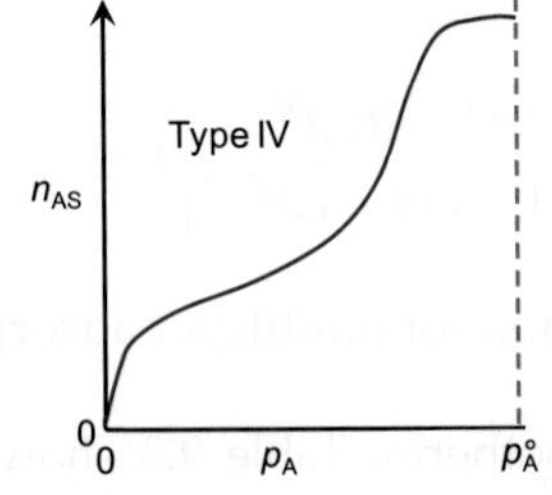

Multi-layer adsorption: $n_{As} = n_{As,N}$

$$= n_{\sigma 1} c \alpha p_A \frac{1-[1+N(1-\alpha p_A)](\alpha p_A)^N}{(1-\alpha p_A)[1-(1-c)\alpha p_A - c(\alpha p_A)^{N+1}]}$$

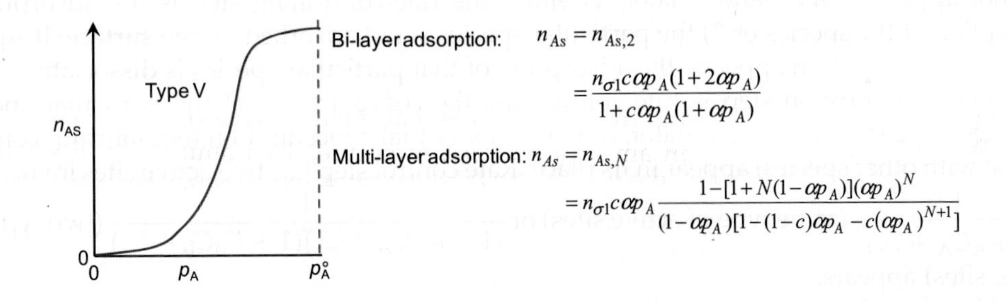

Types IV and V are all multilayer adsorption isotherms. They could be observed for both chemisorptions and physisorptions. For chemisorptions, the multilayer concept is merely an approximation to the different level of interaction energy as a combination of adsorbate–adsorbent and adsorbate–adsorbate interactions. Again, there is a saturation adsorption level, i.e. the adsorption capacity is limited.

For multispecies adsorption on the same sites nonselectively, the coverage of species j on layer i (among the total of N layers) is given by

$$\theta_{ij} = \frac{c(\beta^{i-1} - \beta^N)}{1-(1-c)\beta - \beta^{N+1}} K_j C_j \tag{9.79}$$

where K_j is the adsorption isotherm constant for species j for all layers above the first one layer, c is ratio of the adsorption isotherm constant of the first layer to that of layers above

$$c = \frac{K_{1j}}{K_j}, \tag{9.80}$$

and

$$\beta = \sum_{j=1}^{N_S} K_j C_j \tag{9.81}$$

The total number of species j molecules adsorbed is given by

$$\begin{aligned} n_{js,N} &= n_{\sigma 1} \sum_{i=1}^{N} \theta_{ij} = n_{\sigma 1} c \sum_{i=1}^{N} \frac{\beta^{i-1} - \beta^N}{1 - (1-c)\beta - c\beta^{N+1}} K_j C_j \\ &= n_{\sigma 1} c \frac{\dfrac{1-\beta^N}{1-\beta} - N\beta^N}{1 - (1-c)\beta - c\beta^{N+1}} K_j C_j = n_{\sigma 1} c \frac{1 - [1 + N(1-\beta)]\beta^N}{(1-\beta)[1 - (1-c)\beta - c\beta^{N+1}]} K_j C_j \end{aligned} \tag{9.82}$$

which is the most general adsorption isotherm expression (valid for multilayer adsorption of multispecies mixture on surfaces).

LHHW kinetics is derived from Langmuir adsorption isotherm. Table 9.3 shows some examples of rates with different rate-controlling steps. The terms in the denominator of the rate can tell the type of reaction and/or controlling step. If the concentration of one species did not appear in the denominator, 1) either the rate-controlling step is the adsorption–desorption of the species or 2) the particular species is not adsorbed on the surface. If square root of a concentration appears, the adsorption of that particular species is dissociative. If an adsorption–desorption step is rate controlling, the concentration of the particular species does not appear in the denominator, however, its virtual concentration (equilibrium concentration with other species) appear in its place. Rate control step has two active sites involved if $\frac{1}{(1 + K_A C_A + \ldots)^2}$ (same type of active sites) or $\frac{1}{(1 + K_A C_A + \ldots)(1 + K_B C_B + \ldots)}$ (two types of active sites) appears.

In kinetic analysis, PSSH (on all the intermediates) is more general and a better approximation than equilibrium step assumptions. PSSH can be traced back to the overall effect of all the fluxes on the reaction network or pathway. However, the final rate expressions are quite similar when the rate constants are lumped together. Therefore, there is no difference on the quality of fit to experimental data one may obtain. The difference between the actual (or full solution) and either one of the approximation methods (PSSH or LHHW) is noticeable if the initial time period (at the onset of adsorption and reaction) is considered. After the onset or the start of reaction, the difference between the approximation and full solutions is negligible. Therefore, equilibrium step (or the opposite, rate-limiting step) assumptions are well suited for kinetic analyses or simplification to complex problems.

The rate expression can also appear to be of power-law form if Freundlich isotherm were used or Temkin approximation were applied to UniLan isotherms. The accuracy of LHHW rate expressions can be as accurate as power-law forms even for nonideal surfaces. This is due largely to the fact that the power-law rate forms are approximate and only valid in narrow ranges of concentrations (intermediate). When wide range of concentrations are examined, LHHW rate expressions are not showing larger deviations because of their better agreement at low surface coverages either than Temkin or Freundlich isotherms.

To obtain rate expressions valid at low coverages as well as at high surface coverages, nonideal isotherms must be employed without Freundlich and/or Temkin approximation. ExLan isotherms consider the distribution of available adsorption sites to be exponentially dependent on the interaction energy between adsorbate molecules and adsorbent. When ExLan isotherm is employed to describe nonideal surfaces, some of the reaction rate expressions are shown in Table 9.5. These relations are valid in wide ranges of concentrations and thus have similar quality as LHHW expressions for ideal surfaces.

Similar to the ExLan isotherm, UniLan isotherms consider that the nonideality on the adsorbent surface gives rise to linear distribution of available sites with the interaction energy between the adsorbate molecules and adsorbent. UniLan isotherms can also be employed to describe nonideal surfaces, some of the reaction rate expressions are shown in Table 9.6.

The multilayer adsorption can also be applied to describe reactions on nonideal surfaces as steric interactions and interaction potential differences can be effectively modeled by multilayers. Table 9.7 show some examples of the rate expressions for nonideal surface reactions.

Rate expressions for noncatalytic reactions involving solids can be derived in the same manner as LHHW. The participation of the surface active centers in actual reactions can affect the site balance, either active center renewal or depletion occurs.

For catalytic surfaces, the activity can decrease with increase duration of service. The surface activity decline can be treated the same way as the concentration of a reacting component in the mixture.

Further Reading

Butt, J.B., Petersen, E.E., 1989. *Activation, Deactivation and Poisoning of Catalysts*, Academic Press, Inc. San Diego, CA.
Fogler, H.S., 1999. *Elements of Chemical Reaction Engineering*, (3rd ed.). Prentice Hall PTR, Inc., Upper Saddle River, NJ.
Liu, S., 2011. "A sustainable woody biomass biorefinery", *Journal of Biotechnology Advances*.
Masel, R.I., 1996. *Principles of Adsorption and Reaction on Solid Surfaces*, Wiley & Sons, New York.
Saterfield, C.N., 1991. *Heterogeneous Catalysis in Industrial Practices*, (2nd ed.). McGraw-Hill, New York.
Smil, V., 2001. *Enriching the Earth: Frith Haber, Carl Bosch and the Transformation of World Food Production*, MIT Press.
Somojai, G.A., 1994. *Introduction to surface chemistry and catalysis*, John Wiley & Sons.
White, M.G., 1990. *Heterogeneous Catalysis*, Prentice Hall, Upper Saddle River, NJ.

PROBLEMS

9.1. One way of modeling the multilayer adsorption is to employ the available site distribution function. Assume that there are $n+1$ layers, with equal fraction of available sites in each layer and the excess heat of adsorption decrease each layer by an equal fixed amount. This assumption leads to

$$c = \frac{K_{1,j}}{K_{n+1,j}} = \exp\left(\frac{E_{\max}}{RT}\right); \quad c^{1/n} = \frac{K_{i-1,j}}{K_{i,j}} = \exp\left(\frac{E_{\max}}{nRT}\right)$$

Derive the adsorption isotherm expression similar to the way UniLan isotherm is obtained.

9.2. When deriving at multilayer adsorption isotherms, Eqns (9.80) and (9.82), we have assumed steric interactions: desorption can occur only if the adsorbed molecule is not covered by the layer above it. Rework P9.1 with $n = 2$ (or three layers), however, follow the multilayer adsorption derivation with the additional steric interaction implied.

9.3. The following data were recorded for the adsorption of a gas on a solid:

	Equilibrium Pressure, mmHg		
Volume Adsorbed cm³/g	**$T = 0\,°C$**	**$T = 25\,°C$**	**$T = 100\,°C$**
2	0.12	0.31	5.8
3.5	0.21	0.54	10.3
5	0.31	0.8	14
7	0.48	1.2	21
10	0.8	2.0	32
15	1.7	4.3	56
20	3.1	7.8	91
30	7.7	19	210
40	15	38	380

(a) Plot the three isotherms on a log–log scale.

(b) The heat of adsorption can be related to the equilibrium pressure at constant level of adsorption through Clausius–Clapeyron equation, $\frac{d\ln P}{dT} = -\frac{\Delta H}{RT^2}$. Determine the heat of adsorption and plot the heat of adsorption as a function of surface coverage (or level of adsorption).

(c) Is the Langmuir adsorption isotherm a good assumption? Why? How about Temkin isotherm?

(d) Examine the quality of adsorption isotherm fit with ExLan.

(e) Examine the quality of adsorption isotherm fit with Multilayer model.

9.4. The mechanism proposed by Topchieva (K.V. Topchieva, R. Yun-Pun and LV. Smirnova, *Advan. Catalysis*, 9, 799, 1957) for ethanol dehydration over Al_2O_3, is

(1)

$$C_2H_5OH + \underset{\;}{\overset{OH}{\overset{|}{-Al-}}} \rightleftarrows \overset{OC_2H_5}{\overset{|}{-Al-}} + H_2O$$

(2)

$$\underset{|}{\overset{OC_2H_5}{}}\!\!-Al- \rightleftarrows \underset{|}{\overset{OH}{}}\!\!-Al- \; + C_2H_4$$

The designated active site, $\overset{OH}{\underset{-Al-}{|}}$, is consumed in the first step and regenerated in the second, thus forming a closed sequence. Derive a rate equation for the rate of dehydration of alcohol assuming that

(a) Both reactions occur at the comparable rates.

(b) Reaction (1) is much faster than reaction (2), and (2) is irreversible.

9.5. Methanol synthesis from syn gas

$$2\,H_2 + CO \rightleftarrows CH_3OH \tag{1}$$

May be described by the following mechanism

$$H_2 + \sigma \rightleftarrows H_2{\cdot}\sigma \tag{2}$$

$$CO + \sigma \rightleftarrows CO{\cdot}\sigma \tag{3}$$

$$CO{\cdot}\sigma + H_2{\cdot}\sigma \rightleftarrows HCOH{\cdot}\sigma + \sigma \tag{4}$$

$$HCOH{\cdot}\sigma + H_2{\cdot}\sigma \rightleftarrows CH_3OH{\cdot}\sigma + \sigma \tag{5}$$

Derive a rate expression if the surface is ideal and reaction (4) is rate limiting.

9.6. Synthesis of ammonia from nitrogen and hydrogen over Ru/C catalyst is found to follow the following steps:

$$N_2 + \sigma \rightleftarrows N_2{\cdot}\sigma \tag{1}$$

$$N_2{\cdot}\sigma + \sigma \rightleftarrows 2N{\cdot}\sigma \tag{2}$$

$$H_2 + 2\sigma \rightleftarrows 2H{\cdot}\sigma \tag{3}$$

$$H{\cdot}\sigma + N{\cdot}\sigma \rightleftarrows NH{\cdot}\sigma + \sigma \tag{4}$$

$$H{\cdot}\sigma + NH{\cdot}\sigma \rightleftarrows NH_2{\cdot}\sigma + \sigma \tag{5}$$

$$H{\cdot}\sigma + NH_2{\cdot}\sigma \rightleftarrows NH_3{\cdot}\sigma + \sigma \tag{6}$$

$$NH_3{\cdot}\sigma \rightleftarrows NH_3 + \sigma \tag{7}$$

$$+) = \text{overall} \qquad N + 3\,H_2 \rightleftarrows 2\,NH_3 \tag{8}$$

The adsorption of nitrogen, step (1) is found to be the rate-limiting step. Derive a rate expression that is consistent with the mechanism based on ideal surface.

9.7. Christoph and Baerns (R. Christoph and M. Baerns, *Chem-Ing-Tech.*, 58, 494, 1968) conducted extensive studies on the methanation of CO

$$CO + 3\,H_2 \rightarrow CH_4 + H_2O \tag{1}$$

On supported Ni catalyst in the presence of large excess of H_2 ($H_2/CO > 25$) and temperature of about 500 K. A correlation proposed that fit their kinetic data is given by

$$-r_{CO} = \frac{aC_{CO}^{0.5}C_{\sigma}^{2}}{(d + bC_{CO}^{0.5})^{2}} \tag{2}$$

and the catalyst decay follows

$$-r_{\sigma} = k_d C_{CO} C_{\sigma} \tag{3}$$

Suggest a mechanism for the methanation that is consistent with this rate expression and a mechanism for the decay of the catalyst activity.

9.8. **(a)** For the decomposition of NH_3 (A) on Pt (as catalyst), what is the form of the rate law, according to the Langmuir–Hinshelwood model, if NH_3 (reactant) is weakly adsorbed and H_2 (product) strongly adsorbed on Pt? Explain briefly. Assume N_2 does not affect the rate.

(b) Do the following experimental results, obtained by Hinshelwood and Burk (1925) in a constant-volume batch reactor at 1411 K, support the form used in (a)?

t, s	0	10	60	120	240	360	720
P, kPa	26.7	30.4	34.1	36.3	38.5	40.0	42.7

P is total pressure, and only NH3 is present initially. Justify your answer quantitatively, for example, by using the experimental data in conjunction with the form given in (a). Use partial pressure as a measure of concentration.

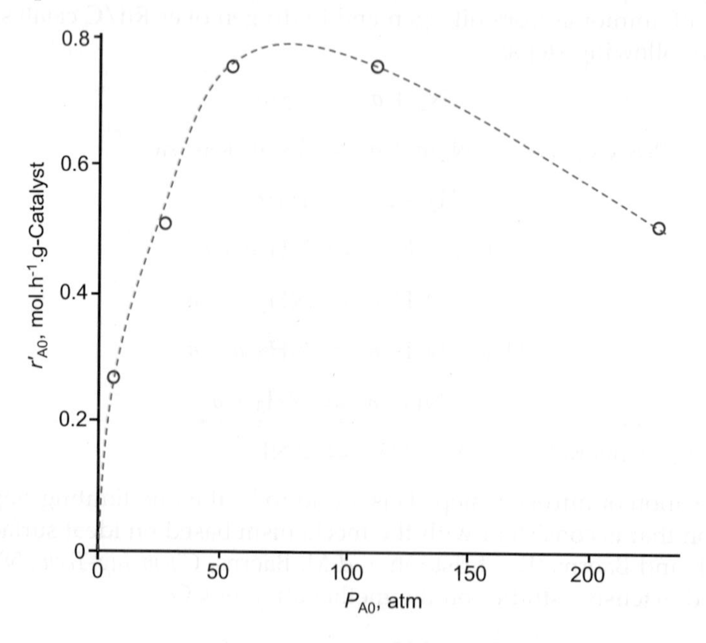

FIGURE P9.9

9.9. Dehydration of alcohol over alumina–silica catalyst can be employed to produce alkenes. The dehydration of *n*-butanol was investigated by J.F. Maurer (PhD thesis, University of Michigan). The data shown in Fig. P9.9 were obtained at 750 °F in a modified differential reactor. The feed consisted of pure butanol.

(a) Suggest a mechanism and rate-controlling step that is consistent with the data

(b) Evaluate the rate law parameters.

9.10. The catalytic dehydration of methanol (M) to form dimethyl ether (DME) and water (W) was carried out over an ion exchange catalyst (K. Klusacek, Collection Czech. *Chem. Commun.*, 49, 170, 1984). The packed bed was initially filled with nitrogen gas (N) and at $t = 0$, a feed of pure methanol vapor entered the reactor at 413 K, 100 kPa, and 0.2×10^{-6} m^3/s. The following partial pressure data were recorded at the exit to the differential reactor containing 1.0 g of catalyst in 4.5×10^{-6} m^3 of reactor volume.

t, s	0	10	50	100	150	200	300
p_N, kPa	100	50	10	2	0	0	0
p_M, kPa	0	2	15	23	25	26	26
p_W, kPa	0	10	15	30	35	37	37
p_{DME}, kPa	0	38	60	45	40	37	37

9.11. In the decomposition of N_2O on Pt, if N_2O is weakly adsorbed and O_2 is moderately adsorbed, what form of rate law would be expected based on an LHHW mechanism? Explain briefly.

9.12. Rate laws for the decomposition of PH_3 (A) on the surface of Mo (as catalyst) in the temperature range 843–918 K are as follows:

Pressure p_A, kPa	**Rate law**
~0	$-r_A = kp_A$
8×10^{-3}	$-r_A = kp_A/(a + bp_A)$
2.6×10^{-2}	$-r_A =$ constant

Interpret these results in terms of an LHHW mechanism.

9.13. Consider the following overall reaction:

$$\frac{1}{2}A_2 + B \rightarrow C + D$$

The mechanism has the following features:

(i) Molecules of A_2 dissociatively adsorb on two type 1 sites (one A atom on each site).

(ii) Molecules of B adsorb on type 2 sites.

(iii) The rate-determining step is the surface reaction between adsorbed A and adsorbed B.

(iv) Molecules of C adsorb on type 1 sites and molecules of D adsorb on type 2 sites Derive an LHHW type rate expression that is consistent with this mechanism.

9.14. The solid-catalyzed exothermic reaction

$$A_2 + 2B \xrightleftharpoons{\text{catalyst}} 2D$$

is virtually irreversible at low temperatures and low product concentrations, and the rate law is given by

$$r = \frac{kC_{A_2}^{1/2}C_B}{(1 + \sqrt{K_{A_2}C_{A_2}} + K_BC_B)^2}$$

(a) How many active sites are involved in the rate-limiting step?
(b) Why is $\sqrt{C_{A_2}}$ appearing in denominator of the rate law? How many species are adsorbed on the catalyst surface?
(c) Suggest a rate law that is valid for a wide range of temperature and concentrations.
(d) Suggest a mechanism for the rate law you have suggested. Identify the rate-limiting step.
(e) Show that your mechanism is consistent with the rate law.

9.15. Synthesis of ammonia from nitrogen and hydrogen over Ru/C catalyst is found to follow the following steps:

$$N_2 + \sigma \rightleftarrows N_2\cdot\sigma \tag{1}$$

$$N_2\cdot\sigma + \sigma \rightleftarrows 2N\cdot\sigma \tag{2}$$

$$H_2 + 2\sigma \rightleftarrows 2H\cdot\sigma \tag{3}$$

$$H\cdot\sigma + N\cdot\sigma \rightleftarrows NH\cdot\sigma + \sigma \tag{4}$$

$$H\cdot\sigma + NH\cdot\sigma \rightleftarrows NH_2\cdot\sigma + \sigma \tag{5}$$

$$H\cdot\sigma + NH_2\cdot\sigma \rightleftarrows NH_3\cdot\sigma + \sigma \tag{6}$$

$$NH_3\cdot\sigma \rightleftarrows NH_3 + \sigma \tag{7}$$

$$+) = \text{overall} \qquad N + 3H_2 \rightleftarrows 2NH_3 \tag{8}$$

The surface reaction step (4) is found to be the rate-limiting step. Derive a rate expression that is consistent with the mechanism based on nonideal surfaces with ExLan isotherm.

9.16. The rate law for the hydrogenation (H) of ethylene (E) to form ethane (A) over a cobalt-molybdenum catalyst is found to be

$$r'_A = kP_EP_H\ln\left(1 + \frac{K_E}{P_E}\right)$$

Suggest a mechanism and rate-limiting step consistent with the rate law. Describe the feature of the catalysts surface.

CHAPTER

10

Cell Metabolism

OUTLINE

Bioprocess Engineering
http://dx.doi.org/10.1016/B978-0-444-59525-6.00010-X

We study cells because we want cells to help us to produce a desired product or accomplish a desired process. How a certain substrate is transported into the cell and converted to the desired product? How cells maintain viable? How cell works?

You have now learned something about how cells are constructed (Chapter 2) and how enzymes function (Chapter 8). We are now ready to move into more complex systems. A cell is like a bag filled with lipids, amino acids, sugars, enzymes, and nucleic acids, which you have been exposed to in Chapter 2. The cell must control how these components are made and modulate how these components interact with each other. The processes involved all have the fundamental bases from Chapters 3, 4, 5, 6, and 9. In this chapter, we explore some examples of metabolic regulations and how the metabolic regulations are reflected through the bioprocess kinetics. It is this ability to coordinate a wide variety of chemical reactions that makes a cell a living cell.

The key to metabolic regulation is the flow and control of information. Humanity is a perfect example to illustrate the importance of the flow and control/manipulation of information. Our full grasp of computers has led the "Information Age." Prior to the invention of paper, scientific discoveries were extremely slow to appear and spread. Our ability to gather and communicate message or information was more or less limited to verbal dialog. The limitation in the scope of learning and assembling of information by individuals hindered the "evolution" of new knowledge, and thus inventions. Our comfortable level of living standards was rising very slowly. Paper had become a convenient means of storing and disseminating information and knowledge since about 200 AD. When books become readily available, literature spreads were faster starting in the 1700s and 1800s. A booming increase in scientific discoveries and our understanding of the universe began to unravel rapidly. A revolutionary change occurred again when computers entered into our daily life. For example, literature is no longer limited to physical contacts and books. Our way of living is no longer limited to individuals. Communication among individuals becomes mechanized and the human society becomes an integrated entity. There are many analogies between human society's need to use and exchange information and a cell's need to use and exchange information between subcellular components. Today, human society depends primarily on electronic signals for information storage, processing, and transmission; cells use chemical signals for the same purposes. Molecular biology is primarily the study of information flow and control. How chemicals or sensors are released and received forms the basis of cell-to-cell and cell to environment interactions. In this chapter, we will learn the biological process of cell growth and fermentation or information and nutrient flow and control in cells.

10.1. THE CENTRAL DOGMA

Almost all living organisms have the same core approach to the storage, expression, and utilization of information. On a grand scale, we can perceive is the human society as depicted in the above section. The modern human society is a good analogy to all the living systems. Information is stored in the DNA molecule in cells as depicted in Fig. 10.1. Like information on a computer disc or drive, the information stored in the DNA can be replicated. It can also be played back or transcribed to produce a message. The message must translate into some action, such as production of RNA, and protein, for the message to carry a profound impact.

Cells operate with an analogous system. Figure 10.2 displays the *central dogma* of biology, further exemplifying from Fig. 10.1. Information is stored on the DNA molecule. The stored information can be *replicated* directly to form a second identical molecule. Further segments of information on the molecule can be *transcribed* to yield RNAs. Using a variety of RNAs,

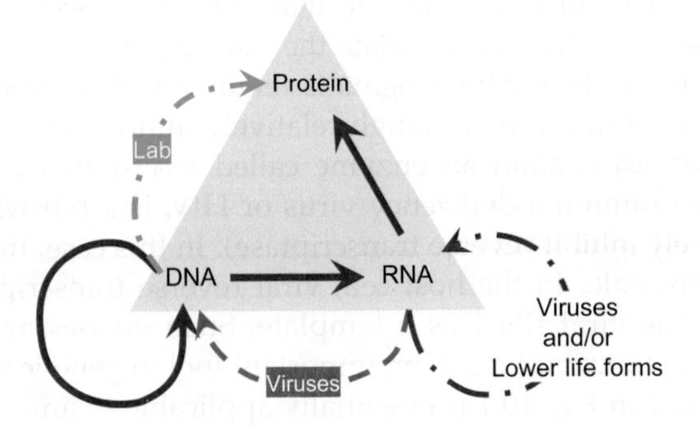

FIGURE 10.1 The flow of biological information in living systems.

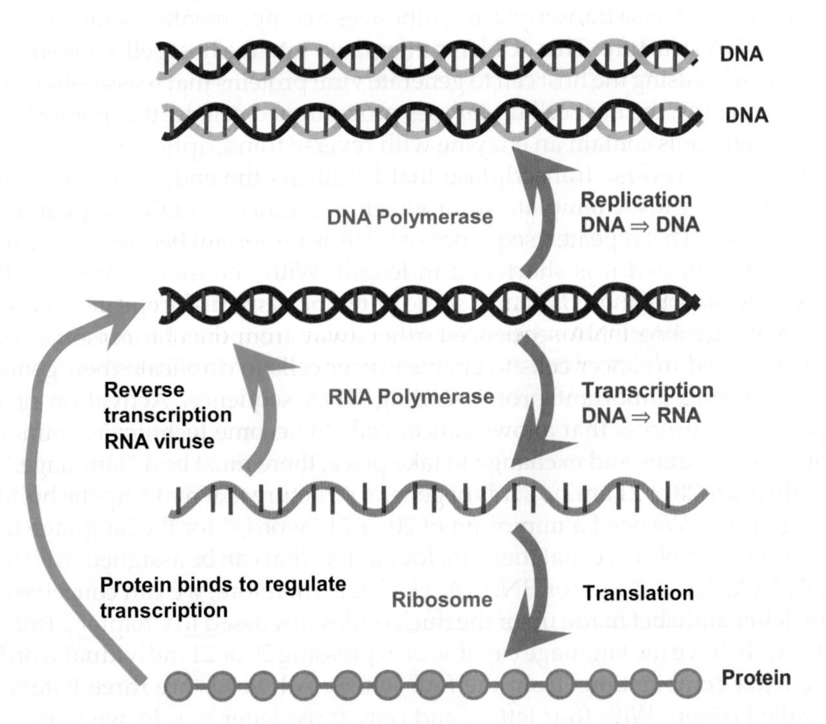

FIGURE 10.2 The central dogma is the primary tenet of molecular biology, which applies to all living organisms. DNA serves as the template for its own replication, as well as transcription to RNA. The information transcribed into the RNA can then be translated into proteins using an RNA template. The information on the DNA molecule is time independent at a timescale much longer than RNA, then protein. The information exists in the form of RNA and more so protein molecules depends on the history and environment of the cell and is more clearly time dependent. Some of the proteins interact with DNA to control which genes are transcribed in response to the environment.

this information is *translated* into proteins. The proteins then perform a structural or enzymatic role, mediating almost all the metabolic functions in the cell. The information content of the DNA molecule is static; changes occur very slowly through infrequent mutations or rearrangements nearly by accidents. Which species of RNA that are present and in what amount varies with time and with changes in culture conditions. Likewise, the proteins that are present will change with time but on a different timescale than for RNA species. Some of the proteins produced in the cell bind to DNA and regulate the transcriptional process to form RNAs.

The important feature of the central dogma is its universality from the simplest to most complex organisms. One important, although relatively minor, deviation is that some RNA tumor viruses (*retroviruses*) contain an enzyme called *reverse transcriptase*. The virus that causes AIDS, the human immunodeficiency virus or HIV, is a retrovirus (one approach to treatment is to selectively inhibit reverse transcriptase). In this case, the virus encodes information on an RNA molecule. In the host cell, viral reverse transcriptase produces a viral DNA molecule using the viral RNA as a template. Such viruses are clinically important and the enzyme, reverse transcriptase, is an important tool in genetic engineering. Nonetheless, the process depicted in Fig. 10.1 is essentially applicable to any cell of importance.

In the case of HIV, reverse transcriptase is responsible for synthesizing a complementary DNA (cDNA) strand to the viral RNA genome. An associated enzyme, ribonuclease H, digests the RNA strand, and reverse transcriptase synthesizes a complementary strand of DNA to form a double-helix DNA structure. This cDNA is integrated into the host cell's genome via another enzyme (integrase) causing the host cell to generate viral proteins that reassemble into new viral particles. Subsequently, the host cell undergoes programmed cell death, apoptosis.

Some eukaryotic cells contain an enzyme with reverse transcription activity called telomerase. Telomerase is a reverse transcriptase that lengthens the ends of linear chromosomes. Telomerase carries an RNA template from which it synthesizes DNA repeating sequence, or "nonsense" DNA. This repeated sequence of DNA is important because every time a linear chromosome is duplicated it is shortened in length. With "nonsense" DNA at the ends of chromosomes, the shortening eliminates some of the nonessential, repeated sequence rather than the protein-encoding DNA sequence farther away from the chromosome end. Telomerase is often activated in cancer cells to enable cancer cells to duplicate their genomes indefinitely without losing important protein-coding DNA sequence. Activation of telomerase could be part of the process that allows cancer cells to become technically immortal.

For information storage and exchange to take place, there must be a "language." As shown in Table 2.5, there are 20 or 21 amino acids of general structure that make up the building blocks for all the organisms. We need a minimum of 20 or 21 "words" for the language to be useful. From Fig. 2.30, one can observe that there are four letters that can be assigned to all the building blocks of DNA (A, T, G, C) and/or RNA (A, U, G, C). Therefore, we can conceive of all life as using a four-letter alphabet made up of the nucleotides discussed in Chapter 2 (that is, A, T, G, and C in DNA). To have the language capable of expressing 20 or 21 individual words, we need to use three letter combinations from the four letters. All words are three letters long; such words are called *codons*. With four letters and only three-letter words, we have a maximum of 64 words, which is more than 20. There are then multiple expressions (words) to describe one particular "meaning." These words, when expressed, represent a particular amino acid or "stop" (when it does not represent a particular amino acid) protein synthesis. This natural "language" design is essential to DNA, RNA, and proteins.

When these words are put into a sequence, they can make a "sentence" (i.e. a *gene*), which when properly transcribed and translated is a protein. Other combinations of words regulate when the gene is expressed. Carrying the analogy to the extreme, we may look at the complete set of information in an organism's DNA (i.e. the *genome*) as a book. (For the human genome, it would be more than 1000 books the size of this one.)

This simple language of 64 words is all that is necessary to summarize the total physical make up of all living organisms at birth and all natural capabilities of a living organism. It is essentially universal, the same for *Escherichia coli* and *Homo sapiens* (humans). This universality has helped us to make great strides in understanding life and is a practical tool in genetic engineering and biotechnology.

Each of the steps in information storage and transfer (Figs 10.1 and 10.2) requires a macromolecular template. Let us next examine how these templates are made and how this genetic-level language is preserved and expressed.

10.2. DNA REPLICATION: PRESERVING AND PROPAGATING THE CELLULAR MESSAGE

The double-helix structure of DNA discussed in Chapter 2 is extremely well suited to its role of preserving genetic information. Information resides simply in the linear arrangement of the four nucleotide letters (A, T, G, and C). *Because* G *can hydrogen-bind only to* C *and A only to T, the strands must be complementary* if an undistorted double helix is to result. Replication is *semiconservative* (see Fig. 2.31); each daughter chromosome contains one parental strand and one newly generated strand.

To illustrate the replication process (see Figs 2.34, 10.3, and 10.4), let us briefly consider DNA replication in *E. coli*. The enzyme responsible for covalently linking the monomers is DNA polymerase. *Escherichia coli* has three DNA polymerases (named Pol I, Pol II, and Pol III). A DNA polymerase is an enzyme that will link deoxynucleotides together to form a DNA polymer. Pol III enzymatically mediates the addition of nucleotides to an RNA primer. Pol I can hydrolyze an RNA primer and duplicates single-stranded regions of DNA; it is also active in the repair of DNA molecules. Pol II enzyme is 90 kDa in size and is coded by the pol B gene. Strains lacking the gene show no defect in growth or replication. Synthesis of Pol II is induced during the stationary phase of cell growth. This is a phase in which little growth and DNA synthesis occurs. It is also a phase in which the DNA can accumulate damage such as short gaps, which act as a block to DNA Pol III. Under these circumstances, Pol II helps to overcome the problem because it can reinitiate DNA synthesis downstream of gaps. Pol II has a low error rate but it is much too slow to be of any use in normal DNA synthesis. Pol II differs from Pol I in that it lacks a C5-to-C3 exonuclease activity and cannot use a nicked duplex template.

In addition to the enzyme, the enzymatic reaction requires activated monomer and the template. The activated monomers are the nucleoside triphosphates. The formation of the C5–C3 phosphodiester bond to link a nucleotide with the growing DNA molecule results in the release of a pyrophosphate, which provides the energy for such a biosynthetic reaction. The resulting nucleoside monophosphates are the constituent monomers of the DNA molecule.

Replication of the chromosome normally begins at a predetermined site, the *origin of replication*, which in *E. coli* is attached to the plasma membrane at the start of replication. Initiator

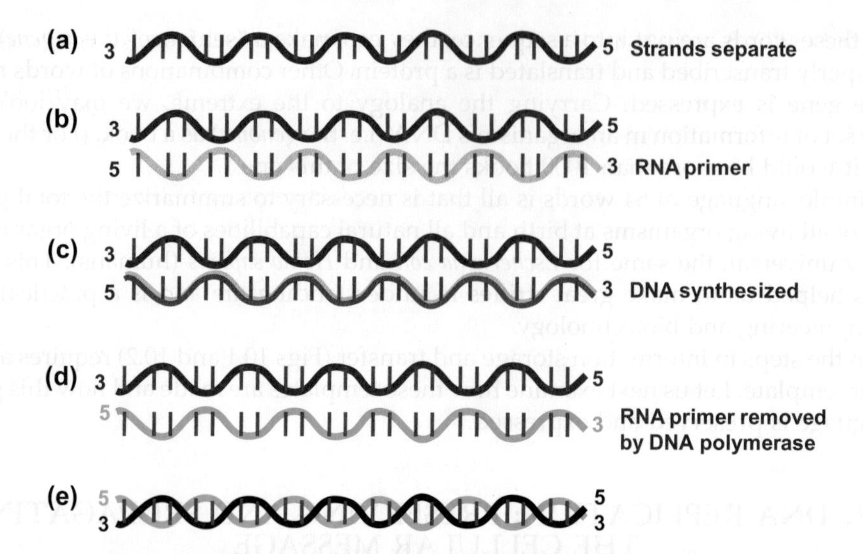

FIGURE 10.3 Initiation of DNA synthesis requires the formation of an RNA primer.

proteins bind to DNA at the origin of replication, break hydrogen bonds in the local region of the origin, and force the two DNA strands apart. When DNA replication begins, the two strands separate to form a Y-shaped structure called a *replication fork*.

Movement of the fork must be facilitated by the energy-dependent action of *DNA gyrase* and *unwinding enzymes*. In *E. coli*, the chromosome is circular. In *E. coli* (but not all organisms),

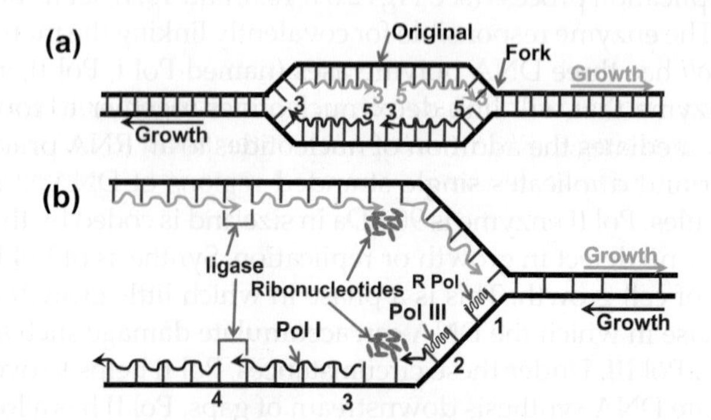

FIGURE 10.4 Schematic of the steps in the replication of the bacterial chromosome. (a) A replicating bacterial chromosome at a stage shortly after replication begun at the origin. The newly polymerized strands of DNA (wavy lines) are synthesized in the C5-to-C3 direction, using the preexisting DNA strands (solid lines) as a template. The process creates two replication forks, which travel in opposite directions until they meet on the opposite side of the circular chromosome, completing the replication process. (b) A detailed view of one replicating fork, showing the process where short lengths of DNA are synthesized and eventually joined to produce a continuous new strand of DNA. For illustration, four short segments of nucleic acid are illustrated at various stages: (1) primer RNA (thickened area) is being synthesized by an RNA polymerase (R Pol); Successively, in (2) DNA is being polymerized to it by DNA polymerase III (pol III); in (3) a preceding primer RNA is being hydrolyzed, while DNA is being polymerized in its place by the exonuclease and polymerase activities of DNA polymerase I (pol I); finally, (4) the completed short segment of DNA is joined to the continuous strand by the action of DNA ligase.

the synthesis of DNA is *bidirectional*. Two forks start at the origin and move in opposite directions until they meet again, approximately 1800 from the origin.

To initiate DNA synthesis, an *RNA primer* is required; RNA polymerase requires no primer to initiate the chain-building process, while DNA polymerase does. We can speculate on why this is so. In DNA replication, it is critical that no mistakes be made in the addition of each nucleotide. The DNA polymerase, Pol III, can *proofread*, in part due to the enzyme's C3 to C5 exonuclease activity, which can remove mismatches by moving backward. On the other hand, a mistake in RNA synthesis is not nearly so critical, so RNA polymerase lacks this proofreading capacity. Once a short stretch of RNA complementary to one of the DNA strands is made, DNA synthesis begins with Pol III. Next, the RNA portion is degraded by Pol I and DNA is synthesized in its place. This process is summarized in Fig. 10.4 (and 2.34).

DNA polymerase works only in the C5-to-C3 direction, which means that the next nucleotide is always added to the exposed C3-OH group of the chain. Thus, one strand (the *leading strand*) can be formed continuously if it is synthesized in the same direction as the replication fork is moving. The other strand (the *lagging strand*) must be synthesized discontinuously. Short pieces of DNA attached to RNA are formed on the lagging strand. These fragments are called *Okazaki fragments*. The whole process is summarized in Figs 2.34 and 10.4. The enzyme, *DNA ligase*, which joins the two short pieces of DNA on the continuous strand, will be very important in our discussions of genetic engineering.

This brief summarizes the essentials of how one DNA molecule is made from another and thus preserves and propagates the genetic information in the original molecule. Now we turn to examine how this genetic information can be transferred.

10.3. TRANSCRIPTION: SENDING THE MESSAGE

Transcription is the process of creating a complementary RNA copy of a sequence of DNA. Therefore, the primary products of transcription are the three major types of RNA we introduced in Chapter 2: messenger RNA (*mRNA*), transfer RNA (*tRNA*), and ribosomal RNA (*rRNA*). Their rates of synthesis determine the cell's capacity to make proteins. Figure 10.5 shows the major factors associated with the transcription process, where prokaryotes and eukaryotes translate differently. In prokaryotes, the transcription has a start and an end location on the template DNA. RNA synthesis from DNA is mediated (or read) by the enzyme, *RNA polymerase*. To be functional, RNA polymerase must have two major subcomponents: the *core* enzyme (consisted of five subunits—two α, one β, one β', and an ω units) and (binds with) the σ (*sigma*) *factor*, as illustrated in Fig. 10.5. The core enzyme contains the catalytic site, while the σ factor is a protein essential to locating the appropriate beginning for the message. The core enzyme plus the σ factor constitutes the *holoenzyme*. While in some case the σ factor would leave after initialization of the transcription, in other cases the σ factor remain bonded to the core enzyme throughout the transcription process.

You may wonder which one of the two strands of DNA is actually transcribed. It turns out that either strand can be read. However, only one is read at a time, which is different from DNA replication. RNA polymerase always reads in the C3 to C5 direction, so the direction of reading will be opposite on each strand. On one part of the chromosome, one strand of DNA may serve as the template or *sense strand*, and on another portion of the chromosome the other strand may serve as a template. During transcription, a DNA sequence is read by

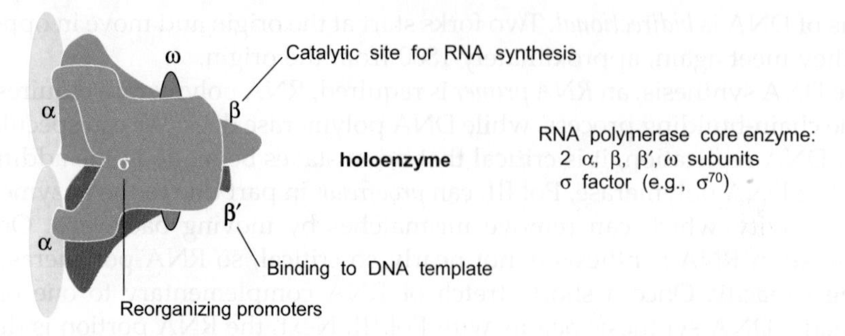

FIGURE 10.5 A schematic of RNA polymerase.

RNA polymerase, which produces a complimentary, antiparallel RNA strand. As opposed to DNA replication, transcription results in an RNA complement that includes uracil (U) in all instances where thymine (T) would have occurred in a DNA complement.

The processes of initiation, propagation, and termination are summarized in Fig. 10.6. A detailed illustration of the propagation is shown in Fig. 10.7. The σ factor plays an

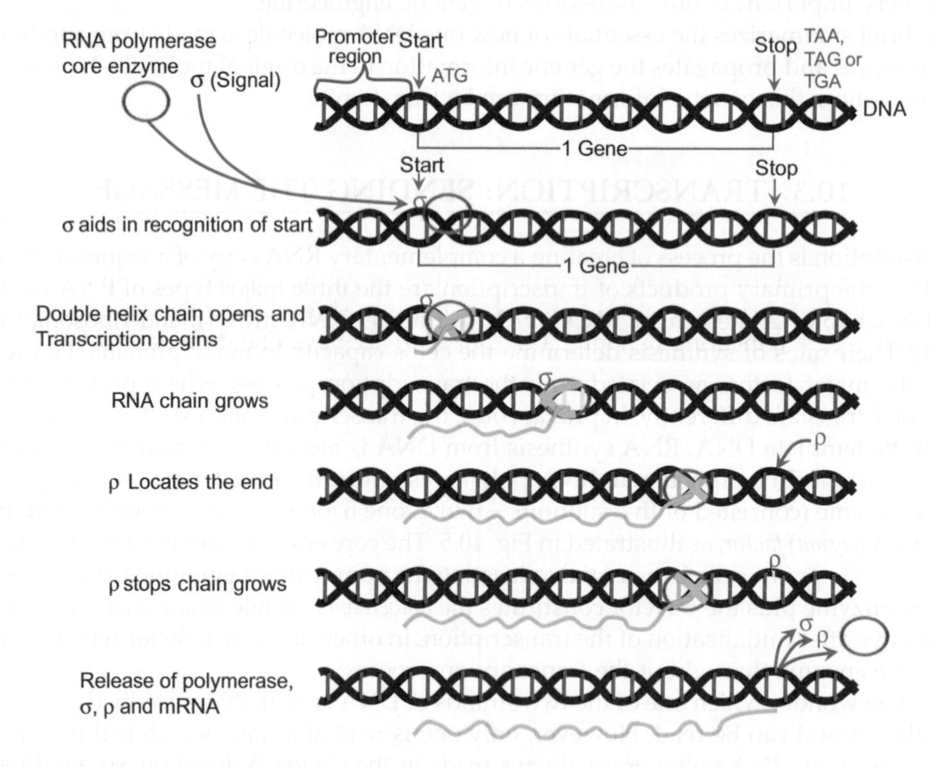

FIGURE 10.6 Steps in mRNA synthesis. The start and stop sites are specific nucleotide sequences on the DNA. RNA polymerase moves down the DNA chain, causing temporary opening of the double helix and transcription of one of the DNA strands. ρ binds to the termination site and stops chain growth; termination can also occur at some sites without ρ.

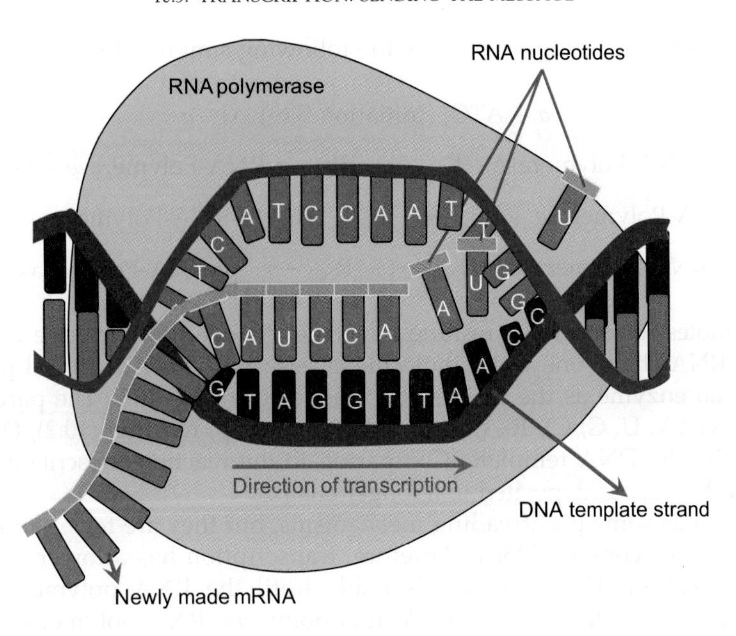

FIGURE 10.7 A schematic of mRNA synthesis as catalyzed by the RNA polymerase.

important role in initiation. The σ factor recognizes a specific sequence of nucleotides on a DNA strand. This sequence is the *promoter region*. Promoters can vary somewhat, and this alters the affinity of the σ factor (and consequently the holoenzyme) for a particular promoter. Table 10.1 shows the promoter sequences in prokaryotes and eukaryotes. As one can observe from Table 10.1, the promoter region starts from 10 to 80 nucleotides prior to the start codon ATG. A strong *promoter* is one with a high affinity for the holoenzyme. The rate of formation of transcripts is determined primarily by the frequency of initiation of transcription, which is directly related to promoter strength. This will be important in our discussions of genetic engineering (Chapter 14). Cells usually have one dominant σ factor that is required to recognize the vast majority of promoters in the cell. However, other σ factors can play important roles under different growth conditions (particularly stress) and are used to initiate transcription from promoters that encode proteins important to the cell for coping with unusual growth conditions or stress.

After the initiation site (a particular ATG codon) is recognized, elongation of the transcript begins. The synthesis of the growing RNA molecule is energy requiring, so activated triphosphate monomers of the ribonucleotides are required.

TABLE 10.1 The Conserved DNA Promoter Binding Sequences in Bacterial and Eukaryotic Polymerases

Cell type	Promoter binding location	Promoter sequence
Prokaryotic	−10	TATAAT
	−35	TTGACA
Eukaryotic	−25	TATA
	−80	CAAT

The transcription can be represented by the following simplified steps:

$$\sigma + \text{ATG}|\ (\text{Initiation Site}) \rightarrow |{-}\sigma \tag{10.1}$$

$$|{-}\sigma\text{-RNA-Polymerase} + \text{R}_{\text{NA}} \rightarrow |{-}\text{R}_{\text{NA}}\text{-}\sigma\text{-RNA-Polymerase} + \text{H}_2\text{O} \tag{10.2}$$

$$|{-}\text{R}_{\text{NA}}\text{-}\sigma\text{-RNA-Polymerase} + \text{R}_{\text{NA}} \rightarrow |{-}\text{R}_{\text{NA}}{-}\text{R}_{\text{NA}}\text{-}\sigma\text{-RNA-Polymerase} + \text{H}_2\text{O} \tag{10.3}$$

$$|{-}(\text{R}_{\text{NA}}{-})_n\sigma\text{-RNA-Polymerase} + \text{R}_{\text{NA}} \rightarrow |{-}(\text{R}_{\text{NA}}{-})_{n+1}\sigma\text{-RNA-Polymerase} + \text{H}_2\text{O} \tag{10.4}$$

where R_{NA} denotes for one RNA residue molecule. As one RNA residue is deposited (or added) to the RNA chain, one water molecule is released. This is a typical polymerization reaction, with an enzyme as the catalyst, as illustrated in Fig. 10.7. The particular type of RNA nucleotides (A, U, G, C), R_{NA}, is added at each step, reaction (10.2), (10.3), or (10.4), is determined by the DNA template. Comparing to the reactions described in Chapter 8, the product in this case is deposited to a longer chain.

Transcription has some proofreading mechanisms, but they are fewer and less effective than the controls for copying DNA; therefore, transcription has a lower copying fidelity than DNA replication. The transcript is made until the RNA polymerase encounters a stop signal or *transcription terminator.* At this point, the RNA polymerase disassociates from the DNA template and the RNA transcript is released. Bacteria use two different strategies for transcription termination: ρ-dependent and ρ-independent transcription terminations. In ρ-independent transcription termination, RNA transcription stops when the newly synthesized RNA molecule forms a G–C-rich hairpin loop followed by a run of Us. When the hairpin forms, the mechanical stress breaks the weak rU–dA bonds, now filling the DNA–RNA hybrid. This pulls the poly-U transcript out of the active site of the RNA polymerase, in effect, terminating transcription. In the "ρ-dependent" type of termination, a protein factor called ρ destabilizes the interaction between the template and the mRNA, thus releasing the newly synthesized mRNA from the elongation complex. Terminators can be strong or weak. If a weak terminator is coupled with a strong promoter, some of the RNA polymerase will *read through* the terminator, creating an artificially long transcript and possibly disrupting subsequent control regions on that DNA strand. We must consider terminator regions and their strength when constructing recombinant DNA systems.

The transcripts that are formed may be roughly lumped as either stable or unstable RNA species. The stable RNA species are *r-RNA* and *t-RNA*. m-RNA is highly unstable (about a 1-min half-life for a typical *E. coli m-RNA*, although *m-RNA* may be considerably more stable in cells from higher plants and animals). Why is *m-RNA* is relatively unstable? The answer should become apparent as we discuss translation and regulation.

Although the general features of transcription are universal, there are some significant differences in transcription between prokaryotic and eukaryotic cells. One example is that in prokaryotes related proteins are often encoded in a row without interspacing terminators. Thus, transcription from a single promoter may result in a *polygenic* message. *Polygenic* indicates many genes; *each single gene encodes a separate protein*. Thus, the regulation of transcription from a single promoter can provide efficient regulation of functionally related proteins; such a strategy is particularly important for relatively small and simple cells. On the other hand, eukaryotic cells do not produce polygenic messages.

In prokaryotic cells, there is no physical separation of the chromosome from the cytoplasma and ribosomes. Often an *m-RNA* will bind to a ribosome and begin translation immediately, even while part of it is still being transcribed! However, in eukaryotes, where the nuclear membrane separates chromosomes and ribosomes, the *m-RNA* is often subject to processing before translation (see Fig. 10.8). The DNA can encode for a transcript with an intervening sequence (called an *intron*) in the middle of the transcript. This intron is then cut out of the transcript at two specific sites. The ends of the remaining fragments are joined by a process called *m-RNA splicing*. The spliced message can then be translated into an actual protein. The part of the transcript forming the intron is degraded and the monomers recycled. When *m-RNA* is recovered from the cytosol it will be in the mature form, while m-RNA within the nucleus has introns. Many eukaryotic genes contain "nonsense DNA," which encodes for the intronic part of the transcript. The word "nonsense" denotes that particular sequence of DNA does not encode for amino acids. The presence of introns complicates the transfer of eukaryotic genes to protein production systems in prokaryotes such as *E. coli*.

As shown in Fig. 10.9, two other *m-RNA* processing steps occur in eukaryotic cells that do not occur in prokaryotes. One is *RNA capping*, in which the C5 end is modified by the addition of a guanine nucleotide with a methyl group attached. The other is *polyadenylation*, in which a string of adenine nucleotides are added to the C3 end. This tail of adenines is often

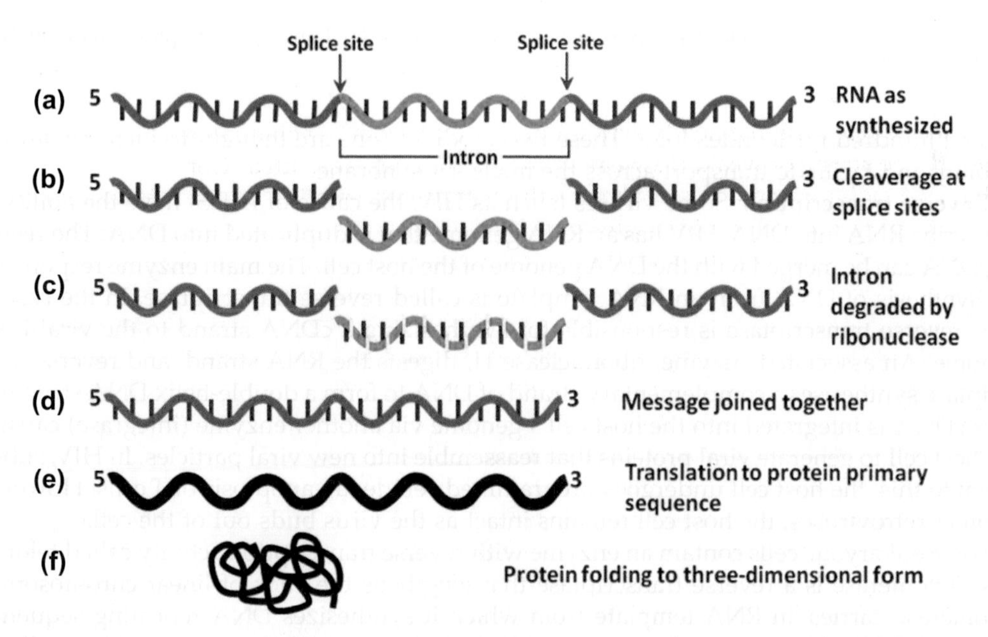

FIGURE 10.8 In eukaryotes, RNA splicing is important. The presence of introns is a complication in cloning genes from eukaryotes to prokaryotes.

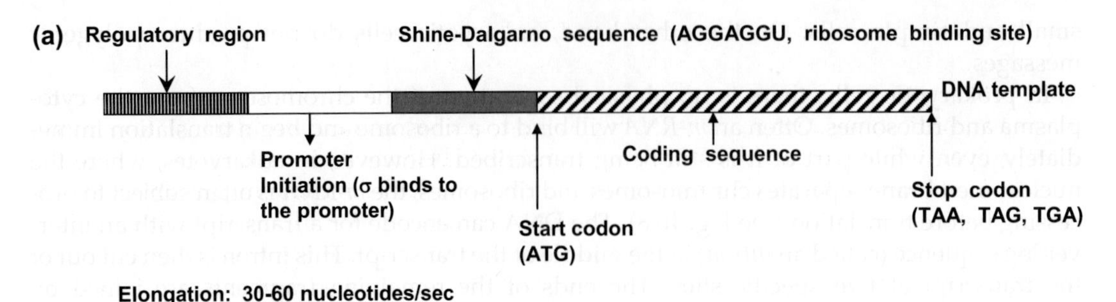

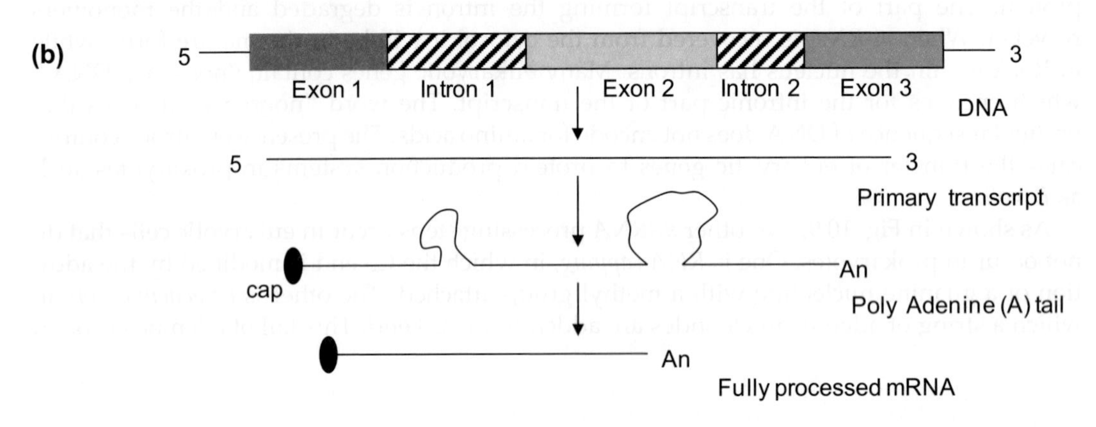

FIGURE 10.9 Translation process in prokaryotes and eukaryotes. (a) Transcription in prokaryotes. (b) Transcription in eukaryotes.

several hundred nucleotides long. These two modifications are thought to increase *m-RNA* stability and facilitate transport across the nuclear membrane.

Reverse transcription. Some viruses (such as HIV, the cause of AIDS) have the ability to transcribe RNA into DNA. HIV has an RNA genome that is duplicated into DNA. The resulting DNA can be merged with the DNA genome of the host cell. The main enzyme responsible for synthesis of DNA from an RNA template is called reverse transcriptase. In the case of HIV, reverse transcriptase is responsible for synthesizing a cDNA strand to the viral RNA genome. An associated enzyme, ribonuclease H, digests the RNA strand, and reverse transcriptase synthesises a complementary strand of DNA to form a double-helix DNA structure. This cDNA is integrated into the host cell's genome via another enzyme (integrase) causing the host cell to generate viral proteins that reassemble into new viral particles. In HIV, subsequent to this, the host cell undergoes programmed cell death, apoptosis of T cells. However, in other retroviruses, the host cell remains intact as the virus buds out of the cell.

Some eukaryotic cells contain an enzyme with reverse transcription activity called telomerase. Telomerase is a reverse transcriptase that lengthens the ends of linear chromosomes. Telomerase carries an RNA template from which it synthesizes DNA repeating sequence, or "junk" DNA. This repeated sequence of DNA is important because, every time a linear chromosome is duplicated, it is shortened in length. With "junk" DNA at the ends of chromosomes, the shortening eliminates some of the nonessential, repeated sequence rather than the protein-encoding DNA sequence farther away from the chromosome end. Telomerase is often activated in cancer cells to enable cancer cells to duplicate their genomes indefinitely without losing important protein-coding DNA sequence. Activation of telomerase could be part of the process that allows cancer cells to become immortal.

Now that we have learned transcription, we can now move to examine translation. RNA molecules are made with a DNA template. The translation of information on *m*RNA into proteins occupies a very large fraction of the cells' resources. Like a large automobile plant, the generation of blueprints and the construction of the manufacturing machinery are worthless until the final product is made.

10.4. TRANSLATION: MESSAGE TO PRODUCT

The central dogma of molecular biology describes the passing of genetic code to protein from DNA as shown in Figs 10.1 and 10.2. Table 10.2 summarizes the process of transferring information from DNA template to proteins. From a DNA template, a complementary RNA strand is made, from which it is translated into protein. Our emphasis now is on the protein formation.

10.4.1. Genetic Code: Universal Message

The blueprint for any living cell is consisted of 20 amino acids as shown in Table 2.4. There are four letters for DNA and/or RNA as shown in Fig. 2.21. With the four letters, a three-letter word is needed to completely expressing the 20 amino acids. Therefore, the genetic code is made up of three-letter words (*codons*) with an alphabet of four letters as discussed earlier. Sixty-four words are possible, but many of these words are redundant (as only 20 individual amino acids needed expression). Even though such a "language" may appear to be simple, it is sufficient to serve as a complete blueprint for the expression of any "message" or "construction" of the reader.

The dictionary for this language is given in Table 10.3, and an illustration of the relationship of nucleotides in the chromosome and *m*RNA to the final protein product is given in Fig. 10.10. The code is *degenerate* in that more than one codon can specify a particular amino acid (for example, UCU, UCC, UCA, and UCG all specify serine). Three codings, UAA, UAG, and UGA, do not encode normally for any amino acids. As a result, these codons act as stop

TABLE 10.2 The Central Dogma of Molecular Biology for Protein Production

DNA, template		RNA		Protein
4 nucleotides (A, C, G, T)	⇒	4 nucleotides (A, C, G, U)	⇒	20 amino acids
ACCGCTTGACTACAC	*Transcription* by polymerase	UGGCGAACUGAUGUG	*Translation* by ribosome	Try-Arg-Thr-Asp-Val
Phosphodiester bond		Phosphodiester bond		Peptide bond

TABLE 10.3 The Genetic Code: Correspondence between RNA Codons and Amino Acids (as in Protein)

First base	Second base U		C		A		G		Third base
U	UUU	phe*	UCU	ser	UAU	tyr	UGU	cys	U
	UUC	Phe	UCC	ser	UAC	tyr	UGC	cys	C
	UUA	Leu	UCA	ser	UAA	end†	UGA	end†	A
	UUG	Leu	UCG	ser	UAG	end†	UGG	try	G
C	CUU	Leu	CCU	pro	CAU	his	CGU	arg	U
	CUC	Leu	CCC	pro	CAC	his	CGC	arg	C
	CUA	Leu	CCA	pro	CAA	gln	CGA	arg	A
	CUG	Leu	CCG	pro	CAG	gln	CGG	arg	G
A	AUU	Ilu	ACU	thr	AAU	asn	AGU	ser	U
	AUC	Ilu	ACC	thr	AAC	asn	AGC	ser	C
	AUA	Ilu	ACA	thr	AAA	lys	AGA	arg	A
	AUG	Met	ACG	thr	AAG	lys	AGG	arg	G
G	GUU	Val	GCU	ala	GAU	asp	GGU	gly	U
	GUC	Val	GCC	ala	GAC	asp	GGC	gly	C
	GUA	Val	GCA	ala	GAA	glu	GGA	gly	A
	GUG	Val	GCG	ala	GAG	glu	GGG	gly	G

** Amino acids are abbreviated as the first three letters in each case (see Table 2.4).*
†The codons UAA, UAG, and UGA are end codons (or nonsense codons); UAA and UAG are called the ochre codon and the amber codon, respectively.

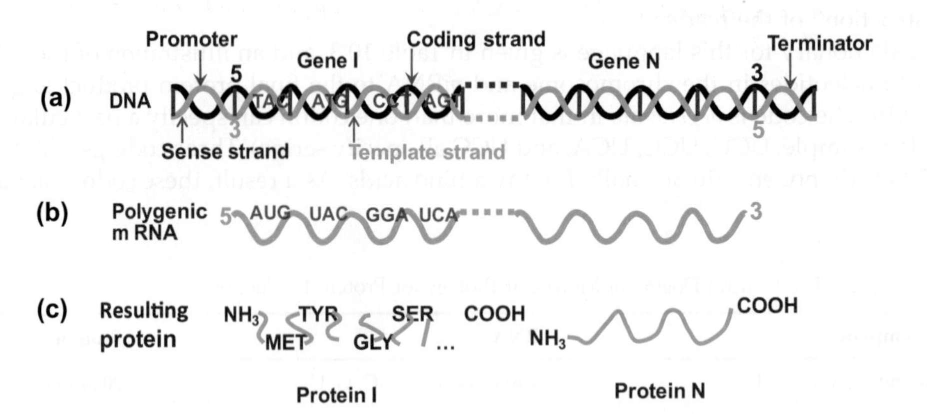

FIGURE 10.10 Overview of the transfer of information from codons on the DNA template to proteins. In prokaryotes, messages are often polygenic, whereas in eukaryotes, polygenic messages are not made and only monogenic messages are constructed.

points in translation. They are encoded at the end of each gene. Thus, they are called *end codons*. Sometime, we also call these codons *nonsense codons* because they have no correspondence to any amino acids.

The genetic code is essentially universal, although some exceptions exist (particularly in the mitochondria and for inclusion of rare amino acids). This essential universality greatly facilitates genetic engineering. The language used to make a human protein is understood in *E. coli* and yeast, and these simple cells will faithfully produce the same amino acid sequence as a human cell.

Knowing the genetic language, we may now examine the mechanism by which proteins are actually constructed.

10.4.2. Translation: How the Machinery Works

Translation is the third stage of protein biosynthesis. In translation, mRNA produced by transcription is decoded by the ribosome to produce a specific amino acid chain, or polypeptide, that will later fold into an active protein. In bacteria, translation occurs in the cell's cytoplasm, where the large and small subunits of the ribosome are located and bind to the mRNA. In eukaryotes, translation occurs across the membrane of the endoplasmic reticulum in a process called vectorial synthesis. The ribosome facilitates decoding by inducing the binding of tRNAs with complementary anticodon sequences to that of the mRNA (Fig. 2.35). The tRNA's carry specific amino acids that are chained together into a polypeptide as the mRNA passes through and is "read" by the ribosome in a fashion reminiscent to that of a stock ticker and ticker tape.

In many instances, the entire ribosome/mRNA complex will bind to the outer membrane of the rough endoplasmic reticulum and release the nascent protein polypeptide inside for later vesicle transport and secretion outside of the cell. Many types of transcribed RNA, such as *t*RNA, *r*RNA, and small nuclear RNA, do not undergo translation into proteins.

The process of translation consists of four primary steps: *activation, initiation, elongation,* and *termination*. In activation, the correct amino acid is covalently bonded to the correct tRNA. The amino acid is joined by its carboxyl group to the C3-OH of the tRNA by an ester bond. When the tRNA has an amino acid linked to it, it is termed "charged." Initiation involves the small subunit of the ribosome binding to the C5-end of mRNA with the help of initiation factors (IFs). All protein synthesis begins with an AUG codon (or GUG) on the *m-RNA*. This AUG encodes for a modified methionine, *N*-formylmethionine. In the middle of a protein, AUG encodes for methionine, so the question is how the cell knows that a particular AUG is an initiation codon or for *N*-formylmethionine. The answer lies about six to nine nucleotides upstream of the AUG, where the ribosome-binding site (Shine–Delgarmo box) is located. For prokaryotes, the consensus sequence is known as Shine–Delgarmo sequence or Shine–Delgarmo box: AGGAGG, a six base sequence just ahead of AUG. For eukaryotes, this is known as the Kozak consensus sequence: (GCC)GCCACCAUGG or (GCC) GCCGCCAUGG. That is, there is one base after the initiation codon AUG for eukaryotes. Ribosome-binding sites can vary in strength and are an important consideration in genetic engineering. The initiation of polymerization in prokaryotes requires an *initiation complex* composed of a 30s ribosomal unit with an *N*-formylmethionine bound to its initiation region, a 50s ribosomal unit, three proteins called IFs (PIF1, PIF2, and PIF3), and the phosphate bond energy from guanosine triphosphate (GTP). In eukaryotes, there are six IFs: EIF1 (AX, AY, 1B), EIF2 (α, β, γ), EIF3 (A, B, C, D, F, G, H, I, J, K, M, S6), EIF4 (A2, A3, B, E1, E2, G1, G2, G3, H), EIF5 (A, A2, 5B), and EIF6.

The elongation of the amino acid chain uses *tRNAs* as decoders. One end of the *tRNA* contains the *anticodon*, which is complementary to the codon on the *mRNA*. The other end of the *tRNA* binds a specific amino acid. The *tRNA* is called *charged* when it is carrying an amino acid. The binding of an amino acid to the *t*RNA molecule requires the energy from two phosphate bonds and enzymes known as *aminoacyl-tRNA synthetases*. Figure 2.32 depicts a *tRNA* molecule.

The basic process of protein production is addition of one amino acid at a time to the end of a protein. This operation is performed by a ribosome. The choice of amino acid type to add is determined by an mRNA molecule. Each amino acid added is matched to a three nucleotide subsequence of the mRNA. For each such triplet possible, only one particular amino acid type is accepted. The successive amino acids added to the chain are matched to successive nucleotide triplets in the mRNA. In this way, the sequence of nucleotides in the template mRNA chain determines the sequence of amino acids in the generated amino acid chain.

The mRNA carries genetic information encoded as a ribonucleotide sequence from the chromosomes to the ribosomes. The ribonucleotides are "read" by translational machinery in a sequence of nucleotide triplets called codons. Each of those triplets codes for a specific amino acid.

The ribosome molecules translate this code to a specific sequence of amino acids. The ribosome is a multisubunit structure containing rRNA and proteins. It is the "factory" where amino acids are assembled into proteins. tRNAs are small noncoding RNA chains (74–93 nucleotides) that transport amino acids to the ribosome. tRNAs have a site for amino acid attachment, and a site called an anticodon. The anticodon is an RNA triplet complementary to the mRNA triplet that codes for their cargo amino acid.

Aminoacyl-tRNA synthetase (an enzyme) catalyzes the bonding between specific tRNAs and the amino acids that their anticodon sequences call for. The product of this reaction is an aminoacyl-tRNA molecule. This aminoacyl-tRNA travels inside the ribosome, where mRNA codons are matched through complementary base pairing to specific tRNA anticodons. The ribosome has three sites for tRNA to bind. They are the aminoacyl site (abbreviated A), the peptidyl site (abbreviated P), and the exit site (abbreviated E). With respect to the mRNA, the three sites are oriented C5-to-C3 E-P-A, because ribosomes move in a C3 to C5 fashion. The A site binds the incoming tRNA with the complementary codon on the mRNA. The P site holds the tRNA with the growing polypeptide chain. The E site holds the tRNA without its amino acid. When an aminoacyl-tRNA initially binds to its corresponding codon on the mRNA, it is in the A site. Then, a peptide bond forms between the amino acid of the tRNA in the A site and the amino acid of the charged tRNA in the P site. The growing polypeptide chain is transferred to the tRNA in the A site. Translocation occurs, moving the tRNA in the P site, now without an amino acid, to the E site; the tRNA that was in the A site, now charged with the polypeptide chain, is moved to the P site. The tRNA in the E site leaves and another aminoacyl-tRNA enters the A site to repeat the process.

After the new amino acid is added to the chain, the energy provided by the hydrolysis of a GTP bound to the translocase EF-G (in prokaryotes) and eEF-2 (in eukaryotes) moves the ribosome down one codon toward the C3 end. The energy required for translation of proteins is significant. The rate of translation varies; it is significantly higher in prokaryotic cells (up to 17–21 amino acid residues per second) than in eukaryotic cells (up to 6–9 amino acid residues per second).

When a stop codon is reached, the protein is released from the ribosome with the aid of a protein *release factor* (RF). Termination of the polypeptide happens when the A site of the ribosome faces a stop codon (UAA, UAG, or UGA). No tRNA can recognize or bind to this codon. Instead, the stop codon induces the binding of a RF protein that prompts the disassembly of the entire ribosome/mRNA complex. The 70s ribosome then dissociates into 30s and 50s subunits. An *mRNA* typically is being read by many (for example, 10 to 20) ribosomes at once; as soon as one ribosome has moved sufficiently far along the message that the ribosome-binding site is not physically blocked, another ribosome can bind and initiate synthesis of a new polypeptide chain.

A number of antibiotics act by inhibiting translation; these include anisomycin, cycloheximide, chloramphenicol, tetracycline, streptomycin, erythromycin, and puromycin, among others. Prokaryotic ribosomes have a different structure from that of eukaryotic ribosomes, and thus antibiotics can specifically target bacterial infections without any detriment to a eukaryotic host's cells.

10.4.3. Posttranslational Processing: Making the Product Useful

Often the polypeptide formed from the ribosome must undergo further processing before it can become truly useful. First, the newly formed polypeptide chain must fold to assume native secondary and tertiary structures, which is known as protein folding. In some cases, several different chains must associate to form a particular enzyme or structural protein. Additionally, *chaperones* are an important class of proteins that assist in the proper folding of peptides. There are distinct pathways to assist in folding polypeptides. The level of chaperones in a cell increases in response to environmental stresses such as high temperature. Misfolded proteins are subject to degradation if they remain soluble. Often misfolded proteins aggregate and form insoluble particles (i.e. inclusion bodies). High levels of expression of foreign proteins through recombinant DNA technology in *E. coli* often overwhelm the processing machinery, resulting in inclusion bodies.

The formation of proteins in inclusion bodies greatly complicates any bioprocess, since in vitro methods to unfold and refold the protein product must be employed. Even when a cell properly folds a protein, additional cellular processing steps must occur to make a useful product. This may include the formation of disulfide bridges or attachment of any of a number of biochemical functional groups, such as acetate, phosphate, various lipids and carbohydrates. Enzymes may also remove one or more amino acids from the leading (amino) end of the polypeptide chain, leaving a protein consisting of two polypeptide chains connected by disulfide bonds.

Many proteins are secreted through a membrane. In many cases, the translocation of the protein across the membrane is done *cotranslationally* (during translation), while in some cases *post translation* movement across the membrane occurs. When proteins move across a membrane, they have a *signal sequence* (about 20 to 25 amino acids). This signal sequence is clipped off during secretion. Such proteins exist in a preform and mature form. The preform is what is made from the *m-RNA*, but the actual active form is the mature form. The preform is the signal sequence plus the mature form.

In prokaryotes, secretion of proteins occurs through the cytoplasmic membrane. In *E. coli* and most gram-negative bacteria, the outer membrane blocks release of the secreted protein into the extracellular compartment. In gram-positive cells, secreted proteins readily pass the cell wall into the extracellular compartment. Whether a protein product is retained in a cell or released has a major impact on bioprocess design.

In eukaryotic cells, proteins are released by two pathways. Both involve *exocytosis,* where *transport vesicles* fuse with the plasma membrane and release their contents. Transport vesicles mediate the transport of proteins and other chemicals from the endoplasmic reticulum (ER) to the Golgi apparatus and from the Golgi apparatus to other membrane-enclosed compartments. Such vesicles bud from a membrane and enclose an aqueous solution with specific proteins, lipids, or other compounds. In the secretory pathway vesicles, carrying proteins bud from the ER, enter the *cis* face of the Golgi apparatus, exit the Golgi *trans* face, and then fuse with the plasma membrane. Only proteins with a signal sequence are processed in the ER to enter the secretory pathway. Two pathways exist. One is the *constitutive exocytosis pathway,* which operates at all times and delivers lipids and proteins to the plasma membrane. The second is the *regulated exocytosis pathway,* which typically is in specialized secretory cells. These cells secrete proteins or other chemicals only in response to specific chemical signals.

Other modifications to proteins can take place, particularly in higher eukaryotic cells. These modifications involve the addition of nonamino acid components (for example, sugars and lipids) and *phosphorylation*. *Glycosylation* refers to the addition of sugars. These modifications can be quite complex and are important considerations in the choice of host organisms for the production of proteins. A bioprocess engineer must be aware that many proteins are subject to extensive processing after the initial polypeptide chain is made.

A particularly important aspect of post translational processing is *N-linked glycosylation.* The glycosylation pattern can serve to target the protein to a particular compartment or to control its degradation and removal from the organism. For therapeutic proteins injected into the human body, these issues are critical ones. A protein product may be ineffective if the *N*-linked glycosylation pattern is not humanlike, as the protein may not reach the target tissue or may be cleared (i.e. removed) from the body before it exerts the desired action. Furthermore, undesirable immunogenic responses can occur if a protein has a nonhumanlike pattern. Thus, the glycoform of a protein product is a key issue in bioprocesses to make therapeutic proteins.

The process of *N*-linked glycosylation occurs *only* in eukaryotic cells and involves both the ER and Golgi. Thus, the use of prokaryotic cells, such as *E. coli,* to serve as hosts for expression of human therapeutic proteins is limited to those proteins where *N*-linked glycosylation is not present or unimportant. However, not all eukaryotic cells produce proteins with humanlike, *N*-linked glycosylation. For example, yeasts, lower fungi, and insect cells often produce partially processed products. Even mammalian cells (including human cells) will show altered patterns of glycosylation when cultured in bioreactors, and these patterns can shift upon scale-up in bioreactor size.

The process of *N*-linked glycosylation is depicted in Fig. 10.11. The pattern shown is "typical," and many variants are possible. The natural proteins in the human body usually

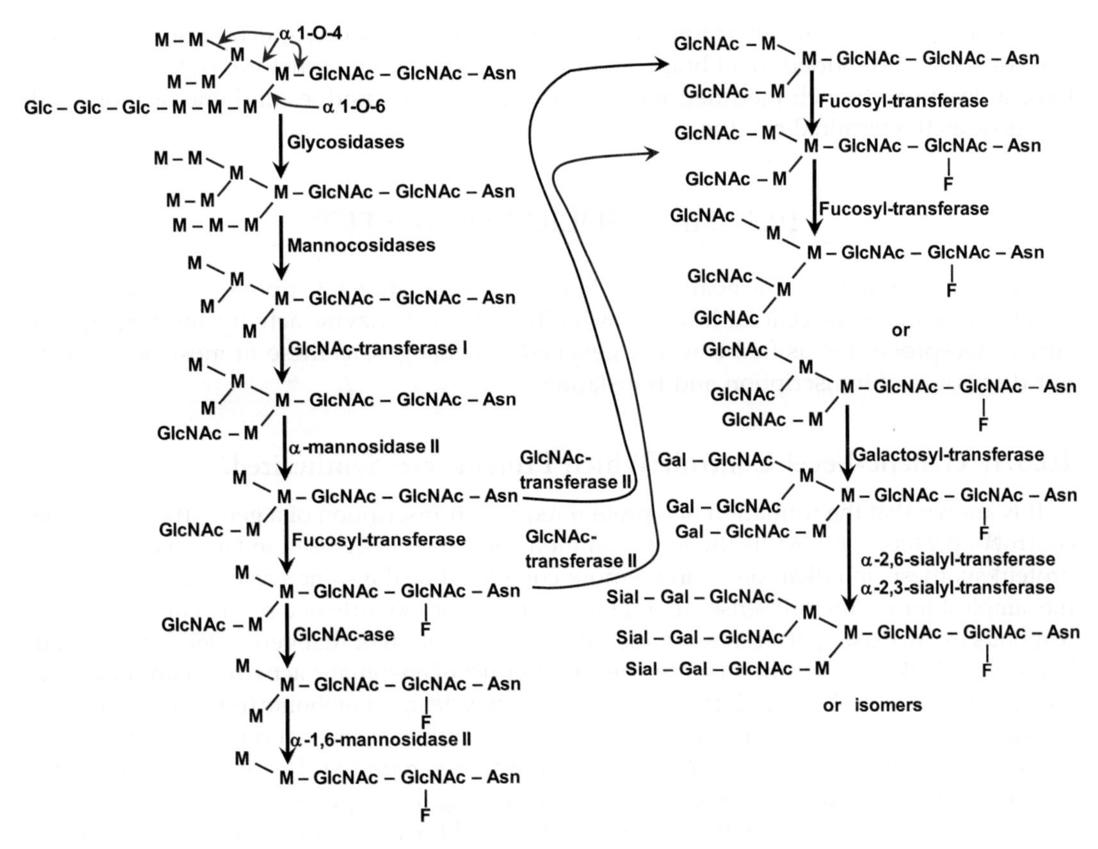

FIGURE 10.11 Example of a *N*-linked glycosylation pathway (Glc = glucose residue, M = mannose residue, GlcNAc = *N*-acetylglucosamine residue, F = fucose residue, Gal = galactose residue, Sial = sialic acid residue). The oligosaccharide side-chain is bound to an asparagine (Asn) of the protein. The upper (and main) arms are connected via α-1-O-4 connection and the lower ones via α-1-O-6. The GlcNAc-ase step is important in insect cells but not mammalian cells.

display a range of glycoforms; a single form is not observed. A simple sequence of three amino acids, of which asparagine must be one, is required for attachment of *N*-linked sugars and amino sugars. The sequence at the attachment site is Asn-Xaa-Ser/Thr, where Xaa is any amino acid and the third amino acid in the sequence must be serine or threonine.

The process of *N*-linked glycosylation begins in the ER, where a preformed branched oligosaccharide (the *dolichol pyrophosphate-oligosaccharide*) with 14 sugars is transferred to the amino group of asparagine. The 14-sugar residue is first "trimmed" by a set of specific glycosidases. In yeast, oligosaccharide processing often stops in the ER, leading to *simple glycoforms* (or high mannose or oligomannose forms). The initial trimming takes place in the ER, followed by transfer to the Golgi apparatus where final trimming occurs, followed by addition of various sugars or amino sugars. These units are added through the action of various glycosyltransferases using nucleotide-sugar cosubstrates as sugar donors. In insect cells, high levels of *N*-acetylglucosaminidase activity results typically in dead-end structures with a mannose cap. *Complex glycoforms* have sugar residues (*N*-acetylglucosamine, galactose, and/or sialic acid) added to all branches of the oligosaccharide structure. *Hybrid glycoforms* have at least one branch modified with one of these sugar residues and one or more with mannose as the terminal residue.

10.5. METABOLIC REGULATION

Metabolic regulation is the heart of any living cell. Regulation takes place principally at the genetic level and at the cellular level (principally, control of enzyme activity and through cell surface receptors). Let us first consider genetic-level changes, as these fit most closely with our discussion of transcription and translation.

10.5.1. Genetic-Level Control: Which Proteins are Synthesized?

It is known that the formation of a protein requires transcription of a gene. Transcriptional control of protein synthesis is the most common control strategy used in bacteria. Control of protein synthesis in eukaryotes can be more complex, but the same basic concepts hold. In the simplest terms, the cell senses that it has too much or too little of a particular protein and responds by increasing or decreasing the rate of transcription of that gene. One form of regulation is *feedback repression*. In this case, the end product of enzymatic activity accumulates and blocks transcription. Another form of regulation is *induction*; a metabolite (often a substrate for a pathway) accumulates and acts as an *inducer* of transcription. These concepts are summarized in Figs 10.12 and 10.13. In both cases, a repressor protein is required. The repressor can bind to the *operator* region and hinder RNA polymerase binding. For repression, a corepressor (typically the end product of the pathway) is required, and the repressor can block transcription only when bound to the corepressor. For induction, the inducer (typically a substrate for a reaction) will combine with the repressor, and the complex is inactive as a repressor.

Figures 10.12 and 10.13 show that several genes are under the control of a single promoter. A set of contiguous genes, encoding proteins with related functions, under the control of

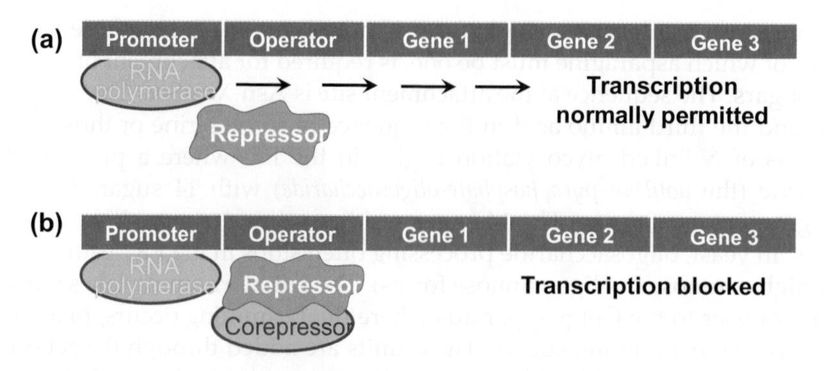

FIGURE 10.12 Process of enzyme repression. (a) Transcription of the operon occurs because the repressor is unable to bind to the operator. (b) After a corepressor (small molecule) binds to the repressor, the repressor now binds to the operator and blocks transcription. *mRNA* and the proteins it codes for are not made.

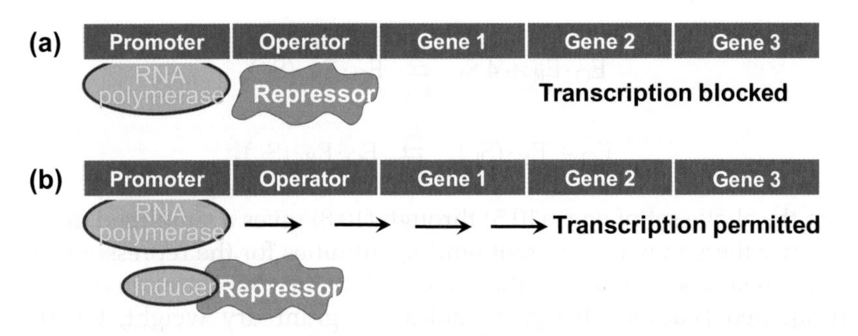

FIGURE 10.13 Process of enzyme induction. (a) A repressor protein binds to the operator region and blocks the action of RNA polymerase. (b) Inducer molecule binds to the repressor and inactivates it. Transcription by RNA polymerase occurs and an *mRNA* for that operon is formed.

a single promoter–operator is called an *operon*. The *operon* concept is central to understanding microbial regulation. Control can be even more complex than indicated in Figs 10.12 and 10.13. *Escherichia coli* is well-studied species in terms of the promoter–operon coordination. The lactose (or lac) operon controls the synthesis of three proteins involved in lactose utilization as a carbon and energy source in *E. coli*. These genes are *lac z* (gene 1), *lac y* (gene 2), and *lac a* (gene 3). The repressor is made on a separate gene called *lac i*. Lac z encodes β-galactosidase (or lactase), which cleaves lactose to glucose and galactose. The lac y protein is lactose *permease*, which acts to increase the rate of uptake of lactose into the cell. *Lac a* is for thiogalactoside transacylase. Lactose is modified in the cell to allolactose, which acts as the inducer. The conversion of lactose to allolactose is through a secondary activity of the enzyme β-galactosidase. Repression of transcription in uninduced cells is incomplete, and a low level (*basal level*) of proteins from the operon is made. Allolactose acts as indicated in Fig. 10.13, but induction by allolactose is not both necessary and sufficient for maximum transcription. Further regulation is exerted through *catabolite repression* (also called the *glucose effect*).

The three genes coding for enzymes necessary for lactose metabolism in *E. coli* are coordinated in a so-called operon, and gene expression is coordinately controlled by two regulatory sites positioned upstream of the genes (see Fig. 10.13): (1) Control at the operator by a repressor protein; (2) Carbon catabolite repression at the promotor. The repressor protein E_R has two binding sites—one site that specifically ensures binding to the operator (E_O) and one site which may bind lactose (S_L). When lactose binds to the repressor protein, its conformation changes so that its affinity for binding to the operator is significantly reduced. Thus, lactose prevents the repressor protein from binding to the operator, and transcription of the genes by RNA polymerase is therefore allowed. Consequently, lactose serves as an inducer of transcription; i.e. expression of the three genes *lacZ*, *lacY*, and *lacA* is not possible unless lactose or another inducer, e.g. isopropyl-13-D-thiogalactoside, abbreviated IPTG, is present. The binding of the repressor protein to lactose and the operator may be described by

$$E_R + 4\,S_L \underset{k_{-1}}{\overset{k_1}{\rightleftarrows}} E_R \cdot (S_L)_4 \tag{10.5}$$

$$E_O + E_R \underset{k_{-2}}{\overset{k_2}{\rightleftarrows}} E_O \cdot E_R \tag{10.6}$$

$$E_O \cdot E_R + 4\,S_L \underset{k_{-3}}{\overset{k_3}{\rightleftarrows}} E_O \cdot E_R \cdot (S_L)_4 \tag{10.7}$$

$$E_O + E_R \cdot (S_L)_4 \underset{k_{-4}}{\overset{k_4}{\rightleftarrows}} E_O \cdot E_R \cdot (S_L)_4 \tag{10.8}$$

The model in the above set of eqns (10.5) through (10.8) gives a simplified description of the true system since there may be different binding affinities for the repressor protein depending on how much lactose is bound to the protein. With the concentration of the species (indicated with squared brackets) being in moles per gram dry weight, the (reciprocals of equilibrium) constants K_i, $i = 1, 2, 3, 4$ are given by:

$$K_1 = \frac{k_{-1}}{k_1} = \frac{[E_R][S_L]^4}{[E_R \cdot (S_L)_4]} \tag{10.9}$$

$$K_2 = \frac{k_{-2}}{k_2} = \frac{[E_R][E_O]}{[E_O \cdot E_R]} \tag{10.10}$$

$$K_3 = \frac{k_{-3}}{k_3} = \frac{[E_O \cdot E_R][S_L]^4}{[E_O \cdot E_R \cdot (S_L)_4]} \tag{10.11}$$

$$K_4 = \frac{k_{-4}}{k_4} = \frac{[E_O][E_R \cdot (S_L)_4]}{[E_O \cdot E_R \cdot (S_L)_4]} \tag{10.12}$$

A macroscopic description can be used to express the influence of the reacting species on the kinetics, i.e. the concentrations of the different components are used. However, microorganisms only contain a few (1–4) copies of one type of operator per cell and the number of repressor proteins per cell is also low (10–20). For such small entities, the meaning of concentrations and of thermodynamic equilibrium is disputable, and it may be more correct to apply a stochastic modeling approach. As in Michaelis–Menten kinetics for enzymes all reactions in (10.6) through (10.8) are assumed to be equilibrium reactions. This is reasonable since the relaxation times for the equilibria are much smaller than for most other cellular reactions.

Balances for the repressor, operator, and inducer are

$$[E_R]_T = [E_R] + [E_R \cdot (S_L)_4] + [E_O \cdot E_R] + [E_O \cdot E_R \cdot (S_L)_4] \tag{10.13}$$

$$[E_O]_T = [E_O] + [E_O \cdot E_R] + [E_O \cdot E_R \cdot (S_L)_4] \tag{10.14}$$

$$[S_L]_T = [S_L] + 4\,[E_R \cdot (S_L)_4] + 4\,[E_O \cdot E_R \cdot (S_L)_4] \tag{10.15}$$

where the subscript T refers to the total concentration. In wild-type *E. coli*, there are 10–20 times more repressor molecules than there are operators, and in this case, the last two terms in Eqn (10.13) can be neglected. That is,

$$[E_R]_T \approx [E_R] + [E_R \cdot (S_L)_4] = [E_R] + K_1 [E_R][S_L]^4 \tag{10.16}$$

Equation (10.15) can be simplified by assuming that the intracellular concentration of inducer molecules is in sufficient excess over repressor molecules, and consequently that $4\,[E_R \cdot (S_L)_4] + 4\,[E_O \cdot E_R \cdot (S_L)_4] << [S_L]$. That is,

$$[S_L] \approx [S_L]_T \tag{10.17}$$

With these simplifications, the fraction of repressor-free operators is found to be

$$\begin{aligned}\frac{[E_O]}{[E_O]_T} &= \frac{[E_O]}{[E_O]+[E_O\cdot E_R]+[E_O\cdot E_R\cdot (S_L)_4]}\\&= \frac{[E_O]}{[E_O]+K_2^{-1}[E_O][E_R]+K_4^{-1}K_1^{-1}[E_O][E_R][S_L]^4}\\&= \frac{1}{1+K_2^{-1}[E_R]+K_4^{-1}K_1^{-1}[E_R][S_L]^4}\\&\approx \frac{1}{1+\dfrac{K_2^{-1}K_1+K_4^{-1}[S_L]_T^4}{K_1+[S_L]_T^4}[E_R]_T}\end{aligned} \tag{10.18}$$

Since the total number of operators of a given type in the cell is very small, it does not make much sense to talk about the fraction of repressor-free operators. However, in a description of enzyme synthesis, one may use Eqn (10.18) as an expression for the probability that the operator is repressor free.

Since the transcription of the three genes in the operon is likely to be determined by the fraction of repressor-free operators, Eqn (10.18) is valuable for description of the synthesis of the enzymes necessary for lactose metabolism that aims at describing diauxic growth on glucose and lactose. The inducer concentration $[S_L]$ likely to be correlated with the extracellular lactose concentration, whereas the total content of repressor protein can be assumed to be constant.

Small molecules that influence the transcription of genes are called effectors, and in the lac-operon, the effector (lactose) is an *inducer*. In other operons, there may, however, be a negative type of control, and here the effector is called an *antiinducer*. With an inducer, the binding affinity to the operator of the tree repressor is much larger than that of the inducer-repressor complex. i.e. $K_2 >> K_4$, whereas with antiinducer it is the other way round. For an antiinducer, the action of repressor-free operators can be found from an expression similar to Eqn (10.18).

The other control mechanism in the lac-operon is the so-called carbon catabolite repression, which ensures that no enzymes necessary for lactose metabolism are synthesized as long as a preferred substrate is available, e.g. glucose. When *E. coli* senses the presence of a carbon-energy source preferred to lactose, it will not use the lactose until the preferred substrate (e.g. glucose) is fully consumed. This control mechanism is exercised through a protein called *CAP* (cyclic-AMP-activating protein). Cyclic-AMP (cAMP, the single phosphate residue is bound on both C3 and C5 positions of the ribose residue) levels increase as the amount of energy available to the cell decreases. Thus, if glucose or a preferred substrate is depleted, the level of cAMP will increase. Under these conditions, cAMP will readily bind to CAP to form a complex that binds near the lac promoter. This complex greatly enhances RNA polymerase binding to the lac promoter. *Enhancer* regions exist in both prokaryotes and eukaryotes.

The site of the binding of the cAMP-CAP complex has been located in several operons that are under carbon catabolite repression, and binding of the complex to DNA has been found to promote helix destabilization downstream. This in turn facilitates the binding of the RNA polymerase and hereby stimulates gene expression. The carbon catabolite repression can be described by the following equilibria:

$$\mathrm{CAP} + m\,\mathrm{cAMP} \underset{k_{-5}}{\overset{k_5}{\rightleftarrows}} \mathrm{CAP}\cdot(\mathrm{cAMP})_m \tag{10.19}$$

$$\mathrm{E_P} + \mathrm{CAP}\cdot(\mathrm{cAMP})_m \underset{k_{-6}}{\overset{k_6}{\rightleftarrows}} \mathrm{E_P CAP}\cdot(\mathrm{cAMP})_m \tag{10.20}$$

where m is a stoichiometric coefficient. Equilibrium between CAP and the promotor (E_P) is not considered, since this binding coefficient is taken to be very small. Again, we apply an assumption of a pseudo-steady state and assume that the concentrations of the individual components can be used. Thus, the association (or rather the dissociation) constants are

$$K_5 = \frac{k_{-5}}{k_5} = \frac{[\mathrm{CAP}][\mathrm{cAMP}]^m}{[\mathrm{CAP}\cdot(\mathrm{cAMP})_m]} \tag{10.21}$$

$$K_6 = \frac{k_{-6}}{k_6} = \frac{[\mathrm{E_P}][\mathrm{CAP}\cdot\mathrm{cAMP}]}{[\mathrm{E_P}\cdot\mathrm{CAP}\cdot\mathrm{cAMP}]} \tag{10.22}$$

and the total balances for CAP and promotor are

$$[\mathrm{CAP}]_\mathrm{T} = [\mathrm{CAP}] + [\mathrm{CAP}\cdot(\mathrm{cAMP})_m] + [\mathrm{E_P}\cdot\mathrm{CAP}\cdot(\mathrm{cAMP})_m] \tag{10.23}$$

$$[\mathrm{E_P}]_\mathrm{T} = [\mathrm{E_P}] + [\mathrm{E_P}\cdot\mathrm{CAP}\cdot(\mathrm{cAMP})_m] \tag{10.24}$$

We can now derive an expression for the fraction of promoters being activated:

$$\frac{[\mathrm{E_P}\cdot\mathrm{CAP}\cdot(\mathrm{cAMP})_m]}{[\mathrm{E_P}]_T} = \frac{[\mathrm{CAP}][\mathrm{cAMP}]^m}{K_5K_6 + [\mathrm{CAP}][\mathrm{cAMP}]^m} \tag{10.25}$$

The ratio in Eqn (10.25) can be used to model the repression effect of glucose, just as the ratio in Eqn (10.18) is used to describe the induction of lactose on gene expression and hereby synthesis of enzymes necessary for lactose metabolism. However, in order to apply Eqn (10.25), one needs to know the intracellular level of CAP (which in a simple model may be assumed to be constant) and also the level of cAMP. There are many routes one may take to model the cAMP level, such as the adenosine triphosphate (ATP) concentration, specific growth rate, and the level of currently utilized substrate concentration. Harder and Roels (1982) suggested the following empirical correlation between [cAMP] and the extracellular glucose concentration $[\mathrm{S_G}]$,

$$[\mathrm{cAMP}] = \frac{K}{K + [\mathrm{S_G}]} \tag{10.26}$$

With Eqn (10.26) [cAMP] is linked up to the glucose concentration in the medium, and the genetic model may be used to describe diauxic growth. Equation (10.26) is a totally empirical description of all the different processes involved in determining the cAMP level in the cell at different glucose concentrations. This illustrates a general problem when a genetically structured model is combined with overall models for cell function: Certain mechanisms may be described in great detail—in this case, the gene expression, whereas other processes are described by completely empirical expressions. Hereby the performance of the overall model is largely determined by the performance of the empirical expressions in the model, and it may be adequate to apply a simpler model for the gene expression.

The real strength of the genetic approach is, however, not its linkage to the overall growth model but rather the possibility offered to analyze the influence of specific model parameters on the process. Thus, using the above model, the importance of the different equilibrium constants, which are related to the binding affinities, e.g. of the repressor to the operator, can be studied in detail. This can be done by comparison with experimental data for the mRNA level, preferably at conditions where the overall cell activity is the same in all experiments.

One should now see how the cellular control strategy emerges and how to model it mathematically. If the cell has an energetically favorable carbon-energy source available, it will not expend significant energy to create a pathway for utilization of a less favorable carbon-energy source. If, however, energy levels are low, then it seeks an alternative carbon-energy source. If and only if lactose is present will it activate the pathway necessary to utilize it.

Catabolite repression is a global response that affects more than lactose utilization. Furthermore, even for lactose, the glucose effect can work at levels other than genetic. The presence of glucose inhibits the uptake of lactose, even when an active uptake system exists. This is called *inducer exclusion*.

The role of global regulatory systems is still emerging. One concept is that of a *regulon*. Many noncontiguous gene products under the control of separate promoters can be coordinately expressed in a regulon. The best-studied regulon is the *heat shock regulon*. The cell has a specific response to a sudden increase in temperature (or other stresses that result in abnormal protein formation or membrane disruption), which results in the elevated synthesis of specific proteins. Evidence now exists that this regulon works by employing the induction of an alternative sigma factor, which leads to high levels of transcription from promoters that do not readily recognize the normal *E. coli* σ factor. Examples of other regulons involve nitrogen and phosphate starvation, as well as a switch from aerobic to anaerobic conditions.

Although many genes are regulated, others are not. Unregulated genes are termed *constitutive*, which means that their gene products are made at a relatively constant rate irrespective of changes in growth conditions. Constitutive gene products are those that a cell expects to utilize under almost any condition; the enzymes involved in glycolysis are an example.

Example 10-1.

Diauxic growth is a term to describe the sequential use of two different carbon-energy sources. Industrially, diauxic growth is observed when fermenting a mixture of sugars, such as those obtained from the hydrolysis of biomass. The classic example of diauxic growth is growth of *E. coli* on a glucose–lactose mixture. Observations on this system led to formulation of the operon hypothesis and the basis for a Nobel prize (for J. Monod and F. Jacob). Consider the plot in Fig. 10.14, where the utilization of glucose and lactose and the growth of a culture are depicted for a batch culture (batch reactor). As we will discuss in more detail in Chapter 11, the amount of biomass in a culture, X, accumulates exponentially. Note that at

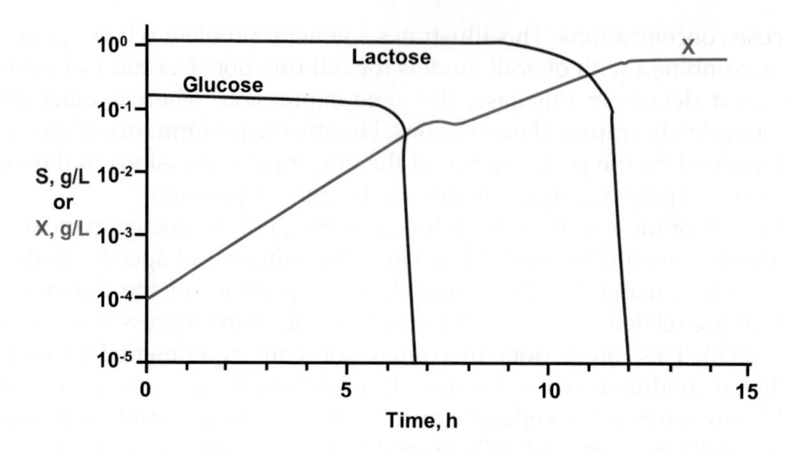

FIGURE 10.14 Diauxic growth curve for *E. coli* on glucose and lactose.

2 h after inoculation, cells are growing rapidly, glucose is being consumed, and lactose is not being utilized. At 7 h, cell mass accumulation is zero. All the glucose has been consumed. At 10 h, the culture is growing and lactose is being consumed, but the rate of growth (cell mass accumulation) is less than at 2 h. Explain what is happening with intracellular control to account for the observations at 2, 7, and 10 h. What rate of β-galactosidase formation would you expect to find in the culture at these times in comparison to the basal rate (which is <1% of the maximum rate)?

Solution:

At 2 h, the lac-operon is fully induced, since lactose converted to allolactose combines with the *lac i* repressor protein, inactivating it. With the repressor protein deactivated, RNA polymerase is free to bind to the promoter but does so inefficiently. Glucose levels are still high, which results in higher levels of ATP and low levels of AMP and cAMP. Consequently, little cAMP-CAP complex is formed, and the interaction of the lac promoter with RNA polymerase is weak in the absence of cAMP-CAP. The rate of β-galactosidase formation would be slightly increased from the basal level—perhaps 5% of the maximal rate.

At 7 h, the glucose has been fully consumed. The cell cannot generate energy, and the level of ATP decreases and cAMP increases. The cAMP-CAP complex level is high, which increases the efficiency of binding RNA polymerase to the lac promoter. This increased binding leads to increased transcription and translation. The rate of β-galactosidase formation is maximal and much higher than the basal rate or the 2 h rate. However, the cells have not yet accumulated sufficient intracellular concentrations of β-galactosidase and lac permease to allow efficient use of lactose and rapid growth.

At 10 h, the intracellular content of proteins made from the lac-operon is sufficiently high to allow maximal growth on lactose. However, this growth rate on lactose is slower than on glucose, since lactose utilization generates energy less efficiently. Consequently, the cAMP level remains higher than when the cell was growing on glucose. The level of production of β-galactosidase is thus higher than the basal or 2-h level.

Irrespective of whether an enzyme is made from a regulated or constitutive gene, its activity in the cell is regulated. Let us now consider control at the enzymatic level.

10.5.2. Metabolic Pathway Control

In Chapter 8, we learned how enzyme activity could be modulated by inhibitors or activators. Here, we discuss how the activities of a group of enzymes (a pathway) can be controlled. The cell will attempt to make the most efficient use of its resources; the fermentation specialist tries to disrupt the cell's control strategy so as to cause the cell to overproduce the product of commercial interest. An understanding of how cells control their pathways is therefore vital to the development of many bioprocesses.

First, consider the very simple case of a linear pathway making a product, P_1. Most often the first reaction in the pathway is inhibited by accumulation of the product (*feedback inhibition* or *end-product inhibition*). The enzyme for the entry of substrate into the pathway would be an allosteric enzyme (as described in Chapter 8), where the binding of the end product in a secondary site distorts the enzyme so as to render the primary active site ineffective. Thus, if the cell has a sufficient supply of P_1 (perhaps through an addition to the growth medium), it will deactivate the pathway so that the substrates normally used to make P_1 can be utilized elsewhere.

This simple concept can be extended to more complicated pathways with many branch points (see Fig. 10.15). Assuming that P_1 and P_2 are both essential metabolites, the cell may use one of several strategies to ensure adequate levels of P_1 and P_2 with efficient utilization of substrates.

One strategy is the use of isofunctional enzymes (*isozymes*). Two separate enzymes are made to carry out the same conversion, while each is sensitive to inhibition by a different end product. Thus, if P_1 is added in excess in the growth medium, it inhibits one of the

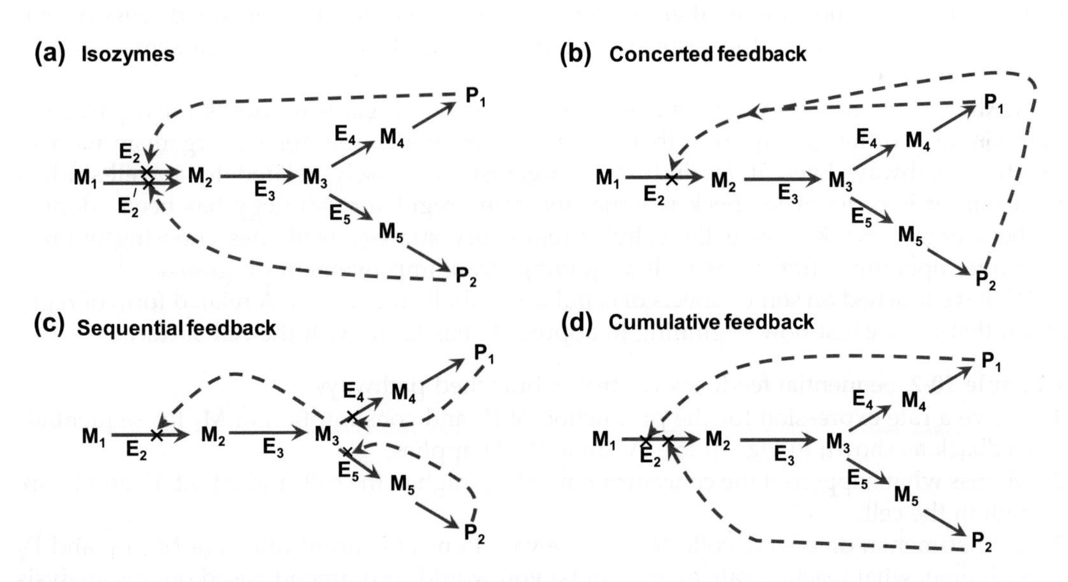

FIGURE 10.15 Examples of feedback control of branched pathways. P_1 and P_2 are the desired end products. M_1, M_2,..., M_j are intermediates, and E_j is the enzyme involved in converting metabolite M_{j-1} to M_j possible paths of inhibition are shown by dashed lines.

isozymes (E_2), while the other enzyme (E_2') is fully active. Sufficient activity remains through isozyme E_2' to ensure adequate synthesis of P_2.

An alternative approach is *concerted feedback inhibition*. Here, a single enzyme with two allosteric binding sites (for P_1 and P_2) controls entry into the pathway. A high level of either P_1 or P_2 is not sufficient by itself to inhibit enzyme E_2, while a high level of both P_1 and P_2 will result in full inhibition.

A third possibility is *sequential feedback inhibition*, by which an intermediate at the branch point can accumulate and act as the inhibitor of metabolic flux into the pathway. High levels of P_1 and P_2 inhibit enzymes E_4 and E_5, respectively. If either E_4 or E_5 is blocked, M_3 will accumulate, but not as rapidly as when both E_4 or E_5 are blocked. Thus, intermediate flux levels are allowed if either P_1 or P_2 is high, but the pathway is inactivated if both P_1 and P_2 are high.

Other effects are possible in more complex pathways. A single allosteric enzyme may have effector sites for several end products of a pathway; each effector causes only partial inhibition. Full inhibition is a cumulative effect, and such control is called *cumulative feedback inhibition* or *cooperative feedback inhibition*. In other cases, effectors from related pathways may also act as activators. Typically, this situation occurs when the product of one pathway was the substrate for another pathway.

One may wonder what are the differences between feedback inhibition and repression. Inhibition occurs at the enzyme level and is rapid; repression occurs at the genetic level and is slower and more difficult to reverse. In bacteria where growth rates are high, unwanted enzymes are diluted out by growth. Would such a strategy work for higher cells in differentiated structures? Clearly not, since growth rates would be nearly zero. In higher cells (animals and plants), the control of enzyme levels is done primarily through the control of protein degradation rather than at the level of synthesis. Most of our discussion has centered on prokaryotes; the extension of these concepts to higher organisms must be done carefully.

Another caution is that the control strategy that one organism adopts for a particular pathway may differ greatly from that adopted by even a closely related organism with an identical pathway. Even if an industrial organism is closely related to a well-studied organism, it is prudent to check whether the same regulatory strategy has been adopted by both organisms. Knowing the cellular regulatory strategy facilitates choosing optimal fermenter operating strategy, as well as guiding strain improvement programs.

We have touched on some aspects of cellular metabolic regulation. A related form of regulation that we are just now beginning to appreciate has to do with the cell surface.

Example 10-2. Sequential feedback control of branched pathways.

1. Derive a rate expression for the production of P_1 and consumption of M_1 for sequential feedback as shown in Fig. 10.15c. Assume PSSH applies.
2. Discuss what happens if the concentration of P_1 is high in the cell, and if both P_1 and P_2 are high in the cell.
3. If experimental data were collected for the variations of concentrations of M_1, P_1, and P_2 with time, what reaction rate expression(s) you would recommend based on this analysis to analyze the measured data?

Solution:

1. To derive a reasonable rate expression from the simplified pathway given in Fig. 10.15c, we first add some details to the reactions (stoichiometry):

$$M_1 + E_2 \underset{k_{-1}}{\overset{k_1}{\rightleftarrows}} M_1 \cdot E_2 \overset{k_{1c}}{\rightarrow} M_2 + E_2 \tag{E10-2.1}$$

$$M_3 + E_2 \underset{k_{-f1}}{\overset{k_{f1}}{\rightleftarrows}} M_3 \cdot E_2 \tag{E10-2.2}$$

$$M_2 + E_3 \underset{k_{-2}}{\overset{k_2}{\rightleftarrows}} M_2 \cdot E_3 \overset{k_{2c}}{\rightarrow} M_3 + E_3 \tag{E10-2.3}$$

$$M_3 + E_4 \underset{k_{-3}}{\overset{k_3}{\rightleftarrows}} M_3 \cdot E_4 \overset{k_{3c}}{\rightarrow} M_4 + E_4 \tag{E10-2.4}$$

$$P_1 + E_4 \underset{k_{-f2}}{\overset{k_{f2}}{\rightleftarrows}} P_1 \cdot E_4 \tag{E10-2.5}$$

$$M_4 \overset{k_{4c}}{\rightarrow} P_1 \tag{E10-2.6}$$

$$M_3 + E_5 \underset{k_{-5}}{\overset{k_5}{\rightleftarrows}} M_3 \cdot E_5 \overset{k_{5c}}{\rightarrow} M_5 + E_5 \tag{E10-2.7}$$

$$P_2 + E_5 \underset{k_{-f3}}{\overset{k_{f3}}{\rightleftarrows}} P_2 \cdot E_5 \tag{E10-2.8}$$

$$M_5 \overset{k_{6c}}{\rightarrow} P_2 \tag{E10-2.9}$$

We have assumed that the intermediate product M_4 and desired product P_1 are essentially the same or required no catalyst to proceed. The same holds for M_5 and P_2. The rate of reaction or rate of generation for species j is given by (Chapter 3),

$$r_j = \sum_{i=1}^{N_R} \nu_{ji} r_i \tag{E10-2.10}$$

where r_j is the reaction rate for species j, N_R is the total number of reactions in the system, ν_{ji} is the stoichiometric coefficient of species j in the reaction i, and r_i is the rate of reaction for the reaction i as written. Based on the reaction system described by Eqns (E10-2.1) through (E10-2.9), the reaction rates can be written as

$$r_{M_1} = -k_1[M_1][E_2] + k_{-1}[M_1E_2] \tag{E10-2.11}$$

$$r_{M_1E_2} = k_1[M_1][E_2] - (k_{-1} + k_{1c})[M_1E_2] \tag{E10-2.12}$$

$$r_{M_3E_2} = k_{f1}[M_3][E_2] - k_{-f1}[M_3E_2] \tag{E10-2.13}$$

$$r_{M_2} = k_{1c}[M_1E_2] - k_2[M_2][E_3] + k_{-2}[M_2E_3] \tag{E10-2.14}$$

$$r_{M_2E_3} = k_2[M_2][E_3] - (k_{-2} + k_{2c})[M_2E_3] \tag{E10-2.15}$$

$$\begin{aligned} r_{M_3} = {} & k_{2c}[M_2E_3] - k_3[M_3][E_4] + k_{-3}[M_3E_4] - k_5[M_3][E_5] \\ & + k_{-5}[M_3E_5] - k_{f1}[M_3][E_2] + k_{-f1}[M_3E_2] \end{aligned} \tag{E10-2.16}$$

$$r_{M_3E_4} = k_3[M_3][E_4] - (k_{-3} + k_{3c})[M_3E_4] \tag{E10-2.17}$$

$$r_{P_1E_4} = k_{f2}[P_1][E_4] - k_{-f2}[P_1E_4] \tag{E10-2.18}$$

$$r_{M_3E_5} = k_5[M_3][E_5] - (k_{-5} + k_{5c})[M_3E_5] \tag{E10-2.19}$$

$$r_{P_2E_5} = k_{f3}[P_2][E_5] - k_{-f3}[P_2E_5] \tag{E10-2.20}$$

$$r_{M_4} = k_{3c}[M_3E_4] - k_{4c}[M_4] \tag{E10-2.21}$$

$$r_{M_5} = k_{5c}[M_3E_5] - k_{6c}[M_5] \tag{E10-2.22}$$

$$r_{P_1} = k_{4c}[M_4] - k_{f2}[P_1][E_4] + k_{-f2}[P_1E_4] \tag{E10-2.23}$$

$$r_{P_2} = k_{6c}[M_5] - k_{f3}[P_2][E_5] + k_{-f3}[P_2E_5] \tag{E10-2.24}$$

The species balances:

$$[M_1]_T = [M_1] + [M_1E_2] \tag{E10-2.25}$$

$$[M_2]_T = [M_2] + [M_2E_3] \tag{E10-2.26}$$

$$[M_3]_T = [M_3] + [M_3E_2] + [M_3E_4] + [M_3E_5] \tag{E10-2.27}$$

$$[M_4]_T = [M_4] \tag{E10-2.28}$$

$$[M_5]_T = [M_5] \tag{E10-2.29}$$

$$[P_1]_T = [P_1] + [P_1E_4] \tag{E10-2.30}$$

$$[P_2]_T = [P_2] + [P_2E_5] \tag{E10-2.31}$$

and the enzyme balances:

$$[E_2]_T = [E_2] + [M_1E_2] + [M_3E_2] \tag{E10-2.32}$$

$$[E_3]_T = [E_3] + [M_2E_3] \tag{E10-2.33}$$

$$[E_4]_T = [E_4] + [M_3E_4] + [P_1E_4] \tag{E10-2.34}$$

$$[E_5]_T = [E_5] + [M_3E_5] + [P_2E_5] \tag{E10-2.35}$$

When the cell is fully functional, i.e. all the pathways reached steady operation, pseudo-steady state assumptions can be applied to all the intermediates: M_2, M_3, M_4, M_5, and $M_1 \cdot E_2$, $M_3 \cdot E_2$, $M_2 \cdot E_3$, $M_3 \cdot E_4$, $P_1 \cdot E_4$, $M_3 \cdot E_5$, $P_2 \cdot E_5$. That is to say, the rates of these species are zero.

$$0 = r_{M_1E_2} = k_1[M_1][E_2] - (k_{-1} + k_{1c})[M_1E_2] \tag{E10-2.36}$$

$$0 = r_{M_3E_2} = k_{f1}[M_3][E_2] - k_{-f1}[M_3E_2] \tag{E10-2.37}$$

$$0 = r_{M_2} = k_{1c}[M_1E_2] - k_2[M_2][E_3] + k_{-2}[M_2E_3] \tag{E10-2.38}$$

$$0 = r_{M_2E_3} = k_2[M_2][E_3] - (k_{-2} + k_{2c})[M_2E_3] \tag{E10-2.39}$$

$$\begin{aligned} 0 = r_{M_3} = & \, k_{2c}[M_2E_3] - k_3[M_3][E_4] + k_{-3}[M_3E_4] - k_5[M_3][E_5] \\ & + k_{-5}[M_3E_5] - k_{f1}[M_3][E_2] + k_{-f1}[M_3E_2] \end{aligned} \tag{E10-2.40}$$

$$0 = r_{M_3E_4} = k_3[M_3][E_4] - (k_{-3} + k_{3c})[M_3E_4] \tag{E10-2.41}$$

$$0 = r_{P_1E_4} = k_{f2}[P_1][E_4] - k_{-f2}[P_1E_4] \tag{E10-2.42}$$

$$0 = r_{M_3E_5} = k_5[M_3][E_5] - (k_{-5} + k_{5c})[M_3E_5] \tag{E10-2.43}$$

$$0 = r_{P_2E_5} = k_{f3}[P_2][E_5] - k_{-f3}[P_2E_5] \tag{E10-2.44}$$

$$0 = r_{M_4} = k_{3c}[M_3E_4] - k_{4c}[M_4] \tag{E10-2.45}$$

$$0 = r_{M_5} = k_{5c}[M_3E_5] - k_{6c}[M_5] \tag{E10-2.46}$$

Equations (E10-2.30) through (E10-2.46) can be employed to determine the intermediate species concentrations in the cell.

Equations (E10-2.43), (E10-2.44), and (10.2-35) yield

$$[E_5] = \frac{K_5[E_5]_T}{K_5 + K_5K_{f3}^{-1}[P_2] + [M_3]} \tag{E10-2.47}$$

Equations (E10-2.41), (E10-2.42), and (10.2-34) yield

$$[E_4] = \frac{K_3[E_4]_T}{K_3 + K_3K_{f2}^{-1}[P_1] + [M_3]} \tag{E10-2.48}$$

Equations (E10-2.39) and (10.2-33) yield

$$[E_3] = \frac{K_2[E_3]_T}{K_2 + [M_3]} \tag{E10-2.49}$$

Equations (E10-2.12), (E10-2.13), and (10.2-32) yield

$$[E_2] = \frac{K_1[E_2]_T}{K_1 + K_1K_{f1}^{-1}[M_3] + [M_1]} \tag{E10-2.50}$$

where

$$K_i = \frac{k_{-i} + k_{ic}}{k_i} \qquad i = 1, 2, 3, \text{ and } 5 \tag{E10-2.51}$$

and

$$K_{fi} = \frac{k_{-fi}}{k_{fi}} \qquad i = 1,2,3 \tag{E10-2.52}$$

Equations (E10-2.38), (E10-2.40), together with Eqns (E10-2.41) and (E10-2.43), give

$$\frac{k_{1c}[\mathrm{M_1}][\mathrm{E_2}]_T}{K_1 + K_1 K_{f1}^{-1}[\mathrm{M_3}] + [\mathrm{M_1}]} = \frac{k_{3c}[\mathrm{M_3}][\mathrm{E_4}]_T}{K_3 + K_3 K_{f2}^{-1}[\mathrm{P_1}] + [\mathrm{M_3}]} + \frac{k_{5c}[\mathrm{M_3}][\mathrm{E_5}]_T}{K_5 + K_5 K_{f3}^{-1}[\mathrm{P_2}] + [\mathrm{M_3}]} \tag{E10-2.53}$$

Therefore, the feedback control has rendered the system nonlinear to the degree that multiple steady states are possible. The intermediate concentration $[\mathrm{M_3}]$ can be determined by solving Eqn (E10-2.53).

The rate of formation for $\mathrm{P_1}$ can be obtained by

$$\begin{aligned} r_{\mathrm{P_1}} &= \sum_{i=1}^{N_R} \nu_{\mathrm{P_1}i} r_i = k_{4c}[\mathrm{M_4}] - k_{f2}[\mathrm{P_1}][\mathrm{E_4}] + k_{-f2}[\mathrm{P_1E_4}] \\ &= k_{4c}[\mathrm{M_4}] = k_{3c}[\mathrm{M_3E_4}] = k_{3c}K_3^{-1}[\mathrm{M_3}][\mathrm{E_4}] \\ &= \frac{k_{3c}[\mathrm{M_3}][\mathrm{E_4}]_\mathrm{T}}{K_3 + K_3 K_{f2}^{-1}[\mathrm{P_1}] + [\mathrm{M_3}]} \end{aligned} \tag{E10-2.54}$$

and the rate of disappearance of $\mathrm{M_1}$ is given by

$$\begin{aligned} -r_{\mathrm{M_1}} &= -\sum_{i=1}^{N_R} \nu_{\mathrm{M_1}i} r_i = k_1[\mathrm{M_1}][\mathrm{E_2}] - k_{-1}[\mathrm{M_1E_2}] \\ &= k_{1c}[\mathrm{M_1E_2}] = k_{1c}K_1^{-1}[\mathrm{M_1}][\mathrm{E_2}] = \frac{k_{1c}[\mathrm{M_1}][\mathrm{E_2}]_\mathrm{T}}{K_1 + K_1 K_{f1}^{-1}[\mathrm{M_3}] + [\mathrm{M_1}]} \end{aligned} \tag{E10-2.55}$$

Also, substituting Eqn (E10-2.53) into (E10-2.55) yields

$$-r_{\mathrm{M_1}} = \frac{k_{3c}[\mathrm{M_3}][\mathrm{E_4}]_T}{K_3 + K_3 K_{f2}^{-1}[\mathrm{P_1}] + [\mathrm{M_3}]} + \frac{k_{5c}[\mathrm{M_3}][\mathrm{E_5}]_T}{K_5 + K_5 K_{f3}^{-1}[\mathrm{P_2}] + [\mathrm{M_3}]} \tag{E10-2.56}$$

2. From Eqn (E10-2.54), one can conclude that if $\mathrm{P_1}$ is accumulated to high levels the rate of formation of $\mathrm{P_1}$ is lowered. If both $\mathrm{P_1}$ and $\mathrm{P_2}$ are accumulated to high levels, the rate for $\mathrm{M_1}$ consumption is to be very low according to Eqn (E10-2.56). Therefore, the sequential feedback control is effective.
3. We have derived two rate expressions as shown in Eqns (E10-2.54) and (10.2-56). However, these two expressions cannot be utilized directly to analyze the measured concentration profile data. In Chapter 8, we learned that rate can be estimated by the rate at any step by adjusting the rate coefficients. Also, the intermediate concentrations can be obtained via

equilibrium to either the products or the reactants (Chapter 9) pending on the step rate were derived. In this case, it is intuitive to rewrite Eqns (E10-2.54) and (E10-2.56) as

$$r_{P_1} = \frac{r_{P_1\max}[M_1]}{K_{M1} + K_{fP1}[P_1] + [M_1]} \tag{E10-2.57}$$

$$-r_{M_1} = \frac{r_{P_1\max}[M_1]}{K_{M1} + K_{fP1}[P_1] + [M_1]} + \frac{r_{P_2\max}[M_1]}{K_{M2} + K_{fP2}[P_2] + [M_1]} \tag{E10-2.58}$$

where $[M_3]$ has been related to $[M_1]$ via equilibrium, all the K's are rate constants.

This example shows that the metabolic pathways can be applied to derive at kinetics of the metabolism.

Example 10-3. Fluxes in Sequential feedback control of branched pathways.

Derive a flux expression for the production of P_1 for sequential feedback as shown in Fig. 10.15c. Assume PSSH is applicable.

Solution:

In the previous example, we have shown how the kinetics can be derived from metabolic pathway via reaction rate approach. In this example, we examine the flux approach to the kinetics. To derive a reasonable flux expression from the simplified pathway given in Fig. 10.15c, we first identify all the nodes and connections as shown in Fig. E10-3.1. We next identify all the fluxes:

$$J_{1'} = J_1 = k_1[M_1][E_2] - k_{-1}[M_1E_2] \tag{E10-3.1}$$

$$J_{2'} = J_2 = k_{1c}[M_1E_2] \tag{E10-3.2}$$

$$J_{3'} = J_3 = k_2[M_2][E_3] - k_{-2}[M_2E_3] \tag{E10-3.3}$$

$$J_{4'} = J_4 = k_{2c}[M_2E_3] \tag{E10-3.4}$$

$$J_5 = J_6 = k_{f1}[M_3][E_2] - k_{-f1}[M_3E_2] \tag{E10-3.5}$$

$$J_{7'} = J_7 = k_3[M_3][E_4] - k_{-3}[M_3E_4] \tag{E10-3.6}$$

$$J_{8'} = J_8 = k_{3c}[M_3E_4] \tag{E10-3.7}$$

$$J_9 = k_4[M_4] \tag{E10-3.8}$$

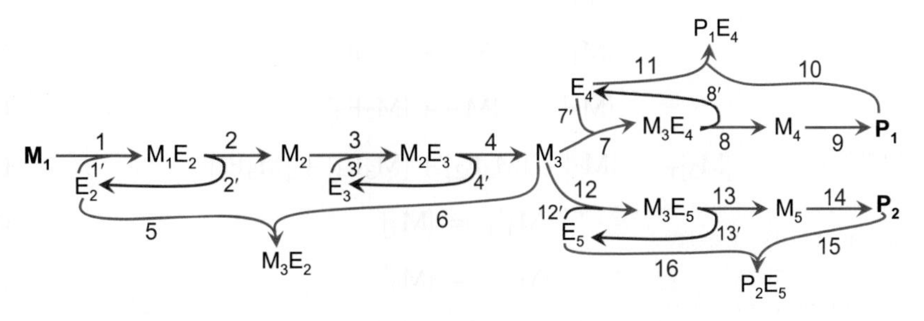

FIGURE E10-3.1 Schematic of a sequential feedback control of branched pathways showing all the nodes and flux connections.

$$J_{10} = J_{11} = k_{f2}[P_1][E_4] - k_{-f2}[P_1E_4] \quad (E10\text{-}3.9)$$

$$J_{12'} = J_{12} = k_5[M_3][E_5] - k_{-5}[M_3E_5] \quad (E10\text{-}3.10)$$

$$J_{13'} = J_{13} = k_{5c}[M_3E_5] \quad (E10\text{-}3.11)$$

$$J_{14} = k_6[M_5] \quad (E10\text{-}3.12)$$

$$J_{15} = J_{16} = k_{f3}[P_2][E_5] - k_{-f3}[P_2E_5] \quad (E10\text{-}3.13)$$

With PSSH, all the net fluxes passing through the internal notes (i.e. E_2, M_1E_2, M_2, E_3, M_2E_3, M_3E_2, E_4, M_3E_4, M_4, P_1E_4, E_5, M_3E_5, M_5, P_2E_5) are zero. That is,

$$E_2 \Rightarrow \quad 0 = -J_{1'} + J_{2'} - J_5 \quad (E10\text{-}3.14)$$

$$M_1E_2 \Rightarrow \quad 0 = J_1 - J_2 \quad (E10\text{-}3.15)$$

$$M_2 \Rightarrow \quad 0 = J_2 - J_3 \quad (E10\text{-}3.16)$$

$$E_3 \Rightarrow \quad 0 = -J_{3'} + J_{4'} \quad (E10\text{-}3.17)$$

$$M_2E_3 \Rightarrow \quad 0 = J_3 - J_4 \quad (E10\text{-}3.18)$$

$$M_3E_2 \Rightarrow \quad 0 = J_5 - J_6 \quad (E10\text{-}3.19)$$

$$E_4 \Rightarrow \quad 0 = -J_{7'} + J_{8'} - J_{11} \quad (E10\text{-}3.20)$$

$$M_3E_4 \Rightarrow \quad 0 = J_7 - J_8 \quad (E10\text{-}3.21)$$

$$M_4 \Rightarrow \quad 0 = J_8 - J_9 \quad (E10\text{-}3.22)$$

$$P_1E_4 \Rightarrow \quad 0 = J_{10} - J_{11} \quad (E10\text{-}3.23)$$

$$E_5 \Rightarrow \quad 0 = -J_{12'} + J_{13'} - J_{16} \quad (E10\text{-}3.24)$$

$$M_3E_5 \Rightarrow \quad 0 = J_{12} - J_{13} \quad (E10\text{-}3.25)$$

$$M_5 \Rightarrow \quad 0 = J_{13} - J_{14} \quad (E10\text{-}3.26)$$

$$P_2E_5 \Rightarrow \quad 0 = J_{15} - J_{16} \quad (E10\text{-}3.27)$$

The species and enzyme balances apply

$$[M_1]_T = [M_1] + [M_1E_2] \quad (E10\text{-}3.28)$$

$$[M_2]_T = [M_2] + [M_2E_3] \quad (E10\text{-}3.29)$$

$$[M_3]_T = [M_3] + [M_3E_2] + [M_3E_4] + [M_3E_5] \quad (E10\text{-}3.30)$$

$$[M_4]_T = [M_4] \quad (E10\text{-}3.31)$$

$$[M_5]_T = [M_5] \quad (E10\text{-}3.32)$$

$$[P_1]_T = [P_1] + [P_1E_4] \quad (E10\text{-}3.33)$$

$$[\mathrm{P_2}]_\mathrm{T} = [\mathrm{P_2}] + [\mathrm{P_2E_5}] \tag{E10-3.34}$$

$$[\mathrm{E_2}]_\mathrm{T} = [\mathrm{E_2}] + [\mathrm{M_1E_2}] + [\mathrm{M_3E_2}] \tag{E10-3.35}$$

$$[\mathrm{E_3}]_\mathrm{T} = [\mathrm{E_3}] + [\mathrm{M_2E_3}] \tag{E10-3.36}$$

$$[\mathrm{E_4}]_\mathrm{T} = [\mathrm{E_4}] + [\mathrm{M_4E_4}] + [\mathrm{P_1E_4}] \tag{E10-3.37}$$

$$[\mathrm{E_5}]_\mathrm{T} = [\mathrm{E_5}] + [\mathrm{M_5E_5}] + [\mathrm{P_2E_5}] \tag{E10-3.38}$$

Further solution of these equations render identical solutions to the problem (for the intermediates) as compared with that from the reaction rate approach as shown in Example 10-2. The fluxes can be obtained as

$$\begin{aligned} J_1 = J_2 &= k_1[\mathrm{M_1}][\mathrm{E_2}] - k_{-1}[\mathrm{M_1E_2}] \\ &= k_{1c}[\mathrm{M_1E_2}] = k_{1c}K_1^{-1}[\mathrm{M_1}][\mathrm{E_2}] \\ &= \frac{k_{1c}[\mathrm{M_1}][\mathrm{E_2}]_\mathrm{T}}{K_1 + K_1K_{f1}^{-1}[\mathrm{M_3}] + [\mathrm{M_1}]} \end{aligned} \tag{E10-3.39}$$

$$\begin{aligned} J_4 = J_3 &= k_2[\mathrm{M_2}][\mathrm{E_3}] - k_{-2}[\mathrm{M_2E_3}] \\ &= k_{2c}[\mathrm{M_2E_3}] = k_{2c}K_2^{-1}[\mathrm{M_2}][\mathrm{E_3}] \\ &= \frac{k_{2c}[\mathrm{M_2}][\mathrm{E_3}]_\mathrm{T}}{K_2 + [\mathrm{M_2}]} \end{aligned} \tag{E10-3.40}$$

$$\begin{aligned} J_8 = J_7 &= k_{3c}[\mathrm{M_3E_4}] = k_{3c}K_3^{-1}[\mathrm{M_3}][\mathrm{E_4}] \\ &= \frac{k_{3c}[\mathrm{M_3}][\mathrm{E_4}]_\mathrm{T}}{K_3 + K_3K_{f2}^{-1}[\mathrm{P_1}] + [\mathrm{M_3}]} \end{aligned} \tag{E10-3.41}$$

$$J_9 = k_{4c}[\mathrm{M_4}] = J_8 = J_7 \tag{E10-3.42}$$

$$J_{13} = J_{12} = \frac{k_{5c}[\mathrm{M_3}][\mathrm{E_5}]_T}{K_5 + K_5K_{f3}^{-1}[\mathrm{P_2}] + [\mathrm{M_3}]} \tag{E10-3.43}$$

$$J_{14} = k_{6c}[\mathrm{M_5}] = J_{13} = J_{12} \tag{E10-3.44}$$

where the upper case K's are defined the same by Eqns (E10-2.51) and (10-2.52). That is,

$$K_i = \frac{k_{-i} + k_{ic}}{k_i} \qquad i = 1, 2, 3, \text{ and } 5 \tag{E10-3.45}$$

and

$$K_{fi} = \frac{k_{-fi}}{k_{fi}} \qquad i = 1, 2, 3 \tag{E10-3.46}$$

Keeping the same notation with reaction rate expressions allows us to see the connections between reaction expressions and the flux expressions.

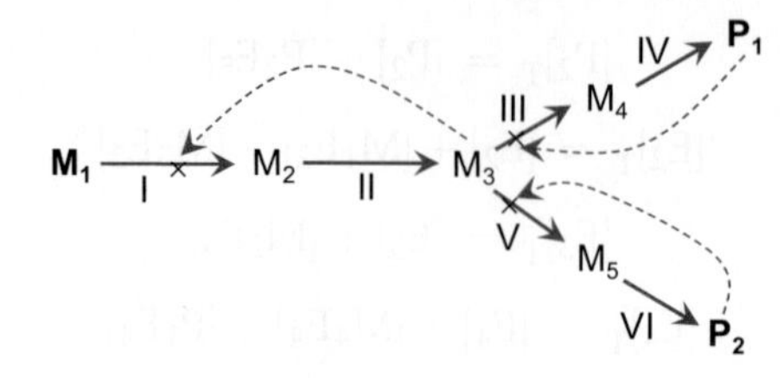

FIGURE E10-3.2 Simplified schematic of the sequential feedback control of branched pathways.

Therefore, the fluxes can be written based on simplified pathways as one usually does. The simplified pathway is shown in Fig. E10-3.2, which is identical to Fig. 10.15c, with each path numbered. The fluxes for each path can be written quite easily based on this example.

From Eqn (E10-3.39),

$$J_{\mathrm{I}} = \frac{k_{1c}[\mathrm{M}_1][\mathrm{E}_2]_{\mathrm{T}}}{K_1 + K_1 K_{f1}^{-1}[\mathrm{M}_3] + [\mathrm{M}_1]} \tag{E10-3.47}$$

From Eqn (E10-3.40),

$$J_{\mathrm{II}} = \frac{k_{2c}[\mathrm{M}_2][\mathrm{E}_3]_{\mathrm{T}}}{K_2 + [\mathrm{M}_2]} \tag{E10-3.48}$$

From Eqn (E10-3.41),

$$J_{\mathrm{III}} = \frac{k_{3c}[\mathrm{M}_3][\mathrm{E}_4]_{\mathrm{T}}}{K_3 + K_3 K_{f2}^{-1}[\mathrm{P}_1] + [\mathrm{M}_3]} \tag{E10-3.49}$$

From Eqn (E10-3.42),

$$J_{\mathrm{IV}} = k_{4c}[\mathrm{M}_4] \tag{E10-3.50}$$

From Eqn (E10-3.43),

$$J_{\mathrm{V}} = \frac{k_{5c}[\mathrm{M}_3][\mathrm{E}_5]_T}{K_5 + K_5 K_{f3}^{-1}[\mathrm{P}_2] + [\mathrm{M}_3]} \tag{E10-3.51}$$

From Eqn (E10-3.44),

$$J_{\mathrm{VI}} = k_{6c}[\mathrm{M}_5] \tag{E10-3.52}$$

This example shows that the fluxes in a complicated pathway can be easily written based on its starting point, whether enzyme is involved (which is the case for almost all the reactions in the cell) and/or regulated by other products or species in the cell. The fluxes are not linear in most cases because of the enzyme catalysis. In general, the flux expression is consistent with the Michaelis–Menten equation (Chapter 8) or any other related form pending on the type of the reaction involved.

10.6. HOW A CELL SENSES ITS EXTRACELLULAR ENVIRONMENT

When cells are placed into a new environment, whether cells respond to the change in the environment depends on whether cells are "aware" of the environment. For the cell to be aware of the environment, substances in the environment must first be moved into the cell.

10.6.1. Mechanisms to Transport Small Molecules across Cellular Membranes

A cell must take nutrients from its extracellular environment if it is to grow or retain metabolic activity. As we discussed in Example 10-1, the rate at which nutrients enter the cell can be important in regulating metabolic activity.

Molecules enter the cell through either *passive diffusion* (i.e. via concentration or Gibbs potential gradient of the nutrients being transported) or *facilitated diffusion* (coordinated reaction and diffusion). While passive diffusion is spontaneous, the facilitated diffusion can be either spontaneous or energy dependant. The energy-dependent uptake mechanisms include *active transport* and *group translocation*.

In passive diffusion, molecules move down a concentration gradient (from high to low concentration) that is thermodynamically favorable. Consequently,

$$J_{\rm A} = \frac{D_A}{\delta} S_A (C_{\rm AE} - C_{\rm AI}) = k_{\rm p}(C_{\rm AE} - C_{\rm AI}) \tag{10.27}$$

where $J_{\rm A}$ is the flux of species A across the membrane, mol/(m^2·s); $D_{\rm A}$ is the diffusivity of species A through the membrane, m^2/s; δ is the effective thickness of the membrane, m; $S_{\rm A}$ is the solubility or "partition coefficient" of species A in the membrane, $k_{\rm p}$ is the permeability, m/s, $C_{\rm AE}$ is the extracellular concentration of species A, mol/m^3; and $C_{\rm AI}$ is the intracellular concentration, mol/m^3. The cytoplasmic membrane consists of a lipid core with perhaps very small pores, thus the permeability and/or diffusivity is inversely related to the molecular size of species A. A collection of permeability coefficients for a few compounds in the cytoplasmic membrane of the plant cell *Chara ceratophylla* is given in Table 10.4. Presence of a polar group can significantly reduce the permeability: an extra hydroxyl group on the molecule decreases the permeability by 100- or 1000-fold. A carboxyl group has an even larger effect. An extra amide group is more or less equivalent to two extra hydroxyl groups. Conversely, an extra methyl group in the compound is likely to increase the permeability 5-fold, while a doubling of molecular volume decreases the permeability 30-fold. Therefore, for charged or large molecules, the value of $k_{\rm p}$ is very low and the flow of material across the membrane is negligible. The cellular uptake of water and oxygen appears to be due to passive diffusion. Furthermore, lipids or other highly hydrophobic compounds have relatively high diffusivities (10^{-12} m^2/s) in cellular membranes, and passive diffusion can be a mechanism of quantitative importance in their transport.

With facilitated transport, a carrier molecule (protein) can combine specifically and reversibly with the molecule of interest. The carrier protein is considered embedded in the membrane. The carrier protein, after binding the target molecule, undergoes conformational changes, which result in release of the molecule on the intracellular side of the membrane. The carrier can bind to the target molecule on the intracellular side of the membrane,

TABLE 10.4 Permeability Coefficients for Compounds in Membranes of the Plant Cell *Chara ceratophylla*

Compound	Permeability, m^2/s
Carbon dioxide	4.5×10^{-5}
Bicarbonate	5.0×10^{-11}
Water	6.6×10^{-8}
Urea	2.8×10^{-11}
Methanol	2.5×10^{-8}
Ethanol	1.4×10^{-8}
Ethanediol	1.7×10^{-9}
Acetamide	1.4×10^{-9}
Formamide	2.0×10^{-9}
Lactamide	1.5×10^{-10}
Butyramide	5.0×10^{-9}
Glucose	5.0×10^{-12}
Glycerol	2.2×10^{-11}

Source: Stein, W.,D., 1990. Channels, Carriers and Pumps. An Introduction to Membrane Transport. Academic Press, San Diego, CA.

resulting in the efflux or exit of the molecule from the cell. Thus, the net flux of a molecule depends on its concentration gradient. The carrier protein effectively increases the solubility of the target molecule in the membrane.

$$A_{(E)} + \text{Protein} \underset{k_{-\text{Eb}}}{\overset{k_{\text{Eb}}}{\rightleftarrows}} \text{A}\cdot\text{Protein} \tag{10.28}$$

$$A_{(I)} + \text{Protein} \underset{k_{-\text{Ib}}}{\overset{k_{\text{Ib}}}{\rightleftarrows}} \text{A}\cdot\text{Protein} \tag{10.29}$$

Assuming that the binding occurs faster than the protein conformational change and moving the molecule into the internal cell side of the membrane, one can consider reactions (10.28) and (10.29) are in equilibrium. Inside the membrane, the total concentration of the carrier protein remains constant:

$$[\text{Protein}] + C_{\text{AM}} = [\text{Protein}]_{\text{M}} \tag{10.30}$$

where C_{AM} is the concentration of target species—carrier protein complex concentration in the membrane and $[\text{Protein}]_M$ is the total concentration of carrier protein present in the membrane. Therefore, the concentration of A inside the membrane at either side of the membrane interface can be computed as

$$C_{\text{AME}} = [\text{A}\cdot\text{Protein}]_{\text{E}} = \frac{C_{\text{AE}}[\text{Protein}]_{\text{M}}}{K_{\text{AE}} + C_{\text{AE}}} \tag{10.31}$$

$$C_{AMI} = [\text{A}\cdot\text{Protein}]_I = \frac{C_{AI}[\text{Protein}]_M}{K_{AI} + C_{AI}} \tag{10.32}$$

where K_{AE} is external binding affinity of the substrate, mol/m^3 and is equal to k_{-Eb}/k_{Eb}; K_{AI} is internal binding affinity of the substrate, mol/m^3 and is equal to k_{-Ib}/k_{Ib}; C_{AMI} is the concentration of species A in the membrane at the internal side interface; and C_{AME} is the concentration of species A in the membrane at the external side interface.

The flux of the target molecule into the cell depends on concentration gradient of species A inside the membrane, that is,

$$J_A = \frac{D_{AM}}{\delta}(C_{AME} - C_{AMI}) = J_{Amax}\left(\frac{C_{AE}}{K_{AE} + C_{AE}} - \frac{C_{AI}}{K_{AI} + C_{AI}}\right) \tag{10.33}$$

where D_{AM} is the diffusivity of the protein carrier bound with species A in the membrane, and J_{Amax} is the maximum flux rate of A, $mol/(m^2\cdot s)$. One can observe from equation (10.33) that $C_{AE} < C_{AI}$ does not necessarily mean a net flux out of the cell. Facilitated transport of sugars and other low-molecular-weight organic compounds is common in eukaryotic cells, but infrequent in prokaryotes. However, the uptake of glycerol in enteric bacteria (such as *E. coli*) is a good example of facilitated transport.

Active transport is one particular type of facilitated transport in that active transport occurs *"against" a concentration gradient*, i.e. $C_{AE} < C_{AI}$. The active transport is effected by $K_{AI} > K_{AE}$. The intracellular concentration of a molecule may be a 100-fold or greater than the extracellular concentration. The movement of a molecule (by itself) up a concentration gradient is thermodynamically unfavorable and will not occur spontaneously; energy must be supplied (or coupled with another reaction) for the binding to occur. In active transport, several energy sources are possible: (1) the electrostatic or pH gradients of the proton-motive force and (2) secondary gradients (for example, of Na^+ or other ions) derived from the proton-motive force by other active transport systems and by the hydrolysis of ATP.

The *proton-motive force* results from the extrusion of hydrogen as protons. The respiratory system of cells (see section 10.7.4) is configured to ensure the formation of such gradients. Hydrogen atoms, removed from hydrogen carriers (most commonly NADH) on the inside of the membrane, are carried to the outside of the membrane, while the electrons removed from these hydrogen atoms return to the cytoplasmic side of the membrane. These electrons are passed to a final electron acceptor, such as O_2. When O_2 is reduced, it combines with H^+ from the cytoplasm, causing the net formation of OH^- on the inside. Because the flow of H^+ and OH^- across the cellular membrane by passive diffusion is negligible, the concentration of chemical species cannot equilibrate. This process generates a pH gradient and an electrical potential across the cell. The inside of the cell is alkaline compared to the extracellular compartment. The cytoplasmic side of the membrane is electrically negative, and the outside is electrically positive. The proton-motive force is essential to the transport of many species across the membrane, and any defect in the cellular membrane that allows free movement of H^+ and OH^- across the cell boundary can collapse the proton-motive force and lead to cell death.

Some molecules are actively transported into the cell without coupling to the ion gradients generated by the proton-motive force. By a mechanism that is not fully understood, the hydrolysis of ATP to release phosphate bond energy is utilized directly in transport (e.g. the transport of maltose in *E. coli*). Another energy-dependent approach to the uptake of nutrients is group translocation.

The key factor here is the chemical modification of the substrate during the process of transport. The best-studied system of this type is the *phosphotransferase system*. This system is important in the uptake of many sugars in bacteria. The biological system itself is complex, consisting of four separate phosphate-carrying proteins. The source of energy is phosphoenolpyruvate (PEP).

Effectively, the process can be represented by:

$$\text{Sugar}_{(\text{extracellular})} + \text{PEP}_{(\text{intracellular})} \rightarrow \text{sugar-P}_{(\text{intracellular})} + \text{pyruvate}_{(\text{intracellular})} \tag{10.34}$$

By converting the sugar to the phosphorylated form, the sugar is trapped inside the cell. The asymmetric nature of the cellular membrane and this process make the process essentially irreversible. Because the phosphorylation of sugars is a key step in their metabolism, nutrient uptake of these compounds by group translocation is energetically preferable to active transport. In active transport, energy would be expended to move the unmodified substrate into the cell and then further energy would be expended to phosphorylate it.

Certainly, the control of nutrient uptake is a critical cellular interface with its extracellular environment. In some cases, however, cells can sense their external environment without the direct uptake of nutrients.

Example 10-4. *Escherichia coli* uptake of lactose is found to be enzyme assisted. At one point of culturing in lactose-limiting medium, the lactose concentration in the fermentation broth is measured to be 0.1 g/L. The lactose consumption rate is determined to be 0.65 g/(L h). If the maximum volumetric lactose uptake flux is $J_{S\max}a = 1.5$ g/(L h) and the corresponding saturation parameters are given by $K_{SE} = 5$ mg/L and $K_{SI} = 0.2$ g/L. Here, a is the specific surface area of the cells, m^2/m^3-culture.

1. Determine the effective concentration of lactose inside the *E. coli* cell body (biotic phase).
2. Does the result obtained in part (a) make sense and why?

Solution. Figure E10-4.1 shows a schematic of the lactose transport and reaction process in the cell. The uptake flux may be computed through Eqn (10.33), or

$$J_S = J_{S\max}\left(\frac{S}{K_{SE} + S} - \frac{S_b}{K_{SI} + S_b}\right) \tag{E10-4.1}$$

where S is the substrate concentration in the medium (or abiotic phase) and S_b is the substrate concentration inside the cell body (biotic phase).

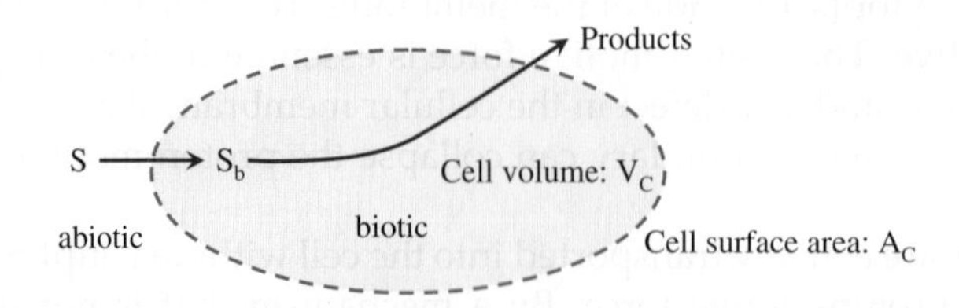

FIGURE E10-4.1 A schematic of substrate uptake and conversion by a cell.

1. Referring to Fig. E10-4.1, mass balance of lactose in the cell (area enclosed by the dotted line) yields:

$$\text{In} - \text{Out} + \text{Generation} = \text{Accumulation}$$

$$J_S A_c - 0 + r_s' V_C = 0 \tag{E10-4.2}$$

where r_s' is the rate of generation of substrate in the cell based on the cell volume. This rate is not convenient rate to use for engineering calculations because of the cell volume use.

For balanced growth, pseudo-steady state holds. There is no accumulation of substrate inside the cell. Therefore, Eqn (E10-4.2) has the out flow and accumulation terms zero. Equation (E10-4.2) can be rearranged to yield

$$J_S A_C = -r_s' V_C = -r_S V \tag{E10-4.3}$$

where V is the volume of the culture (including cell and medium). The rate r_S is a more commonly used rate. Equation (E10-4.3) leads to

$$J_S\, a = -r_S \tag{E10-4.4}$$

where a is specific surface area of the cells,

$$a = \frac{A_C}{V} \tag{E10-4.5}$$

Substituting Eqn (E10-4.1) into (E10-4.4), we obtain

$$J_{Smax} a \left(\frac{S}{K_{SE} + S} - \frac{S_b}{K_{SI} + S_b} \right) = -r_S \tag{E10-4.6}$$

which can be solved to give

$$S_b = \frac{K_{SI}}{\dfrac{1}{\dfrac{S}{K_{SE} + S} + \dfrac{r_S}{J_{Smax} a}} - 1} \tag{E10-4.7}$$

Since $K_{SI} = 0.2$ g/L, $S = 0.1$ g/L, $K_{SE} = 5$ mg/L $= 5 \times 10^{-3}$ g/L, $r_S = -0.65$ g/(L·h), and $J_{Smax} a = 1.5$ g/(L·h), Eqn (E10-4.5) gives $S_b = 0.2158$ g/L.

2. From part (a), we obtained that $S_b = 0.2518$ g/L. The lactose concentration in the biotic phase is more than double that in the medium. One may think that the diffusion flux would force the lactose out of the cell body as the concentration inside the cell body is higher than that outside of the cell (in the medium). However, the mass transfer is controlled by enzyme mediation. This is the reason that the transport of lactose is apparently against the concentration gradient. Thus, the higher concentration of lactose inside the biotic phase than that in the abiotic phase is correct.

10.6.2. Role of Cell Receptors in Metabolism and Cellular Differentiation

Almost all cells have receptors on their surfaces. These receptors can bind a chemical in the extracellular space. Such receptors are important in providing a cell with information about its environment. Receptors are particularly important in animals in facilitating cell-to-cell communication. Animal cell surface receptors are important in transducing signals for growth or cellular differentiation. These receptors are also prime targets for the development of therapeutic drugs. Many viruses mimic certain chemicals (e.g. a growth factor) and use cell surface receptors as a means to entering a cell.

Simpler examples exist with bacteria. Some motile bacteria have been observed to move up concentration gradients for nutrients or down gradients of toxic compounds. This response is called *chemotaxis.* Some microbes also respond to gradients in oxygen (*aerotaxis*) or light (*phototaxis*). Such tactic phenomena are only partially understood. However, the mechanism involves receptors binding to specific compounds, and this binding reaction results in changes in the direction of movement of the flagella. Motile cells move in a random-walk fashion; the binding of an attractant extends the length of time the cell moves on a "run" toward the attractant. Similarly, repellents decrease the length of runs up the concentration gradient.

Microbial communities can be highly structured (e.g. biofilms), and cell-to-cell communication is important in the physical structure of the biofilm. Cell-to-cell communication is also important in microbial phenomena such as bioluminescence, exoenzyme synthesis, and virulence factor production. Basically, these phenomena depend on local cell concentration. How do bacteria count? They produce a chemical known as *quorum sensing molecule,* whose accumulation is related to cell concentration. When the quorum-sensing molecule reaches a critical concentration, it activates a response in all of the cells present. A typical quorum-sensing molecule is an acylated homoserine lactone. The mechanism of quorum sensing depends on an intracellular receptor protein, while chemotaxis depends on surface receptor proteins. With higher cells, the timing of events in cellular differentiation and development is associated with surface receptors. With higher organisms, these receptors are highly evolved. Some receptors respond to steroids (*steroid hormone receptors*). Steroids do not act by themselves in cells but rather the hormone-receptor complex interacts with specific gene loci to activate the transcription of a target gene.

A host of other animal receptors respond to a variety of small proteins that act as *hormones* or *growth factors.* These growth factors are normally required for the cell to initiate DNA synthesis and replication. Such factors are a critical component in the large scale use of animal tissue cultures. Other cell surface receptors are important in the attachment of cells to surfaces. Cell adhesion can lead to changes in cell morphology, which are often critical to animal cell growth and normal physiological function. The exact mechanism by which receptors work is only now starting to emerge. One possibility for growth factors that stimulate cell division is that binding of the growth factor to the receptor causes an alteration in the structure of the receptor. This altered structure possesses catalytic activity (e.g. tyrosine kinase activity), which begins a cascade of reactions leading to cellular division. Surface receptors are continuously internalized, complexes degraded, and receptors recycled to supplement newly formed receptors. Thus, the ability of cells to respond to changes in environmental signals is continuously renewed. Such receptors will be important in our later discussions on animal cell culture.

10.7. MAJOR METABOLIC PATHWAY

We have now learned the mechanisms of cellular information transmissions. We also learned how cells uptake nutrients (substrates). The metabolism of substrates is the key in realizing the passage of the cellular information.

A major challenge in bioprocess development is to select an organism that can efficiently make a given product (from a particular substrate). Before about 1980 only naturally occurring organisms were available. With the advent of genetic engineering, it is possible to remove and add genes to an organism to alter its metabolic functions in a predetermined manner (*metabolic engineering*). In any case, the bioprocess developer must understand the metabolic capabilities of natural organisms either to use them directly or to know how to metabolically engineer them to make a desired, perhaps novel, product, from a particular substrate. Consequently, we turn our focus toward learning about some essential metabolic pathways.

Differences in microbial metabolism can be attributed partly to genetic differences and/or to differences in their responses to changes in their environment. Even the same species may produce different products when grown under different nutritional and environmental conditions. The control of metabolic pathways by nutritional and environmental regulation has become an important consideration in bioprocess engineering. For example, *Saccharomyces cerevisiae* (baker's yeast) produces ethanol when grown under anaerobic conditions. However, the major product is yeast cells (baker's yeast) when growth conditions are aerobic. Moreover, even under aerobic conditions, at high glucose concentrations some ethanol formation is observed, which indicates metabolic regulation not only by oxygen but also by glucose. This effect is known as the *Crabtree effect*.

Ethanol formation during baker's yeast fermentation may be reduced or eliminated by culture with intermittent addition of glucose or by using carbon sources other than sucrose and glucose that support less rapid growth.

The major metabolic pathways and products of various microorganisms will be briefly covered in this chapter. Metabolic pathways are subgrouped as aerobic and anaerobic metabolism. There are two key concepts in our discussion. *Catabolism* is the intracellular process of degrading a compound into smaller and simpler products (e.g. glucose to CO_2 and H_2O). Catabolism produces energy for the cell. *Anabolism* is involved in the synthesis of more complex compounds (e.g. glucose to glycogen) and requires energy.

10.7.1. Bioenergetics

Living cells require energy for biosynthesis, transport of nutrients, motility, and maintenance. This energy is obtained from the catabolism of carbon compounds, mainly carbohydrates. Carbohydrates are synthesized from CO_2 and H_2O in the presence of light by photosynthesis. The sun is the ultimate energy source for the life processes on earth. The only exception is near some thermal vents at the bottom of the ocean, where nonphotosynthetic ecosystems exist independently of sunlight.

Metabolic reactions are fairly complicated and vary from one organism to another. However, these reactions can be classified into three major categories. A schematic diagram of these reactions is presented in Fig. 10.16. The major categories are (1) fueling reactions: degradation of nutrients, (II) biosynthesis of small molecules (amino acids, nucleotides), (III) polymerization reactions: biosynthesis of large molecules, and (IV) assembling reactions. These reactions take place in the cell simultaneously. As a result of metabolic reactions, end products are formed and released from the cells. These end products (organic acids, amino acids, antibiotics) are often valuable products for human and animal consumption.

Energy in biological systems is primarily stored and transferred via ATP, which contains high-energy phosphate bonds. The active form of ATP is complexed with Mg^{2+}. The standard free-energy charge for the hydrolysis of ATP is 30.5 kJ/mol. The actual free-energy release in the cell may be substantially higher because the concentration of ATP is often much greater than that for ADP.

$$\text{ATP} + \text{H}_2\text{O} \rightleftarrows \text{ADP} + \text{H}_3\text{PO}_4, \quad \Delta G^0 = -30.5 \text{ kJ/mol} \tag{10.35}$$

Figure 10.17 shows the chemical structural changes of Eqn (10.35). Biological energy is stored in ATP by reversing this reaction to form ATP from ADP and H_3PO_4. Similarly, ADP dissociates to release energy.

$$\text{ADP} + \text{H}_2\text{O} \rightleftarrows \text{AMP} + \text{H}_3\text{PO}_4, \quad \Delta G^0 = -30.5 \text{ kJ/mol} \tag{10.36}$$

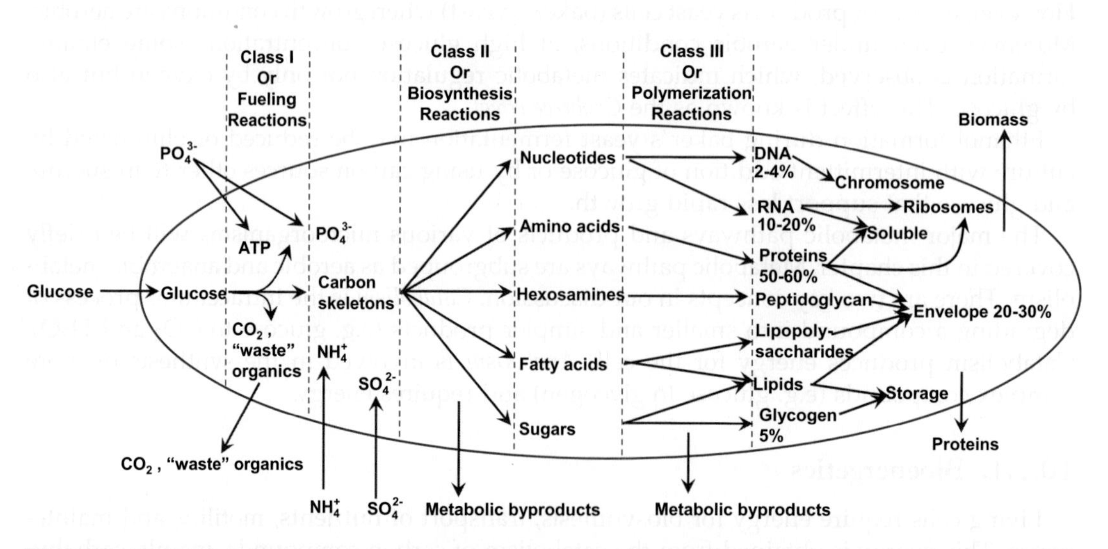

FIGURE 10.16 Schematic diagram of reactions and processes involved in cellular growth and product formation in a bacterial cell. Substrates are taken up by the cells by transport processes and converted into precursor metabolites via fueling reactions. The precursor metabolites (nucleotides, amino acids, hexosamines, fatty acids, and sugars) are converted to building blocks that are polymerized to macromolecules. Finally, macromolecules are assembled into cellular structures like membranes, organelles etc. that make up the functioning cell. Precursor metabolites and building blocks may be secreted to the extracellular medium as metabolites or they may serve as precursors for metabolites that are secreted. The cell may also secrete certain macromolecules—primarily proteins that can act as hydrolytic enzymes, but some cells may also secrete polysaccharides

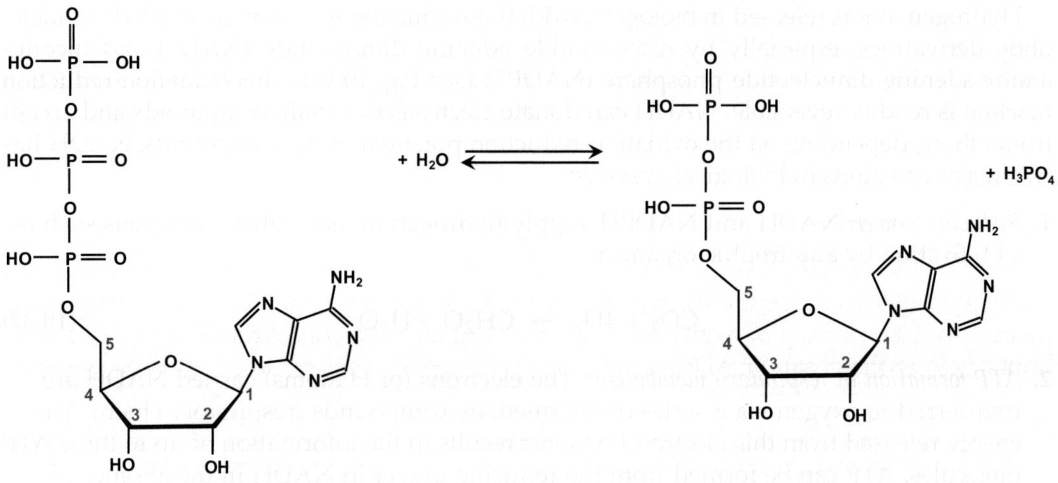

FIGURE 10.17 Structure of ATP and its hydrolysis reaction.

Analog compounds of ATP, such as GTP, uridine triphosphate, and cytidine triphosphate, also store and transfer high-energy phosphate bonds but not to the extent of ATP. High-energy phosphate compounds produced during metabolism, such as PEP and 1,3-biphosphoglycerate, transfer their phosphate group into ATP. Energy stored in ATP is later transferred to lower energy phosphate compounds such as glucose-6-phosphate and glycerol-3-phosphate, as depicted in Fig. 10.18.

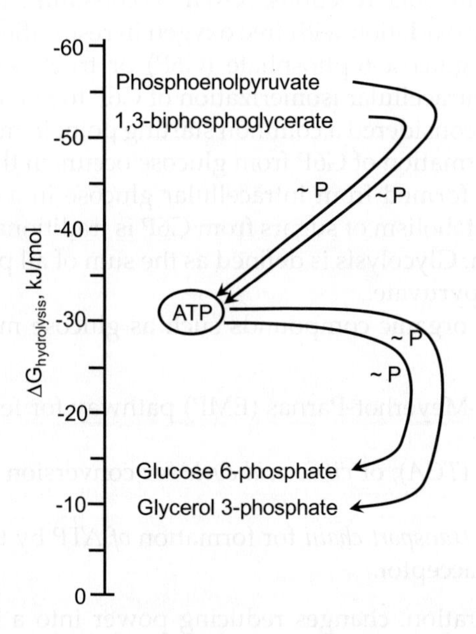

FIGURE 10.18 Transfer of biological energy from high-energy to low-energy compounds via ATP.

Hydrogen atoms released in biological oxidation-reduction reactions are carried by nucleotide derivatives, especially by nicotinamide adenine dinucleotide (NAD^+) and nicotinamide adenine dinucleotide phosphate ($NADP^+$) (see Fig. 10.19). This oxidation-reduction reaction is readily reversible. NADH can donate electrons to certain compounds and accept from others, depending on the oxidation-reduction potential of the compounds. NADH has two major functions in biological systems:

1. *Reducing power*: NADH and NADPH supply hydrogen in biosynthetic reactions such as CO_2 fixation by autotrophic organisms.

$$CO_2 + 4H_2 \rightarrow CH_2O + H_2O \tag{10.37}$$

2. *ATP formation in respiratory metabolism*: The electrons (or H atoms) carried NADH are transferred to oxygen via a series of intermediate compounds (respiratory chain). The energy released from this electron transport results in the information of up to three ATP molecules. ATP can be formed from the reducing power in NADH in the absence of oxygen if an alternative electron acceptor is available (e.g. NO_3^-).

10.7.2. Glucose Metabolism: Glycolysis and the TCA Cycle

The most frequently applied energy source for cellular growth is sugars, in particular glucose, which are converted to metabolic products (e.g. carbon dioxide, lactic acid, acetic acid, and ethanol) with concurrent formation of ATP, NADH, and NADPH. NADH is produced together with NADPH in the catabolic reactions, but whereas NADPH is consumed mainly in the anabolic reactions, NADH is consumed mainly within the catabolic reaction pathways, e.g. by oxidation with free oxygen in respiration (see Section 10.7.4). Most sugars are converted to glucose-6-phosphate (G6P) or fructose-6-phosphate (F6P) before being metabolized. The intracellular isomerization of G6P to F6P is normally in equilibrium, and G6P can therefore be considered a common starting point in many catabolic pathways. In some microorganisms, formation of G6P from glucose occurs in the transport process, but in others this compound is formed from intracellular glucose in a reaction coupled with the hydrolysis of ATP. The catabolism of sugars from G6P is traditionally divided into glycolysis and pyruvate metabolism. Glycolysis is defined as the sum of all pathways by which glucose (or G6P) is converted to pyruvate.

Aerobic catabolism of organic compounds such as glucose may be considered in three different phases:

1. Glycolysis or Embden-Meyerhof-Parnas (EMP) pathway for fermentation of glucose to pyruvate.
2. *Krebs, tricarboxylic acid* (*TCA*), or *citric acid cycle* for conversion of pyruvate to CO_2 and NADH.
3. Respiratory or *electron transport chain* for formation *of* ATP by transferring electrons from NADH to an electron acceptor.

The final phase, respiration, changes reducing power into a biologically useful energy form (ATP). *Respiration* may be aerobic or anaerobic, depending on the final electron acceptor.

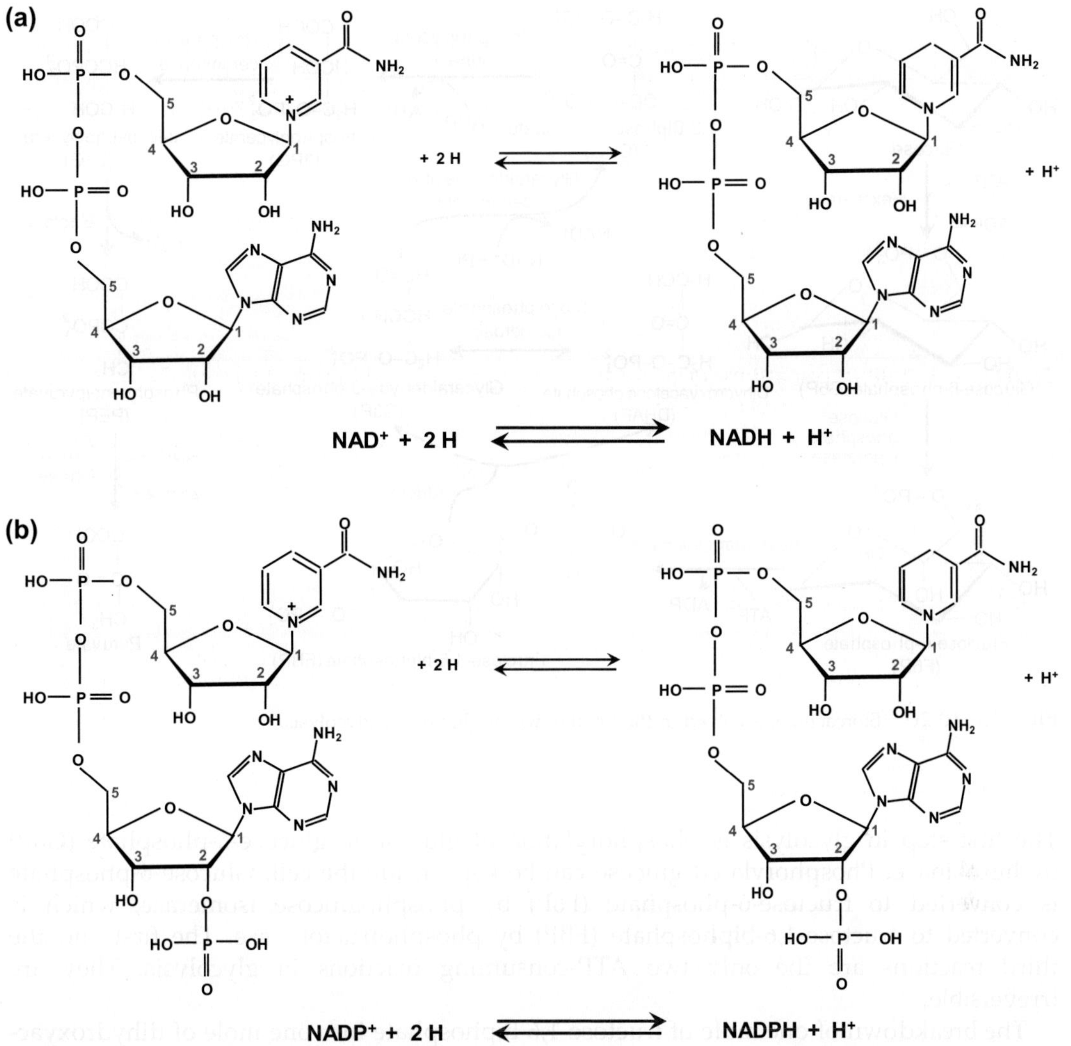

(a)

$NAD^+ + 2H \rightleftarrows NADH + H^+$

(b)

$NADP^+ + 2H \rightleftarrows NADPH + H^+$

FIGURE 10.19 Structure of the oxidation-reduction coenzyme nicotinamide adenine dinucleotide (NAD^+) and nicotinamide adenine dinucleotide phosphate $NADP^+$. (a) $NAD^+ + 2H \rightleftarrows NADH + H^+$. (b) $NADP^+ + 2H \rightleftarrows NADPH + H^+$.

If oxygen is used as final electron acceptor, the respiration is called *aerobic respiration*. When other electron acceptors, such as NO_3^-, SO_4^{2-}, Fe^{3+}, Cu^{2+}, and S, are used, the respiration is termed *anaerobic respiration*.

Glycolysis results in the breakdown of one glucose to two pyruvate molecules. The enzymatic reaction sequence involved in glycolysis is illustrated in Fig. 10.20. Each step may occur at a different part of location of the cell and is assisted by an enzyme.

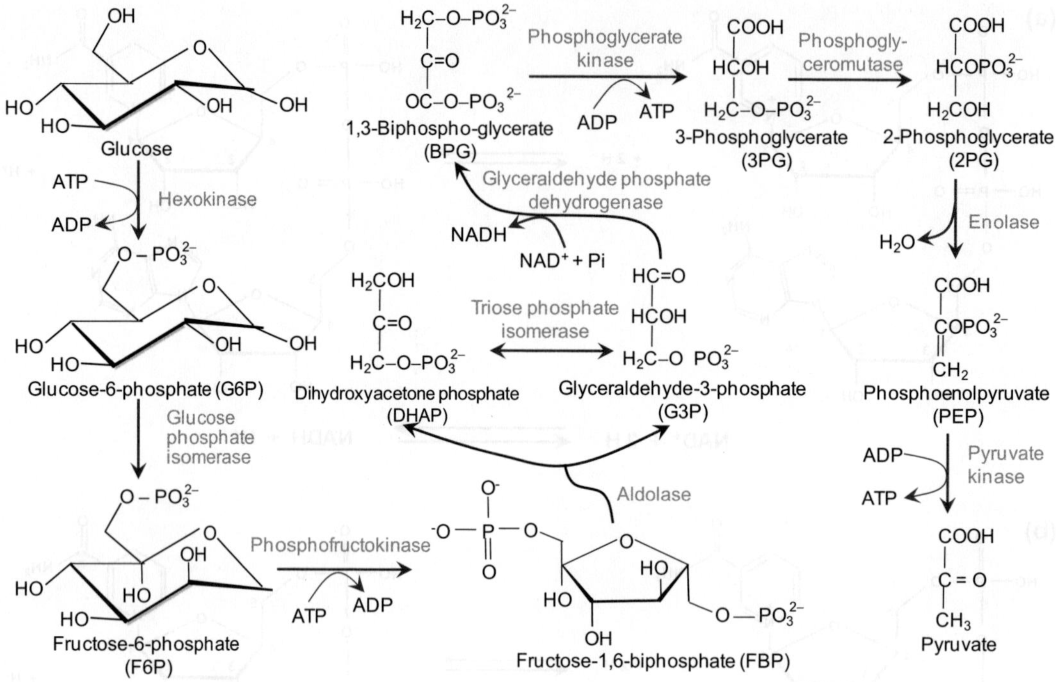

FIGURE 10.20 Bioreactions involved in the breakdown of glucose by glycolysis.

The first step in glycolysis is phosphorylation of glucose to glucose-6-phosphate (G6P) by hexokinase. Phosphorylated glucose can be kept inside the cell. Glucose-6-phosphate is converted to fructose-6-phosphate (F6P) by phosphoglucose isomerase, which is converted to fructose-1,6-biphosphate (FBP) by phosphofructokinase. The first and the third reactions are the only two ATP-consuming reactions in glycolysis. They are irreversible.

The breakdown of one mole of fructose-1,6-biphosphate into one mole of dihydroxyacetone phosphate (DHAP) and one mole of glyceraldehyde-3-phosphate (G3P) by aldolase is one of the key steps in glycolysis (e.g. C_6 to 2 C_3). DHAP and G3P are in equilibrium. As G3P is utilized in glycolysis, DHAP is continuously converted to G3P. One mole of glyceraldehyde-3-phosphate is first oxidized with the addition of inorganic phosphate to 1,3-biphosphoglycerate (BPG) by glyceraldehyde-3-phosphate dehydrogenase. BPG releases one phosphate group to form ATP from ADP and is converted to 3-phosphoglycerate (3PG) by 3-phosphoglycerate kinase. 3PG is further converted to 2-phosphoglycerate (2PG) by phosphoglyceromutase. Dehydration of 2PG to PEP by enolase is the next step. PEP is further dephosphorylated to pyruvate (Pyr) by pyruvate kinase, with the formation of an ATP. Reactions after DHAP and G3P formation repeat twice during glycolysis, i.e. there are two moles passing through to the final product of the glycolysis: pyruvate.

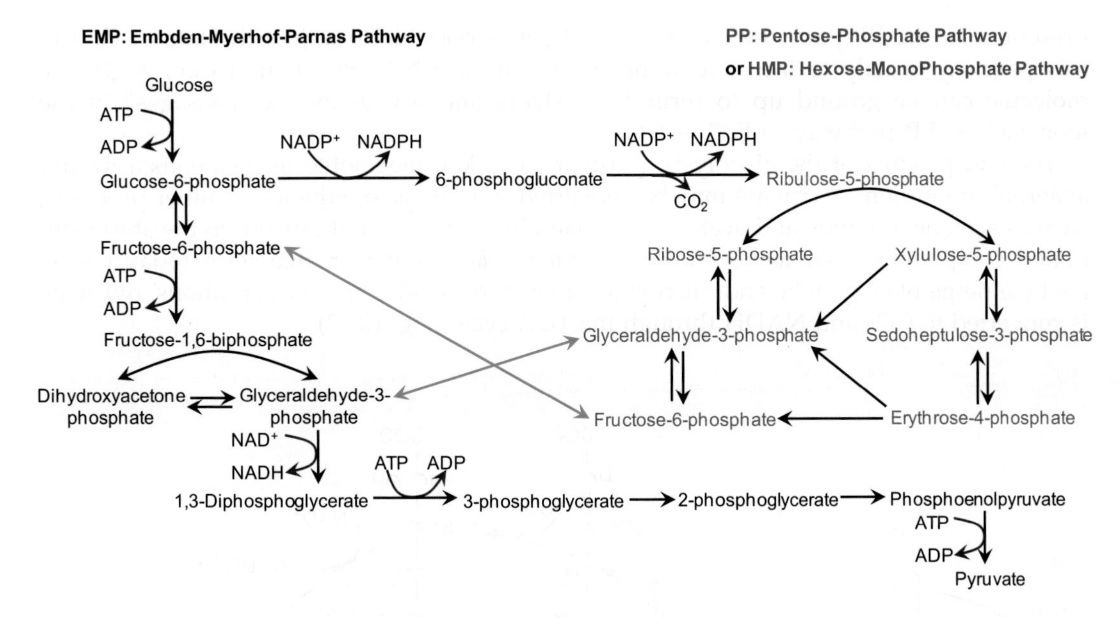

FIGURE 10.21 Embden-Meyerhof-Parnas (EMP) pathway and the pentose phosphate (PP) pathway. Each step is assisted by an enzyme, which has been omitted in the figure for clearance. The scheme is without a PTS transport system. Fructose-6-phosphate and glyceraldehyde-3-phosphate takes part in both pathways and hereby allows recycling of carbon from the PP pathway back to the EMP pathway.

Two major pathways, the EMP pathway and the pentose phosphate (PP) pathway (see Fig. 10.21), are considered as glycolysis pathways as well. For simplicity, we have neglected to identify the enzymes involved in each step. Can you add the enzymes in the schematic? The PP pathway is very closely resembled by the *hexose monophosphate pathway* (HMP). One other important pathway that can be regarded as glycolysis is *Entner-Doudoroff* (ED) pathway, which will be covered later.

In the EMP pathway, G6P is converted to pyruvate, and the overall stoichiometry from glucose is given by

$$\text{Glucose} + 2\,\text{ADP} + 2\,\text{H}_3\text{PO}_4 + 2\,\text{NAD}^+ = 2\,\text{PYR} + 2\,\text{ATP} + 2\,\text{H}_2\text{O} + 2\,\text{NADH} + 2\text{H}^+ \tag{10.38}$$

One reaction (the conversion of F6P to FBP) requires a concomitant hydrolysis of ATP to proceed, but two other reactions which run twice for every molecule of G6P produce enough Gibbs free energy to give a net production of ATP in the pathway. Since ATP (or PEP) is used for formation of G6P from glucose, the net yield of ATP is 2 mol per mole of glucose converted to pyruvate. The four electrons liberated by the partial oxidation of 1 mol glucose to 2 mol pyruvate are captured by 2 mol of NAD^+ leading to formation of 2 mol NADH.

The major function of the PP pathway is to supply the anabolic reactions with reducing equivalents in the form of NADPH and to produce the precursor metabolites ribose-5-phosphate (R5P) and erythrose-4-phosphate (E4P). Due to the branch points presented in the PP pathway (see Fig. 10.21), it is possible to adjust the fate of G6P in this pathway exactly to the cellular need for R5P and NADPH. If necessary a glucose molecule can be ground up to form 12 NADPH and 6 CO_2 by six "passages" in the loop G6P → PP pathway → F6P → G6P.

The end product of the glycolysis: pyruvate, is a key metabolite in metabolism. Under anaerobic conditions, pyruvate may be converted to lactic acid, ethanol, or other products, such as acetone, butanol, and acetic acid. Anaerobic conversion of glucose to the aforementioned compounds used to be known as *fermentation*. However, that term today covers a whole range of enzymatic and microbial conversions. Under aerobic conditions, pyruvate is converted to CO_2 and NADH through the TCA cycle (Fig. 10.22).

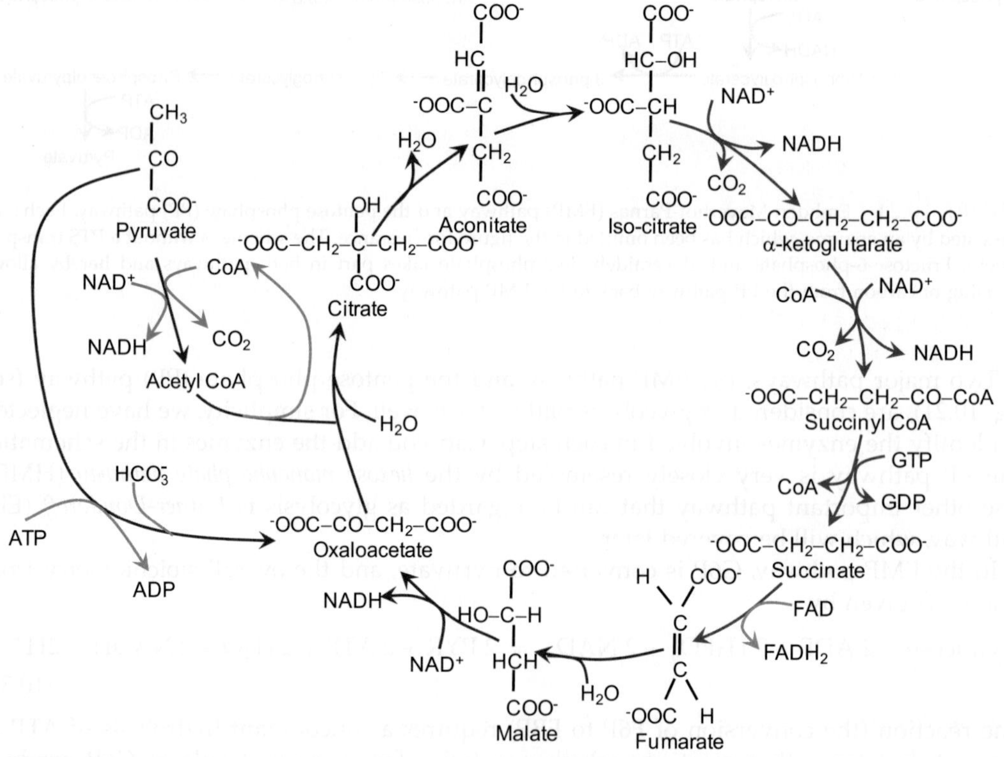

FIGURE 10.22 Tricarboxylic acid (TCA) cycle, also known as Krebs cycle, citric acid cycle, or Szent-Györgyi-Krebs cycle. TCA consists of a series of enzyme-catalyzed chemical reactions, which is of central importance in all living cells that use oxygen as part of cellular respiration. In eukaryotes, TCA occurs in the matrix of the mitochondrion. In aerobic organisms, the TCA is part of a metabolic pathway involved in the chemical conversion of carbohydrates, fats and proteins into carbon dioxide and water to generate a form of usable energy. Other relevant reactions in the pathway include those in glycolysis and pyruvate oxidation before the TCA cycle and oxidative phosphorylation after it. In addition, it provides precursors for many compounds including some amino acids and is therefore functional even in cells performing fermentation.

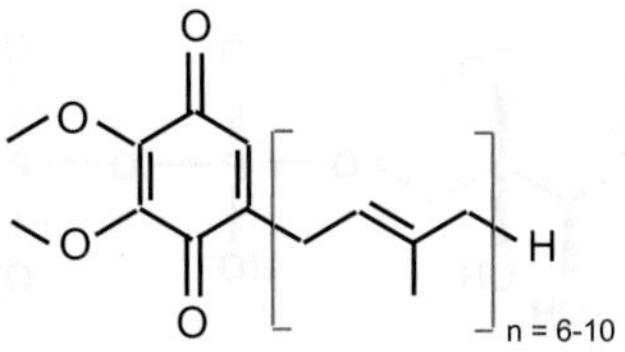

Co Enzyme Ubiquinone: CoQ_n

The pyruvate formed in the glycolysis can be oxidized completely to carbon dioxide and water in the TCA cycle, which is entered via acetyl-CoA. Here, one mole of GTP, an "energy package" equivalent to ATP, and five reduced cofactor molecules are formed for each pyruvate molecule. Four of these are NADH, the fifth is $FADH_2$. A prerequisite for the complete conversion of pyruvate in the TCA cycle is that NAD^+ and FAD can be regenerated from NADH and $FADH_2$. This is done in the respiratory chain (for details, see Section 10.7.4), an oxidative process involving free oxygen and therefore operable only in aerobic organisms. In the respiratory chain, electrons are passed from NADH to a coenzyme called ubiquinone (CoQ or CoQ_n with n being the number of isoprene units) by NADH dehydrogenase. They are carried on from CoQ_n through a sequence of cytochromes (proteins containing a heme group) and are finally donated to oxygen, forming water.

The net ATP yield in glycolysis is 2 mol ATP/glucose under anaerobic conditions. Pyruvate produced in the EMP pathway transfers its reducing power to NAD^+ via the TCA cycle. Glycolysis takes place in cytoplasm, whereas the site for the TCA cycle is the matrix of mitochondria in eukaryotes. In prokaryotes, these reactions are associated with membrane-bound enzymes. Entry into the TCA cycle is provided by the acylation of coenzyme-A by pyruvate.

$$\text{pyruvate} + NAD^+ + \text{CoA-SH} \xrightarrow[\text{}]{\text{Pyruvate dehydrogenase}} \text{acetyl CoA} + CO_2 + NADH + H^+ \quad (10.39)$$

Figure 10.23 shows the structure of CoA or CoA-SH and acetyl-CoA or CoA-S-Ac. Acetyl-CoA is transferred through mitochondrial membrane at the expense of the conversion of the two NADHs produced in glycolysis to 2 $FADH_2$. Acetyl-CoA is a key intermediate in the metabolism of amino acids and fatty acids. Figure 10.24 shows the molecular structures of FAD and $FADH_2$. FAD is an aromatic ring (flavin group) system, whereas $FADH_2$ is not. This means that $FADH_2$ is significantly higher in energy, without the stabilization that aromatic structure provides. $FADH_2$ is an energy-carrying molecule, because, if it is oxidized, it will regain aromaticity and release all the energy represented by this stabilization.

A schematic of reactions in a TCA cycle is presented in Fig. 10.22. Condensation of acetyl-CoA with oxaloacetic acid results in citric acid, which is further converted to isocitric acid and then to α-ketoglutaric acid (α-KGA) with a release of CO_2. α-KGA is decarboxylated and oxidized to succinic acid (SA), which is further oxidized to fumaric acid (FA). Hydration of fumaric acid to malic acid (MA) and oxidation of malic acid to

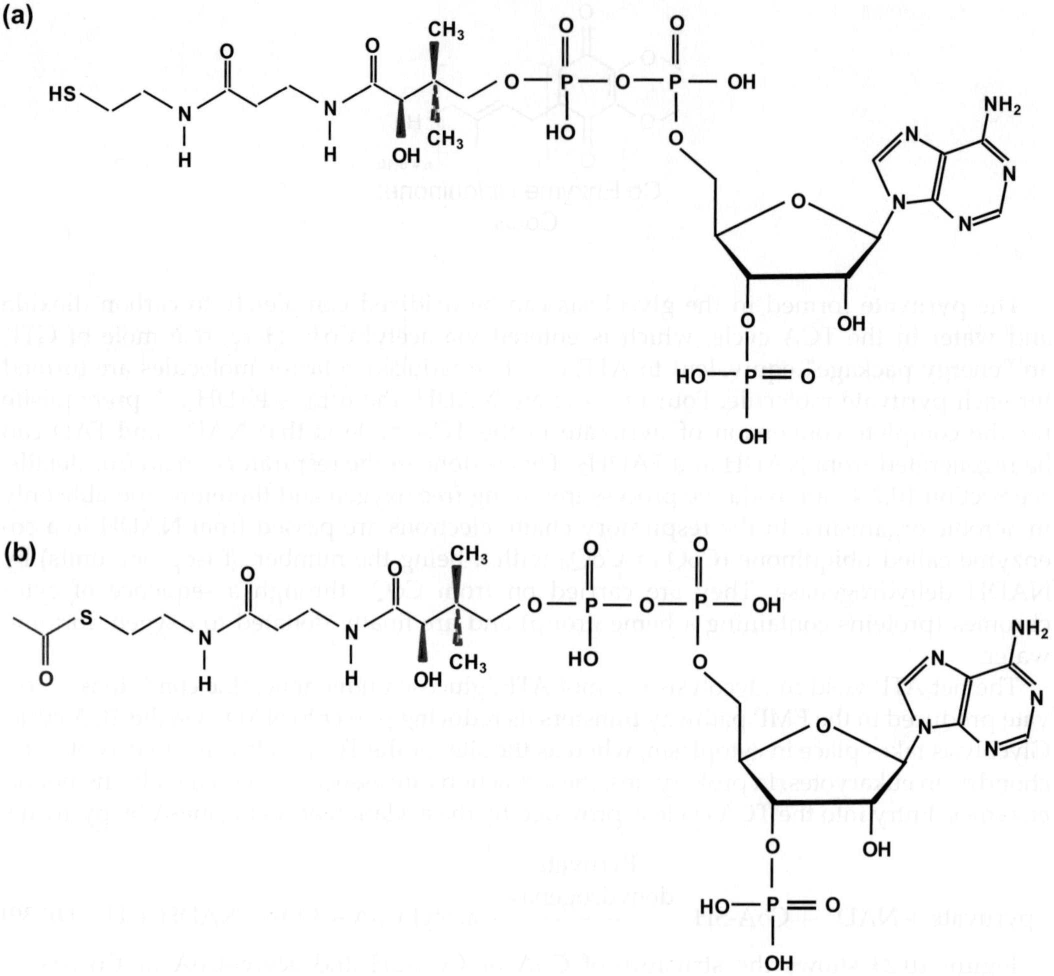

(a)

(b)

FIGURE 10.23 Stereo structures of (a) CoA (or CoA-SH) and (b) Acetyl-CoA (or CoA-S-Ac).

oxaloacetic acid (OAA) are the two last steps of the TCA cycle. For each pyruvate molecule entering the cycle, three CO_2, four $NADH + H^+$, and one $FADH_2$ are produced. The succinate and α-ketoglutarate produced during the TCA cycle are used as precursors for the synthesis of certain amino acids. The reducing power ($NADH + H^+$ and $FADH_2$) produced is used either for biosynthetic pathways or for ATP generation through the electron transport chain.

The overall reaction of the TCA cycle is

$$\text{acetyl-CoA} + 3\,NAD^+ + FAD + GDP + H_3PO_4 + 2H_2O \rightarrow CoA + 3(NADH + H^+) + FADH_2 + GTP + 2\,CO_2 \quad (10.40)$$

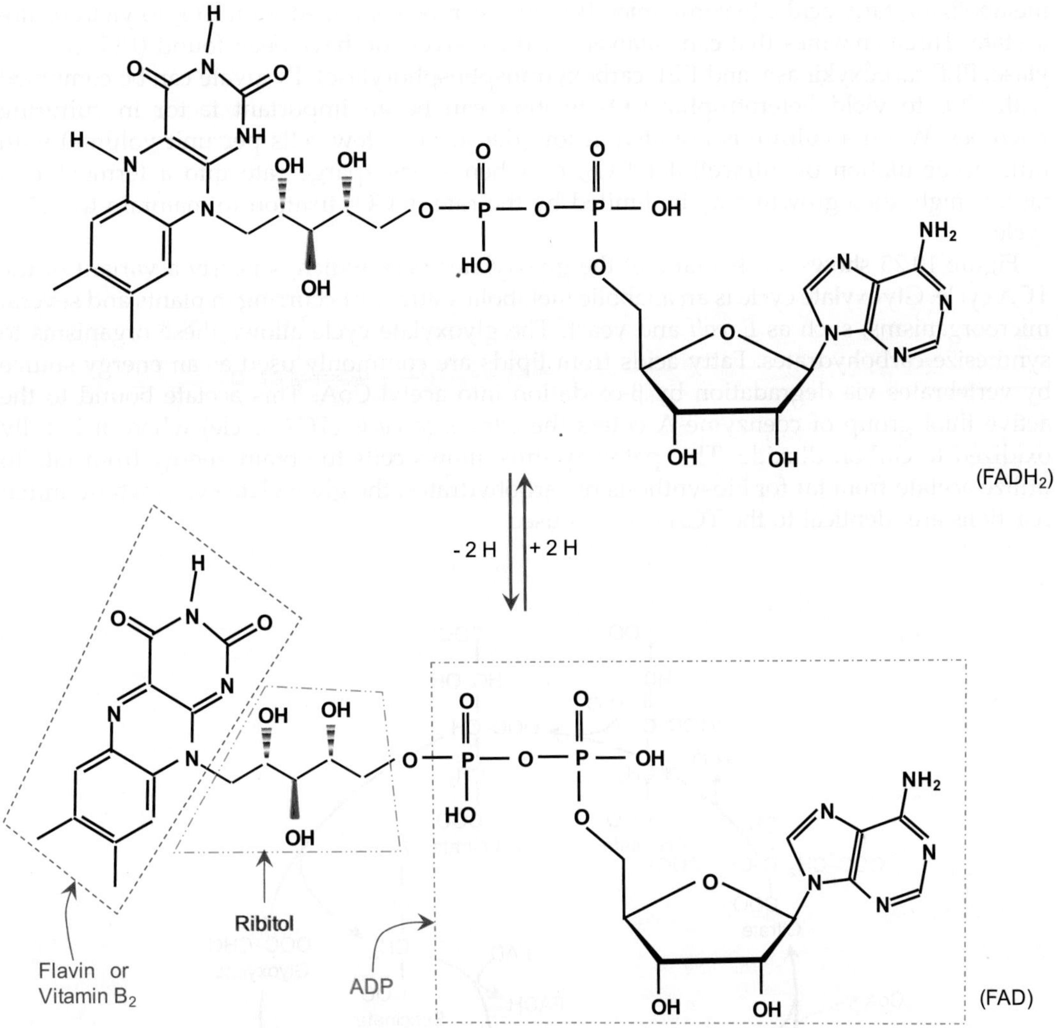

FIGURE 10.24 The redox of flavin adenine dinucleotide (FAD) and $FADH_2$.

Note from Fig. 10.22 that GTP can be converted easily into ATP; some descriptions of the TCA cycle show directly the conversion of ADP plus phosphorus into ATP, as succinyl-CoA is converted to succinate.

The major roles of the TCA cycle are (1) to provide electrons (NADH) for the electron transport chain and biosynthesis, (2) to supply C skeletons for amino acid synthesis, and (3) to generate energy.

Many of the intermediates in the TCA cycle are used extensively in biosynthesis. Removal of these intermediates "short-circuits" the TCA cycle. To maintain a functioning TCA cycle, the cell can fix CO_2 (heterotrophic CO_2 fixation) or supply acetyl-CoA via metabolizing fatty acids. In some microbes, PEP can be combined with CO_2 to yield oxaloacetate. Three enzymes that can catalyze such a conversion have been found (PEP carboxylase, PEP carboxykinase, and PEP carboxytransphosphorylase). Pyruvate can be combined with CO_2 to yield heterotrophic CO_2 fixation can be an important factor in culturing microbes. When a culture is initiated at low density (i.e. few cells per unit volume) with little accumulation of intracellular CO_2, or when a gas sparge rate into a fermentation tank is high, then growth may be limited by the rate of CO_2 fixation to maintain the TCA cycle.

Figure 10.25 shows a schematic of the glyoxylate cycle, which is nearly a variant of the TCA cycle. Glyoxylate cycle is an anabolic metabolic pathway occurring in plants and several microorganisms, such as *E. coli* and yeast. The glyoxylate cycle allows these organisms to synthesize carbohydrates. Fatty acids from lipids are commonly used as an energy source by vertebrates via degradation by β-oxidation into acetyl-CoA. This acetate bound to the active thiol group of coenzyme-A enters the *citric acid cycle* (TCA cycle) where it is fully oxidized to carbon dioxide. This pathway thus allows cells to obtain energy from fat. To utilize acetate from fat for biosynthesis of carbohydrates, the glyoxylate cycle, whose initial reactions are identical to the TCA cycle, is used.

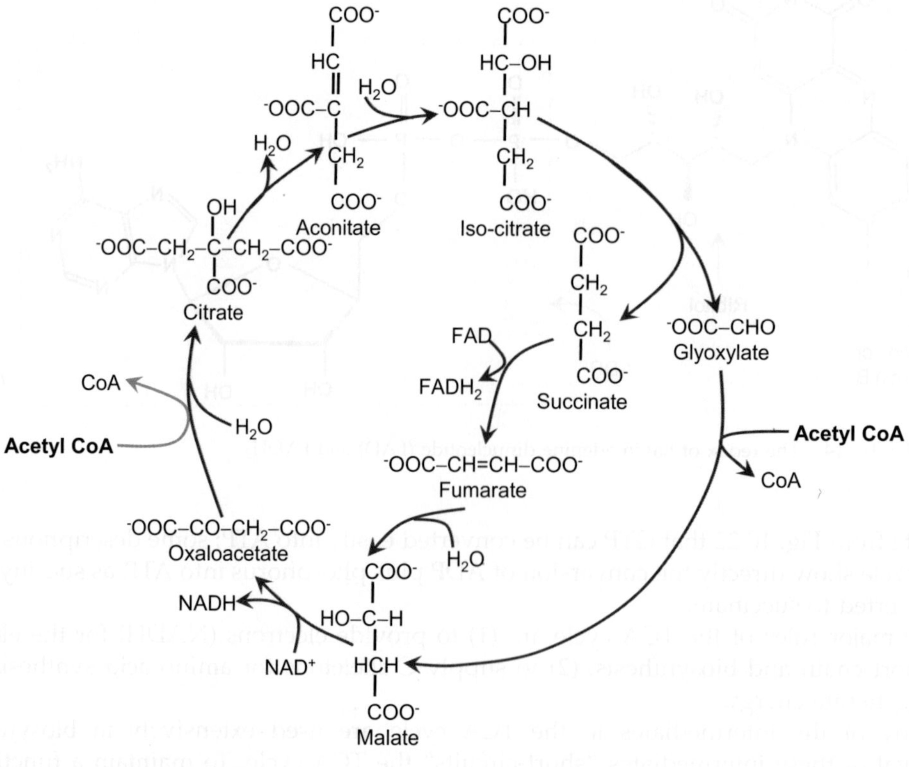

FIGURE 10.25 The glyoxylate cycle.

Cell wall containing organisms, such as plants, fungi, and bacteria, require very large amounts of carbohydrates during growth for the biosynthesis of complex structural polysaccharides, such as cellulose, glucans, and chitin. In these organisms, in the absence of available carbohydrates (for example, in certain microbial environments or during seed germination in plants), the glyoxylate cycle permits the synthesis of glucose from lipids via acetate generated in fatty acid β-oxidation.

The glyoxylate cycle bypasses the steps in the TCA cycle where carbon is lost in the form of CO_2. The two initial steps of the glyoxylate cycle are identical to those in the TCA cycle: *acetate → citrate → isocitrate*. In the next step, catalyzed by the first glyoxylate cycle enzyme, isocitrate lyase, isocitrate undergoes cleavage into succinate and glyoxylate (the latter gives the cycle its name). Glyoxylate condenses with acetyl-CoA (a step catalyzed by malate synthase), yielding malate. Both malate and oxaloacetate can be converted into PEP, which is the substrate of PEP carboxykinase, the first enzyme in gluconeogenesis. The net result of the glyoxylate cycle is therefore the production of glucose from fatty acids. Succinate generated in the first step can enter into the citric acid cycle to eventually form oxaloacetate.

10.7.3. Metabolism of Common Plant Biomass Derived Monosaccharides

Major monomeric sugars obtainable from plant biomass can be categorized as six carbon sugars: glucose, fructose, mannose and galactose, and five carbon sugars: xylose and arabinose. By far, glucose is the preferred substrate to microorganisms. There are few known organisms that can utilize these nonglucose sugars. Table 10.5 shows various natural microorganisms and their natural ability to metabolize these monosaccharides.

Figure 10.26 shows the uptake of six carbon sugars, which replaces the front end of glucose metabolism shown in the previous section. One can observe that the metabolism of fructose and mannose does not go through Glucose-6P intermediate before reaching Fructose-6P. Galactose needs two additional steps to get to the intermediate Glucose-6P.

Figure 10.27 shows the pentose metabolisms. Xylose and arabinose are metabolized into Xylulose-5P, from which enters into the HMP or PP pathways.

TABLE 10.5 Various Natural Microorganisms and Their Ability to Metabolize Monosaccharides

	Natural sugar utilization pathways					Major products	
Organism	**Glucose**	**Mannose**	**Galactose**	**Xylose**	**Arabinose**	**Ethanol**	**Other**
Anaerobic bacteria	Yes	Yes	Yes	Yes	Yes	Yes	Yes
E. coli	Yes	Yes	Yes	Yes	Yes	No	Yes
Z. mobilis	Yes	No	No	No	No	Yes	No
S. cerevisiae	Yes	Yes	Yes	No	No	Yes	No
P. stipitis	Yes	Yes	Yes	Yes	Yes	Yes	No
Filamentous fungi	Yes	Yes	Yes	Yes	Yes	Yes	No

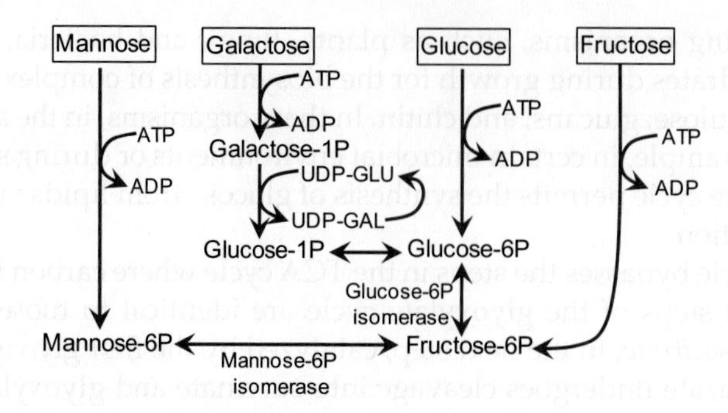

FIGURE 10.26 Six carbon sugar uptake pathways.

10.7.4. Fermentative Pathways

When the oxidative phosphorylation is inactive (due to the absence of oxygen or lack of some of the necessary proteins), pyruvate is not oxidized in the TCA cycle since that would lead to an accumulation of NADH inside the cells. In this situation, NADH is oxidized with simultaneous reduction of pyruvate to acetate, lactic acid, or ethanol. These processes are collectively called *fermentative metabolism*. Fermentative metabolism is not the same in all microorganisms, but there are many similarities.

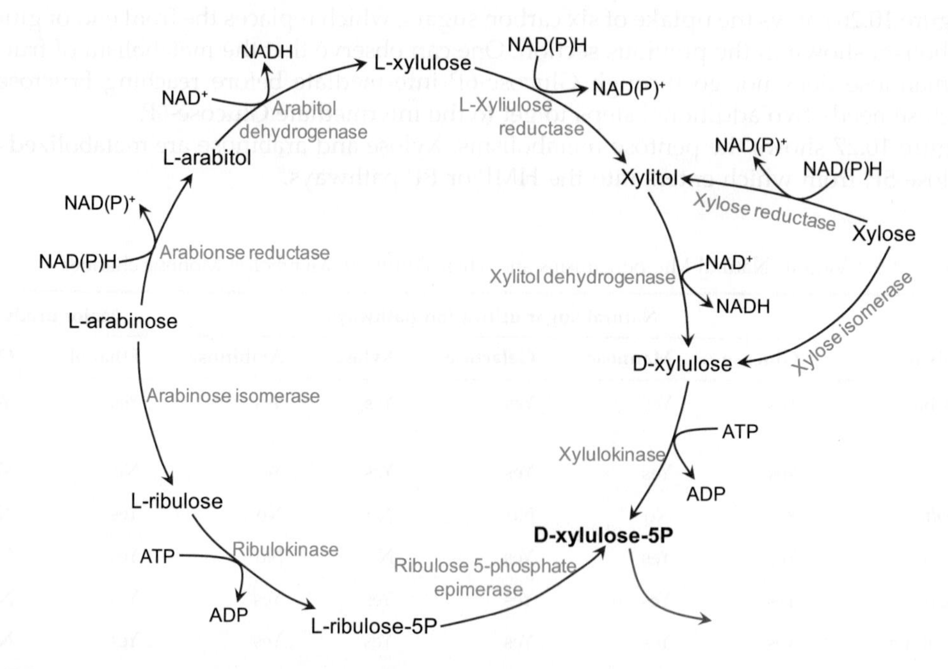

FIGURE 10.27 Pentose metabolism.

Bacteria can regenerate all NAD^+ by reduction of pyruvate to lactic acid in Fig. 10.28a and b. They can also regenerate all NAD^+ by formation of ethanol in the so-called mixed acid fermentation pathway for which the entry point is the compound acetyl-CoA. CoA is a cofactor with a free –SH group that can be acetylated to CH_3CO-S- as illustrated in Fig. 10.23, either directly from acetate or by capturing two of the carbon atoms of pyruvate with the last carbon atom liberated as carbon dioxide or formic acid, HCOOH. Lactic acid bacteria (Fig. 10.28b) have both pathways for conversion of one pyruvate to acetyl-CoA, whereas *E. coli* only has the pyruvate formate lyase catalyzed reaction. In yeast, the fermentative pathway does not proceed via acetyl-CoA but instead by decarboxylation of pyruvate to acetaldehyde. From acetate, cytosolic acetyl-CoA may be synthesized, and this serves as precursor for fatty acid biosynthesis, whereas the mitocondrial acetyl-CoA

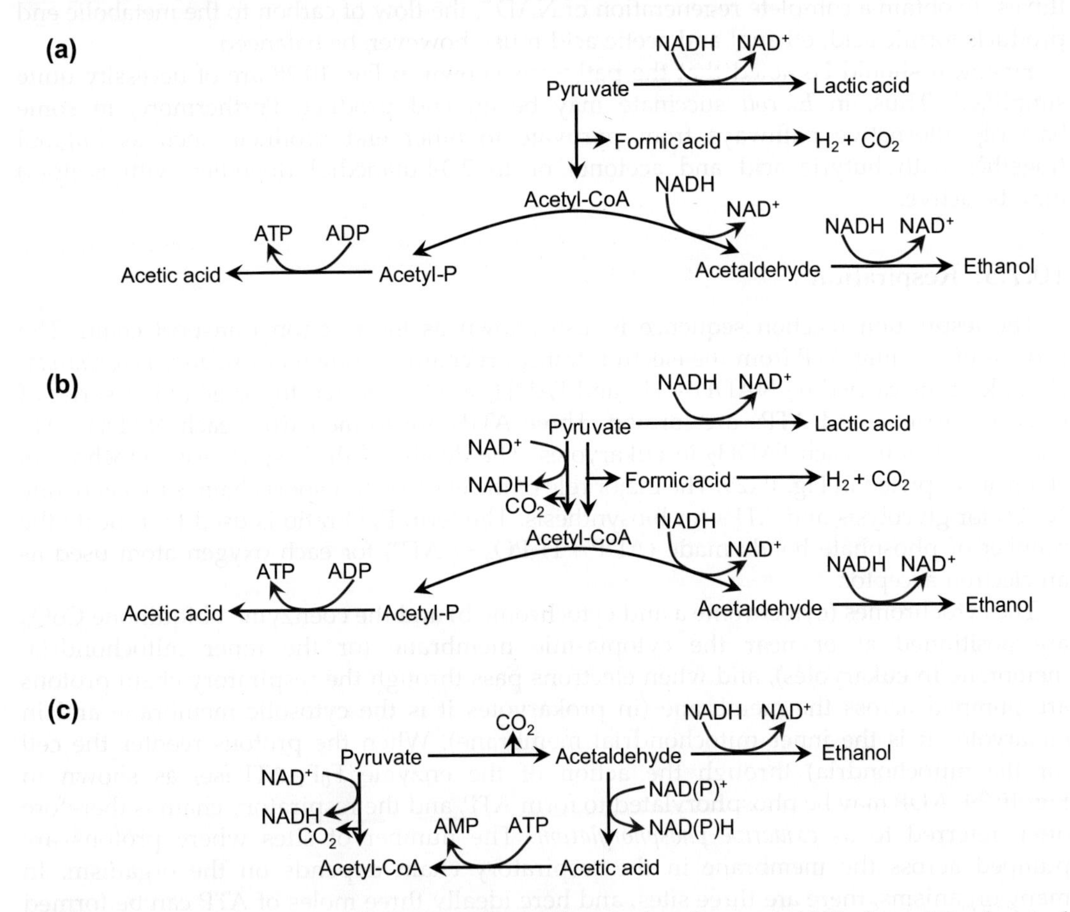

FIGURE 10.28 Different major fermentative pathways for reduction of pyruvate. (a) The fermentative (or mixed acid) metabolism of *Escherichia coli*. (b) The fermentative metabolism of lactic acid bacteria. (c) The fermentative metabolism in the yeast *S. cerevisiae*. Not all reactions occur in the same compartment, i.e. the pyruvate dehydrogenase catalyzed conversion of pyruvate to acetyl-CoA occurs in the mitochondrion whereas the other reactions occur in the cytosol.

that is formed directly from pyruvate serves as an entry point to the TCA cycle. In yeast, the primary metabolic product is ethanol, but even with respiratory growth, where complete reoxidation of NADH is possible by oxidative phosphorylation the pyruvate dehydrogenase complex (Fig. 10.28c), which catalyzes the direct conversion of pyruvate to acetyl-CoA, may be by-passed as indicated. Above a certain glucose uptake rate, the respiratory capacity becomes limiting and this leads to overflow in the by-pass and consequently ethanol is formed. This overflow metabolism is traditionally referred to as the *Crabtree effect*.

Acetyl-CoA can be regarded as an activated form of acetic acid as it can be converted to acetic acid in Fig. 10.28a and b. As seen in the last step of acetic acid formation an ATP is released, hereby doubling the ATP yield by catabolism of glucose from 2 to 4 ATP per glucose molecule. This is the reason why bacteria use the mixed acid pathways at very low glucose fluxes. To obtain a complete regeneration of NAD^+, the flow of carbon to the metabolic end products formic acid, ethanol and acetic acid must, however, be balanced.

Finally, it should be noted that the pathways shown in Fig. 10.28 are of necessity quite simplified. Thus, in *E. coli* succinate may be an end product. Furthermore, in some bacteria, alternative pathways from pyruvate to other end products such as butanol (together with butyric acid and acetone) or to 2,3-butanediol (together with acetoin) may be active.

10.7.5. Respiration

The respiration reaction sequence is also known as the electron transport chain. The process of forming ATP from the electron transport chain is known as *oxidative phosphorylation*. Electrons carried by $NADH + H^+$ and $FADH_2$ are transferred to oxygen via a series of electron carriers, and ATPs are formed. Three ATPs are formed from each $NADH + H^+$ and two ATPs for each $FADH_2$ in eukaryotes. The details of the respiratory (cytochrome) chain are depicted in Fig. 10.29. The major role of the electron transport chain is to regenerate NADs for glycolysis and ATPs for biosynthesis. The term P/O ratio is used to indicate the number of phosphate bonds made ($ADP + H_3PO_4 \rightarrow ATP$) for each oxygen atom used as an electron acceptor.

The cytochromes (cytochrome a and cytochrome b) and the coenzyme ubiquinone CoQ_n are positioned at or near the cytoplasmic membrane (or the inner mitochondrial membrane in eukaryotes), and when electrons pass through the respiratory chain protons are pumped across the membrane (in prokaryotes it is the cytosolic membrane and in eukaryotes it is the inner mitochondrial membrane). When the protons reenter the cell (or the mitochondria) through the action of the enzyme F_0F_1-ATPase, as shown in Fig. 10.29, ADP may be phosphorylated to form ATP, and the respiratory chain is therefore often referred to as *oxidative phosphorylation*. The number of sites where protons are pumped across the membrane in the respiratory chain depends on the organism. In many organisms, there are three sites, and here ideally three moles of ATP can be formed by the oxidation of NADH. $FADH_2$ enters the respiratory chain at CoQ_n. The electrons therefore do not pass the NADH dehydrogenase and the oxidation of $FADH_2$ therefore results only in the pumping of protons across the membrane at two sites. The number of moles of ATP formed for each oxygen atom used in the oxidative phosphorylation is

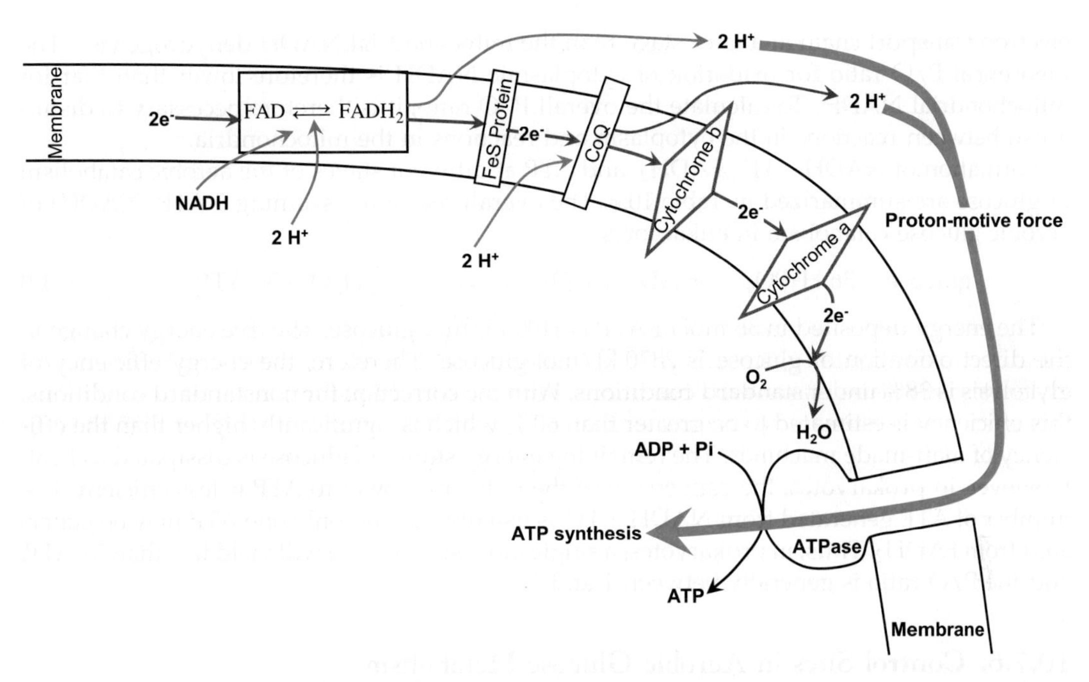

FIGURE 10.29 Electron transport and electron transport phosphorylation. *Top*: Oxidation of NADH and the flow of electrons through the electron transport system, leading to the transfer of protons (II) from the inside to the outside of the membrane. The tendency of protons to return to the inside is called *proton-motive force*. *Bottom*: ATP synthesis occurs as protons reenter the cell. An ATPase enzyme uses the proton-motive force for the synthesis of ATP. The proton-motive force is discussed in Section 10.6.

normally referred to as the *P/O* ratio, and the value of this stoichiometric coefficient indicates the overall thermodynamic efficiency of the process. If NADH was the only coenzyme formed in the catabolic reactions, the theoretical P/O ratio would be exactly 3, but since some $FADH_2$ is also formed the P/O ratio is always less than 3. Furthermore, the proton and electrochemical gradient are also used for solute transport and the overall stoichiometry in the process is therefore substantially smaller than the upper value of 3. As the different reactions in the oxidative phosphorylation are not directly coupled the P/O ratio varies with the growth conditions, and the overall stoichiometry is therefore written as:

$$\mathrm{NADH} + \tfrac{1}{2}\mathrm{O_2} + \mathrm{P/O\ ADP} + \mathrm{H^+} + \mathrm{P/O\ H_3PO_4} = \mathrm{NAD^+} + (1 + \mathrm{P/O})\ \mathrm{H_2O} + \mathrm{P/O\ ATP} \tag{10.41}$$

In many microorganisms, one or more of the sites of proton pumping are lacking, and this of course results in a substantially lower P/O ratio.

Since the electron transport chain is located in the inner mitochondrial membrane in eukaryotes and since NADH cannot be transported from the cytosol into the mitochondrial matrix NADH formed in the cytosol needs to be oxidized by another route. Strain-specific NADH dehydrogenases face the cytosol, and these proteins donate the electrons to the electron transport chain at a later stage than the mitochondrial NADH dehydrogenase. The theoretical P/O ratio for oxidation of cytoplasmic NADH is therefore lower than that for mitochondrial NADH. To calculate the overall P/O ratio, it is therefore necessary to distinguish between reactions in the cytoplasm and reactions in the mitochondria.

Formation of NADH + H^+, $FADH_2$, and ATP at different stages of the aerobic catabolism of glucose are summarized in Table 10.6. The overall reaction (assuming 3 ATP/NADH) of aerobic glucose catabolism in eukaryotes

$$\text{glucose} + 36\ H_3PO_4 + 36\ \text{ADP} + 6\ O_2 \rightarrow 6\ CO_2 + 6\ H_2O + 36\ \text{ATP} \tag{10.42}$$

The energy deposited in 36 mol of ATP is 1100 kJ/mol-glucose. The free energy change in the direct oxidation of glucose is 2870 kJ/mol-glucose. Therefore, the energy efficiency of glycolysis is 38% under standard conditions. With the correction for nonstandard conditions, this efficiency is estimated to be greater than 60%, which is significantly higher than the efficiency of man-made machines. The remaining energy stored in glucose is dissipated as heat. However, in prokaryotes, the conversion of the reducing power to ATP is less efficient. The number of ATP generated from NADH + H^+ is usually ≤ 2, and only one ATP may be generated from $FADH_2$. Thus, in prokaryotes, a single glucose molecule will yield less than 24 ATP, and the P/O ratio is generally between 1 and 2.

10.7.6. Control Sites in Aerobic Glucose Metabolism

Several enzymes involved in glycolysis are regulated by feedback inhibition. The major control site in glycolysis is the phosphorylation of fructose-6-phosphate by phosphofructokinase.

$$\text{fructose-6-phosphate} + \text{ATP} \rightarrow \text{fructose-1,6-diphosphate} + \text{ADP} \tag{10.43}$$

The enzyme phosphofructokinase is an allosteric enzyme activated by ADP and H_3PO_4 but inactivated by ATP.

$$\text{Phosphofructokinase (active)} \underset{\text{ADP}}{\overset{\text{ATP}}{\rightleftarrows}} \text{phosphofructokinase (inactive)} \tag{10.44}$$

At high ATP/ADP ratios, this enzyme is inactivated, resulting in a reduced rate of glycolysis and reduced ATP synthesis. The concentration of dissolved oxygen or oxygen partial

TABLE 10.6 Summary of NADH, $FADH_2$, and ATP Formation During Aerobic Catabolism of Glucose (Based on the Consumption of one mole of Glucose)

	NADH	$FADH_2$	ATP
Glycolysis	2		2
Oxidative decarboxylation of pyruvate	2		
TCA cycle	6	2	2
Total	10	2	4

pressure has a regulatory effect on rate of glycolysis, known as the *Pasteur effect*. The rate of glycolysis under anaerobic conditions is higher than that under aerobic conditions. In the presence of oxygen, ATP yield is high, since the TCA cycle and electron transport chain are operating. As a result of high levels of ATP, ADP and H_3PO_4 become limiting, and phosphofructokinase becomes inhibited. Also, some enzymes of glycolysis with -SH groups are inhibited by high levels of oxygen. A high $NADH/NAD^+$ ratio also reduces the rate of glycolysis.

Certain enzymes of the Krebs cycle are also regulated by feedback inhibition. Pyruvate dehydrogenase is inhibited by ATP, NADH, and acetyl-CoA and activated by ADP, AMP, and NAD^+. Similarly, citrate synthase is inactivated by ATP and activated by ADP and AMP; succinyl-CoA synthetase is inhibited by NAD^+. In general, high ATP/ADP and $NADH/NAD^+$ ratios reduce the processing rate of the TCA cycle.

Several steps in the electron transport chain are inhibited by cyanide, azide, carbon monoxide, and certain antibiotics, such as amytal. Such inhibition is important due to its potential to alter cellular metabolism.

10.7.7. Metabolism of Nitrogenous Compounds

Most of the organic nitrogen compounds have an oxidation level between carbohydrates and lipids. Consequently, nitrogenous compounds can be used as nitrogen, carbon, and energy source. Proteins are hydrolyzed to peptides and further to amino acids by proteases. Amino acids are first converted to organic acids by deamination (removal of amino group). Deamination reaction may be oxidative, reductive, or dehydrative, depending on the enzyme systems involved. A typical oxidative deamination reaction can be represented.

$$R{-}CH(NH_2){-}COOH + H_2O + NAD^+ \rightarrow R{-}CO{-}COOH + NH_3 + NADH + H^+ \quad (10.45)$$

Ammonia released from deamination is utilized in protein and nucleic acid synthesis as a nitrogen source, and organic acids can be further oxidized for energy production (ATP).

Transamination is another mechanism for conversion of amino acids to organic acids and other amino acids. The amino group is exchanged for the keto group of α-keto acid. A typical transamination reaction is

$$\text{glutamic acid} + \text{oxaloacetic acid} \rightarrow \alpha\text{-keto glutaric acid} + \text{aspartic acid} \quad (10.46)$$

Nucleic acids can also be utilized by many organisms such as carbon, nitrogen, and energy source. The first step in nucleic acid utilization is enzymatic hydrolysis by specific nucleases hydrolyzing RNA and DNA. Nucleases with different specificities hydrolyze different bonds in nucleic acid structure, producing ribose/deoxyribose, phosphoric acid, and purines/pyrimidines. Sugar molecules are metabolized by glycolysis and the TCA cycle, producing CO_2 and H_2O under aerobic conditions. Phosphoric acids are used in ATP, phospholipid, and nucleic acid synthesis.

Purines/pyrimidines are degraded into urea and acetic acid and then to ammonia and CO_2. For example, the hydrolysis of adenine and uracil can be represented as follows:

$$\text{adenine} \rightarrow CO_2 + NH_3 + \text{acetic acid} + \text{urea} \rightarrow 5\,NH_3 + 5\,CO_2 \quad (10.47)$$

$$\text{uracil} \rightarrow \text{alanine} + NH_3 + CO_2 \rightarrow 2\,NH_3 + 4\,CO_2 \quad (10.48)$$

10.7.8. Nitrogen Fixation

Certain microorganisms fix atmospheric nitrogen to form ammonia under reductive or microaerophilic conditions. Organisms capable of fixing nitrogen under aerobic conditions include *Azotobacter, Azotomonas, Azotococcus,* and *Biejerinckia*. Nitrogen fixation is catalyzed by the enzyme "nitrogenase," which is inhibited by oxygen. Typically, these aerobic organisms sequester nitrogenase in compartments that are protected from oxygen.

$$N_2 + 6H^+ + 6e^- \rightarrow 2\,NH_3 \tag{10.49}$$

Azotobacter species present in soil provide ammonium for plants by fixing atmospheric nitrogen and some form associations with plant roots. Some facultative anaerobes such as *Bacillus, Klebsiella, Rhodopseudomonas,* and *Rhodospirillum* fix nitrogen under strict anaerobic conditions as well as strict anaerobes such as *Clostridia* can also fix nitrogen under anaerobic conditions. Certain cyanobacteria, such as *Anabaena* sp., fix nitrogen under aerobic conditions. The lichens are *associations* of cyanobacteria and fungi. *Cyanobacteria* provide nitrogen to fungi by fixing atmospheric nitrogen. *Rhizobium* species are heterotrophic organisms growing in the roots of leguminous plants. *Rhizobium* fix atmospheric nitrogen under low oxygen pressure and provide ammonium to plants. *Rhizobium* and *Azospirillum* are widely used for agricultural purposes and are bioprocess products.

10.7.9. Metabolism of Hydrocarbons

The metabolism of aliphatic hydrocarbons is important in some bioprocesses and often critical in applications such as bioremediation. Such metabolism requires oxygen, and only few organisms (e.g. *Pseudomonas, Mycobacteria,* certain yeasts and molds) can metabolize hydrocarbons. The low solubility of hydrocarbons in water is a barrier to rapid metabolism.

The first step in metabolism of aliphatic hydrocarbons is oxygenation by oxygenases. Hydrocarbon molecules are converted to an alcohol by incorporation of oxygen into the end of the carbon skeleton. The alcohol molecule is further oxidized to aldehyde and then to an organic acid that is further converted to acetyl-CoA, which is metabolized by the TCA cycle.

Oxidation of aromatic hydrocarbons takes place by the action of oxygenases and proceeds much slower than those of aliphatic hydrocarbons. Cathecol is the key intermediate in this oxidation sequence and can be further broken down ultimately to acetyl-CoA or TCA cycle intermediates. Aerobic metabolism of benzene is depicted below:

$$\begin{array}{l} \text{benzene} \longrightarrow \text{cathecol} \longrightarrow \text{cis-cis-muconate} \longrightarrow \beta\text{-keto adipate} \\ \qquad\qquad\qquad\qquad\qquad\qquad\qquad\qquad\qquad\downarrow \\ \qquad\qquad\qquad\qquad\qquad\qquad\quad \text{acetyl-CoA} + \text{succinate} \end{array} \tag{10.50}$$

Anaerobic metabolism of hydrocarbons is more difficult. Only a few organisms can metabolize hydrocarbons under *anaerobic* conditions. They cleave the C—C bonds and saturate with hydrogen to yield methane.

10.8. OVERVIEW OF BIOSYNTHESIS

The TCA cycle and glycolysis are critical catabolic pathways and also provide important precursors for the biosynthesis of amino acids, nucleic acids, lipids, and polysaccharides.

Although many additional pathways exist, we will describe just two more, one in the context of biosynthesis and the other under anaerobic metabolism.

The first is the *PP pathway* or HMP (see Fig. 10.20). Although this pathway produces significant reducing power, which could be used, in principle, to supply energy to the cell, its primary role is to provide carbon skeletons for biosynthetic reactions and the reducing power necessary to support anabolism. Normally, NADPH is used in biosynthesis, whereas NADH is used in energy production. This pathway provides an array of small organic compounds with three, four, five, and seven carbon atoms. These compounds are particularly important for the synthesis of ribose, purines, coenzymes, and the aromatic amino acids. The glyceraldehyde-3-phosphate formed can be oxidized to yield energy through conversion to pyruvate and further oxidation of pyruvate in the TCA cycle.

A vital component of biosynthesis, which consumes a large amount of cellular building blocks, is the production of amino acids. Many amino acids are also important commercial products, and the alteration of pathways to induce overproduction is critical to commercial success. The 20 amino acids can be grouped into various families. Figure 10.30 summarizes these families and the compounds from which they are derived. The amino acid, histidine, is not included in Fig. 10.30. Its biosynthesis is fairly complicated and cannot be easily grouped with the others. However, ribose-5-phosphate from HMP is a key precursor in its synthesis.

In addition to the synthesis of amino acids and nucleic acids, the cell must be able to synthesize lipids and polysaccharides. The key precursor is acetyl-CoA (see Fig. 10.22 for

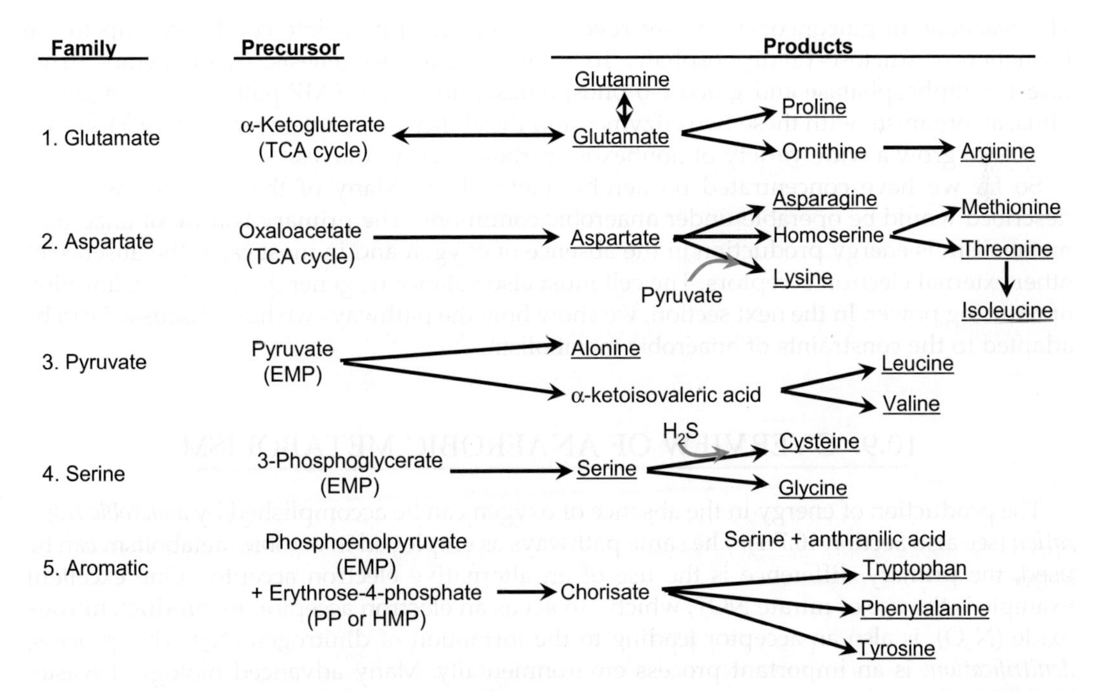

FIGURE 10.30 Summary of the amino acid families and their synthesis from intermediates in the EMP, TCA, and HMP pathways. The amino acids are underlined.

the TCA cycle). Fatty acid synthesis consists of the stepwise buildup of acetyl-CoA. Also, CO_2 is an essential component in fatty acid biosynthesis. Acetyl-CoA and CO_2 produce malonyl-CoA, which is a three-carbon-containing intermediate in fatty acid synthesis. This requirement for CO_2 can lengthen the start-up phase (or lag phase; see Chapter 11) for commercial fermentations if the system is not operated carefully. The requirement for CO_2 can be eliminated if the medium is formulated to supply key lipids, such as oleic acid.

The synthesis of most of the polysaccharides from glucose or other hexoses is readily accomplished in most organisms. However, if the carbon-energy source has less than six carbons, special reactions need to be used. Essentially, the EMP pathway needs to be operated in reverse to produce glucose. The production of glucose is called *gluconeogenesis*.

Since several of the key steps in the EMP pathway are irreversible, the cell must circumvent these irreversible reactions with energy-consuming reactions. Since pyruvate can be synthesized from a wide variety of pathways, it is the starting point. However, in glycolysis, the final step to convert PEP into pyruvate is irreversible. In gluconeogenesis, PEP is produced from pyruvate from

$$\text{pyruvate} + CO_2 + \text{ATP} + H_2O \rightarrow \text{oxaloacetate} + \text{ADP} + H_3PO_4 + 2H^+ \tag{10.51}$$

and

$$\text{oxaloacetate} + \text{ATP} \rightarrow \text{PEP} + \text{ADP} + CO_2 \tag{10.52}$$

or a net reaction of

$$\text{pyruvate} + 2\ \text{ATP} + H_2O \rightarrow \text{PEP} + 2\ \text{ADP} + 2\ H^+ \tag{10.53}$$

The reactions in gluconeogenesis are reversible (under appropriate conditions) up to the formation of fructose-1,6-diphosphate. To complete gluconeogenesis, two enzymes (fructose-1, 6-diphosphatase and glucose-6-phosphatase) not in the EMP pathway are required. Thus, an organism with these two enzymes and the ability to complete reaction 10.53 should be able to grow a wide variety of nonhexose carbon-energy sources.

So far we have concentrated on aerobic metabolism. Many of the reactions we have described would be operable under anaerobic conditions. The primary feature of anaerobic metabolism is energy production in the absence of oxygen and in most cases the absence of other external electron acceptors. The cell must also balance its generation and consumption of reducing power. In the next section, we show how the pathways we have discussed can be adapted to the constraints of anaerobic metabolism.

10.9. OVERVIEW OF ANAEROBIC METABOLISM

The production of energy in the absence of oxygen can be accomplished by *anaerobic respiration* (see also Section 10.7.1). The same pathways as employed in aerobic metabolism can be used; the primary difference is the use of an alternative electron acceptor. One excellent example is the use of nitrate NO_3^-, which can act as an electron acceptor. Its product, nitrous oxide (N_2O), is also an acceptor leading to the formation of dinitrogen (N_2). This process, *denitrification*, is an important process environmentally. Many advanced biological waste-treatment systems are operated to promote denitrification.

Many organisms grow without using the electron transport chain. The generation of energy without the electron transport chain is called *fermentation*. This definition is the exact and original meaning of the term fermentation, although currently it is often used in a broader context. Since no electron transport is used, the organic substrate must undergo a balanced series of oxidative and reductive reactions. This constraint requires that the rates of conversion of NAD^+ and $NADP^+$ to NADH and NADPH must equal the rates of conversion of NADH and NADPH to NAD^+ and $NADP^+$. For example, with the EMP pathway, the 2 mol of NAD reduced in this pathway in the production of pyruvate are reoxidized by oxidation of pyruvate to other products. Two prime examples are lactic acid and ethanol production (see Fig. 10.31). Both lactic acid and ethanol are important commercial products from bioprocesses. Other partially oxidized by-products from fermentation are or have been commercially important [acetone-butanol fermentation, propionic acid, acetic acid (for vinegar), 2,3-butanediol, isopropanol, and glycerol].

Figure 10.31 summarizes common routes to some of these fermentation end products. Pyruvate is a key metabolite in these pathways. In most cases, pyruvate is formed through glycolysis. However, alternative pathways to form pyruvate exist. The most common of these is the *ED pathway* (see Fig. 10.32). This pathway is important in the fermentation of glucose by the bacterium *Zymomonas*. The use of *Zymomonas* to convert glucose into ethanol is of potential commercial interest, because the use of the ED pathway produces only 1 mol of ATP per mole of glucose. This low energy yield forces more glucose into ethanol and less into cell mass than for yeast, which uses glycolysis to produce pyruvate, which yields 2 mol ATP per mole of glucose. No one organism makes all the products indicated in Fig. 10.33. Different organisms will contain different combinations of pathways. Thus, it is important to screen

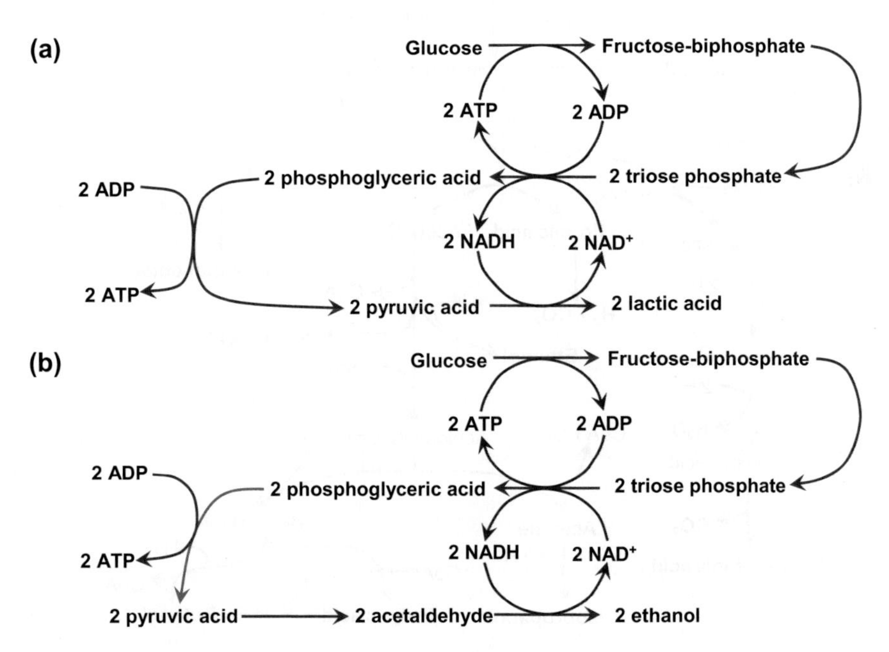

FIGURE 10.31 Comparison between (a) lactic acid and (b) alcoholic fermentations.

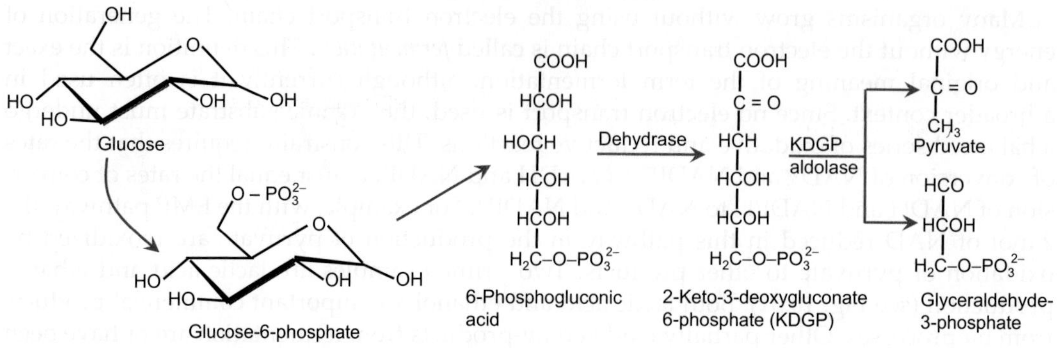

FIGURE 10.32 Entner–Doudoroff pathway.

a wide variety of organisms to select one that will maximize the yield of a desired product, while minimizing the formation of other by-products.

10.10. INTERRELATIONSHIPS OF METABOLIC PATHWAYS

In a given cell, major metabolic pathways we learned so far are synergetically integrated together so that the cell can function in certain way. Figures 10.34 and 10.35 show two examples of such integrations: one for microbial cell and another for mammalian cell.

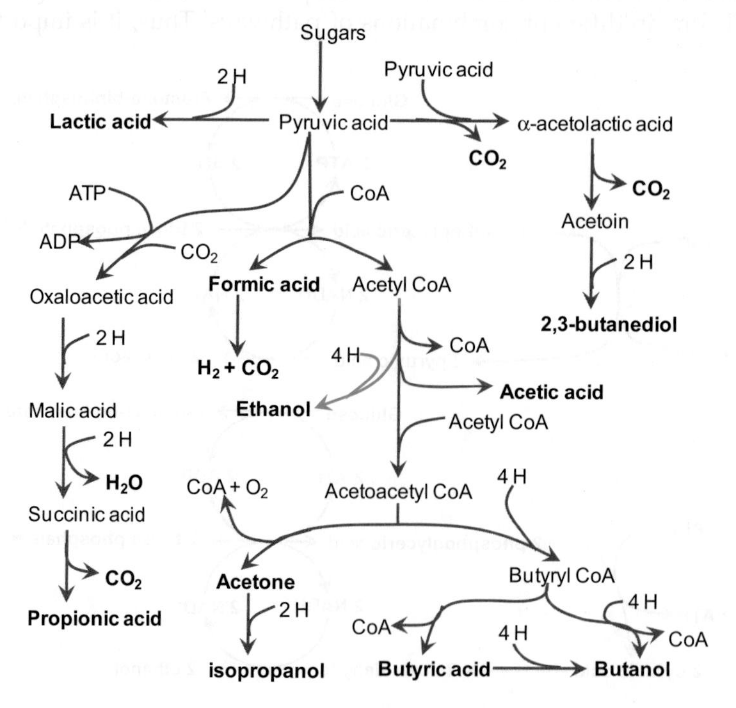

FIGURE 10.33 Derivations of some major end products of the bacterial fermentations of sugars from pyruvic acid. The end products are shown in boldface type.

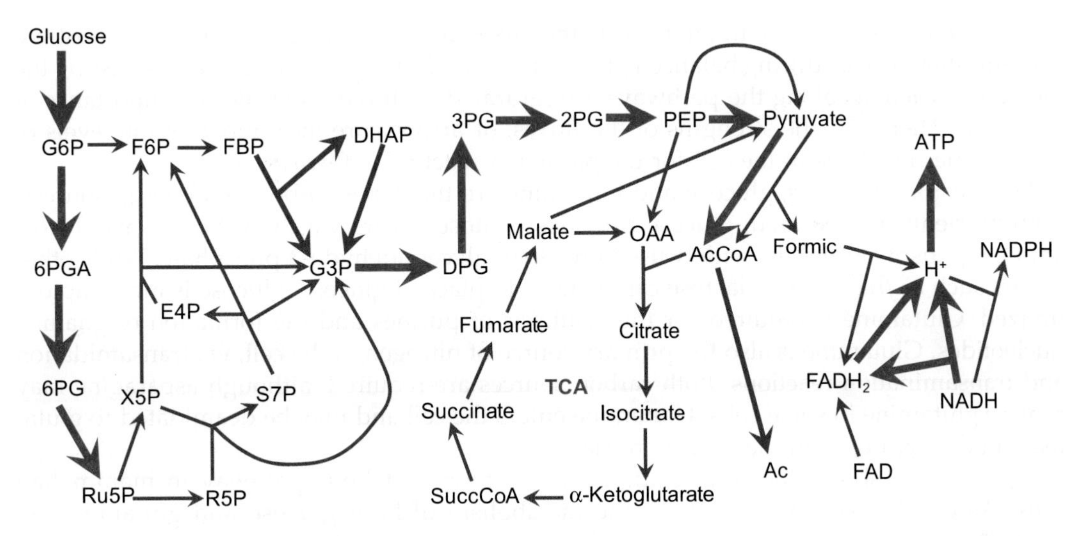

FIGURE 10.34 Interrelationship of major metabolic pathways in *E. coli*. The connecting path thickness represents the strength of the flux through it.

Figure 10.34 shows the interrelationship of major metabolic pathways in *E. coli*. The direction of the arrow indicates the direction of material flow (from the substrate glucose). Glucose enters the cell via glycolysis: EMP and PP and connects to TCA. The width of arrows indicates the strength of the fluxes. There is no net loss of strength of fluxes at each node (molecule) along the metabolic pathways. As shown in Example 10-3, the fluxes from one molecule to another along the metabolic pathways are nonlinear functions of the concentrations. However, due to the relative magnitude of the saturation constants as compared to the

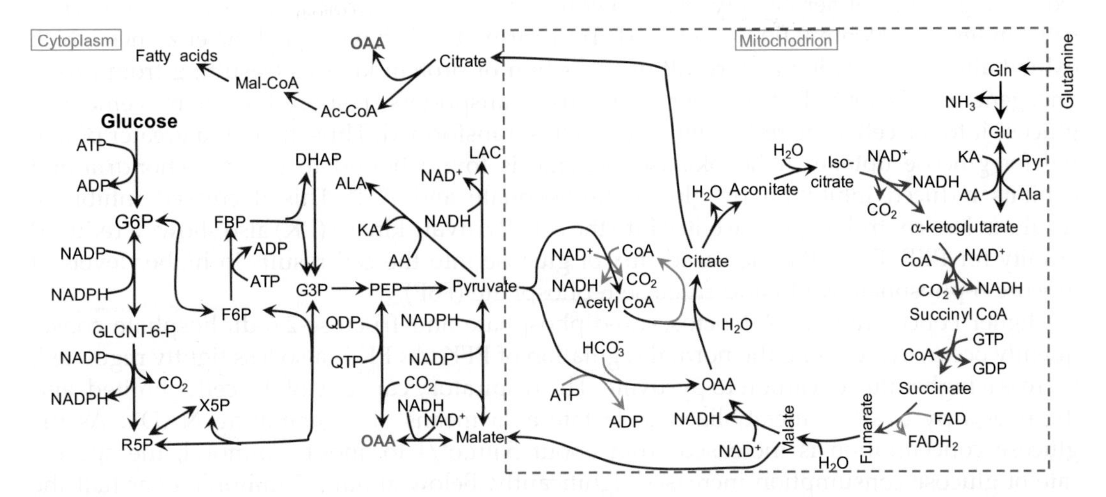

FIGURE 10.35 The major metabolic pathways in mammalian cells. The cytosolic and mitochondrial reactions are shown together with the compounds which can cross from the mitochondria to the cytosol.

concentrations of the molecules in the cell, the fluxes are nearly independent of the substrate concentration at least during balanced growth periods. The enzymes or proteins assisting the metabolic reactions along the pathways are saturated with the molecules of importance at each step. Therefore, the strengths of the fluxes, or arrows, are indications of the levels of the enzymes available in the cell for the particular reaction pathways.

For most animal cells, glucose and glutamine are the major carbon and energy sources. Both nutrients are required; glucose provides pentose sugars via the PP pathway, glucosamine-6-phosphate and the widely used precursor glyceraldehyde-3-phosphate. While other sugars such as *fructose* or galactose can be used in place of glucose, glucose is more rapidly utilized. Glutamine is required for the synthesis of purines and the formation of guanine nucleotides. Glutamine is also the primary source of nitrogen in the cell, via transamidation and transamination reactions. Both carbon sources are required, although asparagine may replace glutamine in some cells. Glutamine enters the cell and may be deamidated to glutamate in the cytosol or in the mitochondria.

Figure 10.35 shows the interrelationship of major metabolic pathway in mammalian cells. As can be seen on Fig. 10.35, the metabolism of both glucose and glutamine are interrelated; however, glutamine typically provides most of the energy required by the cell through respiration. In all mammalian cells, glucose is metabolized to pyruvate. In normal (i.e. nontumor) cells, pyruvate is converted to acetyl-CoA and oxidized via the TCA cycle. The ATP produced by mitochondrial respiration regulates glycolysis as a result of its inhibition of phosphofructokinase (PFK). Glucose-6-phosphate then accumulates and regulates the phosphorylation of *glucose* via its action on hexokinase. When oxygen is less available, the production of ATP in the mitochondria is reduced and PFK is deregulated. More glucose-6-phosphate is consumed, increasing the glucose flux into the cell. As oxidative phosphorylation is restricted at low oxygen concentrations, pyruvate is converted to lactic acid as a means of regenerating NAD^+ from the NADH generated by glycolysis.

In contrast to normal mammalian cells, cultured cells, tumor cells, and proliferating cells exhibit high rates of aerobic glycolysis. High rates of lactate production, similar to normal cells under oxygen limitation, are found. Transformed cells have glycolytic enzymes which exhibit altered regulation as a result of the action of protein kinases (resulting from proto-oncogene expression). The number of glucose transporters, responsible for movement of glucose into the cell, is increased when the cell is transformed. Thus, there is a greater potential for glucose uptake. A hexokinase isozyme is found bound to the mitochondria and exhibits reduced inhibition by glucose-6-phosphate and ATP. This decreased inhibition results in less control of glucose entry into the cell. Pyruvate kinase (PK) also shows a reduced affinity for PEP. Thus, the increased flux of glucose into the cell results in higher levels of glucose-6-phosphate (G6P) and fructose-6-phosphate (F6P).

Higher concentrations of fructose-1,6-diphosphate and fructose-2,6-diphosphate consequently occur, overcoming the normal regulation of PFK. As PK is also less tightly regulated, there is a higher flux of carbon to pyruvate. The respiratory capacity of the cell is limited, and the excess pyruvate is metabolized to lactate as a means of regenerating NAD^+. As the glucose concentration is increased from about 5 μmol/l to about 5 mmol/l, the specific rate of glucose consumption increases significantly. Below about 0.5 mmol/l, over half the glucose consumed by rat hepatomas, for example, is incorporated into nucleotides, but beyond 5 mmol/l over 90% of the glucose is converted to lactate. The metabolism of glutamine is altered in tumor cells and proliferating normal cells.

Many normal cells produce glutamine, but cells which grow in culture show high rates of glutamine consumption. Glutamine metabolism occurs primarily in the TCA cycle, where glutamine enters as α-ketoglutarate. More than half the CO_2 production by normal diploid fibroblasts is derived from glutamine.

10.11. OVERVIEW OF AUTOTROPHIC METABOLISM

Cell growth requires two basic atoms in large quantity: carbon and hydrogen. The function or transfer of hydrogen/proton in cells also leads us to classify hydrogen as electron donor. While cell can obtain hydrogen from organic (*organotroph*) or inorganic (*lithotroph*) compounds, there are two sources for carbon as well: CO_2 or organic compounds. While the source of hydrogen may not be as critical, the source of carbon can make a significant difference in cell metabolism. So far we have been concerned primarily with *heterotrophic growth* (e.g. organic molecules serve as carbon-energy sources). However, *autotrophs* obtain nearly all their carbon from CO_2. Table 10.7 shows a summary of the major characteristics of heterotrophs and autotrophs. Most autotrophs (either photoautotrophs or chemoautotrophs) fix or capture CO_2 by a reaction catalyzed by the enzyme ribulose bisphosphate carboxylase, which converts ribulose-1,5-diphosphate plus CO_2 and H_2O into two molecules of glyceric acid-3-phosphate. This is the key step in the *Calvin cycle* (or Calvin–Benson cycle). This cycle is summarized in Fig. 10.36 and provides the building blocks for autotrophic growth.

Energy for autotrophic growth can be supplied by light (photoautotroph) or chemicals (chemoautotroph). Here, we consider the special case of photoautotrophic growth.

Photosynthesis takes place in two phases. The overall reaction is

$$6\,CO_2 + 6H_2O \xrightarrow{\text{light}} C_6H_{12}O_6 + 6\,O_2 \tag{10.54}$$

The first phase of photosynthesis is known as the *light phase*. Light energy is captured and converted into biochemical energy in the form of ATP and reducing agents, such as NADPH. In this process, hydrogen atoms are removed from water molecules and are used to reduce

TABLE 10.7 Summary of Heterotrophic and Autotrophic Metabolisms

Classification	Carbon source	Energy source	Examples
Photoautotrophs	CO_2	Light	Green plant, algae, cyanobacteria, photosynthetic bacteria
Photoheterotrophs	Organic compounds	Light	Nonsulfur purple bacteria
Chemoautotrophs	CO_2	Oxidation-reduction reaction	Nitrifying bacteria; hydrogen, sulfur, and iron bacteria
Chemoheterotrophs	Organic compounds	Oxidation-reduction reaction	All animals, most microorganisms

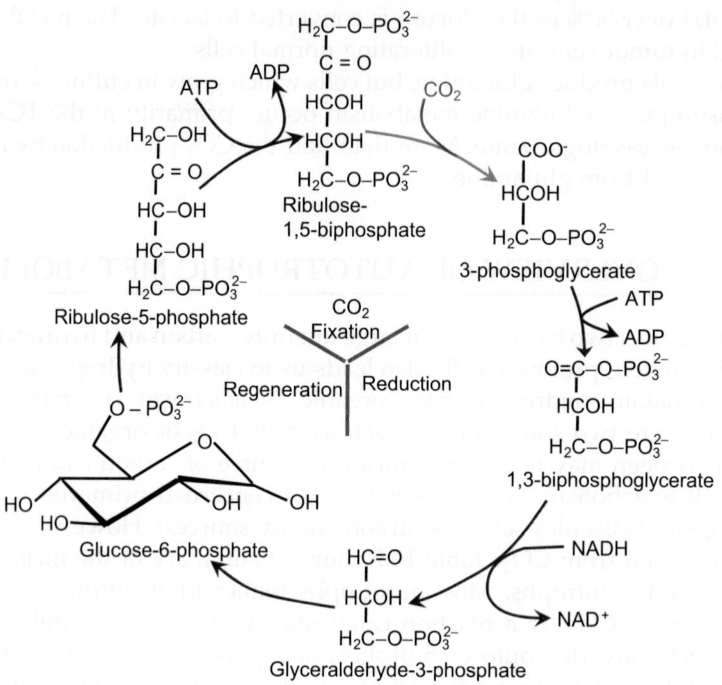

FIGURE 10.36 Schematic representation of the Calvin–Benson cycle, illustrating its three phases: CO_2 fixation, reduction of fixed CO_2, and regeneration of the CO_2 acceptor.

$NADP^+$, leaving behind molecular oxygen. Simultaneously, ADP is phosphorylated to ATP. The light-phase reaction of photosynthesis is

$$H_2O + NADP^+ + H_3PO_4 + ADP \xrightarrow{\text{light}} O_2 + NADPH + H^+ + ATP \tag{10.55}$$

In the second phase, the energy-rich products of the first phase, NADPH and ATP, are used as the sources of energy to reduce the CO_2 to yield glucose (see Fig. 10.36). Simultaneously, NADPH is reoxidized to $NADP^+$, and the ATP is converted into ADP and phosphate. This *dark phase* is described by the following reaction:

$$CO_2 + NADPH + H^+ + ATP \rightarrow \frac{1}{6}\text{glucose} + NADP^+ + ADP + H_3PO_4 \tag{10.56}$$

Both prokaryotic and eukaryotic cells can fix CO_2 by photosynthesis. In prokaryotes (e.g. cyanobacteria), photosynthesis takes place in stacked membranes, whereas in eukaryotes an organelle called the *chloroplast* conducts photosynthesis. Both systems contain chlorophyll to absorb light. Light absorption by chlorophyll molecules results in an electronic excitation. The excited chlorophyll molecule returns to the normal state by emitting light quanta in a process known as *fluorescence*. The excited chlorophyll donates an electron to a sequence of enzymes, and ATP is produced as the electrons travel through the chain. This ATP generation process is called *photophosphorylation*. Electron carriers in this process are ferredoxin and several cytochromes.

The light phase of photosynthesis consists of two photosystems. Photosystem I (PS I) can be excited by light of wavelength shorter than 700 nm and generates NADPH. Photosystem II (PS II) requires light of wavelength shorter than 680 nm and splits H_2O into $\frac{1}{2}\,O_2 + 2\,H^+$. ATPs are formed as electrons flow from PS II to PS I.

10.12. SUMMARY

In this chapter, you have learned some of the elementary concepts of how cells control their composition in response to an ever-changing environment. The essence of an organism resides in the chromosome as a linear sequence of nucleotides that form a language (*genetic code*) to describe the production of cellular components. The cell controls the storage and transmission of such information, using macromolecular templates: DNA or RNA. DNA is responsible for its own *replication* and is also a template for *transcription* of information into RNA species that serve both as machinery and template to *translate* genetic information into proteins. Proteins often must undergo posttranslational processing to perform their intended functions.

The cell controls both the amount and activity of proteins it produces. Many proteins are made on *regulated genes* (e.g. *repressible* or *inducible*), although other genes are *constitutive*. With regulated genes, small effector molecules alter the binding of regulatory proteins to specific sequences of nucleotides in the *operator* or *promoter* regions. Such regulatory proteins can block transcription or in other cases enhance it. A group of contiguous genes under the control of a single promoter-operator is called an *operon*. More global control through *regulons* is also evident. Some gene products are not regulated, and their synthesis is constitutive.

Once a protein is formed, its activity may be continuously modulated through *feedback inhibition*. A number of alternative strategies are employed by the cell to control the flux of material through a pathway. Another form of regulation occurs through the interaction of extracellular compounds with cell surface protein receptors.

Cell senses the availability of substrate(s) due to the transport of substrate(s) from the medium (abiotic phase) into cytoplasm (or biotic phase) as depicted by Fig. 10.16. The transport can be passive diffusion through cell membrane,

$$J_S = k_P(C_{SE} - C_{SI}) \tag{10.27}$$

or by protein-facilitated transport,

$$J_S = J_{S\max}\left(\frac{C_{SE}}{K_{SE} + C_{SE}} - \frac{C_{SI}}{K_{SI} + C_{SI}}\right) \tag{10.33}$$

where C_{SI} is the concentration of substrate inside the cell (biotic phase) and C_{SE} is the concentration of substrate in the medium (abiotic phase). Passive transport (diffusion) requires a positive concentration gradient, i.e. $C_{SE} > C_{SI}$. However, active transport (protein-facilitated transport) can appear to be against the concentration gradient, due to the difference in binding coefficients, or the saturation constants, K_{SE} and K_{SI}.

Cellular metabolism starts with the transport of substrates into the cell and is concerned with two primary functions: *catabolism* and *anabolism*. A summary of the metabolism is shown in Table 10.8. Catabolism involves the degradation of a substrate to more highly

TABLE 10.8 A summary of Metabolism in Cells

General	Metabolic pathway and/or Metabolic network		
Cellular respiration	Aerobic respiration	Glycolysis → pyruvate decarboxylation → citric acid cycle → oxidative phosphorylation (electron transport chain + ATP synthase)	
	Anaerobic respiration	Glycolysis → fermentation (ABE, ethanol, lactic acid)	
Specific paths	Protein metabolism	Protein synthesis and catabolism	
	Carbohydrate metabolism (carbohydrate catabolism and anabolism)	Human	Glycolysis ↔ gluconeogenesis Glycogenolysis ↔ glycogenesis Pentose phosphate pathway; fructolysis; galactolysis glycosylation (N-linked, O-linked)
		Nonhuman	Photoautotroph or Photosynthesis (Carbon fixation) Chemoautotrophs Pentose metabolism
	Lipid metabolism (lipolysis, lipogenesis)	Fatty acid metabolism	Fatty acid degradation (beta oxidation); Fatty acid synthesis
		Other	Steroid metabolism; sphingolipid metabolism; eicosanoid metabolism; ketosis
	Amino acid	Amino acid synthesis; urea cycle	
	Nucleotide metabolism	Purine metabolism; nucleotide salvage; pyrimidine metabolism	
	Other	Metal metabolism (iron metabolism); ethanol metabolism; hydrocarbon metabolism	

oxidized end products for the purpose of generating energy and reducing power. Anabolism is the biosynthesis of more complex compounds from simpler compounds, usually with the consumption of energy and reducing power. The key compound to store and release energy is ATP. Reducing power is stored by *NADH* or *NADPH*.

Three of the most important pathways in the cell are (1) the EMP pathway, or *glycolysis*, which converts glucose into pyruvate; (2) the *TCA cycle* or *citric acid cycle*, which can oxidize pyruvate through acetyl-CoA into CO_2 and H_2O; and (3) the *PP* or HMP pathway, which converts glucose-6-phosphate into a variety of carbon skeletons (C_3, C_4, C_5, C_6, and C_7), with glyceraldehyde-3-phosphate (G3P) as the end product. Although all three pathways can have catabolic and anabolic roles, the EMP pathway and TCA cycle are the primary means for energy generation, and HMP plays a key role in supplying carbon skeletons and reducing power for direct use in biosynthesis. In this chapter, we have briefly considered the relationship of these pathways to amino acid, fatty acid, and polysaccharide biosynthesis. The conversion of pyruvate to glucose, necessary for polysaccharide biosynthesis when the carbon source does not have six carbons, is called *glucogenesis*.

Reducing power can be used to generate ATP through the *electron transport chain*. If oxygen is the final electron acceptor for this reducing power, the process is called *aerobic respiration*. If another electron acceptor is used in conjunction with the electron transport chain, then the process is called *anaerobic respiration*. Cells that obtain energy without using the electron transport chain use *fermentation*. *Substrate-level phosphorylation* supplies ATP. The end products of fermentative metabolism (e.g. ethanol, acetone-butanol, and lactic acid) are important commercially and are formed in response to the cell's need to balance consumption and the production of reducing power.

For most animal cells, glucose and glutamine are the major carbon and energy sources. Both nutrients are required; glucose provides pentose sugars via the PP pathway, glucosamine-6-phosphate and the widely used precursor glyceraldehyde-3-phosphate. While other sugars such as *fructose* or galactose can be used in place of glucose, glucose is more rapidly utilized. Glutamine is required for the synthesis of purines and the formation of guanine nucleotides. Glutamine is also the primary source of nitrogen in the cell, via transamidation and transamination reactions. Both carbon sources are required, although asparagine may replace glutamine in some cells. Glutamine enters the cell and may be deamidated to glutamate in the cytosol or in the mitochondria.

Many normal cells produce glutamine, but cells which grow in culture show high rates of glutamine consumption. Glutamine metabolism occurs primarily in the TCA cycle, where glutamine enters as α-ketoglutarate. More than half the CO_2 production by normal diploid fibroblasts is derived from glutamine.

Autotrophic organisms use CO_2 as their carbon source and rely on the *Calvin* (or *Calvin–Benson*) cycle to incorporate (or fix) carbon from CO_2 into cellular material. Energy is obtained either through light *(photoautotroph)* or oxidation of inorganic chemicals (*chemoautotroph*). Figure 10.36 summarizes the major metabolic pathways and their interrelationship for autotrophs.

Further Reading

Alberts, B., others, 1998. *Essential Cell Biology*, Garland Publishing, Inc., New York.

Alberts, B., Bray, D., Johnson, A., Lewis, J., Raff, M., Roberts, K., Walter, P., 1998. *Essential Cell Biology: An Introduction to the Molecular Biology of the Cell*, Garland Publication, Inc., New York.

Black, I.G., 1996. *Microbiology: Principles and Applications*, 3rd ed., Prentice Hall, Upper Saddle River, NJ.

Cook, P.R., 1999. The Organization of Replication and Transcription, *Science* 284, 1790–1795.

Crueger, W., Crueger, A., 1990. *Biotechnology. A Textbook of Industrial Microbiology* (T. D. Brock. ed., English edition), 2nd ed., Sinauer Associates, Inc., Sunderland, MA.

Eigenbrodt, E., Fister, P., Reinacher, M., 1991. In: Wang, D., Ho, C.S. (Eds.), Animal Cell Bioreactors, Butterworth-Heinemann Press.

Elgard, L., Molinari, M., Helenius, A., 1999. Setting the Standards: Quality Control in the Secretory Pathway, *Science* 286, 1882–1888.

Harder, A. Roels, J.A., 1982. Application of simple structured models in bioengineering, *Adv. Biochem. Eng.*, 21, 55–107.

Kapanidis, A.N., Margeat, E., Laurence, T.A., Doose, S., Ho, S.O., Mukhopadhyay, J., Kortkhonjia, E., Mekler, V., Ebright, R.H., Weiss, S., 2005. Retention of transcription initiation factor sigma70 in transcription elongation: single-molecule analysis. *Mol. Cell* 20 (3) 347–56.

Kelly, M.T., Hoover, T.R., 1999. Bacterial Enhancers Function at a Distance, *Asm News* 65, 484–489.

Kolter, R., Losick, R., 1998. One for All and All for One, *Science* 280, 226–227.

Madigan, M.T., Martinko, J.M., Parker, J., 1997. *Brock Biology of Microorganisms*, 8th ed., Prentice Hall, Upper Saddle River, NJ.
Moran, L.A., Scrimgeour, K.G., Horton, H.R., Ochs, R.S., Rawn, J.D., 1994. *Biochemistry*, 2nd ed., Prentice Hall, Upper Saddle River, NJ.
Neway, J.O., 1989. *Fermentation Process Development of Industrial Organisms*, Marcel-Dekker, Inc., NewYork.
Stanier, R.Y, and others, 1986. *The Microbial World*, 5th ed., Prentice Hall, Englewood Cliffs, NJ.
Stephanopoulos, G.N., Aristidou, A.A., Nielsen, J., 1998. Metabolic Engineering: Principles and Methodologies. Academic Press: San Diego, CA.
Vonhippel, P.H., 1998. An Integrated Model of the Transcription Complex in Elongation, Termination and Editing, *Science* 281, 660–665.
Zeilke, H.R., Ozand, P.T., Tildon, J.T., Sevdalian, D.A., Cornblath, M., 1978. *J Cell Physiology* 9541.

PROBLEMS

10.1. Why is *mRNA* so unstable in most bacteria (half-life of about 1 min)? In many higher organisms, *mRNA* half-lives are much longer (>1 h). Why?

10.2. What would be the consequence of one base deletion at the beginning of the message for a protein?

10.3. S.B. Lee and J.E. Bailey ("Genetically structured models for lac promoter-operator function in the *E. coli* chromosome and in multicopy plasmids: lac promoter function", Biotechnology & Bioengineering, 26: 1381–1389, 1984) modeled the lac-operon by including binding of the repressor to a nonspecific binding site in the chromosome (X_d). Neglecting the binding of inducer to the repressor-operator complex, the equilibria are given by

$$E_r + mS_L \overset{K_1}{\leftrightarrow} E_r(S_L)_m \quad \text{(P10.3-1)}$$

$$E_O + E_r \overset{K_2}{\leftrightarrow} E_oE_r \quad \text{(P10.3-2)}$$

$$E_O + E_r(S_L)_m \overset{K_3}{\leftrightarrow} E_OE_r(S_L)_m \quad \text{(P10.3-3)}$$

$$X_d + E_r \overset{K_4}{\leftrightarrow} X_dE_r \quad \text{(P10.3-4)}$$

$$X_d + E_r(S_L)_m \overset{K_5}{\leftrightarrow} X_dE_r(S_L)_m \quad \text{(P10.3-5)}$$

(a) assuming $[X_d]_T \approx [X_d]$, show

$$\frac{[E_O]}{[E_O]_T} = \frac{1 + K_4[X_d]_T + K_1[S_L]_T^m(1 + K_5[X_d]_T)}{1 + K_4[X_d]_T + K_1[S_L]_T^m(1 + K_5[X_d]_T) + K_2[E_r]_T} \quad \text{(P10.3-6)}$$

where K's are equilibrium constants.

(b) Let $K_1 = 10^7$ mol^{-1} l, $K_2 = 2 \times 10^{12}$ mol^{-1} l, $K_3 = 2 \times 10^9$ mol^{-1} l, $K_4 = 10^3$ mol^{-1} l, $K_5 = 1.5 \times 10^9$ mol^{-1} l, and $[X_d]_T = 4 \times 10^{-2}$ mol/l and $[E_r]_T = 2 \times 10^{-8}$ mol/l. Plot the value of the free to total operator ratio (with $m = 4$), both from Eqn (P10.3-6) and (10.18), as a function of the inducer concentration $[S_L]_T$. Comment on the results.

10.4. Derive rate expressions for the productions of P_1 and P_2 and consumption of M_1 for concerted feedback control of branched pathways as shown in Fig. 10.15b. Assume that PSSH applies. Discuss what happens if the concentrations of P_1 and/or P_2 are high in the medium. Clearly define the symbols you use.

10.5. Derive flux expressions for the productions of P_1 and P_2 and consumption of M_1 for cumulative feedback control of branched pathways as shown in Fig. 10.15d. Assume that PSSH applies. Discuss what happens if the concentrations of P_1 and/or P_2 are high in the medium. If experimental data were collected for the variation of concentrations of M_1, P_1, and P_2 with time, what rate expression(s) you would recommend to use to analyze the experimental data? Clearly define the symbols you use.

10.6. How many ribosomes are actively synthesizing proteins at any instant in an *E. coli* cell growing with a 45-min doubling time? The birth size of *E. coli* is 1 μm in diameter and 2 μm in length. The water content is 75%. About 60% of the dry material is protein, and the rate of amino acid addition per ribosome is 20 amino acids per second. The average molecular weight of free amino acids in *E. coli* is 126.

10.7. Describe simple experiments to determine if the uptake of a nutrient is by passive diffusion, facilitated diffusion, active transport, or group translocation.

10.8. Consider the transport of glucose into cells in a medium containing 1 g/L glucose. The maximum glucose uptake flux is $J_{Smax}a = 2\ g\,l^{-1}\,h^{-1}$, $K_{SE} = 2$ mg/L, $K_{SI} = 0.5$ g/L. Determine

(a) Maximum biotic glucose concentration. Does this concentration make sense?

(b) The concentration of glucose in the biotic fluid if glucose consumption rate is $-r_S = 0.8\ g \cdot L^{-1} \cdot h^{-1}$.

10.9. Consider the transport of xylose into cells in a medium containing 10 g/L xylose. The maximum xyose uptake flux is $J_{Smax}a = 1.8\ g\,l^{-1}\,h^{-1}$, $K_{SE} = 2.5$ mg/L, $K_{SI} = 0.25$ g/L. Determine

(a) Maximum biotic xylose concentration. Does this concentration make sense?

(b) The biotic xylose concentration if xyose consumption rate is $-r_S = 0.5\ g\,L^{-1}\,h^{-1}$.

10.10. For the *m-RNA* nucleotide code below: a) Deduce the corresponding sequence of amino acids. b) What is the corresponding nucleotide sequence on the chromosome? This sequence codes for a part of insulin.

CCG UAU CGA CUU GUA ACA *ACG* CGC

10.11. Identify the enzymes needed in the TCA cycle as shown in Fig. 10.22.

10.12. Identify the enzymes needed in the glyoxylate cycle as shown in Fig. 10.24.

10.13. Explain the difference between feedback inhibition and feedback repression.

10.14. You are asked by your boss to produce a human protein in *E. coli*. Because you have learned some of the differences in the way that prokaryotes and eukaryotes make proteins, you worry about at least two factors that could complicate production of an authentic protein for human use.

(a) What complication might you worry about if the human DNA encoding the protein were placed directly in *E. coli*?
(b) Assume that the correct primary sequence of amino acids has been produced. What posttranslational steps do you worry about and why?

10.15. Consider the process of *N*-linked glycosylation.
(a) What organelles are required?
(b) What is the residual sugar on a glycoprotein that has simple glycosylation?
(c) If glycosylation is complete, what will be the final sugar on the glycoform?
(d) Why may *N*-linked glycosylation be important?

10.16. Cite the ATP-consuming and ATP-generating steps in glycolysis.

10.17. Briefly specify major functions of the TCA cycle.

10.18. What are the major control sites in glycolysis?

10.19. What is the Pasteur effect? Explain in terms of regulation of metabolic flow into a pathway.

10.20. How is glucose synthesized from pyruvate?

10.21. Explain the major functions of the dark and light reaction phases in photosynthesis.

10.22. What are the major differences in photosynthesis between microbes and plants?

10.23. What is transamination? Provide an example.

10.24. Briefly explain the Crabtree Effect.

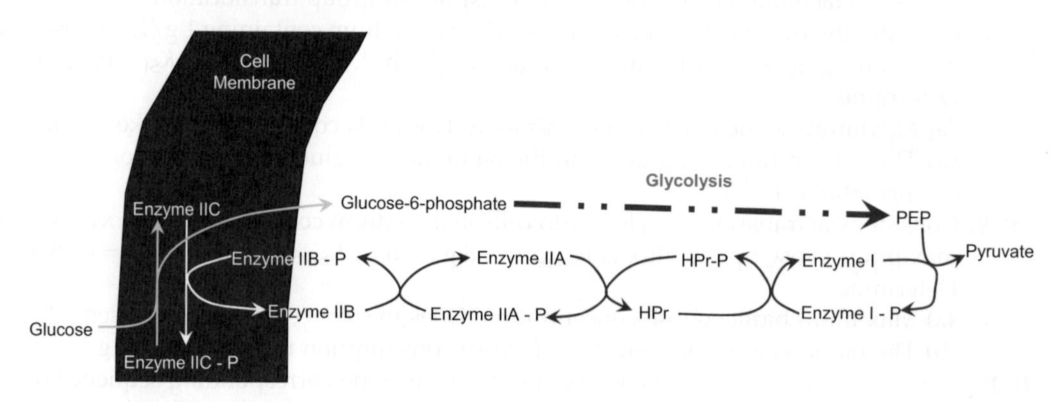

FIGURE P10.27 A schematic of a phosphotransferase system (PTS).

10.25. What are the major steps in aerobic metabolism of hydrocarbons? What are the end products?

10.26. What is nitrogen fixation? Compare the aerobic and anaerobic nitrogen fixation mechanisms.

10.27. Figure P10.27 shows a schematic of the PTS system in *E. coli* as discussed in the text around Eqn (10.32). Glucose is translocated from the medium (abiotic) into the cell (biotic) by a concerted effort of enzymes. This is a typical example of active transport of nutrients into the cell. Derive at a rate expression for the uptake of glucose. Clearly define the symbols you use.

CHAPTER

11

How Cells Grow

OUTLINE

Bioprocess Engineering
http://dx.doi.org/10.1016/B978-0-444-59525-6.00011-1

In biosynthesis, the cells, also referred to as the biomass, consume nutrients to grow and produce more cells and important products. Growth is a result of both replication and change in cell size. Microorganisms can grow under a variety of physical, chemical, and nutritional conditions. In a suitable nutrient medium, organisms extract nutrients from the medium and convert them into biological compounds. This transformation of nutrients to energy and bio-products is accomplished through a cell's use of a number of different enzymes in a series of reactions to produce metabolic products as outlined in Chapter 10. These products can either remain in the cell (intracellular) or be secreted from the cells (extracellular). In the former case, the cells must be lysed (ruptured) and then the product can be purified from the whole broth (reaction mixture).

Theoretically, cell growth is very complicated due to the complicated metabolic pathways as illustrated in Chapter 10. While one may be able to guess how cells grow mathematically by extrapolation from what we have learned in Chapters 8 and 10, we shall return to basics and exam cell growth from experimental observations following the progression of natural or physical observatory development. In this chapter, we will learn how cells grow quantitatively based on experimental observations, how the complicated kinetics may be simplified by approximation, and how cell culture and fermentation are modeled or quantitatively predicted.

11.1. QUANTIFYING BIOMASS

Quantification of cell biomass in a culture medium is essential for the determination of the kinetics of microbial growth. The methods used in the quantification of cell concentration can be direct and indirect. In many cases, the direct methods are not feasible due to the presence of suspended solids or other interfering compounds (for example, color) in the medium. Either cell number or cell mass can be quantified depending on the type of information needed and the properties of the system. Cell mass concentration is often preferred to the measurement of cell number density when only one is measured, but the combination of the two measurements is often desirable.

11.1.1. Cell Number Density

A Petroff–Hausser slide or a *hemocytometer* is often used for direct cell counting. In this method, a calibrated grid is placed over the culture chamber, and the number of cells per grid square is counted using a microscope. To be statistically reliable, at least 20 grid squares must be counted and averaged. The culture medium should be clear and free of particles that could hide cells or be confused with cells. Stains can be used to distinguish between dead and live cells. This method is suitable for nonaggregated cultures. It is difficult to count molds under the microscope because of their mycelial nature.

Plates containing appropriate growth medium gelled with agar (Petri dishes) are used for counting viable or live cells. (The word *viable* used in this context means capable of reproduction.) Culture samples are diluted and spread on the agar surface, and the plates are incubated. Colonies are counted on the agar surface following the incubation period. The results are expressed in terms of colony-forming units. If cells form aggregates, then a single colony may not be formed from a single cell. This method (*plate counts*) is more suitable for bacteria and yeasts and much less suitable for molds. A large number of colonies must be counted to yield a statistically reliable number. Growth media have to be selected carefully, since some media support growth better than others. The *viable count* may vary, depending on the composition of the growth medium. From a single cell, it may require 25 generations to form an easily observable colony. Unless the correct medium and culture conditions are chosen, some cells that are metabolically active may not form colonies.

In an alternative method, an agar-gel medium is placed in a small ring mounted on a microscope slide, and cells are spread on this miniature culture dish. After an incubation period of a few doubling times, the slide is examined with a microscope to count cells. This method has many of the same limitations as plate counts, but it is more rapid, and cells capable of only limited reproduction will be counted.

Automatic cell counters are based on the relatively high electrical resistance of cells. Commercial *particle counters* employ two electrodes and an electrolyte solution. One electrode is placed in a tube containing an orifice. A vacuum is applied to the inner tube, which causes an electrolyte solution containing the cells to be sucked through the orifice. An electrical potential is applied across the electrodes. The voltage applied across the orifice is of the same magnitude as that required for the dielectric breakdown of microbial membranes. Therefore, the voltage must be carefully adjusted. As cells pass through the orifice, the electrical resistance increases and causes pulses in electrical voltage. The number of pulses is a measure of the number of particles; particle concentration is known, since the counter is activated for a predetermined sample volume. The height of the pulse is a measure of cell size. Probes with various orifice sizes are used for different cell sizes. This method is suitable for discrete cells in a particulate-free medium and cannot be used for mycelial organisms.

In an alternative automatic method, the cells are measured via image recognition. When dilute cell culture is passed through an orifice, images are taken continuously (with a fast image capturing camera) and subsequently digitally analyzed on a computer. Special technique such as polarized light may be required to illuminate the cells. This method can measure both cell number and cell sizes.

Alternatively, the number of particles in solution can be determined from the measurement of scattered light intensity with the aid of a phototube (nephelometry). Light passes through the culture sample, and a phototube measures the light scattered by cells in the sample. The intensity of the scattered light is proportional to cell concentration. This method gives best results for dilute cell and particle suspensions.

11.1.2. Cell Mass Concentration

Cell mass holds direct perceivable link to the substrate consumption and product formation. There are two kinds of cell mass quantification methods: direct methods and indirect methods.

11.1.2.1. Direct Methods

Determination of cellular *dry weight* is the most commonly used direct method for determining cell mass concentration and is applicable only for cells grown in solids-free medium. If noncellular solids, such as molasses solids, cellulose, xylan, or corn steep liquor, are present, the dry-weight measurement will be inaccurate. Typically, samples of culture broth are centrifuged or filtered and washed with a buffer solution or water. The washed wet cell mass is then dried at 80 °C for 24 h; then dry cell weight is measured.

Bulk cell volume is used to rapidly but roughly estimate the cell concentration in a fermentation broth (e.g. industrial antibiotic fermentations). Fermentation broth is centrifuged in a tapered graduated tube under standard conditions (revolution per minute and time), and the bulk volume of cells is measured.

Another rapid method is based on the absorption of light by suspended cells in sample culture media. The intensity of the transmitted light is measured using a spectrometer. Turbidity or *optical density* (OD) measurement of the culture medium provides a fast, inexpensive, and simple method of estimating cell density in the absence of other solids or light absorbing compounds. The use of optical methods for medium containing hydrolysates of woody biomass may not be ideal as plant cell fragments, and other particles can interfere in the same were as microbial cells. The extent of light transmission in a sample chamber is a function of cell density and the thickness of the chamber. Light transmission is modulated by both absorption and scattering. Pigmented cells give different results than unpigmented ones. Background absorption by components in the medium must be considered, particularly if absorbing dissolved species are taken into cells. The medium should be essentially particle free. Proper procedure entails using a wavelength that minimizes absorption by medium components (600–700 nm wavelengths are often used), "blanking" against medium, and the use of a calibration curve. The calibration curve relates OD to dry-weight measurements. Such calibration curves can become nonlinear at high OD values (>0.3) and depend to some extent on the physiological state of the cells.

11.1.2.2. Indirect Methods

In many fermentation processes, such as mold fermentations, direct methods cannot be used. In such cases, indirect methods are used, which are based mainly on the measurement of substrate consumption and/or product formation during the course of growth.

Intracellular components of cells such as RNA, DNA, and protein can be measured as indirect measures of cell growth. During a batch growth cycle, the concentrations of these intracellular components change with time. Concentration of RNA (RNA/cell weight) varies significantly during a batch growth cycle; however, DNA and protein concentrations remain fairly constant. Therefore, in a complex medium, DNA concentration can be used as a measure of microbial growth. Cellular protein measurements can be achieved using different methods. Total amino acids, Biuret, Lowry (folin reagent), and Kjeldahl nitrogen measurements can be used for this purpose. Total amino acids and the Lowry method are the most reliable. Recently, protein determination kits from several vendors have been developed for simple and rapid protein measurements. However, many media contain proteins as substrates, which limits the usefulness of this approach.

The intracellular ATP concentration (g-ATP/g-cells) is approximately constant for a given organism. Thus, the ATP concentration in a fermentation broth can be used as a measure of biomass concentration. The method is based on luciferase activity, which catalyzes oxidation of luciferin at the expense of oxygen and ATP with the emission of light.

$$\text{Luciferin} + O_2 + \text{ATP} \xrightarrow{\text{luciferase}} \text{light} \tag{11.1}$$

When oxygen and luciferin are in excess, total light emission is proportional to total ATP present in the sample. Photometers can be used to detect emitted light. Small concentrations of biomass can be measured by this method, since very low concentrations of ATP (10^{-12} g-ATP/L) can be measured by photometers or scintillation counters. The ATP content of a typical bacterial cell is 1 mg-ATP/g-cells, approximately.

Sometimes, nutrients used for cellular mass production can be measured to follow microbial growth. Nutrients used for product formation are not suitable for this purpose. Nitrate, phosphate, or sulfate measurements can be used. The utilization of a carbon source or oxygen uptake rate (OUR) can be measured to monitor cellular growth when cell mass is the major product.

The products of cell metabolism can be used to monitor and quantify cellular growth. Certain products produced under anaerobic conditions, such as ethanol and lactic acid, can be related nearly stoichiometrically to microbial growth. Products must be either growth associated (ethanol) or mixed growth associated (lactic acid) to be correlated with microbial growth. For aerobic fermentations, CO_2 is a common product and can be related to microbial growth. In some cases, changes in the pH or acid–base addition to control pH can be used to monitor nutrient uptake and microbial growth. For example, the utilization of ammonium results in the release of hydrogen ions (H^+) and therefore a drop in pH. The amount of base added to neutralize the H^+ released is proportional to ammonium uptake and growth. Similarly, when nitrate is used as the nitrogen source, hydrogen ions are removed from the medium, resulting in an increase in pH. In this case, the amount of acid added is proportional to nitrate uptake and therefore to microbial growth.

In some fermentation processes, as a result of mycelial growth or extracellular polysaccharide formation, the viscosity of the fermentation broth increases during the course of fermentation. If the substrate is a biodegradable polymer, such as starch or cellulose, then the viscosity of the broth decreases with time as biohydrolysis continues. Changes in the viscosity of the fermentation broth can be correlated with the extent of microbial growth. Although polymeric broths are usually non-Newtonian, the apparent viscosity measured at a fixed rate can be used to estimate cell or product concentration.

11.2. BATCH GROWTH PATTERNS

When a liquid nutrient medium is inoculated with a seed culture (inoculums), the organisms selectively take up dissolved nutrients from the medium and convert them into biomass. A typical batch growth curve includes the following phases: (1) lag phase, (2) logarithmic or exponential growth phase, (3) deceleration phase, (4) stationary phase, and (5) death phase. Figure 11.1 describes a batch microbial growth cycle. The semi-log plot is employed to idealize the growth regimes with the aid of the straight lines drawn.

The *lag phase* occurs immediately after inoculation and is a period of adaptation of cells to a new environment. Microorganisms reorganize their molecular constituents when they are transferred to a new medium. Depending on the composition of nutrients, new enzymes are synthesized, the synthesis of some other enzymes is repressed, and the internal machinery of cells is adapted to the new environmental conditions. These changes reflect the intracellular mechanisms for the regulation of the metabolic processes discussed in Chapter 10. During this phase, cell mass may increase a little, without an increase in cell number density.

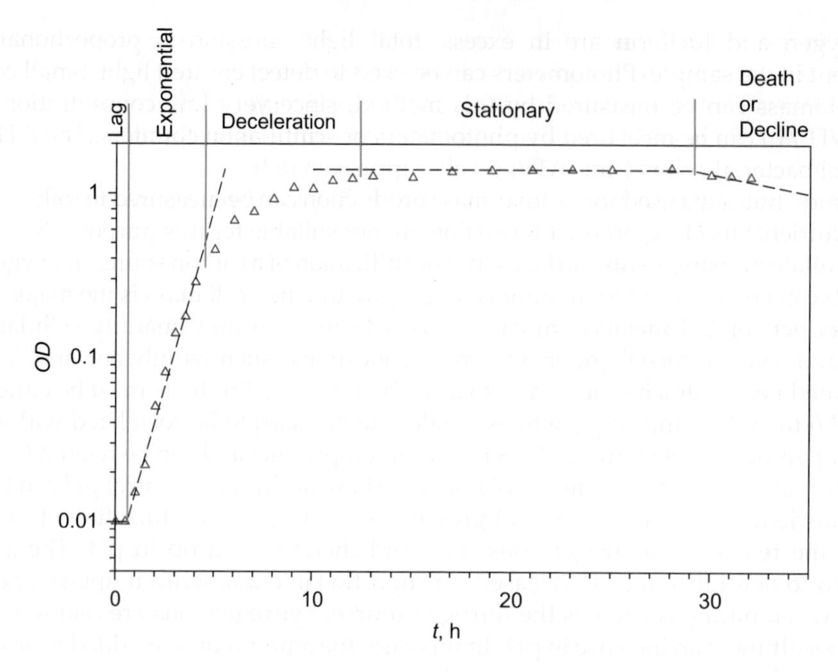

FIGURE 11.1 A typical batch growth pattern. The data points are measurements for *Escherichia coli* fbr5 in a glucose-rich medium.

When the inoculum is small and has a low fraction of cells that are viable, there may be a pseudo-lag phase, which is a result, not of adaptation, but of small inoculums size or poor condition of the inoculum.

Low concentration of some nutrients and growth factors may also cause a long lag phase. For example, the lag phase of *Enterobacter aerogenes* (formerly *Aerobacter aerogenes*) grown in glucose and phosphate buffer medium increases as the concentration of Mg^{2+}, which is an activator of the enzyme phosphatase, is decreased. As another example, even heterotrophic cells require CO_2 fixation (to supplement intermediates removed from key energy-producing metabolic cycles during rapid biosynthesis), and excessive sparging can remove metabolically generated CO_2 too rapidly for cellular restructuring to be accomplished efficiently, particularly with a small inoculum.

The age of the inoculum culture has a strong effect on the length of lag phase. The age refers to how long a culture has been maintained in a batch culture. Usually, the lag period increases with the age of the inoculum. In some cases, there is an optimal inoculums age resulting in minimum lag period. To minimize the duration of the lag phase, cells should be adapted to the growth medium and conditions before inoculation, cells should be young (or exponential phase cells) and active, and the inoculum size should be large (5% to 10% by volume). The nutrient medium may need to be optimized, and certain growth factors are included to minimize the lag phase. Many commercial fermentation plants rely on batch culture; to obtain high productivity from a fixed plant size, the lag phase must be as short as possible.

Multiple lag phases may be observed when the medium contains more than one carbon source. This phenomenon, known as diauxic growth, is caused by a shift in metabolic pathways in the middle of a growth cycle (see Example 10-1). After one carbon source is exhausted, the cells adapt their metabolic activities to utilize the second carbon source. The first carbon source is more readily utilizable than the second, and the presence of more readily available carbon source represses the synthesis of the enzymes required for the metabolism of the second substrate.

The *exponential growth phase* is also known as the *maximum growth phase* and *logarithmic growth phase.* In this phase, the cells have adjusted to their new environment. After this adaptation period, cells can multiply rapidly with maximum rate, and cell mass and cell number density increase exponentially with time. This is a period of *balanced growth,* in which all components of a cell grow at the same rate (pseudosteady state). That is, the average composition of a single cell remains approximately constant during this phase of growth. During balanced growth, the net specific growth rate determined from either cell number or cell mass would be the same. The specific growth rate is constant, from which a phenomenological model is proposed for the exponential growth phase:

$$r_X = \mu_{net} X \tag{11.2}$$

with the net specific growth rate being constant during this growth phase. This simple relation of Eqn (11.2) is called the Malthus growth model. In the batch process, the rate of change of biomass concentration is the same as the rate of generation of biomass (mass balance). Integration of the mass balance equation with Eqn (11.2) as the rate of generation of biomass yields

$$\ln \frac{X}{X_0} = \mu_{net} t \tag{11.3a}$$

or

$$X = X_0 e^{\mu_{net} t} \tag{11.3b}$$

where X and X_0 are cell concentrations at time t and initial time $t = 0$, respectively.

The time required to double the microbial mass can be computed using Eqn (11.3a) as

$$t_d = \frac{\ln 2}{\mu_{net}} \tag{11.4}$$

The doubling time is also the time required for a new generation of cells to appear during exponential growth period.

The *deceleration growth phase* follows the exponential phase. In this phase, growth decelerates due to either the depletion of one or more essential nutrients or the accumulation of toxic by-products of growth. For a typical bacterial culture, these changes occur over a very short period of time. The rapidly changing environment results in *unbalanced growth.* During unbalanced growth, cell composition and size will change. In the exponential phase, the cellular metabolic control system is set to achieve maximum rates of reproduction. In the deceleration phase, the stresses induced by nutrient depletion or waste accumulation cause a restructuring of the cell to increase the prospects of cellular survival in a hostile environment. These observable changes are the result of the molecular mechanisms of repression and induction that we discussed in Chapter 10. Because of the rapidity of these changes, cell physiology under conditions of nutrient limitation is more easily studied in continuous culture, as discussed later in Chapter 12.

Malthus growth model is valid only in the exponential growth phase. A modification of the Malthus model by Verhulst in 1844 included an *apparent biomass inhibition* term:

$$r_X = kX\left(1 - \frac{X}{X_\infty}\right) \tag{11.5}$$

where X_∞ is the carrying capacity of the cells in the medium and k is the carrying capacity coefficient. For a batch growth of constant culture volume, cell balance subjected to growth rate given by Eqn (11.5) gives rise to

$$X = \frac{X_0 e^{kt}}{1 - \frac{X_0}{X_\infty}(1 - e^{kt})} \tag{11.6}$$

Equation (11.6) is also termed the logistic equation. The Verhulst model is able to describe the exponential growth phase, the deceleration phase, and the stationary phase, via Eqn (11.6). Therefore, the Verhulst model (or logistic model) is a more accurate phenomenological model than the Malthus model.

The *stationary phase* starts at the end of the deceleration phase, when the net growth rate is zero (no cell division) or when the growth rate is equal to the death rate. Even though the net growth rate is zero during the stationary phase, cells are still metabolically active and produce secondary metabolites. *Primary metabolites* are growth-related products and *secondary metabolites* are nongrowth related. In fact, the production of certain metabolites is enhanced during the stationary phase (e.g. antibiotics, some hormones) due to metabolite deregulation. During the course of the stationary phase, one or more of the following phenomena may take place:

1. Total cell mass concentration may stay constant, but the number of viable cells may decrease.
2. Cell lysis may occur, and viable cell mass may drop. A second growth phase may occur, and cells may grow on lysis products of lysed cells (cryptic growth).
3. Cells may not be growing but may have active metabolism to produce secondary metabolites. Cellular regulation changes when concentrations of certain metabolites (carbon, nitrogen, phosphate) are low. Secondary metabolites are produced as a result of metabolite deregulation.

During the stationary phase, the cell catabolizes cellular reserves for new building blocks and for energy-producing monomers. This is called *endogenous metabolism.* The cell must always expend energy to maintain an energized membrane (i.e. proton-motive force) and transport of nutrients and for essential metabolic functions such as motility and repair of damage to cellular structures. This energy expenditure is called *maintenance energy.* As such, maintenance energy and endogenous metabolism are not limited to the stationary phase but become dominant in the stationary phase. The maintenance or endogenous expenditure is just a small fraction of the total cell needs during maximum growth. When the primary metabolism diminishes as in the stationary phase, the endogenous metabolism becomes dominant.

The reason for termination of growth may be either exhaustion of an essential nutrient or accumulation of toxic products. If an inhibitory product is produced and accumulates in the medium, the growth rate will slow down, depending on inhibitor production, and at a certain level of inhibitor concentration, growth will stop. Ethanol production by yeast is an example of a fermentation in which the product is inhibitory to growth. Dilution of toxified medium, addition of an unmetabolizable chemical compound complexing with the toxin, or simultaneous removal of the toxin would alleviate the adverse effects of the toxin and yield further growth.

The *death phase* (or decline phase) follows the stationary phase. However, some cell death may start during or even before the stationary phase, and a clear demarcation between these two phases is not always possible. Often, dead cells lyse, and intracellular nutrients released into the medium are used by the living organisms during stationary phase. At the end of the stationary phase, because of either nutrient depletion or toxic product accumulation, the death phase begins. The death rate can be thought of as a first-order reaction. Because S is zero, μ_G is zero starting from the stationary phase:

$$r_X = -k_d X \tag{11.7}$$

where k_d is a first-order rate constant for cell death. Mass balance of the cell biomass in the batch reactor leads to

$$-k_d XV = r_X V = \frac{\mathrm{d}(XV)}{\mathrm{d}t} \tag{11.8}$$

which can be integrated to yield (for constant medium V):

$$X = X_{S0} e^{-k_d t} \tag{11.9}$$

where X_{S0} is the cell mass concentration at the beginning of the stationary phase.

During the death phase, cells may or may not lyse, and the reestablishment of the culture may be possible in the early death phase if cells are transferred into a nutrient-rich medium. In both the death and stationary phases, it is important to recognize that there is a distribution of properties among individuals in a population. With a narrow distribution, cell death will occur nearly simultaneously; with a broad distribution, a subfraction of the population may survive for an extended period. It is this subfraction that would dominate the reestablishment of a culture from inoculum derived from stationary- or death-phase cultures. Thus, using an old inoculum may select for variants of the original strain having altered metabolic capabilities.

While the phenomenological models can describe the batch experiments of cell growth reasonably well, the parameters are not as meaningful for further genetical and more mechanistic evaluations. The regimes, especially the exponential phase, deceleration phase, and stationary phase, change with different loading of the same nutrients. The cell growth is understandably related to the availability of the substrates (or nutrients) in the medium, which may not be due to the biomass inhibition as logistic model depicts. One can imagine that the exponential growth is due to the sufficient supply of nutrients. The stationary phase is due to the exhaustion of the nutrients not necessarily due to cell biomass inhibition. Therefore, by not examining the substrate change, it leads to a noncomplete description of cell growth.

11.3. BIOMASS YIELD

To better describe growth kinetics in a simple fashion, we define some stoichiometrically related parameters. Yield factors are defined based on the amount of consumption of another material (Chapter 3). For example, the growth yield factor in a fermentation is defined as

$$YF_{X/S} = \frac{\mu_G X}{-r_S} \left(= \frac{dX|_{Growth}}{-dS} \right) \tag{11.10}$$

where μ_G is the true specific growth rate of the cells and more conveniently,

$$Y_{X/S} = \frac{X - X_0}{S_0 - S} \tag{11.11}$$

Note that the substrate change in Eqn (11.11) is the total substrate consumption, and the biomass change is total or net change. This definition is of convenience when first used, and it does have merits behind this definition as well. Sometimes, we refer to $Y_{X/S}$ in Eqn (11.11) as the apparent growth yield. The apparent growth yield is easy to understand; however, it is not a constant when a wide range of growth period is considered, in particular when K_S and K_P are not identical, or when cell death also occurs during growth. The fact that the apparent growth yield is not a constant makes its application difficult in kinetic studies. On the other hand, the yield factor as defined in Eqn (11.10) is the true growth yield factor.

At the end of the batch growth period, we have an *apparent growth yield factor* (or growth yield). Because culture conditions can alter patterns of substrate utilization, the apparent growth yield factor is not a true constant. One can observe from Eqn (11.11) that there are two quantities that affect the growth yield: perceived biomass change and the substrate change. These two quantities are exclusively linked with each other. For example, with a compound (such as glucose) that is both a carbon and energy source, substrate may be consumed due to more than one purposes as:

$$\Delta S = \Delta S_{\substack{\text{Conversion}\\ \text{to biomass}}} + \Delta S_{\substack{\text{Growth}\\ \text{energy}}} + \Delta S_{\substack{\text{Maintenance}\\ \text{energy}}} + \Delta S_{\substack{\text{Conversion}\\ \text{to extracellular}\\ \text{products}}} \tag{11.12}$$

although the net effect of each cell function is not independent for a clear distribution of the substrate diversion. A growth yield accounts for the substrate consumption in the first two terms on the right hand side of Eqn (11.12) would be more logical. Maintenance needs, however, are required whether the cell is growing or simply staying functional (or viable), although they can be growth rate dependent in some fashion. Conversion to extracellular products may not be directly related to the cell biomass growth, although it is at least related to maintenance needs. Therefore, if one defines the yield as the substrate consumption directly attributed to the biomass assimilation, it might well be a constant. However, this fictitious growth yield factor is not a factor that can be determined simply by examining the overall biomass yield and substrate consumption.

Cell functions are integral to the cell, and Eqn (11.12) is merely presented to elucidate the various demands of the cell. The division of substrate uptake to biomass assimilation and extracellular product conversion explains only one part of the biomass yield relation. The other part is the biomass change. Cells die when environmental conditions become less favorable or simply due to aging. Because of the complexity in microbial metabolic activities, it is very difficult to separate the different effects on growth yield.

Yield factors based on other substrates or product formation may be defined; for example,

$$YF_{X/O_2} = \frac{dX|_{Growth}}{-d[O_2]} \tag{11.13}$$

$$YF_{P/S} = \frac{dP}{-dS} \tag{11.14}$$

For organisms growing aerobically on glucose, $YF_{X/S}$ is typically 0.4–0.6 g/g for most yeast and bacteria, while YF_{X/O_2} is 0.9–1.4 g/g. Anaerobic growth is less efficient, and the yield factor is reduced substantially (see apparent biomass growth yield illustration on Fig. 11.2). With substrates that are more or less reduced than glucose, the value of the apparent yield will change. For methane, $YF_{X/S}$ would assume values of 0.6–1.0 g/g, with the corresponding YF_{X/O_2} decreasing to about 0.2 g/g. In most cases, the yield of biomass on a carbon-energy source is 1.0 ± 0.4 g biomass per gram of carbon consumed. Table 11.1 lists some examples of $YF_{X/S}$ and YF_{X/O_2} for a variety of substrates and organisms.

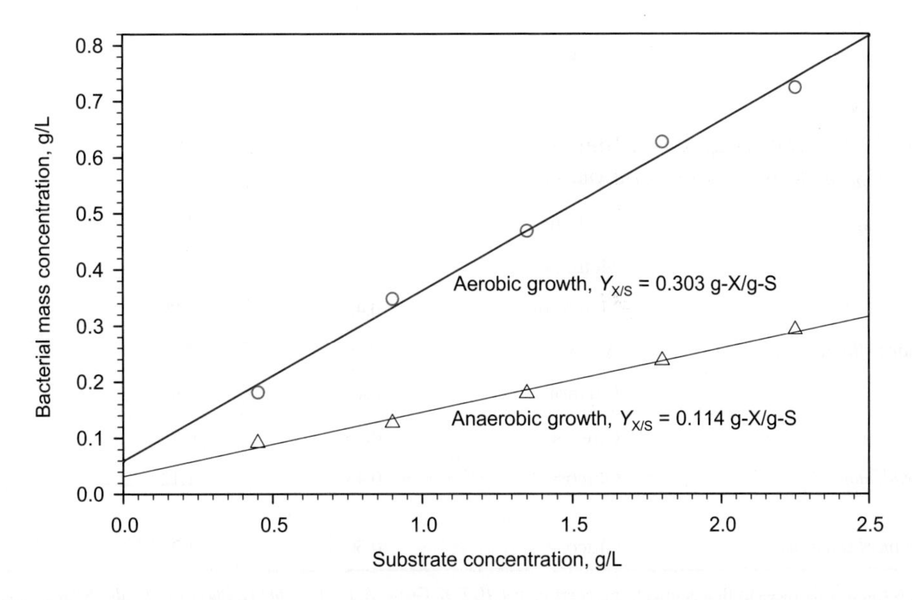

FIGURE 11.2 Aerobic and anaerobic growth yields of *Streptococcus faecalis* in glucose-limited media. The slope of the biomass growth versus substrate concentration line is the biomass growth yield, based on Eqn (11.11). *Data source: B. Atkinson and F. Mavituna,* Biochemical Engineering and Biotechnology Handbook, *Macmillan Inc.: New York, 1983.*

TABLE 11.1 A Collection of Yield Factors for Aerobic Growth of Different Microorganisms on Various Carbon Sources

Organism	Substrate	$YF_{X/S}$ g/g	$YF_{X/S}$ g/g-C	YF_{X/O_2} g/g
Candida utilis	Acetate	0.36	0.90	0.70
	Ethanol	0.68	1.30	0.61
	Glucose	0.51	1.28	1.32
Enterobacter aerogenes	Acetate	0.18	0.43	0.31
	Fructose	0.42	1.05	1.46
	Glucose	0.40	1.01	1.11
	Glycerol	0.45	1.16	0.97
	Lactate	0.18	0.46	0.37
	Maltose	0.46	1.03	1.50
	Mannitol	0.52	1.32	1.18
	Pyruvate	0.20	0.49	0.48
	Ribose	0.35	0.88	0.98
	Succinate	0.25	0.62	0.62
Klebsiella sp.	Methanol	0.38	1.01	0.56
Methylococcus sp.	Methane	1.01	1.34	0.29
	Methanol	0.48	1.28	0.53
Penicillium chrysogenum	Glucose	0.43	1.08	1.35
Pseudomona methanica	Methane	0.56	0.75	0.17
Pseudomona sp.	Methane	0.80	1.06	0.20
	Methane	0.60	0.80	0.19
	Methanol	0.41	1.09	0.44
Pseudomonas fluorescens	Acetate	0.28	0.70	0.46
	Ethanol	0.49	0.93	0.42
	Glucose	0.38	0.95	0.85
Rhodopseudomon spheroids	Glucose	0.45	1.12	1.46
Saccharomyces cerevisiae	Glucose	0.50	1.25	0.97

Source: S. Nagai in Advances in Biochemical Engineering, *vol. II, T. K. Ghose, A. Fiechter, and N. Blakebrough, eds., Springer-Verlag: New York, p. 53, 1979.*

Example 11-1. A strain of mold was grown in a batch culture on glucose and the following data were obtained as shown in Table E11-1. Do the following:

(a) Calculate the maximum net specific growth rate.
(b) Calculate the apparent growth yield.
(c) What maximum cell concentration could one expect if 150 g of glucose were used with the same size inoculum?
(d) How many generations of cells are there in the culture for part c).

TABLE E11-1 Kinetic Data of a Batch Culture

Time, h	Cell concentration, g/L	Glucose concentration, g/L
0	1.0	50.0
10	1.5	48.5
18	2.9	45.2
25	5.5	38.8
33	11.4	24.0
37	16.3	11.8
40	19.2	4.5
44	20.9	0.3

Solution.
(a) To obtain the maximum net specific growth rate, we calculate the rates using finite difference scheme as illustrated in the following table:

t, h	X, g/L	$\frac{\Delta X}{X \Delta t}$, h^{-1}
0	1.0	
10	1.5	0.040
18	2.9	0.085
25	5.5	0.088
33	11.4	0.087
37	16.3	0.088
40	19.2	0.054
44	20.9	0.021

From the table, we find that the maximum specific growth rate, $\mu_{max} = 0.088/h$.

(b) $Y_{X/S} = \frac{\Delta X}{-\Delta S} = \frac{20.9-1.0}{50.0-0.3} = 0.400$

(c) $X_{max} = X_0 + Y_{X/S}S_0 = 1.0 + 0.4(150) = 61.0$ g cells/l

(d) For each increase in generation, cell biomass doubles. That is, $X/X_0 = 2^n$ or $n = \ln(X/X_0)/\ln 2$, Therefore,

$$n = \frac{\ln(X/X_0)}{\ln 2} = \frac{\ln(61.0/1.0)}{\ln 2} = 5.93$$

There are $6 + 1 = 7$ generations of cells in the final culture.

11.4. APPROXIMATE GROWTH KINETICS AND MONOD EQUATION

In Chapter 8, we have learned that enzymatic reactions in general are governed by Michaelis–Menten kinetics or its variations. This same type of kinetic equation is also evident in the DNA and RNA replication and manipulations as one can infer from Chapter 10. In Chapter 10, we also learned that cell metabolism involves numerous groups, pathways, and reaction steps. Each reaction step along the metabolic pathway is an enzymatic reaction. Quantifying cell growth with all the governing parameters following all the genetic steps and metabolic pathways would make the computation tedious if not impossible. To the least, determining all the parameters would be very difficult. Therefore, some simplification of the kinetics is necessary in quantifying cell growth and thus bioreactions in general.

To begin with, let us examine a simple metabolic pathway as shown in Fig. 11.3. Substrate is uptaken into the cell and then converted into two products: P_1 and P_2 after a few intermediate steps. We assume that P_1 is an extracellular product, while P_2 is an intracellular product. The stoichiometries along the pathway illustrated in Fig. 11.3 can be written as:

$$S + E_1 \underset{k_{-1}}{\overset{k_1}{\rightleftarrows}} S \cdot E_1 \overset{k_{1c}}{\rightarrow} M_1 \cdot E_1 \tag{11.15a}$$

$$E_2 + M_1 \cdot E_1 \underset{k_{-2}}{\overset{k_2}{\rightleftarrows}} M_1 \cdot E_2 + E_1 \tag{11.15b}$$

$$M_1 \cdot E_2 \overset{k_{2c}}{\rightarrow} M_2 \cdot E_2 \tag{11.15c}$$

$$M_2 \cdot E_2 + E_3 \underset{k_{-3}}{\overset{k_3}{\rightleftarrows}} M_2 \cdot E_3 + E_2 \tag{11.15d}$$

$$M_2 \cdot E_3 \overset{k_{3c}}{\rightarrow} M_3 \cdot E_3 \tag{11.15e}$$

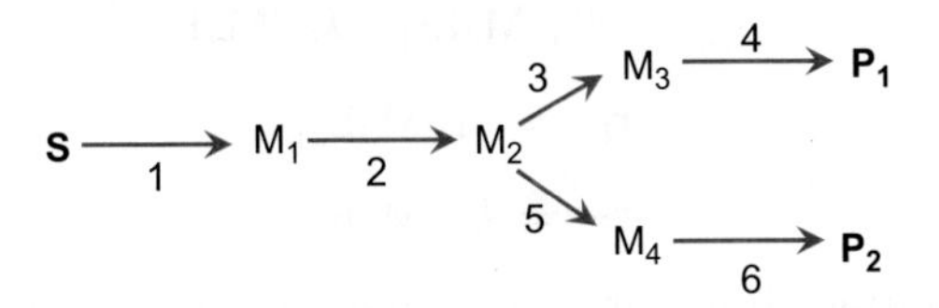

FIGURE 11.3 A simple metabolic pathway producing two products P_1 and P_2 from a single limiting substrate S.

$$M_3 \cdot E_3 \overset{k_{4c}}{\rightarrow} E_3 + P_1 \tag{11.15f}$$

$$M_2 \cdot E_2 + E_5 \underset{k_{-5}}{\overset{k_5}{\rightleftarrows}} M_2 \cdot E_5 + E_2 \tag{11.15g}$$

$$M_2 \cdot E_5 \overset{k_{5c}}{\rightarrow} M_4 \cdot E_5 \tag{11.15h}$$

$$M_4 \cdot E_5 \overset{k_{6c}}{\rightarrow} P_2 + E_5 \tag{11.15i}$$

$$M_4 \cdot E_5 \rightleftarrows {}_{\upsilon E_j} E_j + E_5, \; j = 1, 2, 3, 5 \tag{11.15j}$$

We have assumed that the intermediate product M_3 and product P_1 are essentially the same or required no catalyst to proceed. The same holds for M_4 and P_2. The rate of reaction or rate of generation for species j is given by (Chapter 3),

$$r_j = \sum_{i=1}^{N_R} \upsilon_{ji} r_i \tag{11.16}$$

where r_j is the reaction rate for species j, N_R is the total number of reactions in the system, υ_{ji} is the stoichiometric coefficient of species j in the reaction i, and r_i is the rate of reaction for the reaction i as written. Based on the reaction system described by Eqns (11.15a) through (11.15i), the reaction rates can be written as

$$r_S = -k_1 S[E_1] + k_{-1}[SE_1] \tag{11.17a}$$

$$r_{SE_1} = k_1 S[E_1] - (k_{-1} + k_{1c})[SE_1] \tag{11.17b}$$

$$r_{M_1E_1} = k_{1c}[SE_1] - k_2[E_2][M_1E_1] + k_{-2}[M_1E_2][E_1] \tag{11.17c}$$

$$r_{M_1E_2} = k_2[M_1E_1][E_2] - (k_{-2}[E_1] + k_{2c})[M_1E_2] \tag{11.17d}$$

$$r_{M_2E_2} = k_{2c}[M_1E_2] - k_3[M_2E_2][E_3] + k_{-3}[M_2E_3][E_2] - k_5[M_2E_2][E_5] + k_{-5}[M_2E_5][E_2] \tag{11.17e}$$

$$r_{M_2E_3} = k_3[M_2E_2][E_3] - (k_{-3}[E_2] + k_{3c})[M_2E_3] \tag{11.17f}$$

$$r_{M_2E_5} = k_5[M_2E_2][E_5] - (k_{-5}[E_2] + k_{5c})[M_2E_5] \tag{11.17g}$$

$$r_{M_3E_3} = k_{3c}[M_2E_3] - k_{4c}[M_3E_3] \tag{11.17h}$$

$$r_{M_4E_5} = k_{5c}[M_2E_5] - k_{6c}[M_4E_5] \tag{11.17i}$$

$$r_{P_1} = k_{4c}[M_3E_3] \tag{11.17j}$$

$$r_{P_2} = k_{6c}[M_4E_5] \tag{11.17k}$$

Assume that P_2 is the intracellular products. Since E_1, E_2, E_3, and E_5 are all part of the cellular material, we further simplify Eqn (11.15j) and incorporate it into the enzyme balances lead to:

$$[E_1]_T = [E_1]_0 + \chi_1 P_2 = [E_1] + [SE_1] + [M_1E_1] \tag{11.18a}$$

$$[E_2]_T = [E_2]_0 + \chi_2 P_2 = [E_2] + [M_1E_2] + [M_2E_2] \tag{11.18b}$$

$$[E_3]_T = [E_3]_0 + \chi_3 P_2 = [E_3] + [M_2E_3] + [M_3E_3] \tag{11.18c}$$

$$[E_5]_T = [E_5]_0 + \chi_5 P_2 = [E_5] + [M_2E_5] + [M_4E_5] \tag{11.18d}$$

Mass balances in a batch reactor with constant medium volume lead to

$$\frac{dC_j}{dt} = r_j \tag{11.19}$$

At time $t = 0$, $C_j = 0$ for all j except $S = S_0$. The total enzyme concentrations at time 0 are each assumed to be 2% of the total substrate S_0, except $[E_3]_{T0} = 0.04\,S_0$. Equation (11.19) can be integrated with OdexLims and the solution is shown in Fig. 11.4. In Fig. 11.4, we have assumed that the increase in the amount of each enzyme is 5% of the intercellular product P_2 or $\chi_j = 0.05$, except E_3 is increased by 10% of P_2 or $\chi_3 = 0.1$. One can observe that the substrate

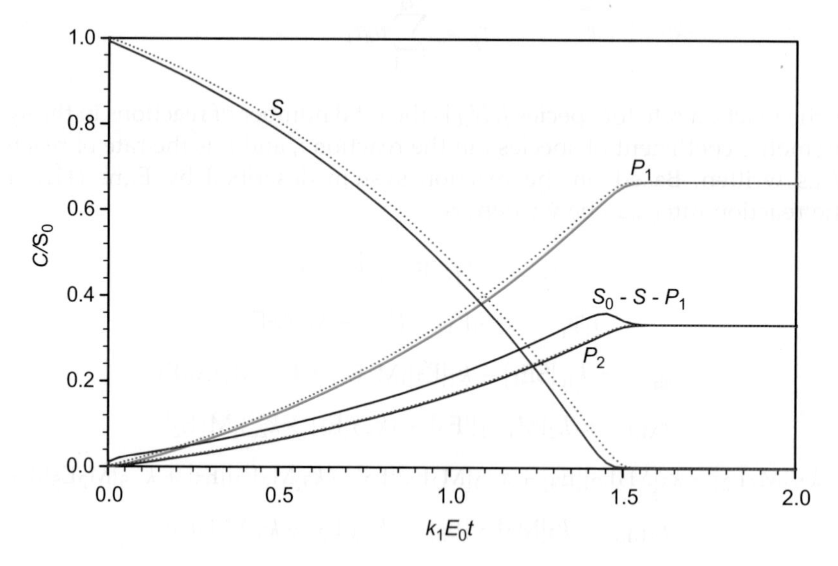

FIGURE 11.4 A comparison of the full solution and approximate solution (single-step Michaelis–Menten equation) for the reaction network showing in Fig. 11.3. The solid lines are based on the full solution, while the dotted lines are based on the approximated model. The kinetic constants are $k_{-j}\,S_0 = k_{jc} = 0.01\,k_j S_0$; $k_j = k_1$, for all j except $j = 1$. Also, $k_{-1} = 0.01\,k_1\,S_0$.

concentrations decrease monotonously while the product concentrations increase monotonously. However, the difference in the initial (fed) substrate concentrations and the sum of the residual substrate and extracellular product concentrations increases initially, reaches a maximum, and then decreases to its final value at long times. This is an interesting and important observation for bioreactions, as the substrate uptake by cells and subsequent conversion to intracellular and extracellular products pass through a number of intermediates. When cell biomass is measured, substrate retained inside the cells are likely to be treated as biomass. Therefore, one can expect a maximum biomass weight before all the substrate is consumed.

As we have learned from Chapters 8 and 9, the reaction system as described by Eqn (11.5) may be simplified by one rate-limiting step (for each branch of parallel reactions) with rate constants altered to fit the whole reaction network. It is not difficult to show that each complete step of conversion from one species to another in Eqn (11.15) can be approximated by the Michaelis–Menten equation, i.e.

$$r_{P1} = \frac{r_{P1\max} S}{K_{P1} + S}(1 + \chi_0 P_2) \tag{11.20a}$$

$$r_{P2} = \frac{r_{P2\max} S}{K_{P2} + S}(1 + \chi_0 P_2) \tag{11.20b}$$

and

$$r_S = -r_{P1} - r_{P2} \tag{11.20c}$$

Utilizing this simplification to approximate the rates for P_1 and P_2, one can solve the problem more easily based on Eqn (11.17) for S, P_1, and P_2. The solutions based on Eqn (11.20) with $r_{P1\max} = 0.20853\ k_1[E_1]_0$, $K_{P1} = 0.014424\ S_0$, $r_{P2\max} = 0.10117\ k_1[E_1]_0$, $K_{P2} = 0.07919\ S_0$, and $\chi_0 = 9.81296/S_0$ are plotted as dotted line in Fig. 11.4.

One can observe from Fig. 11.4 that the approximate model, i.e. Eqn (11.20) gives reasonable prediction for the reaction network in the product formation and the substrate consumption. As one may infer from Chapter 10 that DNA and RNA constructions and manipulations by cells also follow a kinetic equation similar to Eqn (11.20), the approximation may actually be applicable to cell growth and/or metabolism, in general. Therefore, it is reasonable to approximate the growth rate of cells by an equation similar to Eqn (11.20), or

$$\mu_G = \frac{r_X}{X} = \frac{\mu_{\max} S}{K_S + S} \tag{11.21}$$

which is known as the Monod equation of growth. Equation (11.21) is an empirical rate function, and we have now seen its relevance in the kinetics of cell growth from an approximate kinetic behavior point of view. Similarly, for extracellular product formation,

$$\mu_P = \frac{r_P}{X} = \frac{\mu_{P\max} S}{K_P + S} \tag{11.22}$$

Often, K_P and K_S are assumed to be identical, further simplifying the growth kinetics.

However, one can notice the difference between the simple approximation and the full solution in Fig. 11.4. There seemed to have a difference in substrate concentration due to presence of substrate inside the cells (substrate–enzyme complexes) and the intermediates. The intermediates are not able to be captured by the simple approximation. Therefore, the simple approximation is applicable for pseudosteady-state cases. Inclusion of the initial or induction time results in noticeable differences (or errors). The difference between the dashed line and the solid line in Fig. 11.4 exhibits a time lag when matching products formation and substrate consumption. The time lag is due to the inability of the simple model to capture the uptake of substrate in the cell and a "delay" in excrete products. This phenomenon is more pronounced in real cultures as the metabolic pathway is much more complex than that exemplified by Fig. 11.3.

Equation (11.21) indicates that when the limiting substrate concentration is high, i.e. $S \gg K_S$, the specific growth rate $\mu \approx \mu_{max} =$ constant. That is, the growth is at the maximum growth rate. Thus, the exponential growth regime (of the batch cell growth, Fig. 11.1) is also termed maximum growth regime. The change of growth rate is due to the change of substrate concentration. There is no control on the growth. Therefore, the batch exponential growth is also uncontrolled exponential growth.

11.5. CELL DEATH RATE

In section 11.4, cell growth rate is suggested based on metabolic pathway analysis. Cells (or whole microorganisms) die due to environmental conditions (for example heat) or physiological developments. The death rate of cells is proportional to the cell population, and thus the specific death rate is not a function of cell population of concentration, which is confirmed by the experimental observation, Eqn (7). That is,

$$\mu_d = k_d \tag{11.23}$$

In single-celled microorganisms, *cell death* is the point at which reinitiation of division is no longer possible. Dead cells cease nutrient uptake and cell functions stop.

The net specific cell growth rate is the growth rate subtracted cell death rate, that is

$$\mu_{net} = \mu_G - k_d \tag{11.24}$$

During sterilization by heat, cells are destroyed due to excessive heat. The death rate increases with increasing temperature. In normal growth conditions, the death rate is usually very low.

Before we exiting the discussions on the cell growth, let us go back to revisit the biomass yield in §11.3. Solving the mass balance equations of biomass and substrate based on Eqns (11.24), (11.21), (11.10), and (11.11), we obtain the apparent yield in batch cultivations as

$$Y_{X/S} = \frac{X - X_0}{S_0 - S} = YF_{X/S}\left(1 - \frac{k_d}{\mu_{max}} - \frac{k_d}{\mu_{max}}\frac{K_S}{S_0 - S}\ln\frac{S_0}{S}\right) \tag{11.25}$$

That is, the apparent growth yield $Y_{X/S}$ is always less than the growth yield factor $YF_{X/S}$. The higher the death rate in comparison to the growth rate, the lower the apparent growth yield. We note that

$$\frac{K_S}{S_0 - S}\ln\frac{S_0}{S} = \frac{K_S}{(S_0, S)_{log-mean}} \tag{11.26}$$

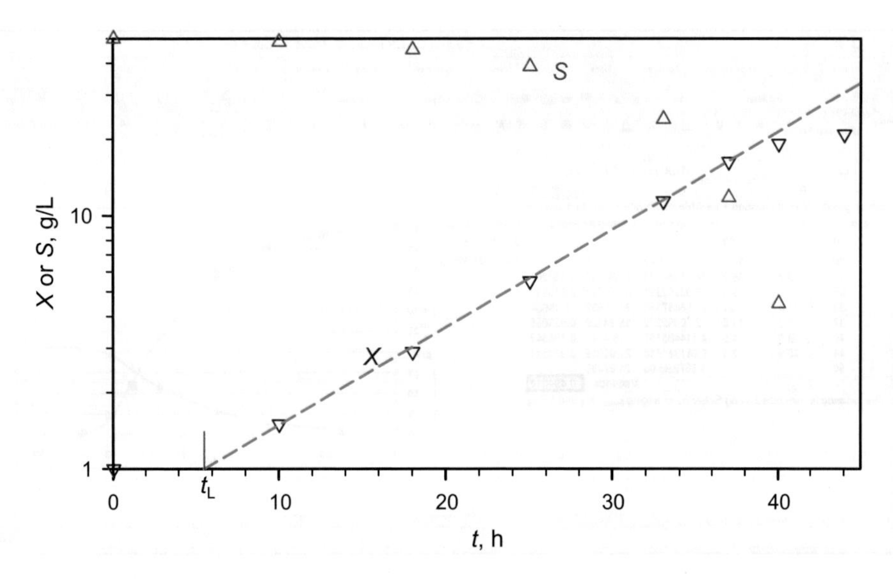

FIGURE E11-2.1 Semi-log plot of the biomass concentration (and substrate concentration) variation with time.

Equation (11.25) also shows that a lower initial substrate concentration gives rise to a lower apparent yield for a given finite specific death rate in the growth kinetics. Usually, $S_0 >> K_S$, the effect of initial substrate concentration on the apparent biomass yield is negligible as indicated by Eqn (11.25).

Example 11-2. Using Monod equation of growth and a constant biomass yield factor to correlate the data in Example 11-1. Determine the maximum growth rate μ_{max}, saturation constant K_S, and yield factor $YF_{X/S}$.

Solution. The Monod equation of growth is only applicable for balanced growth, i.e. when pseudosteady state inside the cells has been established. Therefore, it is not applicable in the lag phase. To be certain of the time to start for using Monod equation of growth, we plotted out the cell growth data on semi-log scale as shown in Fig. E11-2.1. A straight line (dashed line) is drawn as a guide on the cell biomass data. From Fig. 12.2-1, we can observe that there is an apparent lag time of $t_L = 5.5$ h. The cell concentration changes with time becomes exponential after $t = 10$ h. Thus, we correlate the data starting from $t = 10$ h.

Mass balance of the cell biomass in the batch reactor leads to

$$\frac{dX}{dt} = \mu_G X = \frac{\mu_{max} S}{K_S + S} X \tag{E11-2.1}$$

Mass balance on the substrate in the batch reactor leads to

$$\frac{dS}{dt} = -\frac{\mu_G X}{YF_{X/S}} = \frac{\mu_{max} S}{K_S + S} \times \frac{X}{YF_{X/S}} \tag{E11-2.2}$$

Using the OdexLims in Excel to solve the two differential equations, (E11-2.1) and (E11-2.2), while correlating the experimental data, we obtain the kinetic parameters:

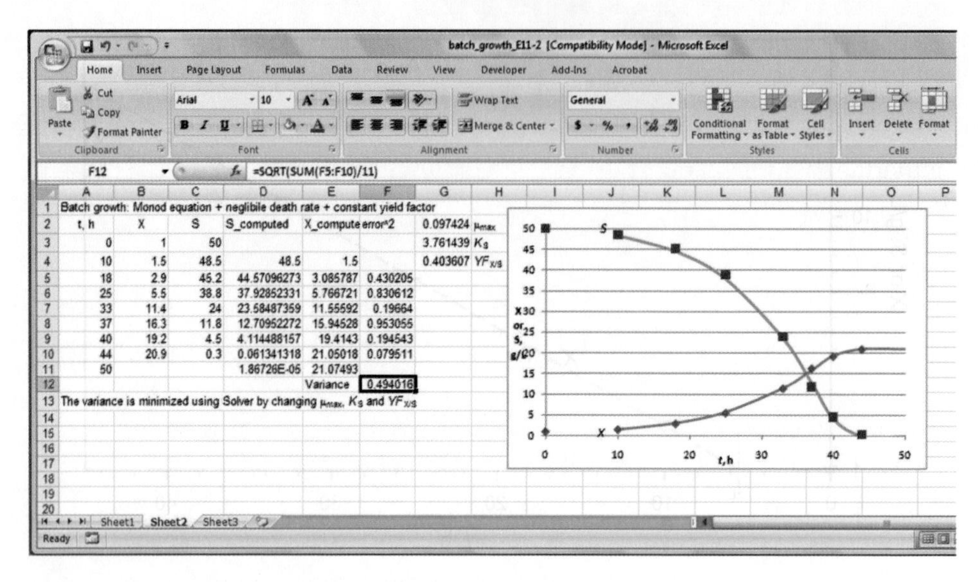

FIGURE E11-2.2 Monod growth equation fit to data in Excel.

$\mu_{max} = 0.0974/h$, $K_S = 3.76$ g/L, and $YF_{X/S} = 0.4036$. The quality of the fit is shown in Fig. E11-2.2. Now that all the kinetic parameters are known, we can calculate or predict the growth behavior of the cells in the culture. The parameters obtained this way are more reliable than that from Example 11-1.

11.6. CELL MAINTENANCE AND ENDOGENOUS METABOLISM

As discussed in Chapter 10, cell metabolism is complicated and simplification is possible for any given focus. In section §11.4, we have learned how a complicated metabolic pathway may be simplified based on our perspective or parameters that can be measured. Cell growth-associated internal cell functions are not easily measurable; however, they play important roles in kinetic behaviors. In this section, we look at simplifying the cell growth-associated functions with a focus on their effects on growth needs.

To harness the free energy produced by catabolic processes in terms of high-energy phosphate bonds, in particular in the form of ATP, for subsequent use in the biosynthesis of biomass constituents in the anabolism, the cellular content of ATP (and ADP) must be controlled quite rigorously. As the turnover time of ATP is low (U. Theobald, J. Mohns, M. Rizzi. Dynamics of orthophosphate in yeast cytoplasm, Biotechnology Letters 18(4): 461–466 APR 1996), there must be tight balancing of the energy-forming reactions (catabolism) and the energy-utilizing reactions (the anabolism) inside the cell. In analogy to the tight balancing of synthesis and consumption of ATP, the cell needs to balance the synthesis and consumption of the cofactors NADH or NADPH, which have a small turnover time. Consequently, the cell must exercise a strict control of the level of these compounds as well.

The balances for ATP, NADH, and NADPH are used to relate the fluxes through different parts of the metabolic network. However, in order to apply the ATP balance, it is important that all ATP forming and consuming reactions are considered; one group of energy-consuming processes inside the cell, namely, maintenance processes is especially important as it is seemingly a net energy drain without an apparent benefit to the system.

Cell maintenance is the consumption of a key substrate under consideration to maintain the desired functionality of the cell in addition to the stoichiometrically quantifiable desired outcome, such as cell growth. The balance of ATP, NADH, and NADPH, for example, requires maintenance energy. *Endogenous metabolism*, on the other hand, refers to the metabolic needs of a cell to stay viable either by consuming nutrients in the medium when available or by converting intracellular materials when starved. Therefore, strictly speaking, cell maintenance is cell growth dependent, while endogenous metabolic needs are often growth independent. Cell maintenance and endogenous metabolic needs are, however, closely related and not easily separated in practice. Therefore, these two are often combined in bioprocess modeling, and both terminologies are used interchangeably at times.

Herbert (D. Herbert. 1959 "Some principles of continuous culture", *Recent Prog. Microb.*, 7: 381–396) showed that it is necessary to consider the "endogenous metabolism" or cell death when the substrate utilization for biomass growth is to be calculated. He assumed that this endogenous metabolism results in a decrease of the amount of biomass, and he described the degradation as a first-order process with a specific rate of biomass degradation μ_e. Restitution of the degraded biomass requires substrate, and the total substrate consumption is therefore:

$$-r_S = (YF_{S/X}\mu_G + YF_{S/X}\mu_e)X \tag{11.27}$$

Equation (11.27) shows that there are two contributions to the substrate utilization: one term which is directly proportional to the observed, net specific growth rate (i.e. a growth-associated part) and another term which counteracts the continuous degradation of the cell mass due to endogenous metabolism. The yield factor $YF_{S/X}$ specifies the yield in the conversion of substrate into biomass. Pirt (S.J. Pirt. 1965 "The maintenance energy of bacteria in growing cultures", *Proc. Royal Soc. London. Series B.* **163**: 224–231) introduced an empirical correlation identical in form to Eqn (11.27), but he collected the product of $YF_{S/X}$ and μ_e in the empirical constant m_S,

$$-r_S = (YF_{S/X}\mu_G + m_S)X \tag{11.28}$$

This empirical constant was called the maintenance coefficient. While strictly speaking, maintenance requirements and endogenous needs are different, we tend to simplify the metabolic system by "equate" the maintenance and endogenous needs. This allows us to lump the two different indirect growth needs to one quantity. The *maintenance coefficient* can then be related to the specific rate of substrate uptake for cellular maintenance, via

$$m_S = \frac{-r_S|_{\text{maintenance}}}{X} = YF_{S/X}k_d \tag{11.29}$$

Maintenance coefficient (m_S) is an important parameter in fermentation process and has great influence on the biomass and product yield. The primary method for the determination of maintenance coefficient is obtained from the linear relation Eqn (11.28). To get an accurate result of m_S, the rates should be precisely measured in a wide range. However, the true substrate consumption rate for maintenance process may be a function of the specific growth rate when both cell maintenance requirements and endogenous metabolic needs are considered. A linear relation between the total or true maintenance coefficient and the cell growth rate has been proposed by Ma et al. (H.W. Ma, X.M. Zhao, X.F. Guo. 2002. "Calculation of empirical and true maintenance coefficients by flux balance analysis", *Chinese J. Chem. Eng.*, **10**(1): 89–92)

$$m_S^{true} = a\mu_G + b \tag{11.30}$$

where m_S^{true} is the true maintenance coefficient (J. Nielsen, J. Villadsen, G. Lidén. 2003 *Bioreaction Engineering Principles*, Plenum Press: New York). However m_S^{true} is difficult to be determined experimentally. We normally drop the superscript true.

Despite its empirical nature, the maintenance coefficient approach, Eqn (11.28) gives a good description of the specific substrate uptake rate for many cellular systems especially at high growth rates. However, the simple linear rate equation does not in a biologically satisfactory way explain what the extra substrate consumed for maintenance is in processes. Not only m_S is a constant, but $YF_{X/S}$ varies apparently with the specific growth rate as well. During the stationary phase where little external substrate is available, endogenous metabolism of biomass components (no substrate consumption) is used for maintenance energy. Cellular maintenance represents energy expenditures to repair damaged cellular components, to transfer some nutrients and products in and out of cells, for motility, and to adjust the osmolarity of the cells' interior volume.

Utilization of energy, and consequently substrate, in all the processes involved with cell maintenance is likely to be a function of the specific growth rate. When the specific growth rate is high, there is a high turnover of macromolecules (eg. mRNA), and with increasing activity level in the cell, it is for example necessary to pump more protons out of the cell. Furthermore, with a higher flux through the cellular pathways, there is a higher loss of energy due to the hydrolysis of high-energy phosphates such as ATP. This is biologically reasonable since when the cells grow under limited conditions (a low specific growth rate), they will try to use the substrate as efficiently as possible, and the maintenance processes are therefore curtailed. The energy expenditure in maintenance processes is therefore likely to be an increasing function of the specific growth rate. Thus, part of the Gibbs free energy spent in these maintenance processes may be included in the overall yield factor $YF_{X/S}$, and only the part of free energy that is spent not directly proportional to the specific growth rate are included in the maintenance coefficient.

Bauchop and Elsden (T. Bauchop, S.R. Esden. 1960 "The growth of microorganisms in relation to their energy supply", *J. Gen. Microb.* **23**: 35–43) introduced the concept of ATP requirements for biomass synthesis via the yield factor $YF_{ATP/X}$ and proposed a balance equation that is analogous to Eqn (11.28):

$$r_{ATP} = YF_{ATP/X}\mu_G + m_{ATP} \tag{11.31}$$

Here r_{ATP} specifies the total formation rate of ATP in catabolic pathways (different from the net formation rate of ATP, which is implicitly assumed to be zero in the equation). From precise measurements of the metabolic products of the anaerobic metabolism, it is possible to calculate the specific formation rate of ATP, i.e. r_{ATP}. This may be used to find experimental values for $YF_{ATP/X}$ and m_{ATP}, as shown in many studies. In aerobic processes, a major part of the ATP formation originates in the respiration, and the yield of ATP in this process is given by the P/O ratio. It is difficult to estimate the operational value of the P/O ratio. Detailed empirical studies (e.g. W.M. van Gulik, J.J. Heijnen. 1995 "A metabolic network stoichiometry analysis of microbial growth and product formation", *Biotechnol. Bioeng.* **48**: 681–698) have indicated an operational P/O ratio of 1.2–1.3, but this will depend on the microorganism and perhaps also on the environmental conditions. The ATP production can therefore not be calculated with the same accuracy in organisms that gain ATP by respiration as for organisms that are only able to produce ATP in fermentative pathways (substrate-level phosphorylation).

In Table 11.2, experimentally determined values for $YF_{ATP/X}$ and m_{ATP} are collected for a number of microorganisms growing at anaerobic conditions where r_{ATP} could be precisely determined. There is a large variation in the experimentally found values. This is partly explained by the fact that $YF_{ATP/X}$ depends both on the applied medium and on the macromolecular composition of the biomass. However, more definitive explanation that lies on the maintenance cost can have a different rate than the cell growth.

Instead of focusing on simple empirical correlations of cell maintenance with cell growth rate, we next examine the cell maintenance from a more mechanistic point of view. As we have learnt that the Monod equation is an approximated growth rate from the complicated metabolic pathways (section §11.4). The same approximation can be applied to be based on a key intermediate (for example ATP), rather than the substrate from the environment. Let us denote this key intermediate as Y, the specific cell growth rate can then be approximated by

$$\mu_G = \frac{r_X}{X} = \frac{\mu_{max} Y}{K_{YG} + Y} \tag{11.32}$$

While Y is the intermediate for cells to add mass (grow), it is consumed to maintain the cell active. For example, one can assume Y to be M_2 for the simple metabolic pathway in Fig. 11.3. The maintenance cost of the intermediate Y can be assumed to be in a fashion similar to any other bioreactions. In other words, the maintenance (or endogenous) cost can be approximated by

$$\mu_e = \frac{r_e}{X} = \frac{\mu_{emax} Y}{K_{Ye} + Y} \tag{11.33}$$

where the saturation constant K_{Ye} needs not to be identical to the saturation constant K_Y in the cell growth rate. K_{Ye} may not be exactly zero either (for which a constant maintenance coefficient prevails). There are two ways to express the cell maintenance cost, either to the cell growth rate or to the substrate availability. It is not difficult to see that

$$\mu_e = \frac{r_e}{X} = \frac{\mu_{emax} S}{K_{Se} + S} \tag{11.34}$$

TABLE 11.2 Experimentally Determined Values of $YF_{ATP/X}$ and m_{ATP}, for Various Microorganisms Grown under Anaerobic Conditions with Glucose as the Energy Source

Microorganism	$YF_{ATP/X}$, mmoles-ATP/g-cells	m_{ATP}, mmoles-ATP/(g-cells·h)	Sources
Aerobacter aerogenes	71.4 56.8	6.8 2.3	A.H. Stouthamer, C. Bettenhaussen. 1973 *Biochim. Biophysics Acta*, **301**: 53–70.
Bacillus clausii PP 473-8	42.0	2.93	T. Christiansen, J. Nielsen. 2002 *Bioprocess and Biosystems Eng.* **24** (5): 329–339.
Candida parapsilosis	80	0.2	B. Atkinson, F. Mavituna. 1983 *Biochemical Engineering and Biotechnology Handbook*, MacMillan, Inc.: New York.
Escherichia coli	97 118	18.9 6.9	W.P. Hempfling, S.E. Mainzer. 1975 *J. Bacteriol.* **123**: 1076–1087.
Lactobacillus casei	41.2	1.5	W. de Vries, et al. 1970 *J. Gen. Microbiol.* **63**: 333–345.
Lactobacillus delbruckii	72	0	N.C. Major, A.T. Bull. 1985. *Biotechol. Letters*, **7**: 401–405.
Lactococcus cremoris	73	1.4	R. Otto, et al. *Prod. Nat. Acad. Sci.* **77**: 5502–5506.
	53	–	W.W. Brown, E.B. Colins. 1977 *Appl. Environ. Microbiol.* **59**: 3206–3211.
	15–50	7–18	S. Benthin, et al. 1994. Chem. Eng. Sci. 49: 589–609.
Lactococcus diacetilactis	47	–	W.W. Brown, E.B. Colins. 1977 *Appl. Environ. Microbiol.* **59**: 3206–3211.
Penicillium chrysogenum	61	1.2	W.M. van Gulik, et al. 2001 *Biotechnol. Bioeng.*, **72**: 185–193.
Saccharomyces cerevisiae	71–91	<1	C. Verduyn, et al. 1990. *J. Gen. Microbiol.* **136**: 405–411.
S. cerevisiae	91 77	0.5 0.25	Atkinson and Mavituna (1983)
S. cerevisiae (petite)	88.5	0.7	Atkinson and Mavituna (1983)

which is a more general expression than the various ways of approximating the cell maintenance and death. Since cell maintenance goes head to tail with cell growth, substituting Eqn (11.32) into (11.33), we obtain

$$\mu_e = \frac{\mu_{emax} K_{YG} \mu_G}{K_{Ye}\mu_{max} + (K_{YG} - K_{Ye})\mu_G} \tag{11.35}$$

Equation (11.35) can be rewritten as

$$\mu_e = \frac{\mu_{e\mu max}\mu_G}{K_{e\mu} + \mu_G} \tag{11.36}$$

Now that we derived at an equation for the cell maintenance, we can observe that the cell maintenance may not be a constant nor it would be a straight line when correlated with the cell growth rate. When a straight line is forced upon the cell maintenance needs, one can expect both the slope (proportionality constant) and the intercept (or the constant "apparent" maintenance coefficient) to vary depending on the range of data collected.

To illustrate the importance of the variable endogenous metabolism with cell growth, we examine the data collected by Benthin et al. (S. Benthin, U. Schulze, J. Nielsen, J. Vlladsen. 1994. Growth energetics of *Lactococcus cremoris* FD1 during energy-, carbon-, and nitrogen-limitation in steady state and transient cultures. Chem. Eng. Sci. 49: 589–609), who conducted an analysis of the cell growth and product formation of *Lactococcus cremoris* (part of the results are shown in Table 11.2). Figure 11.5 shows the specific production rate μ_P versus the specific growth rate μ_G from a batch fermentation of *L. cremoris*. The medium contained 20 g/L of glucose and 7 g/L of a complex N source (a mixture of 50% yeast extract and 50% caseine peptone). The biomass concentration was monitored by flow injection analysis, and the specific total acid production was measured by monitoring the amount of alkali added to keep the pH constant in the bioreactor. Throughout the batch fermentation, the glucose concentration was high, and consequently only lactic acid was produced.

The lactic acid production is closely correlated to the ATP production (1 mole of ATP per mole of lactic acid produced), and Fig. 11.5 can therefore be used to estimate $YF_{X/ATP}$ and μ_{eATP} based on Eqns (11.25) and (11.36). That is,

$$\mu_{ATP} = YF_{ATP/X}(\mu_G + \mu_e) = YF_{ATP/X}\left(\mu_G + \frac{\mu_{e\mu max}\mu_G}{K_{e\mu} + \mu_G}\right) \tag{11.37}$$

The line plotted is with $YF_{ATP/X} = 1.216$ g-lactic acid/g-cells = 13.5 mmol/g-cells; $\mu_{e\mu max} = 1.521\ h^{-1}$; and $K_{e\mu} = 0.083\ h^{-1}$.

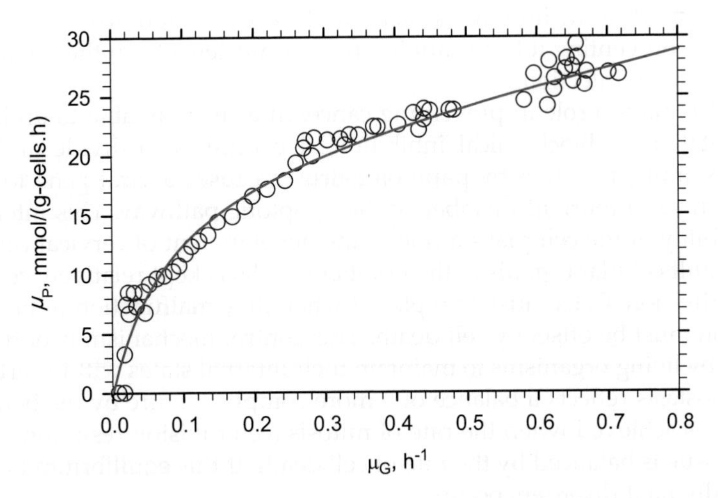

FIGURE 11.5 Specific product (acids) formation rate as a function of growth rate for *Lactococcus cremoris* in a complex medium containing 20 g/L glucose and 7 g/L nitrogen source. *Data source: S. Benthin, U. Schulze, J. Nielsen, J. Vlladsen. 1994. Growth energetics of* Lactococcus cremoris *FD1 during energy-, carbon-, and nitrogen-limitation in steady state and transient cultures. Chem. Eng. Sci. 49: 589–609.*

So far we have been focused on the cell's endogenous needs with single-cell organisms. For multicellular organisms, the endogenous organism needs also include the replacement of dead cells. To certain degree, the cell death and division in multicellular organisms help us understand cell endogenous metabolism needs.

Apoptosis is the process of programmed cell death (PCD) that may occur in multicellular organisms. PCD involves a series of biochemical events that lead to a variety of morphological changes, including blebbing changes to the cell membrane such as loss of membrane asymmetry and attachment, cell shrinkage, nuclear fragmentation, chromatin condensation, and chromosomal DNA fragmentation. Processes of disposal of cellular debris whose results do not damage the organism differentiate apoptosis from necrosis.

In contrast to necrosis, which is a form of traumatic cell death that results from acute cellular injury, apoptosis, in general, confers advantages during an organism's life cycle. For example, the differentiation of fingers and toes in a developing human embryo occurs because cells between the fingers apoptose; the result is that the digits are separate. Between 50 and 70 billion cells die each day due to apoptosis in the average human adult. For an average child between the ages of 8 and 14 years, approximately 20–30 billion cells die a day. In a year, this amounts to the proliferation and subsequent destruction of a mass of cells equal to one's body weight.

Research on apoptosis has increased substantially since the early 1990s. In addition to its importance as a biological phenomenon, defective apoptotic processes have been implicated in an extensive variety of diseases. Excessive apoptosis causes hypotrophy, such as in ischemic damage, whereas an insufficient amount results in uncontrolled cell proliferation, such as cancer.

Apoptosis occurs when a cell is damaged beyond repair, infected with a virus, or undergoing stressful conditions such as starvation. Damage to DNA from ionizing radiation or toxic chemicals can also induce apoptosis via the actions of the tumor-suppressing gene. The "decision" for apoptosis can come from the cell itself, from the surrounding tissue, or from a cell that is part of the immune system. In these cases, apoptosis functions to remove the damaged cell, preventing it from sapping further nutrients from the organism or halting further spread of viral infection.

Apoptosis also plays a role in preventing cancer. If a cell is unable to undergo apoptosis because of mutation or biochemical inhibition, it continues to divide and develop into a tumor. For example, infection by papillomaviruses causes a viral gene to interfere with the cell's protein, an important member of the apoptotic pathway. This interference in the apoptotic capability of the cell plays a role in the development of cervical cancer.

In an adult multicellular organism, the number of cells is kept relatively constant through cell death and division. Cells must be replaced when they malfunction or become diseased, but proliferation must be offset by cell death. This control mechanism is part of the homeostasis required by living organisms to maintain their internal states within certain limits. The related term allostasis reflects a balance of a more complex nature by the body.

Homeostasis is achieved when the rate of mitosis (cell division resulting in cell multiplication) in the tissue is balanced by the rate of cell death. If this equilibrium is disturbed, one of two potentially fatal disorders occurs:

- the cells divide faster than they die, resulting in the development of a tumor.
- the cells divide slower than they die, causing cell loss.

Homeostasis involves a complex series of reactions, an ongoing process inside an organism that calls for different types of cell signaling. Any impairment can cause a disease. For example, dysregulation of signaling pathway has been implicated in several forms of cancer. The pathway, which conveys an antiapoptotic signal, has been found to be activated in pancreatic adenocarcinoma tissues.

PCD is an integral part of both plant and animal tissue development. Development of an organ or tissue is often preceded by the extensive division and differentiation of a particular cell, the resultant mass is then "pruned" into the correct form by apoptosis. Unlike necrosis, cellular death caused by injury, apoptosis results in cell shrinkage and fragmentation. Such shrinkage and fragmentation allow the cells to be phagocytosed and their components reused without releasing potentially harmful intracellular substances such as hydrolytic enzymes into the surrounding tissue.

The process of apoptosis is controlled by a diverse range of cell signals, which may originate either extracellularly (*extrinsic inducers*) or intracellularly (*intrinsic inducers*). Extracellular signals may include toxins, hormones, growth factors, nitric oxide, or cytokines and therefore must either cross the plasma membrane or transduce to effect a response. These signals may positively (i.e. trigger) or negatively (i.e. repress, inhibit, or dampen) affect apoptosis. (Binding and subsequent initiation of apoptosis by a molecule is termed *positive induction*, whereas the active repression or inhibition of apoptosis by a molecule is termed *negative induction*.)

A cell initiates intracellular apoptotic signaling in response to a stress, which may bring about cell suicide. The binding of nuclear receptors by glucocorticoids, heat, radiation, nutrient deprivation, viral infection, hypoxia, and increased intracellular calcium concentration, for example, by damage to the membrane, can all trigger the release of intracellular apoptotic signals by a damaged cell. A number of cellular components, such as poly ADP ribose polymerase, may also help regulate apoptosis.

Before the actual process of cell death is precipitated by enzymes, apoptotic signals must cause regulatory proteins to initiate the apoptosis pathway. This step allows apoptotic signals to cause cell death or the process to be stopped, should the cell no longer need to die. Several proteins are involved, but two main methods of regulation have been identified: targeting mitochondria functionality or directly transducing the signal via adaptor proteins to the apoptotic mechanisms. Another extrinsic pathway for initiation identified in several toxin studies is an increase in calcium concentration within a cell caused by drug activity, which also can cause apoptosis via a calcium-binding protease calpain.

PCD in plants has a number of molecular similarities to animal apoptosis, but it also has differences, notably the presence of a cell wall and the lack of an immune system which removes the pieces of the dead cell. Instead of an immune response, the dying cell synthesizes substances to break itself down and places them in a vacuole which ruptures as the cell dies. Whether this whole process resembles animal apoptosis closely enough to warrant using the name *apoptosis* (as opposed to the more general PCD) is unclear.

One can infer that cell death in multicellular organisms is a means to maintain the overall health of the organism. The energy spent may be termed endogenous metabolism. This is a magnification of endogenous metabolism in single cells.

11.7. PRODUCT YIELD

In general, microbes take nutrients from the environment to maintain the overall health of their species (or to maintain a healthy population). One way or the other, extracellular products produced are related to the endogenous metabolism and/or the cell growth. The products are produced not because the nutrients are there and the microbes have nothing to do. Therefore, the specific rate of microbial products formation can be written as

$$\mu_P = YF_{P/XG}\mu_G + YF_{P/e}\mu_e \tag{11.38}$$

where $YF_{P/XG}$ is the product yield on biomass growth and $YF_{P/e}$ is the product yield on endogenous needs. This is the general form of microbial product rate as related to the growth and maintenance rates. Equation (11.38) is valid in general as the specific growth can be zero (due to the lack of one or more growth required nutrients), but the specific product rate may not be. Therefore, the extracellular product generation needs not be associated with the cell growth.

Equation (11.38) can be reduced into different forms when different growth and maintenance conditions are considered. When cell growth is not zero and the limiting substrate to cell growth is also the limiting substrate for the extracellular product generation, three simple forms of product formation rates have been shown in the literature:

1. Growth-associated products are produced simultaneously with microbial growth. The specific rate of product formation is proportional to the specific rate of growth, μ_G.

$$\mu_P = \frac{r_P}{X} = YF_{P/X}\mu_G \tag{11.39}$$

The production of a constitutive enzyme is an example of a growth-associated product. It is obtained from Eqn (11.38) when $YF_{P/e} = 0$ or the endogenous metabolism can be neglected. This case is applicable in the slow growth phase.

2. Nongrowth-associated product formation takes place during the stationary phase when the growth rate is zero due to the lack of at least one necessary substrate for growth. This case also occurs in the fast growth regime where endogenous metabolism has reached maximum rate. The specific rate of product formation is constant.

$$\mu_P = \beta = \text{constant} \tag{11.40}$$

Many secondary metabolites, such as antibiotics (for example, penicillin) production at high cell growth rate phase and during stationary phase, are nongrowth-associated products. Equation (11.40) is obtained from Eqn (11.38) when $\mu_G = 0$.

3. *Luedeking–Piret* equation. This is the case when $K_\mu = 0$ when Eqn (11.38) is applied. It is often the approximated equation based on part of the experimental data during the slow growth and stationary phases. In this case, the specific rate of product formation is given by the:

$$\mu_P = \beta + \alpha\mu_G \tag{11.41}$$

If $\alpha = 0$, the product is only nongrowth associated, and if $\beta = 0$, the product would be only growth associated, and consequently α would then be equal to $YF_{P/XG}$.

As we have already observed from Fig. 11.5 that the growth- and endogenous metabolism-associated product formation may be more general and the three cases listed above can be simplified from it, i.e. Eqn (11.38). Only when the substrate limiting the product generation is the same as that limiting the cell growth, the three simplified cases prevail. In most industrial applications, this is not the case.

11.8. OXYGEN DEMAND FOR AEROBIC MICROORGANISMS

Dissolved oxygen (DO) is an important substrate in aerobic fermentations and may be a limiting substrate, since oxygen gas is sparingly soluble in water. At high cell concentrations, the rate of oxygen consumption may exceed the rate of oxygen supply, leading to oxygen limitations. When oxygen is the rate-limiting factor, specific growth rate varies with dissolved-oxygen concentration according to Monod equation, just like any other substrate-limited case.

Above a *critical oxygen concentration*, the growth rate becomes independent of the dissolved-oxygen concentration. Figure 11.6 depicts the variation of specific growth rate with dissolved-oxygen concentration in a rich medium (no other substrate limitation). Oxygen is a growth rate-limiting factor when the DO level is below the critical DO concentration. In this case, another medium component (e.g. glucose, ammonium) becomes growth-extent limiting. For example, with *Azotobacter vinelandii* at a DO = 0.05 mg/L, the growth rate is about 50% of maximum even if a large amount of glucose is present. However, the maximum amount of cells formed is not determined by the DO, as oxygen is continually resupplied. If glucose were totally consumed, growth would cease even if DO = 0.05 mg/L. Thus, the extent of growth (mass of cells formed) would depend on glucose, while the growth rate for most of the culture period would depend on the value of DO.

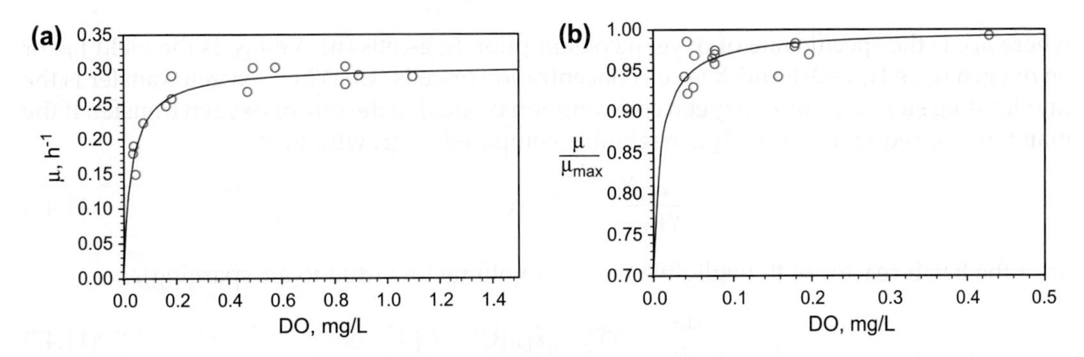

FIGURE 11.6 Growth-rate dependence on DO for aerobic (a) and facultative organisms (b). The lines are Monod equation fit to the data (symbols). *Data source: J. Chen, A.L. Tannahill and M.L. Shuler, Biotechnol. Bioeng., 27: 151, 1985. (a) Strictly aerobic organism:* Azotobacter vinelandii. *(b) Facultative organism (*Escherichia coli*).*

As shown in Fig. 11.6, the dependence of DO for aerobic and facultative organisms on cell growth follows the Monod growth equation. For aerobic organisms

$$\mu = \frac{\mu_{max} DO}{K_{DO} + DO} \tag{11.42}$$

and for facultative organisms,

$$\mu = \mu_{max0} + \frac{(\mu_{max} - \mu_{max0}) DO}{K_{DO} + DO} \tag{11.43}$$

where μ_{max0} is the maximum specific growth rate in anaerobic conditions. Facultative organisms grow with or without oxygen. For anaerobic organisms, there is no growth if oxygen is present.

The critical oxygen concentration is about 5% to 10% of the saturated DO concentration for bacteria and yeast and about 10% to 50% of the saturated DO concentration for mold cultures, depending on the pellet size of molds. Saturated DO concentration in water at 25 °C and 1 atm pressure is about 7 ppm. The presence of dissolved salts and organics can alter the saturation value, while increasingly high temperatures decrease the saturation value.

Oxygen is usually introduced to the fermentation broth by sparging air through the broth. Oxygen transfer from gas bubbles to cells is usually limited by oxygen transfer through the liquid film surrounding the gas bubbles. The rate of oxygen transfer from the gas to liquid phase is given by

$$N_{O_2} = k_L a (C^* - C_L) = \text{OTR} \tag{11.44}$$

where k_L is the oxygen transfer coefficient (m/h), a is the gas–liquid interfacial area (m^2/m^3), C^* is saturated DO concentration (g/L), C_L is the actual DO concentration in the broth (g/L), and the N_{O_2} is the rate of oxygen transfer (g/L/h). Also, the term *oxygen transfer rate* (OTR) is used.

The rate of oxygen uptake is denoted as OUR and

$$\text{OUR} = \mu_{O_2} X = \frac{\mu_G X}{YF_{X/O_2}} \tag{11.45}$$

where μ_{O_2} is the specific rate of oxygen consumption (g g-cells/h), YF_{X/O_2} is the yield factor on oxygen (g-cells/g-O_2), and X is cell concentration (g-cells/L). When oxygen transfer is the rate-limiting step, the rate of oxygen consumption is equal to the rate of oxygen transfer. If the maintenance requirement of O_2 is negligible compared to growth, then

$$\frac{\mu_G X}{YF_{X/O_2}} = k_L a (C^* - C_L) \tag{11.46}$$

or in the batch reactor with negligible medium volume loss (due to air sparging),

$$\frac{dX}{dt} = YF_{X/O_2} k_L a (C^* - C_L) \tag{11.47}$$

Growth rate varies nearly linearly with the OTR under oxygen-transfer limitations. Among the various methods used to overcome DO limitations are the use of oxygen-enriched air or pure oxygen and operation under high atmospheric pressure (2–3 atm). Oxygen transfer has a big impact on reactor design.

The maximum or saturation oxygen concentration is a function of temperature, oxygen pressure, as well as medium compositions. Electrolytes have a strong effect on oxygen solubility and transport. Quicker et al. (G. Quicker, A. Schumpe, B. König and W.-D. Deckwer. 1981. Comparison of measured and calculated oxygen solubility in fermentation media. *Biotechnol. Bioeng.*, 23: 635–650) gave a simple correlation between the saturation oxygen concentration (C^*) and medium ionic and nonionic solute concentration:

$$\log\frac{C_0^*}{C^*} = \frac{1}{2}\sum_{j=1}^{\text{Ionic species}} H_j Z_j^2 C_j + \sum_{j=1}^{\text{nonionic species}} H_j C_j \tag{11.48}$$

where C_0^* is the oxygen saturation concentration in pure water (Table 11.3), C^* is the oxygen saturation concentration in the medium, H_j is the oxygen solubility interaction constants (Table 11.4), Z_j is the ionic charge of ionic species j, and C_j is the concentration of species j in the fermentation medium.

TABLE 11.3 Solubility of Oxygen in Pure Water

Temperature, °C	Oxygen solubility in pure water when contacting with air at 1 atm, $kg \cdot m^{-3}$	Henry's law constant, atm-O_2 $m^3 \cdot kg^{-1}$	Density of water, kg/m^3
0	1.46×10^{-2}	14.4	999.839
5	1.28×10^{-2}	16.4	999.964
10	1.14×10^{-2}	18.4	999.699
15	1.02×10^{-2}	20.5	999.099
20	0.929×10^{-2}	22.6	998.204
25	0.849×10^{-2}	24.7	997.045
30	0.782×10^{-2}	26.9	995.647
35	0.731×10^{-2}	28.7	994.032
40	0.692×10^{-2}	30.4	992.215
45	0.656×10^{-2}	32.0	990.213
50	0.627×10^{-2}	33.5	988.037
60	0.583×10^{-2}	36.0	983.200
70	0.550×10^{-2}	38.2	977.771
80	0.528×10^{-2}	39.8	971.799
90	0.515×10^{-2}	40.8	965.321
100	0.510×10^{-2}	41.2	958.365

Source: Calculated from International Critical Tables, 1928, vol. III, p. 257. McGraw-Hill: New York.

TABLE 11.4 Oxygen Solubility Interaction Constants at 25 °C

Cation	H_j, 10^{-4} m³/mol	Anion	H_j, 10^{-4} m³/mol	Sugar	H_j, 10^{-4} m³/mol
H^+	−7.74	OH^-	9.41	Glucose	1.19
K^+	−5.96	Cl^-	8.44	Lactose	1.97
Na^+	−5.50	CO_3^{2-}	4.85	Sucrose	1.49
NH_4^+	−7.20	SO_4^{2-}	4.53		
NHt_4^+	−9.12	NO_3^-	8.02		
Mg^{2+}	−3.14	HCO_3^-	10.58		
Ca^{2+}	−3.30	$H_2PO_4^-$	10.37		
Mn^{2+}	−3.11	HPO_4^{2-}	4.85		
		PO_4^{3-}	3.20		

11.9. EFFECT OF TEMPERATURE

Temperature is an important factor affecting the performance of cells. Table 11.5 shows the classification of microorganisms according to their temperature optima.

As the temperature is increased toward optimal growth temperature, the growth rate approximately doubles for every 10 °C increase in temperature. Above the optimal temperature range, the growth rate decreases and thermal death may occur. The growth rate decrease is due in part to the enzymes (protein denaturing) become less active at high temperatures. The endogenous metabolism or maintenance needs also increase as temperature is increased beyond optimum range, which leads to a decrease in the apparent biomass yield.

TABLE 11.5 Classification of Microorganisms Based on Thermal Endurance (after H.W. Blanch and D.S. Clark. 1996 Biochemical Engineering, Marcel Dekker, Inc.: New York).

Thermal preference classification	Growth temperature range, °C		
	Lower limit	Optimum range	Upper limit
Psychrophiles	−5 (to 5)	15–18	19–22
Mesophiles	10 (to 15)	30–45	35–45
Thermophiles	25	45–75	60–80
Extreme thermophiles	50	60–75	75–95
Hyperthermophiles			100 and over

At high temperatures, the thermal death rate exceeds the growth rate, which causes a net decrease in the concentration of viable cells.

$$\mu_{\text{net}} = \mu_{\text{G}} - k_d \tag{11.24}$$

Thermal death is more sensitive to temperature changes than microbial growth. Temperature also affects product formation. However, the temperature optimum for growth and product formation may be different. The yield factor is also affected by temperature due to the change in the endogenous metabolism requirements as shown in Eqn (11.24). An increase in temperature at high temperatures results in a decrease in yield factor is expected. In some cases, such as single-cell protein production, temperature optimization to maximize the yield factor ($YF_{X/S}$) is critical. When temperature is increased above the optimum temperature, the maintenance or endogenous metabolism requirements of cells increase. That is, the endogenous metabolism increases with increasing temperature with an activation energy of 60–85 kJ/mol, resulting in a decrease in the apparent yield factor.

Temperature also may affect the rate-limiting step in a fermentation process. At high temperatures, the rate of bioreaction might become higher than the diffusion rate, and diffusion would then become the rate-limiting step (for example, in an immobilized cell system). The activation energy of molecular diffusion is about 25 kJ/mol. The activation energy for most bioreactions is more than 48 kJ/mol, so diffusional limitations must be carefully considered at high temperatures. Figure 11.7 depicts a typical variation of the net maximum growth rate with temperature. One can observe that there is a growth rate maximum at

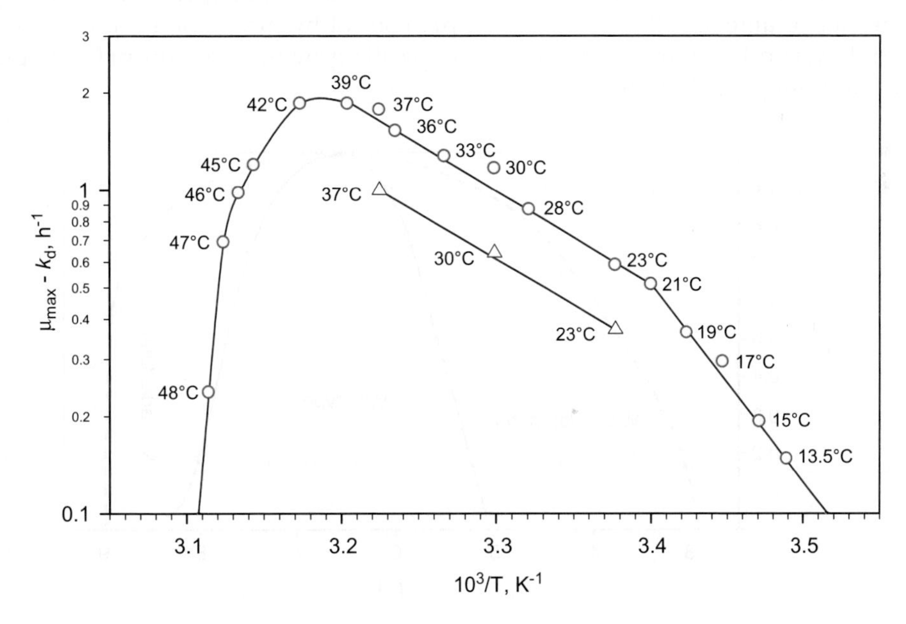

FIGURE 11.7 Variation of net specific maximum growth rate with temperature for *Escherichia coli* B/r. Circles are growth in a glucose-rich medium and triangles are growth in a glucose-minimal medium. *Data source: S.L. Herendeen et al. 1979 J. Bacteriology, 139:185–194.*

optimum temperature. The profile is quite similar to that of an enzyme-catalyzed reaction in Chapter 8.

11.10. EFFECT OF pH

Hydrogen-ion concentration (pH) affects the activity of enzymes and therefore the microbial growth rate. The optimal pH for growth may be different from that for product formation. Generally, the acceptable pH range varies about the optimum by 1–2 pH units. Different organisms have different pH optima: the pH optimum for many bacteria ranges from pH = 3–8; for yeast, pH = 3–6; for molds, pH = 3–7; for plant cells, pH = 5–6; and for animal cells, pH = 6.5–7.5. Many organisms have mechanisms to maintain intracellular pH at a relatively constant level in the presence of fluctuations in environmental pH. When pH differs from the optimal value, the maintenance energy requirements increase. One consequence of different pH optima is that the pH of the medium can be used to select one organism over another.

In most fermentations, pH can vary substantially. Often the nature of the nitrogen source can be important. If ammonium is the sole nitrogen source, hydrogen ions are released into the medium as a result of the microbial utilization of ammonia, resulting in a decrease in pH. If nitrate is the sole nitrogen source, hydrogen ions are removed from the medium to reduce nitrate to ammonia, resulting in an increase in pH. Also, pH can change because of the production of organic acids, the utilization of acids (particularly amino acids), or the production of bases. The evolution or supply of CO_2 can alter pH greatly in some systems (e.g. seawater or animal cell culture). Thus, pH control by means of a buffer or an active pH control system is important. Variation of specific growth rate with pH is depicted in Fig. 11.8, indicating a pH optimum.

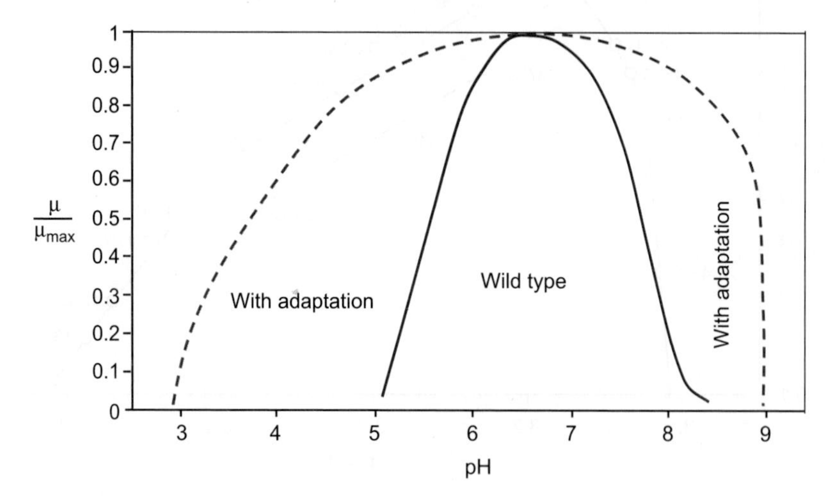

FIGURE 11.8 A fictitious variation of specific growth rate with pH. With some microbial cultures, it is possible to adapt cultures to a wider range of pH values if pH changes are made in small increments from culture transfer to transfer.

11.11. EFFECT OF REDOX POTENTIAL

The redox potential is an important parameter that affects the rate and extent of many oxidative–reductive reactions. In a fermentation medium, the redox potential is a complex function of DO, pH, and other ion concentrations, such as reducing and oxidizing agents. The electrochemical potential of a fermentation medium can be expressed by the following equation:

$$E_h = E_0 + \frac{RT}{4F} \ln p_{O_2} + \frac{RT}{F} \ln[H^+] = E_0 + \frac{RT}{4F} \ln p_{O_2} - \frac{RT}{F} \text{pH} \ln 10 \tag{11.49}$$

where F is the Farady constant, the electrochemical potential is measured in millivolts by a pH/voltmeter, and p_{O_2} is in atmospheres.

The redox potential of a fermentation media can be reduced by passing nitrogen gas or by the addition of reducing agents such as cysteine, HCl, or Na_2S. Oxygen gas can be passed or some oxidizing agents can be added to the fermentation media to increase the redox potential.

Dissolved carbon dioxide (DCO_2) concentration may have a profound effect on performance of organisms. Very high DCO_2 concentrations may be toxic to some cells. On the other hand, cells require a certain DCO_2 level for proper metabolic functions. The DCO_2 concentration can be controlled by changing the CO_2 content of the air supply and the agitation speed.

11.12. EFFECT OF ELECTROLYTES AND SUBSTRATE CONCENTRATION

The ionic strength of the fermentation media affects the transport of certain nutrients in and out of cells, the metabolic functions of cells, and the solubility of certain nutrients, such as DO. The ionic strength is given by the following equation:

$$I = \frac{1}{2} \sum_{j=1}^{N_j} C_j Z_j^2 \tag{11.50}$$

where C_j is the molar concentration of ionic species j, Z_j is the charge of ionic species j, and I is the ionic strength of the medium.

High substrate concentrations that are significantly above stoichiometric requirements are inhibitory to cellular functions. Inhibitory levels of substrates vary depending on the type of cells and substrate. Glucose may be inhibitory at concentrations above 200 g/L (e.g. ethanol fermentation by yeast), probably due to a reduction in water activity. Certain salts such as NaCl may be inhibitory at concentrations above 40 g/L due to high osmotic pressure. Some refractory compounds, such as phenol, toluene, and methanol, are inhibitory at much lower concentrations (e.g. 1 g/L). Typical maximum noninhibitory concentrations of some nutrients are glucose, 100 g/L; ethanol, 50 g/L for yeast, much less for most organisms; ammonium, 5 g/L; phosphate, 10 g/L; and nitrate, 5 g/L. Substrate inhibition can be overcome by intermittent addition of the substrate to the medium.

11.13. HEAT GENERATION BY MICROBIAL GROWTH

About 40% to 50% of the energy stored in a carbon and energy source is converted to biological energy (ATP) during aerobic metabolism, and the rest of the energy is released as heat. For actively growing cells, the maintenance requirement is low, and heat evolution is directly related to growth.

The heat generated during microbial growth can be calculated using the heat of combustion of the substrate and of cellular material. A schematic of an enthalpy balance for microbial utilization of substrate is presented in Fig. 11.9. The heat of combustion of the substrate is equal to the sum of the metabolic heat and the heat of combustion of the cellular material.

$$\frac{\Delta H_{c,S}}{YF_{X/S}} = \frac{\Delta H_{c,P}}{YF_{X/S}} YF_{P/S} + \Delta H_{c,X} + YF_{H/X} \tag{11.51}$$

where $\Delta H_{c,S}$ is the heat of combustion of the substrate (kJ/g-substrate), $YF_{X/S}$ is the biomass yield factor (g-cell/g-substrate), $\Delta H_{c,X}$ is the heat of combustion of cells (kJ/g-cells), $YF_{P/S}$ is the extracellular product yield factor (g-P/g-substrate), $\Delta H_{c,P}$ is the heat of combustion of extracellular products (kJ/g-P), and $YF_{H/X}$ is the heat yield factor on biomass or the metabolic heat evolved per gram of cell mass produced (kJ/g-cells).

Equation (11.51) can be rearranged to yield

$$YF_{H/X} = \frac{\Delta H_{c,S} - YF_{X/S}\Delta H_{c,X} - YF_{P/S}\Delta H_{c,P}}{YF_{X/S}} \tag{11.52}$$

$\Delta H_{c,S}$, $\Delta H_{c,P}$, and $\Delta H_{c,X}$ can be determined from the combustion of substrate, extracellular products, and cells. When these data are not available, one can estimate them via energy regulations (Chapter 3). Typical ΔH_c values for bacterial cells are 20–25 kJ/g-cells. Typical values of $YF_{H/X}$ are glucose, 10 kJ/g; malate, 14 kJ/g; acetate, 20 kJ/g; ethanol, 23 kJ/g; methanol, 35 kJ/g; and methane, 69 kJ/g. Clearly, the degree of oxidation of the substrate has a strong effect on the amount of heat released.

The total rate of heat evolution in a batch fermentation is

$$\Delta H_G = \frac{V_L \mu_{net} X}{YF_{X/H}} \tag{11.53}$$

where V_L is the liquid volume (L) and X is the cell concentration (g/L).

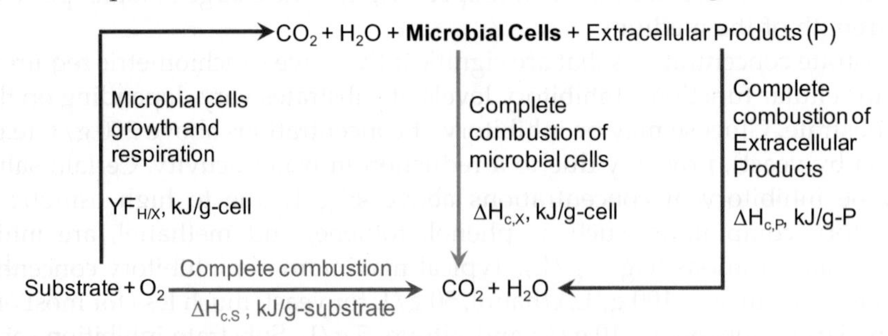

FIGURE 11.9 Enthalpy balance on substrate combustion and with microbial and extracellular product utilizations.

In aerobic fermentations, the rate of metabolic heat evolution can roughly be correlated to the rate of oxygen uptake, since oxygen is the final electron acceptor.

$$\Delta H_G = 4\Delta H_\gamma \frac{V_L \mu_{O_2} X}{M_{O_2}} \tag{11.54}$$

where ΔH_γ is the heat of combustion for one unit of degree of reduction, see Eqn (3.94).

Metabolic heat released during fermentation can be removed by circulating cooling water through a cooling coil or cooling jacket in the fermenter. Often, temperature control (adequate heat removal) is an important limitation on reactor design (see Chapter 10). The ability to estimate heat-removal requirements is essential to proper reactor design.

11.14. OVERVIEW OF MICROBIAL GROWTH KINETIC MODELS

We have described key concepts and kinetics in the growth of cultures based on cell metabolism and cell generation. To bring about a mathematical description of cell growth, we often resort to approximations, as illustrated in Fig. 11.10. A successful mathematical description is using the least amount of computation to capture the maximum amount of physical behaviors. To this extent, the Monod equation was commonly used.

Cellular composition and biosynthetic capabilities change in response to new growth conditions (*unbalanced growth*), although a constant cellular composition and balanced growth can predominate in steady and pseudosteady growth (e.g. the maximum growth during batch growth) phase. If the decelerating growth phase (or growth rate is lower than maximum) is due to substrate limitation or depletion rather than inhibition by toxins, the growth rate decreases in relation to decreasing substrate concentrations. In the stationary and death phases, the distribution of properties among individuals is important (e.g. cryptic death).

Although these kinetic ideas are evident in batch culture, they are equally evident and important in other modes of culture (e.g. continuous culture). Clearly, the complete description of the growth kinetics of a culture would involve recognition of the complete metabolic pathway and genetic construction of cell. However, the whole metabolic pathway involves

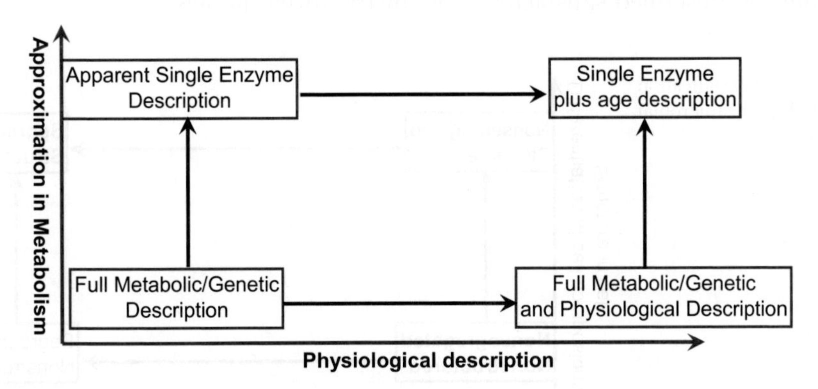

FIGURE 11.10 Simplifications in microbial kinetic description.

a large number of parameters and intercellular components. Full kinetic description can be extremely demanding. While on the first instances mathematical description via simplification of metabolic pathway by approximation is desirable, sometimes we resort to phenomenological models that may or may not reflect directly the metabolic pathway. Models that can describe wide range of growth behaviors involve recognition of the *structured* nature of each cell and the *segregation* of the culture into individual units (cells) that may differ from each other.

A compositionally structured phenomenological model divides the cell mass into components. A fully structured model would be the one able to mimic the complete metabolism and cell generation and physiology. If the ratio of the individual cell components can change in response to perturbations in the extracellular environment, then the structured model is behaving analogously to a cell changing its composition in response to environmental changes. Consider in Chapter 10 our discussion of cellular regulation, particularly the induction of whole pathways. Any of these metabolic responses results in changes in intracellular structure. Furthermore, if a model of a culture is constructed from discrete units, it begins to mimic the segregation observed in real cultures whereby cell physiology can be modeled. As shown in Fig. 11.11, models may be structured and segregated, structured and nonsegregated, unstructured and segregated, and unstructured and nonsegregated. Models containing both structure and segregation can be the most realistic, but they are also computationally complex.

The degree of realism and complexity required in a phenomenological model depends on what is being described; the modeler should always choose the simplest model that can adequately describe the desired system. An unstructured model assumes fixed cell composition, which is equivalent to assuming pseudosteady state or *balanced growth.* The balanced growth assumption is valid primarily in single-stage, steady-state continuous culture and the exponential phase of batch culture; it fails during any transient conditions. How fast the cell responds to perturbations in its environment and how fast these perturbations occur determine whether pseudobalanced growth can be assumed. If cell response is fast compared to external changes and if the magnitude of these changes is not too large (e.g. a 10% or 20% variation from initial conditions), then the use of unstructured models can be justified, since the deviation from balanced growth may be small. Culture response to large or rapid perturbations cannot be described satisfactorily by unstructured models.

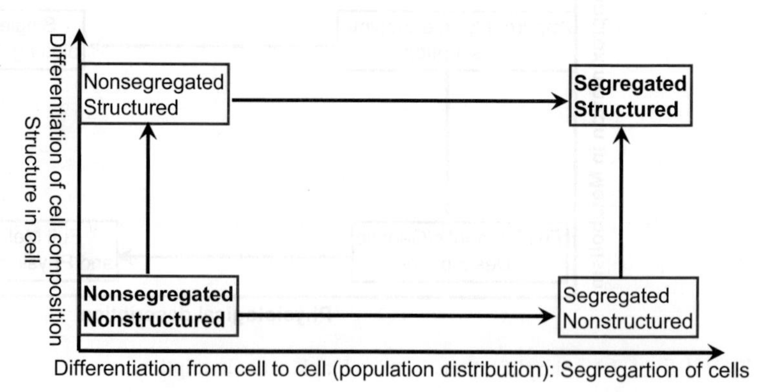

FIGURE 11.11 Classification of phenomenological microbial kinetic models.

For many systems, segregation is not a critical component of culture response, so nonsegregated models will be satisfactory under many circumstances. An important exception is the prediction of the growth responses of plasmid-containing cultures.

In this text, we focus more on the metabolic and genetic approaches and their simplification/approximations. Therefore, our discussions in this text will be confined to very simple phenomenological models only.

11.14.1. Unstructured Growth Models

The simplest growth kinetic equations are unstructured models. These models view the cell as a single species in solution and attempt to describe the kinetics of cell growth based on cell and nutrient concentration profiles. The simplest model is that of Malthus (§11.2):

$$r_X = \mu_{net} X \tag{11.2}$$

Upon examining Eqn (11.2), one may conclude that this is the definition for specific growth rate and thus valid in general. However, this is not the case in the context of Malthus model, as μ_{net} is assumed to be constant, not dependent on substrate concentration. This is based on the empirical observation of batch growth during the maximum growth phase (§11.2).

It is clear that the application of Malthus model is limited as it provides no limit to the cell growth. The only limit would be the exhaust of substrate, which is not built into the model. Even for the simplest batch growth case, the deceleration phase would not be fully described with the Malthus model. The relation to the substrate can be found via the growth yield.

To provide means to limit growth, Verhulst model inserted an apparent biomass inhibition term to the Malthus equation:

$$r_X = kX(1 - X/X_\infty) \tag{11.5}$$

which is also known as the logistic equation. The Verhulst model can describe the batch growth quite accurately for a wide range of growth periods.

Apart from the ability of the logistic equation to correlate the deceleration and stationary phases on top of the Malthus model, it has the appeal that the maximum cell concentration can be considered. Although the carrying capacity X_∞ was a parameter related to the maximum nutrient level available in the medium, it can also be the maximum (packing) density of the cells as well (when the nutrients are unlimited).

11.14.2. Simple Growth Rate Model: Monod Equation

The simple growth rate model can mechanistically describes microbial growth in close approximation is the one that approximates the whole metabolic pathway and cell generation with a single rate-limiting step. In this case, the Monod equation prevails. This is also the simplest model that incorporates the effects of both the cell concentration and substrate concentration:

$$\mu_G = \frac{r_X}{X} = \frac{\mu_{max} S}{K_S + S} \tag{11.21}$$

TABLE 11.6 Typical Values of μ_{max} and K_S for Various Organisms and Substrates at Optimum Growth Temperature

Microorganism	Limiting substrate	μ_{max}, h^{-1}	K_S, mg/L
Escherichia coli at 37 °C	Glucose	0.8–1.4	2–4
E. coli at 37 °C	Glycerol	0.87	2
E. coli at 37 °C	Lactose	0.8	20
Saccharomyces cerevisiae at 30 °C	Glucose	0.5–0.6	25
Candida tropicalis at 30 °C	Glucose	0.5	25–75
Candida sp.	Oxygen	0.5	0.045–0.45
	Hexadecane	0.5	
Klebsiella aerogenes	Glucose	0.85	9
Aerobacter aerogenes	Glucose	1.22	1–10

Source: H.W. Blanck and D.S. Clark, Biochemical Engineering, 1996, Marcel Dekker, Inc: New York.

and a general product formation rate of

$$\mu_P = \frac{r_P}{X} = \frac{\mu_{P\max} S}{K_P + S} \tag{11.22}$$

This is the most commonly used microbial growth model. As we have discussed in §11.4, it performs well in pseudosteady state (or balanced growth) cases. Table 11.6 shows typical values of μ_{max} and K_S.

In Chapters 8, 9 10 and §11.4, we learned that the rate form may be taken on any individual step in particular when the mathematical forms are similar. To show Monod equation is truly an approximation to microbial growth, we further consider the effect of external diffusion (or mass transfer) on the growth rate. In this case, the equation of mass transfer rates is different mathematically from the enzymatic reaction rate. More extensive coverage on the mass transfer effects is found in Chapter 17. Let us consider that the bulk medium contains S g/L of substrate and the substrate concentration in the medium just outside of the cell membrane is S_c. The substrate concentration just outside of the cell membrane is the concentration that the cell can make use of. Therefore:

$$\mu_G = \frac{r_X}{X} = \frac{\mu_{max} S_c}{K_S + S_c} \tag{11.55}$$

The substrate uptake rate is thus given by

$$r_S = \frac{r_X}{YF_{X/S}} = \frac{X}{YF_{X/S}} \frac{\mu_{max} S_c}{K_S + S_c} \tag{11.56}$$

Mass transfer flux between the bulk medium and the microbial cells is given by

$$N_{S_c} = k_L a_c \frac{X}{\rho_{cell}} (S - S_c) \tag{11.57}$$

where k_L is the mass transfer coefficient in the liquid medium, a_c is the cell surface area per unit volume of the cell, and ρ_{cell} is the density of the cells. At pseudosteady state, the substrate uptake rate is identical to the substrate transfer rate to the cells. Therefore,

$$X\mu_G = \frac{\mu_{max}S_c}{K_S + S_c}X = YF_{X/S}N_{S_c} = YF_{X/S}k_L a_c \frac{X}{\rho_{cell}}(S - S_c) \tag{11.58}$$

which yields,

$$S = \frac{K_S \mu_G}{\mu_{max} - \mu_G} + \frac{\rho_{cell}\mu_G}{YF_{X/S}k_L a_c} \tag{11.59}$$

Rearranging Eqn (11.59) in the explicit form of growth rate μ_G, we obtain

$$\mu_G = \frac{S + K_S + \dfrac{\rho_{cell}\mu_{max}}{YF_{X/S}k_L a_c}}{2\dfrac{\rho_{cell}}{YF_{X/S}k_L a_c}}\left[1 - \sqrt{1 - \frac{4S\dfrac{\rho_{cell}\mu_{max}}{YF_{X/S}k_L a_c}}{\left(S + K_S + \dfrac{\rho_{cell}\mu_{max}}{YF_{X/S}k_L a_c}\right)^2}}\right] \tag{11.60}$$

which is the exact specific rate of growth when external diffusion to the cells are considered. However, this equation may be approximated by noting

$$\left[S + K_S + \frac{\rho_{cell}\mu_{max}}{YF_{X/S}k_L a_c}\right]^2 > \left[S + \frac{\rho_{cell}\mu_{max}}{YF_{X/S}k_L a_c}\right]^2 = \left[S - \frac{\rho_{cell}\mu_{max}}{YF_{X/S}k_L a_c}\right]^2 + 4S\frac{\rho_{cell}\mu_{max}}{YF_{X/S}k_L a_c} \tag{11.61}$$

since all the parameters are positive. Equation (11.61) leads to

$$\frac{4S\dfrac{\rho_{cell}\mu_{max}}{YF_{X/S}k_L a_c}}{\left(S + K_S + \dfrac{\rho_{cell}\mu_{max}}{YF_{X/S}k_L a_c}\right)^2} < 1 \tag{11.62}$$

Thus, the first order approximation to Eqn (11.60) gives

$$\mu_G = \frac{S + K_S + \dfrac{\rho_{cell}\mu_{max}}{YF_{X/S}k_L a_c}}{2\dfrac{\rho_{cell}}{YF_{X/S}k_L a_c}} \times \frac{4S\dfrac{\rho_{cell}\mu_{max}}{YF_{X/S}k_L a_c}}{2\left(S + K_S + \dfrac{\rho_{cell}\mu_{max}}{YF_{X/S}k_L a_c}\right)^2} \tag{11.63}$$

That is,

$$\mu_G = \frac{\mu_{max}S}{S + K_S + \dfrac{\rho_{cell}\mu_{max}}{YF_{X/S}k_L a_c}} = \frac{\mu_{max}S}{S + K_S'} \tag{11.64}$$

TABLE 11.7 Values of Monod Saturation Constant for Oxygen Limited Growth of Several Types of Cells

Microorganism	T, °C	Cell size, μm	K_S, mmol/L-O_2
Micrococcus candicans	20.2	0.5	1.1×10^{-5}
Aerobacter aerogenes	19.0	0.6	3.1×10^{-5}
Escherichia coli	19.2	0.6	2.22×10^{-5}
Serratia marescens	18.8	0.7	3.60×10^{-5}
Azotobacter indicum	19.6	1.6	3.00×10^{-4}
Bacillus megatherium	19.2	2.0	5.97×10^{-4}
Bacillus megatherium (LiCl)	20.0	2.4	7.07×10^{-4}
Acetobacter suboxydans	19.2	2.7	1.57×10^{-3}
Bacillus megatherium (glycine)	20.6	4.0	3.12×10^{-3}

Data source: J. Longmuir, Biochem. J., 57: 81, 1954.

In other words, Monod equation still holds. However, the saturation constant K_S is modified. The saturation constant is higher when mass transfer effect is pronounced. Apart from the discussion in §11.4, this derivation gives us a clue why the Monod equation is the approximate growth rate equation for a complicated metabolic pathway when pseudosteady state (balanced growth) holds.

Since the mass transfer coefficient increases with increasing agitation (convection), temperature, and particle (cell) size (surface area decrease with cell size), one can expect the (apparent) saturation constant K_S to vary with these parameters. Table 11.7 shows typical values of saturation constant for oxygen limited growth as a function of cell size. One does observe a trend in cell size dependence.

While Monod equation is the most widely used cell growth model, it has its limitations. For example, balanced growth conditions (pseudosteady state), dilute substrate concentrations, dilute cell concentration, no inhibitory substances present in the medium, and single limiting substrate (with all other required substrates in excess) are the most severe limitations. Some of these limitations can be relaxed by adding additional terms.

11.14.2.1. *Modification of Monod Equation with Growth Inhibitors*

At high concentrations of substrate or product and in the presence of inhibitory substances in the medium, growth becomes inhibited, and growth rate depends on inhibitor concentration. The inhibition pattern of microbial growth is analogous to enzyme inhibition. If a single-substrate enzyme-catalyzed reaction is the rate-limiting step in microbial growth, then kinetic constants in the rate expression are biologically meaningful. Often, the underlying mechanism is complicated, and kinetic constants do not have biological meanings and are obtained from experimental data by curve fitting.

11.14.2.1.1. SUBSTRATE INHIBITION

At high substrate concentrations, microbial growth rate is inhibited by the substrate. As in enzyme kinetics, substrate inhibition of growth may be competitive or noncompetitive.

If a single-substrate enzyme-catalyzed reaction is the rate-limiting step in microbial growth, then inhibition of the enzyme activity results in inhibition of microbial growth by the same pattern. Since the Monod equation is an approximate growth rate equation, one is not able to differentiate the maximum growth rate and saturation constant from the noninhibited case. The kinetic constants are merely correlation coefficients. Therefore, only the noncompetitive substrate inhibition is presented here:

$$\mu_G = \frac{\mu_{max}}{\left(1+\frac{K_S}{S}\right)\left(1+\frac{S}{K_I}\right)} \tag{11.65}$$

which is most general form of substrate inhibited growth rate equation if Monod growth prevails.

11.14.2.1.2. PRODUCT INHIBITION

High concentration of extracellular product can be inhibitory for microbial growth. Product inhibition may be competitive or noncompetitive, and in some cases when the underlying mechanism is not known, the inhibited growth rate is approximated to exponential or linear decay expressions.

Competitive product inhibition:

$$\mu_G = \frac{\mu_{max} S}{K_S\left(1+\frac{P}{K_P}\right)+S} \tag{11.66}$$

Noncompetitive product inhibition:

$$\mu_G = \frac{\mu_{max} S}{(K_S+S)\left(1+\frac{P}{K_P}\right)} \tag{11.67}$$

Ethanol fermentation from glucose by yeasts is a good example of noncompetitive product inhibition, and ethanol is the inhibitor at concentrations above about 5%. Other rate expressions used for ethanol inhibition are

$$\mu_G = \frac{\mu_{max} S}{K_S+S}\left(1-\frac{P}{P_m}\right)^n \tag{11.68}$$

where P_m is the product concentration at which growth stops, or

$$\mu_G = \frac{\mu_{max} S}{K_S+S} e^{-P/K_P} \tag{11.69}$$

where K_P is the product inhibition constant.

11.14.2.1.3. CELL INHIBITION

Perhaps, the most common inhibition is the cells themselves. In most cases, there is no limitation on the space for the cells to occupy; however, it can become an issue for batch growth. Before cells can divide, it needs to have space available for the new cells. Just like the reactants in an elementary reaction, the free space is necessary as one cell will take one cell's space. Therefore, the effect of cell inhibition can be added the same way as the logistic equation as it reflects the concentration of free space in terms of the (imaginary) cells (available):

$$\mu_G = \frac{\mu_{max} S}{K_S + S}\left(1 - \frac{X}{X_\infty}\right) \tag{11.70}$$

where X_∞ is the maximum cell concentration or the packing density of the cells. The value of X_∞ depends on the type of cells: size, shape, and physiological conditions. When the cell concentration reaches its maximum packing density, cell growth stops.

11.14.2.1.4. INHIBITION BY TOXIC COMPOUNDS

Toxic compounds can affect the metabolic behavior of cells via poisoning and/or rendering the necessary enzymes less effective. While poisoning can be modeled with cell death in extreme cases, the deactivation of enzymes is similar to inhibition in enzymatic reactions. The following rate expressions are used for competitive, noncompetitive, and uncompetitive inhibition of growth in analogy to enzyme inhibition.

Competitive inhibition:

$$\mu_G = \frac{\mu_{max} S}{K_S\left(1 + \frac{I}{K_I}\right) + S} \tag{11.71}$$

Noncompetitive and uncompetitive inhibitions:

$$\mu_G = \frac{\mu_{max} S}{(K_S + S)\left(1 + \frac{I}{K_P}\right)} \tag{11.72}$$

In some cases, the presence of toxic compounds in the medium results in the inactivation of cells or death.

11.14.2.2. Multiple Limiting Substrates

So far, we have been focused on cases where only one substrate is limiting. When more than one substrate is limiting, the microbial growth rate changes with the concentrations of these substrates that can change significantly in the medium.

11.14.2.2.1. COMPLEMENTARY SUBSTRATES

When two or more substrates that are complimentary, all these substrates are necessary for the microbial growth. In this case, product rule applies:

$$\mu_G = \mu_{max} \prod_{j=1}^{N_{SC}} \frac{S_j}{K_{S_j} + S_j} \tag{11.73}$$

where N_{SC} is the number of limiting substrates that are complementary. For example, energy source, nitrogen source, sulfur source, and carbon source can be complementary, if only one of each is supplied and are not in excess.

11.14.2.2.2. SUBSTITUTABLE SUBSTRATES

When two or more substrates of similar functionality are limiting, the contributions of the substrates to the microbial growth are additive:

$$\mu_G = \sum_{j=1}^{N_{SS}} \alpha_j \frac{\mu_{\max j} S_j}{K_{S_j} + S_j} \tag{11.74}$$

where N_{SS} is the number of limiting substrates that are substitutive and α_j is the fractional rate contribution of substrate j. For example, glucose, xylose, and mannose are substitutive. The quantity α_j is a function of the concentrations of the substrate mixture and

$$\sum_{j=1}^{N_{SS}} \alpha_j = 1 \tag{11.75}$$

That is, the total amount of enzymes in a cell is constant. However, the distribution of the enzymes that can assist the uptake and conversion of each substrate can change according to the growth and medium conditions.

11.14.2.2.3. MIXED TYPES OF SUBSTRATES

When both complimentary and substitutive substrates are present, the overall growth rate is more completed and will depend on the combination of the substrates. For example, with one type of substrate being substitutive and all the others being complementary, the microbial growth rate is given by:

$$\mu_G = \prod_{j=1}^{N_{SC}} \frac{S_j}{K_{S_j} + S_j} \sum_{l=1}^{N_{SS}} \alpha_l \frac{\mu_{\max l} S_l}{K_{S_l} + S_l} \tag{11.76}$$

11.14.3. Simplest Reaction Network (or Simplest Metabolic) Model

The simplest reaction network that has the potential to capture the transitional effects (or unbalanced growth) is given below

$$S + \mathrm{E} \underset{k_{-1}}{\overset{k_1}{\rightleftarrows}} S\cdot\mathrm{E} \overset{k_{1c}}{\rightarrow} \mathrm{YF}_{P/S}P + \mathrm{YF}_{X/S}X + \mathrm{E} \tag{11.77a}$$

$$X \underset{k_{-2}}{\overset{k_2}{\rightleftarrows}} \nu_{\mathrm{E}}\mathrm{E} \tag{11.77b}$$

This is the simplest approximation to a metabolic pathway. It has the potential to describe balanced as well as unbalanced growth.

The approximation is not only on the number of steps involved in metabolism and cell generation but also on the elementary steps. Clearly, at least two steps in Eqn (11.77) are not elementary, where stoichiometrical coefficients are not restricted to integers between 0 and 3.

Besides the substrate S, extracellular product P, and biomass X, there are two intermediate species (that are part of the biomass): E and S·E. The net rates of the system are given by

$$r_E = -k_1 S[E] + (k_{-1} + k_{1c})[S\cdot E] + \nu_E(k_2 X - k_{-2}[E]) \tag{11.78a}$$

$$r_{S\cdot E} = k_1 S[E] - (k_{-1} + k_{1c})[S\cdot E] \tag{11.78b}$$

$$r_S = -k_1 S[E] + k_{-1}[S\cdot E] \tag{11.78c}$$

$$r_P = YF_{P/S} k_{1c}[S\cdot E] \tag{11.78d}$$

$$r_X = YF_{X/S} k_{1c}[S\cdot E] \tag{11.78e}$$

By setting $0 = r_E$ and $0 = r_{S\cdot E}$, the simplest reaction network results in the same rate expression as the Monod equation. However, without the pseuosteady-state (or balanced growth) assumption, the rate Eqn (11.78) describes the temporal variations of the enzyme and thus the lag phase in substrate consumption and biomass production.

11.14.4. Simplest Metabolic Pathway

The simplest metabolic pathway that can capture the lag phase and temporal transitional effects is shown in Fig. 11.12. Substrate uptake occurs as the cell converts intracellular-bound substrate into an intermediate Y, and then to an extracellular product P and an intracellular product P_2, which is integrated into the cell biomass X. The enzyme required for each step is also produced as part of P_2. The stoichiometries along the pathway illustrated in Fig. 11.12 can be written as:

$$S + E_1 \underset{k_{-1}}{\overset{k_1}{\rightleftarrows}} S\cdot E_1 \overset{k_{1c}}{\rightarrow} Y\cdot E_1 \tag{11.79a}$$

$$E_2 + Y\cdot E_1 \underset{k_{-2}}{\overset{k_2}{\rightleftarrows}} Y\cdot E_2 + E_1 \tag{11.79b}$$

$$Y\cdot E_2 \overset{k_{2c}}{\rightarrow} P\cdot E_2 \tag{11.79c}$$

$$P\cdot E_2 \underset{k_{-P}}{\overset{k_P}{\rightleftarrows}} P + E_2 \tag{11.79d}$$

$$Y\cdot E_1 + E_3 \underset{k_{-3}}{\overset{k_3}{\rightleftarrows}} Y\cdot E_3 + E_1 \tag{11.79e}$$

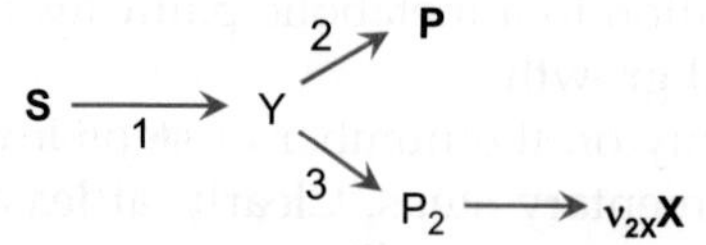

FIGURE 11.12 The simplest metabolic pathway for cell growth with one limiting substrate S.

$$Y \cdot E_3 \xrightarrow{k_{3c}} P_2 \cdot E_3 \tag{11.79f}$$

$$P_2 \cdot E_3 \xrightarrow{k_X} \nu_{2X} X + E_3 \tag{11.79g}$$

$$X \underset{k_{-4}}{\overset{k_4}{\rightleftarrows}} \nu_{Ej} E_j \tag{11.79h}$$

This is a set of reaction network based on the simplest metabolic pathway approximation. It is slightly more complex than the simplest reaction network. The brunching of extracellular and intracellular products formation can capture the difference in rates (product and biomass) as observed in many microbial systems.

The rate expressions for all the species in the simplest metabolic pathway are given by

$$r_S = k_1 S[E_1] + k_{-1}[SE_1] \tag{11.80a}$$

$$r_{SE_1} = k_1 S[E_1] - (k_{-1} + k_{1c})[SE_1] \tag{11.80b}$$

$$\begin{aligned} r_{E_1} &= k_{-1}[SE_1] - k_1 S[E_1] + k_2[YE_1][E_2] - k_{-2}[YE_2][E_1] \\ &\quad + k_3[YE_1][E_3] - k_{-3}[YE_3][E_1] + \nu_{E_1}(k_4 X - k_{-4}[E_1]) \end{aligned} \tag{11.80c}$$

$$r_{YE_1} = k_{1c}[SE_1] - k_2[E_2][YE_1] + k_{-2}[E_1][YE_2] - k_3[E_3][YE_1] + k_{-3}[E_1][YE_3] \tag{11.80d}$$

$$r_{YE_2} = k_2[E_2][YE_1] - k_{-2}[YE_2][E_1] - k_{2c}[YE_2] \tag{11.80e}$$

$$r_{PE_2} = k_{2c}[YE_2] + k_{-P}[E_2][P] - k_P[PE_2] \tag{11.80f}$$

$$r_{E_2} = -k_2[E_2][YE_1] + k_{-2}[YE_2][E_1] + k_P[PE_2] - k_{-P}[P][E_2] + \nu_{E_2}(k_4 X - k_{-4}[E_2]) \tag{11.80g}$$

$$r_{YE_3} = k_3[YE_1][E_3] - k_{-3}[YE_3][E_1] - k_{3c}[YE_3] \tag{11.80h}$$

$$r_{P_2E_3} = k_{3c}[YE_3] - k_X[P_2E_3] \tag{11.80i}$$

$$r_{E_3} = -k_3[E_3][YE_1] + k_{-3}[YE_3][E_1] + k_X[P_2E_3] + \nu_{E_3}(k_4 X - k_{-4}[E_3]) \tag{11.80j}$$

$$r_P = k_P[PE_2] - k_{-P}[P][E_2] \tag{11.80k}$$

$$r_X = k_X \nu_X [P_2E_3] \tag{11.80l}$$

The metabolic pathway usually results in a set in excess of 12 equations.

11.14.5. Cybernetic Models

Another modeling approach has been developed primarily to predict growth under conditions when several substrates are available. Simple systems have been outlined in §11.14.2.2. These substrates may be complementary (e.g. carbon or nitrogen) or substitutable. However, there have been no models given for the fractional rate contribution α_j's in Eqns (11.74) through (11.76). Multiple substrate medium is common. For example, glucose and lactose would be substitutable, as these compounds both supply carbon and energy. We discussed the diauxic phenomenon for sequential use of glucose and lactose in Chapter 10. That experimental observation led us to an understanding of regulation of the *lac* operon and catabolite repression. This metabolic regulation was necessary for the transition from one primary pathway to another. You might infer that the culture had as its objective function the maximization of its growth rate.

One approach to modeling growth on multiple substrates is *cybernetic*. Cybernetic means that a process is goal seeking (e.g. maximization of growth rate when substrate level is high). While this approach was initially motivated by a desire to predict the response of a microbial culture to growth on a set of substitutable carbon sources, it has been expanded to provide an alternative method of identifying the regulatory structure of a complex biochemical reaction network (such as cellular metabolism) in a simple manner. Typically a single objective, such as maximum growth rate, is chosen and an objective-oriented mathematical analysis is employed. This analysis is similar to many economic analyses for resource distribution. For many practical situations, this approach describes satisfactorily growth of a culture on a complex medium. However, the potential power of this approach is in metabolic engineering and in relating information on DNA sequences in an organism to physiologic function.

This approach has limitations, as the objective function for any organism is maximizing its long-term survival as a species. Maximization of growth rate or of growth yield is really subobjectives which can dominate under some environmental conditions for example substrate level is high and the population is sparse; these conditions are often of great interest to the bioprocess engineer. Consequently, the cybernetic approach is often a valuable tool. A generation of this approach leads to our discussion in the next section.

11.14.6. Computational Systems Biology

As a progression of the kinetic models presented in the previous sections, we are moving to the next level: system-level understanding of cellular cultures. As the need for a complete quantitative description (holism) in biology is recognized, the understanding develops that living systems cannot be understood by studying just individual parts. Computational systems biology aims at a system-level understanding by analyzing biological data using computational techniques. The fast progress of genome sequencing in multiple fronts and massive amounts of data generated by high-throughput experiments in DNA microarrays, proteomics, and metabolomics advances have lead to a leap in biological system modeling. The approaches outlined so far are approximations of cellular systems at various degrees of simplifications. A system-wide understanding will help in simplifying systems at different input and/or environmental conditions and provide guidance to altering cellular systems for a desired goal.

11.15. PERFORMANCE ANALYSIS OF BATCH CULTURE

Cultivation of cells is commonly performed in batch mode. Bioreactions are commonly applied in the production of drugs, food, and waste treatment. Apart from waste treatment, the product value is usually high and the prime directive is thus quality control. Bioreactors in pharmaceuticals and food industries are commonly operated in batch mode, eliminating the potential for cross-contaminations and loss of productivity due to the loss of desired cells.

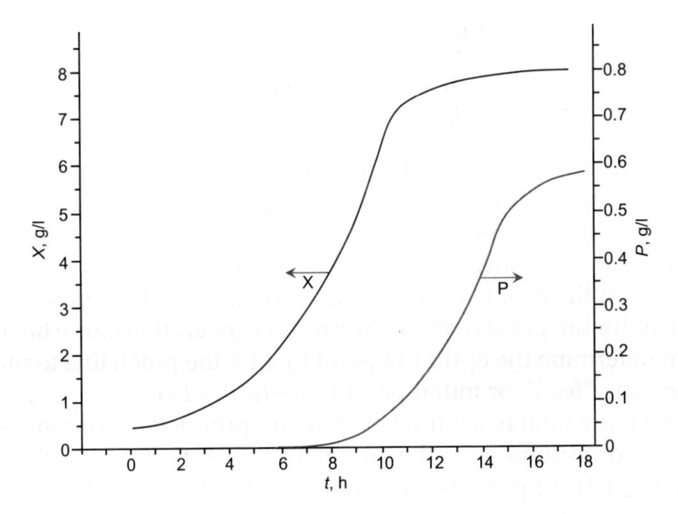

FIGURE E11-3.1

Batch operations are not controlled operations. There is no control being exerted on to the system after fermentation started other than external environment. In the same time, there is less chance of introducing unwanted material into the system. This is also the reason that drug productions are usually batch. We have learnt how to solve a batch reactor problem in Chapter 4. In this section, we shall use an example to refresh our understanding on batch fermentation.

Example 11-3. Optimum Reactor Size
Production of a secondary metabolite has been characterized using a small batch reactor and the kinetic data is shown in Fig. E11-3.1. You are to design a reactor to produce 2 Mg/year of the product P. Batch production mode is chosen based on the approved drug production method. Identical reaction conditions (same seed culture concentrations, pH, and temperature) will be used as those for generating the data in Fig. E11-3.1. Experience is that for each batch of operations, there are 6 h additional time needed for reactor loading, preparation, unloading after reaction, and reactor cleaning. Determine the minimum reactor size required for this production.

Solution. The kinetic data have not been treated to obtain mathematical expressions. We shall attempt to use a graphical method to solve this problem. Minimizing the reactor size is equivalent to maximize the productivity of P. The productivity of P is given by

$$P_P = \frac{P - P_0}{t_B} \tag{E11-3.1}$$

where P is the product concentration at a total batch time t_B (the sum of reaction time t and preparation time t_P), while P_0 is the product concentration in the feed (or initial stream). To maximize P_P, we set

$$0 = \left.\frac{dP_P}{dt_B}\right|_{t_{Bmin}} = \left.\frac{t_B \dfrac{dP}{dt_B} - (P - P_0)}{t_B^2}\right|_{t_{Bmin}} \tag{E11-3.2}$$

Equation (E11-3.2) can be reduced to

$$\left.\frac{dP}{dt_B}\right|_{t_{Bmin}} = \left.\frac{P - P_0}{t_B}\right|_{t_{Bmin}} \quad \text{(E11-3.3)}$$

Equation (E11-3.3) implies that the production rate (based on overall time required by the process) at the time of discharge (each batch) and the average production rate (based on total batch time required by the process) are identical when the production rate is maximized (or process time at minimum). In other words, the line connects ($t = t_B - t_P = -t_P$, $P = P_0$) and the optimum point (t, P) on the product generation curve, and the tangential line (in terms of t_B and P) passing the optimum point (t, P) on the product generation curve have the same slope. Therefore, one can determine the optimum point by plot the pinch line to the product generation curve passing the "feed" or initial point ($t = -t_P$, $P = P_0$).

The initial point I has a total batch time of zero and production concentration of zero. The total batch time zero corresponding to the growth time of $-t_p$, here t_p is the total preparation time. Therefore, in Fig. E11-3.1 provided, the initial point is ($t = -6$ h, $P = 0$). We plot the pinch line passing point I ($t = -6$ h, $P = 0$), the pinch point is then the optimum point for the fermentation discharge. The graphical solution is illustrated in Fig. E11-3.2. Therefore, we can read out the fermentation time and the concentrations obtained from a batch operation:

$$P_{max} = 0.562\ \text{g/L},\ t_f = 16.66\ \text{h}\ (t = 22.66\ \text{h}),\ \text{and}\ X_{max} = 8\ \text{g/L}.$$

The production rate is given by

$$F_P = \frac{PV}{t} \quad \text{(E11-3.4)}$$

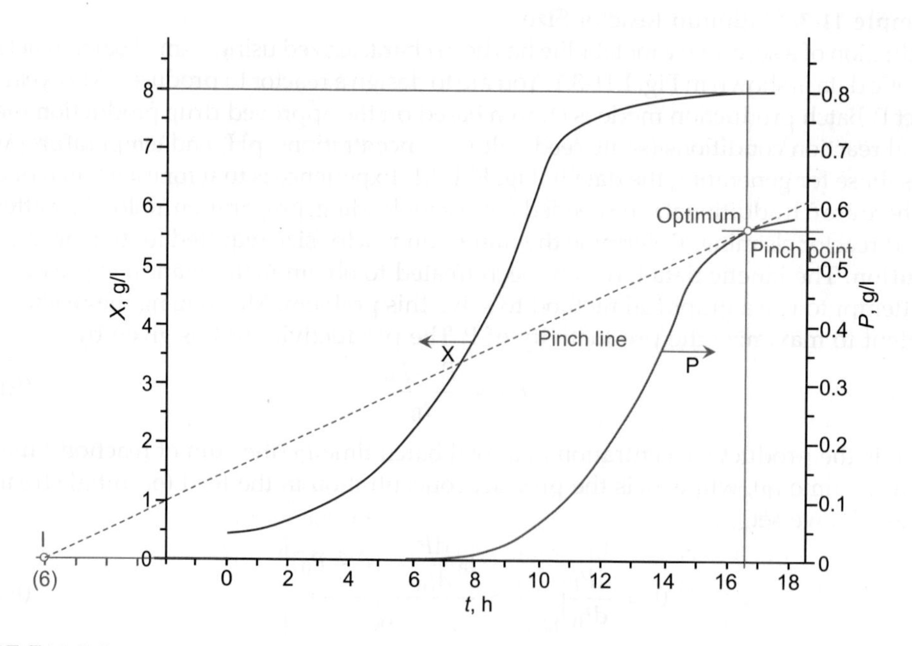

FIGURE E11-3.2

Since $F_P = 2$ Mg/year, we have

$$V = \frac{F_P t}{P} = \frac{2 \times 10^6}{365 \times 24} \times \frac{22.66}{0.562} L = 9205.54 L$$

11.16. SUMMARY

The kinetics of cell growth and product generation is the combined effects of cell metabolism and cell duplication. Metabolic pathways, cell physiology, and duplication are all important in the overall kinetic behavior. The complete description of the kinetic behavior requires system-wide analysis (e.g. computational systems biology). In normal applications, we deal with balanced (or pseudosteady state) growth or metabolism and thus simplification can be applied. Multiple substrates are required for growth and fermentation; however, we normally have many substrates in excess as compared with others. The simple growth and product formation rate equations for the case limited by a single substrate are of Michaelis–Menten form or the Monod equation:

$$\mu_G = \frac{r_X}{X} = \frac{\mu_{max} S}{K_S + S} \tag{11.21}$$

which is the Monod equation of growth. Similarly, for extracellular product formation,

$$\mu_P = \frac{r_P}{X} = \frac{\mu_{Pmax} S}{K_P + S} \tag{11.22}$$

which can also be expressed as

$$\mu_P = YF_{P/X} G\mu_G + YF_{P/e}\mu_e \tag{11.38}$$

In other words, the generation of extracellular product is almost always related to the endogenous metabolism of the cells and/or growth. Traditionally, there are three growth and product rates well-known, namely, growth-associated product formation, nongrowth-associated product formation, and mixed growth-related product formation. These three cases are all results of piece-wise interpretation (i.e. only in narrow range of growth rates) of the growth and product formation.

Simplification or utilization of simple growth and product formation kinetic models is valid for balanced growth (or pseudosteady state). However, there is an apparent time lag between substrate consumption and product formation due to the inability of the simple model to capture the uptake of substrate in the cell and a "delay" in execration of products. This "delay" can be significant resulting in the product emerging in the fermentation broth long after substrate had been consumed due to a "long route" of metabolic pathway.

The extracellular product generation needs not be directly associated with growth since the growth can be limited or diminished by the lack of one or more growth required nutrients. Cells can still be active other than replication. The endogenous metabolic rate also follows the Monod rate law

$$\mu_e = \frac{r_e}{X} = \frac{\mu_{emax} S}{K_{Se} + S} \tag{11.34}$$

However, if the substrate limiting the growth is also the one being converted to the extracellular product, the specific endogenous metabolic rate can be expressed as

$$\mu_e = \frac{\mu_{e\mu max} \mu_G}{K_{e\mu} + \mu_G} \tag{11.36}$$

Cells die (physiological development) due to harsh environment (high temperature, pH, or harmful chemicals) or simply due to aging. The death rate is usually modeled by a first-order relation:

$$\mu_d = k_d \tag{11.23}$$

In single-celled microorganisms, *cell death* is the point at which reinitiation of division is no longer possible. Dead cells cease nutrients uptake. Cell functions stop even other cells continue to function normally.

The net specific cell growth rate is the growth rate subtracted cell death rate, that is

$$\mu_{net} = \mu_G - k_d \tag{11.24}$$

To this end, we have the necessary simple growth model equations to characterize cell growth and product formation.

During batch cultivation, a population of cells typically exhibits several different growth phases. During the lag phase, the cell builds the biosynthetic pathways necessary for maximal growth rates in the fresh medium. The lag phase is a period when cells attempt to establish pseudosteady-state metabolic functions. Once pseudosteady state (balanced growth) is established, cell growth is the fastest. During *maximum growth,* cell replication rate is maximal, and the chemical composition of the cell population is nearly constant (e.g. balanced growth). Total cell mass increases exponentially with time, which is the reason this phase also termed *exponential growth.* Because of the exponential increase of cell biomass with time, experimental data can be presented on semi-log plot to better illustrate the various phases of growth. When substrate is nearly exhausted or when toxic metabolic by-products have built to a critical level, the growth rate begins to drop rapidly, causing significant changes in biosynthetic pathways. In the *stationary phase,* there is no net growth; cells now reorient their metabolic machinery to increase the probability of long-term survival. At some point, some cells can no longer obtain enough energy from their reserves or enough of another critical resource, and the culture enters the *death phase.* Dead cells do not have an energized membrane and often lyse (or break apart). Nutrients released by lysed cells can be utilized by survivors, allowing cryptic growth. Products formed by cells can be related to this batch-culture growth cycle. Primary products are growth associated. Secondary products are nongrowth associated and are made in the stationary phase and/or death phase. Some products have both growth- and nongrowth-associated components.

Batch cultivations are commonly applied in pharmaceutical and food productions. Strict quality control up to the detailed process flow sheet by Food and Drug Administration and the commonly low production rate are the main reasons for batch operations, among others.

Reading Materials

Aiba S., Humphrey, A.E., Millis, N.F., 1973. *Biochemical Engineering,* 2nd ed., Academic Press, New York.

Atkinson B., Mavituna F., 1983. *Biochemical Engineering and Biotechnology Handbook,* MacMillan, Inc.: New York.

Bailey, J.E., 1998. Mathematical modeling and analysis in biochemical engineering: past accomplishments and future opportunities, *Biotechnol. Prog.* 14, 8.

Bailey, J.E., Ollis, D.F., 1986. *Biochemical Engineering Fundamentals,* 2nd ed., Mc-Graw-Hill Book Co., New York.

Blanch, H.W., Clark, D.S., 1996. *Biochemical Engineering*. Marcel Dekker, Inc., New York.

Frederickson, A.G., Megeeill, R.D., Tsuchiyam, H., 1970. Mathematical models for fermentation processes, *Adv. Appl. Microbiol.* 23, 419.

Gadden, E.L., Jr., 1955. Fermentation kinetics and productivity, *Chem. 1nd. Rev.* (London), p. 154.

Kriete, A., Eils, R., 2005. Computational Systems Biology, Elsevier.

Liu, Y.H., Bi, J-X., Zeng, A-P., Yuan, J.Q., 2008. A cybernetic model to describe the dynamics of myeloma cell cultivations, App. Math. Comp. 205, 84–97.

Shuler, M.L., Kargi F., 2006. Bioprocess Engineering, Basic Concepts. 2nd ed., Prentice Hall: Upper Saddle River, NJ.

Straight, J.V., Ramkrishna, D., 1994. Cybernetic modeling and regulation of metabolic pathways, growth on complementary nutrients, *Biotechnol. Prog.* 10, 574.

PROBLEMS

11.1. A simple, batch fermentation of an aerobic bacterium growing on methanol gave the results shown in Table P11.1. Calculate:

(a) Maximum growth rate (μ_{max})
(b) Yield on substrate ($YF_{X/S}$)
(c) Mass doubling time (t_d)
(d) Saturation constant (K_S)
(e) Specific growth rate (μ_{net}) at $t = 10$ h

TABLE P11.1

Time, h	X, g/L	S, g/L	Time, h	X, g/L	S, g/L
0	0.20	9.23	12	3.20	4.60
2	0.21	9.21	14	5.60	0.92
4	0.31	9.07	16	6.15	0.08
8	0.98	8.03	18	6.20	0
10	1.77	6.80			

11.2. The data in Table P11.2 were obtained for *Pyrodictium occultum* at 98 °C. Run 1 was carried out in the absence of yeast extract and run 2 with yeast extract. Both runs initially contained Na_2S. The vol % of the growth product H_2S collected above the broth was reported as a function of time as shown in Table P11.2.

(a) What is the lag time with and without the yeast extract?
(b) What is the difference in the maximum specific growth rates, μ_{max}, of the bacteria with and without the yeast extract?

TABLE P11.2

Run 1	Time (h)	0	10	15	20	30	40	50	60	70
	Cell density, cells/L	0.27	0.28	1.5	7.0	40.0	60.0	71.5	60.0	52.5
	% H_2S	0.5	0.8	1.0	1.2	6.8	4.7	7.5	8.0	8.2
Run 2	Time (h)	0	5	10	15	20	30	40	50	60
	Cell density, cells/L	0.27	0.70	1.1	8.0	25.0	35.0	35.0	25.0	
	% H_2S	0.1	0.7	0.7	0.8	1.2	4.3	7.5	11.0	12.3

(c) How long is the stationary phase?

(d) During which phase does the majority production of H_2S occur?

11.3. It is desired to model the growth of an *individual* bacterium. The cell transports S_1 into the cell enzymatically, and the permease is subject to product inhibition. S_1 is converted into precursors, P, that are converted finally into the macromolecular portion of the cell, M. The catalyst of all reactions is M.

(1) $S_1^* \underset{M}{\rightarrow} S_1$ (per unit surface area), where S^* = outside concentration of S

(2) $S_1 \underset{M}{\rightarrow} P$

(3a) $\left.\begin{array}{l} \text{Energy} + P \underset{M}{\rightarrow} M \\ S_1 + \underset{M}{\rightarrow} \text{Energy} \end{array}\right\}$ coupled reaction

(3b) $S_1 + P \underset{M}{\rightarrow} M$

The dry weight of the cell is T and is equal to

(4) $T = S_1 + P + M_1 = \rho V$, where ρ = cell density and V = cell volume

Write the equations and define all symbols necessary to describe the changes in S_1, P, M, and T within the cell. Remember that the cell volume is always changing.

11.4. The data in Table P11.4 were obtained for the effect of temperature on the fermentative production of lactic acid by a strain of *Lactobacillus delbrueckii*. From these data, calculate the value of the activation energy for this process. Is the value of the activation energy typical of this sort of biological conversion?

TABLE P11.4

Temperature, °C,	Rate constant, mol·L^{-1}·h^{-1}
40.4	0.0140
36.8	0.0112
33.1	0.0074
30.0	0.0051
25.1	0.0036

11.5. The production of glycerol from corn amylum/asylum is to be carried out by fermentation using yeast cells. The specific growth rate is given by

$$\mu_G = \frac{\mu_{max} S}{K_S + S + S^2/K_I}\left(1 - \frac{X}{X_\infty}\right)\exp\left(-K_{PI}P\right)$$

with $YF_{P/S} = 1.33$ g-P/g-S, $\mu_{max} = 0.25$/s, $K_S = 0.018$ g/L, $K_I = 11.8$ g/L, $X_\infty = 32.4$ g/L, $K_{PI} = 0.06$ L/g. The product generation is growth associated, $\mu_P = \alpha\mu_G + \beta$, here $\alpha = 34.5$ and $\beta = -0.147$/s.

Plot the concentration of cells, substrate, and product as a function of time for an initial concentration of cells of 10^{-8} g/L and a substrate concentration of 50 g/L.

11.6. The production of L-malic acid (used in medicines and food additives) was produced over immobilized cells of *Bacillus flavum* MA-3.

$$\text{HOOCCH{=}CHCOOH} + H_2O \xrightarrow{\text{fumarase}} \text{HOOCCH}_2\text{CH(OH)COOH}$$

The following rate law was obtained for the rate of formation of product:

$$r_P = \frac{r_{max} S}{K_S + S}\left(1 - \frac{P}{P_\infty}\right)$$

where $r_{max} = 76$ mol·L^{-1}·day^{-1}, $K_S = 0.048$ mol/L, and $P_\infty = 1.69$ mol/L. Design a batch reactor to process 10 m^3/day of 1.5 mol/L of fumaric acid (S). The required conversion of fumaric acid is 99%. The total preparation time (loading, unloading, and cleaning) is 3 h for each batch.

11.7. A biochemical engineer has determined in her laboratory that the optimal productivity of a valuable antibiotic is achieved when the carbon nutrient, in this case molasses, is metered into the fermenter at a rate proportional to the growth rate. However, she cannot implement her discovery in the antibiotic plant, since there is no reliable way to measure the growth rate r_X or biomass concentration (X) during the course of the fermentation. It is suggested that an oxygen analyzer be installed on the plant fermenters so that the OUR, g/L-h, may be measured.

(a) Derive expressions that may be used to estimate X and r_X from OUR and time data, assuming that a simple yield and maintenance model may be used to describe the rate of oxygen consumption by the culture.

(b) Calculate values for the yield (YF_{X/O_2}) and maintenance (m_{O_2}) parameters from the data in Table P11.7:

TABLE P11.7

Time	OUR, g/h	X, g/L	Time	OUR, g/h	X, g/L
0	0.011	0.60	11	1.12	9.40
1	0.008	0.63	12	1.37	11.40
2	0.084	0.63	13	1.58	12.22

(*Continued*)

TABLE P11.7—Cont'd

Time	OUR, g/h	X, g/L	Time	OUR, g/h	X, g/L
3	0.153	0.76	14	1.26	13.00
4	0.198	1.06	15	1.58	13.37
5	0.273	1.56	16	1.26	14.47
6	0.393	2.23	17	1.12	15.37
7	0.493	2.85	18	1.20	16.12
8	0.642	4.15	19	0.99	16.18
9	0.915	5.37	20	0.86	16.67
10	1.031	7.59	21	0.90	17.01

11.8. Formation of lactic acid from glucose is realized in a batch reactor using *Streptococcus lactis*. The reactor is initially charged with 5 L medium containing 5 g/L glucose and 0.1 g/L cell biomass. There is no lactic acid present initially. The following information was obtained from experimental studies.

$$\mu_{max} = 0.2\ h^{-1},\ K_S = 200\ mg/L,\ k_d = 0.002\ h^{-1},\ YF_{X/S} = 0.4\ g\text{-}X/g\text{-}S,\ \mu_P = 0.1\ \mu_G.$$

(a) Plot the variations of S, X, and P with reaction time.
(b) Determine the maximum production rate of lactic acid in g/(day·L) if with each batch a reactor loading, unloading, and sterilization time of 3.5 h is needed.

11.9. The kinetics of microbial growth, substrate consumption, and mixed growth-associated product formation for a batch culture are given by the following equations:

$$r_X = \frac{\mu_{max} S}{K_S + S} X$$

$$r_S = -\frac{\mu_{max} S}{K_S + S} \frac{X}{YF_{X/S}}$$

$$r_P = \alpha \frac{\mu_{max} S}{K_S + S} X + \beta X$$

The kinetic parameters are $\mu_{max} = 0.7\ h^{-1}$, $K_S = 20$ mg/L, $YF_{X/S} = 0.5$ g-X/g-S, $\alpha = 0.1$, $\beta = 0.02\ h^{-1}$. The reactor is initially charged with a medium containing 1 g/L of substrate and 0.02 g/L cells. It takes 4 h to prepare, load, and unload the reactor. Determine the maximum production rate of P in g/(L·h).

11.10. The data on the specific growth rate and specific rate of penicillin synthesis with glucose as the limiting substrate, are given in Table P11.10 below (D.D.Y. Ryu and J. Hospodka, 1980 "Quantitative Physiology of Penicillium Chrysogenum in Penicillin Fermentation", Biotechnol. Bioeng., 22(2): 289-298.)

Determine the relationship between the product rate and the specific growth rate.

TABLE P11.10

Specific growth rate (μ_G), h^{-1}	The ratio of product rate to its maximum rate	Specific growth rate (μ_G), h^{-1}	The ratio of product rate to its maximum rate
0.0055	0.360	0.0139	1.063
0.0041	0.243	0.0137	0.891
0.0052	0.522	0.0151	0.996
0.0065	0.364	0.0167	1.117
0.0065	0.708	0.0180	0.944
0.0073	0.541	0.0191	1.030
0.0085	0.423	0.0201	1.103
0.0087	0.549	0.0230	1.169
0.0092	0.700	0.0215	0.976
0.0096	0.910	0.0243	0.896
0.0104	0.792	0.0265	1.017
0.0120	0.920	0.0742	1.035
0.0118	0.782	0.0770	0.948
0.0116	0.598		

11.11. Ethanol formation from glucose is accomplished in a batch culture of *Saccharomyces cerevisiae* with certain amount of a complex medium (nitrogen, energy, and minerals) to produce biomass from the small inoculums. The following data (Table P11.11) were obtained.

TABLE P11.11

Time (*t*), h	Glucose (*S*), g/L	Biomass (*X*), g/L	Ethanol (*P*), g/L
0	100	0.5	0.0
2	95	1.0	2.5
5	85	2.1	7.5
10	58	4.8	20.0
15	30	7.7	34.0
20	12	9.6	43.0
25	5	10.4	47.5
30	2	10.7	49.0

(a) Correlating the data with the logistic equation, determine the carrying capacity, and carrying capacity coefficient.

(b) Consider that glucose is the only substrate for the product (ethanol) generation while some glucose also consumed for the cell growth. Correlate the ethanol product rate with Monod model. Determine the specific maximum product formation rate, saturation coefficient, and the yield factors $YF_{P/S}$ and $YF_{X/S}$.

11.12. Production of a secondary metabolite has been characterized using a small batch reactor, and the kinetic data are shown in Fig. P11.12. You are to design a reactor to produce 5 Mg/year of the product P. Batch production mode is chosen based on the approved drug production method. Identical reaction conditions (same seed culture concentrations, pH, and temperature) will be used as those for generating the data in Fig. P11.12. Experience is that for each batch of operations, there are 2 h additional time needed for reactor loading, preparation, unloading after reaction, and reactor cleaning. Determine the minimum reactor size required for this production.

FIGURE P11.12

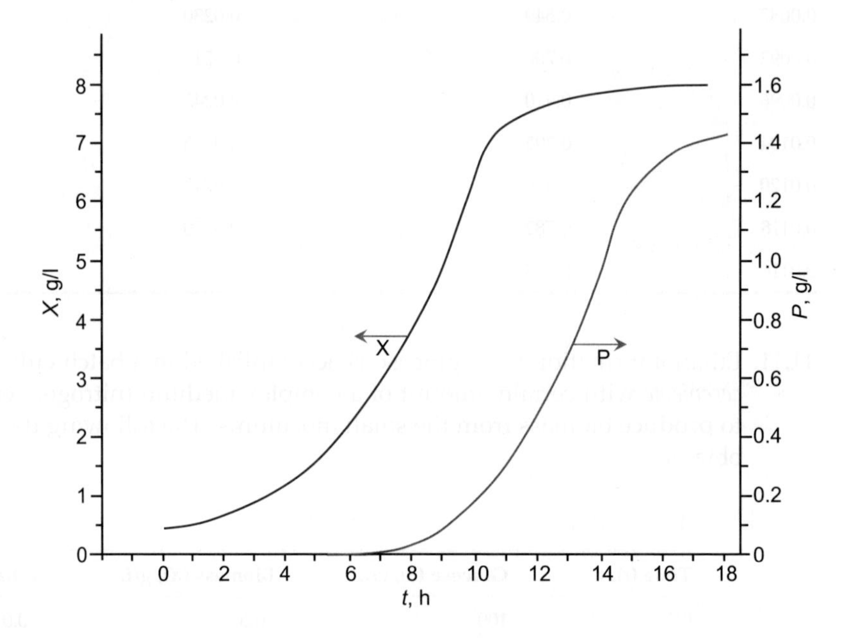

11.13. The production of biomass is actually desired for the case of Fig. P11.12. Batch production mode is chosen based on the approved drug production method. Identical reaction conditions (same seed culture concentrations, pH, and temperature) will be used as those for generating the data in Fig. P11.12. Experience is that for each batch of operations, there are 2 h additional time needed for reactor loading, preparation, unloading after reaction, and reactor cleaning. Determine the maximum production rate for biomass.

CHAPTER

12

Continuous Cultivation

OUTLINE

Cell growth and/or fermentation in different conditions can render significantly different rate for the production of the desired primary product. Difference in trace elements/electrolytes can alter the growth and fermentation pattern. Macronutrient concentration changes affect the rates in a more measurable manner. In some cases, we have limitations on the type of reactor and/or operating strategies. In other cases, our limitation is only the highest efficiency achievable. An important decision for selecting or designing any biological or chemical process concerns the configuration the reactor system should take. The choice of reactor and operating strategy determine product concentration, number and types of impurities, degree of substrate conversion, yields, and whether sustainable, reliable performance can be achieved. The reactor section represents a very major component (usually >40%) of the total capital expenditures, which is comparable to separation needs. Choices at the reactor level and of the biocatalyst determine the difficulty of the separation. Thus, our choice of reactor must be made in the context of the total process: substrate, biocatalyst, reactor, and separation and purification train. In Chapter 11, while we were discussing the kinetics of cell

Bioprocess Engineering
http://dx.doi.org/10.1016/B978-0-444-59525-6.00012-3

growth, we have learned how to analyze batch growth. We can infer that there is no control being exerted in batch growth other than the initial substrate addition and maintaining the reactor temperature. In this chapter, we shall focus more on the controlled growth where control can be exerted on the growth more than the simple substrate/inoculums addition.

12.1. CONTINUOUS CULTURE

The medium conditions change continually in a batch culture due to cell metabolism and lack of control. Growth, product formation, and substrate utilization terminate after a certain time interval, whereas, in a continuous culture as it implies, fresh nutrient medium is continually supplied to a well-mixed (or more precisely uniform) culture, and products and cells are simultaneously withdrawn. Growth and product formation can be maintained for prolonged periods in a continuous culture. After a certain period of time, the system reaches a steady state where cell, product, and substrate concentrations remain constant. Continuous culture provides constant culture environmental conditions for growth and product formation and supplies uniform quality product. Therefore, continuous culture is a controlled culture. Continuous culture is an important tool to determine the response of microorganisms to their environment and to produce the desired products under optimal environmental conditions.

12.1.1. Chemostat Devices for Continuous Culture

The primary type of continuous cultivation devices is the *chemostat* (with many variations pending on the feedback control mechanism: *cytostat*, *turbidostat*, and *perfusion reactor* are some of the classic chemostats equipped with different external peripherals or recycle capabilities) although plug flow reactors (PFRs) are also used. In some cases, these units are modified by recycle of cells (perfusion reactor). Figure 12.1 is a schematic of a continuous culture

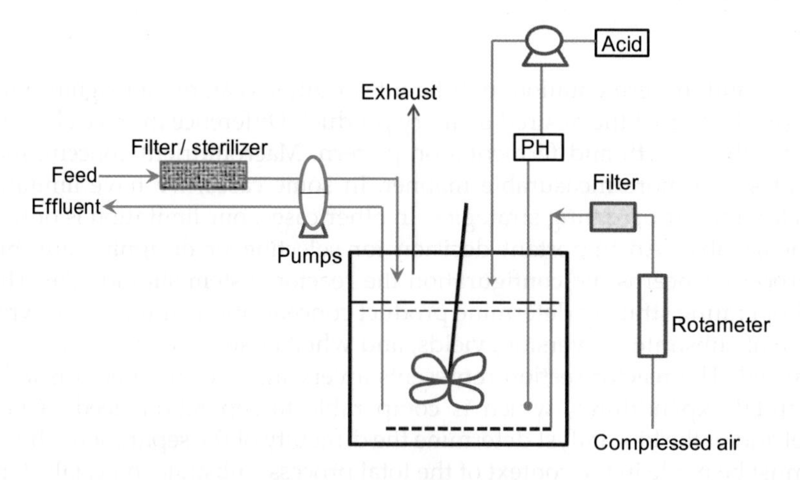

FIGURE 12.1 A continuous-culture laboratory setup (chemostat).

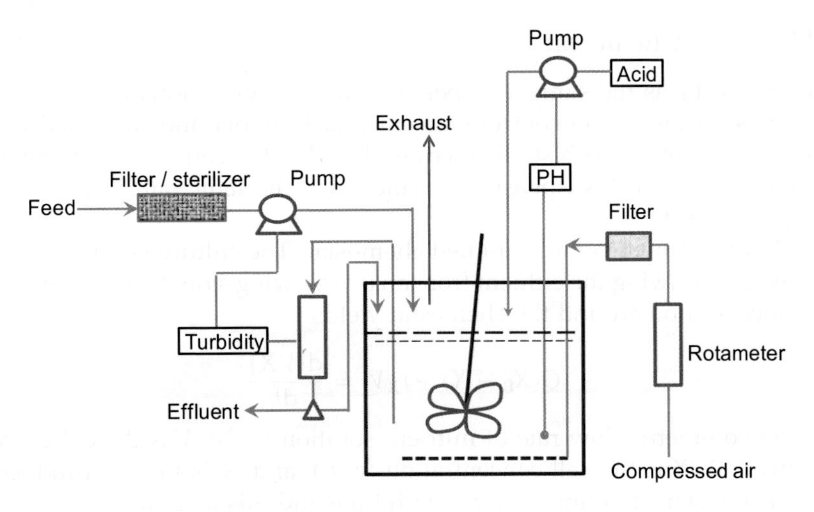

FIGURE 12.2 Typical laboratory setup for a turbidostat.

device (chemostat). Chemostat is the continuous stirred-tank reactor (CSTR) as described in Chapters 3 and 5, however, for cell culture applications. Cellular growth is usually limited by one essential nutrient, and other nutrients are in excess. As we will show, when a chemostat is at steady state, the nutrient, product, and cell concentrations are constant. For this reason, the name *chemostat* refers to constant chemical environment (for cell culture).

Figure 12.2 is a schematic of a turbidostat in which the cell concentration in the culture vessel is maintained constant by monitoring the optical density of the culture and controlling the feed flow rate. When the turbidity of the medium exceeds the set point, a pump is activated and fresh medium is added. The culture volume is kept constant by removing an equal amount of culture fluid. Therefore, turbidostat is a chemostat with a particular control mechanism, via the turbidity of the culture. As discussed in Chapter 11, cell concentration affects the optical density and thus turbidity can be correlated to the cell concentration. Turbidostats can be very useful in selecting subpopulations able to withstand a desired environmental stress (for example, high-ethanol concentrations), because the cell concentration is maintained constant. The selection of variants or mutants with desirable properties is very important.

A PFR can also be used for continuous cultivation purposes. Since there is no backmixing in an ideal PFR, fluid elements containing active cells cannot inoculate other fluid elements at different axial positions. Therefore, strict PFR is only applicable for fermentations where cells are fixed along the reactor (immobilized and supported, for example packed beds). Liquid recycle is required for continuous inoculation of nutrient media for cell growth cultivation. In a PFR, substrate and cell concentrations vary with axial position in the vessel. An ideal PFR resembles a batch reactor in which distance along the fermentor replaces incubation time in a batch reactor as discussed in Chapters 4 and 5. In waste treatment, some units approach PFR behavior, and multistage chemostats tend to approach PFR dynamics if the number of stages is large (CSTR train, Chapter 5).

12.1.2. The Ideal Chemostat

An ideal chemostat is the same as a perfectly mixed continuous-flow reactor or CSTR. Most chemostats require some control elements, such as pH and dissolved oxygen (DO) control units, to be useful. Fresh sterile medium is fed to the completely mixed and aerated (if required) reactor, and cell suspension is removed at the same rate. Liquid volume in the reactor is kept constant.

Figure 12.3 is a schematic of a simplified chemostat. The culture volume in the reactor is maintained by withdrawing the effluent from an overflowing side device. A material balance on the cell concentration around the chemostat yields

$$Q(X_0 - X) + r_X V = \frac{d(VX)}{dt} \tag{12.1}$$

where Q is the volumetric flow rate of nutrient solution (L/h), V is the culture volume (L) (assumed constant), X is the cell concentration (g/L), and r_X is the net production rate of biomass. At steady state, nothing changes with time and this includes

$$\frac{d(VX)}{dt} = 0 \tag{12.2}$$

Dividing Eqn (12.1) by reactor volume V and substituting in Eqn (12.2), we obtain the cell mass balance equation for an ideal chemostat:

$$D(X - X_0) = r_X \tag{12.3}$$

where D is *dilution rate* and $D = Q/V$. D is the reciprocal of space time. Figure 12.4 shows a schematic of cell mass balance on the cell mass concentration vs cell growth rate plane. Clearly, the mass balance is a straight line. The intercept(s) are the solutions for the chemostat for the given cell growth curve.

The net growth rate can be expressed as

$$r_X = \mu_{net} X \tag{12.4}$$

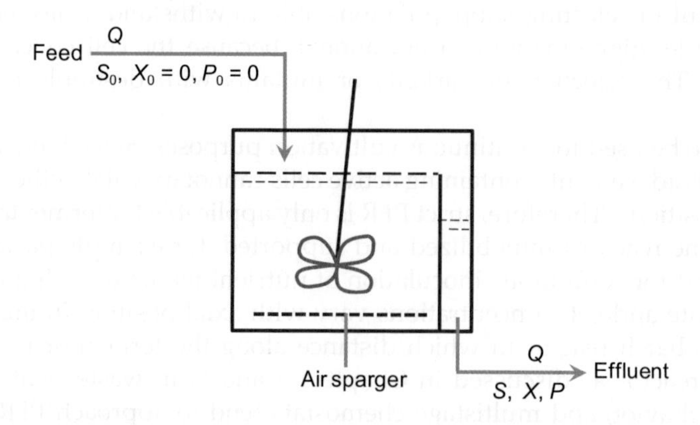

FIGURE 12.3 A schematic of a chemostat.

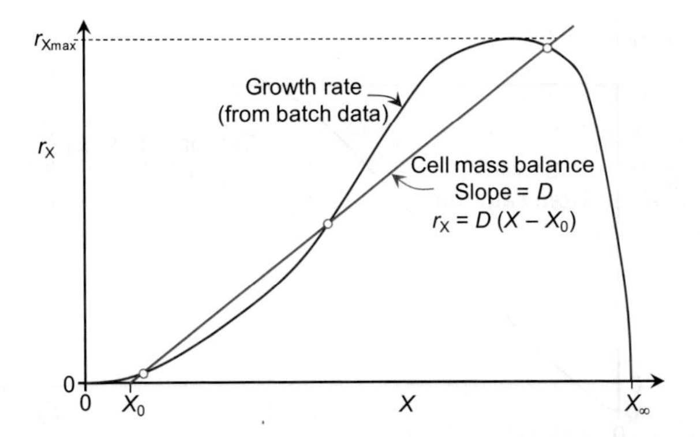

FIGURE 12.4 A sketch of cell mass balance on the cell mass concentration vs cell growth rate plane.

where μ_{net} is the net specific growth rate, which is given by

$$\mu_{net} = \mu_G - k_d \tag{12.5}$$

μ_G and k_d are growth and death rate constants, respectively (h^{-1}). Equation (12.3) can be rearranged as

$$D(X - X_0) = (\mu_G - k_d)X \tag{12.6}$$

Usually, the feed media are sterile, $X_0 = 0$, thus Eqn (12.6) gives rise to two solutions

$$X = 0 \tag{12.7}$$

or

$$D = \mu_{net} = \mu_G - k_d \tag{12.8}$$

Since we built the reactor to culture the cells, the trivial solution Eqn (12.7) is not a desired solution. More often, this trivial solution is omitted. However, as we will see later, this solution could be the only solution realizable in some cases, for example when the flow rate is too high (washout).

Figure 12.5 shows a schematic of the cell mass balance on the μ_{net} vs S plane. Clearly, the cell mass balance line is a horizontal line with fixed net specific growth rate equal to the dilution rate. Figures 12.4 and 12.5 show that cell mass balance can be represented differently depending on the rate data available.

Furthermore, if the endogenous metabolism or death rate is negligible as compared to the growth rate ($k_d << \mu_G$)

$$D = \mu_G \tag{12.9}$$

Therefore, cells are removed in a chemostat at a rate equal to their (net) growth rate, and the (net) growth rate of cells equals the dilution rate. *This property allows the investigator to manipulate net growth rate as an independent parameter* and makes the chemostat a powerful experimental tool. In simple terms, the growth rate can be controlled by the dilution rate.

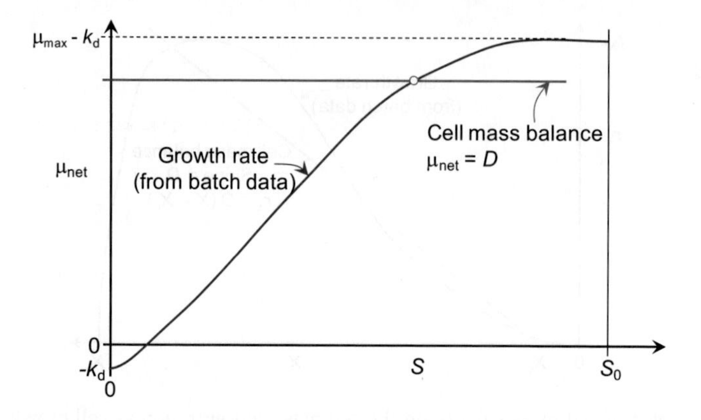

FIGURE 12.5 A sketch of cell mass balance on the substrate concentration vs specific cell growth rate plane.

Since growth rate is limited by at least one substrate in a chemostat, a simple description of chemostat performance can be made by substituting the Monod equation, Eqn (11.10) for μ_G in Eqn (12.9):

$$D = \mu_G - k_d = \frac{\mu_{max} S}{K_S + S} - k_d \tag{12.10}$$

where S is the steady-state limiting substrate concentration (g/L). If D is set at a value greater than $\mu_{max} - k_d$, Eqn (12.10) or (12.8) cannot be satisfied. The culture cannot reproduce quickly enough to maintain itself and is *washed out*. Equation (12.7) is then the only answer to the culture.

Using Eqn (12.10), we can relate effluent substrate concentration to dilution rate for $D < \mu_{max} - k_d$

$$S = \frac{K_S (D + k_d)}{\mu_{max} - D - k_d} \tag{12.11}$$

which is the intercept shown in Fig. 12.5.

A material balance on the limiting substrate in the absence of endogenous metabolism yields

$$Q(S_0 - S) + r_S V = \frac{d(VS)}{dt} \tag{12.12}$$

where S_0 and S are feed and effluent substrate concentrations (g/L), r_S is the rate of generation of substrate. Again, at steady state, nothing changes with time or

$$\frac{d(VS)}{dt} = 0 \tag{12.13}$$

Dividing Eqn (12.12) by the reactor volume V, we obtain

$$D(S_0 - S) = -r_S \tag{12.14}$$

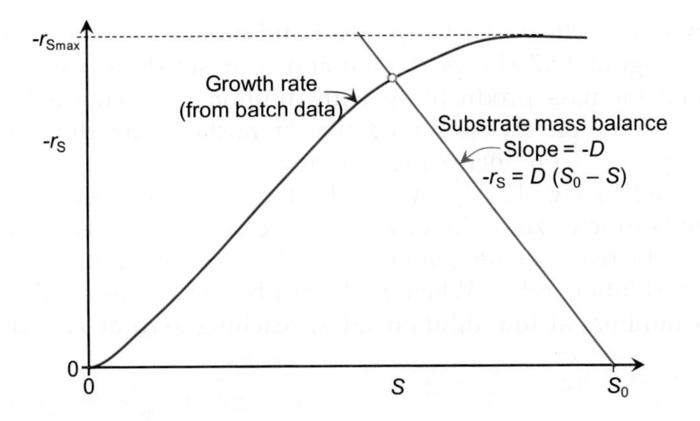

FIGURE 12.6 A sketch of substrate mass balance on the substrate concentration vs substrate consumption rate plane.

which is the general mass balance for substrate over an ideal chemostat. Figure 12.6 shows a schematic of substrate mass balance on the substrate concentration vs substrate disappearance rate plane. Clearly, substrate mass balance is a straight line passing through ($S = S_0$, $-r_S = 0$) with a negative slope of $-D$. The nontrivial solution is the intercept of the mass balance line and the substrate consumption curve (by the cells). The substrate consumption rate can be obtained through stoichiometry (or yield factor) by

$$-r_S = \frac{\mu_G X}{YF_{X/S}} \tag{12.15}$$

where $YF_{X/S}$ is the yield factors (g-cell/g-S). If no cell growth and an extracellular product is generated due to the consumption of substrate, stoichiometry leads to

$$-r_S = \frac{\mu_P X}{YF_{P/S}} \tag{12.16}$$

where μ_P is the specific rate of extracellular product formation, g-P/(L · g-cells h), and $YF_{P/S}$ is the yield factor (g-P/g-S).

In most cases, cell growth is apparent, Eqn (12.14) is reduced to

$$D(S_0 - S) = \frac{\mu_G X}{YF_{X/S}} \tag{12.17}$$

Since $D = \mu_{net} = \mu_G - k_d$ at steady state,

$$X = \frac{D}{D + k_d} YF_{X/S}(S_0 - S) \tag{12.18}$$

Using Eqn (12.11), the steady-state cell concentration can be expressed as

$$X = YF_{X/S} D \left(\frac{S_0}{D + k_d} - \frac{K_S}{\mu_{max} - D - k_d} \right) \tag{12.19}$$

The productivity of a chemostat for product and biomass can be found from DP and DX, respectively. Figure 12.7 shows the variations of substrate concentration, biomass concentration, and biomass productivity with dilution rate. Figure 12.7(a) shows that substrates are nearly completely consumed in a chemostat at low dilution rates. Substrate concentration increases with increasing dilution rate. Different endogeneous growth needs are illustrated in Fig. 12.7: growth rate dependent or growth rate independent. When death rate is exactly zero, the cell biomass concentration is maximum at low (or zero) dilution rate. Increasing endogenous needs decreases the cell biomass concentration especially at low dilution rates. When finite death rate is observed, the cell biomass concentration is minimal at low dilution rates, reaching zero at zero dilution rate. The

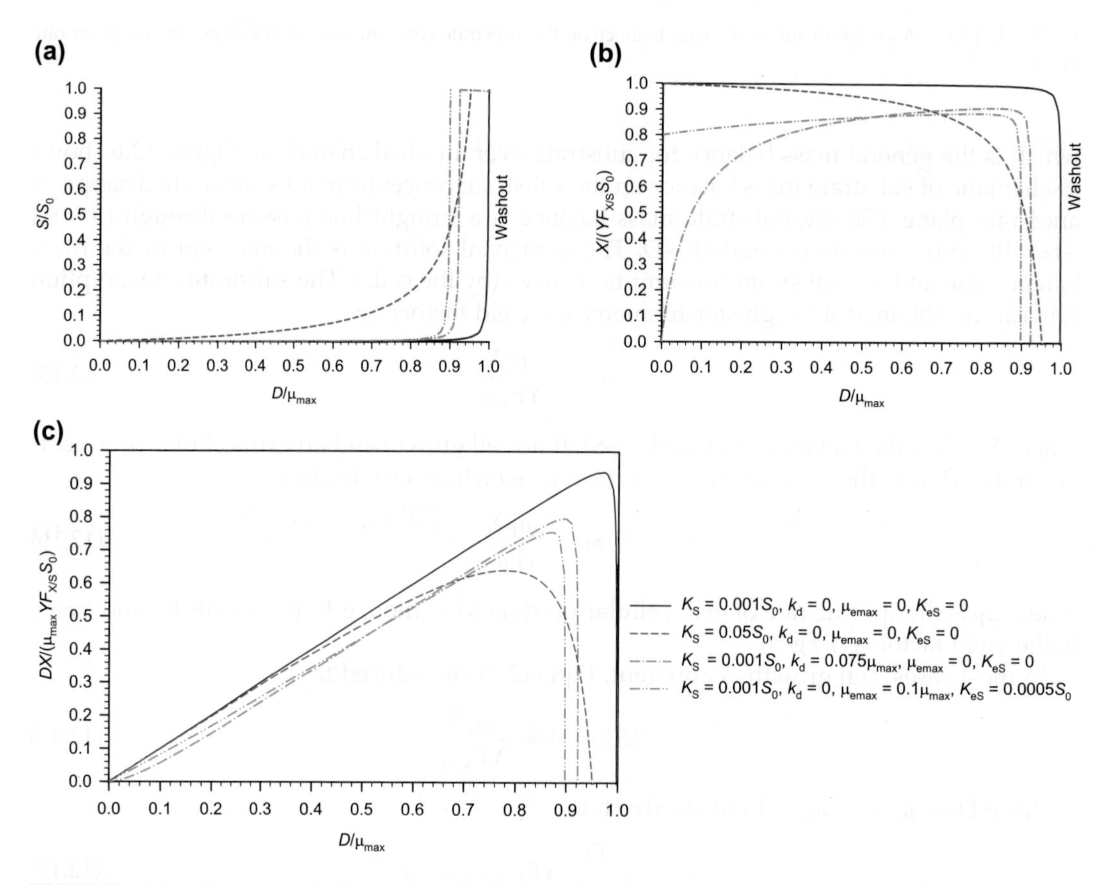

FIGURE 12.7 Variations of substrate concentration (a), biomass concentration and (b), biomass productivity (c) with dilution rate in a chemostat where growth kinetics is given by $\mu_{net} = \mu_G - \mu_e$ with $\mu_G = \frac{\mu_{max} S}{K_S + S}$ and $\mu_e = \frac{\mu_{e\,max} S}{K_{eS} + S} + k_d$. The solid line is the base case with the growth parameters shown, whereas the dashed lines are with the change of one parameter from the base case.

cell biomass concentration decreases monotonously with dilution although more sharply near washout to zero when no endogenous needs required for cell growth (Fig. 12.7b). The decrease is more pronounced when the saturation coefficient is increased at lower dilution rates. However, the cell biomass concentration increases with increasing dilution rate, reaches a maximum before decreases sharply to zero at washout (near $D = \mu_{max} - \mu_{e\,max} - k_d$) when the endogenous needs are not exactly zero (Fig. 12.7b). Increasing cell death rate and/or endogenous needs decreases the biomass productivity and washout limit dilution rate for a given feed (Fig. 12.7c). An increase in the saturation coefficient (K_S) also decreases the washout limit of dilution rate as well as the cell biomass productivity. One can also observe that there is a maximum cell productivity that varies with growth parameters.

Cytostat and turbidostat are designed to control the cell density (or biomass concentration) in the reactor. As one can observe from Fig. 12.7b, the cell biomass concentration depends on the dilution rate weakly, especially between $0.4\mu_{max} < D < 0.8\mu_{max}$. Therefore, controlling cell density by adjusting the flow rate (or dilution rate) is not effective in medium dilution rates. Normally, the cell density control by varying flow rate is operated at high throughput, $0.8\mu_{max} < D < 0.95\mu_{max}$, and when the productivity is near maximum (Fig. 12.7c).

The dilution rate that maximizes productivity is found by differentiating DP or DX with respect to D and setting the derivative equal to zero. The optimal value of D, D_{opt}, will depend on whether endogenous metabolism and/or product formation is considered. Eqn (12.19) gives

$$DX = \frac{D^2 YF_{X/S}}{D + k_d}\left(S_0 - K_S\frac{D + k_d}{\mu_{max} - D - k_d}\right) \tag{12.20}$$

By setting

$$0 = \frac{d(DX)}{dD} = \frac{D(D + 2k_d)}{(D + k_d)^2} S_0 YF_{X/S} - K_S YF_{X/S}\frac{D(2\mu_{max} - D - 2k_d)}{(\mu_{max} - D - k_d)^2} \tag{12.21}$$

we obtain the optimum dilution rate, D in Eqn (12.21), or

$$S_0(\mu_{max} - D_{opt(DX)} - k_d)^2(D_{opt(DX)} + 2k_d) = K_S(D_{opt(DX)} + k_d)^2(2\mu_{max} - D_{opt(DX)} - 2k_d) \tag{12.22}$$

Since k_d is usually small, $D_{opt(DX)}\,(D_{opt(DX)} + 2k_d) \approx (D_{opt(DX)} + k_d)^2$ and Eqn (12.22) is approximated by

$$D_{opt(DX)} \approx (\mu_{max} - k_d)\left(1 - \sqrt{\frac{K_S}{K_S + S_0}}\right) \tag{12.23}$$

Since S_0 is usually much greater than K_S, $D_{opt(DX)}$ will approach $D = \mu_{max} - k_d$ or the washout point. Stable chemostat operation with $D \approx \mu_{max} - k_d$ is very difficult, unless the flow rate and liquid volume can be maintained exactly constant. Consequently, a value of D slightly less than $D_{opt(DX)}$ may be a good compromise between stability and biomass productivity.

Furthermore, when $k_d = 0$, Eqn (12.22) is reduced to

$$D_{opt(DX)} = \mu_{max}\left(1 - \sqrt{\frac{K_S}{K_S + S_0}}\right) \tag{12.24}$$

It should also be apparent that $D_{opt(DX)}$ for biomass formation will not necessarily be optimal for product formation. Example 12-1 illustrates the use of these equations to characterize the performances of chemostats.

Example 12-1. A new strain of yeast is being considered for biomass production. Table E12-1.1 shows data obtained from a chemostat with a sterile feed. The substrate feed concentration was 800 mg/L and an excess of oxygen was used at a pH of 5.5 and $T = 35$ °C. Determine μ_{max}, K_S, $YF_{X/S}$, k_d, and m_S, assuming $\mu_{net} = \frac{\mu_{max} S}{K_S + S} - k_d$.

TABLE E12-1.1

Dilution rate, h^{-1}	Carbon substrate concentration, mg/L	Cell concentration, mg/L
0.05	9.6	301
0.1	16.7	366
0.2	33.5	407
0.3	59.4	408
0.4	101	404
0.5	169	371
0.6	298	299
0.7	702	59

Solution. This is a case of parametric estimation as μ_{max}, K_S, $YF_{X/S}$, k_d, and m_S are all kinetic parameters needing to be determined from the experimental data set. Mass balance of the biomass inside the chemostat leads to:

$$\frac{dX}{dt} = D(X_0 - X) + (\mu_G - k_d)X \tag{E12-1.1}$$

where D is *dilution rate* and $D = Q/V$. Since the feed medium is sterile, $X_0 = 0$, and the system is at steady state ($dX/dt = 0$), then Eqn (E12-1.1) gives rise to

$$X = 0 \tag{E12-1.2}$$

or

$$D = \mu_{net} = \mu_G - k_d \tag{E12-1.3}$$

Combine with the Monod equation

$$\mu_G = \frac{\mu_{max} S}{K_S + S} \tag{E12-1.4}$$

we obtain

$$S = \frac{K_S(D + k_d)}{\mu_{max} - D - k_d} \tag{E12-1.5}$$

Thus, from the mass balance of the cells in the chemostat, we are able to relate the substrate concentration with the dilution rate with the given kinetic model (Monod equation).

We next perform a mass balance on the substrate in the chemostat:

$$Q(S_0 - S) - \frac{\mu_G X}{YF_{X/S}} V = \frac{d(VS)}{dt} \tag{E12-1.6}$$

Again at steady state, nothing would change with time,

$$X = DYF_{X/S} \frac{S_0 - S}{\mu_G} \tag{E12-1.7}$$

Substitute Eqns (E12-1.3) and (E12-1.5) into Eqn (E12-1.7), we obtain

$$X = \frac{DYF_{X/S}}{D + k_d}\left(S_0 - K_S \frac{D + k_d}{\mu_{max} - D - k_d}\right) \tag{E12-1.8}$$

Equations (E12-1.5) and (E12-1.8) define the chemostat operation. Now it is a matter of fitting the experimental data to these two equations to obtain the kinetic parameters.

TABLE E12-1.2 Parametric Estimation Results

D, h^{-1}	S, mg/L	X, mg/L	S_C calculated from Eqn (E12-1.5), g/L	X_c calculated from Eqn (E12-1.8), g/L	Error^2 or $(S - S_C)^2\,\omega^2 + (X - X_c)^2$	Error weighting factor, ω
0			3.394824	0		
0.02			5.770941	193.014		
0.05	9.6	301	9.575349	301.1293	0.077482	10
0.08			13.70043	349.0995		
0.1	16.7	366	16.64925	368.0817	4.59119	10
0.2	33.5	407	34.38288	407.2729	78.02232	10
0.3	59.4	408	59.32796	412.1521	17.75862	10
0.4	101	404	97.00599	400.4078	28.85616	1
0.5	169	371	160.5069	369.4652	74.48863	1

(Continued)

TABLE E12-1.2 Parametric Estimation Results—Cont'd

D, h^{-1}	S, mg/L	X, mg/L	S_C calculated from Eqn (E12-1.5), g/L	X_c calculated from Eqn (E12-1.8), g/L	Error² or $(S - S_C)^2 \omega^2 + (X - X_c)^2$	Error weighting factor, ω
0.55			211.9521	341.5247		
0.575			246.5724	322.1526		
0.6	298	299	290.2169	297.37	63.23377	1
0.625			346.9428	264.7917		
0.65			423.668	220.3428		
0.675			533.2326	156.4519		
0.7	702	59	702.4604	57.29264	3.12706	1
0.710082			800	−3.4E-07		
			$\sqrt{\sum(S - S_C)^2\omega^2 + (X - X_c)^2}$	= 16.43404		

The strategy here is to make the error between Eqns (E12-1.5) and (E12-1.8) and the experimental data minimum. Before we look at the error between the model prediction and the data, we should examine the potential errors in the data set. Examining the data set, we can see that the errors of S and X are not uniform. While the errors for all the data on biomass concentration X may be regarded uniform (e.g. ±1), however, the errors of S may be ±1 for $S > 100$ and ±0.1 for $S < 100$. Therefore, when we calculate the error we need to scale the errors to the same level so that the final parameters are the best estimates from the data. A scaling factor ω is thus needed to include the errors of the substrate concentrations. Table E12-1.2 shows the results. When minimizing $\sqrt{\sum(S - S_C)^2\omega^2 + (X - X_c)^2}$ by altering μ_{max}, K_S, $YF_{X/S}$, and k_d, we obtain $\mu_{max} = 0.8223\ h^{-1}$, $K_S = 88.30$ mg/L, $YF_{X/S} = 0.6129$ g-cells/g-S, $k_d = 0.0304\ h^{-1}$, and $\sqrt{\sum(S - S_C)^2\omega^2 + (X - X_c)^2} = 16.434$.

Now we are still missing the maintenance coefficient m_S. To compute the maintenance coefficient, we need to go back to definition Eqn (11.27) or

$$-r_S = \left(YF_{S/S}\,\mu_{net} + m_s\right)X \tag{E12-1.9}$$

When carrying out mass balance, we have used

$$-r_S = YF_{S/S}\,\mu_G X = \left(YF_{S/S}\,\mu_{net} + m_s\right)X \tag{E12-1.10}$$

Therefore,

$$-r_S = YF_{S/S}\,\mu_G X = \left[YF_{S/S}\left(\mu_G - k_d\right) + m_s\right]X \tag{E12-1.11}$$

That is

$$m_S = YF_{S/S}\,k_d = k_d/YF_{X/S} \tag{E12-1.12}$$

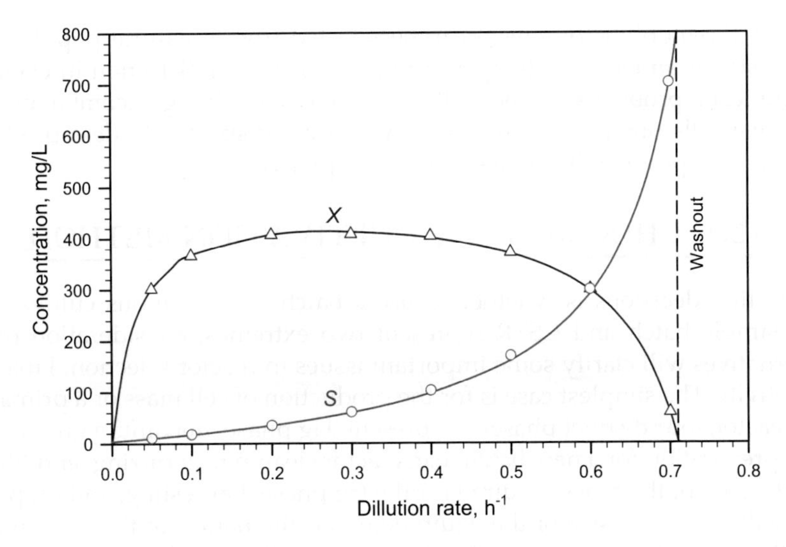

FIGURE E12-1.1 Variations of biomass and substrate concentrations with dilution rate in a chemostat.

We can then calculate the maintenance coefficient, which is given by $m_S = k_d / YF_{X/S} = 0.04967/\text{h}$.

Figure E12-1.1 shows the agreement between the data set (symbols) and the model predictions (lines). One can clearly see the match between the experimental data and the model predictions. The washout condition is shown on the right.

12.1.3. The Chemostat as a Tool

The chemostat can be used as a tool to study the mutation and selection of cultures and also to study the effect of changes in the environment on cell physiology. The molecular aspects of mutation and selection will be discussed in Chapter 14.

Natural or induced *mutations* can take place in a chemostat culture. Errors in DNA replication take place with an average frequency of about 10^{-6} to 10^{-8} genes per generation. With a cell concentration of 10^{12} cells/L in culture, the probability is high in a chemostat that a wide variety of mutant cells will be formed. The vast majority of natural mutations in a chemostat are of little significance, unless the mutation alters the function of a protein involved in growth in the chemostat environment. If the specific growth rate of the mutant is larger than that of the wild type, then the mutant outgrows the wild type in a chemostat. This selection for a variant cell type can be accomplished by creating a more favorable environment for growth of the mutant organism.

A chemostat culture can be used for the selection of special organisms. Selection or enrichment nutrient media need to be used for this purpose. For example, if it is desired to select an organism growing on ethanol, a nutrient medium containing ethanol and mineral salts is used as a feed to a chemostat culture. An organism capable of oxidizing some toxic refractory compounds can be selected from a mixed culture by slowly feeding this compound to a chemostat. A thermophilic organism can be selected from a natural population by operating a chemostat at an elevated temperature (e.g. 50–60 °C). Selection in chemostats also presents significant problems in the culture of cells containing recombinant DNA. The most productive cells often grow more slowly and are displaced by less productive cells. We will discuss this problem in more detail in Chapter 16.

12.2. CHOOSING THE CULTIVATION METHOD

One of the first decisions is whether to use a batch or continuous cultivation scheme. Although a simple batch and CSTR represent two extremes, consideration of these two extreme alternatives will clarify some important issues in reactor selection. First to consider is the productivity. The simplest case is for the production of cell mass or a primary product. For a batch reactor, four distinct phases are present: lag phase, maximum growth phase, harvesting, and preparation for a new batch (e.g. reactor cleaning, sterilizing, and filling). Let us define t_P as the sum of the times required for the lag phase, harvesting, and preparation. The value for t_P will vary with size of the equipment and the nature of the fermentation but is normally in the range of several hours (3–10 h). Thus, the total time to complete a batch cycle, t_B, assuming growth rate is not limited by nutrients,

$$t_B = \frac{1}{\mu_{net}} \ln \frac{X}{X_0} + t_P \tag{12.25}$$

where μ_{net} is the specific growth rate in maximum growth regime ($\mu_{net} = \mu_{max} - k_d$), X is the maximal attainable cell concentration and X_0 is the cell concentration at inoculation. In arriving at Eqn (12.25), we have assumed that the fermentation will not go beyond the maximum growth rate regime.

The total amount of cell mass produced comes from knowing the total amount of growth extent-limiting nutrient present and its yield factor:

$$X - X_0 = YF_{X/S} S_0 \tag{12.26}$$

The rate of cell mass production in one batch cycle (P_{XB}) is

$$P_{XB} = \frac{X - X_0}{t_B} = \frac{YF_{X/S} S_0}{\mu_{net}^{-1} \ln \frac{X}{X_0} + t_P} = \frac{YF_{X/S} S_0}{\frac{1}{\mu_{net}} \ln\left(1 + \frac{YF_{X/S} S_0}{X_0}\right) + t_P} \tag{12.27}$$

The maximum productivity of a chemostat is found by differentiating DX with respect to D and setting $\frac{d(DX)}{dD} = 0$. From Eqns (12.19) and (12.23),

$$P_{XC} = (DX)_{opt} = YF_{X/S}(\mu_{max} - k_d)\left[1 - \sqrt{\frac{K_S}{S_0 + K_S}}\right]^2 \left[\frac{S_0}{1 - \sqrt{\frac{K_S}{S_0 + K_S} + \frac{k_d}{\mu_{max} - k_d}}} - \sqrt{K_S(S_0 + K_S)}\right] \tag{12.28}$$

Under normal circumstances $S_0 >> K_S$, so the rate of chemostat biomass production, P_{XC}, is approximately

$$P_{XC} = (DX)_{opt} \approx (\mu_{max} - k_d) YF_{X/S} S_0 \tag{12.29}$$

$$\frac{P_{XC}}{P_{XB}} = \ln\frac{X}{X_0} + t_P(\mu_{max} - k_d) \tag{12.30}$$

Most commercial fermentations operate with $X/X_0 = 10$–20. Thus, we would expect continuous systems to always have a significant productivity advantage for primary products. For example, an *Escherichia coli* fermentation with $X/X_0 = 20$, $t_P = 5$ h, and $\mu_{max} - k_d = 1.0$/h would yield $P_{XC}/P_{XB} = 8$ as in the maximum growth regime, $\mu_{net} = \mu_{max} - k_d$.

Figure 12.8 shows a comparison of (a) batch and (b) continuous cultivations of *Saccharomyces cerevisiae* LBG H 1022 (ATCC 3216) in 4 m^3 air-lift reactor with a glucose-limited medium. There are noticeable differences in the growth and by-product (ethanol) formation between the two cultivation techniques. For batch cultivation (Fig. 12.8a), there is a noticeable lag phase observed (for the first 5–8 h). Both ethanol concentration and cell biomass concentration increase as glucose is consumed after the lag phase and until 16 h. After glucose is completely consumed, the cells turned to ethanol as the substrate, leading to the decrease in ethanol concentration and further increase in the cell biomass concentration. There is a noticeable *diauxic* phase between the batch cultivation time of 16 and 19 h. The secondary growth is pronounced after 19 h. For the continuous cultivation (Fig. 12.8b), the cell biomass concentration is at maximum when the dilution rate is low ($D < 0.17$/h) or at long residence times ($\tau = D^{-1} > 5.9$ h). Almost all the glucose is consumed in the reactor and there is no ethanol produced. When the dilution rate is increased beyond 0.17 h^{-1}, glucose concentration increases in the reactor. The Crabtree effect is observed and a sudden increase in the ethanol concentration in the reactor. The cell biomass concentration decreases as the dilution rate is increased. When the dilution rate is increased beyond the maximum growth rate of the yeast cells, the glucose concentration rise to its initial feed value and the cells are washed out. The productivity of the continuous cultivation is significantly higher than that of the batch cultivation. The maximum cell dry mass concentration is reached after 26 h of batch cultivation, whereas the residence time in the continuous cultivation is 5.9 h.

Based on this productivity advantage, we might be surprised to learn that most commercial bioprocesses are batch systems. Why? There are several answers. The first is that Eqn (12.30) applies only to growth-associated products. Many secondary products are not made by growing cells; growth represses product formation. Secondary metabolites are produced when cells are under stress and lacking one or more nutrients. Under such circumstances, product is made only at very low dilution rates, far below those values optimal for biomass formation. For secondary products, the productivity in a batch reactor may significantly exceed that in a simple *single* chemostat. Another primary reason for the choice of batch systems over chemostats is *genetic instability*. The biocatalyst in most bioprocesses has undergone extensive selection. These highly "bred" organisms often grow less well than the parental strain. A chemostat imposes strong selection pressure for the most rapidly growing cell. Back mutation from the productive specialized strain to one similar to the less productive parental strain (i.e. a revertant) is always present. In the chemostat, the less

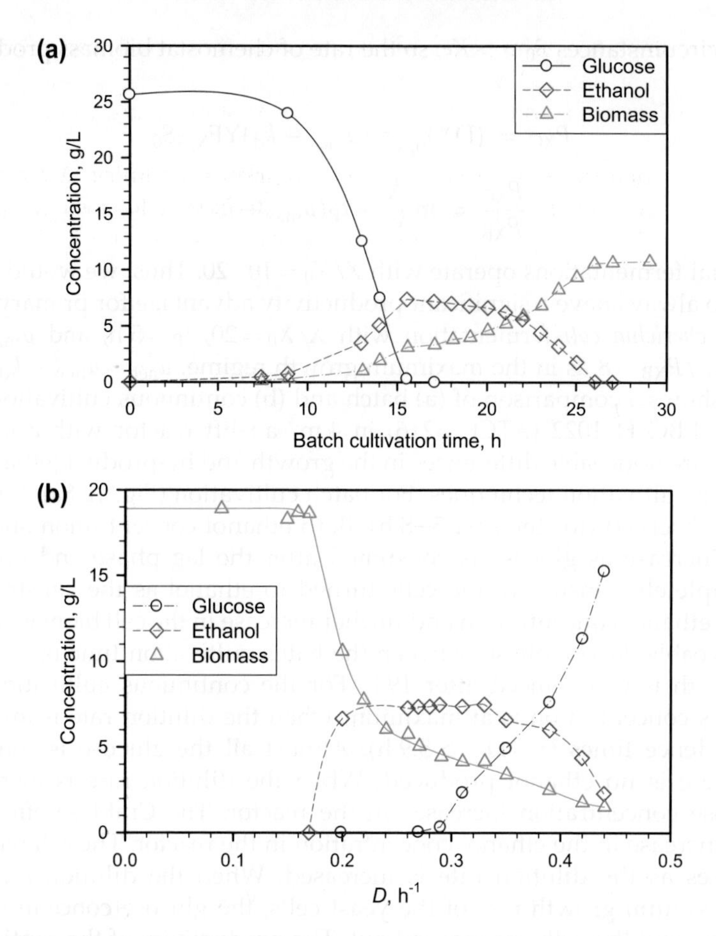

FIGURE 12.8 Variations of total cell (viable and dead) dry biomass, glucose, and ethanol concentrations during (a) batch and (b) continuous cultivations of *S. cerevisiae* LBG H 1022 (ATCC 3216) in a 4 m^3 air-lift reactor with a glucose-limited medium. The data are from "Lotz M. 1986 Untersuchungen zur Hefekultivierung auf Nebenprodkten der Stärkegewinnung in einer Pilotanglage, PhD Dissertation, University of Hannover and Lotz M., Fröhlich S., Matthes R., Schügerl K. and Seekamp M. 1991 Bakers' yeast cultivation on by-products and wastes of potato and wheat starch production on a laboratory and pilot plant scale. *Process Biochem.* 26: 301–311."

productive variant will become dominant, decreasing productivity. In the batch culture, the number of generations available is usually less than 25 (from slant cultures to a commercial-scale fermentor) for the revertant cell to outgrow the more productive strain is limited. Cells at the end of the batch are not reused (though resulting in higher cost). These considerations of genetic stability are very important for cells with recombinant DNA and are discussed in detail in Chapter 16.

Another consideration is operability and reliability. Batch cultures can suffer great variability from one run to another. Variations in product quality and concentration create problems in downstream processing and are undesirable. However, long-term continuous culture can be problematic; pumps may break, controllers may fail, and so on. Maintenance of sterility (absence of detectable foreign organisms) can be very difficult to achieve for periods of months, and the consequences of a loss of sterility are more severe than with batch culture.

One other factor determining reactor choice is market economics. A continuous system forms the basis of a dedicated processing system dedicated to a single product. Many fermentation products are required in small amounts (especially for high-value products), and demand is difficult to project. Batch systems provide much greater flexibility. The same reactor can be used for 2 months to make product A and then for the next 3 months for product B and the rest of the year for product C.

Most bioprocesses are based on batch reactors. Continuous systems are used to make single-cell protein (SCP), and modified forms of continuous culture are used in waste treatment, in ethanol production, and for some other large-volume, growth-associated products such as lactic acid. Let us consider some modifications to these reactor modes.

12.2.1. Chemostat with Recycle

Microbial conversions are autocatalytic, and the rate of conversion increases with cell concentration. To keep the cell concentration higher than the normal steady-state level in a chemostat, cells in the effluent can be recycled back to the reactor. Cell recycle increases the rate of conversion (or productivity) and also increases the stability of some systems (e.g. wastewater treatment) by minimizing the effects of process perturbation. Cells in the effluent stream are either centrifuged, filtered, or settled in a conical tank for recycling.

Consider the chemostat system with cell recycle as depicted in Fig. 12.9. A material balance on cell (biomass) concentration around the fermentor yields the following equation:

$$QX_0 + RQC_RX - (1+R)QX + V\mu_{net}X = \frac{d(VX)}{dt} \tag{12.31}$$

where R is the recycle ratio based on volumetric flow rates, C_R is the concentration factor or ratio of cell concentration in the cell recycle stream to the cell concentration in the reactor

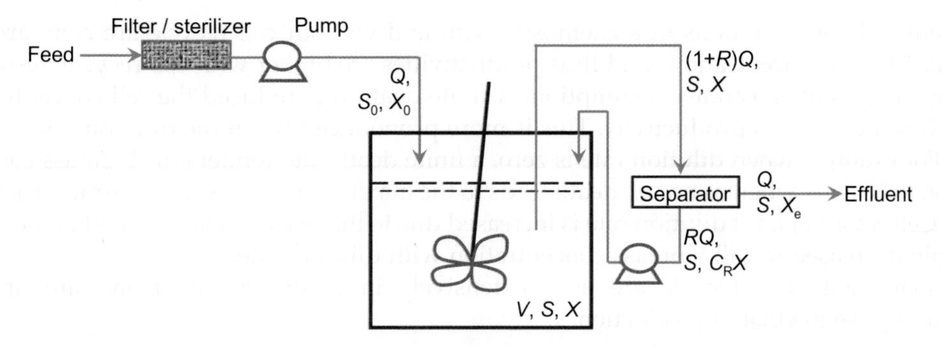

FIGURE 12.9 A schematic of a chemostat with cell recycle or sometimes called perfusion reactor. The cell separator could be a sedimentation tank, a centrifuge, a microfiltration, or a device.

effluent, Q is nutrient flow rate, V is culture volume, X_0 and X are cell concentrations in feed and recycle streams, and X_e is cell concentration in effluent from the cell separator.

At steady state and if $\frac{d(VX)}{dt} = 0$ and $X_0 = 0$ (that is, sterile feed), then Eqn (12.31) becomes

$$\mu_{net} = (1 + R - RC_R)D = [1 + R(1 - C_R)]D \tag{12.32}$$

Since $C_R > 1$ and $R(1 - C_R) < 0$, then $\mu_{net} < D$. That is, *a chemostat can be operated at dilution rates higher than the specific growth rate when cell recycle is used*.

A material balance for growth-limiting substrate around the fermentor yields

$$QS_0 + RQS - (1 + R)QS - V\frac{\mu_G X}{YF_{X/S}} = \frac{d(SV)}{dt} \tag{12.33}$$

At steady state, $\frac{d(VS)}{dt} = 0$ and

$$X = \frac{D}{\mu_G} YF_{X/S}(S_0 - S) \tag{12.34}$$

Substitution of growth rate into Eqn (12.34) yields

$$X = YF_{X/S} \frac{S_0 - S}{1 + R(1 - C_R) + k_d/D} \tag{12.35}$$

Therefore, the steady-state cell concentration in a chemostat is increased by a factor of $\frac{1}{1 + R(1 - C_R) + k_d/D}$ by cell recycle. The substrate concentration in the effluent is determined from Eqn (12.35) and the Monod Eqn (6.30) and is

$$S = \frac{K_S[(1 + R - RC_R)D + k_d]}{\mu_{max} - [(1 + R - RC_R)D + k_d]} \tag{12.36}$$

Then Eqn (12.35) becomes

$$X = \frac{YF_{X/S}}{1 + R(1 - C_R) + k_d/D}\left[S_0 - K_S \frac{(1 + R - RC_R)D + k_d}{\mu_{max} - (1 + R - RC_R)D - k_d}\right] \tag{12.37}$$

Effluent cell concentrations in a chemostat with and without cell recycle are compared in Fig. 12.10. Cell concentrations and thus productivities are higher with cell recycle, resulting in higher rates of substrate consumption. A finite death rate reduced the cell concentration and thus the biomass productivity. This is more pronounced when the dilution rate is very low. For example when dilution rate is zero, a finite death rate renders the biomass concentration to be zero, whereas no cell death leads to the maximum biomass concentration achievable. Cell washout limit dilution rate is increased due to the recycle. The washout is shown as sharply decreased in cell biomass concentration with dilution rate.

Systems with cell recycle are used extensively in waste treatment and are finding increasing use in ethanol production.

Example 12-2. In a chemostat with cell recycle, as shown in Fig. 12.2, the feed flow rate and culture volumes are $Q = 1$ mL/min and $V = 1000$ mL, respectively. The system is operated

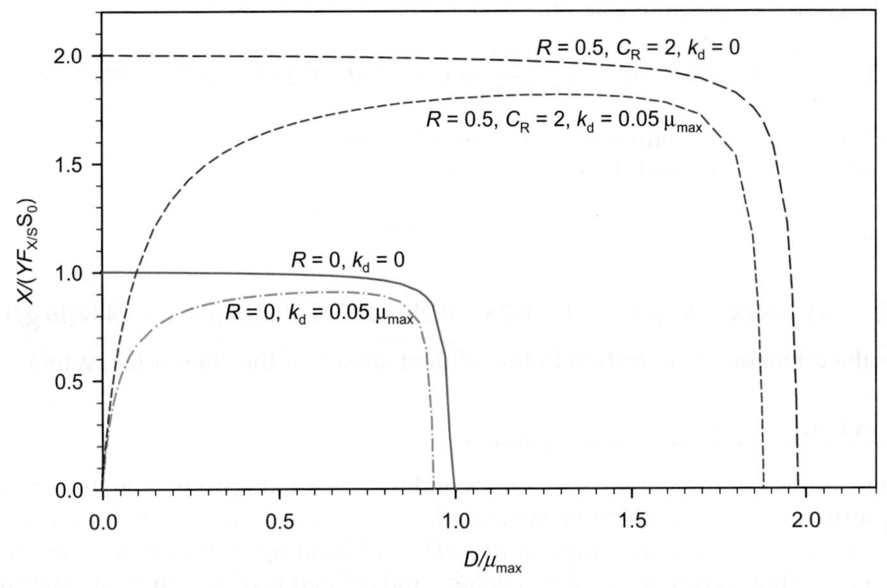

FIGURE 12.10 Comparison of biomass concentrations in steady states of chemostat cultures with and without recycle. The saturation parameter is $K_S = 0.01\,S_0$.

under glucose limitation, and the yield factor, $YF_{X/S}$, is 0.5 g-cells/g-substrate. Glucose concentration in the feed is $S_0 = 50$ g glucose/L. The kinetic constants of the organisms are $\mu_{max} = 0.2\ h^{-1}$, $K_S = 1$ g glucose/L. The value of C_R is 2.5, and the recycle ratio is $R = 0.25$. The system is at steady state.

(a) Find the substrate concentration in the recycle stream (S).
(b) Find the specific growth rate (μ_{net}) of the organisms.
(c) Find the cell (biomass) concentration in the recycle stream.
(d) Find the cell concentration in the centrifuge effluent (X_e).

Solution. In this solution, we will use the derivations already shown in the proceeding section. For students, you are expected to follow the steps from the beginning with mass balances. Using Eqn (12.32), we determine μ_{net}.

$$\mu_{net} = (1 + R - RC_R)D = (1 + 0.25 - 0.25 \times 2.5) \times 1/1000\ \text{min}^{-1} = 0.000625\ \text{min}^{-1}$$
$$= 0.0375\ \text{h}^{-1}$$

Since the endogenous maintenance is negligible, we have

$$\mu_{net} = \mu_G = \frac{\mu_{max} S}{K_S + S}$$

which can be rearranged to give

$$S = \frac{K_S \mu_{net}}{\mu_{max} - \mu_{net}} = \frac{1 \times 0.0375}{0.2 - 0.0375}\ \text{g/L} = 0.23077\text{g/L}$$

Mass balance of the substrate leads to

$$X = \frac{D}{\mu_G} YF_{X/S}(S_0 - S) = \frac{1/1000}{0.000625} \times 0.5 \times (50 - 0.23077)\ \text{g/L} = 39.815\ \text{g/L}$$

which is the biomass concentration in the recycle stream.

A biomass balance around the separator yields

$$(1 + R)QX = RC_RQX + QX_e$$

Thus,

$$X_e = (1 + R)X - RC_RX = (1 + 0.25 - 0.25 \times 2.5) \times 39.815\ \text{g/L} = 24.8846\ \text{g/L}$$

which is the biomass concentration in the effluent stream of the chemostat system.

12.2.2. Multistage Chemostat Systems

In some fermentations, particularly for secondary metabolite production, the growth and product formation steps need to be separated, since optimal conditions for each step are different. Conditions such as temperature, pH, and limiting nutrients may be varied in each stage, resulting in different cell physiology and cellular products in multistage systems.

An example of a multistage system that may be beneficial is in the culture of genetically engineered cells. To improve genetic stability, a plasmid-carrying recombinant DNA usually uses an inducible promoter to control production of the target protein (see Chapter 14). In the induced state, the plasmid-containing cell grows at nearly the same rate as the cell that loses the plasmid (a revertant), so the plasmid-free cell holds little growth advantage over the plasmid-containing cell. However, if the inducer is added, the plasmid-containing cells will make large quantities of the desired protein product but will have greatly reduced growth rates. Thus, a single-stage chemostat would not be suitable for the production of the target protein because of resulting problems in genetic stability.

A multistage system can circumvent this problem. In the first stage, no inducer is added and the plasmid-containing cell can be maintained easily (usually an antibiotic is added to kill plasmid-free cells; see Chapter 14 for a more complete discussion). In the second stage, the inducer is added and large quantities of product are made. Cells defective in product synthesis should not overtake the culture (at least not completely), because fresh genetically unaltered cells are being continuously fed to the reactor. Thus, the two-stage system can allow the stable continuous production of the target protein when it would be impossible in a simple chemostat.

Perhaps an easier situation to consider is the production of a secondary product (e.g. ethanol or an antibiotic). Here, we worry not so much about a mixture of subpopulations, but that conditions that promote growth completely repress product formation. A very large-scale multistage system for ethanol production is currently in use. A multistage system of CSTR approaches PFR behavior. A PFR mimics the batch system, where space time (the time it takes the culture fluid to reach a specific location in the PFR) replaces culture time. A multistage system is much like taking the batch growth curve and dividing it into sections, with each section being "frozen" in a corresponding stage of the multistage system. As in the batch reactor, the culture's physiological state progresses from one stage to the next.

The mathematical analysis of the multistage system that we present here is imperfect. Growth in the second and subsequent stages is intrinsically unbalanced growth, even though it is steady-state growth. New cells entering the second or subsequent stage are continuously adapting to the new conditions in that stage. Consequently, unstructured models are not expected to give completely accurate predictions. However, we use unstructured models here due to their simplicity and to illustrate at least some aspects of multistage systems.

A two-stage chemostat system is depicted in Fig. 12.11. Biomass and substrate balances on the first stage yield the following equations (ignoring endogeneous metabolism):

$$S_1 = \frac{K_S(D_1 + k_d)}{\mu_{max} - D_1 - k_d} \tag{12.38}$$

$$X_1 = \frac{YF_{X/S}}{1 + k_d/D_1}\left[S_0 - K_S\frac{D_1 + k_d}{\mu_{max} - D_1 - k_d}\right] \tag{12.39}$$

The biomass balance for the second stage yields

$$QX_1 - Q_2X_2 + V_2\mu_{net2}X_2 = \frac{d(V_2X_2)}{dt} \tag{12.40}$$

At steady state, Eqn (12.40) becomes

$$\frac{Q}{Q_2}D_2X_1 - D_2X_2 + \mu_{net2}X_2 = 0 \tag{12.41}$$

which can be rearranged to yield

$$X_2 = \frac{Q}{Q_2}\frac{D_2X_1}{D_2 - \mu_{net2}} = \frac{Q}{Q_2}\frac{D_2X_1}{D_2 - \mu_{G2} + k_d} \tag{12.42}$$

The substrate balance for the limiting substrate in the second stage is

$$QS_1 + (Q_2 - Q)S_{02} - Q_2S_2 - V_2\frac{\mu_{G2}X_2}{YF_{X/S}} = \frac{d(S_2V_2)}{dt} \tag{12.43}$$

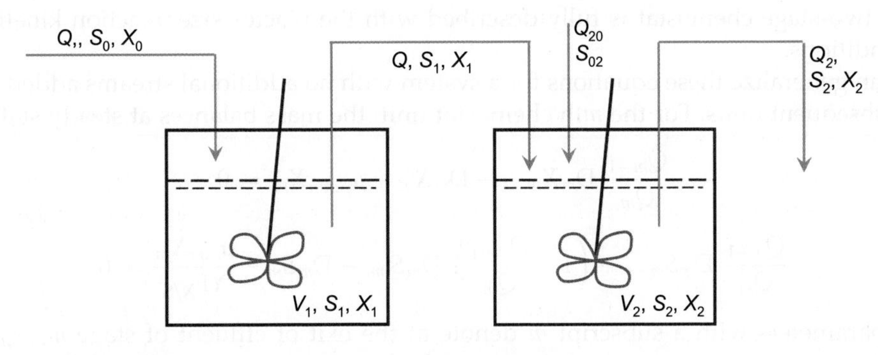

FIGURE 12.11 A schematic of a two-stage chemostat system.

At steady state,

$$\frac{Q}{Q_2}D_2S_1 + \left(1 - \frac{Q}{Q_2}\right)D_2S_{02} - D_2S_2 - \frac{\mu_{G2}X_2}{YF_{X/S}} = 0 \tag{12.44}$$

where

$$\mu_{G2} = \frac{\mu_{max}S_2}{K_S + S_2} = \mu_{net2} + k_d \tag{12.45}$$

Substitute Eqn (12.42) into Eqn (12.44) and rearrange, one can obtain

$$\mu_{G2} = \frac{\frac{Q}{Q_2}D_2S_1 + \left(1 - \frac{Q}{Q_2}\right)D_2S_{02} - D_2S_2}{\frac{Q}{Q_2}\frac{D_2X_1}{YF_{X/S}} + \frac{Q}{Q_2}D_2S_1 + \left(1 - \frac{Q}{Q_2}\right)D_2S_{02} - D_2S_2}(D_2 + k_d) = 0 \tag{12.46}$$

Combining Eqns (12.46) and (12.45) and solving for S_2,

$$S_2 = \frac{b - \sqrt{b^2 - 4D_2(\mu_{max} - D_2 - k_d)(D_2 + k_d)\left[\frac{Q}{Q_2}D_2S_1 + \left(1 - \frac{Q}{Q_2}\right)D_2S_{02}\right]}}{2D_2(\mu_{max} - D_2 - k_d)} \tag{12.47}$$

where

$$b = (D_2 + k_d)D_2K_S + \mu_{max}\frac{Q}{Q_2}\frac{D_2S_1}{YF_{X/S}} + (\mu_{max} - D_2 - k_d)\left[\left(1 - \frac{Q}{Q_2}\right)D_2S_{02} + \frac{Q}{Q_2}D_2S_1\right] \tag{12.48}$$

Substituting Eqn (12.46) into (12.42), one obtain

$$X_2 = YF_{X/S}\frac{\frac{Q}{Q_2}\frac{D_2X_1}{YF_{X/S}} + \frac{Q}{Q_2}D_2S_1 + \left(1 - \frac{Q}{Q_2}\right)D_2S_{02} - D_2S_2}{D_2 + k_d} \tag{12.49}$$

Thus, a two-stage chemostat is fully described with the reactor size, reaction kinetics, and feed conditions.

We can generalize these equations for a system with no additional streams added or with more subsequent units. For the mth chemostat unit, the mass balances at steady state yield:

$$\frac{Q_{m-1}}{Q_m}D_mX_{m-1} - D_mX_m + \mu_{netm}X_m = 0 \tag{12.50}$$

$$\frac{Q_{m-1}}{Q_m}D_mS_{m-1} + \left(1 - \frac{Q_{m-1}}{Q_m}\right)D_mS_{0m} - D_mS_m - \frac{\mu_{Gm}X_m}{YF_{X/S}} = 0 \tag{12.51}$$

where parameters with a subscript m denote at the exit of effluent of stage m, S_{0m} is the substrate concentration in the fresh (or extra) feed stream to stage m. The difference of the effluent volumetric flow rates: $Q_m - Q_{m-1}$ is the volumetric fresh feed rate to stage m. The specific growth rates:

$$\mu_{Gm} = \frac{\mu_{max} S_m}{K_S + S_m} = \mu_{netm} + k_d \tag{12.52}$$

The substrate and biomass concentrations can be solved one stage after another.

$$S_m = \frac{b_m - \sqrt{b_m^2 - 4D_m(\mu_{max} - D_m - k_d)(D_m + k_d)\left[\frac{Q_{m-1}}{Q_m} D_m S_{m-1} + \left(1 - \frac{Q_{m-1}}{Q_m}\right) D_m S_{0m}\right]}}{2D_m(\mu_{max} - D_m - k_d)} \tag{12.53}$$

where

$$b_m = (D_m + k_d) D_m K_S + \mu_{max} \frac{Q_{m-1}}{Q_m} \frac{D_m S_{m-1}}{Y F_{X/S}} + (\mu_{max} - D_m - k_d) \times \left[\left(1 - \frac{Q_{m-1}}{Q_m}\right) D_m S_{0m} + \frac{Q_{m-1}}{Q_m} D_m S_{m-1}\right] \tag{12.54}$$

Substituting Eqn (12.52) into Eqn (12.50), one obtain

$$X_m = Y F_{X/S} \frac{\frac{Q_{m-1}}{Q_m} \frac{D_m X_{m-1}}{Y F_{X/S}} + \frac{Q_{m-1}}{Q_m} D_m S_{m-1} + \left(1 - \frac{Q_{m-1}}{Q_m}\right) D_m S_{0m} - D_m S_m}{D_m + k_d} \tag{12.55}$$

Example 12-3. Data for the production of a secondary metabolite from a small-scale batch reactor are shown in Fig. E12-3.1. There is a stream of substrate available at 120 L/h of the same medium as that generating the batch fermentation data. Assume that two reactors, each with 800-L working volume, are available. You will use exactly the same culture conditions (medium, pH, temperature, and so on) as in the batch reactor.

(a) Determine the outlet concentration of the product.

(b) Compare that obtained in part (a) to the value predicted if a single 1600-L reactor was used.

Solution. This is a chemostat problem. Mass balance for biomass over the ith chemostat at steady state yields:

$$QX_{i-1} - Q\,Xi + r_{Xi} V_i = 0 \tag{E12-3.1}$$

Dividing through by V_i, we obtain

$$r_{Xi} = D_i(X_i - X_{i-1}) \tag{E12-3.2}$$

where r_{Xi} is the rate of biomass production inside the ith chemostat and X_i is the biomass concentration in the effluent stream of the ith chemostat, which is the same as that inside the ith chemostat. Therefore, to solve the chemostat problem, we will need the rate of biomass production.

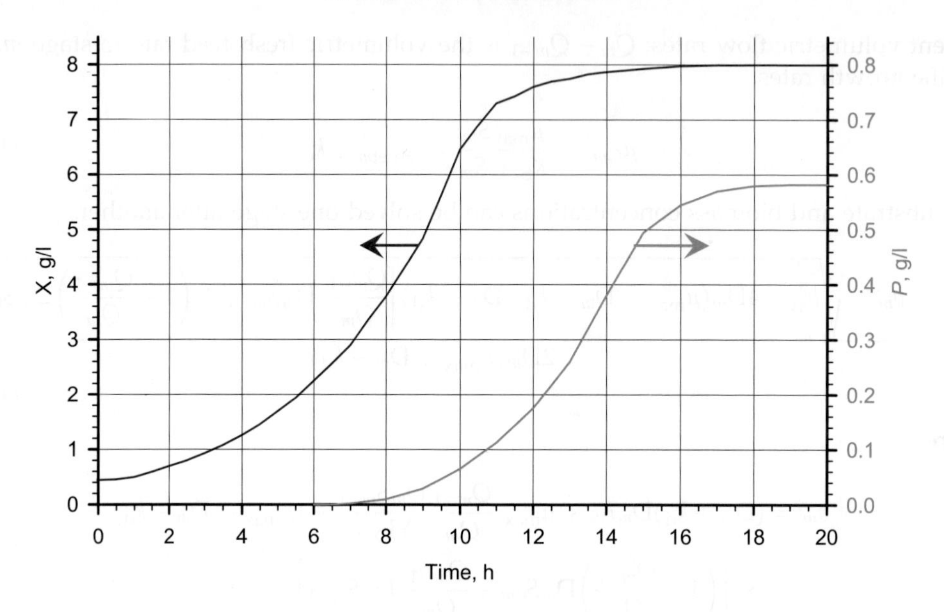

FIGURE E12-3.1 Biomass concentration and the concentration of a secondary metabolite in a batch culture.

Mass balance of the secondary metabolite P over the ith chemostat at steady state gives:

$$Q\,P_{i-1} - Q\,P_i + r_{Pi}V_i = 0 \tag{E12-3.3}$$

Dividing through by V_i, we obtain

$$r_{Pi} = D_i(P_i - P_{i-1}) \tag{E12-3.4}$$

Eqns (E12-3.4) and (E12-3.2) are similar, in that the rate of formation of the secondary metabolite is a straight line on the rate vs concentration plane passing through the feed point ($P = P_{i-1}$, $r_P = 0$) with a slope of D_i, intercepts with the fermentation rate curve at ($P = P_i$, $r_P = r_{Pi}$). Therefore, if the rate functions are known, one can solve the problem easily (as we have been doing). Alternatively, we can solve the problem graphically based on the property as mentioned.

Therefore, to solve the problem, we must produce the rate curves. For the batch data, there were minimum measurements available: only the concentrations of biomass and product change with time. Fortunately, this is enough to produce the rate curves. In batch operations, mass balance yields

$$r_j = \frac{dC_j}{dt} \tag{E12-3.5}$$

Thus, the rate of production can be obtained by differentiating the concentration curve (either measure the slopes of tangential lines or via central difference). These curves are shown in Figs E12-3.2 and E12-3.3. The quality or smoothness of the curves in Figs E12-3.2 and E12-3.3 is noticeably poor, which is due to the differentiation of data. The error in the data is magnified and distorted because of the differentiation (see Chapter 7).

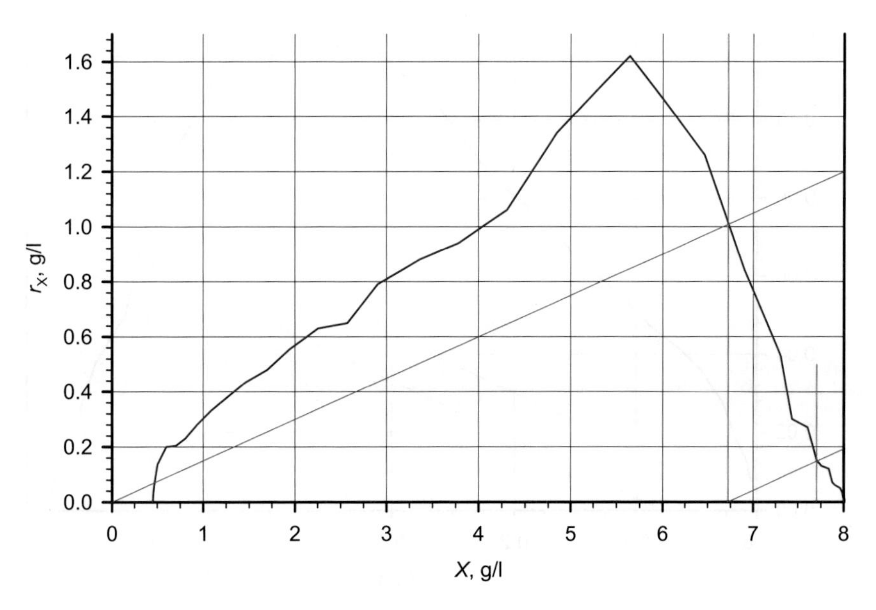

FIGURE E12-3.2 Rate of production of biomass based on the batch fermentation data.

(a) Two chemostats of equal volume in series. $D_1 = D_2 = 120/800\ h^{-1} = 0.15\ h^{-1}$.
Figure E12-3.2 shows the solutions of biomass. We overlay the mass balance, Eqn (E12-3.2) on top of the rate curve obtained from Fig. E12-3.1. In the feed to the first reactor, the medium is sterile ($X_0 = 0$). The two lines all have slopes of 0.15/h. The intercepts occur at the biomass concentration of $X_1 = 6.72$ g/L and $X_2 = 7.70$ g/L. We ignored the one of the two intercepts for the first reactor, $X_1 = 0.45$ g/L. The reason is that this is the starting condition for the batch data where lag phase present. In chemostat operation, this point is easily avoided by stating the withdrawing of culture after the biomass growth established.

We next compute the concentration of the secondary metabolite. At this point, one may use the values of biomass concentration obtained already and read off corresponding values of secondary metabolite concentration from Fig. E12-3.1 since the medium is identical. If we did that, we obtain $P_1 = 0.079$ g/L and $P_2 = 0.23$ g/L. We know that the feed to the first reactor $P_0 = 0$. Clearly, these three values of P do not satisfy Eqn (E12-3.4) and the secondary metabolite rate data in Fig. E12-3.3. If we use the rate data in Fig. E12-3.3 and Eqn (E12-3.4), we would get a different set of values of P. Which one is correct?

The batch data did not give the substrate concentration nor we know the stoichiometry. This is a drawback. We know that for the secondary metabolite to be produced, there must be 1) large quantity of cell biomass and 2) one of more of the key growth-required substrate concentration is low. Therefore, the first reactor is not really producing secondary metabolite as the substrates are all in excess and there is no cell biomass in the feed. Therefore, the value of P_1 is correct as it reads off from Fig. E12-3.1. However, the rate of formation of secondary metabolite does agree with that of the intercept of Eqn (E12-3.4) and the curve in Fig. E12-3.3.

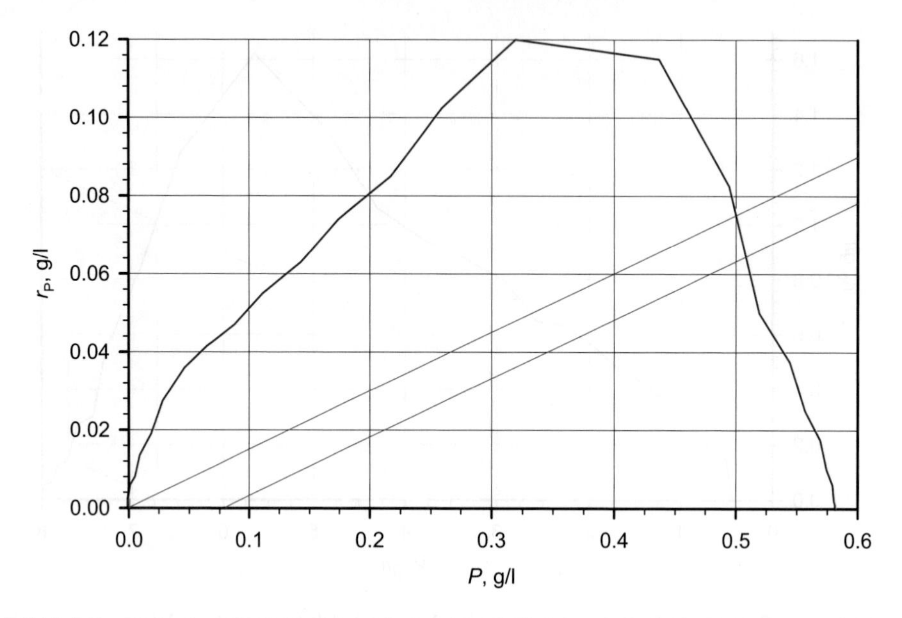

FIGURE E12-3.3 Rate of production of secondary metabolite based on the batch fermentation data.

For the second reactor, there is high cell biomass already in the feed, and the key substrate for cell growth is limiting. Therefore, growth in the second reactor is suppressed, while secondary metabolite production is amplified. Therefore, we use Eqn (E12-3.4) and Fig. E12-3.3 to find the concentration for the secondary metabolite coming out of the second reactor. Figure E12-3.3 shows that the line passing through ($P = P_1 = 0.079$ g/L, $r_P = 0$) with slope of $D_2 = 0.15$/h intercepts secondary metabolite generation curve at $P_2 = 0.505$ g/L. Figure E12-3.4 shows a schematic of the overall procedure we have used to determine P_2. The production rate of the secondary metabolite is then $Q\,P_2 = 51.6$ g/h.

(b) Based on the discussions in part (a), a single chemostat would produce biomass rather than secondary metabolite. Therefore, Fig. E12-3.2 can be employed to determine the biomass concentration, and then use Fig. E12-3.1 to determine the secondary metabolite concentration. $D = 120/1600$/h $= 0.075$/h. We overlay the mass balance, Eqn (E12-3.2) on top of the rate curve obtained from Fig. E12-3.1. In the feed to the first reactor, the medium is sterile ($X_0 = 0$). There two intercepts and only one is used $X = X_1 = 7.29$ g/L. The corresponding $P = 0.115$ g/L. The production rate of the secondary metabolite is then $Q\,P_2 = 13.8$ g/h.

Therefore, two stages of chemostats increase the secondary metabolite concentration from 0.115 g/L to 0.505 g/L or the secondary metabolite production from 13.8 g/h to 51.6 g/h.

Example 12-4. In Example 12-3, the solution to the chemostat problem was solved by differentiating the batch fermentation data. As one can observe from Figs E12-3.2 and E12-3.3 that the rate obtained contain higher error and it gives one less confidence on the

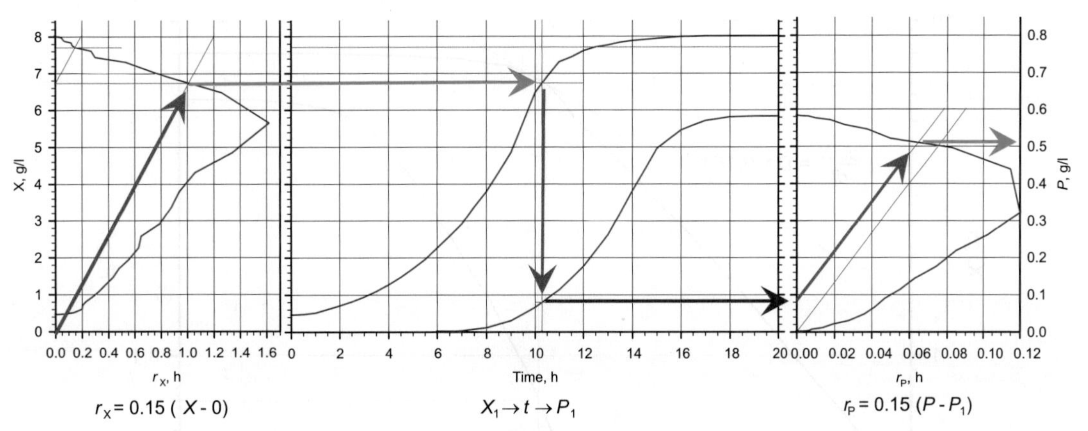

FIGURE E12-3.4 A schematic of graphical solution procedure for secondary metabolite in two chemostats in series.

solution. Use an alternative graphical solution to solve the chemostat problem of Example E12-3 without differentiating the batch fermentation data.

Solution. One can either find the rate model (via methods in Chapter 7) or re-evaluate the mass balance equations to find alternative format of plots. The mass balance Eqns (E12-3.2) and (E12-3.4) can be written as

$$\frac{r_j}{C_j - C_{jF}} = D \tag{E12-4.1}$$

where C_{jF} is the concentration of species j in the feed stream. Since the rates of reaction are not known, we need to find a way to circumvent the rate requirement.

For the batch data, the concentration change with time is measured. Therefore, one can obtain the rate through

$$r_j = \frac{dC_j}{dt} \tag{E12-3.5}$$

From Eqn (E12-4.1), we need the rate divided by the concentration difference. Rather than finding the rates and then do the conversion, we divide Eqn (E12-3.5) also by the concentration difference,

$$\frac{r_j}{C_j - C_{jF}} = \frac{1}{C_j - C_{jF}}\frac{dC_j}{dt} = \frac{d\ln(C_j - C_{jF})}{dt} \tag{E12-4.2}$$

Therefore, the left hand side of Eqn (E12-4.1) is the same as the slope of the tangent on the batch experimental data having a value of $C_j - C_{jF}$ if the batch data were plotted on a semilog paper of $C_j - C_{jF}$ vs t. Thus, we can avoid determining the rates from the batch data. This has been illustrated in § 5.11.

Figure E12-4.1 shows the semilog plots for the cell concentration and secondary metabolite concentration change with time from the batch data (replotted from Fig. E12-3.1). Since the

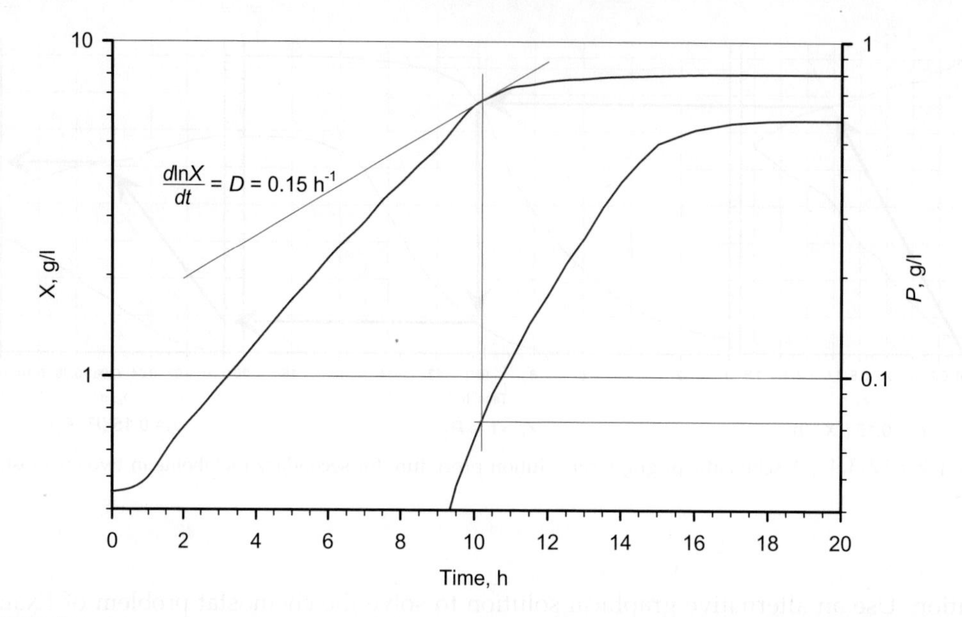

FIGURE E12-4.1 A semilog plot of biomass concentration and the concentration of a secondary metabolite in a batch culture. Chemostat culture can be determined by the tangential line (tangent) with its slope equal to the dilution rate.

feed to the first chemostat is sterile, therefore, we can determine the outlet concentration directly from this graph by plotting a line with a slope of 0.15/h/ln10 that is tangent to the batch growth data (for concentration higher than the initial culture). From this graph, we can read off the effluent conditions as $X_1 = 6.66$ g/L and $P_1 = 0.73$ g/L (at the tangent point).

To determine the secondary metabolite concentration in the second chemostat, we replot the batch for $P - P_1$ on a semilog plot as shown in Fig. E12-4.2. One can follow the same procedure to plot the tangent. We obtain from the tangent point at which $P_2 = P_1 + (P_2 - P_1) = 0.073 + 0.435$ g/L $= 0.508$ g/L.

Looking back at Examples 12-3 and 12-4, we learned that a continuous culture problem can be solved based on batch data without elaborate data processing. By examining the mass balance equations, one can devise simple procedures for solving continuous culture problems without obtaining the growth or reaction rates explicitly. Avoid differentiation of data also leads to quality solution. In fact, the solution in Example 12-4 seemed to be simpler than that in Example 12-3, for the exact same problem.

12.3. WASTEWATER TREATMENT PROCESS

Waste materials generated in a society can be classified in three major categories:

(1) Industrial wastes are produced by various industries, and waste characteristics vary greatly from one industry to another. Industrial wastes usually contain hydrocarbons,

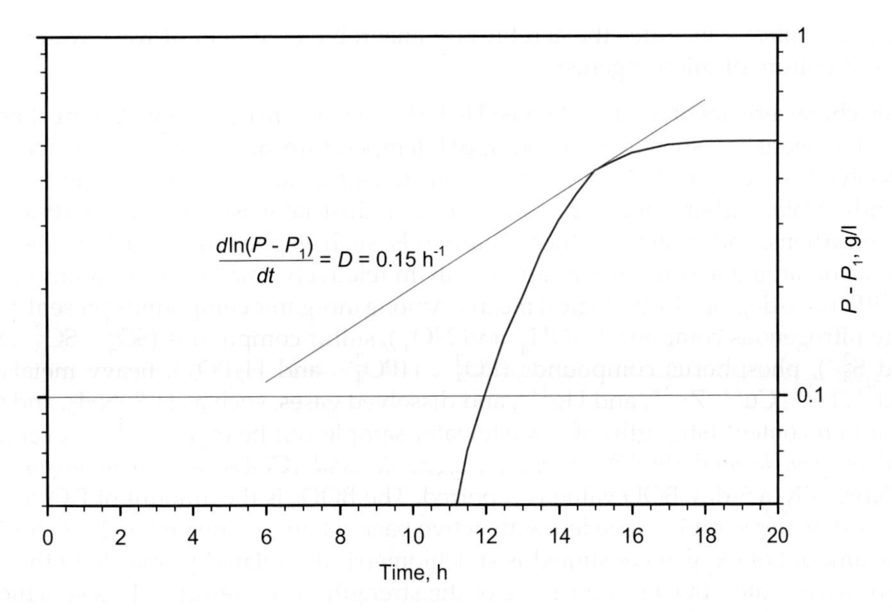

FIGURE E12-4.2 A semilog plot of the concentration difference of a secondary metabolite (to the feed concentration) in a batch culture. Chemostat culture can be determined by the tangent with its slope equal to the dilution rate.

carbohydrates, alcohols, lipids, and aromatic organics. Industrial wastes are rich in carbon compounds and usually deficient in nitrogen (high C/N ratio); therefore, the biological treatment of industrial wastes usually requires supplemental addition of nitrogen compounds and other nutrients. The presence of potentially toxic compounds must be carefully considered in devising a treatment strategy.

(2) Domestic wastes are treated by municipalities and derived from humans and their daily activities. They include ground garbage, laundry water, excrement, and often some industrial wastes that have been sewered into the municipal system. Domestic waste varies significantly with time in terms of flow and composition due to the periodic nature of human activity (e.g. flow decreases at night when most people sleep).

(3) Agricultural wastes are produced by farm animals (e.g. manure) and include waste plants, such as straws. Agricultural wastes are usually carbon rich because of high-cellulosic material content, although some wastes, such as poultry manure, are high in nitrogen.

Each of these waste materials has its own characteristics and treatment methods vary depending on these characteristics.

Three major waste treatment methods are:

(1) *Physical treatment* includes screening, flocculation, sedimentation, filtration, and flotation, which are usually used for the removal of insoluble materials.

(2) *Chemical treatment* includes chemical oxidations (chlorination, ozonation) and chemical precipitation using $CaCl_2$, $FeCl_3$, $Ca(OH)_2$, or $Al_2(SO_4)_3$.

(3) *Biological treatment* includes the aerobic and anaerobic treatment of wastewater by a mixed culture of microorganisms.

Certain characteristics of wastewater need to be known before treatment. Among them are 1) physical characteristics, such as color, odor, pH, temperature, and solid contents (suspended and dissolved solids) and 2) chemical characteristics, such as organic and inorganic compounds. Major carbon compounds in a typical industrial waste are carbohydrates, lipids oils, hydrocarbons, and proteins. Other compounds, such as phenols, surfactants, herbicides, pesticides, and aromatic compounds, are usually in relatively small concentrations ($\ll 1$ g/L) but are difficult to degrade by biological means. Among inorganic compounds present in wastewater are nitrogenous compounds (NH_4^+ and NO_3^-), sulfur compounds (SO_4^{2-}, SO_3^{2-}, S^0, S^{2-}, S_2^{2-}, and S_3^{2-}), phosphorus compounds (PO_4^{3-}, HPO_4^{2-}, and $H_2PO_4^-$), heavy metals (Ni^{2+}, Pb^{2+}, Cd^{2+}, Fe^{2+}, Cu^{2+}, Zn^{2+}, and Hg^{2+}), and dissolved gases, such as H_2S, NH_3, and CH_4.

The carbon content (strength) of a wastewater sample can be expressed in several ways: *biological oxygen demand* (BOD), *chemical oxygen demand* (COD), and *total organic carbon* (TOC). Normally, a 5-day BOD value is reported. The BOD_5 is the amount of DO consumed when a wastewater sample is seeded with active bacteria and incubated at 20 °C for 5 days. Since the amount of oxygen consumed is stoichiometrically related primarily to the organic content of wastewater, BOD is a measure of the strength of wastewater. This stoichiometric coefficient is not always known, since the composition of the organics is usually unknown. Also, some nitrogen-containing or inorganic compounds will exert an oxygen demand. If the only organic compound is glucose, oxygen consumption can be easily related to the carbon content of wastewater under aerobic conditions.

$$C_6H_{12}O_6 + 6\,O_2 \longrightarrow 6\,CO_2 + 6\,H_2O \tag{12.56}$$

According to the stoichiometry of this reaction 1.07 g of oxygen is required for the oxidation of 1 g of glucose.

Samples of wastewater need to be properly diluted to obtain an accurate BOD_5 measurement, seeded with active bacteria and incubated at 20 °C for 5 days along with an unseeded blank. BOD_5 is calculated using the following equation:

$$BOD_5 = [(DO)_{t=0} - (DO)_{t=5\,day}]_{sample} - [(DO)_{t=0} - (DO)_{t=5\,day}]_{blank} \tag{12.57}$$

BOD measurements have some shortcomings. This method is applicable only to biodegradable, soluble organics and requires a high concentration of active bacteria preadapted to this type of waste. Moreover, if organic compounds are refractory, 5 days of incubation may not suffice, and 20 days of incubation (BOD_{20}) may be required.

COD is a measure of the concentration of chemically oxidizable organic compounds present in wastewater. Organic compounds are oxidized by a strong chemical oxidant, and using the reaction stoichiometry, the organic content is calculated. Almost all organic compounds present in wastewater are oxidized by certain strong chemical oxidants. Therefore, the COD content of a wastewater sample usually exceeds the measured BOD ($COD > BOD_5$).

A typical chemical oxidation reaction is

$$3\,CH_2O + 16\,H^+ + 2\,Cr_2O_7^{2-} \xrightarrow{heat} 4\,Cr^{3+} + 3\,CO_2 + 11\,H_2O \tag{12.58}$$

Dichromate may be used as an oxidizing agent, and by a redox balance, the amount of oxygen required to oxidize organic compounds can be calculated. This method is faster (order of 3 h), easier, and less expensive than BOD measurements.

The TOC content of wastewater samples can be determined by using a TOC analyzer. After proper dilutions, samples are injected into a high-temperature (680–1,350 °C) furnace and all organic carbon compounds are oxidized to CO_2, which is measured by an infrared analyzer. To determine the TOC content, wastewater samples should be acidified to remove inorganic carbon compounds (mainly carbonates). The total carbon content of wastewater can be determined before and after acidification, and the difference is inorganic carbon content.

The nitrogen content of wastewater samples is usually measured by total Kjeldahl nitrogen determination. Other key nutrient concentrations, such as phosphate, sulfur, and toxic compounds, should be determined before waste streams are treated.

The concentration of biomass in a waste treatment system using suspended cells is measured as combustible solids at 600 °C (CS600) or some referred to as the mixed-liquor volatile suspended solids (MLVSS). Basically wastewater of known volume is filtered and the collected solids dried and weighed to give mixed-liquor suspended solids. This material is then "volatilized" by burning in air at 600 °C. The weight of the remaining noncombustible inorganic material is the "fixed" solids. The difference between the original mass prior to combustion and the fixed solids is the combustible or "volatile" portion at 600 °C. The CS600 or MLVSS is assumed to be primarily microbes, although carbonaceous particles are included in the measurement. A typical waste treatment operation employing biological treatment includes the following steps:

(1) Primary treatment includes the removal of coarse solids and suspended matter (screening, sedimentation, and filtration) and conditioning of the wastewater stream by pH adjustment and nutrient additions (e.g. PO_4^{3-} and NH_4^+).
(2) Secondary treatment is the major step in biological treatment; it includes biological oxidation or anaerobic treatment of soluble and insoluble organic compounds. Organic compounds are oxidized to CO_2 and H_2O by organisms under aerobic conditions. Unoxidized organic compounds and solids from aerobic treatment (e.g. cell wall material, lipids—fats) are decomposed to a mixture of CH_4, CO_2, and H_2S under anaerobic conditions. A *sludge* of undecomposed material must be purged from either system.
(3) Tertiary treatment includes the removal of the remaining inorganic compounds (phosphate, sulfate, and ammonium) and other refractory organic compounds by one or more physical separation methods, such as carbon adsorption, deep-bed filtration, and in some cases membrane-based techniques, such as reverse osmosis or electrodialysis.

Biological wastewater treatment usually employs a mixed culture of organisms whose makeup varies with the nature of the waste. Biological treatment may be aerobic or anaerobic. The major aerobic processes (or reactor types) used in wastewater treatment are 1) activated sludge, 2) trickling filter, 3) rotating biological contractors, and 4) oxidation ponds.

A schematic of a typical wastewater treatment flow sheet is shown in Fig. 12.12. *Activated sludge* processes include a well-agitated and aerated continuous-flow reactor and a settling tank. Depending on the physical design of the tank and how feed is introduced into the tank, it may approximate either a PFR or CSTR. A long narrow tank with single feed

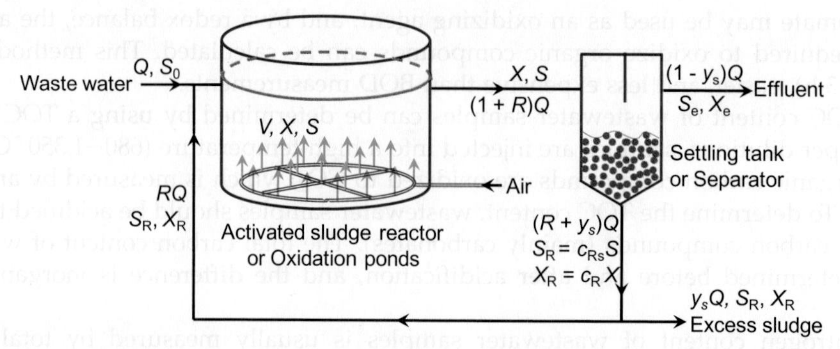

FIGURE 12.12 Schematic diagram of a typical wastewater processing unit.

approaches PFR behavior: circular tanks approach CSTR. The concentrated cells from the settling tank are recycled back to the stirred-tank reactor. Usually, a mixed culture of organisms is utilized in the bioreactor. Some of these organisms may produce polymeric materials (polysaccharides), which help the organisms to agglomerate. Floc formation is a common phenomenon encountered in activated sludge processes, which may impose some mass transfer limitations on the biological oxidation of soluble organics; but good floc formation is essential for good performance of the system, since large dense floes are required in the sedimentation step. Cell recycle from the sedimentation unit improves the volumetric rate of biological oxidation (i.e. high-density culture) and therefore reduces the residence time or volume of the sludge reactor for a given feed rate. The recycle maintains the integrity of biocatalysts (microbials) in the process in case of minor upsets or fluctuations. The recycle ratio needs to be controlled to maximize BOD removal rate.

The selection of aerator and agitators is a critical factor in the design of activated sludge processes. The aeration requirements vary depending on the strength of the wastewater and cell concentration. Oxygen requirements for a typical activated sludge process are about 30–60 m^3-O_2/kg-BOD removed. Various aeration devices with and without mechanical agitation can be used in activated sludge units. Mechanical surface aerators are widely used for shallow activated sludge units. Surface aerators consist of partially submerged impellers attached to motors mounted on fixed structures. Surface aerators spray liquid and create rapid changes at the air–water interface to enhance oxygen transfer. Pure oxygen may be used for high-strength wastewater treatment. Also, stagewise operation with pure oxygen has been found to be a very effective method of wastewater treatment. The UNOX Process, first developed by Union Carbide, is based on this concept. Other forms of aeration include bubble aerators and fixed turbines.

The activated sludge system faces many uncontrolled disturbances in input parameters, such as waste flow and composition. Such disturbances can lead to system failure (less than adequate treatment of the waste stream). One type of disturbance is referred to as *shock loading*. A shock load indicates the sudden input (pulse) of a high concentration of a toxic compound. A CSTR design, of course, is less affected by such inputs than a PFR design.

One response to disturbances is sludge *bulking*. A *bulking sludge* has flocs that do not settle well, and consequently cell mass is not recycled. *Bulking* sludge often results from a change in the composition of the microbial population in the treatment unit. For example, filamentous bacteria may dominate the normal floc-forming cells, leading to small, light flocs.

Various modifications of activated sludge processes have been developed. Two examples are the following:

(1) *Step feed process*: The feed stream is distributed along the length of the reactor. Such a configuration converts a conventional PFR system to more CSTR-like behavior, which provides greater stability and more effective distribution and utilization of oxygen and oxygen transfer.

(2) Solids reaeration (*contact stabilization*): In the conventional activated sludge process, the dissolved organics are quickly adsorbed onto (or into) the flocs, while the actual conversion to CO_2 and H_2O proceeds much more slowly. In contact stabilization, two tanks are used: one (about 1-h residence time) is used to promote the uptake of the organics and the second (3- to 6-h residence time) is used for reaeration and the final conversion of the organic material. By concentrating the sludge before oxidation, the total required tank volume for aeration is reduced by 50% in comparison to the conventional system.

A summary of typical values for the kinetic parameters in biological waste treatment is shown in Table 12.2. Despite all simplifying assumptions, the pure culture model seems to fit steady-state experimental data reasonably well, although it does not predict the dynamic performance very well.

Example 12.5. An industrial waste with an inlet BOD_5 of 800 mg/L must be treated to reduce the exit BOD_5 level to below 20 mg/L. The inlet flow rate is 400 m^3/h. Kinetic parameters have been estimated as $\mu_{max} = 0.20$/h, $K_S = 50$ mg-BOD_5/L, $YF_{X/S} = 0.5$ g-CS600/g-BOD_5, and $k_d = 0.005\ h^{-1}$. A waste treatment unit of 3200 m^3 is available for the process. Assume a recycle ratio of $R = 0.40$ and the separation is complete, $X_e = 0$. If you operate at a concentration ratio c_R of 2.5, find the BOD_5 at the exit and determine if sufficient BOD_5 removal is attained to meet specifications assuming that the activated sludge process is well mixed. What will be the concentration of biomass exiting the reactor, X, and the sludge production rate from the process?

TABLE 12.2 Typical Monod Model Parameters for the Activated Sludge Process

Waste source	μ_{max}, h^{-1}	K_S, mg/L	$YF_{X/S}$, g-cells/g-waste	k_d, h^{-1}	Basis
Domestic	0.4–0.55	50–120	0.5–0.67	0.002–0.003	BOD_5
Shell finish processing	0.43	96	0.58	0.058	BOD_5
Yeast processing	0.038	680	0.88	0.0033	BOD_5
Phenol	0.46	1.66	0.85		Phenol
		$K_I = 380$			
Plastic processing	0.83	167	0.30	0.0033	COD

Data from Sundstrom DW and Klei HE, Wastewater Treatment, Pearson Education, Upper Saddle River, NJ, 1979.

Solution. Assume the waste is not being concentrated during the separation phase of the biomass after the sludge reactor. Refer to Fig. 12.12 with $S_R = S_e = S$, mass balance over the sludge reactor for the biomass at steady state yields

$$Rc_RQX - (1+R)QX + V\mu_{net}X = \frac{d(VX)}{dt} = 0 \tag{E12-5.1}$$

Since $X \neq 0$, Eqn (E12-5.1) gives

$$Rc_RQ - (1+R)Q + V\mu_{net} = 0 \tag{E12-5.2}$$

That is,

$$\mu_{net} = \frac{Q}{V}[1 + R(1 - c_R)] \tag{E12-5.3}$$

Thus

$$\frac{\mu_{max}S}{K_S + S} = \mu_G = \mu_{net} + k_d = \frac{Q}{V}[1 + R(1 - c_R)] + k_d \tag{E12-5.4}$$

or

$$S = \frac{K_S(\mu_{net} + k_d)}{\mu_{max} - \mu_{net} - k_d} = K_S \frac{\frac{Q}{V}[1 + R(1 - c_R)] + k_d}{\mu_{max} - \frac{Q}{V}[1 + R(1 - c_R)] - k_d} \tag{E12-5.4}$$

Substituting the kinetic and operating parameters into Eqn (E12-5.4), we obtain

$$S = K_S \frac{\frac{Q}{V}[1 + R(1 - c_R)] + k_d}{\mu_{max} - \frac{Q}{V}[1 + R(1 - c_R)] - k_d}$$

$$S = 50 \times \frac{\frac{400}{3200}[1 + 0.4 \times (1 - 2.5)] + 0.005}{0.2 - \frac{400}{3200}[1 + 0.4 \times (1 - 2.5)] - 0.005} \text{ mg-BOD}_5\text{/L}$$

$$= 18.97 \text{ mg-BOD}_5\text{/L}$$

Therefore, the operation meet the specification as $S = 18.97$ mg/L < 20 mg/L.

We next compute the biomass concentration. Mass balance of the substrate (BOD_5) over the sludge reactor at steady state leads to

$$QS_0 + RQS - (1+R)QS - V\frac{\mu_G X}{YF_{X/S}} = \frac{d(SV)}{dt} = 0 \tag{E12-5.5}$$

which gives

$$X = \frac{Q}{V}\frac{S_0 - S}{\mu_G}YF_{X/S} = \frac{S_0 - S}{1 + R(1 - c_R) + k_d\frac{V}{Q}}YF_{X/S} \tag{E12-5.6}$$

Substituting the kinetic and operating parameters into Eqn (E12-5.6), we obtain

$$X = \frac{S_0 - S}{1 + R(1 - c_R) + k_d \dfrac{V}{Q}} YF_{X/S} = \frac{800 - 18.97}{1 + 0.4 \times (1 - 2.5) + 0.005 \times \dfrac{3200}{400}} \times 0.5 \text{ mg/L}$$

$$= 887.53 \text{ mg/L}$$

And the total sludge production G_X,

$$G_X = (1 + R)QX - c_R RQX = [1 + R(1 - c_R)]QX \quad \text{(E12-5.7)}$$

$$G_X = [1 + 0.4 \times (1 - 2.5)] \times 400 \times 887.53 \text{ g/h} = 142005 \text{ g/h} = 142 \text{ kg-CS600/h}$$

12.4. IMMOBILIZED CELL SYSTEMS

Immobilization of cells as biocatalysts are almost as common as enzyme immobilization. Immobilization is the restriction of cell mobility within a defined space. Immobilized cell cultures have the following potential advantages over suspension cultures:

(1) Immobilization provides high cell concentrations.
(2) Immobilization provides cell reuse and eliminates the costly processes of cell recovery and cell recycle.
(3) Immobilization eliminates cell washout problems at high dilution rates.
(4) The combination of high cell concentrations and high flow rates (no washout restrictions) allows high volumetric productivities.
(5) Immobilization may also provide favorable microenvironmental conditions (i.e. cell–cell contact, nutrient-product gradients, and pH gradients) for cells, resulting in better performance of the biocatalysts (e.g. higher product yields and rates).
(6) In some cases, immobilization improves genetic stability.
(7) For some cells, protection against shear damage is important.

The major limitation on immobilization is that the product of interest should be excreted by the cells. A further complication is that immobilization often leads to systems for which diffusional limitations are important. In such cases, the control of microenvironmental conditions is difficult, owing to the resulting heterogeneity in the system. With living cells, growth and gas evolution present significant problems in some systems and can lead to significant mechanical disruption of the immobilizing matrix.

In Chapter 8, we discussed enzyme immobilization. Figure 8.16 provides a useful summary of immobilization strategies. Many of the ideas in enzyme immobilization have a direct counterpart in whole cells. However, the maintenance of a living cell in such a system is more complex than maintaining enzymatic activity. The primary advantage of immobilized cells over immobilized enzymes is that immobilized cells can perform multistep, cofactor-requiring, biosynthetic reactions that are not practical using purified enzyme preparations.

12.4.1. Active Immobilization of Cells

Active immobilization is entrapment or binding of cells by physical or chemical forces. The two major methods of active immobilization are entrapment and binding.

Physical entrapment within porous matrices is the most widely used method of cell immobilization. Various matrices can be used for the immobilization of cells. Among these are porous polymers (agar, alginate, K-carrageenan, polyacrylamide, chitosan, gelatin, and collagen), porous metal screens, polyurethane, silica gel, polystyrene, and cellulose triacetate.

Polymer beads should be porous enough to allow the transport of substrates and products in and out of the bead. They are usually formed in the presence of cells and can be prepared by one of the following methods:

(1) *Gelation of polymers*: Gelatin and agar beads may be prepared by mixing the liquid form of these polymers with cell suspensions and using a template to form beads. Reduction of temperature in the templates causes solidification of the polymers with the cells entrapped. Gel beads are usually soft and mechanically fragile. However, we can use a hard core (glass and plastic) and a soft gelatin shell with entrapped cells to overcome some mechanical problems associated with polymer beads. Because of diffusional limitations, the inner core of such beads is often not active, so this approach does not necessarily decrease the amount of product made per bead.

(2) *Precipitation of polymers*: Cells are dispersed in a polymer solution, and by changing the pH or the solvent, the polymer can be precipitated. The starting solution of the polymer has to be prepared with an organic solvent or a water-solvent mixture. Ethanol and acetone are examples of water-miscible solvents. Polymers used for this purpose are polystyrene, cellulose triacetate, and collagen. The direct contact of cells with solvents may cause inactivation and even the death of cells.

(3) *Ion-exchange gelation*: Ion-exchange gelation takes place when a water-soluble polyelectrolyte is mixed with a salt solution. Solidification occurs when the polyelectrolyte reacts with the salt solution to form a solid gel. The most popular example of this kind of gelation is the formation of Ca-alginate gel by mixing Na-alginate solution with a $CaCl_2$ solution. Some other polymers obtained by ion-exchange gelation are Al-alginate, Ca/Al carboxymethyl cellulose, Mg pectinate, K-carrageenan, and chitosan polyphosphate. Alginate and K-carrageenan are the most widely used polymers for cell immobilization purposes. Ionic gels can be further stabilized by covalent cross-linking.

(4) *Polycondensation*: Epoxy resins are prepared by polycondensation and can be used for cell immobilization. Polycondensation produces covalent networks with high chemical and mechanical stability. Usually, liquid precursors are cured with a multifunctional component. Functional groups usually are hydroxy, amino, epoxy, and isocyanate groups. Some examples of polymer networks obtained by polycondensation are epoxy, polyurethane, silica gel, gelatin-glutaraldehyde, albumin-glutaraldehyde, and collagen-glutaraldehyde. Severe reaction conditions (high temperature and low or high pH values) and toxic functional groups may adversely affect the activity of cells.

(5) *Polymerization*: Polymeric networks can be prepared by cross-linking copolymers of a vinyl group containing monomers. Polyacrylamide beads are the most widely used polymer beads, prepared by copolymerization of acrylamide and bisacrylamide. Several different monomers can be used for polymer formation; acrylamide, methacrylamide, and 2-hydroxyethyl methacrylate are the most widely used. Cross-linking is usually initiated by copolymerization with a divinyl compound, such as methylenebisacrylamide.

Immobilization by polymerization is a simple method. The polymerizing solution is mixed with the cell suspension, and polymerization takes place to form a polymeric block, which is pressed through a sieve plate to obtain regular-shaped particles. Suspension or emulsion polymerization can also be used to form polymeric beads for cell entrapment.

Encapsulation is another method of cell entrapment. Microcapsules are hollow, spherical particles bound by semipermeable membranes. Cells are entrapped within the hollow capsule volume. The transport of nutrients and products in and out of the capsule takes place through the capsule membrane. Microcapsules have certain advantages over gel beads. More cells can be packed per unit volume of support material into capsules, and intraparticle diffusion limitations are less severe in capsule due to the presence of liquid cell suspension in the intracapsule space. Various polymers can be used as capsule membranes. Among these are nylon, collodion, polystyrene, acrylate, polylysine-alginate hydrogel, cellulose acetate, ethyl cellulose, and polyester membranes. Different membranes (composition and molecular weight [MW] cutoff) may need to be used for different applications in order to retain some high-MW products inside capsules and provide passage to low-MW nutrients and products.

Another form of entrapment is the use of macroscopic membrane-based reactors. The simplest of these is the hollow fiber reactor. This device is a mass transfer analog of the shell- and tube-heat exchanger in which the tubes are made of semipermeable membranes. Typically, cells are inoculated on the shell side and are allowed to grow in place. The nutrient solution is pumped through the insides of the tubes. Nutrients diffuse through the membrane and are utilized by the cells, and metabolic products diffuse back into the flowing nutrient stream. Owing to diffusional limitations, the unmodified hollow fiber unit does not perform well with living cells. Modifications involving multiple membrane types (for example, for gas exchange or extractive product removal) or changes to promote convective flux within the cell layer have been proposed. Several commercial reactors for animal cell cultivation use membrane entrapment. In addition to entrapment or encapsulation, cells can be bound directly to a support. Immobilization of cells on the surfaces of support materials can be achieved by physical adsorption or covalent binding. Adsorption of cells on inert support surfaces has been widely used for cell immobilization. The major advantage of immobilization by adsorption is direct contact between nutrient and support materials. High cell loadings can be obtained using microporous support materials. However, porous support materials may cause intraparticle pore diffusion limitations at high cell densities, as is also the case with polymer-entrapped cell systems. Also, the control of microenvironmental conditions is a problem with porous support materials. A ratio of pore to cell diameter of 4 to 5 is recommended for the immobilization of cells onto the inner surface of porous support particles. At small pore sizes, accessibility of the nutrient into inner surfaces of pores may be the limiting factor, whereas at large pore sizes, the specific surface area may be the limiting factor. Therefore, there may be an optimal pore size, resulting in the maximum rate of bioconversion.

Adsorption capacity and strength of binding are the two major factors that affect the selection of a suitable support material. Adsorption capacity varies between 2 mg/g (porous silica) and 250 mg/g (wood chips). Porous glass carriers provide adsorption capacities (10^8-10^9 cells/g) that are less than or comparable to those of gel-entrapped cell concentrations (10^9-10^{11} cells/mL). The binding forces between the cell and support surfaces may vary, depending on the surface properties of the support material and the type of cells. Electrostatic forces are dominant when positively charged support surfaces (ion-exchange resins and gelatin) are used. Cells also adhere on negatively charged surfaces by covalent binding or H bonding. The adsorption of cells on neutral polymer support surfaces may be mediated by chemical bonding, such as covalent bonding, H bonds or van der Waals forces. Some specific chelating agents may be used to develop stronger cell–surface interactions. Among the support materials used for cell adsorption are porous glass, porous silica, alumina, ceramics, gelatin, chitosan, activated carbon, wood chips, polypropylene ion-exchange resins (DEAE-Sephadex, CMC-), and Sepharose. Adsorption is a simple, inexpensive method of cell immobilization. However, limited cell loadings and rather weak binding forces reduce the attractiveness of this method. Hydrodynamic shear around adsorbed cells should be very mild to avoid the removal of cells from support surfaces. Covalent binding is the most widely used method for enzyme immobilization. However, it is not as widely used for cell immobilization. Functional groups on cell and support material surfaces are not usually suitable for covalent binding. Binding surfaces need to be specially treated with coupling agents (e.g. glutaraldehyde or carbodiimide) or reactive groups for covalent binding. These reactive groups may be toxic to cells. A number of inorganic carriers (metal oxides such as titanium and zirconium oxide) have been developed that provide satisfactory functional groups for covalent binding. Covalent binding forces are stronger than adsorption forces, resulting in more stable binding. However, with growing cells, large numbers of cell progeny must be lost. Support materials with desired functional groups are rather limited. Among the support materials used for covalent binding are CMC plus carbodiimide; carriers with aldehyde, amine, epoxy, or halocarbonyl groups; Zr(IV) oxide; Ti(IV) oxide; and cellulose plus cyanuric chloride. Support materials with $-OH$ groups are treated with CNBr, with $-NH_2$ are treated with glutaraldehyde, and with COOH groups are treated with carbodiimide for covalent binding with protein groups on cell surfaces.

The direct cross-linking of cells by glutaraldehyde to form an insoluble aggregate is more like cell entrapment than binding. However, some cells may be cross-linked after adsorption onto support surfaces. Cross-linking by glutaraldehyde may adversely affect the cell's metabolic activity and may also cause severe diffusion limitations. Physical cross-linking may also be provided by using polyelectrolytes, polymers such as chitosan and salts [$CaC1_2$, $Al(OH)_3$, $FeC1_3$]. Direct cross-linking is not widely used because of the aforementioned disadvantages.

Some examples of cell immobilization by entrapment and by surface attachment (binding) are summarized in Tables 12.3 and 12.4, respectively. A good support material should be rigid and chemically inert, should bind cells firmly, and should have high loading capacity. In the case of gel entrapment, gels should be porous enough and particle size should be small enough to avoid intraparticle diffusion limitations. The effect of particle size and permeability inside the particle is discussed in Chapter 17.

TABLE 12.3 Examples of Cell Immobilization by Entrapment Using Different Support Materials

Cells	Support matrix	Conversion
S. cerevisiae	K-Carrageenan or polyacrylamide	Glucose to ethanol
Enterobacter aerogenes	K-Carrageenan	Glucose to 2,3-butanediol
E. coli	K-Carrageenan	Fumaric acid to aspartic acid
Trichoderma reesei	K-Carrageenan	Cellulose production
Zymomonas mobilis	Ca-alginate	Glucose to ethanol
Acetobacter sp.	Ca-alginate	Glucose to gluconic acid
Morinda citrifolia	Ca-alginate	Anthraquinone formation
Candida trapicalis	Ca-alginate	Phenol degradation
Nocardia rhodocraus	Polyurethane	Conversion of testosterone
E. coli	Polyurethane	Penicillin G to G-APA
Catharantus roseus	Polyurethane	Isocitrate dehydrogenase activity
Rhodotorula minuta	Polyurethane	Menthyl succinate to menthol

TABLE 12.4 Examples of Cell Immobilization by Surface Attachment

Cells	Support surface	Conversion
Lactobacillus sp.	Gelatin (adsorption)	Glucose to lactic acid
Clostridium acetobutylicum	Ion-exchange resins	Glucose to acetone, butanol
Streptomyces	Sephadex (adsorption)	Streptomycin
Animal cells	DEAE-sephadex/cytodex (adsorption)	Hormones
E. coli	Ti(IV) oxide (covalent binding)	
Bacillus subtilis	Agarose-carbodiimide (covalent binding)	
Solanum aviculare	Polyphenylene oxide-glutaraldehyde (covalent binding)	Steroid glycoalkaloids formation

12.4.2. Passive Immobilization: Biological Films

Biological films are the multilayer growth of cells on solid support surfaces. The support material can be inert or biologically active. Biofilm formation is common in natural and industrial fermentation systems, such as biological wastewater treatment and mold fermentations. The interaction among cells and the binding forces between the cell and support material may be very complicated.

In mixed culture microbial films, the presence of some polymer-producing organisms facilitates biofilm formation and enhances the stability of the biofilms. Microenvironmental conditions inside a thick biofilm vary with position and affect the physiology of the cells.

In a stagnant biological film, nutrients diffuse into the biofilm and products diffuse out into liquid nutrient medium. Nutrient and product profiles within the biofilm are important factors affecting cellular physiology and metabolism. Biofilm cultures have almost the same advantages as those of the immobilized cell systems over suspension cultures.

The thickness of a biofilm is an important factor affecting the performance of the biotic phase. Thin biofilms will have low rates of conversion due to low biomass concentration, and thick biofilms may experience diffusionally limited growth, which may or may not be beneficial depending on the cellular system and objectives. Nutrient-depleted regions may also develop within the biofilm for thick biofilms. In many cases, an optimal biofilm thickness resulting in the maximum rate of bioconversion exists and can be determined. In some cases, growth under diffusion limitations may result in higher yields of products as a result of changes in cell physiology and cell–cell interactions. In this case, improvement in reaction stoichiometry (e.g. high yield) may overcome the reduction in reaction rate, and it may be more beneficial to operate the system under diffusion limitations. Usually, the most sparingly soluble nutrient, such as DO, is the rate-limiting nutrient within the biofilm.

Immobilized cell culture offers more freedom in terms of methods of cultivation. When cells are immobilized, the fermentation can be carried out in batch and flow reactors. Fluidized bed (close to CSTR or chemostat) and packed bed (close to PFR) reactors can be employed such that cells are retained in the reactor. The cost to cell immobilization and some loss of efficiency (effectiveness) can be justified by the saving from cell recycle (or with minor loss only).

Example 12.6. Xylose (S) is converted to ethanol (P) in a packed bed by a genetically altered *S. cerevisiae* (X) cells immobilized via entrapment in Ca-alginate beads. Ethanol production rate follows Monod/Michaelis–Menten equation. The maximum specific rate of formation of ethanol $\mu_{P\max} = 0.25$ g-P/(g-X·h) and the saturation constant is 0.0018 g/L. The average cell loading achieved in the bed is $\overline{X} = 20$ g/L. Assume that cell growth is negligible and the bead size is small enough and the flow condition is turbulent enough that the overall effectiveness factor is 1. That is, the reaction rate is not affected by the immobilization. The xylose feed concentration is 120 g/L and the ethanol yield factor $YF_{P/S} = 0.48$. If the desired xylose conversion is 99%, determine

(a) Required dilution rate.
(b) Ethanol concentration in the effluent.

Solution. (a) A packed bed reactor can be approximated by a PFR. Mass balance of the substrate (xylose) in a differential volume of the reactor leads to

$$QS|_V - QS|_{V+dV} + r_S dV = \frac{d(SdV)}{dt} \tag{E12-6.1}$$

At steady-state operation, nothing changes with time: 0

Equation (E12-6.1) is reduced to

$$-QdS = -r_S \, dV \tag{E12-6.2}$$

From stoichiometry,

$$r_S = \frac{-r_P}{YF_{P/S}} \tag{E12-6.3}$$

whereas

$$r_P = \frac{\mu_{P\max} S}{K_S + S}\overline{X} \tag{E12-6.4}$$

Thus, Eqn (E12-6.2) is reduced to

$$-Q dS = \frac{\mu_{P\max} S}{K_S + S}\frac{\overline{X}}{YF_{P/S}} dV \tag{E12-6.5}$$

Separation of variables

$$-Q\frac{K_S + S}{S} dS = \frac{\mu_{P\max}\overline{X}}{YF_{P/S}} dV \tag{E12-6.6}$$

and integrating

$$-\int_{S_0}^{S} Q\frac{K_S + S}{S} dS = \int_0^V \frac{\mu_{P\max}\overline{X}}{YF_{P/S}} dV \tag{E12-6.7}$$

we obtain

$$Q\left(K_S \ln\frac{S_0}{S} + S_0 - S\right) = \frac{\mu_{P\max}\overline{X}}{YF_{P/S}} V \tag{E12-6.8}$$

The conversion of substrate is defined as

$$f_S = \frac{QS_0 - QS}{QS_0} = \frac{S_0 - S}{S_0} \tag{E12-6.9}$$

Thus, the dilution rate can be obtained by substituting Eqn (E12-6.9) into Eqn (E12-6.8) and rearranging,

$$D = \frac{Q}{V} = \frac{\mu_{P\max}\overline{X}}{YF_{P/S}[S_0 f_S - K_S \ln(1 - f_S)]} \tag{E12-6.10}$$

Therefore,

$$D = \frac{\mu_{P\max}\overline{X}}{YF_{P/S}[S_0 f_S - K_S \ln(1 - f_S)]} = \frac{0.25 \times 20}{0.48 \times [120 \times 0.99 - 0.0018 \times \ln(1 - 0.99)]}\ \text{h}^{-1}$$

$$= 0.08768\ \text{h}^{-1}$$

(b) Ethanol concentration can be obtained via stoichiometry,

$$P = YF_{P/S}(S_0 - S) = 0.48 \times 120 \times 0.99\ \text{g/L} = 57.02\ \text{g/L}$$

12.5. SOLID SUBSTRATE FERMENTATIONS

Our focus so far has been on the liquid media fermentations with very little discussion on solid substrates. Solid substrate fermentations imply a general method of fermentations in which moisture content may or may not need to be low, but the substrate is in the form of solid particles, where the media can be in liquid phase. Bacterial ore leaching (i.e. growth and microbial oxidation on surfaces of mineral sulfide particles) or fermentation of rice in a packed column with circulating liquid media is an example of solid substrate fermentations. When the solid substrate is submerged in the liquid medium, the fermentation is usually referred to as submerged fermentation (SmF). However, when no free liquid presents in the system, the fermentation is usually referred to as solid-state fermentation (SSF).

SSFs are a special form of solid substrate fermentations for which the substrate is solid and the moisture level is low, which usually refers to as no free flowing water in the medium. The water content of a typical SmF is more than 90%. The water content of a solid mash in SSF often varies between 40% and 80%. SSFs are usually employed for the fermentation of agricultural products or foods, such as rice, wheat, barley, durum, oat, peas, millet, corn, broad beans, and soybeans. The unique characteristic of SSFs is operation at very low moisture levels, which provides a selective environment for the growth of mycelial organisms, such as molds. In fact, most SSFs are mold fermentations producing extracellular enzymes on moist agricultural substrates. Since bacteria and yeasts cannot tolerate low moisture levels (water activities), the chances of contamination of fermentation media by bacteria or yeast are greatly reduced in SSF. Although most SSFs are mold fermentations, SSFs based on bacteria and yeast operating at relatively high moisture levels (75–90%) are also used. SSFs are used widely in Asia for food products, such as tempeh, miso, or soy sauce fermentations, and also for enzyme production.

The choice of using SSF was quite intuitive at the dawn of food processing. Tofu and grains go "bad" under moisture and our ancestors discovered that they could be turned to tasty food. The major advantages of SSF over SmF systems are 1) small volume of fermentation mash or reactor volume to deal with for the same amount of final product, leading to low capital and operating costs, 2) a lower chance of contamination by unwanted microorganisms due to low moisture levels, 3) easy product recovery, 4) energy efficiency, 5) the allowing of the development of fully differentiated structures, which is critical in some cases to product formation, and 6) easy to implement with simple capital structure and minimum operation requirements. The major disadvantage of SSFs is the heterogeneous nature of the media due to poor mixing characteristics, which result in poor ability to control the conditions (pH, DO, and temperature) within the fermentation mash. To eliminate these control problems, fermentation media are usually mixed either continuously or intermittently. For large fermentation mash volumes, the concentration gradients may not be eliminated at low agitation speeds, and mycelial cells may be damaged at high agitation speeds. Usually, a rotating drum fermentor is used for SSF systems, and the rotational speed needs to be optimized for the best performance.

Table 12.5 lists some of the traditional food products produced via aerobic SSF. The *koji process* is an SSF system that employs molds (*Aspergillus*, *Rhizopus*) growing on grains or foods (wheat, rice, and soybean). A typical SSF process involves two stages. The first and

TABLE 12.5 Some Traditional Food Fermentations

			Thermal processing			Incubation		
Product	Primary genus	Common substrate	Temperature, °C	Time, min	Initial moisture, %	Time, h	Temperature, °C	Further processing
Soy sauce	*Aspergillus*	Soybean, wheat	110	30	45	72	30	Yes
Miso	*Aspergillus*	Rice, soybean	100	40	35	44	30	Yes
Tempeh	*Rhizopus*	Soybean	100	30	40	22	32	No
Hamanatto	*Aspergillus*	Soybean, wheat				36		Yes
Sufu	*Actinomucor*	Tofu	100	10	74		15	Yes

the primary stage is an aerobic, fungal, solid-state fermentation of grains called the *koji*. The second stage is an anaerobic SmF with a mixed bacterial culture called the *moromi*. The moromi process may be realized by using the natural flora, or, usually, with externally added bacteria and yeasts.

Some strains of *Saccharomyces, Torulopsis*, and *Pediococcus* are used as flavor producers in soy sauce manufacture. The moromi is usually fermented for 8–12 months. However, the processing time can be reduced to 6 months by temperature profiling. The final product is pressed to recover the liquid soy sauce and is pasteurized, filtered, and bottled.

The major industrial use of the koji process is for the production of enzymes by fungal species. Fungal amylases are produced by SSF of wheat bran by *Aspergillus oryzae* in a rotating drum fermentor. Wheat bran is pretreated with formaldehyde, and the initial pH of the bran is adjusted to pH = 3.5–4.0 to reduce the chance of contamination. Usually, perforated pans, rotating drums, or packed beds with air ventilation are used. Enzymes other than amylases, such as cellulase, pectinase, protease, and lipases, can be produced by rotary drum fermentations. *Trichoderma viride* species have been used for the production of cellulases from wheat bran in a rotary tray fermentor.

Some secondary metabolites, such as antibacterial agents, are produced by *Rhizopus* and *Actinomucor* species in some koji processes. Certain mycotoxins, such as aflatoxins, were produced by SSF of rice (40% moisture) by *Aspergillus parasiticus*. Ochratoxins were also produced by *Aspergillus* species on wheat in a rotary drum fermentor. Microbial degradation of lignocellulosics can also be accomplished by solid-state fermentations for waste treatment purposes or in biopulping of wood chips for use in paper manufacture. Spores from some molds have found use as insecticides. Proper spore formation is difficult to obtain in submerged culture, and SSF must be used.

Major process variables in SSF systems are moisture content (water activity), inoculum density, temperature, pH, particle size, and aeration/agitation. Optimization of these parameters to maximize product yield and rate of product formation is the key in SSF systems and depends on the substrate and organism used. Most natural substrates (e.g. grains) require pretreatment to make the physical structure of substrates more susceptible to mycelial penetration and utilization. Solid substrates are usually treated with antimicrobial agents, such as formaldehyde, and are steamed in an autoclave. Nutrient media addition, pH adjustment, and the adjustment of moisture level are realized before inoculation of the fermentation mash. Koji fermentations are usually realized in a controlled humidity air environment with air ventilation and agitation. Many solid-state mycelial fermentations are shear sensitive due to disruption of the mycelia at high agitation/rotation speeds. At low agitation rates, oxygen transfer and CO_2 evolution rates become limiting. Therefore, an optimal range of agitation rate or rotation speed needs to be determined. Similarly, there is a minimum level of moisture content (−30% by weight) below which microbial activity is inhibited. At high moisture levels (>60%), solid substrates become sticky and form large aggregates. Moreover, moisture level affects the metabolic activities of cells. Optimal moisture level needs to be determined experimentally for each cell-substrate system. For most of the koji processes, the optimal moisture level is about $40 \pm 5\%$. Particle size should be small enough to avoid any oxygen–CO_2 exchange or other nutrient transport limitations. Porosity of the particles can be improved by pretreatment to provide a larger intraparticle surface to volume ratio for microbial action.

Most of the SSF processes are realized using a rotary tray type of reactor in a temperature- and humidity-controlled chamber where controlled humidity air is circulated through stacked beds of trays containing fermented solids. Rotary drum fermentors are used less frequently because of the shear sensitivity of mycelial cells.

12.6. SUMMARY

The primary form of continuous culture is a steady-state CSTR or *chemostat*. A chemostat ensures a time-invariant chemical environment for the cell cultivation. The net specific growth rate is equal to the dilution rate, which is determined by the flow rate to the chemostat. Thus, the growth rate can be manipulated by the investigator. This is a typical method of controlling the cell growth (and/or production formation rate). A constant dilution rate gives rise to a constant specific growth rate, which is equivalent to a fixed exponential growth rate. Another benefit is the control of substrate concentration in the reactor at a given (low) value, which can promote a desired product formation. A *cytostat* (or *turbidostat*) adjusts flow rate to maintain a constant cell density (via turbidity). Cell density control via adjusting flow rate is not effective except at high flow rates. A turbidostat operates well at high flow rates (near the washout point) and is useful in selecting cellular subpopulations that have adapted to a particular stress.

Continuous culturing is more productive than batch culturing. The productivity of chemostat increases with increasing dilution rate to a maximum before sharply decreases near the washout limit. Higher endogenous needs and/or death rate decreases cell biomass concentration and productivity. The cell biomass concentration is maximum at zero dilution rate if there are no endogenous requirements and the death rate is zero. A finite death rate gives rise to a zero viable cell biomass concentration at zero dilution rate. Increasing endogenous needs decrease cell biomass concentration especially at low dilution rates. There is a maximum cell biomass concentration near the washout limit either if there are endogenous requirements or if the death rate is not zero.

The growth and/or product formation patterns can be different between batch and continuous cultivations. In a batch system, lag phase is commonly observed which is absent in a continuous system. On the other hand, Crabtree effect can be observed with changing flow rates in a continuous system, which is absent in a batch cultivation curve.

Bioreactors using suspended cells can be operated in many modes intermediate between a batch reactor and a single-stage chemostat. Although a chemostat has potential productivity advantages for primary products, considerations of genetic instability, process flexibility, low quantities of product demand, and process reliability (such as biocontamination and biostability) have greatly limited the use of chemostat units. The use of cell recycle with a CSTR increases volumetric productivity and has found use in large-volume, consistent production demand and low-product value processes (e.g. waste treatment and fuel-grade ethanol production).

Multistage continuous systems improve the potential usefulness of continuous processes for the production of secondary metabolites and for the use of genetically unstable cells. The perfusion system is another option that is particularly attractive for animal cells.

Immobilized cell systems offer a number of potential processing advantages, and the commercialization of such systems is proceeding rapidly where cell culture is expensive and difficult (e.g. animal cell tissue culture). Physical entrapment or encapsulation is used in most cases, although adsorption onto surfaces or covalent binding of cells to surfaces is possible.

In some cases, self-immobilization on surfaces is possible and a biofilm is formed. Biofilm reactors can apply to tissue culture, mold, and bacterial systems. Biofilm-based reactors are very important in waste treatment applications and in natural ecosystems. The analysis of immobilized cell reactors is analogous to that for immobilized enzyme reactors except for the feature of biocatalyst replication.

Solid-state fermentations share some characteristics with immobilized cell systems but differ in that no discernible liquid is present. SSFs have found important uses in the production of some traditional fermented foods and may have use in upgrading agricultural or forest materials and in the production of mold products requiring full mold differentiation.

Further Reading

Bailey, J.E., 1998. Mathematical Modeling and Analysis in Biochemical Engineering: Past Accomplishments and Future Opportunities, *Biotechnol. Prog.* 14:8.

Bailey, J.E., Ollis, D.F., 1986. *Biochemical Engineering Fundamentals,* 2nd ed. Mc-Graw-Hill Book Co., New York.

Blanch, H.W., Clark, D.S., 1996. *Biochemical Engineering.* Marcel Dekker, Inc., New York.

Herbert, D.R., Ellsworth, R., Telling, R.C., 1956. The Continuous Culture of Bacteria: A Theoretical and Experimental Study, *J. Gen. Microbiol.* 14:601.

Mitchell, D.A., Krieger, N., Berovic, M., (Eds.). 2006. *Solid State F ermentation Bioreactors: Fundamentals of Design and Operation,* Springer.

Pandey, A., Soccol, C.R., Larroche, C., (Eds.). 2008. *Current Developments in Solid State Fermentation,* Springer.

Shuler, M.L., Kargi, F., 2006. Bioprocess Engineering, Basic Concepts. 2nd ed. Prentice Hall: Upper Saddle River, NJ.

PROBLEMS

12.1. *Pseudomonas sp.* has a mass doubling time of 2.4 h when grown on acetate. The saturation constant using this substrate is 1.3 g/L (which is unusually high), and cell yield on acetate is 0.46 g cell/g acetate. If the feed stream to a chemostat contains 38 g/L acetate, determine:
(a) Maximum dilution rate,
(b) Cell concentration when the dilution rate is one-half of the maximum,
(c) Substrate concentration when the dilution rate is 0.8 D_{max},
(d) Cell productivity at 0.8 D_{max}

12.2. Consider a 1000-L CSTR in which biomass is being produced with glucose as the substrate. The microbial system follows a Monod relationship with $\mu_{max} = 0.4\ h^{-1}$, $K_S = 1.5$ g/L (an unusually high value), and the yield factor $YF_{X/S} = 0.5$ g-biomass/g-substrate consumed. If normal operation is with a sterile feed containing 10 g/L glucose at a rate of 100 L/h:
(a) What is the specific biomass production rate ($g \cdot L^{-1} \cdot h^{-1}$) at steady state?
(b) If recycle is used with a recycle stream of 10 L/h and a recycle biomass concentration five times as large as that in the reactor exit, what would be the new specific biomass production rate?
(c) Explain any difference between the values found in parts (a) and (b).

12.3. Table P12.3 was obtained in a chemostat for the growth of *E. aerogenes* on a glycerol-limited growth medium.

For this system, estimate the values of:
(a) K_S, g-glycerol/L
(b) $\mu_m \cdot h^{-1}$
(c) $YF_{X/S}$, g-cells/g-glycerol
(d) m_S, g-glycerol/(g-cell · h)

TABLE P12.3

Dilution rate D, h^{-1}	Glycerol concentration S, g/L	Cell concentration X, g/L
0.05	0.012	3.2
0.10	0.028	3.7
0.20	0.05	4.0
0.40	0.10	4.4
0.60	0.15	4.75
0.70	0.176	4.9
0.80	0.80	4.5
0.84	10.00	0.5

Note: $S_0 = 10$ g/L.

12.4. The kinetics of microbial growth, substrate consumption, and mixed-growth-associated product formation for a chemostat culture are given by the following equations:

$$r_X = \frac{\mu_{max} S}{K_S + S} X$$

$$r_S = \frac{1}{YF_{X/S}} \frac{\mu_{max} S}{K_S + S} X$$

$$r_P = \alpha r_X + \beta X = (\alpha \mu_G + \beta) X$$

The kinetic parameter values are $\mu_{max} = 0.7\ h^{-1}$, $K_S = 20$ mg/L, $YF_{X/S} = 0.5$ g-cells/g-substrate, $YF_{P/X} = 0.15$ g-P/g-cells, $\alpha = 0.1$, $\beta = 0.02\ h^{-1}$, and $S_0 = 1$ g/L.

(a) Determine the optimal dilution rate maximizing the productivity of product formation (*PD*).

(b) Determine the optimal dilution rate maximizing the productivity of cell (biomass) formation (DX).

12.5. In a two-stage chemostat system, the volumes of the first and second reactors are $V_1 = 500$ L and $V_2 = 300$ L, respectively. The first reactor is used for biomass production and the second is for a secondary metabolite formation. The feed flow rate to the first reactor is $Q = 100$ L/h, and the glucose concentration in the feed is $S_0 = 5.0$ g/L. Use the following constants for the cells.

$$\mu_{max} = 0.3\ h^{-1},\ K_S = 0.1\ g/L,\ YF_{X/S} = 0.4\ \text{g-cells/g-glucose}$$

(a) Determine cell and glucose concentrations in the effluent of the first stage.

(b) Assume that growth is negligible in the second stage and the specific rate of product formation is $\mu_P = 0.02$ g-P/(g-cell·h) and $YF_{P/S} = 0.6$ g-P/g-S. Determine the product and substrate concentrations in the effluent of the second reactor.

12.6. Ethanol is to be used as a substrate for SCP production in a chemostat. The available equipment can achieve an oxygen transfer rate of 10 g-O_2/L of liquid per hour. Assume the kinetics of cell growth on ethanol is of the Monod type, with $\mu_m = 0.5$/h, $K_S = 30$ mg/L, $YF_{X/S} = 0.5$ cells/g-ethanol, and $YF_{O_2/S} = 2$ g-O_2/g-EtOH. We wish to operate the chemostat with an ethanol concentration in the feed of 22 g/L. We also wish to maximize the biomass productivity and minimize the loss of unused ethanol in the effluent. Determine the required dilution rate and whether sufficient oxygen can be provided.

12.7. Figure P12.7 shows a special two-stage chemostat system where the second chemostat is simply drawing its feed from the first chemostat and returning the contents back into the first chemostat. This is a convenient model to describe the nonideal chemostat operations where a stagnant region presents in a chemostat. Derive at a relationship for *S* and *X* as functions of the feed and operating conditions, based on Monod growth equation with a finite cell death rate.

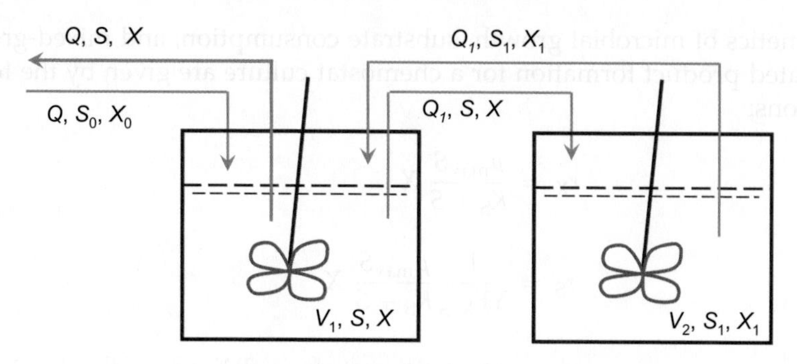

FIGURE P12.7 A schematic of a two-stage chemostat system.

12.8. In a chemostat you know that if a culture obeys the Monod equation, the residual substrate is independent of the feed substrate concentration. You observe that in your chemostat an increase in S_0 causes an increase in the residual substrate concentration. Your friend suggests that you consider whether the Contois equation may describe the situation better. The Contois equation is:

$$\mu = \frac{\mu_{max} S}{K_{SX} X + S}$$

(a) Derive an expression for S in terms of D, μ_{max}, K_{SX}, and X for a steady-state CSTR (chemostat).

(b) Derive an equation for S as a function of S_0, D, K_{SX}, $YF_{X/S}$, and μ_{max}.

(c) If S_0 increases twofold, by how much will S increase?

12.9. Plot the response of a culture to diauxic growth on glucose and lactose based on the following:
$\mu_{glucose} = 1.0\ h^{-1}$; $\mu_{lactose} = 0.6/h$; $YF_{glucose} = YF_{lactose} = 0.5$; enzyme induction requires 30 min to complete. Plot cell mass, glucose, and lactose concentrations, assuming initial values of 2 g/L glucose, 3 g/L lactose, and 0.10 g/L cells.

12.10. *Pseudomonas putida* with $\mu_{max} = 0.5\ h^{-1}$ is cultivated in a continuous culture under aerobic conditions where $D = 0.28\ h^{-1}$. The carbon and energy source in the feed is lactose with a concentration of $S_0 = 2$ g/L. The effluent lactose concentration is desired to be $S = 0.1$ g/L. If the growth rate is limited by oxygen transfer, by using the following information:

$$YF_{X/S} = 0.45\ \text{g-X/g} - \text{S},\ YF_{X/O_2} = 0.25\ \text{g} - \text{X/g} - O_2 \text{ and } C^* = 8\ \text{mg/L}$$

(a) Determine the steady-state biomass concentration (X) and the specific rate of oxygen consumption (μ_{O2}).

(b) What should be the oxygen transfer coefficient ($k_L a$) in order to overcome oxygen transfer limitation (i.e. $C_L = 2$ mg/L)?

12.11. Table P12.11 shows data obtained from oxidation of pesticides present in wastewater by a mixed culture of microorganisms in a continuously operating aeration tank.

TABLE P12.11

D, h^{-1}	Pesticides S, mg/L	X, mg/L
0.05	15	162
0.11	25	210
0.24	50	250
0.39	100	235
0.52	140	220
0.7	180	205
0.82	240	170

Assuming the pesticide concentration in the feed wastewater stream as $S_0 = 500$ mg/L, determine $YF_{X/S}$, k_d, μ_{max}, and K_S.

12.12. The maximum growth yield factor for *B. subtilis* growing on methanol is 0.4 g-X/g-S. The heat of combustion of cells is 21 kJ/g-cells and for substrate it is 30.5 kJ/g. Determine the metabolic heat generated by the cells per unit mass of methanol consumption.

12.13. Calculate the productivity (i.e. DP) of a chemostat under the following conditions:

(1) Assume Monod kinetics apply. Assume that negligible amounts of biomass must be converted to product (<1%).

(2) Assume the Luedeking–Piret equation for product formation applies, i.e.

$$r_P = \alpha r_X + \beta X = (\alpha \mu_G + \beta) X$$

(3) Assume steady state:

$S_0 = 1000$ mg/L; $D = 0.8\ \mu_{max}$; $\mu_{max} = 1.0\ h^{-1}$; $K_S = 10$ mg/L; $YF_{X/S} = 0.5$ g-X/g-S; $\alpha = 0.4$ mg-P/g-X; $\beta = 0.5\ h^{-1}$ mg-P/g-X

12.14. Consider a chemostat. You wish to know the *number* of cells in the reactor and the *fraction* of the cells that are viable (i.e. alive as determined by ability to divide).

(a) Write an equation for viable cell number (n_v). Assume that

$$\mu_{net} = \frac{\mu_{max} S}{K_S + S} - k_d$$

where μ_{net} = net specific replication rate, μ_{max} = maximum specific replication rate, and k_d = death rate. K_S is the saturation parameter.

(b) Derive an expression for the value of S at steady state.

(c) Write the number balance in the chemostat on dead cells (n_d).

(d) Derive an expression for the fraction of the total population which are dead cells.

12.15. *Escherichia coli* is cultivated in continuous culture under aerobic conditions with a glucose limitation. When the system is operated at $D = 0.2$/h, determine the effluent glucose and biomass concentrations by using the following equations ($S_0 = 5$ g/L):

(a) Monod equation: $\mu_G = \frac{\mu_{max} S}{K_S + S}$, with $\mu_{max} = 0.25\ h^{-1}$, $K_S = 100$ mg/L.

(b) Tessier equation: $\mu_G = \mu_{max}[1 - \exp(-KS)]$, with $\mu_{max} = 0.25\ h^{-1}$, $K = 0.005/mg/L$.

(c) Moser equation: $\mu_G = \dfrac{\mu_{max} S^n}{K_S + S^n}$, with $\mu_{max} = 0.25\ h^{-1}$, $K_S = 100$ mg/L, $n = 1.5$.

(d) Contois equation: $\mu_G = \dfrac{\mu_{max} S}{K_{SX} X + S}$, with $\mu_{max} = 0.25\ h^{-1}$, $K_{SX} = 0.04$, $YF_{X/S} =$ 0.4 g/g.

Compare and comment on the results.

12.16. Formation of lactic acid from glucose is realized in a continuous culture by *Streptococcus lactis*. The following information was obtained from experimental studies.

$S_0 = 5$ g/L, $\mu_{max} = 0.2\ h^{-1}$, $K_S = 200$ mg/L, $k_d = 0.002\ h^{-1}$, $YF_{X/S} = 0.4$ g-X/g-S, $\mu_P = 0.1$ g-P/(g-X/h).

(a) Plot the variations of S, X, P, DX, and DP with dilution rate.

(b) Determine (graphically) the optimum dilution rate maximizing the productivities of biomass (DX) and the product (DP).

12.17. In a two-stage chemostat system, the volumes of the first and second reactors are $V_1 = 500$ L and $V_2 = 300$ L, respectively. The first reactor is used for biomass production and the second is for a secondary metabolite formation. The feed flow rate to the first reactor is $Q = 100$ L/h, and the glucose concentration in the feed is $S = 5.0$ g/L. Use the following constants for the cells: $\mu_{max} = 0.3\ h^{-1}$, $K_S = 0.1$ g/L, $YF_{X/S} = 0.4$ g-cells/g-glucose. Assuming that the endogenous metabolism rate is proportional to the growth rate and the yield factor includes the substrate consumption due to extracellular product formation as a result of the endogenous metabolism.

(a) Determine cell and glucose concentrations in the effluent of the first stage.

(b) Assume that growth is negligible in the second stage due to the exhaustion of minor nutrients required for cell growth and the specific rate of product formation is $\mu_P = 0.02$ g-P/(g-cell·h) and $YF_{P/S} = 0.6$ g-P/g-S. Determine the product and substrate concentrations in the effluent of the second reactor.

12.18. An industrial wastewater stream is fed to a stirred-tank reactor continuously and the cells are recycled back to the reactor from the bottom of the sedimentation tank placed after the reactor. The system parameters are given by: $Q = 100$ L/h; $S_0 = 5000$ mg/L; $\mu_{max} = 0.25\ h^{-1}$; $K_S = 200$ mg/L; R (recycle ratio) $= 0.6$; c_R (cell concentration factor) $= 2$; $YF_{X/S} = 0.4$. The effluent concentration is desired to be 100 mg/L.

(a) Determine the required reactor volume.

(b) Determine the cell concentration in the reactor and in the recycle stream.

(c) If the residence time is 2 h in the sedimentation tank, determine the volume of the sedimentation tank and cell concentration in the effluent of the sedimentation tank.

12.19. Consider the batch growth data in Table P12.19 with a complex medium. You have available three tanks of different volumes: 900, 600, and 300 L. Given a flow rate of 100 L/h, what configuration of tanks would maximize the production of the secondary metabolite P?

TABLE P12.19

Time, h	X, g/L	P, g/L
0	0.3	<0.01
3	1.0	<0.01
6	2.3	<0.01
8	4.0	0.010
9	5.1	0.025
10	6.5	0.060
10.5	7.0	
11	7.4	0.10
12	7.7	0.17
13	7.8	0.26
14		0.36
15	8.0	0.47
16	8.0	0.54
17		0.58
18		0.60

12.20. A wastewater stream of $Q = 1\ m^3/h$ with substrate at 2000 mg/L is treated in an upflow packed bed containing immobilized bacteria in the form of biofilm on small ceramic particles. The effluent substrate level is desired to be 30 mg/L. The rate of substrate removal is given by the following equation:

$$r_S = -\frac{r_{max}XS}{K_S + S}$$

The particles are very small and the immobilized bacteria are of a very thin film and thus the effectiveness factor can be considered to be 100%. By using the following information, determine the required height of the column (H) for a bed diameter of 2 m.

$$r_{max} = 0.5\ h^{-1},\ X = 0.1\ g/m^2,\ K_S = 200\ mg/L,\ a = 100\ m^2/m^3$$

12.21. Table P12.21 shows data for the production of a secondary metabolite from a small-scale batch reactor. There is a stream of substrate available at 250 L/h of the same medium as that generating the batch fermentation data. Assume that two reactors, each with 2000-L working volume, are available. You will use exactly the same culture conditions (medium, pH, temperature, and so on) as in the batch reactor.

(a) Determine the outlet concentration of the product.

(b) Compare that obtained in part (a) to the value predicted if a single 4000-L reactor was used.

TABLE P12.21

Time, h	X, g/L	P, g/L
0	0.25	
1	0.28	
2	0.57	
3	0.87	
4	1.29	
5	1.85	
6	2.56	0
7	3.40	0.004
8	4.53	0.019
9	5.89	0.054
10	7.97	0.120
11	9.05	0.207
12	9.44	0.324
13	9.63	0.481
14	9.78	0.703
15	9.86	0.916
16	9.93	1.008
17	9.95	1.055
18	9.95	1.073
19	9.95	1.077
20	9.95	1.077

12.22. The BOD_5 (Biological Oxygen Demand in 5 days) value of a wastewater feed stream to an activated sludge unit is $S_0 = 0.30$ g/L, and the effluent is desired to be $S = 0.03$ g/L. The feed flow rate is $Q = 2 \times 10^7$ L/day. For the recycle ratio of $R = 0.5$ and a steady-state biomass concentration of $X = 5$ g/L, calculate the following:

(a) Required reactor volume (V).

(b) Biomass concentration in recycle (X_R).

(c) Solids concentration ratio c_R.

(d) Determine the daily oxygen requirement.

Use the following kinetic parameters:

$$\mu_{max} = 1.5\ \text{day}^{-1};\ K_S = 0.4\ \text{g/L},\ YF_{X/S} = 0.50\ \text{g-X/g-BOD},\ k_d = 0.07\ \text{day}^{-1}$$

12.23. For the activated sludge unit shown in Fig. P12.23, the specific growth rate constants of cells are given by $\mu_{max} = 1\ h^{-1}$, $K_S = 0.01$ g/L, $YF_{X/S} = 0.50$ g-X/g-S, $k_d = 0.05$/h, and the feed conditions are $Q = 500$ L/h, $R = 0.4$, $y_s = 0.1$, $X_e = 0$, $V = 1500$ L, and $S_0 = 1$ g/L.
(a) Calculate the substrate concentration (S) in the reactor at steady state.
(b) Calculate the cell concentration(s) in the reactor.
(c) Calculate X_R and S_R in the recycle stream.

12.24. Wastewater containing terephthalic acid (TA) is treated using two aerobic sludge tanks in series. The first tank was 12 L in size and the second was 24 L. It is determined to reduce the TA concentration from 5 g-COD/L to below 0.1 g-COD/L. The Monod growth parameters are given by $\mu_{max} = 1.61$/day and $K_S = 0.25$ g/L. The results of the experiments were reported in the following manner:

$$\text{Tank 1:} \frac{X}{D(S_0 - S)} = \frac{0.16}{S} + 0.62$$

$$\text{Tank 2:} \frac{X}{D(S_0 - S)} = \frac{0.3}{S} + 5.4$$

Design a CSTR sludge system to handle a wastewater flow of 1000 m^3/day with a loading of 5.6 kg-COD/m^3.

12.25. An industrial waste with an inlet BOD_5 of 0.8 g/L must be treated to reduce the exit BOD_5 level to no greater than 0.02 g/L. The inlet flow rate is 400 m^3/h. Kinetic parameters have been estimated for waste as $\mu_{max} = 0.20\ h^{-1}$; $K_S = 0.05$ g-BOD_5/L, $YF_{X/S} = 0.50$ g-CS600/g-BOD_5, $k_d = 0.005\ h^{-1}$. A waste treatment unit of 3200 m^3 is available. Assume a recycle ratio of 0.40 and $X_e = 0$. If you operate the concentrator at $c_R = 2$, find S and determine if sufficient BOD_5 removal is attained in a well-mixed activated sludge process to meet specifications. What will be X (or CS600) and the sludge production rate from this process?

12.26. Consider a well-mixed waste treatment system (Fig. P12.26). The system is operated with a reactor of 1000 L and flow rate of 100 L/h. The separator concentrates biomass by a factor of 2. The recycle ratio is 0.7. The kinetic parameters are $\mu_{max} = 0.5\ h^{-1}$; $K_S = 0.2$ g/L, $YF_{X/S} = 0.50$ g-X/g-S, $k_d = 0.05$/h. What is the exit substrate concentration for $S_0 = 1$ g/L?

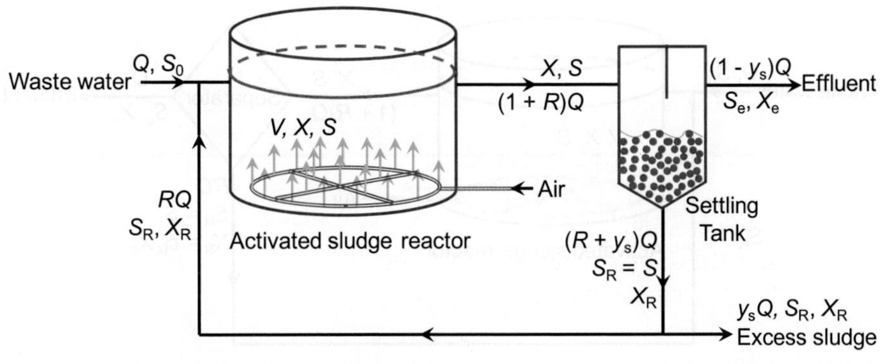

FIGURE P12.23 A schematic of an activated sludge unit.

12.27. A CSTR is being operated at steady state. The cell growth follows the Monod growth law without inhibition. The exiting substrate and cell concentrations are measured as a function of the dilution rate, and the results are shown in Table P12.27. Of course, measurements are not taken until steady state is achieved after each change in the flow rate. Neglect substrate consumption for maintenance and the death rate and assume that $YF_{P/S}$ is zero. For run 4, the entering substrate concentration was 50 g/L and the volumetric flow rate of the substrate was 2 L/s.

TABLE P12.27

Run	S, g/L	D, s^{-1}	X, g/L
1	1	1	0.9
2	3	1.5	0.7
3	4	1.6	0.6
4	10	1.8	4

(a) Determine the Monod growth parameters: μ_{max} and K_S.
(b) Estimate the yield factor, $YF_{X/S}$ and $YF_{S/X}$.

12.28. The growth of bacterium *Stepinpoopi* can be described by the logistic growth law

$$\mu_G = \mu_{max}\left(1 - \frac{X}{X_\infty}\right)$$

with the maximum specific growth rate $\mu_{max} = 0.5\ h^{-1}$ and the carrying capacity $X_\infty = 20$ g/L. The substrate is in excess.
(a) The cell growth is to be carried out in a 2-L batch reactor. Plot the growth rate and cell concentration (g/L) as functions of time after inoculation of 0.4 g of cells into the reactor (ignore the lag phase).
(b) The batch vessel in part (a) is to be turned into a chemostat. Derive an equation for the washout rate. Plot the cell concentration as a function of dilution rate.

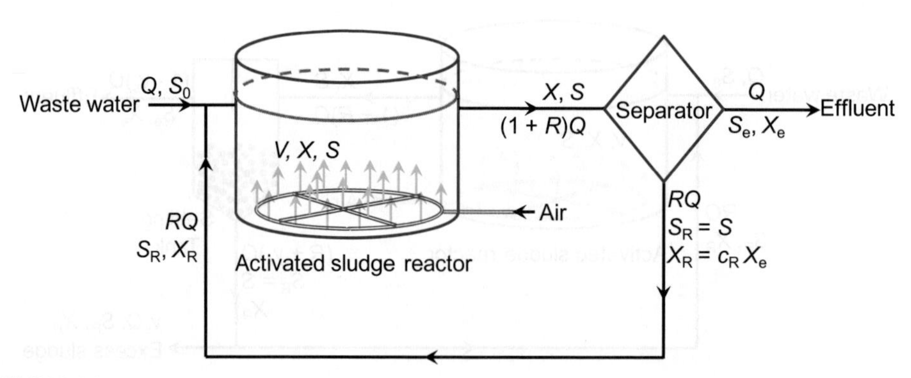

FIGURE P12.26 A schematic of waste treatment system.

12.29. Cell growth with uncompetitive substrate inhibition is taking place in a chemostat. The cell growth rate law for this system is

$$\mu_G = \frac{\mu_{max} S}{K_S + S(1 + S/K_I)}$$

with $\mu_{max} = 1.5\ h^{-1}$, $K_S = 1\ g/L$, $K_I = 50\ g/L$, $S_0 = 30\ g/L$, $YF_{X/S} = 0.08$ g-cell/g-S, $X_0 = 0.5\ g/L$.

(a) Make a plot of the steady-state cell concentration X as a function of D.

(b) Make a plot of the substrate concentration S as a function of D on the same graph as that used for part (a).

12.30. The data in Table P12.30 were obtained for *Pyrodictium occultum* at 98 °C. Run 1 was carried out in the absence of yeast extract and run 2 with yeast extract. Both runs initially contained Na_2S. The vol % of the growth product H_2S collected above the broth was reported as a function of time as shown in Table P12.30.

TABLE P12.30

Run 1	Time, h	0	10	15	20	30	40	50	60	70
	Cell Density, cells/L	0.27	0.28	1.5	7.0	40.0	60.0	71.5	60.0	52.5
	$\%H_2S$	0.5	0.8	1.0	1.2	6.8	4.7	7.5	8.0	8.2
Run 2	Time, h	0	5	10	15	20	30	40	50	60
	Cell Density, cells/L	0.27	0.70	1.1	8.0	25.0	35.0	35.0	25.0	
	$\%H_2S$	0.1	0.7	0.7	0.8	1.2	4.3	7.5	11.0	12.3

(a) What is the lag time with and without the yeast extract?

(b) What is the difference in the maximum specific growth rates, μ_{max}, of the bacteria with and without the yeast extract?

(c) How long is the stationary phase?

(d) During which phase does the majority production of H_2S occur?

(e) The liquid reactor volume in which these batch experiments were carried out was 0.2 L. If this reactor were converted to a chemostat, what would be the corresponding washout rate?

CHAPTER

13

Fed-Batch Cultivation

OUTLINE

The fed-batch technique was originally devised by yeast producers in the early 1900s to regulate the growth in batch culture of *Saccharomyces cerevisiae*. It was observed that in the presence of high concentrations of malt, an undesired by-product, ethanol, was produced,

http://dx.doi.org/10.1016/B978-0-444-59525-6.00013-5

while at low concentrations of malt, the yeast growth was limited. The sudden change in the production of ethanol is due to the overflow metabolism of the cells and also known as Crabtree effect in Chapters 10 and 12. The problem was then solved by a controlled feeding regime, so that yeast growth remained high but under substrate-limited conditions.

The fedbatch concept was then extended to the production of other products, such as some enzymes, antibiotics, growth hormones, microbial cells, vitamins, polyhydroxyalkanoate, amino acids, and other organic acids. Basically, cells are grown under a batch regime for some time (seed culture preparation), usually until close to the end of the exponential growth phase. At this point, the reactor is fed with a solution of substrates, without the removal of culture fluid. This feed is balanced to keep the growth of the microorganisms at a desired specific growth rate, while reduces simultaneously the production of undesired by-products (especially that can be growth or product production inhibitory and make the system less effective). These by-products may also affect the culture environment in such a way that might lead to early cell death even though sufficient nutrients are available or are still being provided. A fed-batch is useful in achieving high concentration of products as a result of high concentration of cells for a relative large span of time. Two cases can be considered: the production of a growth-associated product and the production of a non-growth-associated product. In the first case, it is desirable to extend the growth phase as much as possible, minimizing the changes in the fermentor as far as specific growth rate, production of the product of interest and avoiding the production of by-products.

For non-growth-associated products, the fed-batch would be having two phases: a growth phase in which the cells are grown to the required concentration and then a production phase in which a carbon source and other requirements for production are fed to the fermentor. This case is also of particular interest for recombinant inducible systems: the cells are grown to high concentrations and then induced to express the recombinant product.

Also, considering that plasmid stability (Chapter 15) is very often guaranteed by the presence of an antibiotic marker gene and that the lifetime of this antibiotic in a fermentor can be limited, it might be of interest to use the fed-batch concept to feed this same antibiotic continuously so that the presence of the plasmid in the cells is more of a reliable fact. Fed-batch fermentations can be the best option for some systems in which the nutrients or any other substrates are only sparingly soluble or are too toxic to add the whole requirement for a batch process at the start.

Finally, in fermentations such as mycelial culture, the increase of viscosity with time can be compensated by the addition of relatively small quantity of water during the fermentation time, although the efficacy of this protocol is controversial among researchers. Many factors are involved in the regulation of a fed-batch reactor. As an example, however, the feed rate can be varied to control the concentrations of nutrients in the bioreactor.

Fig. 13.1 shows a schematic of fed-batch reactor operation. Fed-batch reactor operation is also commonly seen when a continuous reactor is being charged (i.e. start-up of chemostat). To ensure that a favorable steady state is achieved, a well mixed continuous flow reactor (commonly known as CSTR for chemical transformations and chemostat for biotransformations) must be run in a semi-batch mode until the desired reaction conditions are reached inside the reactor before the full continuous operation is implemented. This is a control strategy for CSTR operation. In other cases, fed-batch operation is an alternative to continuous operations. This can occur in bioprocess industry where batch operations are common. Batch growth is an uncontrolled growth. To implement control on cell growth, fed-batch becomes a viable option.

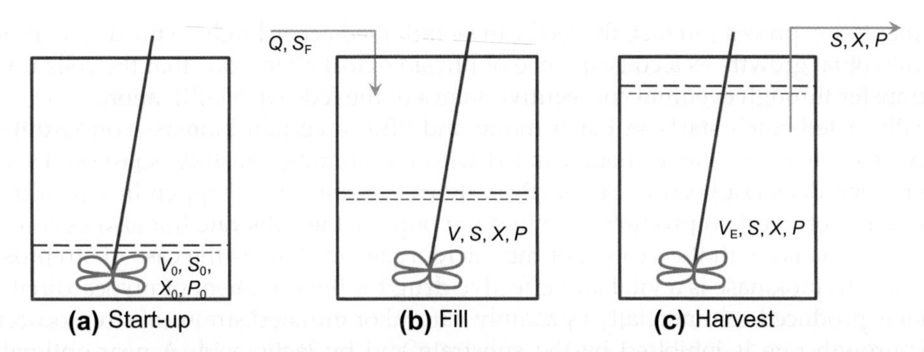

FIGURE 13.1 A schematic of fed-batch reactor operation. (a) Reactor preparation, seed culture ready; (b) reactor filling with a sterile concentrated substrate; (c) harvest both before starting the next round of filling operation.

In Chapter 11, we learned how cells grow in a batch reactor and microbial growth kinetics. In a batch reactor, one is not exerting any control on the system other than the environmental conditions such as temperature. In Chapter 12, we learned cell growth and fermentation in chemostats, where cell growth and/or fermentation is actively controlled by the feed of the substrate(s) into and products withdrawing from the reactor. Continuous fermentation is only suitable for cases where mass production is warranted, such as fuel ethanol fermentation. In most bioreactor operations for food, medicine, and specialty chemical production, batch operations are preferred due to the relatively small production demands and the concern over uncertainty in feed variation. How do we exert control over a batch reactor? The alternative is by modifying the batch operation with a gradual feeding or withdrawing scheme as was discovered by the yeast producers in the early 1900s. In this chapter, we shall focus on the control scheme for batch reactors and provide means to increase productivity up to a modest level.

While batch operation may be desired for extremely valuable product handling, the lack of control in batch operations can significantly reduce the productivity and product yield. In this case, fed-batch operation is desired. For example, when cells are strongly inhibited by the substrate, low substrate concentration is desired in the reactor. However, low substrate concentration also means low biomass concentration is achievable. To counter this conflict, one can feed rich medium gradually into the reactor to maintain growth at low substrate concentrations. The controlled addition of the nutrient directly affects the growth rate of the culture and allows the avoidance of overflow metabolism (or Crabtree effect: formation of side metabolites, such as acetate for *Escherichia coli*, lactic acid in cell cultures, ethanol in *S. cerevisiae*) and oxygen limitation (anaerobiosis). Therefore, fed-batch operation can be employed to control the growth and/or desired product yield.

The feeding mode influences a fed-batch fermentation by defining the growth rate of the microorganisms and the effectiveness of the carbon cycle for product formation and minimization of by-product formation. Inherently related with the concept of fed-batch, the feeding mode allows many variances in how substrate and/or medium is introduced into the reactor and consequently better control over inhibitory effects of the substrate and/or product. The feed mode can be defined based on an open loop, if an exact mathematical model is at disposal (not very common and usually insufficient), a feedback control (e.g. pH or DO) or in any other way depending on the specific kinetics of each fermentation and even within the time frame of the fermentation process. In fact, the feed can be modified accordingly to the different phases of the microbial growth, as a consequence of physiological alterations that the cells undergo upon transfer through eventual consecutive stages of the fed-batch cultivation.

Usually, a fed-batch starts in batch mode and after a certain biomass concentration or substrate consumption, the fermentor is fed with the limiting substrate solution. However, that approach does not need to be the absolute rule. Some cases happen in which the rate of production of a certain product is limited not only by the substrate but also by a primary product, associated with the growth of the microorganism. That is the case of streptokinase formation. Streptokinase is a vital and effective drug for the treatment of myocardinal infection that is produced commercially by mainly natural or mutated strains of streptococci. The specific growth rate is inhibited by the substrate and by lactic acid. A near-optimal feed policy based on a chemotaxis algorithm has been established that defines an initial decreasing feeding phase, followed by a batch fermentation with no more added substrate in the medium. The starting point was the data provided by the batch fermentations and the feed was defined as being a polynomial function of time. By iterative calculations and having the maximum allowable volume of the fermentor as time limits, a feed strategy was defined yielding a 12% increase in streptokinase activity over batch fermentations. This type of approach has also been suggested for ethanol production by *S. cerevisiae* that follows the same kinetics.

Finally, the feed can be continuous, can be provided in pulses, as a shot feeding, single or multisubstrate, increasing linearly, be exponential or constant with time. The design of the feed solution may follow a conventional approach – in which the nutrients are more concentrated as compared with the growing medium in the fermentor – or follows a quantitative design in such a way that depletion or accumulation of nutrients can be avoided or reduced.

Substrate limitation offers the possibility to control the reaction rates to avoid technological limitations connected to the cooling of the reactor and oxygen transfer. Substrate limitation also allows the metabolic control, to avoid osmotic effects, catabolite repression, and overflow metabolism of side products. Fig. 13.2 shows the feed rate as a function of time for fed-batch operations. There are many ways of implement control on the fermentation via feed and at least three different operation strategies for fed-batch are useful: 1) constant

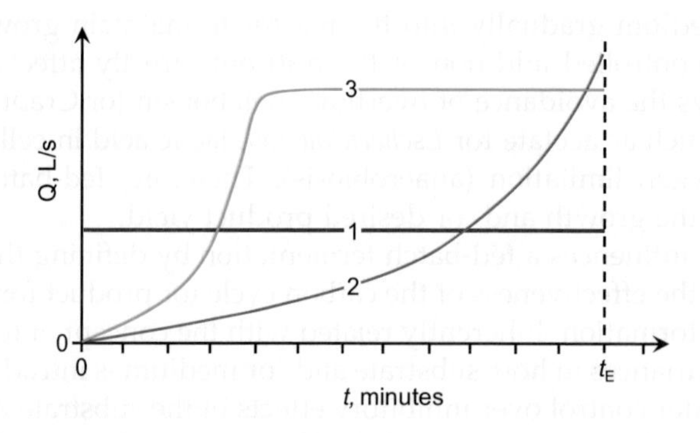

FIGURE 13.2 A schematic commonly employed feed rate strategies for a fed-batch reactor operation. 1) Constant feed rate, this is the easiest one to implement and control; 2) exponential feed rate; and 3) exponential – constant feed strategy.

feed rate, 2) exponential feed rate, and 3) exponential and then constant feed rate strategy. The constant rate is the easiest control strategy and commonly used. The exponential feed operation can be at any rate, up to the maximum rate in the exponential growth phase of a batch growth. This is the case that closely resembles a chemostat operation (Chapter 12). The exponential feed requires the feed rate to increase exponentially and can be demanding for the feeding system. One way to alleviate the difficulty is to feed exponentially first to increase the feed rate at an acceptable level and then maintain a constant feed. Usually, maximum growth rate is not optimal as by-product production can be high, which is the main drawback of batch fermentation.

During fed-batch operations, besides the substrate and product concentrations change with time in the reactor, the total reaction mixture (volume) also changes with time. Therefore, comparing to common desired batch and/or flow reactors, there are at least three balance equations needing to be dealt with before the problem can be solved.

13.1. DESIGN EQUATIONS

Evaluation of batch reactor performance relies on extensive mass and energy balances. We have learned in Chapter 3 how mass and energy balances work. Let us apply the mass and energy balances in this section for a fed-batch reactor. The control volume is shown in Fig. 13.3.

13.1.1. Overall Mass Balance in the Reactor

$$\rho_F Q - 0 + 0 = \frac{d(\rho V)}{dt} \tag{13.1}$$

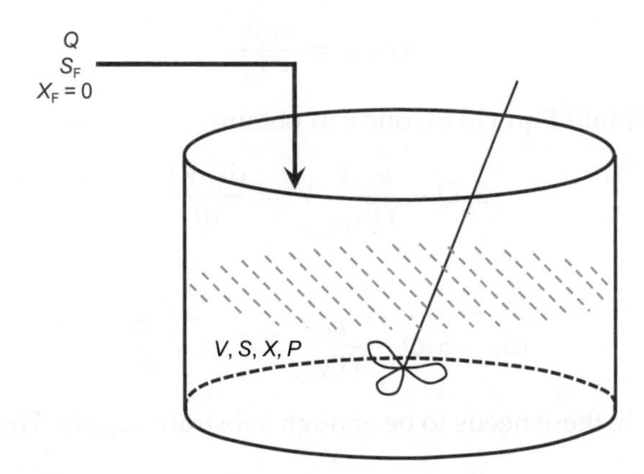

FIGURE 13.3 A schematic of fed-batch reactor. The feed volumetric rate is Q, which is sterile $X_F = 0$ and contains the substrate at a concentration of S_F. The volume of the media in the batch reactor is V, with the biomass concentration being X, substrate concentration being S and a cellular product concentration of P.

Assuming that the density of the feed and that in the reactor are identical, i.e. $\rho_F = \rho$, we have

$$V = V_0 + \int_0^t Q\mathrm{d}t \tag{13.2}$$

where V_0 is the volume of the culture in the fermentor at time $t = 0$. If the feed rate is constant,

$$V = V_0 + Qt \tag{13.3}$$

To mimic the maximum growth, one may resort to exponential feed, i.e.

$$Q = Q_0 \exp(bt) \tag{13.4}$$

where b is a constant. Substituting Eqn (13.4) into Eqn (13.2), we obtain the volume change for an exponential feed,

$$V = V_0 + \frac{Q_0}{b}\left(e^{bt} - 1\right) \tag{13.5}$$

For any other elaborate feeding scheme, one can integrate Eqn (13.2) to obtain the change of culture volume with time.

13.1.2. Mass Balance of the Substrate in the Reactor

$$S_F Q - 0 + r_S V = \frac{\mathrm{d}(SV)}{\mathrm{d}t} \tag{13.6}$$

where S_F is the substrate concentration in the feed. Assuming that all the substrate consumed is for cells to grow, the yield factor is defined as

$$YF_{X/S} = \frac{\mu_G X}{-r_S} \tag{13.7}$$

Substituting Eqn (13.7) into Eqn (13.6), one can obtain

$$S_F Q - \frac{\mu_G X}{YF_{X/S}} V = \frac{\mathrm{d}(SV)}{\mathrm{d}t} \tag{13.8}$$

or

$$(S_F - S)Q - \frac{\mu_G}{YF_{X/S}} XV = V\frac{\mathrm{d}S}{\mathrm{d}t} \tag{13.9}$$

To maintain cell growth, there needs to be enough substrate supply. Thus, Eqn (13.8) implies that

$$S_F Q - \frac{\mu_G X}{YF_{X/S}} V \geq 0 \tag{13.10}$$

or

$$S_F Q \geq \mu_G \frac{XV}{YF_{X/S}} \tag{13.11}$$

If we neglect the cell maintenance cost or cell death, the yield factor can account for all the substrate consumption. From the definition of the yield factor, we obtain

$$YF_{X/S} = \frac{\text{total biomass generated}}{\text{total substrate utilized}} = \frac{XV - X_0 V_0}{S_0 V_0 + \int_0^t S_F Q dt - SV} \tag{13.12}$$

where S_0 and X_0 are the concentrations of the substrate and biomass at time $t = 0$ inside the reactor. Eqn (13.12) can be reduced to

$$XV = YF_{X/S}[(S_F - S)V + (S_0 - S_F)V_0] + X_0 V_0 \tag{13.13}$$

Thus, combining Eqns (13.13) and (13.9), we can solve for the cell biomass and substrate concentrations. Substituting Eqn (13.13) into Eqn (13.9), we obtain

$$\frac{dS}{dt} = \frac{(S_F - S)Q - \mu_G \left[\left(S_F - S)V + (S_0 - S_F)V_0 + \frac{X_0 V_0}{YF_{X/S}} \right] \right.}{V} \tag{13.14}$$

Eqn (3.14) is applicable when cell maintenance or cell death is zero. If the cell maintenance or cell death is not negligible, we then need to perform a separate cell mass balance.

13.1.3. Mass Balance on the Cell Biomass

$$X_F Q - 0 + r_X V = \frac{d(XV)}{dt} \tag{13.15}$$

where X_F is the concentration of cells in the feed and is usually zero or sterile. Thus, Eqn (13.15) can be reduced to

$$(\mu_G - k_d)XV = \mu_{net}XV = r_X V = \frac{d(XV)}{dt} = X\frac{dV}{dt} + V\frac{dX}{dt} \tag{13.16}$$

or

$$\frac{dX}{dt} = \left(\mu_G - k_d - \frac{Q}{V} \right) X \tag{13.17}$$

13.1.4. Mass Balance on Extracellular Products

$$P_F Q - 0 + r_P V = \frac{d(PV)}{dt} \tag{13.18}$$

which can be reduced to

$$\frac{d(PV)}{dt} = r_P V + P_F Q \tag{13.19a}$$

or

$$\frac{dP}{dt} = r_P + \frac{Q}{V}(P_F - P) \tag{13.19b}$$

13.1.5. Energy Balance in the Reactor

Eqn (3.133) is the universal energy balance equation:

$$\sum_{j=1}^{N_S} F_{j0}(H_j - H_{j0}) + V\sum_{i=1}^{N_R} r_i \Delta H_{Ri} + \sum_{j=1}^{N_S} C_{Pj} n_j \frac{dT}{dt} - \frac{d(pV)}{dt} = \dot{Q} - \dot{W}_s \tag{3.133}$$

The reaction mixture is slurry (cells suspended in the liquid medium). We assume that the heat capacities are constant (or we use the average heat capacities) and the pressure remains unchanged, then Eqn (3.133) is reduced to

$$\rho_F Q C_{PF}(T - T_F) + Vr\Delta H_R + C_P \rho V \frac{dT}{dt} - p\frac{dV}{dt} = \dot{Q} - \dot{W}_s \tag{13.20}$$

Furthermore, the heat transfer into the reactor is given by

$$\dot{Q} = UA(T_c - T) \tag{13.21}$$

where T_c is the temperature of the fluid outside of the reactor, U is the heat transfer coefficient, and A is the heat transfer area. The shaft work is given by

$$\dot{W}_s = -Q_{E,\text{Stirrer}} \tag{13.22}$$

where $Q_{E,\text{Stirrer}}$ is the energy input rate of the stirrer. Substituting Eqns (13.22), (13.21), and (13.1) into Eqn (13.20), we obtain

$$C_P \rho V \frac{dT}{dt} = -\rho_F Q C_{PF}(T - T_F) - Vr\Delta H_R + p\frac{\rho_F Q - V\frac{d\rho}{dt}}{\rho} + UA(T_c - T) + Q_{E,\text{Stirrer}} \tag{13.23}$$

Assuming $\rho_F = \rho$, we have

$$C_P \rho V \frac{dT}{dt} = -\rho Q C_{PF}(T - T_F) - Vr\Delta H_R + pQ + UA(T_c - T) + Q_{E,\text{Stirrer}} \tag{13.24}$$

Therefore, the temperature in the reactor is affected by the feed, heat of reaction, reactor outside temperature, and the stirrer input power.

13.2. IDEAL ISOTHERMAL FED-BATCH REACTORS

Each balance equation governs the change of composition for one component (or temperature) in the reactor. These compositions affect each other in the reactor due to the work of the cells as well as the feed in an interactive manner. Therefore, Eqns (13.9), (13.17), and (13.19) need to be solved simultaneously to determine the cell biomass, substrate, and extracellular product concentrations in the reactor. An automatic integrator such as the ODExLIMS is useful in this regard.

Figs. 13.4 through 13.8 show how the biomass production (or accumulation) XV, substrate accumulation SV, and the concentrations of the substrate S and biomass X in the reactor for different feed (constant feed rate vs exponential feed rate), growth (without maintenance or a constant specific death rate), and initial conditions. These figures can help us understand how the growth can be controlled by a feed stream.

Fig. 13.4 shows the reactor contents change for a constant feed rate equal to $\mu_{max}V_0$. Here μ_{max} is the maximum growth rate in the Monod growth equation, which is assumed to be valid. The saturation constant $K_S = 0.05\,S_F$. At the start, the concentrations of the biomass

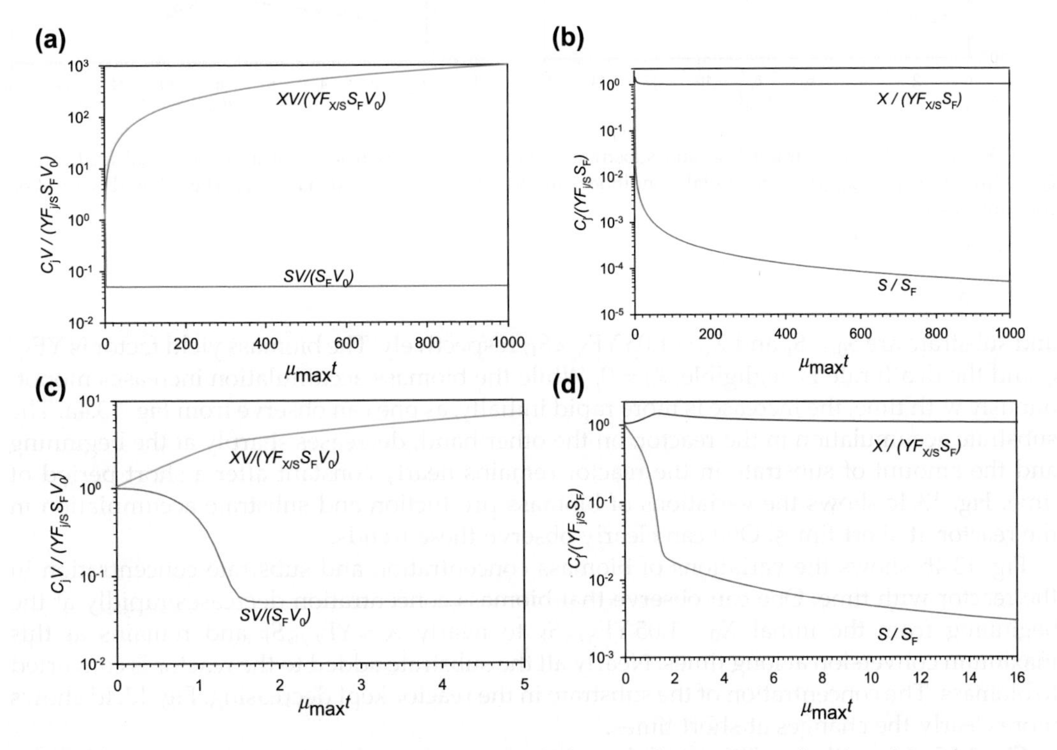

FIGURE 13.4 Biomass production and substrate accumulation in the reactor as a function of time for constant feed rate of $Q = \mu_{max}V_0$. The initial conditions are $S_0 = S_F$ and $X_0 = 1.05\,YF_{X/S}S_F$. The Monod saturation constant $K_S = 0.05\,S_F$.

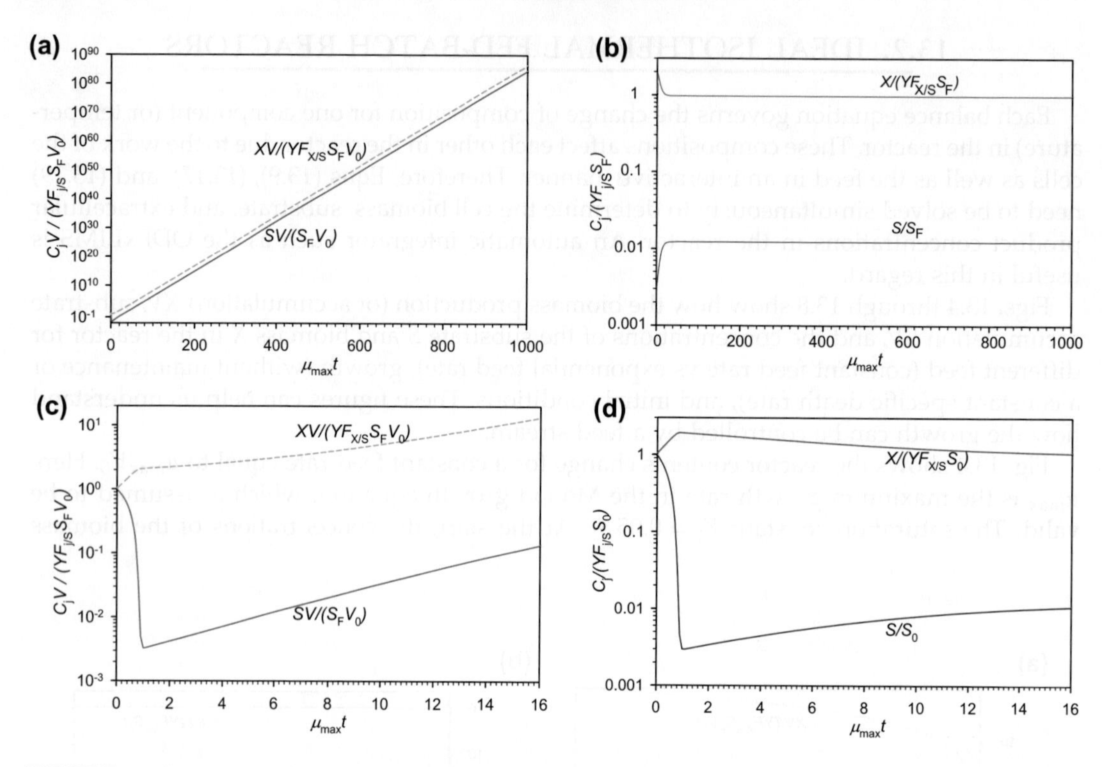

FIGURE 13.5 Biomass production and substrate accumulation in the reactor for an exponential feed rate of $Q = 0.1\mu_{max}V_0 \exp(0.2\mu_{max}t)$. The initial conditions are $S_0 = S_F$ and $X_0 = 1.05\,YF_{X/S}S_F$. The Monod saturation constant $K_S = 0.05\,S_F$.

and substrate are $S_0 = S_F$ and $X_0 = 1.05\,YF_{X/S}S_F$, respectively. The biomass yield factor is $YF_{X/S}$, and the death rate is negligible, $k_d = 0$. While the biomass accumulation increases monotonously with time, the increase is more rapid initially, as one can observe from Fig. 13.4a. The substrate accumulation in the reactor, on the other hand, decreases sharply at the beginning and the amount of substrate in the reactor remains nearly constant after a short period of time. Fig. 13.4c shows the variations of biomass production and substrate accumulation in the reactor at short times. One can clearly observe these trends.

Fig. 13.4b shows the variations of biomass concentration and substrate concentration in the reactor with time. One can observe that biomass concentration decreases rapidly at the beginning from the initial $X_0 = 1.05\,YF_{X/S}S_F$ to nearly $X = YF_{X/S}S_F$ and remains at this maximum conversion at long times. Nearly all the substrate added to the reactor is converted to biomass. The concentration of the substrate in the reactor kept decreasing. Fig. 13.4d shows more clearly the changes at short times.

Fig. 13.5 shows the variations of the reactor contents as functions of time for the same initial and growth conditions as those shown in Fig. 13.4. However, the feed rate is exponential at $Q = 0.1\mu_{max}V_0 \exp(0.2\mu_{max}t)$. This feeding rate is less than that the maximum growth

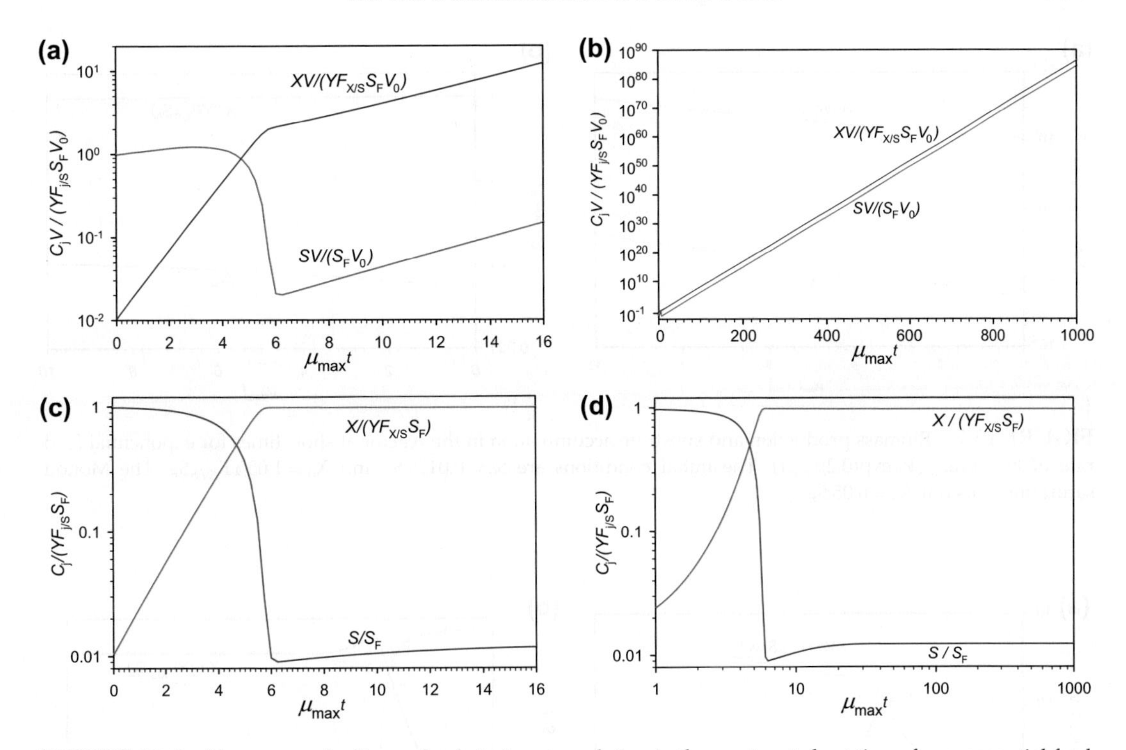

FIGURE 13.6 Biomass production and substrate accumulation in the reactor at short times for exponential feed rate of $Q = 0.1\mu_{max} V_0 \exp(0.2\mu_{max} t)$. The initial conditions are $S_0 = S_F$ and $X_0 = 0.0105\, YF_{X/S} S_F$. The Monod saturation constant $K_S = 0.05\, S_F$.

can consume. Fig. 13.5a shows that the biomass production increases sharply initially, while maintains increasing at a low rate at long time. This is similar to the constant feed rate case shown in Fig. 13.4a. The amount of the substrate in the reactor, on the other hand, decreases sharply at start (Fig. 13.5c) and then increases with time. This is different from the constant feed rate case shown in Fig. 13.4a and c. The increasing trend remains at long time as shown in Fig. 13.5a.

Fig. 13.5b and d shows the variation of substrate and biomass concentrations with time. One can observe that the biomass concentration increases sharply initially to over $2\, YF_{X/S} S_F$ (Fig. 13.5d) and then decreases to the "steady" value ~$YF_{X/S} S_F$ (Fig. 13.5b). The substrate concentration, on the other hand, decreases sharply at start from $S_0 = S_F$ to below $0.002\, S_F$ and then recovers slowly to a steady value of $S \approx 0.0125\, S_F$.

Fig. 13.6 shows the variations of the reactor contents as functions of time for the same feed and growth conditions as shown in Fig. 13.5. However, the initial biomass concentration is lowered from $1.05\, YF_{X/S} S_F$ to $0.0105\, YF_{X/S} S_F$. One can observe that the trends are similar to those in Fig. 13.6. The only differences are that the biomass concentration increases sharply at start, and it take longer to reach "steady values" of biomass and substrate concentrations.

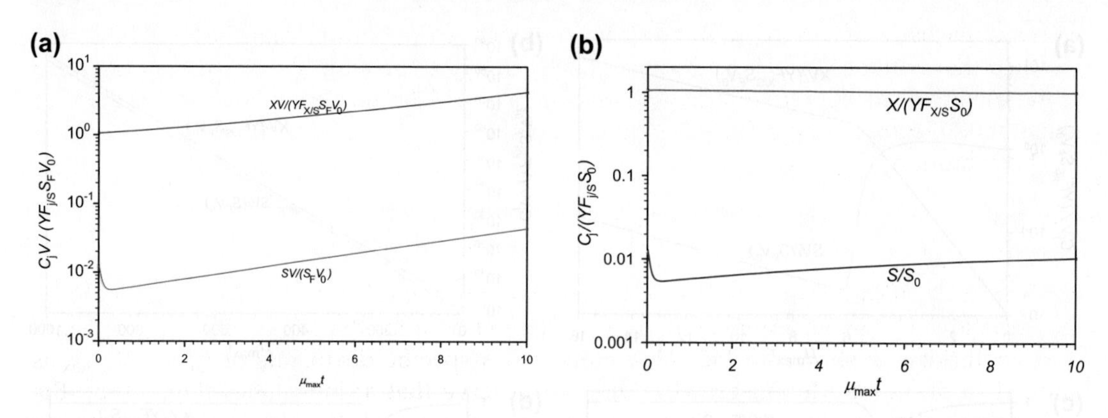

FIGURE 13.7 Biomass production and substrate accumulation in the reactor at short times for exponential feed rate of $Q = 0.1\mu_{max}V_0\exp(0.2\mu_{max}t)$. The initial conditions are $S_0 = 0.0125\,S_F$ and $X_0 = 1.05\,YF_{X/S}S_F$. The Monod saturation constant $K_S = 0.05\,S_F$.

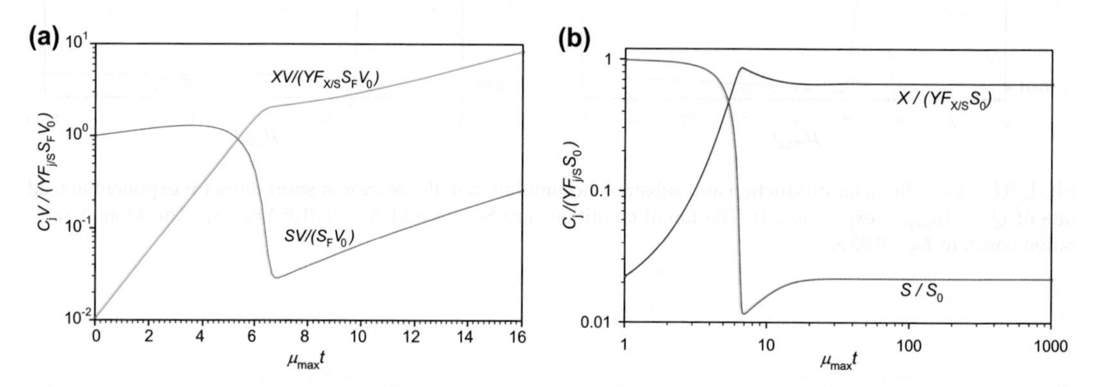

FIGURE 13.8 Biomass production and substrate accumulation in the reactor at short times for exponential feed rate of $Q = 0.1\mu_{max}V_0\exp(0.2\mu_{max}t)$ and $k_d = 0.1\,\mu_{max}$. The initial conditions are $S_0 = S_F$ and $X_0 = 0.0105\,YF_{X/S}S_F$. The Monod saturation constant $K_S = 0.05\,S_F$.

Fig. 13.7 shows the variations of the reactor contents as functions of time for the same feed and growth conditions as shown in Fig. 13.5. However, the initial substrate concentration is lowered from $S_0 = S_F$ to $S_0 = 0.0125\,S_F$. This is particularly an interesting case since one of applications of fed-batch reactor is to produce high biomass concentration for cells that do not grow in concentrated media. In this case, the biomass concentration decreases very slowly from $1.05\,YF_{X/S}S_F$ to the steady value of ~$YF_{X/S}S_F$. The substrate concentration decreases rapidly to below $0.006\,S_F$ before recovering slowly.

Fig. 13.8 shows the variations of the reactor contents as functions of time for the same feed and initial conditions as shown in Fig. 13.6. However, the specific death rate of the cells is of a finite value, at $k_d = 0.1\mu_{max}$ to $S_0 = 0.0125\,S_F$. One can observe that the trends of this case are nearly identical to those with negligible cell death rate. However, the concentration of biomass reaches a maximum and then decreases to a lesser "steady value" of 0.652308 $YF_{X/S}S_F$ than that with negligible death rate of 0.9875 $YF_{X/S}S_F$ substrate show. The concentration of the substrate reaches a minimum and recovers ~0.0214286 S_F as compared with the steady value of 0.0125 S_F for negligible cell death.

The condition of inequality

$$S_F Q \geq \mu_G \frac{XV}{YF_{X/S}} \tag{13.11}$$

can have a significant impact on fed-batch growth with a specific death rate. Fig. 13.9 shows the variations of the reactor contents as functions of time for the same initial and constant feed conditions as shown in Fig. 13.4. However, a specific death rate of $k_d = 0.01\mu_{max}$ is applied to the same Monod growth. One can observe that at long times (Fig. 13.9a), the cell accumulation in the reactor is nearly unchanged, whereas the substrate accumulation kept increasing slightly. The concentration of the substrate in the reactor, on the other hand, remains nearly unchanged, while cell concentration kept decreasing (Fig. 13.9b).

Fig. 13.9c and d shows the reactor content variations at short times. One can observe that while the cell mass accumulation increases with time, the substrate accumulation

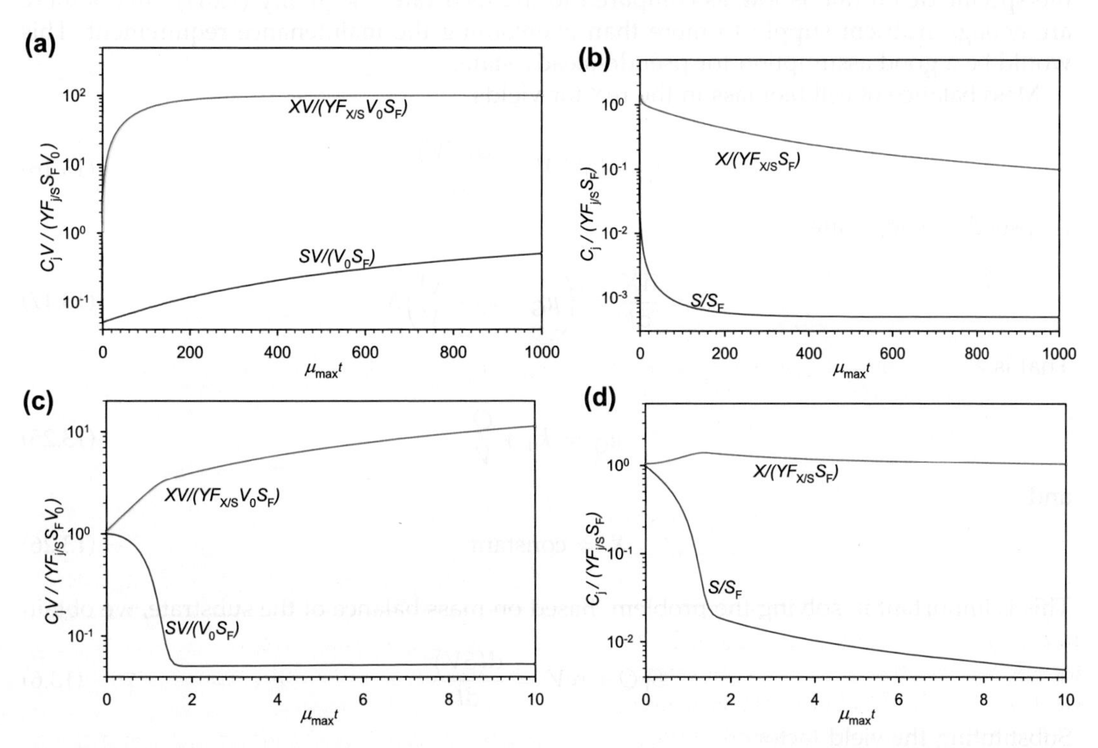

FIGURE 13.9 Biomass production and substrate accumulation in the reactor for constant feed rate of $Q = \mu_{max} V_0$. The initial conditions are $S_0 = S_F$ and $X_0 = 1.05\, YF_{X/S} S_F$. The Monod saturation constant $K_S = 0.05\, S_F$. Specific death rate $k_d = 0.01\mu_{max}$.

decreases rapidly initially and remains nearly constant (or increasing very slowly) after a short period of time (Fig. 13.9c). These trends look identical to Fig. 13.4c, where the specific death rate is zero. Fig. 13.9d show quite similar trends with Fig. 13.4d, in that the concentration of the substrate decreases monotonously, while the cell concentration reaches a plateau shortly after start and remains nearly unchanged. One can conclude based on Fig. 13.9, as compared with Fig. 13.4, that the cell concentration remains unchanged for cell growth in a fed-batch reactor with constant feed rate until the substrate supply is lower than the growth and maintenance requirement. The condition is set by Eqn (13.11).

13.3. ISOTHERMAL PSEUDO-STEADY STATE FED-BATCH GROWTH

When the fed-batch is a purpose operation for a long period of time, intuitively one would imagine that a pseudo-steady state would exist in a large reactor. However, this pseudo-steady state can be different for different initial conditions, feed, and growth kinetics. As one can infer from the previous discussions, at long times biomass concentration in the reactor is "nearly" unchanged. The constant biomass concentration at long times holds if the specific death rate is low as compared to the feed rate, inequality (13.11), that is there are enough nutrient supply to more than overcoming the maintenance requirement. This would be a good assumption for pseudo-steady state.

Mass balance of cell biomass in the reactor yields

$$(\mu_G - k_d)XV = \frac{d(XV)}{dt} \tag{13.16}$$

At pseudo-steady state,

$$0 = \frac{dX}{dt} = \left(\mu_G - k_d - \frac{Q}{V}\right)X \tag{13.17}$$

That is,

$$\mu_G = k_d + \frac{Q}{V} \tag{13.25}$$

and

$$X = \text{constant} \tag{13.26}$$

This is important in solving the problem. Based on mass balance of the substrate, we obtain

$$S_F Q + r_S V = \frac{d(SV)}{dt} \tag{13.6}$$

Substituting the yield factor

$$YF_{X/S} = \frac{\mu_G X}{-r_S} \tag{13.7}$$

into Eqn (13.6), we obtain

$$S_F Q - \frac{\mu_G}{YF_{X/S}} XV = \frac{d(SV)}{dt} \tag{13.8}$$

Substituting Eqn (13.25) into Eqn (13.8) and rearranging, we obtain

$$\frac{d(SV)}{dt} = \left(S_F - \frac{X}{YF_{X/S}}\right) Q - \frac{X}{YF_{X/S}} k_d V \tag{13.27}$$

We know that

$$V = V_0 + \int_0^t Q dt \tag{13.2}$$

Eqn (13.27) can be integrated to give

$$SV - S_0 V_0 = \left(S_F - \frac{X}{YF_{X/S}}\right)(V - V_0) - \frac{X}{YF_{X/S}} k_d \int_0^t V dt \tag{13.28}$$

which can be solved to give

$$\frac{XV}{YF_{X/S}} = \frac{(S_F - S)V - (S_F - S_0)V_0}{1 - \dfrac{V_0}{V} + \dfrac{k_d}{V}\displaystyle\int_0^t V dt} \tag{13.29}$$

Therefore, Eqns (13.25) and (13.29) can be employed to compute both XV and SV for pseudo-steady state fed-batch operations.

If Monod equation is applicable, we have

$$\mu_G = \frac{\mu_{max} S}{K_S + S} \tag{13.30}$$

Substituting into Eqn (13.30), we obtain

$$S = \frac{K_S\left(k_d + \dfrac{Q}{V}\right)}{\mu_{max} - k_d - \dfrac{Q}{V}} \tag{13.31}$$

Substituting Eqn (13.36) into Eqn (13.34), we obtain the biomass concentration. Table 13.1 shows some of the pseudo-steady state solutions for fed-batch operations.

Fig. 13.10 shows the suitability of the pseudo-steady state solution as an approximation to fed-batch operations for various cases of kinetic and feed/initial conditions. The

TABLE 13.1 Pseudo-steady state solution for fed-batch reactors when $S_F Q \geq \mu_G \frac{XV}{YF_{X/S}}$

Q	Constant feed rate: Q_0	Exponential feed: $Q_0 e^{bt}$
V	$V_0 + Q_0 t$	$V_0 + \frac{Q_0}{b}(e^{bt} - 1)$
μ_G	$k_d + \frac{Q_0}{V_0 + Q_0 t}$	$k_d + \frac{Q_0}{(V_0 - Q_0 b^{-1})e^{-bt} + Q_0 b^{-1}}$
	$k_d + \frac{Q_0}{V}$	$k_d + \frac{Q_0 - bV_0}{V} + b$
S (Monod growth)	$\frac{K_S\left(k_d + \frac{Q_0}{V_0 + Q_0 t}\right)}{\mu_{max} - k_d - \frac{Q_0}{V_0 + Q_0 t}}$	$\frac{K_S\left(k_d + \frac{Q_0}{(V_0 - Q_0 b^{-1})e^{-bt} + Q_0 b^{-1}}\right)}{\mu_{max} - k_d - \frac{Q_0}{(V_0 - Q_0 b^{-1})e^{-bt} + Q_0 b^{-1}}}$
	$\frac{K_S\left(k_d + \frac{Q_0}{V}\right)}{\mu_{max} - k_d - \frac{Q_0}{V}}$	$\frac{K_S\left(k_d + \frac{Q_0 - bV_0}{V} + b\right)}{\mu_{max} - k_d - \frac{Q_0 - bV_0}{V} - b}$
$\frac{X}{YF_{X/S}}$	$\frac{V_0(S_0 - S) + (S_F - S)Q_0 t}{Q_0 t\left(1 + \frac{1}{2}k_d t\right) + V_0 k_d t}$	$\frac{Q_0(S_F - S) + [V_0 b(S_0 - S) - Q_0(S_F - S)]e^{-bt}}{Q_0(1 + k_d b^{-1}) - [Q_0 - V_0 b k_d t + k_d b^{-1}(1 + bt)Q_0]e^{-bt}}$
	$\frac{V(S_F - S) - (S_F - S_0)V_0}{V\left(1 + \frac{1}{2}k_d t\right) - V_0\left(1 - \frac{1}{2}k_d t\right)}$	$\frac{V(S_F - S) - (S_F - S_0)V_0}{V(1 + k_d b^{-1}) - V_0[1 - k_d(t - b^{-1})] - Q_0 b^{-1} K_d t}$
PV	$P_0 V_0 + \mu_P X(V_0 + \frac{1}{2}Q_0 t)t + P_F Q_0 t$	$P_0 V_0 + \mu_P X[V_0 t + b^{-2}Q_0(e^{bt} - bt - 1)] + P_F Q_0 b^{-1}(e^{bt} - 1)$
	$P_0 V_0 + \frac{V_0 + V}{2}\mu_P X t + p_F(V - V_0)$	$P_0 V_0 + \mu_P X[(V_0 - b^{-1}Q_0)t + b^{-1}(V - V_0)] + P_F(V - V_0)$

pseudo-steady state approximations are shown as dashed lines, whereas the solid lines are full solutions. In all cases shown (constant feed rate, exponential feed, and variable initial conditions), the dashed lines are the asymptotes to the full solutions. One can observe that the agreement of the pseudo-steady state solution improves as the time of operation increases. If the initial substrate or cell biomass concentrations are far away from the pseudo-steady state conditions, a longer time (induction time) is needed. Therefore, one can feel confident that the pseudo-steady state approximation can be applied to provide a quick estimate to the batch operations. At short times, however, full solutions are still more appropriate.

In the pseudo-steady state approximation, we have used constant biomass concentration as the asymptotic condition. When cells require substantial maintenance to remain active and the feed rate is low, the asymptotic condition will eventually fail. Fig. 13.11 shows the constant feed rate for a Monod growth with a constant specific death rate. One can observe that the pseudo-steady state approximation is only valid for a relatively short period of time after the induction time. At short time, there is a difference between the full solution (solid lines) and the pseudo-steady state approximation (dashed lines) as shown in Fig. 13.11a. After the induction time, the pseudo-steady state approximation, especially the biomass accumulation, agrees reasonably well with the full solutions. However, at long times (Fig. 13.11b), the two solutions grow apart.

When feed is limited and maintenance is needed for the cells to be active, the pseudo-steady state approximation can overestimate the biomass production as shown in Fig. 13.11. When feed is limiting, the first reaction is that net cell growth stops. That is,

$$\mu_{net} = \mu_G - k_d = 0 \tag{13.32}$$

and

$$XV = \text{constant} \tag{13.33}$$

Eqn (13.32) can be rewritten as

$$\mu_G = k_d \tag{13.34}$$

To maintain this condition, the substrate concentration remains constant, that is

$$S = \text{constant} \tag{13.35}$$

Combining Monod equation (13.30) with Eqn (13.34), we obtain

$$S = \frac{K_S k_d}{\mu_{max} - k_d} \tag{13.36}$$

Since mass balance of the substrate in the reactor gives

$$(S_F - S)Q - \frac{\mu_G}{YF_{X/S}} XV = V\frac{dS}{dt} \tag{13.9}$$

we have

$$(S_F - S)Q - \frac{\mu_G}{YF_{X/S}} XV = V\frac{dS}{dt} = 0 \tag{13.37}$$

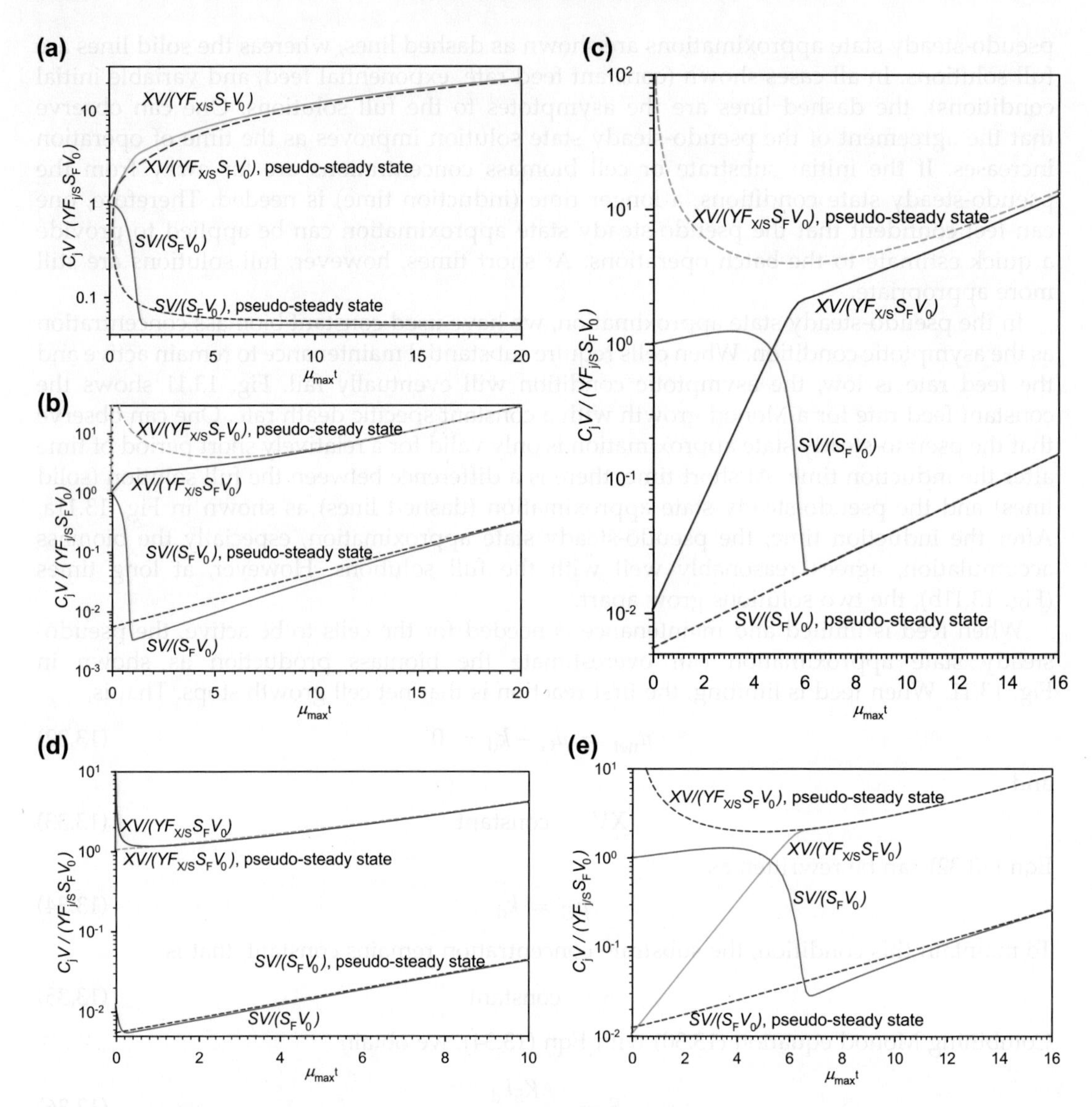

FIGURE 13.10 Suitability of pseudo-steady state assumption for biomass production in the reactor at short times with (a) a constant feed rate of $Q = \mu_{max} V_0$ and initial conditions of $S_0 = S_F$ and $X_0 = 1.05\,YF_{X/S}S_F$; (b) an exponential feed rate of $Q = 0.1\mu_{max}V_0\exp(0.2\mu_{max}t)$ and initial conditions of $S_0 = S_F$ and $X_0 = 1.05\,YF_{X/S}S_F$; (c) an exponential feed rate of $Q = 0.1\mu_{max}V_0\exp(0.2\mu_{max}t)$ and initial conditions of $S_0 = S_F$ and $X_0 = 0.0105\,YF_{X/S}S_F$; (d) an exponential feed rate of $Q = 0.1\mu_{max}V_0\exp(0.2\mu_{max}t)$ and initial conditions of $S_0 = 0.0125\,S_F$ and $X_I = 1.05\,YF_{X/S}S_F$; (e) an exponential feed rate of $Q = 0.1\mu_{max}V_0\exp(0.2\mu_{max}t)$ and initial conditions of $S_0 = S_F$ and $X_0 = 0.0105\,YF_{X/S}S_F$. In the last case (e), there is a death rate of $k_d = 0.1\mu_{max}$. In all cases, the Monod saturation constant $K_S = 0.05\,S_F$.

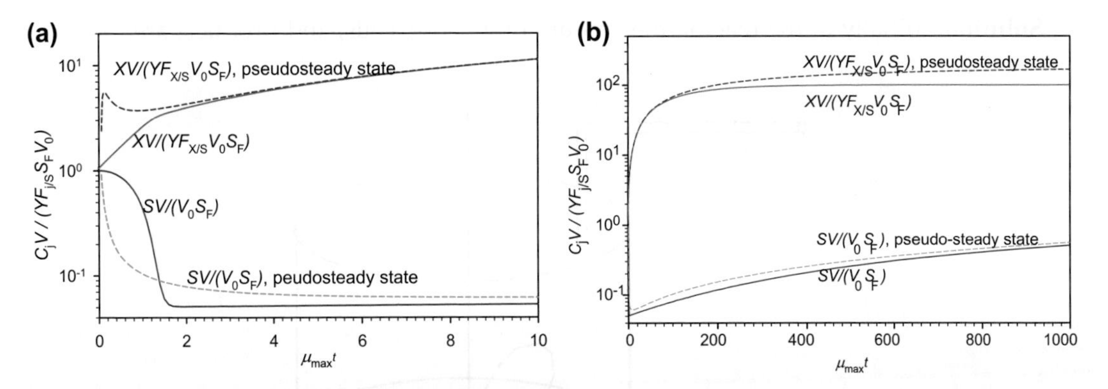

FIGURE 13.11 Suitability of pseudo-steady state assumption for biomass production in the reactor at short times for constant feed rate of $Q = \mu_{max}V_0$. The initial conditions are $S_0 = S_F$ and $X_0 = 1.05\,YF_{X/S}S_F$. The growth constants are $K_S = 0.05\,S_F$ and $k_d = 0.01\mu_{max}$.

from which the cell biomass accumulation can be obtained

$$\frac{XV}{YF_{X/S}} = \frac{(S_F - S)}{\mu_G}Q = \frac{(S_F - S)}{k_d}Q \tag{13.38}$$

Substituting Eqn (13.36) into Eqn (13.37), we obtain

$$\frac{XV}{YF_{X/S}} = \left(S_F - \frac{K_S k_d}{\mu_{max} - k_d}\right)\frac{Q}{k_d} \tag{13.39}$$

For the case shown in Fig. 13.11, Eqns (13.39) and (13.36) gave

$$\frac{XV}{S_F V_0 YF_{X/S}} = \left(1 - \frac{0.05 \times 0.01}{1 - 0.01}\right)\frac{1}{0.01} = \frac{98.95}{0.99} \approx 99.95$$

$$\frac{S}{S_F} = \frac{0.05 \times 0.01}{1 - 0.01} = \frac{0.05}{99} \approx 5.0505 \times 10^{-4}$$

Example 13-1. Penicillin is produced by *Penicillium chrysogenum* in a fed-batch culture with the intermittent addition of glucose solution to the culture medium. The initial culture volume is $V_0 = 200$ L, and glucose-containing nutrient solution is added with a flow rate of $Q = 30$ L/h. Glucose concentration in the feed solution and the initial concentrations in the reactor are $S_F = 300$ g/L, $S_0 = 1$ g/L, and $X_0 = 20$ g/L. The kinetic and yield factors of the organism are $\mu_{max} = 0.2$/h, $K_S = 0.5$ g/L, and $YF_{X/S} = 0.3$ g-dw/g-glucose. Using the pseudo-steady state approximation, we determine

(a) the culture volume at $t = 24$ h;
(b) the concentration of glucose at $t = 24$ h;
(c) the concentration and total amount of cells when $t = 24$ h;
(d) the product (penicillin) concentration in the vessel at 24 h, if $\mu_P = 0.05$ g-product/(g-cells h) and $P_0 = 0.1$ g/L.

Solution: Initially in the reactor, the amount of glucose, cells, and products are:

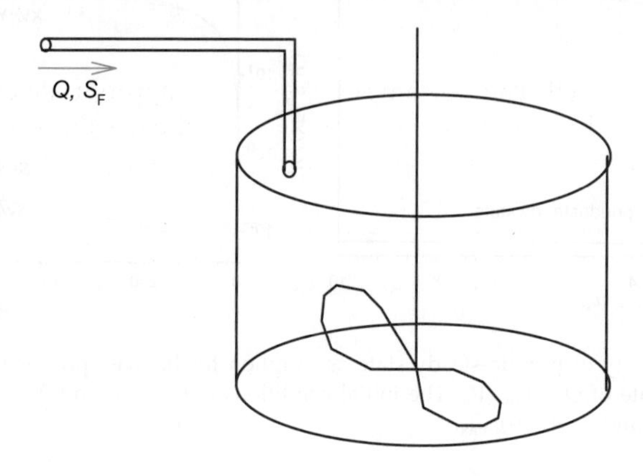

$$S_0V_0 = 1 \times 200 \text{ g} = 200 \text{ g}$$

$$X_0V_0 = 20 \times 200 \text{ g} = 400 \text{ g}$$

$$P_0V_0 = 0.1 \times 200 \text{ g} = 20 \text{ g}$$

(a) Overall mass balance of the medium in the fermentor yields

$$\rho_F Q - 0 + 0 = \frac{d(\rho V)}{dt}$$

Assuming that the density of the culture is the same as that of the feed, $\rho_F = \rho$, integration and rearrangement of the overall mass balance equation lead to

$$V = V_0 + Qt$$

$$V = 200 + 30 \times 24 \text{ L} = 920 \text{ L}$$

(b) At pseudo-steady state, the concentration of cells remains constant. From the mass balance of cells in the reactor, we obtain (13.17),

$$0 = \frac{dX}{dt} = \left(\mu_G - k_d - \frac{Q}{V}\right)X$$

Combining with Monod growth equation and negligible death rate, Eqn (13.15) gives the pseudo-steady state glucose concentration

$$S = \frac{K_S Q/V}{\mu_{max} - Q/V}$$

Therefore,

$$S = \frac{K_S}{\mu_{max} V/Q - 1} = \frac{0.5}{0.2 \times (920/30) - 1} \text{ g/L} = 0.09740 \text{ g/L}$$

(c) The concentration of cells can be computed using an appropriate equation from Table 13.1, which is derived by mass balance of glucose in the reactor. Alternatively, as there is no cell death, we can directly use yield factor from all the glucose converted in the reactor. The total amount of glucose fed to the reactor is

$$Q\, S_F\, t = 30 \times 300 \times 24 \text{ g} = 216{,}000 \text{ g}$$

Glucose in the reactor at 24 h = $VS = 920 \times 0.09740$ g = 89.61 g.
Therefore, the amount of glucose converted is

$$S_0 V_0 + Q\, S_F\, t - VS = 200 + 216{,}000 - 89.61 \text{ g} = 216{,}110.39 \text{ g}$$

which produces 0.3 ($YF_{X/S}$) × 216,110.39 g = 64,833.12 g cells.
Therefore, the total cells in the reactor is

$$XV = 4000\,(X_0 V_0) + 64{,}833.12 \text{ g} = 68{,}833.12 \text{ g}$$

Finally, the concentration of cells is

$$X = \frac{XV}{V} = \frac{68{,}833.12 \text{ g}}{920 \text{ L}} = 74.8186 \text{ g/L}$$

(d) Mass balance on the extracellular products,

$$\frac{d(VP)}{dt} = 0 - 0 + r_P V$$

which leads to

$$\frac{d(VP)}{dt} = \mu_P X(V_0 + Qt)$$

Thus,

$$P = \frac{P_0 V_0 + \mu_P X\left(V_0 + \frac{1}{2} Qt\right)t}{V} = \frac{P_0 V_0 + \frac{1}{2}\mu_P X(V_0 + V)t}{V}$$

$$P = \frac{P_0 V_0 + \frac{1}{2}\mu_P X(V_0 + V)t}{V}$$

$$= \frac{0.1 \times 200 + \frac{1}{2} \times 0.05 \times 74.8186 \times (200 + 920) \times 24}{920} \text{ g/L}$$

$$= 54.67 \text{ g/L}$$

An example of fed-batch culture is its use in some antibiotic fermentations, where a glucose solution is intermittently added to the fermentation broth due to the repression or inhibition of pathways for the production of secondary metabolites caused by high initial glucose concentrations. Fed-batch operations can be applied to other secondary metabolite fermentations such as lactic acid and other plant cell and mammalian cell fermentations, where the rate of product generation is maximal at low concentrations while chemostat is not suitable.

Fed-batch culturing is an important technique for *E. coli* cultivation to make proteins from recombinant DNA technology. To make high concentration of product, high substrate (glucose) is needed. However, with unlimited supply of substrate or at high glucose concentration, *E. coli* will grow at a maximum rate but produce organic acids (e.g. acetic acid) as by-products. The accumulation of these by-products inhibits growth. If glucose is fed at a rate that sustains the growth rate at slightly less than optimal, *E. coli* uses the glucose more efficiently and makes less by-products. Very high cell densities (50−100 g/L) can be achieved.

Fed-batch fermentations, due to an inherent flexibility of the method, provide a valuable tool in biotechnology, not only to study microorganism physiology but also to commercially produce valuable components. The higher productivities of fed-batch as compared with batch and the technical problems of continuous cultures, fed-batch seems to be a technique with increasing importance in bioreactor operations.

13.4. ADVANTAGES AND DISADVANTAGES OF FED-BATCH OPERATIONS

As we have seen that fed-batch fermentation is a production technique in between batch and continuous fermentation. A proper feed rate, with the right component constitution, is required during the process.

Fed-batch offers many advantages over batch and continuous cultures. From the concept of its implementation, it can be easily concluded that under controllable conditions and with the required knowledge of the microorganism involved in the fermentation, the feed of the required components for growth and/or other substrates required for the production of the product can never be depleted and the nutritional environment can be maintained approximately constant during the course of the batch. The production of by-products that are generally related to the presence of high concentrations of the substrate can also be avoided by limiting its concentration to the level that are required solely for the production of the desired biochemical. When high concentrations of the substrate are present, the cells get "overloaded", that is, the oxidative capacity of the cells is exceeded, and due to the Crabtree effect, products other than the one of interest are produced, reducing the efficacy of the carbon flux. Moreover, these by-products "contaminate" the desired product, such as ethanol production in baker's yeast production and to impair the cell growth reducing the fermentation time and its related productivity.

Sometimes, controlling the substrate is also important due to catabolic repression. Since this method usually permits the extension of the operating time, high cell concentrations can be achieved, and thereby, improved productivity (mass of the product produced per unit volume per unit time). This aspect is greatly favored in the production of growth-associated products.

Fed-batch operation allows the replacement of water loss by evaporation and decrease of the viscosity of the broth such as in the production of dextran and xanthan gum, by addition of a water-based feed. Also, fed-batch might be the only option for fermentations dealing with toxic or low-solubility substrates.

Comparing with chemostat operations, fed-batch operation offers a continued presence of certain substances in the reactor. When dealing with recombinant strains, fed-batch mode can guarantee the presence of an antibiotic throughout the course of the fermentation, with the intent of keeping the presence of an antibiotic-marked plasmid. Since the growth can be regulated by the feed, and knowing that in many cases a high growth rate can decrease the expression of encoded products in recombinant products, the possibility of having different feeds and feed modes makes fed-batch an extremely flexible tool for control in these cases.

Because the feed can also be multisubstrate, the fermentation environment can still be provided with required protease inhibitors that might degrade the product of interest, metabolites, and precursors that increase the productivity of the fermentation.

Finally, in a fed-batch fermentation, no special piece of equipment is required in addition to that one required by a chemostat, even considering the operating procedures for sterilization and the preventing of contamination.

A cyclic fed-batch culture has an additional advantage: the productive phase of a process may be extended under controlled conditions. The controlled periodic shifts in growth rate provide an opportunity to optimize product synthesis, particularly if the product of interest is a secondary metabolite whose maximum production takes place during the deceleration in growth.

Advantages:

- Production of high cell densities due to extension of working time (particularly important in the production of growth-associated products)
- Controlled conditions in the provision of substrates during the fermentation, particularly regarding the concentration of specific substrates as for example the carbon source
- Control over the production of by-products or catabolite repression effects due to limited provision of substrates solely required for product formation
- The mode of operation can overcome and control deviations in the growth pattern as found in batch fermentation
- Allows the replacement of water loss by evaporation
- Alternative mode of operation for fermentations leading with toxic substrates (cells can only metabolize a certain quantity at a time) or low-solubility compounds
- Increase of antibiotic-marked plasmid stability by providing the correspondent antibiotic during the time span of the fermentation
- No additional special piece of equipment is required as compared with the continuous fermentation mode of operation

Disadvantages:

- It requires previous analysis of the microorganism, its requirements, and the understanding of its physiology with the productivity

- It requires a substantial amount of operator skill for the setup, definition, and development of the process
- In a cyclic fed-batch culture, care should be taken in the design of the process to ensure that toxins do not accumulate to inhibitory levels and that nutrients other than those incorporated into the feed medium become limiting. Also, if many cycles are run, the accumulation of non-producing or low-producing variants may result
- The quantities of the components to control must be above the detection limits of the available measuring equipment.

13.5. CONSIDERATIONS IN IMPLEMENTING FED-BATCH OPERATIONS

Fed-batch operations can be implemented to mimic CSTR operations or to control culture variations. Before considering fed-batch operations, one should learn from a batch fermentation:

- Optimum abiotic conditions such as temperature, light, agitation, pH, growth medium, etc.
- Specific needs of precursors, inducers or other enrichment factors
- The different growth phases and the consumed (substrate) and produced components (product of interest and by-product)
- The relationship between the biomass and product formation (growth- or non-growth-associated product) and the oxygen uptake rates
- Limiting substrate for growth and the relationship between the specific growth rate and the limiting substrate concentration
- Eventual inhibitions from the substrate and/or product. Fed-batch is ideal for substrate-inhibited systems, whereas not proper for product-inhibited systems.

Fed-batch operation is ideal for high production rate needs, yet unsuitable for continuous cultivation, for example, due to microorganism instability. For example, cultivation of genetically engineered organism is commonly conducted with fed-batch operations to increase productivity.

13.6. EXAMPLES OF FED-BATCH USE IN INDUSTRY

The use of fed-batch culture by the fermentation industry takes advantage of the fact that the concentration of the limiting substrate may be maintained at a very low level, similar to a CSTR or a chemostat; thus,

- Avoiding repressive effects of high substrate concentration
- Controlling the organism's growth rate and consequently controlling the oxygen demand of the fermentation.

Saccharomyces cerevisiae is industrially produced using the fed-batch technique so as to maintain the glucose at very low concentrations, maximizing the biomass yield and minimizing the production of ethanol (due to Crabtree effect), the chief by-product.

Hepatitis B surface antigen (HbsAg) used as a vaccine against type B hepatitis has been purified from human plasma and expressed in recombinant yeast, being now produced commercially. Again, the production of the recombinant protein is achieved using fed-batch culture techniques very similar to that developed for *S. cerevisiae*. A cyclic method is used due to reports of superior productivity.

Penicillin production is an example for the use of fed-batch in the production of a secondary metabolite. The fermentation is divided in two phases: the rapid-growth phase during which the culture grows at the maximum specific growth rate and the slow-growth phase in which penicillin is produced. During the rapid-growth phase, an excess of glucose causes an accumulation of acid and a biomass oxygen demand greater than the aeration capacity of the fermentor, whereas glucose starvation may result in the organic nitrogen in the medium being used as a carbon source, resulting in a high pH and inadequate biomass formation. During the production phase, the feed rates utilized should limit the growth rate and oxygen consumption such that a high rate of penicillin synthesis is achieved and sufficient dissolved oxygen is available in the medium.

Some other examples are the production of thiostrepton from *Streptomyces laurentii* and the production of cellulase by *Trichoderma reesei*. The production of thiostrepton uses pH feedback control and the production of cellulase utilizes carbon dioxide production as a control factor.

13.7. PARAMETERS TO BE CONTROLLED OR MONITORED DURING FED-BATCH OPERATIONS

The ultimate aim of a fed-batch fermentation is to maximize the growth rate, the flow through the central carbon metabolism, or to reduce the overflow of carbon source to metabolic by-products. Fed-batch reactor can be controlled by a simple one-step method in which only one of the parameters is used or it can be by a dual-level control in which two parameters are used. For example, some processes require the control of different parameters at different stages of the fermentation. High-density bacterial fermentation, the production of baker's yeast and penicillin, is such an example. In these cases, two phases can be distinguished: 1) a phase in which the substrate needs to be controlled so as to avoid by-products formation and 2) a second stage in which, due to the high cell density, oxygen transfer is limiting and so, dissolved oxygen (DO) is the one to be controlled above a critical value, under which the cellular metabolism changes. The constraints switch from specific growth rate to DO content after some critical period of time in the fermentation process. The choice of each parameter is system dependent and the decision should be based on convenience and experimental data.

13.7.1. Calorimetry

Calorimetry is an excellent tool for monitoring and controlling microbial fermentations. Its main advantage is the generality of this parameter, since microbial growth is always accompanied by heat production, and the measurements are performed continuously online without introducing any disturbances to the culture. Moreover, the rate of heat production is stoichiometrically related to the rate of substrate consumption and product, including biomass formation. In many cases, it can be replaced by exhaust gas analysis, although this approach cannot be considered in anaerobic processes which proceed without formation of gaseous products.

This technique has been proved successful to indirectly determine the substrate and product concentrations continuously during aerobic batch growth of *S. cerevisiae* with glucose as the carbon and energy source. In the presence of this substrate, this yeast shows diauxic growth by initially consuming the glucose with concomitant production of ethanol and then, once glucose is depleted, using the produced ethanol as an energy source. Calorimetry can then be used to control the feed rate in such a way that ethanol formation is avoided.

Another interesting description of a temperature-based controlled reactor follows a stability criterion. The range of operation is controlled by the reactant feed temperature, which can be controlled by the flow rate of the cooling medium. Although the study has been performed in a chemical reactor, the concepts can be easily extended to a biotransformation process.

13.7.2. Specific Growth Rate

For the production of a growth-associated product, the production of a certain product is related with the specific growth rate of the producing microorganism. This is a case where chemostat (or CSTR) cultivation could be optimum should all the stability conditions met. Consequently, it is of interest to feed the fermentor in such a way that the specific growth rate remains constant. Such is the case of the production of hepatitis B surface antigen by *S. cerevisiae*. The yield of the antigen can be a factor of 10 times that of the fed-batch cultivation for the same final volume and total substrate added. Care should be given to the value of the chosen specific growth rate, because cells may not be "activated" easily, stress proteases can be produced that may degrade the product and also there might be a threshold value of specific growth rate above which there is production of by-products.

13.7.3. Substrate (Carbon and Nitrogen Source)

Substrate is a particularly important parameter to control due to eventually associated growth inhibitions and to increase the effectiveness of the carbon flux, by reducing the amount of by-products formed and the amount of carbon dioxide evolved.

13.7.4. By-product concentration

We refer a by-product as a primary product from a side reaction. Therefore, the production of by-products is undesirable because it reduces the efficacy of the carbon flux in a fermentation. The production of these components takes place whenever the substrate is provided in quantities that exceed the oxidative capacity of the cells. This approach has been used in the fermentation of *S. cerevisiae*, in which acid production rate is used to provide online estimates of the specific growth rate. Also, in modern fed-batch processes for yeast production, the feed is strictly under control based on the measurement of traces of ethanol in the exhaust gas of the fermentor.

13.7.5. Inductive, Enhancer or Enrichment Components

In certain fermentations, it is of interest to continuously add either an inductive or fast consumed components and not just a limiting substrate. An example is the continuous addition of an antibiotic in recombinant microorganims bearing an antibiotic marked plasmid. Genetically altered microorganisms often belong to this category. Another example is given by the production of glutathione by high-glutathione-accumulating *S. cerevisiae*, the microorganims commonly used for commercial production. Cysteine was found to be the only amino acid that enhanced glutathione formation. However, the growth inhibition occurred and it was related to the concentration of cysteine. This problem was then resolved by an adequate addition of cysteine in exponential fed-batch culture without growth inhibition.

Fed-batch operation is an appropriate mode of fermentation in microorganisms that are producing heterologous proteins and whose elevated protein expression results in product degradation by activation of proteases. A general insight on this subject was the study of a recombinant *E. coli* for production of chloramphenicol acetyltransferase. A gradual induction with Isopropyl-β-D-thio-galactoside (IPTG) and phenylalanine (rate-limiting precursor) addition strategies were able to reduce the physiological burden imposed on the bacterium, thereby avoiding cellular stress responses and enhancing bioreactor productivity. In this case, IPTG and phenylalanine were the driving parameters that dominated the feed.

The addition of precursors or inducers should take into account if the product of interest is growth associated or not. For example, the use of a tyrosine-deficient strain of *E. coli* in the production of phenylalanine requires a balanced feed of tyrosine that, if not provided in low quantities, is used as carbon source with subsequent production of excessive biomass synthesis at the expense of phenylalanine synthesis. This limitation on biomass production is possible because the phenylalanine production was not growth associated.

13.7.6. Respiratory Quotient

Gas analyzers, especially mass spectrophotometers, are relatively fast. Respiratory quotient (RQ), the ratio between the moles of carbon evolved per moles of oxygen consumed, has been a general method used to determine indirectly the lack of substrate in the growth medium. It is a fairly rapid method of measurement that is useful because the gas analyses can be related to crucial process variables. The method is not "universal" to all bioprocesses since some biosystems can produce by-products that affect the productivity of the process without affecting the RQ, such as the production of acetic acid by *E. coli*.

Usually, the signal is characterized by a sharp rise in dissolved oxygen. Based on the concept of RQ, there are the so-called DO-stats, in which the feed is regulated in accordance with the dissolved oxygen. The analysis of the dissolved oxygen or carbon dioxide evolution rate can also be used to control or prevent the production of by-products. The RQ is often analyzed to study the carbon flux, that is, the feed should be conditioned in such a way that it should prevent excess of carbon dioxide evolution caused by unnecessary severe substrate limitation.

13.7.7. General Feeding Mode

The feeding mode influences a fed-batch fermentation by defining the growth rate of the microorganisms and the effectiveness of the carbon cycle for product formation and minimization of by-product formation. Inherently related with the concept of fed-batch, the feeding mode allows many variances in substrate or other components constitution and provision modes and, consequently, better control over inhibitory effects of the substrate and/or product. The feed can be modified accordingly to the different phases of the microbial growth, as a consequence of physiological alterations that the cells undergo upon transfer through eventual consecutive stages of the fed-batch cultivation.

Usually, a fed-batch starts as a batch mode and after a certain biomass concentration or substrate consumption, the fermentor is fed with the limiting substrate solution. However, that approach does not need to be the absolute rule. Some cases happen in which the rate of production of a certain product is limited not only by the substrate but also by a primary product, associated with the growth of the microorganism. That is the case of streptokinase formation. Streptokinase is a vital and effective drug for the treatment of myocardinal infection that is currently produced in industry by mainly natural or mutated strains of streptococci. The specific growth rate is inhibited by the substrate and by lactic acid. A near-optimal feed policy based on a chemotaxis algorithm has been established that defines an initial decreasing feeding phase, followed by a batch fermentation with no more added substrate in the medium. The starting point was the data provided by the batch fermentations and the feed was defined as being a polynomial function of time. By iterative calculations and having the batch time fermentation or the maximum allowable volume of the fermentor as time limits, a feed strategy was defined yielding a 12% increase in streptokinase activity over batch fermentations. This type of approach has been previously suggested also for ethanol production by *S. cerevisiae* that follows the same kinetics.

Finally, the feed can be continuous, can be provided in pulses, as a shot feeding, single or multisubstrate, increasing linearly, be exponential or constant with time. The design of the feed solution may follow a conventional approach – in which the nutrients are more concentrated as compared with the growing medium in the fermentor – or follows a quantitative design in such a way that depletion or accumulation of nutrients can be avoided or reduced.

13.7.8. Proton Production

A less common type of controlling process parameters is the proton production to estimate online the specific growth rate in a fed-batch culture and, indirectly, the substrate concentration. The amount of proton produced during the fermentation can be measured based on the volume of base added to the fermentor to control the pH at a preset value.

13.7.9. Fluorescence

A common parameter to monitor cell culture is optical density. A linear relationship exists between the culture fluorescence and the dry cell weight concentration up to 30 g-dwc/L, due to the optical interference of the intracellular NAD(P)H pool. Thus, fluorescence can be used to estimate online the biomass concentration and be a controlling parameter in the feed provision.

13.8. PARAMETERS TO START AND FINISH THE FEED AND STOP THE FED-BATCH FERMENTATION

The times at which the feeding should start and finish, as well as the criteria to stop a fed-batch fermentation is very much dependent on the specific cultivation kinetics and the operator's interest. For example, in substrate-limited processes, the feed should start immediately after the substrate reached the low limit, otherwise the process may be difficult to control, for example, because of a lag phase due to previous starvation. The most commonly used criterion to start the feed is the depletion of the substrate, which can be measured by a multitude of techniques, from specific enzymatic assays, HPLC (high-performance liquid chromatography) and NMR (Nuclear Magnetic Resonance) spectroscopy to indirect methods such as the exhaust gas analysis. Still related with the amount of the substrate in the medium, the operator might not find necessary to reach the complete depletion but to be below a predetermined set point (eventually related with historical data, growth models and known yields).

The fed-batch fermentation should be halted when the production slows down because of cell death, because the metabolic potential of the culture becomes inadequately low or because by-product excretion starts at significant levels. Some other criteria can be an increase in viscosity that implies an increased oxygen demand until the oxygen limitation is achieved, which is the case for penicillin production.

13.9. SUMMARY

Batch operations are not controllable as all the substrate is added into the reactor at the start. Fed-batch reactor is based on feeding of a growth-limiting nutrient substrate to a culture. Cell growth and fermentation can be controlled by the feeding strategy. The fed-batch strategy is typically used in bio-industrial processes to reach a high cell density in the bioreactor. Mostly the feed solution is highly concentrated to avoid dilution of the bioreactor. In essence, fed-batch reactor is applied in such a fashion that a chemostat or CSTR is simulated with a seemingly batch operation. The controlled addition of the nutrient directly affects the growth rate of the culture and allows avoiding overflow metabolism (formation of side metabolites, such as acetate for *E. coli*, lactic acid in cell cultures, ethanol in *S. cerevisiae*) and oxygen limitation (anaerobiosis).

Substrate limitation offers the possibility to control the reaction rates to avoid technological limitations connected to the cooling of the reactor and oxygen transfer. Substrate limitation also allows the metabolic control to avoid osmotic effects, catabolite repression and overflow metabolism of side products. Therefore, there are different operation strategies for fed-batch: 1) constant feed rate or constant growth/fermentation rate; 2) exponential feed rate or constant specific growth rate. The exponential growth with fed-batch operation can be at any rate, up to the maximum rate in the exponential growth phase of a batch growth. This is the case that closely resembles a chemostat operation. Usually, maximum growth rate is not wanted because the undesired by-product production can be high at maximum growth.

Analysis of fed-batch reactors is more complex than either chemostat or batch reactor. Solutions of differential equations are usually required. When long operation time is employed, a pseudo-steady state may be assumed and thus simplifying the analysis. The pseudo-steady state is found to correspond to biomass steady state or $\frac{dX}{dt} = 0$. Some solutions for the biomass concentration and product formation are shown in Table 13.1 for constant feed and exponential feed at pseudo-steady state conditions.

Further Reading

Curless, C., Fu, K., Swank, R., Menjares, A., Fieschko, J., Tsai, L., 1991. Design and Evaluation of a 2-Stage, Cyclic, Recombinant Fermentation Process, *Biotechn. Bioeng.* 38 (9) 1082–1090.

Hewitt, C.J., Nienow, A.W., 2007. The scale-up of microbial batch and fed-batch fermentation processes. *Adv. Appl. Microbiol.* 62, 105–135.

Wlaschin, K.F., Hu, W.S., 2006. Fedbatch culture and dynamic nutrient feeding. *Cell Culture Engineering* 101, 43–74.

Shiloach, J., Fass, R., 2005. Growing *E. coli* to high cell density–a historical perspective on method development. *Biotechnol. Adv.* 23, 345–357.

Liden, G., 2002. Understanding the bioreactor. *Bioprocess and Biosystems Engineering* 24, 273–279.

Lee, J., Lee, S.Y., Park, S., Middelberg, A.P., 1999. Control of fed-batch fermentations. *Biotechnol. Adv.* 17, 29–48.

Lee, S.Y., 1996. High cell-density culture of *Escherichia coli*. *Trends Biotechnol* 14, 98–105.

Mendozavega, O., Sabatie, J., Brown, S.W., 1994. Industrial-Production of Heterologous Proteins by Fed-Batch Cultures of the Yeast *Saccharomyces-Cerevisiae*. *Fems Microbiology Reviews* 15, 369–410.

Yee, L., Blanch, H.W., 1992. Recombinant protein expression in high cell density fed-batch cultures of *Escherichia coli*. *Biotechnology (NY)* 10, 1550–1556.

Riesenberg, D, Schulz, V., 1991. High-cell-density cultivation of *Escherichia coli*. *Curr. Opin. Biotechnol.* 2, 380–384.

PROBLEMS

13.1. Penicillin is produced by *P. chrysogenum* in a fed-batch culture with the intermittent addition of glucose solution to the culture medium. The initial culture volume is $V_0 = 200$ L, and glucose-containing nutrient solution is added with a flow rate of $Q = 30$ L/h. Glucose concentration in the feed solution and the initial concentrations in the reactor are $S_F = 300$ g/L, $S_0 = 1$ g/L, and $X_0 = 20$ g/L. The kinetic and yield factors of the organism are $\mu_{max} = 0.2$ h^{-1}, $K_S = 0.5$ g/L, and $YF_{X/S} = 0.3$ g-dw/g-glucose. Without invoking the pseudo-steady state approximation, determine and compare with Example 13-1:

(a) the culture volume at $t = 24$ h;

(b) the concentration of glucose at $t = 24$ h;

(c) the concentration and total amount of cells when $t = 24$ h;
(d) the product (penicillin) concentration in the vessel at 24 h, if $\mu_P = 0.05$ g-product/(g-cells h) and $P_0 = 0.1$ g/L.

13.2. *Lactobacillus casi* is propagated under essentially anaerobic conditions to provide a starter culture for manufacture of Swiss cheese. The culture produces lactic acid as a by-product of endogenous metabolism. The growth parameters are given by $YF_{X/S} = 0.23$ g-X/g-S, $K_S = 0.15$ g/L, $\mu_{max} = 0.33$ h^{-1}, $k_d = 0.03$ h^{-1}. A stirred tank fermentor is operated in fed-batch mode at pseudo-steady state with a feed flow of 4000 L/h and feed substrate concentration of 80 g/L. The feed is started such that pseudo-steady state is reached from time zero. After 8 h, the liquid volume is 40,000 L.
(a) What was the initial culture volume?
(b) What is the concentration of cell biomass at pseudo-steady state?
(c) What is the mass of cells produced after 8 h fed-batch operation?
(d) What is the substrate concentration in the reactor after 8 h fed-batch operation?

13.3. In a fed-batch culture operating with the intermittent addition of glucose solution, the initial culture volume is $V_0 = 1$ L, and glucose-containing nutrient solution is added exponentially with a flow rate of $Q = 0.2 \exp(0.1 \text{ h}^{-1} \times t)$ L/h. Glucose concentration in the feed solution and the initial concentrations in the reactor are $S_F = 200$ g/L, $S_0 = 1$ g/L, and $X_0 = 50$ g/L. The kinetic and yield factors of the organism are $\mu_{max} = 0.3$ h^{-1}, $K_S = 0.1$ g/L, and $YF_{X/S} = 0.5$ g-dw/g-glucose. Using the pseudo-steady state approximation, determine:
(a) the culture volume at $t = 48$ h;
(b) the concentration of glucose at $t = 48$ h;
(c) the concentration and total amount of cells when $t = 48$ h;
(d) the product (penicillin) concentration in the vessel at 48 h, if $\mu_P = 0.1$ g-product/(g-cells h) and $P_0 = 0$ g/L.

13.4. In a fed-batch culture operating with the intermittent addition of glucose solution, the initial culture volume is $V_0 = 1$ L and glucose-containing nutrient solution is added exponentially with a flow rate of $Q = 0.1 \exp(0.2 \text{ h}^{-1} \times t)$ L/h. Glucose concentration in the feed solution and the initial concentrations in the reactor are $S_F = 300$ g/L, $S_0 = 0.1$ g/L, and $X_0 = 100$ g/L. The kinetic and yield factors of the organism are $\mu_{max} = 0.3$ h^{-1}, $K_S = 0.1$ g/L, $k_d = 0.001$/h, and $YF_{X/S} = 0.5$ g-dw/g-glucose. Using the pseudo-steady state approximation, determine:
(a) the culture volume at $t = 36$ h;
(b) the concentration of glucose at $t = 36$ h;
(c) the concentration and total amount of cells when $t = 36$ h;
(d) the product (penicillin) concentration in the vessel at 36 h, if $\mu_P = 0.02$ g-product/(g-cells h) and $P_0 = 0$ g/L.

13.5. A solution containing bacteria at a concentration of 0.001 g/L was fed to a semibatch reactor. The nutrient was in excess. The reactor was empty at the start of the experiment. If the concentration of bacteria in the reactor at the end of 2 h is 0.025 g/L, what is the net specific growth rate μ_{net} in min^{-1}?

13.6. Cell growth with uncompetitive substrate inhibition is taking place in a chemostat. The cell growth rate law for this system is

$$\mu_G = \frac{\mu_{max} S}{K_S + S(1 + S/K_I)}$$

with $\mu_{max} = 1.5\ h^{-1}$, $K_S = 1$ g/L, $K_I = 50$ g/L, $S_0 = 30$ g/L, $YF_{X/S} = 0.08$ g-cells/g-S, and $X_0 = 0.5$ g/L.

Initially, 0.5 g/L of bacteria was placed in the reactor containing the substrate (equal to the feed) and the flow to the tank started. Plot the concentrations of bacteria and substrate as functions of time.

13.7. In a fed-batch culture operating with the intermittent addition of glucose solution, the initial culture volume is $V_0 = 0.1$ L and glucose-containing nutrient solution is added exponentially with a flow rate of $Q = 0.1 \exp(0.1\ h^{-1} \times t)$ L/h. Glucose concentration in the feed solution and the initial concentrations in the reactor are $S_F = 200$ g/L, $S_0 = 1$ g/L, and $X_0 = 50$ g/L. The growth kinetics is governed by

$$\mu_G = \frac{\mu_{max} S}{K_S + S(1 + S/K_I)}$$

with $\mu_{max} = 1.5\ h^{-1}$, $K_S = 1$ g/L, $K_I = 50$ g/L. The yield factor $YF_{X/S} = 0.5$ g-dw/g-glucose. Using the pseudo-steady state approximation, determine:

(a) the culture volume at $t = 24$ h;

(b) the concentration of glucose at $t = 24$ h;

(c) the concentration and total amount of cells when $t = 24$ h;

(d) the product (penicillin) concentration in the vessel at 24 h, if $\mu_P = 0.1$ g-product/(g-cells h) and $P_0 = 0$ g/L.

13.8. *Nicotiana tabacum* cells are cultivated to high density for production of polysaccharide gum. The reactor used is a stirred tank, with an initial medium volume of 15 L. The maximum specific growth rate of the culture is 0.01 h^{-1}, the saturation constant is 0.1 g/L and the biomass yield factor is $YF_{X/S} = 0.5$ g-X/g-S. The concentration of growth-limiting substrate in the medium is 3% (w/v), for both the initial medium in the reactor and the feed. The reactor is inoculated with 1.0 g/L cells and operated in batch until the substrate is virtually consumed ($S < 0.5$ mg/L); medium flow is then started at a constant rate of 0.2 L/h. Assume that fed-batch operation reaches pseudo-steady conditions rapidly.

(a) Estimate the batch culture time and final biomass concentration.

(b) Fed-batch operation is carried out for 1000 h. What is the final mass of cells in the reactor?

(c) The fermentor is available 300 days per year with a downtime between runs of 24 h. How much plant cell biomass is produced annually?

CHAPTER

14

Evolution and Genetic Engineering

OUTLINE

Bioprocess Engineering
http://dx.doi.org/10.1016/B978-0-444-59525-6.00014-7

Living organisms (unicellular and multicellular; prokaryotic or eukaryotic) utilize nucleic acids (deoxyribonucleic acid or DNA and ribonucleic acid or RNA) for transferring genetic information from one generation to the next and also to decode genetic information into messenger molecules (from DNA to RNA) and then to effecter molecules (proteins), as we have learned in Chapter 10. All prokaryotic and eukaryotic cells/organisms use DNA as their genetic material. Some viruses (called retroviruses), like HIV, use messenger RNA (mRNA) for transferring genetic information to their next generation. To transfer genetic information, DNA is replicated into an exact copy and is passed on to the next generation of cells/organisms. If the genetic material is RNA (usually mRNA), it is first converted to DNA (through reverse transcription); copies of RNA are generated from this DNA, and are then passed on to the next generation. In the passing of genetic information, errors can occur. Despite active self-repairs, some mistakes can carry to the next generation. Some individuals can receive additional genetic information through natural or artificial means. Organisms evolve via genetic mistakes and accidental acquiring of foreign genes as selected by the environment. Therefore, genetic information can be manipulated to produce new cells/organisms with a purpose, which leads to genetic engineering.

To create effecter molecules (proteins) from genetic code (DNA), DNA is first transcribed into messenger RNA and then this message is translated into a protein molecule (Central Dogma of biology). We start the discussions from the passing of genetic information to the next generation and their potential errors.

14.1. MUTATIONS

Although the cell has a well-developed system to prevent errors in DNA replication and an active repair system to correct damage to a DNA molecule, mistakes occur. These mistakes are called mutations. The genetic contents (DNA or RNA) of a cell/organism are called its genotype, and the characteristics that are expressed by the organism (by virtue of its genotype) is called phenotype.

The alterations in the genotype of a cell/organism are called mutations and the altered phenotype (consequent to the alterations in genotype) is called a mutant. The majority of phenotypic changes in response to environmental factors (e.g. darkening of human skin after exposed to sunlight or tanning) are reversible and are produced by the already existing genotypic structure or mechanisms. On the other hand, the phenotypic changes that occur as a consequence of genotypic changes are usually irreversible. Similarly, the genotypic changes or alterations in the genotype (mutations) are permanent and mostly irreversible.

Mutations may involve a single nucleotide base or a single nucleotide base pair (bp). These small changes usually affect a single gene, its coded protein or the expression of a gene. Other mutations may involve large sections of DNA. These mutations result in the duplication of a section of DNA, deletion and loss of a segment of DNA, relocation of a segment of DNA from one part of the genome to another, or rearrangements of the segments of DNA in relation to the others.

Some larger mutations also involve duplication or loss of an entire chromosome. In some cases, especially in plants, a whole set of chromatin or chromosomes are duplicated, resulting in triploid, tetraploid, or polyploid generations.

14.1.1. What Causes Genetic Mutations?

Mutations can occur due to the internal flaws in DNA replication mechanisms, due to external/environmental factors or both working together. For example, an environmental factor (e.g. UV light or DNA-reactive chemicals) can create a small alteration in the components of DNA, and internal mechanisms, in an effort to repair it, can create a permanent change or mutation in the genotype of a cell. Exposure to certain chemicals like mustard gas, alkylating agents, etc. can cause DNA damage that can result into mutations. Table 14.1 illustrates common causes of mutations.

TABLE 14.1 Common Causes of Mutations

Common causes of mutations	Description
Spontaneous	
Aberrant recombination	Abnormal crossing over may cause deletions, duplications, translocations, and inversions.
Aberrant segregation	Abnormal chromosomal segregation may cause aneuploidy or polyploidy.
Errors in DNA replication	A mistake by DNA polymerase may cause a point mutation.
Toxic metabolic products	The products of normal metabolic processes may be chemically reactive agents that can alter the structure of DNA.
Transposable elements	Transposable elements can insert themselves into the sequence of a gene.
Depurination	On rare occasions, the linkage between purines (i.e. adenine and guanine) and deoxyribose can spontaneously break. If not repaired, it can lead to mutation.
Deamination	Cytosine and 5-methylcytosine can spontaneously deaminate to create uracil or thymine.
Tautomeric shifts	Spontaneous changes in base structure can cause mutations if they occur immediately prior to DNA replication.
Induced	
Chemical agents	Chemical substances may cause changes in the structure of DNA.
Physical agents	Physical phenomena such as UV light and X rays damage the DNA.

The large mutations involving whole chromosomes or sets of chromosomes usually occur during cell division due to malfunctioning of the mitotic mechanism (e.g. spindle fibers malfunctioning or centromere nondisjunction, etc.). Certain chemicals like Colchicine inhibit the formation of a mitotic spindle, creating polyploid cells.

Depending upon the cause of mutations, there are two types: spontaneous and induced mutations.

14.1.1.1. *Spontaneous Mutations*

Spontaneous mutations occur randomly in the genetic material of an organism and are a result of natural molecular decay or damage. There are four causes to these type of mutations:

1. Tautomerism—A base is changed by repositioning of a hydrogen atom, altering the hydrogen bonding pattern of that base, resulting in an incorrect base pairing during replication.
2. Depurination—Loss of a purine base (A or G) creating a purinic site.
3. Deamination—Hydrolysis can change a normal base to an atypical base containing a keto group in place of the original amine group. For example, a conversion of cytosine to uracil and adenine to hypoxanthine can be corrected by DNA repair. Conversion of 5-methylcytosine to thymine cannot be corrected because thymine is a natural base.
4. Slipped strand mispairing—Denaturation of the new strand from the template during replication, followed by renaturation in a different spot is called "slipping". It creates "hairpin" like loops of DNA sections with unpaired bases. Repair of this defect can result in deletions.

Natural (or spontaneous) mutation rates vary greatly from gene to gene (10^{-3} to 10^{-9} per cell division), with 10^{-6} mutations in a gene per cell division being typical. Chemical agents (*mutagens*) or radiation is often used in the laboratory to increase mutation rates. Mutagens are nonspecific and may affect any gene.

14.1.1.2. *Induced Mutations*

Induced mutations are results of environmental damages to DNA caused by chemical or physical agents. There are three causes to these mutations:

1. Base analogs, alkylating reagents, DNA-adduct-forming chemicals, DNA-intercalating agents, and DNA-cross linkers are examples of chemical damage to DNA.
2. Oxidative damage caused by free-radical-generating chemicals and radiations is another source of induced mutations.
3. DNA damage caused by UV radiations (non-ionizing) and ionizing radiations is an example of physical agents that can result into various types of mutations.

14.1.2. Types of Mutations

The genetic mutations can be classified into four types: (1) germ-line and somatic mutations; (2) lethal, non-lethal, and neutral mutations; (3) point mutations; and (4) large-scale mutations.

14.1.2.1. *Germ-Line Mutations and Somatic Mutations*

In multicellular organisms with dedicated reproductive cells, mutations can be categorized into two broad categories. Germ-line mutations are those that occur in the reproductive cells and can be passed on to the next generation via the reproduction process.

Somatic mutations involve the cells outside the reproductive system and usually are not transmitted to the next generation, unless the organism is reproducing asexually.

14.1.2.2. *Lethal, Non-Lethal, and Neutral Mutations*

Lethal mutations are harmful mutations or damage to DNA that leads to the death of the mutant organism. These mutations do not have any long-term effects on the populations.

Non-lethal mutations may be harmful, beneficial, or neutral mutations. These mutations accumulate within the gene pool and increase the genetic variations. These mutations are the basis of evolution through natural selection.

Neutral mutations are defined as the mutations that neither have any impact on the function or performance of the product of a gene nor do they influence the fitness of the organism. These mutations can accumulate over time due to genetic drift.

14.1.2.3. *Point Mutations*

Small changes in the DNA molecule are called point mutations and involve a single base or a single base pair. These type of mutations may either have no effect or may be weakly beneficial, but majority of them (about 70%) are harmful. Due to this damaging effect of these mutations, cells and organisms have evolved mechanisms to repair or remove mutations.

Point mutations are caused either by mistakes in the DNA replication process or by chemicals (called mutagens). There are three causes of point mutations: (1) transitions; (2) insertions; and (3) deletions.

14.1.2.3.1. TRANSITIONS OR TRANSVERSIONS

Exchange or substitution of a purine for purine (adenine for guanine and vice versa) or pyrimidine for a pyrimidine (cytosine for thymine and vice versa) are the most common transition mutations. It can be caused by a base mismatching during replication or by chemicals like nitrous acid and base analogs like 5-bromo-2-deoxyuridine. For example:

$$\begin{array}{l} 5\rightarrow \ \text{AACGC}\mathbf{T}\text{AGATC} \ \rightarrow 3 \\ 3\leftarrow \ \text{TTGCG}\mathbf{A}\text{TCTAG} \ \leftarrow 5 \end{array} \longrightarrow \begin{array}{l} 5\rightarrow \ \text{AACGC}\mathbf{G}\text{AGATC} \ \rightarrow 3 \\ 3\leftarrow \ \text{TTGCG}\mathbf{C}\text{TCTAG} \ \leftarrow 5 \end{array}$$

where on the sixth base pair position, the base on the upper strand has its T substituted by G, whereas the lower strand has its base A substituted by base C. This only occurs on one single point.

Point mutations occurring within a protein-coding region of a gene can have three different results: silent mutations; missense mutations; and nonsense mutations.

Silent mutations—The mutated genetic code still codes for the same amino acid. For example: mRNA codon UUU (codes for phenylalanine) is coded by DNA codon AAA. If third "A" is exchanged for "G," resulting mRNA codon UUC will still code for phenylalanine. As shown in Table 14.2, in multiple instances, the change in the third base of a codon

TABLE 14.2 mRNA Codons and Resulting Protein Expressed

First letter	Second letter: U		C		A		G		Third letter
U	UUU	Phe	UCU	Ser	UAU	Tyr	UGU	Cys	U
	UUC		UCC		UAC		UGC		C
	UUA	Leu	UCA		UAA	Stop	UGA	Stop	A
	UUG		UCG		UAG	Stop	UGG	Trp	G
C	CUU	Leu	CCU	Pro	CAU	His	CGU	Arg	U
	CUC		CCC		CAC		CGC		C
	CUA		CCA		CAA	Gin	CGA		A
	CUG		CCG		CAG		CGG		G
A	AUU	Ile	ACU	Thr	AAU	Asn	AGU	Ser	U
	AUC		ACC		AAC		AGC		C
	AUA		ACA		AAA	Lys	AGA	Arg	A
	AUG	Met	ACG		AAG		AGG		G
G	GUU	Val	GCU	Ala	GAU	Asp	GGU	Gly	U
	GUC		GCC		GAC		GGC		C
	GUA		GCA		GAA	Glu	GGA		A
	GUA		GCA		GAA		GGA		G

does not alter the amino acid that it codes. To code for arginine, if first two bases are "C and G" third base can be any one out of all the four RNA bases. In addition, both AGA and AGG also code for arginine.

Missense mutations—Exchange of one nucleotide base with another one results in a codon that codes for a different amino acid. For example, in codon "CGU" (arginine), exchanging cytosine with uracil (U) will result in codon UGU (cysteine).

Nonsense mutations—One type of point mutation that usually has a profound effect results in a nonsense or stop codon. For example, the codon "UGU," exchanging the third base "U" with an "A," will result in a codon "UGA" that codes for a stop and can truncate the protein molecule before completion. This results in the premature termination of translation and an incompletely formed protein.

14.1.2.3.2. INSERTIONS

Addition of one or more extra nucleotides or nucleotide pairs into the DNA of an organism is called insertion. The insertion elements are usually about 700–1400 bp (base pairs) in length; in *Escherichia coli* about five different insertion sequences are known and are present on the chromosome. These elements can move on the chromosome from essentially any site to another. Often they will insert in the middle of a gene, totally destroying its function. Single base pair insertions usually occur due to errors in DNA replication or replication of repeating sections of DNA (e.g. AT base pair repeats). Larger insertions involving long sections of DNA are caused by transposable elements. Insertions in the coding region of a gene (even a single base pair insertion) cause a shift in the reading frame (frameshift). Insertions can also result in the altered splicing of the mRNA, because posttranscriptional splicing of mRNA requires specific sequences of nucleotides. Both of these effects can alter the gene product very significantly and are mostly deleterious.

Example:

```
5→ AACGCTAGATC  →3      5→ AACAGTCGCTAGATC  →3
3← T TGCGATCTAG ←5  ──▶ 3← T TGTCAGCGATCTAG ←5
```

where AGTC bases were inserted between the third and fourth letters in the upper strand, and TCAG bases were inserted into the lower strand between the third and fourth letters.

Insertion of a base pair into an mRNA gene can cause changes to the resulting protein that it expresses. For example:

mRNA from a gene before addition of single base pair:

```
5→ -A-U-G - A-C-C - G-A-C - C-C-G - A-A-A - G-G-G - A-C-C - →3
     Met  -  Thr  -  Asp  -  Pro  -  Lys  -  Gly  -  Thr  -
```

mRNA after addition of G: (frameshift)

```
5→ -A-U-G - A-C-C - G-A-C - G-C-C - G-A-A - A-G-G - G-A-C-C - →3
     Met  -  Thr  -  Asp  -  Ala  -  Glu  -  Arg  -  Asp  -
```

14.1.2.3.3. DELETIONS

Removal of a single base pair or a section of DNA is called deletion. Deletions have similar effects as insertions that have profound effects on cellular metabolism. By deleting or adding one or more bases, we can alter the whole composition of a protein, not just a single amino acid. A deletion can shift the *reading frame* when translating the resulting mRNA.

Back mutations or *reversions* are possible. Sometimes a deletion may get reversed by an addition or vice versa. Revertants are cells for which the original wild-type phenotype has been restored. Restoration of a function can occur due to a direct change at the original mutation (e.g. if the original mutation was CAA to UAA, then a second mutation for UAA to CAA restores the original genotype and phenotype). Second-site revertants can occur that restore phenotype (*suppressor mutations*) but not genotype (e.g. a second deletion mutation that restores the gene to the normal reading frame or a mutation in another gene that restores the wild-type phenotype).

14.1.3. Large-Scale Mutations

14.1.3.1. Chromosomal Structural Mutations

Large-scale mutations involve changes of large sections of DNA (Deletions, insertions, inversions, etc.) within the same chromosome or inter-chromosomal exchange of DNA material.

Deletion of large segments of chromosomes can result in a loss of a gene/genes from the genome of an organism. If deletion involves the regions of DNA that control the expression of a gene/group of genes, the entire group of genes may stop expression or their expression may go out of control. Insertion and inversion can occur during replication and cause major effects.

Amplifications occur due to the duplication of segments of DNA during replication. Some segments of DNA are duplicated several times, leading to multiple copies of the chromosomal regions. This process increases the dosage of certain genes, called gene amplification.

Zygotes produced from gametes involving duplications are often viable and may or may not have any serious problems. For example various sorts of duplications are related to color vision conditions, many of which are quite subtle in their effects, as are certain anemias involving abnormal hemoglobin called the thalassemias.

Chromosomal translocations involve a relocation of a segment of chromosome. Intra-chromosomal translocations move a segment within the same chromosome. Inter-chromosomal translocations move a segment of a chromosome to a non-homologous chromosome. Chromosomal translocations happen during early phases of mitosis or meiosis. The involved chromosomes come in close contact in a process called "crossing-over"; DNA strands of two chromosomes break at a certain point and then relegate, causing a transfer of a DNA segment from one chromosome to another. This process can very adversely affect the gene expression of the transferred genes. Several genetically inheritable disorders result from these translocations. Certain types of Down syndrome involve translocations between chromosome 14 and chromosome 21.

Chromosomal inversion describes a segment of DNA chopped from the parent molecule and inserted after being flipped over by end to end (180°). The effect of DNA inversions is unpredictable and can vary from disastrous effects to no effect. These sorts of inversions are important in reshuffling genes on a chromosome.

Transposable elements are stretches of DNA which can insert themselves into new regions of a chromosome. Because of this ability they are often called jumping genes. The simplest transposable element, called an insertion element, consists of a gene for an enzyme called transposase which is required for the insertion process. This gene is flanked by special sequences called inverted repeats which the enzyme must recognize for insertion to take place.

More complex transposable elements have other genes and carry these genes along with them. Such transposable elements are called transposons.

Transposons can be of benefit to the organism by providing a mechanism for insertion of beneficial genes. For instance, the genes that confer resistance to antibiotics in bacteria are carried by transposable elements to other nonresistant bacteria.

Transposable elements may also insert themselves into the middle of genes in which case the gene sequence is disrupted. For instance, the allele for wrinkled seeds in peas studied by Gregor Mendel is actually the gene for round peas into which a transposon has inserted itself.

14.1.3.2. Changes in Chromosome Number

Aneuploidy is a condition that a normally diploid individual ends up either with extra copies of homologous chromosomes or fewer than the normal diploid number. This happens when homologous chromosomes fail to segregate properly during meiosis. This failure of homologous chromosomes to segregate is called nondisjunction.

There are a number of different types of aneuploidy. The most common types are monosomy in which the diploid individual has only one member of a certain homologous chromosome.

The other common type of aneuploidy is called trisomy because the individual has three copies of the chromosome. Aneuploidy leads to a number of syndromes in humans. For example, trisomy 21 leads to Down syndrome, characterized by mental retardation and other abnormalities.

Aneuploidy involving the sex chromosomes is common. XYY males are normal but XXY males and XXXY males have a syndrome called Klinefelter syndrome. These males are often actually intersexed or hermaphroditic with partially developed sexual organs of both genders. These individuals are sterile and are often subjected to hormones and surgery to bring them into conformance with social gender roles.

Polyploidy refers to a genome consisting of more sets of chromosomes than usual in a nucleus. Polyploidy can happen because of a failure of the spindle fibers in mitosis or meiosis to segregate chromosomes into separate groups. Many organisms have specialized polyploid tissues, even organisms we typically consider as diploid. For example, in plants, a so called double fertilization leads to the genesis of a diploid zygote from the union of two gametes produced by the haploid gametophytes but also a specialized triploid tissue (3N) called endosperm. This tissue is produced when a male gamete fertilizes special diploid tissue from the flower.

In mammals, cells of the liver are typically polyploid. Some organisms are completely polyploid including many plant species and some fish and amphibians. For example, domestic wheat is hexaploid (6N). "Seedless" plants are usually triploid (3N). Polyploidy is believed to be an important mechanism in the development of new species and a common pattern in plants is to find populations of two species both of which might be diploid.

14.2. SELECTION

14.2.1. Natural Selection

Natural selection is the process that results in an increase in the number of those individuals of a population that have a variation (or mutation) in a particular trait (or traits) that provide the bearers with an advantage for survivability and reproducibility. These variants or mutants and their offspring survive and reproduce more succesfully, and will increase in number overtime.

Natural selection works with the phenotypic or observable characteristics of an organism. The genetic basis of the phenotypic change becomes more prevalent in the population overtime, resulting in the adaptations that specialize organisms for particular ecological niches and eventually may result in the emergence of a new species.

Conversely, if a genetic variation or mutation has resulted in a phenotypic change that makes a particular individual less survivable or less fit for the environment, due to this natural selection process, the chances of survival and reproduction for that individual are reduced, resulting in the elimination of the genetic change overtime.

An adaptation method of *E. coli* to wood extract hydrolyzates has been described by Liu et al. (T. Liu, L. Lin, Z. Sun, R. Hu, S. Liu. 2010 "Bioethanol fermentation by robust recombinant *E. coli* FBHW using hot-water wood extract hydrolyzate as substrate" J. Biotech. Adv., 28: 602–608.) as shown in Fig. 14.1. Wood extract hydrolyzate is a complex mixture of sugars (xylose, glucose, mannose, arabinose, etc), phenolic derivatives (from lignin), and electrolytes. Initially, *E. coli* fbr5 does not grow in the wood extract hydrolyzate or to produce ethanol. After the natural adaption, *E. coli* fbr5 mutant strains become productive.

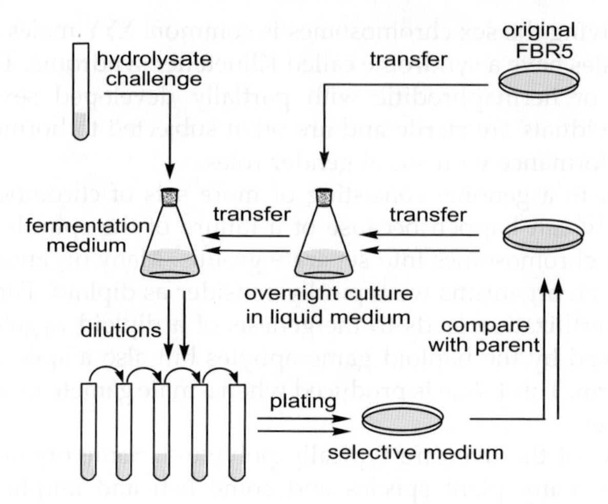

FIGURE 14.1 Schematic diagram of strain adaptation (Liu et al. 2010).

A well-known example of natural selection is the development of antibiotic resistance in microorganisms and development of insecticide resistance in insects overtime. The individual organisms in the natural populations of bacteria contain considerable genetic variations, including genes that confer resistance against antibiotics. In the presence of antibiotics, the bacterial cells that do not have genetic (and thereby phenotypic) capability of inactivating antibiotics die out quickly, leaving behind a population of cells that can survive in the presence of antibiotics. These surviving bacteria will reproduce to generate a next generation of bacterial cells that are resistant to the antibiotic agent.

14.2.2. Artificial Selection (Selection of Mutants with Useful Mutations)

Scientists have exploited the natural process of genetic variations and selection to better understand the cell physiology, workings of the cellular processes, and to control the regulation of biological processes for industrial benefits. Methods to induce mutations and then select for mutants are important tools for catalyst development in bioprocessing.

The selection of a mutant with desirable properties is no easy task. Mutations are classified as selectable or unselectable.

Selectable mutations provide an organism with characteristics that increase its survival under certain specific sets of environmental conditions, such that the mutants can survive but the wild type cannot. An example is the survival of antibiotic-resistant bacteria in the presence of antibiotics. Wild-type bacteria will be killed by the antibiotic. A selectable mutation confers upon the mutant an advantage for growth or survival under a specific set of environmental conditions; thus, only mutants with the desired characteristics will remain (e.g. green pigment).

Unselectable mutations do not provide a survival advantage to the bearer individuals. Selecting individuals (or organisms) with a desirable but unselectable mutation from the wild type is extremely difficult and requires special techniques. Even with mutagens, the frequency of mutation is sufficiently low to prohibit a brute force screening effort for most unselectable mutants.

1. One technique to isolate, for example, cells that cannot synthesize the amino acid histidine is called replica plating. Cells or microbes are cultured on complete media to form distinct colonies; then, a replica of this master is made on (1) a complete medium, and (2) on a minimal medium lacking histidine. The colonies that do not grow on the minimal medium but grow on the complete medium are the ones that cannot synthesize histidine, as illustrated in Fig. 14.2.
2. Recombinant technology with replica plating—in this method, a population of cells are infected with a desired unselectable gene segment combined with a vector DNA containing antibiotic-resistance genes (called recombinant DNA or rDNA). The recombinant strains are then selected using either a direct selection technique or the replica plating technique.

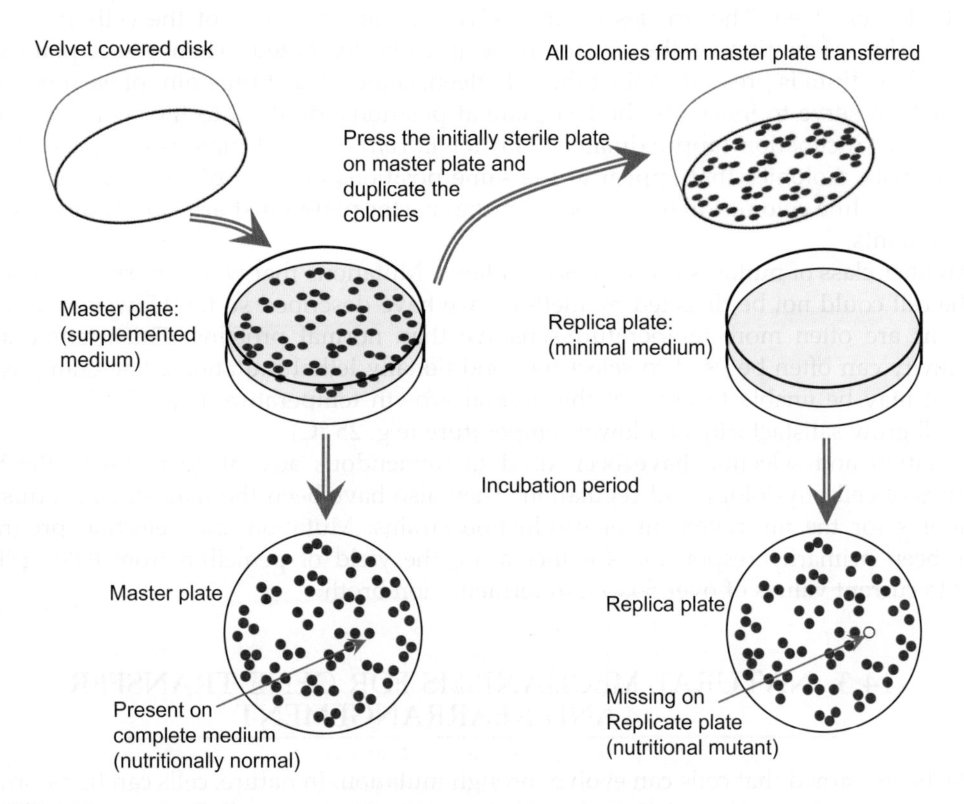

FIGURE 14.2 Duplicate plating method for detecting nutritional mutants.

Selection can be direct or indirect. An example of direct selection would be to find mutants resistant to an antibiotic or toxic compound. A culture fluid containing 10^8–10^{10} cells/mL is subjected to a mutagenic agent. A few drops of culture fluid are spread evenly on a plate, with the antibiotic incorporated into the gelled medium. Only antibiotic-resistant cells can grow, so any colonies that form must arise from antibiotic-resistant mutants. If one in a million cells has this particular mutation, we would expect to find about 10–100 colonies per plate if 0.1 mL of culture fluid was tested.

Indirect selection is used for isolating mutants that are deficient in their capacity to produce a necessary growth factor (e.g. an amino acid or a vitamin). Wild-type *E. coli* grows on glucose and mineral salts. *Auxotrophic* mutants would not grow on such a simple medium unless they were supplemented with the growth factor that the cell could no longer make (e.g. a lysine auxotroph has lost the capacity to make lysine, so lysine must be added to the glucose and salts to enable the cell to grow). The wild-type cell that needs no supplements to a minimal medium is called a *prototroph*. Consider the selection of a rare mutant cell that is auxotrophic for lysine from a population of wild-type cells. This cannot be done directly, since both cell types would grow in the minimal medium supplemented with lysine. A method that facilitated selection greatly is called *replica plating* (see Fig. 14.2). A master plate using a lysine-supplemented medium will grow both the auxotroph and wild-type cells. Once colonies are well formed on the master plate, an imprint is made on sterile velveteen. The bristles on the velveteen capture some of the cells from each colony. The orientation of the master plate is carefully noted. Then a test plate with minimal medium is pressed against the velveteen; some cells at the point of each previous colony then serve to inoculate the test plate at positions identical to those on the master plate. After incubation (approximately 24 h for *E. coli*), the test plate is compared to the master plate. Colonies that appear at the same positions on both plates arise from wild-type cells, while colonies that exist only on the master plate must arise from the auxotrophic mutants.

Another class of mutants is *conditional* mutants. Mutations that would normally be lethal to the cell could not be detected by methods we have described so far. However, mutated proteins are often more temperature-sensitive than normal proteins. Thus, temperature sensitivity can often be used to select for conditionally lethal mutations. For example, the mutant may be unable to grow at the normal growth temperature (e.g. 37 °C for *E. coli*) but will grow satisfactorily at a lower temperature (e.g. 25 °C).

Mutation and selection have been used to tremendous advantage to probe the base features of cell physiology and regulation. They also have been the mainstay of industrial programs for the improvement of production strains. Mutation and selection programs have been primarily responsible for increasing the yield of penicillin from 0.001 g/L in 1939 to current values of over 50 g/L in fermentation broth.

14.3. NATURAL MECHANISMS FOR GENE TRANSFER AND REARRANGEMENT

We have learned that cells can evolve through mutation. In nature, cells can transform by receiving genes from other organisms in their surroundings as well. Bacteria can gain and express wholly different biochemical capabilities (e.g. the ability to degrade an antibiotic or detoxify a hazardous chemical in their environment) literally overnight. These alterations cannot be explained through inheritance and small evolutionary changes in the chromosome. Rather, they arise from gene transfer from one organism to another and/or large rearrangements in chromosomal DNA. In this section, we will discuss genetic recombination, gene transfers, and genetic rearrangements—all mechanisms that can be exploited to genetically engineer cells.

14.3.1. Genetic Recombination

Genetic recombination is a process that brings genetic elements from two different genomes into one unit, resulting in new genotypes in the absence of mutations. Genetic recombination can occur naturally in the absence of human intervention. Genetic recombination in prokaryotes is a rare event but sufficiently frequent to be important industrially and ecologically. The three main mechanisms for gene transfer are *transformation, transduction, and conjugation*. Transformation is a process in which free DNA is taken up by a cell. Transduction is a process in which DNA is transferred by a bacteriophage, and conjugation is DNA transfer between intact cells that are in direct contact with one another.

Once *donor* DNA enters inside a cell, the mechanism for recombination is essentially independent of how the donor DNA entered. Fig. 14.3 summarizes the molecular-level events in general recombination. The donor DNA must be homologous, or nearly so, to a segment of DNA on the recipient DNA. Under the right conditions, cellular enzymes cut out the homologous section of recipient DNA, allow insertion of the donor DNA, and then ligate or join the ends of the donor DNA to the recipient DNA. Pieces of donor DNA that a cell recognizes as foreign are usually degraded by enzymes called *restriction endonucleases* (these enzymes are

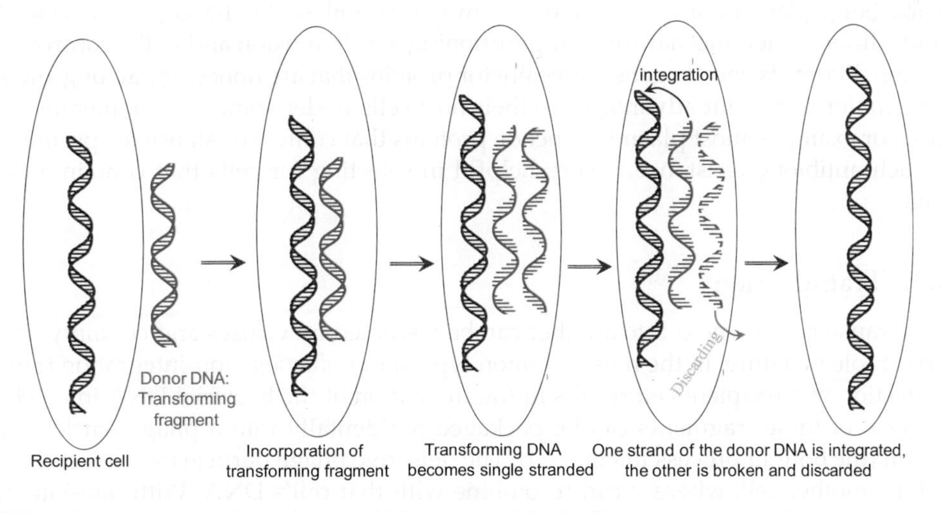

FIGURE 14.3 Integration of transforming DNA into a recipient cell.

essential in genetic engineering). A cell marks its own DNA (e.g. through methylation of certain purine or pyrimidine bases) to distinguish it from foreign DNA. These modifications block the action of a cell's own restriction endonucleases on its own DNA. Under natural conditions, gene transfer is effective only if the donor DNA is from the same or closely related species.

The entrance of donor DNA into a cell holds the key for genetic recombination. The three mechanisms of foreign DNA entering a cell are discussed in the following three sections.

14.3.2. Transformation

The uptake of naked DNA cannot be done by all genera of bacteria. Even within transformable genera, only certain strains are transformable (*competent*). Competent cells have a much higher capacity for binding DNA to the cell surface than do noncompetent cells. Competency can depend on the physiological state of the cell (current and previous growth conditions). Even in a competent population, only a small fraction of cells are transformable. Typically, about 0.1–1.0% is transformable.

Noncompetent cells may be rendered competent under special conditions (a genetic engineering tool). *Escherichia coli* are not normally competent, but their importance to microbial genetics has led to the development of empirical procedures to induce competency. This procedure involves treating *E. coli* with a high concentration of calcium ions coupled with temperature manipulations. The competency of treated cells varies among strains of *E. coli*, but is typically rather low (about one in a million cells becomes successfully transformed). With the use of selective markers, this frequency is still high enough to be quite useful.

Transformation is useful only when the information that enters the cell can be propagated. When doing transformation, we typically use a vector called a *plasmid*. This element forms the basis for most industrially important fermentations with recombinant DNA. A plasmid is an autonomous, self-replicating, double-strand piece of DNA that is normally extrachromosomal. Some plasmids are maintained as low copy number (20–100 copies per cell). These plasmids differ in their mechanisms for partitioning at cell division and in the control of their replication. Plasmids encode genes typically for proteins that are nonessential for growth, but that can confer important advantages to their host cells under some environmental circumstances. For example, most plasmids encode proteins that confer resistance to specific antibiotics. Such antibiotic resistance is very helpful in selecting for cells that contain a desired plasmid.

14.3.3. Transduction

DNA transfer from one cell to another can be mediated by viruses and certainly plays an important role in nature. In the most common type of *transduction*, non-integration transduction, infection of a recipient cell results in fragmentation of the bacterial DNA into 100 or so pieces. One of these fragments can be packaged accidentally into a phage particle during formation (the bottom process in Fig. 14.4). The defective phage particle then injects bacterial DNA into another cell, where it can recombine with that cell's DNA. With non-integration transduction, any bacterial gene may be transferred.

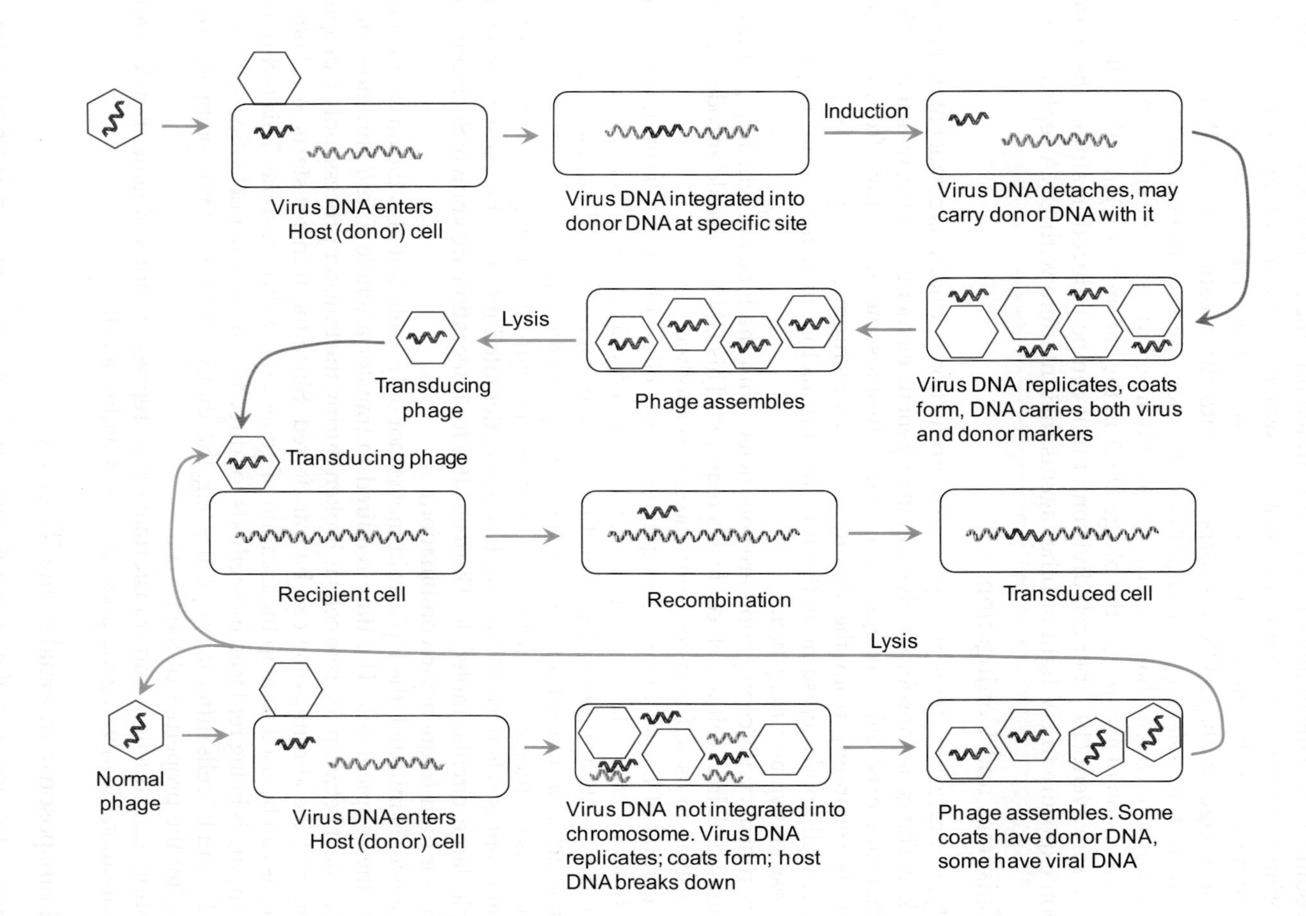

FIGURE 14.4 Transduction: the transfer of genetic material from donor to recipient via virus particles. Two processes are shown: upper one is the integration transduction and the bottom one is the common non-integration transduction.

Another method of transfer, which is far more specific with respect to the genes that are transferred, is integration transduction. Here, the phage incorporates into specific sites in the chromosome, where the phage's DNA is integrated into the host's DNA. The frequency of transduction of a gene is related to its distance away from the site of incorporation. The process is summarized by the upper process shown in Fig. 14.4. *A lysogenic cell* is one carrying a prophage or phage DNA incorporated into chromosomal DNA. Phage λ is an example of such a *temperate phage* (a phage that can either lyse a cell or become incorporated into the chromosome). Such phages almost invariably insert at a specific site in the chromosome. The conversion of a *prophage* (the phage DNA in the chromosome) into the lytic cycle is normally a rare event (10^{-4} per cell division), but it can be induced in almost the whole culture upon exposure to UV light or other agents that interfere with DNA replication.

14.3.4. Episomes and Conjugation

A third type of gene transfer is analogous to reproduction sextually as contact of two intact cells is the key. The gene transfer involves another genetic element: *episome*, which is a DNA molecule that may exist either integrated into the chromosome or separate from it. When episome exists separately from the chromosome (extrachromosomally), it is essentially a plasmid. A well-known episome is the F or fertility factor. Such factors are responsible for the process known as *conjugation*.

Most experiments with conjugation are conducted with the F factor, which is present in low copy number. Direct cell-to-cell contact is required. This DNA molecule encodes at least 13 genes involved in its self-transfer from one cell to another.

In a population of *E. coli*, there are frequently some cells with the F plasmid, which are termed F^+ (male). Other cells are F^- (female). F^+ cells encode proteins to make a *sex pilus*. When F^+ and F^- cells are mixed together, the sex pilus connects an F^+ to an F^- cell. The sex pilus may act as a conduit for the transfer of a copy of the F plasmid.

This process is normal and does not involve transfer of chromosomal genes or recombination. A rarer event is when the F plasmid has been integrated into the chromosome itself to form a single, large, circular molecule. Thirteen sites for integration are known. Such cells are termed Hfr (for high-frequency recombination).

When transfer is initiated, the F plasmid moves not only itself, but also the attached chromosome, to the recipient cell. The time required to transfer a whole *E. coli* chromosome is 100 min. If contact between the two cells is broken during the transfer process, only a proportional amount of the chromosome can be transferred. Since the transfer starts at a known point, Hfr cells can be used to map the location of genes on the chromosome. This technique for gene mapping is being replaced by methods for directly sequencing nucleotide sequences in DNA. If F^+ and F^- cells differ in properties (e.g. the ability to make lysine), conjugation can be used to alter the properties of the F^- cell.

Conjugation, transduction, and transformation all represent forms of gene transfer from one cell to another. However, gene transfer occurs within a cell.

14.3.5. Transposons: Internal Gene Transfer

We discussed the presence of *insertion elements* on the chromosome, e.g. integration transduction. A closely related phenomenon is a *transposon*, which refers to a gene or genes that have the ability to "jump" from one piece of DNA to another or to another position independently of any homology with the recipient piece of DNA. Transposons differ from insertion sequences in that they code for proteins. Transposons appear to arise when a gene becomes bounded on both sides by insertion sequences. Many of the transposons encode antibiotic resistance.

Transposons are important because (1) they can induce mutations when they insert into the middle of a gene, (2) they can bring once separate genes together, and (3) in combination with plasmid- or vital-mediated gene transfer, they can mediate the movement of genes between unrelated bacteria (e.g. multiple antibiotic resistances on newly formed plasmids). Transposon mutagenesis can be a very powerful tool in altering cellular properties.

14.4. TECHNIQUES OF GENETIC ENGINEERING

Genetic engineering is also known as recombinant DNA technology. Genetic recombination is a process of combining genetic elements from two different genomes to form a new genotype in the absence of mutations, which also occur naturally as discussed in the previous section.

In this section, we will focus on the techniques that are used by the genetic engineers to manipulate the genetic material for academic, research, and industrial purposes:

14.4.1. Gene Synthesis

The key to genetic engineering is finding the desired gene to be incorporated into the host to obtain the desired property. It is possible to chemically synthesize a gene in the lab by laboriously joining nucleotides together in the correct order. Automated machines can now make this much easier, but only up to a limit of about 30 bp, so very few real genes could be made this way (anyway it is usually much easier to make complimentary DNA [cDNA]). The genes for the two insulin chains and for the hormone somatostatin (42 bp) have been synthesized this way. It is very useful for making gene probes.

14.4.2. Complimentary DNA

cDNA is a DNA made from mRNA. This makes use of the enzyme reverse transcriptase, which does the reverse of transcription: it synthesizes DNA from an mRNA template. It is produced naturally by a group of viruses called the retroviruses (which include HIV), and it helps them to invade cells.

In genetic engineering, reverse transcriptase is used to make an artificial gene of cDNA (Fig. 14.5). cDNA has helped to solve different problems in genetic engineering. It makes genes much easier to find. There are some 70,000 genes in the human genome, and finding one gene out of this many is a very difficult (though not impossible) task. However, a given cell only expresses a few genes, so only makes a few different kinds of mRNA molecule. For example, the B cells of the pancreas make insulin, so make lots of mRNA molecules coding for insulin. This mRNA can be isolated from these cells and used to make cDNA of the insulin gene.

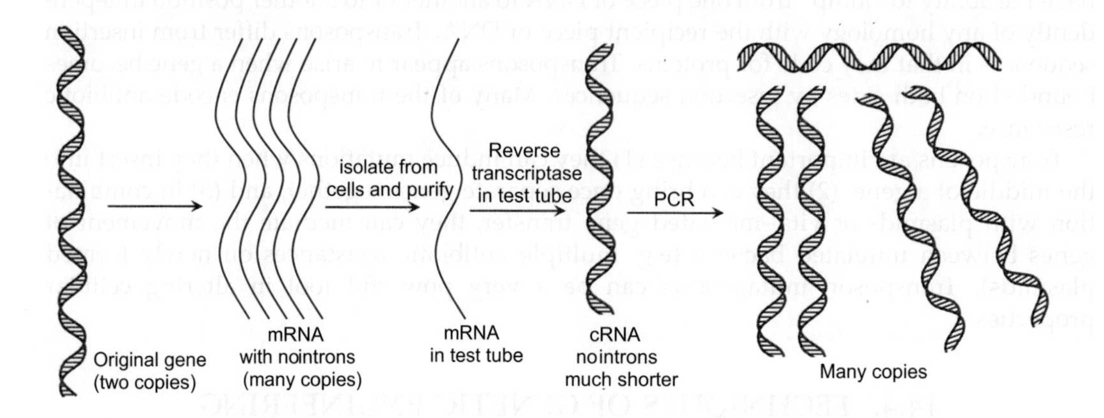

FIGURE 14.5 Method of producing cDNAs.

14.4.3. Cloning Genes into a Plasmid

Once a desired gene is isolated or created, it can be cloned by inserting it into a plasmid as shown in Fig. 14.6.

14.4.4. Polymerase Chain Reaction

Genes can be cloned by cloning the bacterial cells that contain them, but this requires quite a lot of DNA in the first place. Polymerase chain reaction (PCR) can clone (or amplify) DNA samples as small as a single molecule. It is a newer technique, having been developed in 1983 by Kary Mullis, for which discovery he won the Nobel prize in 1993. The PCR is simply DNA replication in a test tube. If a length of DNA is mixed with the four nucleotides (A, T, C, and G) and the enzyme DNA polymerase in a test tube, then the DNA will be replicated many times (Fig. 14.7).

Each original DNA molecule has now been replicated to form two molecules. The cycle is repeated from step 2 and each time the number of DNA molecules doubles. This is why it is called a chain reaction, since the number of molecules increases exponentially, like an explosive chain reaction. Each cycle the PCR is run, the number of DNA molecules doubles. For an n-PCR cycles, the increase in DNA molecules would be 2n times. See if we start out from one DNA strand, each successive PCR cycle would lead to an increase by 100%, or 2, $2^2 = 4$, $2^3 = 8$, $2^4 = 16$. In just 10 cycles, the number of DNA strands becomes 1024. In 20 cycles, the number of DNA strands becomes 1,048,576. Typically, PCR is run for 20–30 cycles as shown.

14.4.5. Vectors and Plasmids

Once a desired gene is isolated or created, it is inserted into a carrier DNA called vector. Most often plasmids are used as vectors, although viruses can also be used for carrying the

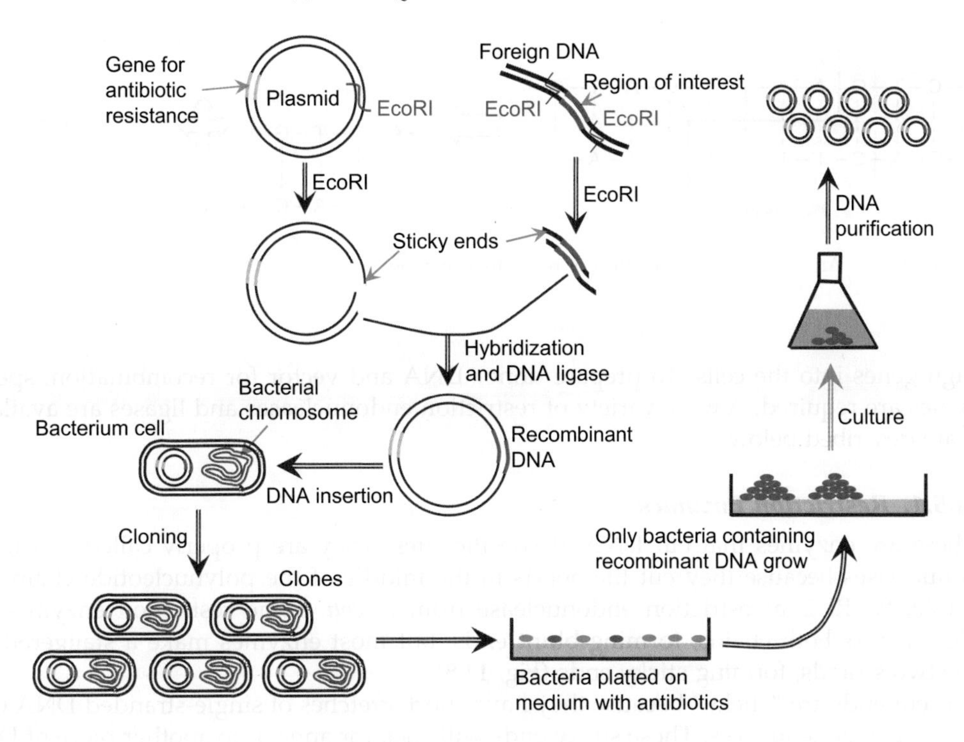

FIGURE 14.6 Method of producing genetically altered DNA.

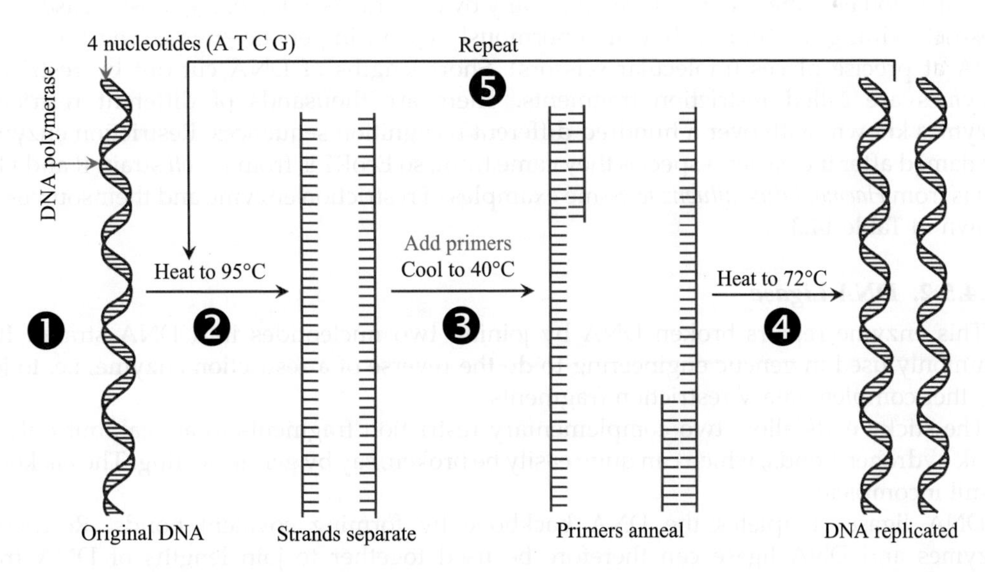

FIGURE 14.7 Procedure of cloning DNA.

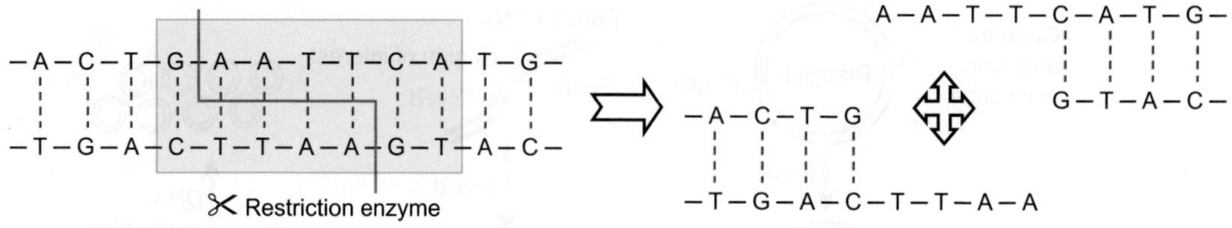

FIGURE 14.8 An illustration of the effect of restrictive enzyme.

foreign genes into the cells. To prepare donor DNA and vector for recombination, special enzymes are required. A wide variety of restriction endonucleases and ligases are available and are described below.

14.4.5.1. Restriction Enzymes

These are enzymes that cut DNA at specific sites. They are properly called restriction endonucleases because they cut the bonds in the middle of the polynucleotide chain. For example, EcoRI is a restriction endonuclease from *E. coli*. Some restriction enzymes cut straight across both chains, forming blunt ends, but most enzymes make a staggered cut in the two strands, forming sticky ends (Fig. 14.8).

The cut ends are "sticky" because they have short stretches of single-stranded DNA with complementary sequences. These sticky ends will stick (or anneal) to another piece of DNA by complementary base pairing, but only if they have both been cut with the same restriction enzyme. Restriction enzymes are highly specific and will only cut DNA at specific base sequences, 4–8 base pairs long, called recognition sequences.

Restriction enzymes are produced naturally by bacteria as a defense against viruses (they "restrict" viral growth), but they are enormously useful in genetic engineering for cutting DNA at precise places (molecular scissors). Short lengths of DNA cut out by restriction enzymes are called restriction fragments. There are thousands of different restriction enzymes known, with over a hundred different recognition sequences. Restriction enzymes are named after the bacteria species they came from, so EcoR1 is from *E. coli* strain R and HindIII is from *Haemophilus influenzae*. Some examples of restriction enzyme and their sources are shown in Table 14.3.

14.4.5.2. DNA Ligase

This enzyme repairs broken DNA by joining two nucleotides in a DNA strand. It is commonly used in genetic engineering to do the reverse of a restriction enzyme, i.e. to join together complementary restriction fragments.

The sticky ends allow two complementary restriction fragments to anneal, but only by weak hydrogen bonds, which can quite easily be broken, say by gentle heating. The backbone is still incomplete.

DNA ligase completes the DNA backbone by forming covalent bonds. Restriction enzymes and DNA ligase can therefore be used together to join lengths of DNA from different sources (Fig. 14.9).

TABLE 14.3 Examples of Restriction Enzymes

Restriction enzyme	Source	Recognition sequence and location of cuts
AluI	*Arthrobacter luteus*	5→ –A–G↓C–T– →3 3← –T–C↑G–A– ←5
HaeIII	*Haemophilus aegyptius*	5→ –G–G↓C–C– →3 3← –C–C↑G–G– ←5
BamHI	*Bacillus amyloliquefaciens*	5→ –G↓G–A–T–C–C– →3 3← –C–C–T–A–G↑G– ←5
HindIII	*H. influenzae*	5→ –A↓A–G–C–T–T– →3 3← –T–T–C–G–A↑A– ←5
EcoRI	*E. coli*	5→ –G↓A–A–T–T–C– →3 3← –C–T–T–A–A↑G– ←5

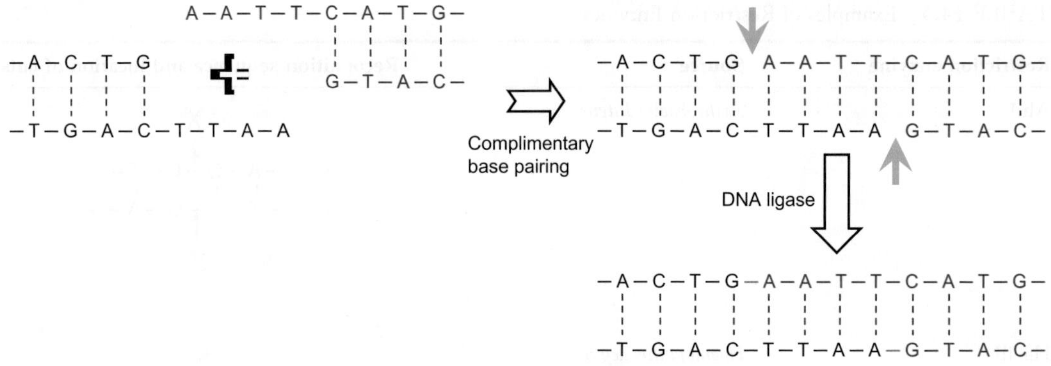

A–A–T–T–C–A–T–G–

–A–C–T–G + G–T–A–C–

–T–G–A–C–T–T–A–A

Complimentary base pairing

–A–C–T–G A–A–T–T–C–A–T–G–

–T–G–A–C–T–T–A–A G–T–A–C–

DNA ligase

–A–C–T–G–A–A–T–T–C–A–T–G–

–T–G–A–C–T–T–A–A–G–T–A–C–

FIGURE 14.9 Attaching a foreign gene onto a DNA molecule (cut by restrictive enzyme).

A vector is needed because a length of DNA containing a gene on its own will not actually do anything inside a host cell. Since it is not part of the cell's normal genome, it will not be replicated when the cell divides, it will not be expressed, and in fact it will probably be broken down pretty quickly. A vector gets around these problems by having these properties:

- It is big enough to hold the gene we want (plus a few others) but not too big.
- It is circular (or more accurately a closed loop), so that it is less likely to be broken down (particularly in prokaryotic cells where DNA is always circular).
- It contains control sequences, such as a replication origin and a transcription promoter, so that the gene will be replicated, expressed, or incorporated into the cell's normal genome.
- It contains marker genes, so that cells containing the vector can be identified.

Many different vectors have been made for different purposes in genetic engineering by modifying naturally occurring DNA molecules, and these are now available off the shelf. Different kinds of vector are also available for different lengths of DNA insertion (Table 14.4).

14.4.5.3. *Plasmids*

Plasmids are by far the most common kind of vector, so we shall look at how they are used in detail. Plasmids are short circular bits of DNA found naturally in bacterial cells. A typical plasmid contains three to five genes and there are usually around 10 copies of a plasmid in a bacterial cell. Plasmids are copied separately from the main bacterial DNA when the cell

TABLE 14.4 Gene Insertion Length into DNA Molecule as a Function of the Vector

Type of vector	Maximum length of DNA insertion
Plasmid	10 kbp
Virus of phage	30 kbp
Bacterial artificial chromosome (BAC)	500 kbp

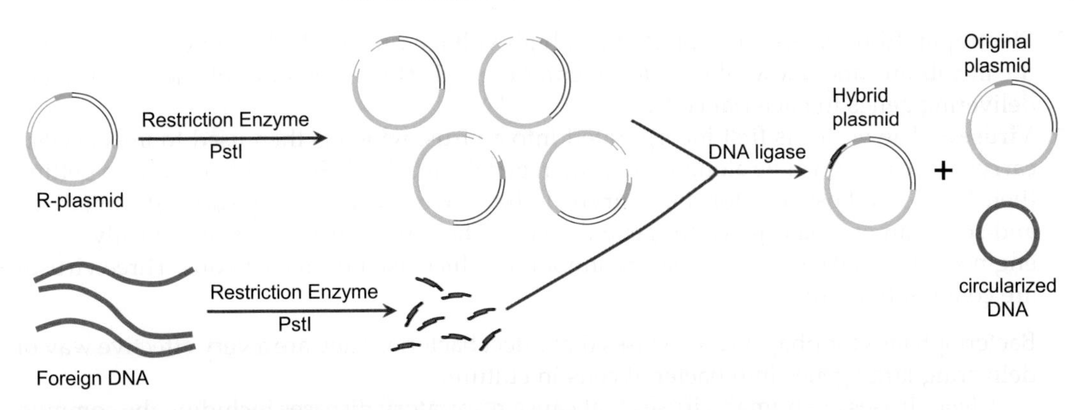

FIGURE 14.10 Insertion of a DNA gene into a plasmid.

divides, so the plasmid genes are passed on to all daughter cells. They are also used naturally for exchange of genes between bacterial cells (the nearest they get to sex), so bacterial cells will readily take up a plasmid. Because they are so small, they are easy to handle in a test tube, and foreign genes can quite easily be incorporated into them using restriction enzymes and DNA ligase.

One of the most common plasmids used is the R-plasmid (or pBR322). This plasmid contains a replication origin, several recognition sequences for different restriction enzymes (with names like PstI and EcoRI), and two marker genes, which confer resistance to different antibiotics (ampicillin and tetracycline).

Fig. 14.10 shows how DNA fragments can be incorporated into a plasmid using restriction and ligase enzymes. The restriction enzyme used here (PstI) cuts the plasmid in the middle of one of the marker genes (we will see why this is useful later). The foreign DNA anneals with the plasmid and is joined covalently by DNA ligase to form a hybrid vector (in other words a mixture or hybrid of bacterial and foreign DNA). Several other products are also formed: some plasmids will simply reanneal with themselves to reform the original plasmid, and some DNA fragments will join together to form chains or circles. These different products cannot easily be separated, but it does not matter, as the marker genes can be used later to identify the correct hybrid vector.

14.4.5.4. Gene Transfer

Vectors containing the genes we want must be incorporated into living cells so that they can be replicated or expressed. The cells receiving the vector are called host cells, and once they have successfully incorporated the vector, they are said to be transformed. Vectors are large molecules which do not readily cross cell membranes, so the membranes must be made permeable in some way. There are different ways of doing this depending on the type of host cell.

1. **Heat shock**—Cells are incubated with the vector in a solution containing calcium ions at 0 °C. The temperature is then suddenly raised to about 40 °C. This heat shock causes some of the cells to take up the vector, though no one knows why. This works well for bacterial and animal cells.

2. **Electroporation**—Cells are subjected to a high-voltage pulse, which temporarily disrupts the membrane and allows the vector to enter the cell. This is the most efficient method of delivering genes to bacterial cells.
3. **Viruses**—The vector is first incorporated into a virus, which is then used to infect cells, carrying the foreign gene along with its own genetic material. Since viruses rely on getting their DNA into host cells for their survival, they have evolved many successful methods and so are an obvious choice for gene delivery. The virus must first be genetically engineered to make it safe, so that it cannot reproduce itself or make toxins. Three viruses are commonly used:

   Bacteriophages (or phages) are viruses that infect bacteria. They are a very effective way of delivering large genes into bacterial cells in culture.

   Adenoviruses are human viruses that cause respiratory diseases including the common cold. Their genetic material is double-stranded DNA, and they are ideal for delivering genes to living patients in gene therapy. Their DNA is not incorporated into the host's chromosomes, so it is not replicated, but their genes are expressed (Fig. 14.11).
4. **Gene gun**—This extraordinary technique fires microscopic gold particles coated with the foreign DNA at the cells using a compressed air gun. It is designed to overcome the problem of the strong cell wall in plant tissue, since the particles can penetrate the cell wall and the cell and nuclear membranes and deliver the DNA to the nucleus, where it is sometimes expressed.

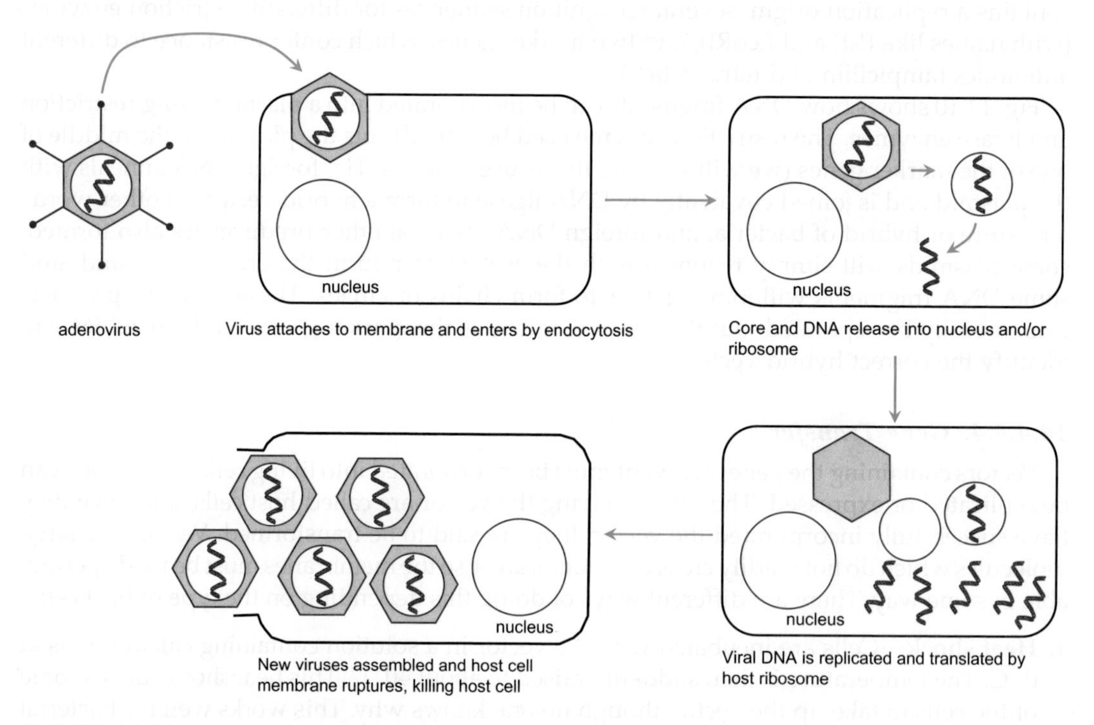

FIGURE 14.11 Replication of adenovirus.

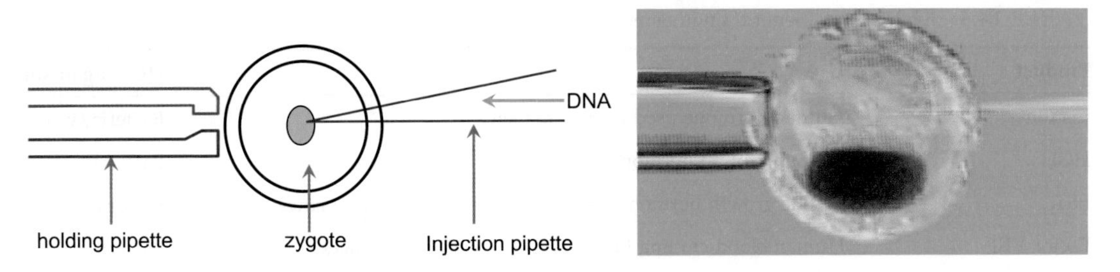

FIGURE 14.12 Microinjection. A DNA molecule is injected into a cell nucleus.

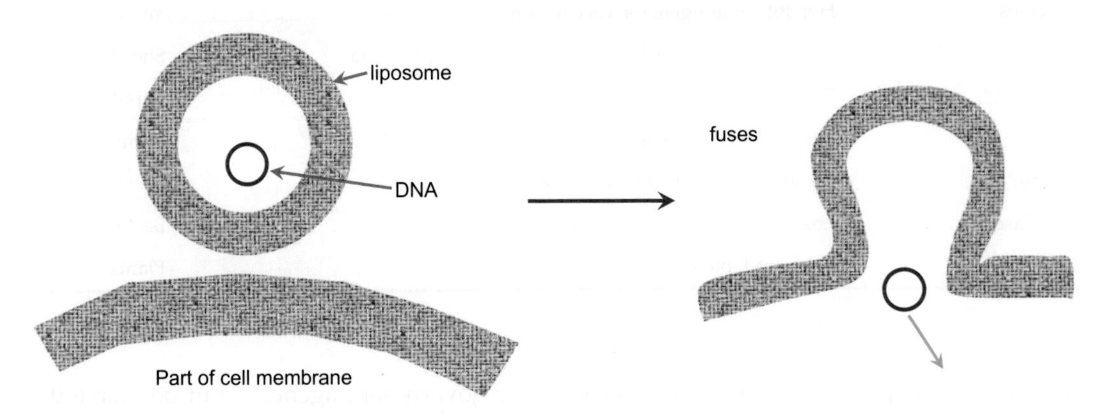

FIGURE 14.13 Delivering genes to cell in vivo via liposome.

5. **Microinjection**—A cell is held on a pipette under a microscope and the foreign DNA is injected directly into the nucleus using an incredibly fine micropipette (Fig. 14.12). This method is used where there are only a very few cells available, such as fertilized animal egg cells. In the rare successful cases, the fertilized egg is implanted into the uterus of a surrogate mother and it will develop into a normal animal, with the DNA incorporated into the chromosomes of every cell.
6. **Liposomes**—Vectors can be encased in liposomes, which are small membrane vesicles (Fig. 14.13). The liposomes fuse with the cell membrane (and sometimes the nuclear membrane too), delivering the DNA into the cell. This works for many types of cell but is particularly useful for delivering genes to cell in vivo (such as in gene therapy).

14.5. APPLICATIONS OF GENETIC ENGINEERING

By far the most applications are as research tools, and the techniques above are helping geneticists to understand complex genetic systems. Genetic engineering still has few successful commercial applications. When dealing with genetic engineering, a bioprocess engineer must be extremely prudent on the safety and long-term effects it may bring, not just to satisfy

TABLE 14.5 Examples of Genetic Engineered Cells

Product	Use	Host organism
Insulin	Human hormone used to treat diabetes	Bacteria/yeast
HGH	Human growth hormone, used to treat dwarfism	Bacteria
BST	Bovine growth hormone, used to increase milk yield of cows	Bacteria
Factor VIII	Human blood clotting factor, used to treat hemophiliacs	Bacteria
Anti-thrombin	Anti-blood clotting agent used in surgery	Goats
Penicillin	Antibiotic, used to kill bacteria	Fungi/bacteria
Vaccines	Hepatitis B antigen, for vaccination	Yeast
AAT	Enzyme used to treat cystic fibrosis and emphysema	Sheep
β-glucosidase	Enzyme used to treat Pompe's disease	Rabbits
DNase	Enzyme used to treat cystic fibrosis	Bacteria
Rennin	Enzyme used in manufacture of cheese	Bacteria/yeast
Cellulase	Enzyme used in paper production	Bacteria
PHB	Biodegradable plastic	Plants

the hype in the public and regulations brought by government agencies, but one have the professional responsibility to maintain a sustainably safe environment for the society. The successes of genetic engineering and its applications are increasing each year as our understanding of the genetic systems and their effects on the overall health of the living organisms as a whole. The applications so far can be considered in three groups.

Gene products—Using genetically modified organisms (usually microbes) to produce chemicals, usually for medical or industrial applications. The biggest and most successful kind of genetic engineering is the production of gene products. These products are of medical, agricultural, or commercial value. Table 14.5 shows a few of the examples of genetically engineered products that are already available.

New phenotypes—Using gene technology to alter the characteristics of organisms (usually farm animals or crops). This is an extremely sensitive area. The progress is limited not only by the perfection of methods but by our understanding of the effects they may bring, as well as public perception.

Gene therapy—Using gene technology on humans to treat a disease. Safety is paramount and the uncertainty has prevented many potential applications. This is the most sensitive area and has the least successful applications. Nevertheless, there have been cases of attempts since 1970s. The first approved gene therapy case in the United States took place on September 14, 1990, at the National Institute of Health. It was performed on a 4-year-old girl named Ashanti DeSilva. It was a treatment for a genetic defect that left her with an immune system deficiency. The effects were only temporary, but successful. In 1992, Doctor Claudio Bordignon working at the Vita-Salute San Raffaele University, Milan, Italy performed the first procedure of gene therapy using hematopoietic stem cells as vectors to deliver genes intended to correct hereditary diseases.

Scientists at the National Institutes of Health (NIH) (Bethesda, Maryland) have successfully treated metastatic melanoma in two patients using killer T cells genetically retargeted to attack the cancer cells. This study constitutes the first demonstration that gene therapy can be effective in treating cancer (Morgan RA, Dudley ME, Wunderlich JR, et al. "Cancer regression in patients after transfer of genetically engineered lymphocytes". *Science* 314 (5796): 126–129, 2006).

In March 2006, an international group of scientists announced the successful use of gene therapy to treat two adult patients for a disease affecting myeloid cells (Ott MG, Schmidt M, Schwarzwaelder K, "Correction of X-linked chronic granulomatous disease by gene therapy, augmented by insertional activation of MDS1-EVI1, PRDM16 or SETBP1". *Nat. Med.* 12 (4): 401–409, 2006).

In November 2006, Preston Nix from the University of Pennsylvania School of Medicine reported on VRX496, a gene-based immunotherapy for the treatment of human immunodeficiency virus (HIV) that uses a lentiviral vector for delivery of an antisense gene against the HIV envelope. In the phase I trial enrolling five subjects with chronic HIV infection who had failed to respond to at least two antiretroviral regimens, a single intravenous infusion of autologous CD4 T cells genetically modified with VRX496 were safe and well tolerated. All patients had stable or decreased viral load; four of the five patients had stable or increased CD4 T cell counts. In addition, all five patients had stable or increased immune response to HIV antigens and other pathogens. This was the first evaluation of a lentiviral vector administered in U.S. Food and Drug Administration-approved human clinical trials for any disease (Levine BL, Humeau LM, Boyer J, et al. "Gene transfer in humans using a conditionally replicating lentiviral vector". *Proc. Natl Acad. Sci. U S A* **103** (46): 17372–17377, 2006). Data from an ongoing phase I/II clinical trial were presented at CROI 2009.

We now turn to discussions on how to apply genetic engineering and/or genetically engineered cells in bioprocesses with a focus on gene products.

14.6. THE PRODUCT AND PROCESS DECISIONS

Genetically engineering cells can be aimed to make two major classes of products: proteins and nonproteins. Nonprotein products can be made by metabolically engineering cells, inserting DNA-encoding enzymes that generate new pathways or pathways with an enhanced capacity to process the precursors to a desired metabolite. This is an area of increasing interest because of our desire for sustainably renewable chemicals, materials, and energy. However, most industrial emphasis traditionally has been on proteins. Table 14.6 lists some of these examples. In 2011, the global market for industrial proteins is estimated at $77 billion annually by RNCOS. The majority of these proteins are human therapeutics, but proteins that can be used in animal husbandry, in food processing, or as industrial catalysts are of interest. To a large extent, this has been driven by the value or price of the product.

With therapeutic proteins that are injectable, the prime concern is the clinical efficiency of the product. Such products must be highly pure, since strong immunogenic reactions by

TABLE 14.6 Key Biopharmaceutical Products

Product	End use
Hormones and peptide factors	
Human insulin	Diabetes
Factor VIII-C	Hemophilia
Human growth hormone	Growth deficiency
Erythropoietin	Anemia, chronic renal failure
Interferon-alpha 2a	Hairy cell leukemia, AIDS-related cancer
Interferon-alpha 2b	Hairy cell leukemia, Herpes
Interferon-beta	Cancer
Interferon-gamma	Cancer, venereal warts, infectious disease
Interleukin-2	Cancer immunotherapy, AIDS
Muromonab-CD3	Acute kidney transplant rejection
Granulocyte colony stimulating factor (G-CSF)	Chemotherapy effects, AIDS
Granulocyte macrophage-colony stimulating factor (GM-CSF)	Autologous bone marrow transplant
Enzymes	
Tissue plasminogen activator	Acute myocardial infarction, stroke
Pro-urokinase/urokinase	Heart attack
DNase	Pulmonary treatment
Glucocerebrosidase	Gaucher
Vaccines	
Hepatitis B	Hepatitis B vaccine
Herpes	Herpes
Monoclonal antibodies	
	Wide range of different antibodies for diagnostics
	Prevention of blood clots
	Breast cancer
	Lung cancer

patients or other side effects can be disastrous. Large molecules are extremely difficult to identify. Minor difference in structural form or functional groups can result in significantly different properties. Therefore, the authenticity of the product is often critical. Correct or near correct posttranslational processing of the protein (e.g. glycosylation or phosphorylation) is sometimes essential to its therapeutic action. Any variant forms of the protein (e.g. the modification of side groups on amino acids) are highly undesirable and present very difficult purification problems.

The processing challenges in making therapeutic proteins are to ensure product quality and safety. Structural differences, for example folding, can be effected by different process conditions. Process efficiency to reduce manufacturing cost, although important, is of less concern, since these products are required in relatively small amounts. They can command high prices, and the selling price is determined by the costs of process development and regulatory approvals, particularly clinical trials. Thus, for large molecular therapeutic products, the choice of biological system and processing equipment is dictated by the need to produce highly purified material in an absolutely consistent manner.

Other protein products are acquired strictly on an economic basis, and manufacturing costs play a much more critical role in the viability of a proposed process. In this case, regulatory demands are of lesser importance than in the production of therapeutic proteins. For animal vaccines or animal hormones, the products must be very pure and render favorable cost ratios. For example, the use of bovine somatropin to increase milk production requires that the increased value of the milk produced be substantially greater than the cost of the hormone and any increase in feed costs due to increased milk production.

For food use, product safety is important, while purity requirements are less stringent than for an injectable therapeutic product. The volume of the required product is often substantial, at minimum several metric tons per year. The price is critical because alternative products from natural sources may be available. Proteins used as specialty chemicals (e.g. adhesives and enzymes for industrial processes) usually can tolerate the presence of contaminating proteins and compounds. The manufacturing costs for such proteins will greatly influence the market penetration.

For nonprotein products based on metabolically engineered cells, processing costs compared to costs of other routes of manufacture (usually nonbiological) will determine the success of such a process. Another important factor is the process safety and environmental impacts. Public perception and acceptance can also influence how a product is produced.

The constraints on production can vary widely from one product class to another. These constraints determine which host cells, vectors, genetic constructions, processing equipment, and processing strategies are selected.

14.7. HOST–VECTOR SYSTEM SELECTION

While overall optimization for a product manufacture is the ultimate goal, most if not all of the bioprocesses today are still based on heuristic approaches. The success or failure of a process often hinges on the initial choice of host organism and expression system. These choices must be made in the context of a processing strategy. Table 14.7 summarizes many of the salient features of common host systems. The most important initial judgment must be whether posttranslational modifications of the product are necessary. If they are, then an animal cell host system must be chosen. If some simple posttranslational processing is required (e.g. some forms of glycosylation), yeast or fungi may be acceptable. Whether posttranslational modifications are necessary for proper activity of a therapeutic protein cannot always be predicted with certainty, and clinical trials may be necessary.

Another important consideration is whether the product will be used in foods. For example, some yeasts (e.g. *Saccharomyces cerevisiae*) are on the FDA GRAS list (generally regarded as safe), which would greatly simplify obtaining regulatory approval for a given

TABLE 14.7 Characteristics of Selected Host Systems for Protein Production from Recombinant DNA (E = Excellent; VG = Very Good; G = Good; F = Fair; P = Poor)

	Organism				
Characteristic	***E. coli***	***S. cerevisiae***	***Pichia pastoris***	**Insect**	**Mammalian**
High growth rate	E	VG	VG	P-F	P-F
Availability of genetic systems	E	G	F	F-G	F-G
Expression levels	E	VG	E	G-E	P-G
Low-cost media available	E	E	E	P	P
Protein folding	F	F-G	F-G	VG-E	E
Simple glycosylation	No	Yes	Yes	Yes	Yes
Complex glycosylation	No	No	No	Yes*	Yes
Low levels of proteolytic degradation	F-G	G	G	VG	VG
Excretion or secretion	P normally, VG in special cases	VG	VG	VG	E
Safety	VG	E	VG	E	G

* *Glycosylation patterns differ from mammalian cells.*

product. In some cases, edible portions of transgenic plants can be used to deliver vaccines or therapeutic proteins.

14.7.1. Escherichia coli

If posttranslational modifications are not necessary, *E. coli* is most often the first choice as the host. The main reason for the popularity of *E. coli* is the broadly available knowledge base for it. *E. coli* physiology and its genetics are probably far better understood than any other living organisms. A wide range of host backgrounds (i.e. combinations of specific mutations) are available, as well as vectors and promoters. This large knowledge base helps to facilitate sophisticated genetic manipulations. The well-defined vectors and promoters greatly speed the development of an appropriate biological catalyst.

The relatively high growth rates for *E. coli* coupled with the ability to grow *E. coli* to high cell concentrations (>50 g/L) and with the high expression levels possible from specific vector-promoter combinations (about 25–50% or more of total protein) can lead to extremely high volumetric productivities. Also, *E. coli* will grow on simple and inexpensive media. These factors give *E. coli* many economic advantages.

An important engineering contribution was the development of strategies to grow cultures of *E. coli* to high cell densities. The build-up of acetate and other metabolic by-products can significantly inhibit the growth of *E. coli*. Controlled feeding of glucose so as to prevent the accumulation of large amounts of glucose in the medium prevents overflow metabolism and the formation of acetate. Glucose feeding can be coupled to consumption rate if the consumption rate can be estimated on-line or predicted. However, *E. coli* is not a perfect host. The major problems result from the fact that *E. coli* does not normally secrete proteins. When proteins are retained intracellularly and produced at high levels, the amount of soluble active protein present is usually limited due to either proteolytic degradation or insolubilization into *inclusion bodies*.

The production of large amounts of foreign protein may trigger a *heat-shock* response. One response of the heat-shock regulon is increased proteolytic activity. In some cases, intracellular proteolytic activity results in product degradation at a rate nearly equal to the rate of production. More often, the target protein forms an inclusion body. Although the heterologous protein predominates in an inclusion body, other cellular material is also often included. The protein in the inclusion body is misfolded. The misfolded protein has no desirable biological activity and is thus of no value. If the inclusion bodies are recovered from the culture, the inclusion bodies can be resolubilized and the activity (and value) can be restored. Resolubilization can vary tremendously in difficulty from one protein to another. When resolubilization is straightforward and recoveries are high, the formation of inclusion bodies can be advantageous, as it simplifies the initial steps of recovery and purification. It is important that during resolubilization the protein be checked by several analytical methods to ensure that no chemical modifications have occurred. Even slight changes in a side group can alter the effectiveness of the product.

Other consequences of cytoplasmic protein production can be important. The intracellular environment in *E. coli* might not allow the formation of disulfide bridges. Also the protein will usually start with a methionine, whereas that methionine would have been removed in normal posttranslational processing in the natural host cell. If the product is retained intracellularly, then the cell must be lysed during recovery. Lysis usually results in the release of endotoxins (or pyrogens) from *E. coli.* Endotoxins are lipopolysaccharides (found in the outer membrane) and can result in undesirable side effects (e.g. high fevers) and death. Thus, purification is an important consideration.

Many of the limitations on *E. coli* can be circumvented with protein secretion and excretion. *Secretion* is defined here as the translocation of a protein across the inner membrane of *E. coli. Excretion* is defined as release of the protein into the extracellular compartment. About 20% of all protein in *E. coli* is translocated across the inner membrane into the periplasmic space or incorporated into the outer membrane. As we have learned in Chapter 10, secreted proteins are made with a signal or leader sequence. The presence of a *signal sequence* is a necessary (but not sufficient) condition for secretion. The signal sequence is a sequence of amino acids attached to the mature protein, and the signal sequence is cleaved during secretion.

Many benefits are possible if a protein is secreted. Secretion eliminates an undesired methionine from the beginning of the protein. Secretion also offers some protection from proteolysis. Periplasmic proteases exist in *E. coli* but usually at a low level. They are most active in alkaline environments. With pH control the target protein degradation can be reduced. The environment in the periplasmic space promotes the correct protein folding in some cases (including the formation of disulfide bridges). Proteins in the periplasmic space can be released by gentle osmotic shock, so that fewer contaminating proteins are present than if the whole cell was lysed.

Extracellular release of target proteins is most preferable. Normally, *E. coli* does not excrete protein (colicin and hemolysin are the two exceptions), but a variety of schemes to obtain excretion in *E. coli* are being developed. Strategies usually involve either trying to disrupt the structure of the outer membrane or attempting to use the colicin or hemolysin excretion systems by constructing a fusion of the target protein with components of these excretion systems. Excretion without cell lysis can simplify recovery and purification even more than secretion alone, while achieving the same advantages as secretion with respect to protein-processing. Excretion also facilitates the potential use of continuous immobilized cell systems.

Excretion of normally cytoplasmic or human-designed proteins is problematic. There are reports for the excretion of normally cytoplasmic proteins, but the general principles for the extension of excretion to cytoplasmic proteins are still being developed. The excretion of normally secreted proteins can be obtained in *E. coli* (and other cells) even when the protein is derived from animal cells. However, extension to nonsecreted proteins is difficult.

The lack of established excretion systems in *E. coli* has led to interest in alternative expression systems. Also, in some cases, patent considerations may require the use of alternative hosts.

14.7.2. Gram-Positive Bacteria

The gram-positive bacterium, *Bacillus subtilis*, is the best studied bacterial alternative to *E. coli*. Since it is gram positive, it has no outer membrane, and it is a very effective excreter of proteins. Many of these proteins, amylases and proteases, are produced commercially using *B. subtilis*. If heterologous proteins could be excreted as efficiently from *B. subtilis*, then *B. subtilis* would be a very attractive production system. However, *B. subtilis* has a number of problems that have hindered its commercial adoption. A primary concern has been that *B. subtilis* produces a large amount and variety of proteases. These proteases can degrade the product very rapidly. Mutants with greatly reduced protease activity have become available, but even these mutants may have sufficient amounts of minor proteases to be troublesome. *Bacillus subtilis* is also much more difficult to manipulate genetically than *E. coli* because of a limited range of vectors and promoters.

Also, the genetic instability of plasmids (Chapter 15) is more of a problem in *B. subtilis* than in *E. coli*. Finally, the high levels of excretion that have been observed with native *B. subtilis* proteins have not yet been obtainable with heterologous protein (i.e. foreign proteins produced from recombinant DNA).

Other gram-positive bacteria that have been considered as hosts include *Streptococcus cremoris* and *Streptomyces* sp. These systems are less well characterized than *B. subtilis*.

Both gram-negative and gram-positive bacteria have limitations on protein-processing that can be circumvented with eukaryotic cells.

14.7.3. Lower Eukaryotic Cells

The yeast, *S. cerevisiae*, has been used extensively in food and industrial fermentations and is among the first organisms harnessed by humans. It can grow to high cell densities and at a reasonable rate (about 25% of the maximum growth rate of *E. coli* in similar medium). Yeast is larger than most bacteria and can be recovered more easily from a fermentation broth.

Further advantages include the capacity to do simple glycosylation of proteins and to secrete proteins. However, *S. cerevisiae* tends to hyperglycosylate proteins, adding large numbers of mannose units. In some cases, the hyperglycosylated protein may even be inactive.

These organisms are also on the GRAS list, which simplifies regulatory approval and makes yeast particularly well suited to production of food-related proteins. Generally, the limitations on *S. cerevisiae* are the difficulties of achieving high-protein expression levels, hyperglycosylation, and good excretion. Although the genetics of *S. cerevisiae* are better known than for any other eukaryotic cell, the range of genetic systems is limited, and stable high-protein expression levels are more difficult to achieve than in *E. coli*. Also, the normal capacity of the secretion pathways in *S. cerevisiae* is limited and is a bottleneck on excreted protein production, even when high expression levels are achieved.

The methylotrophic yeasts, *P. pastoris* and *Hansenula polymorpha*, are very attractive hosts for some proteins. These yeasts can grow on methanol as a carbon energy source; methanol is also an inducer for the AOX 1 promoter, which is typically used to control expression of the target protein. Very high cell densities (e.g. up to 100 g/L) can be obtained. Due to high densities and, for some proteins, high expression levels, the volumetric productivities of these cultures can be higher than with those *E. coli*. Protein folding and secretion are, also, often better than those in *E. coli*. These yeasts make simple glycosylation and are less likely to hyperglycosylate than *S. cerevisiae*. Like many host systems, their effectiveness is often a function of the target protein. The disadvantages of the methylotrophic yeast are due to the high cell density and rate of metabolism, which creates high levels of metabolic heat that must be removed and high oxygen demand. Effective induction of expression, while maintaining cell activity, requires very good process control due to methanol's dual functions as growth substrate and inducer. Furthermore, high levels of methanol are inhibitory (i.e. substrate inhibition), which also demands good process control. Scale-up to large reactors often is very challenging, since heat removal, oxygen supply, and process control are typically more difficult in large reactors with longer mixing times. Also, methanol is flammable and handling large volumes of methanol is a safety concern. Nonetheless, these methylotrophic yeasts are of increasing importance.

Fungi, such as *Aspergillus nidulans* and *Trichoderma reesei*, are also potentially important hosts. They generally have greater intrinsic capacity for protein secretion than *S. cerevisiae*. Their filamentous growth makes large-scale cultivation somewhat more difficult. However, commercial enzyme production from these fungi is well established, and the scale-up problems have been addressed. The major limitation has been the construction of expression and secretion systems that can produce as large amounts of extracellular heterologous proteins as some of the native proteins. A better understanding of the secretion pathway and its interaction with protein structure is critical for this system to reach its potential.

All these lower eukaryotic systems are inappropriate when complex glycosylation and posttranslational modifications are necessary. In such cases, animal cell tissue culture has been employed.

14.7.4. Mammalian Cells

Mammalian cell culture is the prime choice of host if the virtual authenticity of the product protein is complete. Authenticity implies not only the correct arrangement of all amino acids but also that all posttranslational processing is identical to that in the whole animal. In some cases, the cells in culture may not do the posttranslation modifications identically to those done by the same cell while in the body. But for bioreactor processes, mammalian cell tissue culture provides the product closest to its natural counterpart. Another advantage is that most proteins of commercial interest are readily excreted.

Slow growth, expensive media, and low protein expression levels all make mammalian cell tissue culture very expensive. A wide variety of reactor systems can be used with animal cell cultures. Although many of these can improve efficiency significantly, processes based on mammalian cells remain very expensive. Several cell lines have been used as hosts for the production of proteins using recombinant DNA. The most popular hosts are probably lines of CHO (Chinese hamster ovary) cells.

In addition to the cost of production, mammalian cells face other severe constraints. Normal cells from animals are capable of dividing only a few times; these cell lines are *mortal.* Some cells are *immortal* or *continuous* and can divide continuously, just as a bacterium can. Continuous cell lines are *transformed* cells. Cancer cells are also transformed (i.e. have lost the inhibition of cell replication). The theoretical possibility that a cancer promoting substance could be injected along with the desired product necessitates extreme care in the purification process. It is particularly important to exclude nucleic acids from the product. The use of transformed cells also requires cautions to ensure worker safety. Additionally, the vectors commonly used with mammalian cell cultures have been derived from primate viruses. Again, there is concern about the reversion of such vectors back to a form that could be pathogenic in humans.

Most of these vectors cannot give high expression levels of the target protein in common host cells (usually $<5\%$ of total protein). However, higher levels of expression can be obtained (e.g. >100 mg/L of secreted, active protein) through amplification of number of gene copies. It may take 6 months with a CHO cell line to achieve stable high-level expression. It is often easier to obtain high titers (or product concentration) when producing monoclonal antibodies from hybridoma cultures.

While the quality of the protein product may change upon scale-up with any system, this issue is particularly important with animal cell cultures. This contention is due, in part, to the fact that animal cell cultures are used primarily because authenticity of the protein product is a major concern. Since culture conditions (shear, glucose, amino sugars, dissolved oxygen, etc.) can change upon scale-up, the efficiency of cellular protein-processing can change, altering the level of posttranslational processing. Furthermore, protein quality may change with harvest time in batch cultures. This change may be due to alterations in intracellular machinery, but often it is due to release of proteases and siladase (an enzyme that removes the silalic acid cap from glycosylated proteins) from dead cells. Also, excessive levels of protein production may saturate the intracellular protein-processing organelles (i.e. ER and Golgi), leading to incompletely processed proteins. These problems can significantly impact process strategy. For example, harvest up to 24-h early may be required to maintain the silalic acid/protein ratio specified for the product. Early harvest resulted, however, can result in significant (up to 30%) loss in protein concentration. Strategies to reduce such problems include selection of cell lines or genetic manipulation of cell lines with reduced levels of siladase production or enhanced protein-processing capacity. Redesign of medium can be beneficial; chemicals that inhibit undesirable extracellular enzyme activity can be added or precursors added (e.g. amino sugars) to improve processing. Cell lysis can be reduced by adding genes (e.g. *bel* 2) to the host cell that reduces apotosis. An engineering solution is to remove the product from the medium as it is formed. For example, perfusion (i.e. chemostat or CSTR) systems with an integrated product capture step can be used.

14.7.5. Insect Cell-Baculovirus System

A popular alternative for protein production at small (<100 L) or laboratory scale is the insect cell-baculovirus system. This system is particularly attractive for rapidly obtaining biologically active protein for characterization studies. Typical host cell lines come from the fall armyworm (*Spodoptera frugiperda*) and the cabbage looper (*Trichoplusia ni*). The baculovirus, *Autographa californica* nuclear polyhedrosis virus (Ac NPV), is used as a vector for insertion of recombinant DNA into the host cell. This virus has an unusual biphasic replication cycle in nature. An insect ingests the occluded form, in which multiple virus particles are embedded in a protein matrix. The protein matrix protects the virus when it is on a leaf from environmental stresses (e.g. UV radiation). This protein matrix is from the polyhedrin protein. In the midgut of the insect, the matrix dissolves, allowing the virus to attack the cells lining the insect's gut; this is the primary infection. These infected cells release a second type of virus; it is nonoccluded (no polyhedrin matrix) and buds through the cell envelope. The nonoccluded virus (NOV) infects other cells throughout the insect (secondary infection).

In insect cell culture, only NOVs are infectious, and the polyhedrin gene is unnecessary. The polyhederin promoter is the strongest known animal promoter and is expressed late in the infection cycle. Replacing the polyhederin structural gene with the gene for a target protein allows high-level target protein production (up to 50% of cellular protein). Proteins that are secreted and glycosylated are often made at much lower levels than nonsecreted proteins.

In addition to high expression levels, the insect-baculovirus system offers safety advantages over mammal-retrovirus systems. The insect cell lines derived from ovaries or embryos are continuous but not transformed. The baculovirus is not pathogenic toward either plants or mammals. Thus, the insect-baculovirus system offers potential safety advantages. Another important advantage is that the molecular biology and high-level expression of correctly folded proteins can be achieved in less than a month. This system also has the cellular machinery to do almost all the complex posttranslational modifications that mammalian cells do. However, even when the machinery is present, at least some of the proteins produced in the insect cell-baculovirus system are not processed identically to the native protein. In some cases, their slight variations may be beneficial (e.g. increased antigenic response in the development of an AIDS vaccine), while in others they may be undesirable. While complex glycoforms (including silaic acid) have been made, it is more common to observe only simple glycoforms. Production of complex forms requires special host cell lines and is sensitive to culture conditions.

The insect cell-baculovirus system is a good system to illustrate an overall schematic perspective on heterologous protein production. Any bioprocess for protein production is complex, consisting of the nonlinear interaction of many subcomponents. Thus, the optimal process is not simply the sum of individually optimized steps. Fig. 14.14 presents a schematic view for the insect cell-baculovirus system. Because of the viral component, this system is

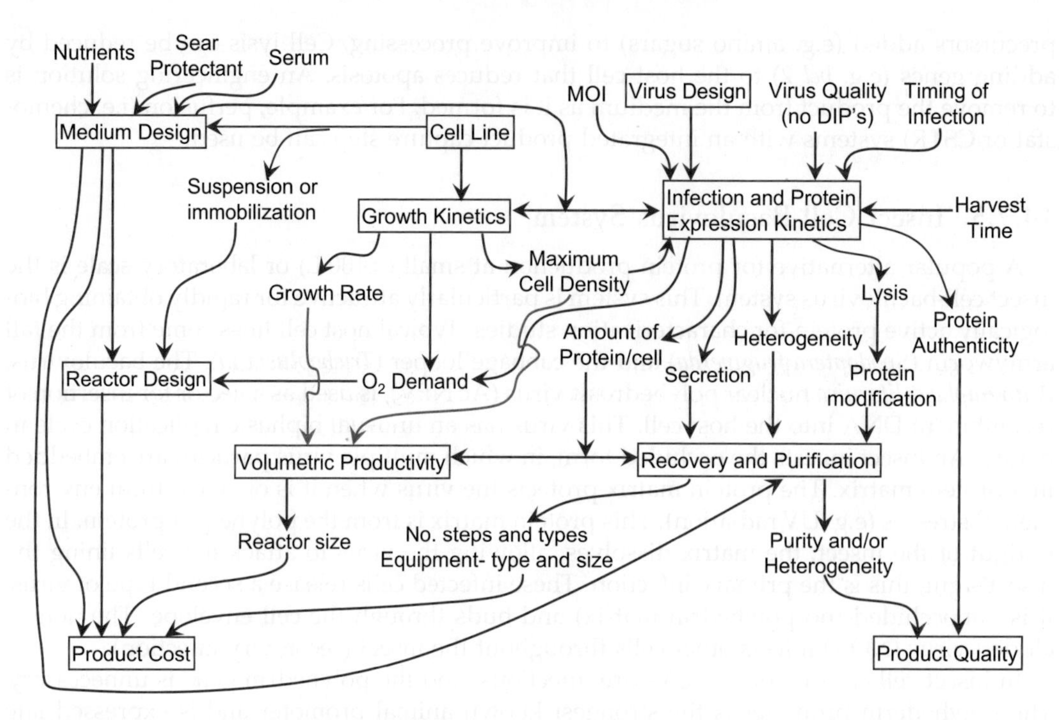

FIGURE 14.14 An overall process consideration for heterologous protein production with the baculovirus expression system.

even more complex than most other bioprocesses, as the infection process and resulting protein expression kinetics must be considered. One factor is the ratio of infectious particles to cells (e.g. multiplicity of infection or MOI), which alters the synchrony of infection and the resulting protein expression kinetics. Another is the genetic design of the virus (which shares many of the general features of vector design). Also, the quality of the virus stock is important; if the virus stock is maintained incorrectly, mutant virus can form. One example is the formation of *defective interfering particles* that reduce protein expression in the culture by 90% when high MOIs are used.

When designing a bioprocess of cell culture, one should work from the bottom of Fig. 14.14 toward the top. What is the tolerance on the desired product quality? What is the potential of the product worth? The answers to these questions then guide the selection of bioprocess strategies to achieve the cost and quality desired. To develop that strategy requires an understanding of the basic kinetics and capabilities of the biological system. Understanding these requirements guides selection of the specific host cell line, the medium, and the molecular design of the virus. For example, the addition of serum to the medium of some *Tini* cell lines results in production of proteins with complex N-linked glycosylation, including a sialic acid cap, which may be a requirement for product quality. However, the use of serum alters growth kinetics, expression levels (often less), and the difficulty of purification, which may alter cost. Such trade-offs need to be considered with respect to alternative approaches (e.g. development of a genetically engineered host that could perform the same reactions but in serum-free medium). Ideally, an overall optimization is most desirable and it is within reach today.

14.7.6. Transgenic Animals

In some cases, proteins with necessary biological activity cannot be made in animal cell culture. While posttranslational protein processes, such as N-linked glycosylation, can be done in cell culture, other more subtle forms of posttranslational processing may not be done satisfactorily. An alternative to cell culture is the use of transgenic animals. Animals are engineered to express the protein and release it into specific fluids, such as milk or urine. High concentrations of complex proteins can be achieved, and such approaches can be cost effective for complex proteins. In these cases, the role for the bioprocess engineer is in protein recovery and purification, although significant issues exist for agricultural engineers and animal scientists in devising appropriate systems to obtain the protein containing fluid (e.g. pig milking stations). While transgenic animals can be developed from many mammals, sheep, goats, and pigs are the primary species used commercially.

There are significant limitations on the transgenic animal technology. In some cases, the protein of interest will cause adverse health problems in the producing animal. The use of animals raises safety concerns with respect to virus or prion transmission. The process to generate and screen for high-producing animals is inefficient and costly (e.g. $100,000 for a goat and $500,000 for a cow). Perhaps surprisingly, not all of the complex posttranslational processing steps necessary to achieve the desired product occur when the protein is expressed in milk, urine, or blood. Nonetheless, transgenic animals will be critical to production of some proteins.

14.7.7. Transgenic Plants and Plant Cell Culture

Proteins, including many complex protein assemblies, such as antibodies and virus-like particles (as vaccines), can be made inexpensively in plants. Transgenic plants offer many potential advantages in addition to cost. Since plant viruses are not infective for humans, there are no safety concerns with respect to endogenous viruses or prions. Scale-up is readily accomplished by planting more acreage. The protein can be targeted for sterile, edible compartments, either reducing the need for rigorous purification or making it an ideal vehicle for oral delivery of a therapeutic protein. Indeed, development of edible vaccines for use in developing countries is being actively pursued.

The disadvantages of transgenic plants are that expression levels are often low (1% of total soluble protein is considered good), N-linked glycosylation is incomplete, and some other mammalian posttranslational processing is missing. While inexpensive, with easy scale-up, it takes 30 months to test and produce sufficient seed for unlimited commercial use. Such long lead times are undesirable. Further, environmental control on field grown crops is difficult, so the amount (and possibly quality) of the product can vary from time to time and place to place.

While many crops could be used, much of the commercial interest centers on transgenic corn. Some corn products are used in medicinals, so there exist some FDA guidelines (e.g. contamination with herbicides and mycotoxins), and there is considerable processing experience. Production costs vary with degree of desired purity. For high purity material (95% pure), a cost of about \$4–\$8/g can be expected. For higher purity material (99%) with full quality assurance and control, a cost of about \$20–\$30/g is reasonable.

At least two enzymes are being produced commercially from transgenic plants. Large-scale production of monoclonal antibodies (e.g. 500 kg/year) for topical uses is being considered.

The use of plant cell cultures is also being explored. The primary advantage of such cultures over transgenic plants is the much higher level of control that can be exercised over the process. Plant cell cultures, compared to animal cell cultures, grow to very high cell density, use defined media, and are intrinsically safer.

14.7.8. Comparison of Strategies

The choice of host–vector system is complicated. The characteristics desired in the protein product and the cost are the critical factors in the choice. The dominant systems for commercial production are *E. coli* and CHO cell cultures. The process economics of these two systems for production of tissue plasminogen activator, tPA, has been given by Datar, Cartwright, and Rosen (*Biotechnology* 11:349, 1993). Their analysis was for plants making 11 kg/year of product. The CHO cell process was assumed to produce 33.5 mg/L of product, while *E. coli* made 460 mg/L. The CHO cell product was correctly folded, biologically active, and released into the medium. The *E. coli* product was primarily in the form of inclusion bodies and thus biologically inactive, misfolded, and insoluble. The process to resolubilize and refold the *E. coli* product into active material requires extra steps. The recovery process for the CHO cell material requires five steps, while 16 steps are required for the *E. coli* process. The larger the number of steps, the greater the possibility of yield loss. Total recovery of 47% with the CHO-produced material was possible compared to only 2.8% for the *E. coli*-produced material.

The extra steps in the *E. coli* process are for cell recovery, cell breakage, recovery of inclusion bodies, resolubilization of inclusion bodies, concentration, sulfination, refolding, and concentration of the renatured protein. The difficulty of these processes depends on the nature of the protein; tPA is particularly difficult. With tPA the concentration of tPA had to be maintained at 2.5 mg/L or less, and refolding is slow, requiring 48 h. A 20% efficiency for renaturation was achieved. Many proteins can be refolded at higher concentrations (up to 1 g/L) and much more quickly. For tPA, the result is unacceptably large tanks and very high chemical usage. In this case, 5 tons of urea and 26 tons of guanidine would be necessary to produce only 11 kg of active tPA.

For tPA, the required bioreactor volumes were 14,000 L for the CHO process and 17,300 L for the *E. coli* process. The capital costs were \$11.1 million for the CHO process and \$70.9 million for the *E. coli* process, with 75% of that capital cost being required for the refolding tanks. Under these conditions, the unit production costs are \$10,660/g for the CHO process versus \$22,000/g for the *E. coli* process. The rate of return on investment (ROI) for the CHO process was 130% versus only 8% for the *E. coli* process. However, if the refolding step yield was 90% instead of 20%, the overall yield would improve to 15.4%, and the unit production cost would fall to \$7530 with an ROI of 85% for the improved *E. coli* process at production of 11 kg/year. If the *E. coli* plant remained the original size (17,300-L fermentor) so as to produce 61.3 kg/year, the unit production cost would drop to \$4400/g. The cost of tPA from the CHO process is very sensitive to cost of serum in the medium. If the price of media dropped from

$10.5/1 to $2/1 (e.g. 10–2% serum in the medium), the cost of the CHO cell product would drop to $6500/g.

A primary lesson from this exercise is the difficulty of making choices of host–vector systems without a fairly complete analysis. The price will depend on the protein, its characteristics, and intended use. Changes in process technology (e.g. low serum medium for CHO cells or protein secretion systems in *E. coli*) can have dramatic effects on manufacturing costs and choice of the host–vector system.

14.8. REGULATORY CONSTRAINTS ON GENETIC PROCESSES

When genetic engineering was first introduced, there was a great deal of concern over whether the release of genetically modified cells could have undesirable ecological consequences.

Reports in the popular press led to fears of "genetic monsters" growing in our sewers, on our farmlands, or elsewhere. Consequently, the use of genetic engineering technology is strictly regulated. The degree of regulatory constraint varies with the nature of the host, vector, and target protein. For example, consider a scenario where serious harm might arise. The gene for a highly toxic protein is cloned into *E. coli* to obtain enough protein to study that protein's biochemistry. Assume that a plasmid that is *promiscuous* (i.e. the plasmid will shuttle across species lines) is used. Also assume that laboratory hygiene is not adequate and a small flying insect enters the laboratory and comes into contact with a colony on a plate awaiting destruction. If that insect leaves the laboratory and returns to its natural habitat, then the target gene is accidentally released into the environment. Laboratory strains of *E. coli* are fragile and usually will not survive long in a natural environment. However, a very small probability exists that the plasmid could cross over species lines and become incorporated into a more hardy soil bacterium (e.g. *Pseudomonas* sp.). The plasmid would most certainly contain antibiotic-resistance factors as well. The newly transformed soil bacterium could replicate. Many soil bacteria are opportunistic pathogens. If they enter the body through a wound, they can multiply and cause an infection. If, in addition, the bacterium makes a toxic protein, the person or animal that was infected could die from the toxic protein before the infection was controlled. If the plasmid also confers antibiotic resistance, the infection would not respond to treatment by the corresponding antibiotic, further complicating control of the spread of the gene for the toxin.

This scenario requires that several highly improbable events occur. No case of significant harm to humans or the environment due to the release of genetically modified cells has been documented. However, the potential for harm is real. Cell recombination can also occur naturally §14.3 when chance presents. For example, the discovery of NDM-1 (New Delhi metallo-beta-lactamase 1) that dubbed as "superbug" has made headlines in 2010. The NDM-1 is a gene that produces an enzyme that deactivates basically all antibiotics. The drug resistance gene NDM-1 can pass from one kind of bacteria to another.

Regulations controlling genetic engineering concentrate on preventing the accidental release of genetically engineered organisms. The deliberate release of genetically engineered cells is possible, but an elaborate procedure must be followed to obtain permission for such experiments.

TABLE 14.8 Minimum Laboratory Containment Standards for Working with Cells with Recombinant DNA

Biosafety Level 1 (BL1)

1. *Standard microbiological practices*
   a. Access to the laboratory is limited or restricted at the discretion of the laboratory director when experiments are in progress.
   b. Work surfaces are decontaminated once a day and after any spill of viable material.
   c. All contaminated liquid or solid wastes are decontaminated before disposal.
   d. Mechanical pipetting devices are used; mouth pipetting is prohibited.
   e. Eating, drinking, smoking, and applying cosmetics are not permitted in the work area. Food may be stored in cabinets or refrigerators designated and used for this purpose only.
   f. Persons wash their hands after they handle materials involving organisms containing recombinant DNA molecules, animals, and before leaving the laboratory.
   g. All procedures are performed carefully to minimize the creation of aerosols.
   h. It is recommended that laboratory coats, gowns, or uniforms be worn to prevent contamination or soiling of street clothes.

2. *Special practices*
   a. Contaminated materials that are to be decontaminated at a site away from the laboratory are placed in a durable, leakproof container that is closed before being removed from the laboratory.
   b. An insect and rodent control program is in effect.

3. *Containment equipment*
   a. Special containment equipment is generally not required for manipulations of agents assigned to biosafety level.

4. *Laboratory facilities*
   a. The laboratory is designed so that it can be easily cleaned.
   b. Bench tops are impervious to water and resistant to acids, alkalis, organic solvents, and moderate heat.
   c. Laboratory furniture is sturdy. Spaces between benches, cabinets, and equipment are accessible for cleaning.
   d. Each laboratory contains a sink for handwashing.
   e. If the laboratory has windows that open, they are fitted with fly screens.

The degree of containment required depends on (1) the ability for the host to survive if released, (2) the ability for the vector to cross species lines or for a cell to be transformed by a piece of naked DNA and then have it incorporated into the chromosome via recombination, and (3) the nature of the genes and gene products being engineered. Experiments involving overproduction of *E. coli* proteins in *E. coli* using plasmids derived from wild populations are readily approved and do not require elaborate containment procedures (see Table 14.8). Experiments that would move the capacity to produce a toxin from a higher organism into bacteria or yeast would be subjected to a much more thorough evaluation, and more elaborate control facilities and procedures would be required.

The National Institutes of Health (NIH) have guidelines that regulate the use of recombinant DNA technology. Special regulations apply to large-scale systems (defined as >10 L). There are three different levels of containment: BLl-LS, BL2-LS, and BL3-LS. BLl-LS (biosafety level 1, large-scale) is the least stringent. Table 14.9 compares the requirements for the three containment levels.

In all cases, no viable organisms can be purposely released. Gas vented from the fermenter must be filtered and sterilized. All cells in the liquid effluent must be killed. The latter can

TABLE 14.9 Physical Containment Requirements for Large-scale Fermentations Using Organisms Containing Recombinant DNA Molecules

Item no.	Description	BL1-LS	BL2-LS	BL3-LS
1	Closed vessel	×	×	×
2	Inactivation of cultures by validated procedure before removing from the closed system	×	×	×
3	Sample collection and addition of material in a closed system	×	×	×
4	Exhaust gases sterilized by filters before leaving the closed system	×	×	×
5	Sterilization by validated procedures before opening for maintenance or other purposes	×	×	×
6	Emergency plans and procedures for handling large losses	×	×	×
7	No leakage of viable organisms from rotating seals and other mechanical devices		×	×
8	Integrity evaluation procedure: monitors and sensors		×	×
9	Containment evaluation with the host organism before introduction of viable organisms		×	×
10	Permanent identification of closed system (fermentor) and identification to be used in all records		×	×
11	Posting of universal biohazard sign on each closed system and containment equipment when working with a viable organism		×	×
12	Posting of universal biohazard sign on entry doors when work is in progress			×
13	Operations to be in a controlled area:			×
	Separate specified entry			×
	Double doors, air locks			×
	Walls, ceiling, and floors to permit ready cleaning and decontamination			×
	Utilities and services (process piping and wiring) to be protected against contamination			×
	Handwashing facilities and shower facilities in close proximity			×
	Area designed to preclude release of culture fluids outside the controlled area in the event of an accident			×
	Ventilation: movement of air, filtration of air			×

With permission, from R. J. Giorgiou and J. J. Wu, Trends in Biotechnology *4:198 (1986).*

present some operating issues, since the inactivation of the host cell must be done in such a way as not to harm what are often fragile products. Emergency plans and devices must be on hand to handle any accidental spill or loss of fluid in the fermentation area. These extra precautions increase manufacturing costs.

The issue of the regulation of cells and recombinant DNA will undoubtedly undergo further refinement with time. Both laboratory and manufacturing personnel need to keep abreast of any such changes.

14.9. METABOLIC ENGINEERING

Metabolic or pathway engineering uses the tools of genetic engineering to endow an organism to make a totally new pathway, amplify an existing pathway, disable an undesired pathway, or alter the regulation of a pathway. The principle motivations for metabolic engineering are the production of specialty chemicals (e.g. indigo, biotin, and amino acids), utilization of alternative substrates (e.g. pentose sugars from hemicellulose), or degradation of hazardous wastes such as benzoates or trichlorethylene. The same concepts form the basis for gene therapy.

One may ask why genetically engineered organisms should be used instead of natural isolates. The potential advantages over natural isolates are as follows:

- Can put an "odd-ball" pathway under the control of a regulated promoter. The investigator can turn on the pathway in situations where the pathway might normally be suppressed (e.g. degradation of a hazardous compound to a concentration lower than necessary to induce the pathway in the natural isolate).
- High levels of enzymes in desired pathways can be obtained with strong promoters; only low activity levels may be present in the natural isolate.
- Pathways moved from lower eukaryotes to bacteria can be controlled by a single promoter; in lower eukaryotes, each protein has a separate promoter.
- Several pathways can be combined in a single organism by recruiting enzymes from more than one organism.
- Can move a pathway from an organism that grows poorly to one that can be more easily cultured.
- The genetically engineered cell can be proprietary property.

Cells that have engineered pathways face many of the same limitations that cells engineered to produce proteins face. Two issues that perhaps assume greater importance with metabolic engineering are stability and regulatory constraints.

Protein products are of high value and can be made in batch culture. Instability is avoided by inducing overproduction only at the end of the culture cycle. The productive phase is too short for nonproducers to grow to a significant level, and cells are not reused. With metabolically engineered cells, the same strategy is untenable. Lower product values necessitate cell reuse or, at least, extended use. The use of antibiotics as selective agents may be undesirable because of contamination of product or cost. For a culture with a maximum growth rate of $\mu_{max} = 0.45\,h^{-1}$ and a 20-h batch cycle, a continuous system has a 14-fold advantage in productivity over a batch system. Although the levels of protein overproduction are lower in metabolically engineered cells, they can experience as high a level of metabolic burden as "protein producers" because of the diversion of cellular building blocks to nonessential metabolites. Also, if the cells are used to treat hazardous compounds, the genetically engineered cells will face competition from a natural flora.

In addition to the need for extra efforts in engineering design to ensure genetic stability, regulatory approval may be more difficult. If a genetically engineered cell is to be used to treat hazardous wastes, containment of the engineered organism is difficult or impossible. Pump-and-treat scenarios for leachates allow the possibility of control. In situ use of such organisms would have to satisfy the constraints for deliberate release.

In addition to these two problems, engineering pathways require good quantitative information on the flow of metabolites in a cell. Detailed kinetic models of cells (Chapter 10) can be used in conjunction with experiments to optimize the design of new pathways. Metabolic engineering has been a fertile area for engineering contributions. Metabolic engineering (and gene therapy) require a delicate balance of activities and are a problem of quantitative optimization rather than simple maximization of expression of a gene.

A goal of the engineering approach has been to develop rational design techniques for metabolic engineering. Due to the highly nonlinear, dynamic nature of a cell and its metabolism, uninformed changes intended to improve production of a specific compound often fail to give the desired result. The problem of metabolic engineering is to express appropriate genes in the "exact" amount needed. Too much of a key enzyme may result in little change, if it is not a rate-influencing step, as there is insufficient reactant to increase the flow of substrate (or *flux*) into the reaction product. If it is rate-influencing, the increased reaction of the substrate will alter fluxes of precursors in other pathways; sometimes these changes compromise the cell's ability to grow or to provide co-reactants when needed.

The limitation of analytical and computational methods had been a hindrance in metabolic engineering and kinetic modeling. Simplifications have been employed to circumvent the computational and analytic demand. *Metabolic control theory* and the closely allied activity of *metabolic flux analysis* are mathematical tools that can be applied to such problems. A flux balance equation consists of the product of a stoichiometric matrix and an intracellular flux vector to yield an overall rate vector. Typically such equations are underdetermined and require assumptions (e.g. on energy stoichiometry) that may not be justified for a metabolically engineered cell. However, improved experimental techniques to measure the intracellular flux vector (e.g. mass spectrometry) coupled with genomic/proteomic information may provide the data to allow complete solution of the flux balance equations. One caution is that analysis of pathways in isolation can be misleading. An assumption of such analysis is that the products of the pathway do not influence inputs into that pathway. Given the complexity of a cell, it is difficult to assure that such an assumption is satisfied.

Metabolic control theory is based on a sensitivity analysis to calculate the response of a pathway to changes in the individual steps in a pathway. This approach allows calculations of flux control coefficients, which are defined as the fractional change of flux expected for a fractional change in the amount of each enzyme. This process involves a linearization, so that flux coefficients can vary significantly if growth conditions and the cell's physiological step change. An important result of the application of this theory to many cases is that it is rare for a single enzyme step to be rate controlling. Typically several enzymatic steps influence rate. Maximization of flux through a particular pathway would require several enzyme activities to be altered simultaneously. The potential of such analysis to contribute to rational design of microbes is clear but not yet routinely applicable.

Real progress has been made toward the industrial use of metabolically engineered cells. Processes to convert glucose from cornstarch into 1,3-propanediol, an important monomer in the polymer, polytrimethylene terepthalate, is poised for commercialization. A process to make 2-keto-L-gluconic acid as a precursor for vitamin C production is in the pilot stage (30,000 L), using metabolically engineered bacteria with glucose as a substrate. Other products from metabolically engineered cells may be new polyketides, modified polyhydroxyalkanoates (as biodegradable polymers), indigo, xylitol, and hybrid antibiotics.

14.10. PROTEIN ENGINEERING

Not only can cells be engineered to make high levels of naturally occurring proteins or to introduce new pathways, but we can also make novel proteins. It is possible to make synthetic genes encoding for totally new proteins. We are beginning to understand the rules by which a protein's primary structure is converted into its three-dimensional form. We are just learning how to relate a protein's shape to its functional properties, stability, and catalytic activity. It may become possible to customize protein design to a particular well-defined purpose.

Protein engineering at present mainly involves the modification of existing proteins to improve their stability, substrate and inhibitor affinity and specificity, and catalytic rate. Generally, the protein structure must be known from X ray crystallography. Key amino acids in the structure are selected for alteration based on computer modeling, on interactions of the protein with substrates, or by analogy to proteins of related structure. The technique used to generate genes encoding the desired changes in protein structure is called *site-directed mutagenesis*. Using this approach, any desired amino acid can be inserted precisely into the desired position.

Site-directed mutagenesis is preferred to simple mutation-selection procedures. One reason is that mutation followed by selection for particular properties may be difficult when the alterations in protein properties are subtle and confer no advantages or disadvantages on the mutant cell. A second reason is that site-directed mutagenesis can be used to generate the insertion of an amino acid in a particular location, while a random mutation giving the same result would occur so infrequently as to be unobtainable. To make this point more evident, consider the degenerate nature of the genetic code. Each codon consists of three letters. The odds for mutation in one of these three letters are about 10^{-8} per generation. The odds that two letters would simultaneously be altered are much lower (order of 10^{-16}). The codon UAC (for tyrosine) could be altered by single letter substitutions to give AAC (asparagine), GAC (aspartate), CAC (histidine), UCC (serine), UUC (phenylalanine), UGC (cysteine), UAA (stop signal), UAG (stop signal), and UAU (tyrosine). Random mutants in this case are very unlikely to carry substitutions for 13 of the 20 amino acids. Thus, most of the potential insertions can be generated reliably only by using site-directed mutagenesis.

The above approaches are directed toward the rational design of proteins. An alternative, and often complementary, approach is that of *directed evolution*. This process is based on random mutagenesis of a gene and the subsequent selection of proteins with desired properties. Large libraries of mutant genes must be made so that the rare beneficial forms are present. A rapid screen or selection must be available to select those mutants with the desired function or characteristics. One technique to generate mutants is the use of "error-prone"

PCR. Another approach is DNA shuffling, which requires genes from homologous proteins. Segments from the genes are recombined randomly to form chimeric genes. Proteins are typically selected for improved stability, binding strength, catalytic activity, or solubility. In some cases, the screen is for new activities based on ability to bind other molecules not normally bound by the native protein. These techniques combined with improved biochemical methods are leading to a better understanding of the relation of protein structure to function. Also, these techniques support the extension of protein catalysis to unusual environments, such as in organic media rather than in aqueous solutions.

14.11. SUMMARY

A cell's *genotype* represents the cell's genetic potential, whereas its *phenotype* represents the expression of a culture's potential. The genotype of a cell can be altered by mutations. Examples of mutations are *point mutations, deletions,* and *additions*. Additions are usually the result of *insertion sequences* that "jump" from one position to another.

Mutations may be *selectable* or *unselectable*. The rate of mutation can be enhanced by the addition of chemicals called mutagens or by radiation. *Auxotrophs* are of particular use in genetic analysis and as a basis for some bioprocess. Another useful class of mutants is conditional mutants.

Gene transfer from one cell to another augments genetic information in ways that are not possible through mutation only. *Genetic recombination* of different DNA molecules occurs within most cells. Thus, genetic information transferred from another organism may become a permanent part of the recipient cell. The three primary modes of gene transfer in bacteria are *transformation, transduction, and conjugation*. Self-replicating, autonomous, extrachromosomal pieces of DNA called *plasmids* play important roles in transformation. *Episomes*, which are closely related to plasmids, are the key elements in conjugation. Bacteriophages are critical to *generalized* transduction, while *temperate phages* are the key to *specialized* transduction. Internal gene transfer can occur due to the presence of *transposons*, which probably also play a role in the assembly of new plasmid.

We can use gene transfer in conjunction with *restriction enzymes* and *ligases* to genetically engineer cells. In vitro procedures to recombine isolated donor DNA genes with *vector* DNA (for example plasmids, temperate phages, or modified viruses) are called recombinant DNA *techniques*. Once the vector with the DNA donor insert has been constructed, it can be moved to a recipient cell through any natural or artificial method of gene transfer. Although transformation is the most common technique in bacteria, a large variety of artificial methods have been developed to insert foreign DNA into a host cell.

The application of recombinant DNA technology at the commercial level requires a judicious choice of the proper host–vector system. *E. coli* greatly facilitates sophisticated genetic manipulations, but process or product considerations may suggest alternative hosts. *S. cerevisiae* is easy to culture and is already on the GRAS list, simplifying regulatory approval, although productivities are low with some proteins and hyperglycosylation is a problem. *Pichia stipitis* can produce very high concentrations of proteins, but the use of methanol presents challenges in reactor control and safety. *Bacillus* and the lower fungi may have well-developed secretion systems that would be attractive if they can be harnessed.

Animal cell culture is required when posttranslational modifications are essential. Mammalian cells offer the highest degree of fidelity to the authentic natural product. Insect cell systems potentially offer high expression levels and greater safety than mammalian cells at the cost of a potential decrease in the fidelity of posttranslational processing. Transgenic animals are good alternatives for complex proteins requiring extensive posttranslational processing. Transgenic plants and plant cell cultures are emerging as production systems for high-volume protein products. Plants are well suited to produce proteins for oral or topical delivery.

The vector must be designed to optimize a desired process. Factors to be considered include vector copy number, promoter strength and regulation, the use of fusion proteins, signal sequences and secretion, genes providing selective pressure, and elements enhancing the accuracy of vector partitioning.

The engineer must be aware of the regulatory constraints on the release of cells with recombinant DNA. These are particularly relevant in plant design, where guidelines for physical containment must be met. Deliberate release of genetically modified cells is possible, but extensive documentation will be required. Two increasingly important applications of genetic engineering are metabolic or pathway engineering for the production or destruction of nonproteins and protein engineering for the production of novel or specifically modified proteins.

Further Reading

Shuler, M.L., Kargi, F. *Bioprocess Engineering – Basic Concepts*, Prentice Hall, Upper Saddle River, NJ, 2006.

Carroll, S.B., Grenier, J., Weatherbee, S.D. *From DNA to Diversity: Molecular Genetics and the Evolution of Animal Design*. 2nd ed. Wiley-Blackwell, 2005.

Liu, T., Lin, L., Sun, Z., Hu, R., Liu, S., 2010. *J. Biotech. Adv.*, 28, 602–608.

http://www.baculovirus.com/

http://staff.jccc.net/PDECELL/evolution/mutations/mutation.html

http://www.biologymad.com/master.html?http://www.biologymad.com/GeneticEngineering/GeneticEngineering.htm

PROBLEMS

14.1. Would a cell with a point mutation or a deletion mutation be more likely to revert back to the original phenotype? Why?

14.2. You wish to isolate temperature-sensitive mutants (e.g. those able to grow at 25 °C but not at 37 °C). Describe experiments to isolate such a cell.

14.3. An important method for screening for carcinogens is called the *Ames test*. The test is based on the potential for mutant cells of a microorganism to revert to a phenotype similar to the nonmutant. The rate of reversion increases in the presence of a mutagen. Many compounds that are mutagens are also carcinogens and vice versa. Describe how you would set up an experiment and analyze the data to determine if nicotine is mutagenic.

14.4. How many different hybridization probes must you make to ensure that at least one corresponds to a set of four codons encoding the amino acid sequence cal-leu-trp-lys?

14.5. You wish to develop a genetically engineered *E. coli* producing a peptide hormone. You know the amino acid sequence of the peptide. Describe the sequence of steps you would use to obtain a culture expressing the gene as a peptide hormone.

14.6. You wish to develop a genetically engineered *E. coli* to produce a particular known protein. The protein converts a colorless substrate into a blue product. You have access to a high-copy-number plasmid with a penicillin-resistant gene and normal reagents for genetic engineering. Describe how you would engineer *E. coli* to produce this protein. Consider: source of donor DNA; regulatory elements that need to be included; how the donor and vector DNA are combined; how the vector DNA is inserted; and how you would select for a genetically engineered cell to use in production.

14.7. You wish to express a particular peptide in *E. coli* using a high-copy-number plasmid. You have the amino acid sequence for the peptide.

a. Explain the experimental process for generating and selecting the genetically engineered *E. coli* using restriction enzymes, ligase, *E. coli*, plasmid with neomycin resistance, and the known amino acid sequence.

b. What control elements would you place on the plasmid to regulate expression and to prevent read-through?

14.8. **a.** There are three primary methods for obtaining donor DNA when performing genetic engineering. Briefly describe those methods.

b. You need to produce a protein from humans in *E. coli*. You do not know the primary amino acid sequence. You suspect that introns are present. Which method will you use to obtain the donor DNA?

14.9. What is the difference between "transduction" and "transformation" when discussing genes transfer to bacteria?

CHAPTER

15

Sustainability: Humanity Perspective

OUTLINE

Music, to create harmony, must investigate discord

Plutarch

While all the materials or substances on earth play different roles in the ecological systems, water, O_2, N_2, and CO_2 are noticeably the most significant agents for life (Fig. 15.1). The sun provides the driving force (energy) powering the never-ending cycle. Plants, animals, organic matters, oceans and soils, and atmosphere are the various sheltering points (or nodes). Ocean and soil (including rocks) are the largest "reservoirs" for CO_2 and water. Atmospheric CO_2 and water are of very small amount due to the chemical and physical properties of these gases. Yet, it is the small amount of these gases, especially CO_2, in the atmosphere that have attracted most attention. Water, O_2, and CO_2 are also carriers or catalysts for energy and materials on earth. For example, the phase behavior of water entails the changing levels of energy it stores and thus buffers the earth's surface temperature around 14 °C with the high latent energies of condensation/vaporization, freezing/melting, and deposition/sublimation, slowing down the change of temperature.

Bioprocess Engineering
http://dx.doi.org/10.1016/B978-0-444-59525-6.00015-9

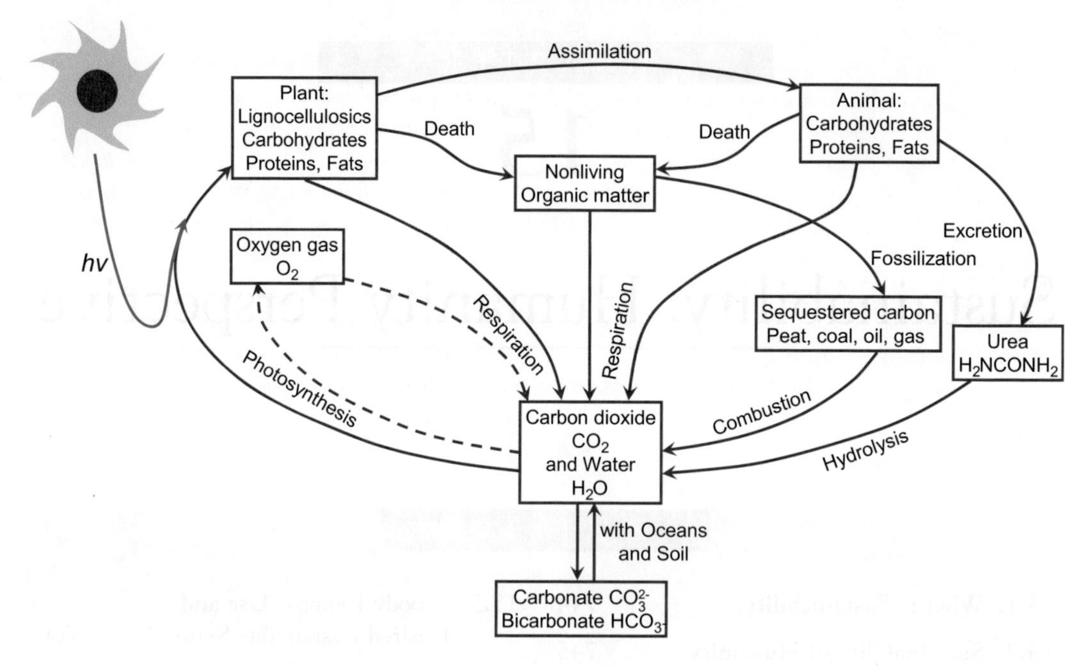

FIGURE 15.1 A simplified schematic of biological H_2O, CO_2, and O_2 cycle in nature.

Water vapor is the dominant greenhouse gas (GHG), followed by carbon dioxide with less than half the effect of water vapor, in the atmosphere, absorbing radiant heat from the sun. Life is supported by water, O_2, and CO_2 with energy from the radiant heat of the sun. Therefore, the sustainable or steady levels of these agents are of the critical concern for the intelligent life form on earth. While continuity or longevity is a universal concern: every process, every product, and every raw material we use, water and CO_2, are two key substances in the cycle of life.

In this chapter, we shall focus on the narrow perceptions of sustainability based on humanity, especially in regards to the basic ingredient for life: water and CO_2. As such, energy, chemical and material source and/or energy carrier forms part of the discussion in this chapter. However, more fundamental understanding of bioprocess sustainability is discussed in Chapter 16.

15.1. WHAT IS SUSTAINABILITY?

Sustainability is the capacity to endure. In a more general scientific sense, sustainability is equivalent to continuum or ability to continue the course without termination. Therefore, sustainability is compatible with the existence of universe and it is the ability to maintain a definite "stable" outcome. The evolution to a sustainable state is predictable. However, the form or state that is sustainable can be changed with intelligence or systematic intervention during the course of evolution.

Sustainability refers to processes and objects or matters. Sustainability is incompatible with monotonous increase or decrease of amounts of a matter. Sustainability exists between competing forces of increase and decrease. Monotonous increase of the amount of one matter leads to the exhaustion of a limited surrounding (that contains the matter) or depletion of source that provides the increase of the matter, while monotonous decrease of the amount of a matter leads to the eventual exhaustion of the matter. In bioprocesses, sustainability is compatible with steady state.

Example 15-1. Bottomless Lake.

Medicine Lake in the Jasper National Park of Canada is a typical glacier lake, except that there is no visible draining outlet. Water from upstream pouring into the lake in a typical summer day at 0.1 m^3/s. In the summer, the lake is full of water. However, in the winter, the lake is completely dry. The Natives call it the Medicine Lake because of this unique feature. We learned that for the lake to be sustainable, one cannot just have an inlet supplying water into the lake without water leaving the lake. Upon close examination, one finds that water is leaking out from the porous bottom. Assume that the rate of water leaking out of the Lake is $0.032\sqrt{h}$ m^3/s with the water level in the lake h in meters. Further assume that the evaporation loss of water from the lake surface is 0.001 m^3/s. Determine the sustainable level of water in the lake in the summer.

Solution. The sustainable level of water in the lake is the level of water at steady state. Material balance of the liquid water around the lake (rate of increasing water amount and rate of decreasing lake water is balanced) leads to

$$Q_F - Q_E - Q_{Evaporation} = 0 \tag{E15-1.1}$$

where Q_F is the rate of water flowing into the lake from upstream, Q_E is the rate of water leaking out of (or exiting) the lake, and $Q_{Evaporation}$ is the rate of liquid water evaporated into the air (as vapor). Substituting the flow rates, we obtain

$$0.1 - 0.032\sqrt{h} - 0.001 = 0 \tag{E15-1.2}$$

Solving Eqn (E15-1.2), we obtain

$$h = \left(\frac{0.1 - 0.001}{0.032}\right)^2 \text{m} = 9.57 \text{ m} \tag{E15-1.3}$$

The sustainable (liquid) water level is impressive in the summer.

15.2. SUSTAINABILITY OF HUMANITY

There is only one type of sustainability: the sustainability of human in existence that is of interest in this chapter. This significantly narrows the definition of sustainability. However, sustainability is necessarily neither unique nor quantitatively invariable. Since the 1980s *sustainability* has been used more in the sense of human sustainability on planet Earth and this has resulted in the most widely quoted definition of sustainability and sustainable development, that of the Brundtland Commission of the United Nations on March 20, 1987: "sustainable development is development that meets the needs of the present without

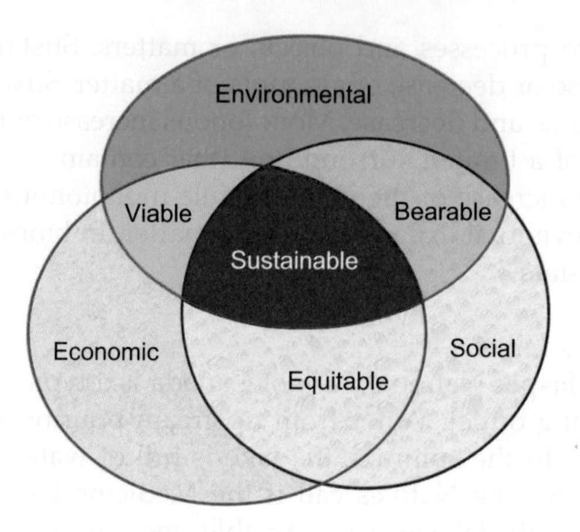

FIGURE 15.2 The three dimensions of sustainability.

compromising the ability of future generations to meet their own needs." [United Nations General Assembly (March 20, 1987). *"Report of the World Commission on Environment and Development: Our Common Future*; Transmitted to the General Assembly as an Annex to document A/42/427—Development and International Co-operation: Environment; Our Common Future, Chapter 2: Towards Sustainable Development; Paragraph 1."]. By default, when we discuss sustainability, we mean sustainability in human terms.

In ecology, the word sustainability describes how biological systems remain (qualitatively) diverse and productive over time, preferably indefinitely. Long-lived and healthy wetlands and forests are examples of sustainable biological systems. For humans, sustainability is the potential for long-term maintenance of well-being, which has three key dimensions: environmental, economic, and social dimensions (Fig. 15.2).

Healthy ecosystems and environments provide vital goods (chemicals, materials, and energy) and services to humans and other organisms. The presence of humans, like any other living organisms that are part of the ecosystem, contributes or affects the sustainability of the ecosystem on earth. Higher comfortability levels or optimum living conditions are demanded by all the organisms in the ecosystem. The optimum living conditions are different for different organisms and thus adverse effects on other organisms can develop if one organism is capable of achieving its ultimate comfortability. Human is the dominant life form and thus human needs are first to be met. Corresponding to the three dimensions of sustainability, there are three major ways of reducing "negative" human impact and enhancing ecosystem services (Fig. 15.3). The first is process and/or product optimization; this approach ensures the minimum impact to the ecosystem we are living in. Process optimization is a significant part of this text for bioprocesses and bio-products, although not directly discussed in this chapter. The second is environmental management; this approach is based largely on information gained from earth science, environmental science, and conservation biology. This text has some coverage in engineering aspect for environmental engineering processes. The third approach, and equally important one, is management of human consumption of resources, which is based largely on information gained from social

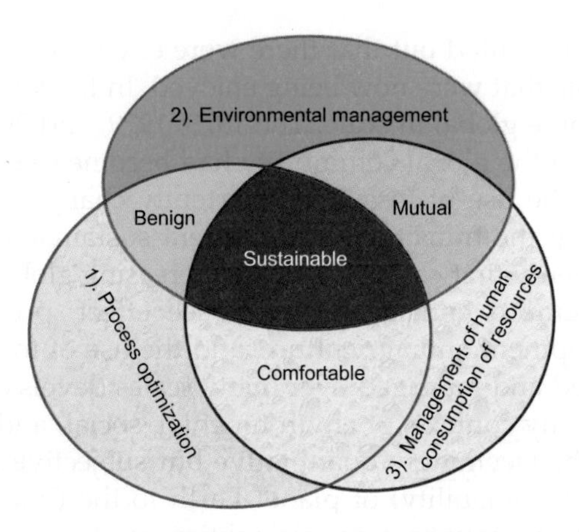

FIGURE 15.3 The three major approaches to reduce negative impacts of human activities and enhance ecosystem services.

and economic requirements. In this chapter, the second approach is focused, while the third approach is out of the scope of this text.

Sustainability interfaces with economics through the social and ecological consequences of economic activity. Sustainability economics involves ecological economics where social, cultural, health-related, and monetary/financial aspects are integrated. Moving toward sustainability is also a social challenge that entails international and national law, urban planning and transport, local and individual lifestyles, and ethical consumerism. Ways of living more sustainably can take many forms from reorganizing living conditions (e.g. ecovillages, eco-municipalities, and sustainable cities), reappraising economic sectors (permaculture, green building, and sustainable agriculture), or work practices (sustainable architecture), using science to develop new technologies (green technologies and renewable energy), to adjustments in individual lifestyles that be renewably and minimize or conserve nonrenewable natural resources.

The awareness of sustainability can be drawn from human-dominated ecological systems from the earliest civilizations to the present. The increased regional success of a particular society, followed by crises that were either resolved, producing sustainability, or not, leading to decline.

Sustainable state is not unique and improved sustainable state is continually being sought either intelligently or inadvertently in the past. In early human history, the use of fire and desire for specific foods may have altered the natural composition of plant and animal communities. Between 8000 and 10,000 years ago, Agrarian communities emerged which depended largely on their environment and the creation of a "structure of permanence". Agriculture is the dominant process to supply the food for human societies today. The ecosystem is completely altered with the advent of agriculture.

The western industrial revolution of the seventeenth to nineteenth centuries tapped into the vast growth potential of the energy in fossil fuels. Coal was used to power ever more efficient engines and later to generate electricity. Modern sanitation systems and advances in medicine protected large populations from disease. In the mid-twentieth century, a gathering environmental movement pointed out that there were environmental costs associated with the many material benefits that were now being enjoyed. In the late twentieth century, environmental problems became global in scale. The 1973, 1979, and 2008 energy crises demonstrated the extent to which the global community had become dependent on nonrenewable energy resources. While the use of fossils inadvertently changed the sustainable state, or more accurately is making the transition to a different sustainable state, fossil use itself is not sustainable. In the twenty first century, there is increasing global awareness of the threat posed by the human-induced enhanced greenhouse effect, produced largely by forest clearing for urban development and agriculture, and the use of fossil fuels.

Sustainability is studied and managed over many scales (levels or frames of reference) of time and space and in many contexts of environmental, social, and economic organization. The focus ranges from the (seemingly quantitative but subjective and able to manipulate) total carrying capacity (sustainability) of planet Earth to the (qualitative) sustainability of economic sectors, ecosystems, countries, municipalities, neighborhoods, home gardens, individual lives, individual goods and services, occupations, lifestyles, behavior patterns, and so on. In short, it can entail the full compass of biological and human activity or any part of it.

15.3. WATER

We have taken water as granted: it is vastly available on earth. Water covers 70.9% of the Earth's surface. Water had been the cause of destruction and prosperity for ancient civilizations. Legends have it how our ancestors tamed the waterways and made land fertile to agriculture.

Water is dependent on by all known forms of life. It is the best solvent and energy carrier for humanity. The importance of water is due to its physical and chemical properties. Fig. 15.4 shows the property of water. What makes water special is that under normal atmospheric

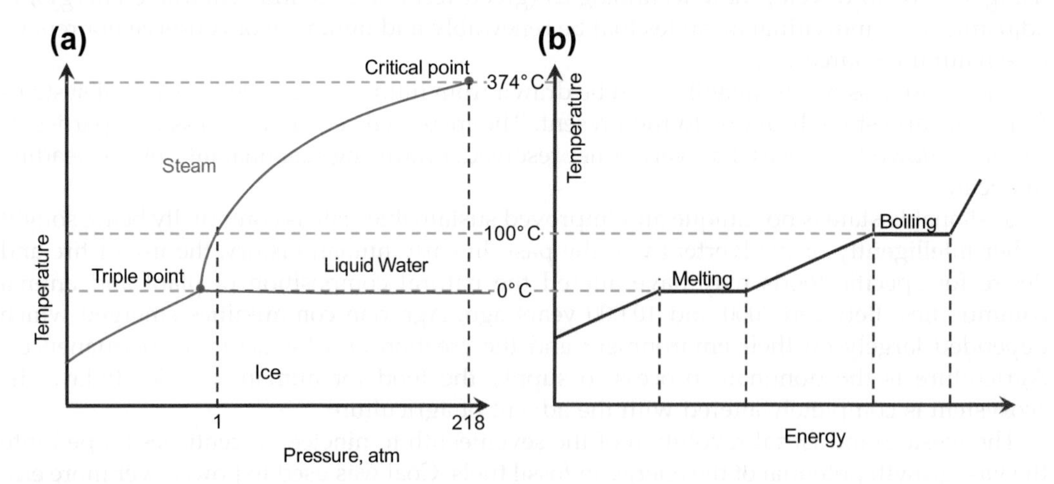

FIGURE 15.4 Phase change of water with temperature and pressure. (a) Phase diagram of water. (b) Internal energy change of water with temperature at 1 atmosphere.

TABLE 15.1 Availability and Distribution of Water on Earth (based on Igor Shiklomanov's Chapter "World fresh water resources" in Peter H. Gleick, ed., 1993, *Water in Crisis: A Guide to the World's Fresh Water Resources*, Oxford University Press, New York)

Type or form of water	Storage, Eg
Fresh water	
Clouds	12.9
Surface water	
Rivers	2.12
Swamps	11.5
Lakes	91
Ground water	
Soil moisture	16.5
Subterranean reserves	10,500
Ice	24,365
Salt water	
Oceans	1,340,000
Lakes	85.4
Aquifer	13,000
Biological water	1.12

conditions, water exists in three states: vapor, liquid, and solid. Altering among the three states, water is able to buffer the temperature on earth surface to be around 14 °C by absorbing radiant heat energy from the sun and releasing to the surroundings when it cools or condenses. Comfortable level of temperature is the key supporting the life on earth.

Table 15.1 shows the availability of water on earth and its distributions. The abundance of water on earth makes the use of water in bioprocesses less hazardous than the use of any other agents that can be found or made on earth. The amount of water we need for bioprocesses is a very small fraction of water on earth. Water is in air, on land, and in oceans. Care must be taken when redistribution of water on earth is to be made, while use of water does not harm the environment as a whole.

Table 15.2 shows the properties of water based on the steam table. From Table 15.2, we observe that the change of state (from solid ice to vapor, from solid ice to liquid water, and from liquid water to vapor) for water results in significant change in internal energy or enthalpy. The change of state occurring on earth and its atmosphere modulates the temperature, intercepts, and stores radiation energy. It plays a key part in the nature cycle as depicted in Fig. 15.1.

TABLE 15.2 Saturated Water Ice (for temperature below 0 °C), Liquid Water (for temperature above 0 °C), and Vapor. Compiled from fundamentals. American Society of Heating, Refrigerating, and Air-Conditioning Engineers, 1967 and 1972, and 1967 ASME Steam Tables

Temperature			Specific volume		Enthalpy		Entropy, J/(kg·K)	
°C	°F	Vapor pressure, kPa	Condensed state, 10^{-3} m^3/kg	Vapor, m^3/kg	Condensed state, J/kg	Vapor, 10^6 J/kg	Condensed state	Vapor
−101.111	−150	1.117×10^{-6}	1.076	7.111×10^{7}	-5.0897×10^{5}	2.3139	−2010.1	14396.9
−95.556	−140	3.398×10^{-6}	1.076	2.412×10^{7}	-5.0122×10^{5}	2.3241	−1965.7	13942.3
−90.000	−130	9.673×10^{-6}	1.077	8.740×10^{6}	-4.9329×10^{5}	2.3344	−1921.7	13516.5
−84.444	−120	2.590×10^{-5}	1.078	3.362×10^{6}	-4.8515×10^{5}	2.3447	−1877.8	13117.0
−78.889	−110	6.562×10^{-5}	1.079	1.367×10^{6}	-4.7678×10^{5}	2.3550	−1834.2	12741.9
−73.333	−100	1.580×10^{-4}	1.079	5.838×10^{5}	-4.6817×10^{5}	2.3653	−1790.7	12389.0
−67.778	−90	3.627×10^{-4}	1.080	2.613×10^{5}	-4.5936×10^{5}	2.3755	−1747.1	12056.1
−62.222	−80	7.977×10^{-4}	1.081	1.220×10^{5}	-4.5031×10^{5}	2.3858	−1703.6	11741.7
−56.667	−70	1.684×10^{-3}	1.081	5.931×10^{4}	-4.4103×10^{5}	2.3961	−1660.0	11444.9
−51.111	−60	3.428×10^{-3}	1.083	2.989×10^{4}	-4.3151×10^{5}	2.4064	−1616.9	11163.5
−45.556	−50	6.740×10^{-3}	1.083	1.558×10^{4}	-4.2179×10^{5}	2.4167	−1573.4	10897.2
−42.778	−45	9.335×10^{-3}	1.084	1.138×10^{4}	-4.1684×10^{5}	2.4218	−1552.0	10769.5
−40.000	−40	1.283×10^{-2}	1.084	8.384×10^{3}	-4.1184×10^{5}	2.4270	−1530.3	10644.8
−37.222	−35	1.751×10^{-2}	1.084	6.218×10^{3}	-4.0677×10^{5}	2.4321	−1508.9	10523.4
−34.444	−30	2.372×10^{-2}	1.085	4.645×10^{3}	-4.0165×10^{5}	2.4372	−1487.1	10405.3
−31.667	−25	3.190×10^{-2}	1.086	3.493×10^{3}	-3.9648×10^{5}	2.4424	−1465.8	10289.7
−28.889	−20	4.262×10^{-2}	1.086	2.645×10^{3}	-3.9125×10^{5}	2.4475	−1444.0	10177.1
−26.111	−15	5.656×10^{-2}	1.086	2.015×10^{3}	-3.8597×10^{5}	2.4527	−1422.7	10067.4
−23.333	−10	7.460×10^{-2}	1.087	1.545×10^{3}	-3.8064×10^{5}	2.4578	−1401.3	9960.7
−20.556	−5	9.784×10^{-2}	1.087	1.192×10^{3}	-3.7525×10^{5}	2.4629	−1379.5	9856.0
−17.778	0	1.275×10^{-1}	1.087	9.246×10^{2}	-3.6978×10^{5}	2.4681	−1358.2	9753.8
−15.000	5	1.652×10^{-1}	1.088	7.210×10^{2}	-3.6427×10^{5}	2.4732	−1336.8	9645.8
−12.222	10	2.128×10^{-1}	1.089	5.656×10^{2}	-3.5871×10^{5}	2.4783	−1315.5	9557.1
−9.444	15	2.728×10^{-1}	1.089	4.460×10^{2}	-3.5308×10^{5}	2.4834	−1293.7	9462.0
−8.889	16	2.865×10^{-1}	1.089	4.256×10^{2}	-3.5197×10^{5}	2.4845	−1289.5	9443.2
−7.778	18	3.158×10^{-1}	1.089	3.877×10^{2}	-3.4969×10^{5}	2.4865	−1281.1	9405.9
−6.667	20	3.478×10^{-1}	1.089	3.535×10^{2}	-3.4741×10^{5}	2.4886	−1272.3	9369.1

TABLE 15.2 Saturated Water Ice (for temperature below 0 °C), Liquid Water (for temperature above 0 °C), and Vapor. Compiled from fundamentals. American Society of Heating, Refrigerating, and Air-Conditioning Engineers, 1967 and 1972, and 1967 ASME Steam Tables—*Cont'd*

Temperature			Specific volume		Enthalpy		Entropy, J/(kg·K)	
°C	°F	Vapor pressure, kPa	Condensed state, 10^{-3} m^3/kg	Vapor, m^3/kg	Condensed state, J/kg	Vapor, 10^6 J/kg	Condensed state	Vapor
−5.556	22	3.828×10^{-1}	1.090	3.225×10^2	-3.4513×10^5	2.4897	−1264.0	9332.7
−4.444	24	4.209×10^{-1}	1.090	2.945×10^2	-3.4282×10^5	2.4926	−1255.2	9296.7
−3.333	26	4.625×10^{-1}	1.090	2.691×10^2	-3.4052×10^5	2.4947	−1246.8	9260.6
−2.222	28	5.078×10^{-1}	1.090	2.462×10^2	-3.3820×10^5	2.4967	−1238.0	9225.1
−1.111	30	5.571×10^{-1}	1.091	2.252×10^2	-3.3587×10^5	2.4988	−1229.6	9189.9
−0.556	31	5.834×10^{-1}	1.091	2.156×10^2	-3.3471×10^5	2.4998	−1225.5	9172.3
0.000	32	6.107×10^{-1}	1.091	2.063×10^2	-3.3354×10^5	2.5008	−1220.9	9155.1
0.010	32.018	6.112×10^{-1}	1.0002	2.062×10^2	0.	2.5016	0	9157.2
1.667	35	6.889×10^{-1}	1.0001	1.840×10^2	6.983×10^3	2.5046	25.5	9113.3
4.444	40	8.386×10^{-1}	1.0000	1.527×10^2	1.867×10^4	2.5097	67.8	9040.8
7.222	45	1.0166	1.0001	1.272×10^2	3.0340×10^4	2.5148	109.7	8970.5
10.000	50	1.2270	1.0003	1.064×10^2	4.1993×10^4	2.5200	151.1	8901.8
12.778	55	1.4749	1.0005	8.940×10^1	5.3634×10^4	2.5251	191.8	8834.9
15.556	60	1.7658	1.0009	7.539×10^1	6.5267×10^4	2.5300	232.4	8769.5
18.333	65	2.1060	1.0014	6.381×10^1	7.6889×10^4	2.5351	272.6	8705.9
21.111	70	2.5022	1.0020	5.421×10^1	8.8508×10^4	2.5402	311.9	8643.5
23.889	75	2.9623	1.0026	4.622×10^1	1.0012×10^5	2.5453	351.3	8582.8
26.667	80	3.4945	1.0033	3.954×10^1	1.1173×10^5	2.5502	390.2	8523.8
29.444	85	4.1081	1.0042	3.394×10^1	1.2334×10^5	2.5553	428.7	8466.0
32.222	90	4.8134	1.0050	2.922×10^1	1.3495×10^5	2.5604	466.8	8409.5
35.000	95	5.6216	1.0060	2.525×10^1	1.4655×10^5	2.5653	504.9	8354.2
37.778	100	6.5013	1.0070	2.187×10^1	1.5816×10^5	2.5704	542.2	8300.2
43.333	110	8.7908	1.0091	1.657×10^1	1.8138×10^5	2.5802	616.3	8196.4
48.889	120	1.1671×10^1	1.0116	1.269×10^1	2.0462×10^5	2.5902	689.1	8096.7
54.444	130	1.5327×10^1	1.0143	9.822	2.2785×10^5	2.6000	760.7	8001.7
60.000	140	1.9920×10^1	1.0171	7.677	2.5095×10^5	2.6097	831.1	7910.8
65.556	150	2.5637×10^1	1.0203	6.060	2.7435×10^5	2.6193	900.1	7823.3

(*Continued*)

TABLE 15.2 Saturated Water Ice (for temperature below 0 °C), Liquid Water (for temperature above 0 °C), and Vapor. Compiled from fundamentals. American Society of Heating, Refrigerating, and Air-Conditioning Engineers, 1967 and 1972, and 1967 ASME Steam Tables—*Cont'd*

Temperature			Specific volume		Enthalpy		Entropy, J/(kg·K)	
°C	°F	Vapor pressure, kPa	Condensed state, 10^{-3} m³/kg	Vapor, m³/kg	Condensed state, J/kg	Vapor, 10^6 J/kg	Condensed state	Vapor
71.111	160	3.2691×10^1	1.0235	4.824	2.9763×10^5	2.6288	968.4	7740.0
76.667	170	4.1317×10^1	1.0270	3.874	3.2091×10^5	2.6381	1035.4	7659.6
82.222	180	5.1786×10^1	1.0307	3.135	3.4424×10^5	2.6474	1101.5	7582.6
87.778	190	6.4397×10^1	1.0346	2.557	3.6760×10^5	2.6565	1166.8	7508.5
93.333	200	7.9469×10^1	1.0386	2.100	3.9097×10^5	2.6656	1230.9	7437.3
98.889	210	9.7374×10^1	1.0429	1.737	4.1437×10^5	2.6742	1294.1	7368.7
100.000	212	1.0133×10^2	1.0437	1.673	4.1907×10^5	2.6760	1306.7	7355.3

15.3.1. Water Cycle

The water cycle (known scientifically as the **hydrologic cycle**) refers to the continuous exchange of water within the hydrosphere, between the atmosphere, soil water, surface water, ground water, and plants. Fig. 15.5 shows a schematic of the water movement on Earth. Water moves perpetually through each of these regions in the *water cycle* consisting of following transfer processes:

- Evaporation from oceans, lakes, rivers, and other water bodies into the air and transpiration from land plants and animals into air.
- Precipitation from water vapor condensing from the air and falling onto the Earth's surface: land or ocean.
- Runoff from the land usually reaching the sea.

Water evaporation rate depends on the temperature, humidity in the air, and turbulence near the water surface. In general, the water evaporation rate is given by

$$N_A = k_p(p_A^0 - p_A) \tag{15.1}$$

where N_A is the flux of water vapor leaving the water surface, k_p is the mass transfer coefficient, p_A^0 is the saturation water vapor pressure, and p_A is the average vapor pressure in the air.

The mass transfer coefficient k_p is a function of the water vapor diffusivity (in air), temperature gradient, wind conditions, and turbulence in the air (especially near the water surface). Waves on water also increase the evaporation rate as the effective surface area increases.

Advection of water vapor in atmosphere is strongly dependent on the wind or pressure/temperature differences between locations. Macromotion of air causes extensive mixing in

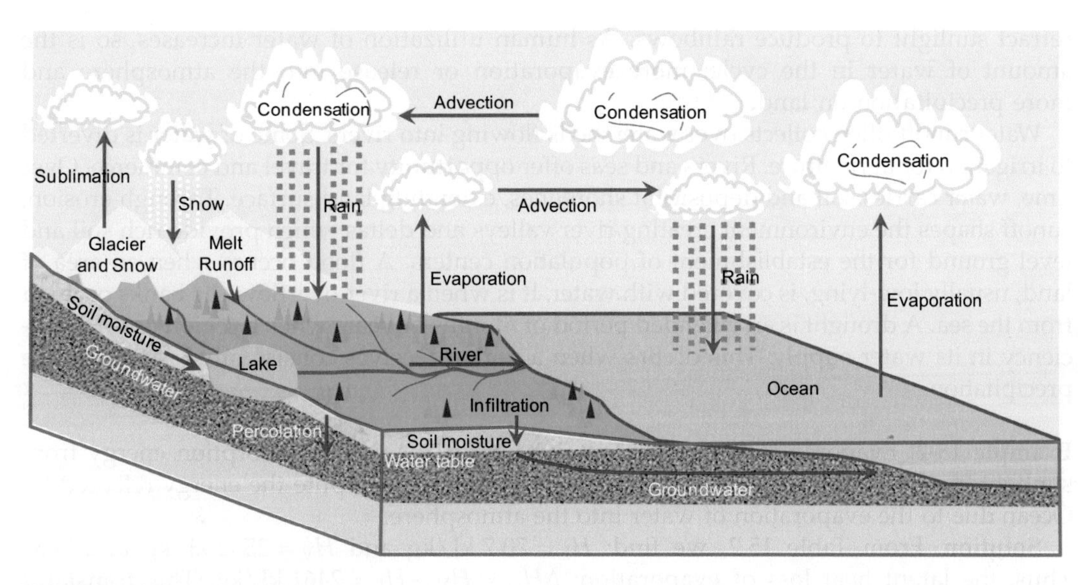

FIGURE 15.5 A schematic of water cycle.

the air and thus moves water vapor from more concentrated area (i.e. above water bodies) to more arid areas (e.g. over mountains). When air temperatures cool down or water vapor is transported to cooler areas, water vapor precipitates into liquid droplets to maintain a vapor pressure at the saturation level (p_A^0) as shown in Table 15.2. Liquid water is much denser (or heavier) than air. As shown in Table 15.2, the specific volume of liquid water is orders of magnitude greater than the specific volume of water vapor. Water droplets fall toward earth surface, forming rain.

Table 15.1 shows the approximate amount of water at each key nodes of along the water transport cycle. The largest reservoir is the interconnected oceans that contain about 96.5% of the total water. Table 15.3 shows the water fluxes. Most water vapor over the oceans returns to the oceans, but winds carry water vapor over land at the same rate as runoff into the sea, about 36 Eg (or 36×10^{15} kg)/year. This is the sustainable level we are used to. Any large fluctuation over or below the 36 Eg causes alarm, as it interacts with (influences or is influenced by) the temperature change on Earth's atmosphere. Over land, evaporation and transpiration contribute another 71 Eg/year. Precipitation, at a rate of 107 Eg/year over land, has several forms: most commonly rain, snow, and hail, with some contribution from fog and dew. Condensed water in the air may also

TABLE 15.3 Hydrological Cycle of Water on Earth

Geological location	Evaporation into atmosphere, Eg/year	Receiving from rainfall, Eg/year
Oceans	434	398
Land	71	107

refract sunlight to produce rainbows. As human utilization of water increases, so is the amount of water in the cycle: more evaporation or release into the atmosphere and more precipitation on land.

Water runoff often collects over watersheds flowing into rivers. Some of water is diverted to irrigation for agriculture. Rivers and seas offer opportunity for travel and commerce. Over time, water carries soil and deposits at shorelines, extending land surface. Through erosion, runoff shapes the environment creating river valleys and deltas which provide rich soil and level ground for the establishment of population centers. A flood occurs when an area of land, usually low-lying, is covered with water. It is when a river overflows its banks or flood from the sea. A drought is an extended period of months or years when a region notes a deficiency in its water supply. This occurs when a region receives consistently below average precipitation.

Example 15-2. Evaporation from Ocean at 398 Eg/year is due to absorption energy from sunlight. Assume an average water temperature of 290 K, compute the energy released by Ocean due to the evaporation of water into the atmosphere.

Solution. From Table 15.2, we find: $H_L = 70.7$ kJ/kg and $H_V = 2532$ kJ/kg at 290 K. Thus, the latent heat loss of evaporation: $\Delta H_{ev} = H_V - H_L = 2461$ kJ/kg. This translates to the energy release from the ocean of $2461 \times 398 \times 10^{15}$ kJ/year $= 9.80 \times 10^{20}$ kJ/year.

It is equivalent to $\dfrac{9.80 \times 10^{20}}{365 \times 24 \times 3600}$ kW $= 3.11 \times 10^{13}$ kW $= 31.1$ PW.

15.3.2. Utilization of Hydro Energy

The sustainable level of water on the land surface is a result of the solar energy exerted on earth's surface. As depicted in Fig. 15.5, evaporation of water vapor from ocean is due to the thermal energy provided by the Sun. Some of the condensation is carried over land, by wind (advection). Again, wind is generated by the solar energy. Sunlight warms up regions of atmosphere where water vapor is denser, causing a pressure differential. Wind is generated because of the rotation of planet Earth as well as the pressure differentials. Precipitation falls far inland, collecting together forming streams and rivers or waterways. The water flowing in the river can be employed to generate electricity as depicted by Fig. 15.6. Worldwide, an installed capacity of 777 GW supplied 2998 TWh of hydroelectricity in 2006, which represented a significant amount of renewable energy.

Hydropower has been used since ancient times to grind flour and perform other tasks. In the mid-1770s, a French engineer Bernard Forest de Bélidor published Architecture Hydraulique which described vertical- and horizontal-axis hydraulic machines. By the late nineteenth century, the electrical generator was developed and could now be coupled with hydraulics. In 1878, the world's first house powered with hydroelectricity was Cragside in Northumberland, England. The old Schoelkopf Power Station No. 1 near Niagara Falls in the U.S. side began to produce electricity in 1881. The first Edison hydroelectric power plant—the Vulcan Street Plant—began operating September 30, 1882, in Appleton, Wisconsin, with an output of about 12.5 kW. By 1886, there were about 45 hydroelectric power plants in the U.S. and Canada. By 1889, there were 200 in the U.S. The development of hydropower was rapid as the source of energy, water flowing through the waterway, never ends.

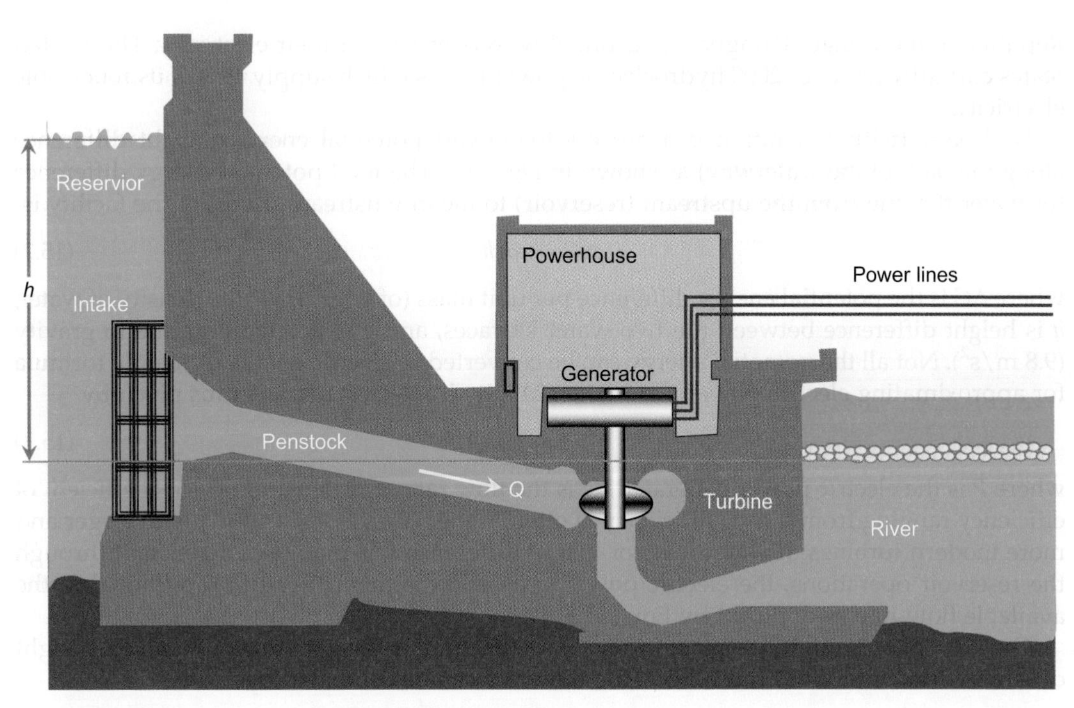

FIGURE 15.6 A schematic of a hydropower plant.

At the beginning of the twentieth century, a large number of small hydroelectric power plants were being constructed by commercial companies in the mountains that surrounded metropolitan areas. By 1920 as 40% of the power produced in the United States was hydroelectric, the Federal Power Act was enacted into law. The Act created the Federal Power Commission whose main purpose was to regulate hydroelectric power plants on federal land and water. As the power plants became larger, their associated dams developed additional purposes to include flood control, irrigation, and navigation. Federal funding became necessary for large-scale development and federally owned corporations like the Tennessee Valley Authority (1933) and the Bonneville Power Administration (1937) were created. Additionally, the Bureau of Reclamation which had began a series of western U.S. irrigation projects in the early twentieth century was now constructing large hydroelectric projects such as the 1928 Boulder Canyon Project Act. The U.S. Army Corps of Engineers was also involved in hydroelectric development, completing the Bonneville Dam in 1937 and being recognized by the Flood Control Act of 1936 as the premier federal flood control agency.

Hydroelectric power plants continued to become larger throughout the twentieth century. After the Hoover Dam's initial 1345 MW power plant became the world's largest hydroelectric power plant in 1936, it was soon eclipsed by the 6809 MW Grand Coulee Dam in 1942. Brazil's and Paraguay's Itaipu Dam opened in 1984 as the largest, producing 14,000 MW but was surpassed in 2008 by the Three Gorges Dam in China with a production capacity of 22,500 MW. Hydroelectricity would eventually supply countries like Norway, Democratic

Republic of the Congo, Paraguay, and Brazil with over 85% of their electricity. The United States currently has over 2000 hydroelectric power plants which supply 49% of its renewable electricity.

Hydroelectricity generation is a process to convert potential energy (height difference along the path of the waterway) as shown in Fig. 15.6. The total potential energy difference for water flowing from the upstream (reservoir) to the downstream (river) of the facility is

$$\Delta G = \rho g h \tag{15.2}$$

where ΔG is the potential energy difference per unit mass (of water), ρ is the density of water, h is height difference between the two water surfaces, and g is acceleration due to gravity (9.8 m/s^2). Not all the potential energy can be converted to electric energy. A simple formula for approximating electric power production at a hydroelectric plant is thus given by

$$P = \eta_P \rho g h Q \tag{15.3}$$

where P is the electric power generated, Q is the flow rate of water, and η_P is a coefficient of efficiency ranging from 0 to 1. Efficiency is often higher (that is, closer to 1) with larger and more modern turbines. If water level or height difference h is maintained constant through the reservoir operations, the electric power generation is then directly proportional to the available flow rate as depicted by Eqn (15.3).

The flow rate through the penstock is also a function of the gate opening and the height difference. Based on fluid mechanics, the flow rate can be estimated by

$$Q = c_S A_G (gh)^{1/2} \tag{15.4}$$

where A_G is the open cross-sectional area of intake gate and c_S is a constant that depends on the penstock pipe construction, intake gate, the turbine, and also weakly on the flow rate. Therefore, the power generation can be related to the height or the flow rate via

$$P = \eta_P c_S A_G \rho (gh)^{3/2} \tag{15.5}$$

or

$$P = \frac{\eta_P}{c_S^2 A_G^2} \rho Q^3 \tag{15.6}$$

The electric energy production is proportional to the water height difference to the power of one and half, or proportional to the cube of the flow rate, if the gate opening remains the same. The power and flow rate relationship can be different if the water level can be controlled independently. This is particularly true for large dam/reservoirs as constant water level is desirable for maximum electric power output as given by Eqn (15.3). Fig. 15.7 shows the typical seasonal flow rate variation for the Three Gorges Dam, China. One can observe that the water flow rate is highest during the summer months and lowest during the winter months.

Example 15-3. A hydroelectricity facility was built below a mountainous area. Owing to the weather changes from summer to winter, the available water flow changes significantly. In 1 year, the water flow rate in a low day was just one-tenth of that in a high flow summer day. Determine the available electricity generation variation.

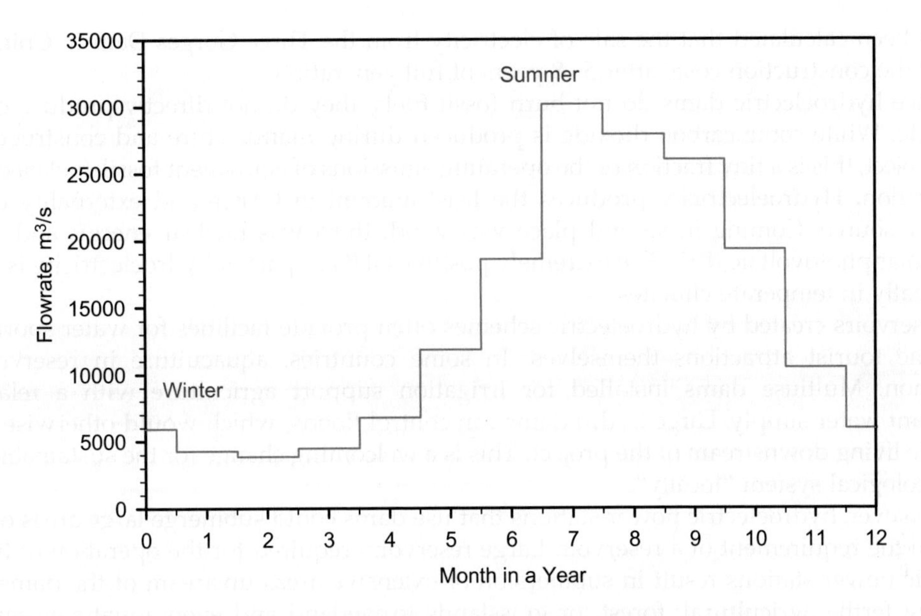

FIGURE 15.7 A typical seasonal flow rate variation for the Three Gorges Dam, China.

Solution. The electricity production is a function of the available water flow rate. If the water flow is used at maximum when available or the penstock gate opening is constant, Eqn (15.6) leads to

$$\frac{P_1}{P_2} = \left(\frac{Q_1}{Q_2}\right)^3$$

assuming the efficiency and flow rate constant are constants. Therefore, a drop of water flow rate by a factor of 10, would result in an available power production by a factor of 1000.

If the Penstock gate opening is controlled to maintain constant water level, then Eqn (15.3) leads to

$$\frac{P_1}{P_2} = \frac{Q_1}{Q_2}$$

assuming the efficiency and flow rate constant are constants. Therefore, a drop of water flow rate by a factor of 10 would only result in an available power production by a factor of 10. This is highly desirable as compared to a constant penstock gate opening.

The major advantage of hydroelectricity is renewability: elimination of the cost of fuel. Hydroelectric plants also tend to have longer economic lives than fuel-fired generation, with some plants now in service, which were built 50–100 years ago. Operating labor cost is also usually low, as plants are automated and have few personnel on site during normal operation.

Where a dam serves multiple purposes, a hydroelectric plant may be added with relatively low construction cost, providing a useful revenue stream to offset the costs of dam operation.

It has been calculated that the sale of electricity from the Three Gorges Dam in China will cover the construction costs after 5–8 years of full generation.

Since hydroelectric dams do not burn fossil fuels, they do not directly produce carbon dioxide. While some carbon dioxide is produced during manufacture and construction of the project, this is a tiny fraction of the operating emissions of equivalent fossil-fuel electricity generation. Hydroelectricity produces the least amount of GHGs and externality of any energy source. Coming in second place was wind, third was nuclear energy, and fourth was solar photovoltaic (PV). The extremely positive GHG impact of hydroelectricity is found especially in temperate climates.

Reservoirs created by hydroelectric schemes often provide facilities for water sports and become tourist attractions themselves. In some countries, aquaculture in reservoirs is common. Multiuse dams installed for irrigation support agriculture with a relatively constant water supply. Large hydro dams can control floods, which would otherwise affect people living downstream of the project. This is a welcoming change for the sustainability of the ecological system "locally".

However, hydroelectric power stations that use dams could submerge large areas of land due to the requirement of a reservoir. Large reservoirs required for the operation of hydroelectric power stations result in submersion of extensive areas upstream of the dams, converting fertile agricultural, forest, or grasslands to wetland and even aquatic system. As such, biologically rich and productive lowland and riverine valley forests, marshland, and grasslands are forever lost to an entirely different ecological system: wetland. The loss of land is often exacerbated by the fact that reservoirs cause habitat fragmentation of surrounding areas. One can imagine the consequences of shifting from one sustainable ecological system to another entirely different ecological system. Still, the change in sustainable state is not limited to simply the small "dry" area that converted to "wet" area but to a larger area around the reservoir.

Especially for large hydroelectric facilities, a reservoir stores large amount of water and occupies a large area of land surface. The ecological change is also associated with a potential climate change. As more evaporation is from the reservoir surface than from "dry" land surface with plant coverage, more precipitation is expected in the surrounding area. The increase in precipitation and its affected area depend on the size of the reservoir. Thus, there is the potential to alter the local climate from more arid to more temperate moist. Again the landscape or ecological system surrounding the large reservoir is altered because of the water storage.

Hydroelectric projects can be disruptive to surrounding aquatic ecosystems both upstream and downstream of the plant site. For instance, studies have shown that dams along the Atlantic and Pacific coasts of North America have reduced salmon populations by preventing access to spawning grounds upstream, even though most dams in salmon habitat have fish ladders installed. Salmon spawn is also harmed on their migration to sea when they must pass through turbines. This has led to some areas transporting smelt downstream by barge during parts of the year. In some cases, dams, such as the Marmot Dam, have been demolished due to the high impact on fish. Turbine and power plant designs that are easier on aquatic life are an active area of research. Mitigation measures such as fish ladders may be required at new projects or as a condition of relicensing of existing projects.

Generation of hydroelectric power changes the downstream river environment. Water exiting a turbine usually contains very little suspended sediment, which can lead to scouring of riverbeds and loss of riverbanks. Since turbine gates are often opened intermittently, rapid or even daily fluctuations in river flow are observed. For example, in the Grand Canyon, the daily cyclic flow variation caused by Glen Canyon Dam was found to be contributing to erosion of sand bars. Dissolved oxygen content of the water may change from pre-construction conditions. Depending on the location, water exiting from turbines is typically much warmer than the pre-dam water, which can change aquatic faunal populations, including endangered species, and prevent natural freezing processes from occurring. Some hydroelectric projects also use canals to divert a river at a shallower gradient to increase the head of the scheme. In some cases, the entire river may be diverted leaving a dry riverbed.

The ecological and "local" climate change can bring changes that may or may not be wanted, especially during the transition from one sustainable state (before water storage) to another sustainable state (when storage reached steady state). The reservoirs of hydropower plants in tropical regions may produce substantial amounts of methane. This is due to plant material in flooded areas decaying in an anaerobic environment and forming methane, a very potent GHG. According to the 2010 World Commission on Dams report, where the reservoir is large compared to the generating capacity (less than 100 W/m^2 of surface area) and no clearing of the forests in the area was undertaken prior to impoundment of the reservoir, GHG emissions from the reservoir may be higher than those of a conventional oil-fired thermal generation plant. Although these emissions represent carbon already in the biosphere, not fossil deposits that had been sequestered from the carbon cycle, there is a greater amount of methane due to anaerobic decay, causing greater damage than would otherwise have occurred had the forest decayed naturally.

In boreal reservoirs of Canada and Northern Europe, however, GHG emissions are typically only 2%–8% of any kind of conventional fossil-fuel thermal generation. The carbon emission due to reservoir displacing vegetation land can be significantly reduced with proper management. A new class of underwater logging operation that targets drowned forests can mitigate the effect of forest decay.

In 2007, International Rivers accused hydropower firms for cheating with fake carbon credits under the Clean Development Mechanism (CDM), for hydropower projects already finished or under construction at the moment they applied to join the CDM. These carbon credits—of hydropower projects under the CDM in developing countries—can be sold to companies and governments in developed countries, in order to comply with the Kyoto protocol.

To embrace the change in sustainable state, there is a need to relocate the people living where the reservoirs are planned. Change of sustainable state is not a process that can be implemented without sacrifice. With any change, there are permanent losses of values. In February 2008, it was estimated that 40–80 million people worldwide had been physically displaced as a direct result of dam construction. In many cases, no amount of compensation can replace ancestral and cultural attachments to places that have spiritual value to the displaced population. Additionally, historically and culturally important sites can be flooded and lost. Such problems have arisen at the Aswan Dam in Egypt between 1960 and 1980, the Three Gorges Dam in China, the Clyde Dam in New Zealand, and the Ilisu Dam in Turkey.

Colossal industrial accidents are rare and could bring noticeable harm to humanity. The most damaging of all is a dam failure. Dam failures have accounted for the most serious industrial accidents ever known today. Because large conventional dammed-hydro facilities hold back large volumes of water at high potential energy, a failure due to poor construction, terrorism, or other causes can be catastrophic to downriver settlements and infrastructure. Dam failures have been some of the largest man-made disasters in history. Also, good design and construction are not an adequate guarantee of safety. Dams are tempting industrial targets for wartime attack, sabotage, and terrorism, such as Operation Chastise in World War II.

The failure of a system of dams including Banqiao Dam and Shimantan Dam in Henan, China, directly resulted in the deaths of 85,000 people in 1975 (Yi S, The World's Most Catastrophic Dam Failures: The August 1975 Collapse of the Banqiao and Shimantan Dams, in Dai Q, *The River Dragon Has Come!*, M.E. Sharpe, New York, 1998). Millions were left homeless. Also, the creation of a dam in a geologically inappropriate location may cause disasters like the one of the Vajont Dam in Italy, where almost 2000 people died, in 1963.

Smaller dams and micro hydro facilities create less risk but can form continuing hazards even after they have been decommissioned. For example, the small Kelly Barnes Dam failed in 1967, causing 39 deaths with the Toccoa Flood, 10 years after its power plant was decommissioned in 1957.

15.4. CO_2 AND BIOMASS

As shown in Fig. 15.1, the amount of CO_2 in the atmosphere is not variable over time as a close loop is formed in nature. Sustainability is not disturbed if no net sink or source is brought into the system.

Although humanity started in harmony with nature sustainably with using exclusively biomass as the source of materials, chemicals, and energy, fossils have overtaken the role as the dominant materials, energy, and chemical source since the industrial revolution. Petroleum, natural gas, and coal have been regarded as toxic waste materials from the distant past. They have been the cheapest sources of energy, chemicals, and materials for over half a century. Valorization of these waste materials has been the focus of research and development and the achievements have been remarkable. The comfortable living standards of humanity have been raised to a significantly high level especially in developed nations. Our living standards today are not compatible with the primitive way of utilization of natural resources. Simply "turning back the clock" is not an option. New sustainable state must be found or will be evolved into. The choice we have is whether to choose one we like to be with.

While fossils have been fueling the raising comfortable standards of human living, humanity has recognized the danger of utilizing fossils bring. For one, the amount of fossil deposits on the Earth is finite. The time for the complete depletion of fossils is now predictable and lies in the foreseeable future despite new discoveries of deposits. Looking for resources that we are used and away from the Earth is not foreseeable option. The continuum or sustainability is thus at risk. The second, equally as important is that material flow is not balanced in utilizing fossils. For example, CO_2 is generated when fossils are used as energy source. Obtaining fossils from the "deep" underneath the earth and sending carbon dioxide "up into" the atmosphere are the essence of fossil utilization. This is not a closed loop. The "one-way traffic" only designed to bring carbon dioxide into the atmosphere from

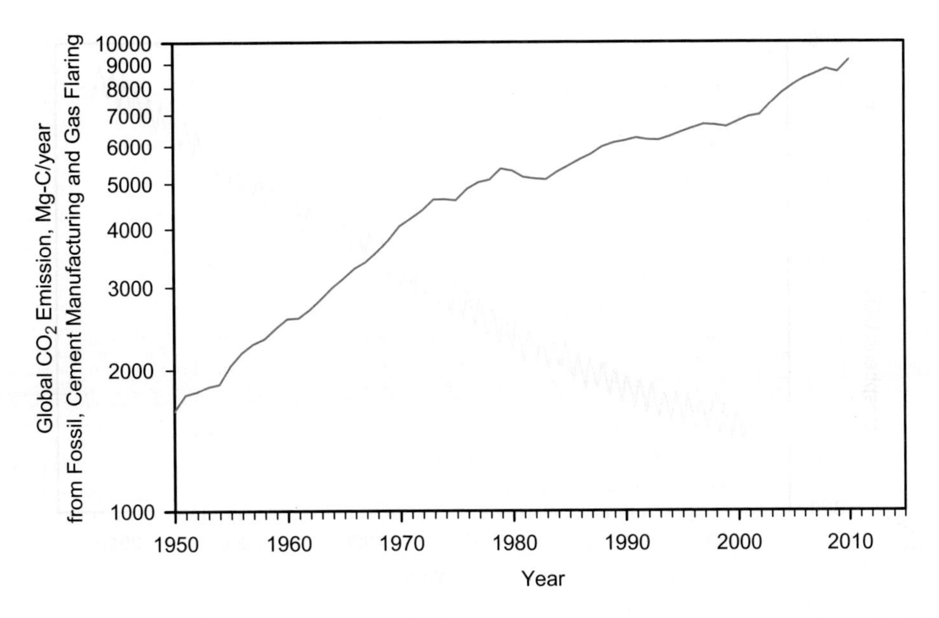

FIGURE 15.8 Global CO_2 emission rate from fossil burning, cement manufacturing, and gas flaring. Data from Carbon Dioxide Information Analysis Center.

underneath earth. By virtue, using fossil energy is not a sustainable process. Fig. 15.8 shows the global fossil CO_2 emission, while Fig. 15.9 shows the CO_2 concentration in atmosphere. Fig. 15.8 shows that the emission rate of CO_2 (log scale) into atmosphere due to fossil energy use increases exponentially with two distinctive periods: from 1950 to 1978 and then from 1982 to 2007. The exponential pace of CO_2 rate increase is lower at the later period. The net rate of CO_2 emission (as a source) is alarming. Fig. 15.9 shows that the concentration of CO_2 (log scale) in atmosphere increases monotonously when seasonal effect is taken out. The seasonal change is due to the equilibrium concentration change with temperature change in the oceans (water) and soil. The concentration change in the atmosphere can be estimated by a mass balance

$$r_{e,CO_2} - YF_{CO_2/X}\frac{\mu_{max}C_{CO_2}}{K_{CO_2} + C_{CO_2}}XS_B = (V_{At} + V_W^* S_{WA})\frac{dC_{CO_2}}{dt} \tag{15.7}$$

where $YF_{CO_2/X}$ is the yield factor of CO_2 on plant biomass, μ_{max} is the average maximum specific overall growth rate of plant biomass, K_{CO_2} is the Monod saturation coefficient of CO_2 for the average growth of plant biomass, X is the standing (plant) biomass, S_B is the area of earth surface on which plant biomass grows, V_{At} is the effective volume of atmosphere, V_W^* is the effective volume of the water bodies, S_{WA} is the effective CO_2 saturation in water, r_{e,CO_2} is the net emission rate of CO_2, and C_{CO_2} is the concentration of CO_2 in atmosphere. One can observe that the increase in CO_2 in the atmosphere since 1970 is exponential except a short period of time between 1992 and 1994 as expected from the corresponding CO_2 emission data in Fig. 15.8. However, the CO_2 emission from fossil

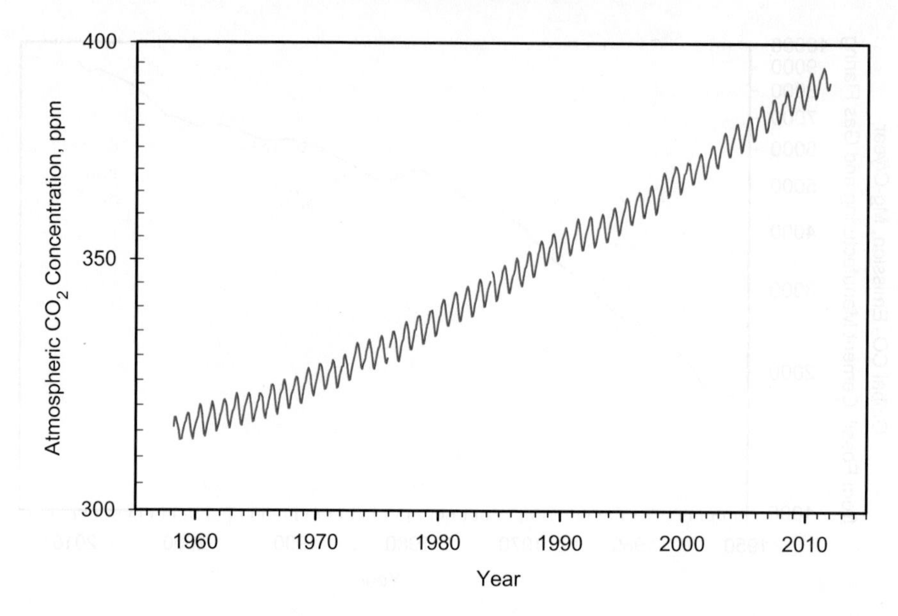

FIGURE 15.9 Mole fraction of CO_2 in atmosphere from 1958 to 2011. Data from Mauna Loa Carbon Dioxide Record.

sources may not be directly correlated to the atmospheric CO_2 level increase as depicted by Eqn (15.7). The growth rate of biomass may be dependent on the biomass density and utilization of biomass also plays a role in the atmospheric CO_2 change.

The net effect of sending CO_2 into the atmosphere has been recognized by humanity. As shown in Fig. 15.9, atmospheric CO_2 increases monotonously with time. It affects the very living environment, which brings a constantly and monotonously changing earth. Net emission of CO_2 into atmosphere (Fig. 15.9) is the cause of atmospheric CO_2 increase. Changing does not automatically mean bad, but monotonous change is definitely not sustainable. Soils and waters on earth can absorb/adsorb some of the CO_2, relieving some load in the atmosphere. Carbon sequestration through compressing CO_2 and sending it "deep" under the earth where the fossils come from could be a temporal option. However, these are still not sustainable processes. Rising level of carbonate in water or soil does not bring any positive benefits that we can perceive. It is not difficult to imagine that compressed CO_2 storing underneath earth is not a permanent solution. These are also dead ends to CO_2. As demonstrated in Figs 15.8 and 15.9, there is no sustainable state (or steady constant CO_2 level in the atmosphere) in sight if the fossil energy consumption continued.

If we have a long enough time scale, sustainability prevails eventually as matter and energy are conserved. Everything is recyclable/renewable. However, there is an acceptable time scale for the continuity in the existence of humanity and this time scale is not long enough for fossils to be renewable. Therefore, it is imperative to find alternatives to fossil sources since the time scale for fossils to recycle or naturally replenish is, at best, on the order of 280 million years, as shown in Table 15.4. Fossils are replenished when a carbonaceous age

TABLE 15.4 Recycle Times and Productivities of Chemical/Energy Feedstock (Liu SJ, Woody Biomass: Niche Position as a Source of Sustainable Renewable Chemicals and Energy and Kinetics of Hot-Water Extraction/Hydrolysis. *J. Biotech. Adv.* 2010; 28: 563–582.)

Feed stock	Recycle time	Standing biomass, tons/ha or 10^{-1} kg/m^2	Biomass production, tons/(ha year) or 10^{-1} kg/m^2/year
Algae	1 month	0.9	11.25
Agricultural crops	3 months– 1 year	4.5	2.93
Temperate grasses	1 year	7.2	2.70
Savanna	1 year	18.0	4.05
Shrubs	1–5 years	27.0	3.15
Tropical forest	5–25 years	202.5	9.90
Tropical season forest	5–25 years	157.5	7.20
Boreal forest	25–80 years	90.0	3.60
Temperate deciduous	10–50 years	135.0	5.40
Temperate evergreen	10–80 years	157.5	5.85
Oil, gas, and coal	*280 million years*	(38.4×10^{21} J)	(0.1371 PJ/year)

occurs on the Earth, preserving a large amount of organic matter. Given the advanced forms of life existing now, the chances of such an event occurring are unlikely. Nevertheless, the 280 million years rotation is far too long and the amount of possible reserves is negligible compared to the recharge duration from a human use (or need) standpoint, even if mankind could survive a fossil replenishment era. If fossil replenishment was possible without interrupting the continuity of humanity, it would be renewable only if the utilization rate was no greater than 0.1371 PJ/year or 4.348 MW, which was six or seven orders of magnitude too small as compared to the current human needs. Thus, fossil resources in general are deemed nonrenewable. Societal awareness of environmental impact as well as problems in the stability and sustainability of the energy supply have made the development and implementation of bio-based chemicals and energy urgent and in the same time, more questions were raised. Regional energy security and rural economies both benefit from a plant biomass-derived chemical/energy economic base. Reverting to reliance on biomass as chemical and energy source is thus our destiny.

Woody biomass is the most abundant organic source on Earth, with an annual production in the biosphere of about 5.64×10^{10} Mg-C (Field CB, Behrenfeld MJ, Randerson JT and Falkowski P. Primary production of the Biosphere: Integrating Terrestrial and Oceanic Components. *Science*. 1998; 281: 237–240). Of the 5.64×10^{10} Mg-C biomass production each year, only 4.8% or 2.7×10^9 Mg-C/year was utilized by mankind, including food (1.7×10^9 Mg-C), pulp, paper, energy, furniture and construction materials (0.9×10^9 Mg-C), and the rest as clothing and chemicals (Thoen J. and Busch R. Industrial chemicals from biomass – industrial

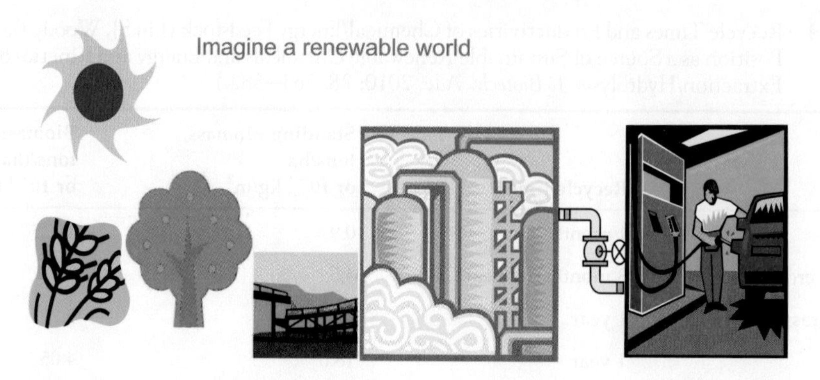

FIGURE 15.10 Energy flow from the Sun to power the needs of humans (Liu SJ. Woody Biomass: Niche Position as a Source of Sustainable Renewable Chemicals and Energy and Kinetics of Hot-Water Extraction/Hydrolysis. *J. Biotech. Adv.* 2010; 28: 563–582).

concepts. In: Kamm, B., Gruber, P.R., and Kamm, M. ed, *Biorefineries – industrial processes and products: Status Quo and Future Directions*. Vol 2. Wiley-VCH, Weinheim, Germany 13: 978-3-527-31027-2, 2006). Tapping into the chemical energy of woody biomass and reclaiming the historically important position of woody biomass in chemicals, energy, and transportation is imperative to the sustainability of the world economy. Rich resources in forest are unparallel to other types of biomass sources. Forests cover about 9.5% of the Earth's surface or about 32% of the land area but account for 89.3% of the total standing biomass, producing 73×10^9 Mg/year or 42.9% of the total annual biomass production. The distant second on the list is savanna and grasses, which account for 11% of total biomass production. Plants synthesize chemicals from solar energy. The chemical energy stored by the biomass can be converted to energy and chemicals that mankind can utilize. A futuristic flow of energy for a plant biomass-based economy is illustrated in Fig. 15.10. Plants grow, die, and regrow naturally even *without human intervention*. Dedicated or managed energy crops (agriforest and/or agricultural biomass) can further increase biomass availability.

Utilization of woody biomass does not mean destroy the forest (or plant biomass) on the planet. However, it does mean that trees will be harvested to allow for conversion to usable energy, chemicals and materials, and to free the space for new trees to grow. There is a change of sustainability, from a relatively invariant none productive forest to a fluctuating productive forest. Fig. 15.11 illustrates the time evolution of total biomass in a given area when left untouched and when utilized by humans. Trees, shrubs, grasses, and algae grow with the CO_2 available in the atmosphere and H_2O in or on the ground. However, the density of biomass on a mass per unit surface area is in the order of highest to lowest: trees, shrubs, then grasses, and algae are similar, as shown in Table 15.4. The high density of trees makes forest biomass most attractive for large-scale industrial development. The biomass production rate, however, is highest for algae, followed by trees, shrubs, and grasses. The order could be changed for the biomass production rate if intensive cultivation and harvesting techniques were employed at different levels. The intensive cultivation can shorten the recycle time and increase the yield. The combined effects could make the shorter rotation plants produce much more incremental biomass than the longer rotation plants. The key

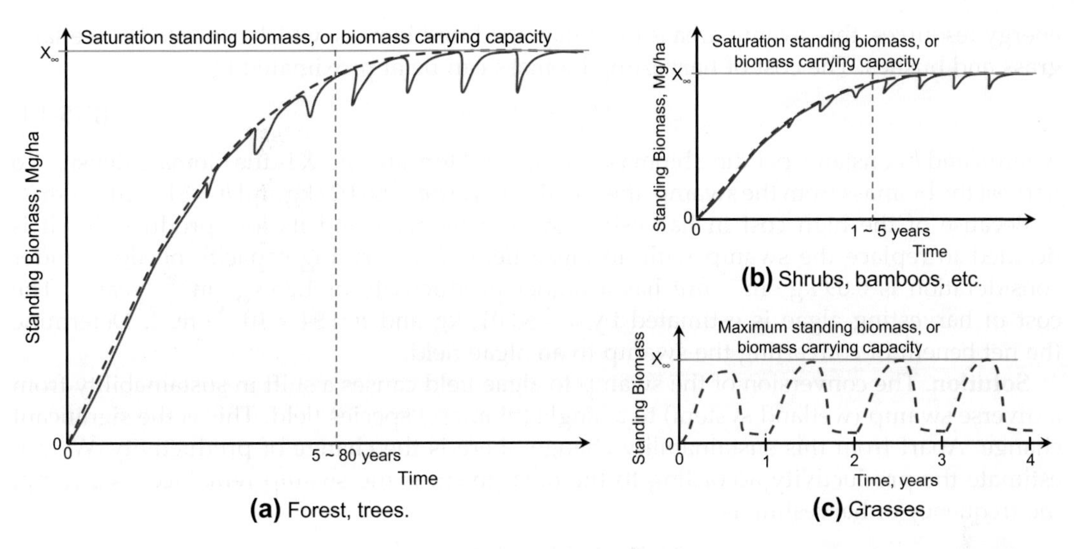

FIGURE 15.11 A schematic of the above ground standing biomass accumulation as a function of time in a given area. The dotted lines represent no disturbances, whereas the solid line is drawn to show the impact of periodic minor disturbances (Liu SJ. Woody Biomass: Niche Position as a Source of Sustainable Renewable Chemicals and Energy and Kinetics of Hot-Water Extraction/Hydrolysis. *J. Biotech. Adv.* 2010; 28: 563–582).

for realizing the potential of woody biomass is to harvest (at least before it decomposes back to CO_2 and H_2O) and make room for new growth.

When intensive cultivation is an option, one needs to consider the net gain or the sustainability of the cultivation process and the impact of the conversion process, as well as the benefits to a regional and global economy. However, there is an upper limit on how much biomass the earth can "host", which limits the conversion site arrangement. If the earth was saturated with plant biomass, no more net additional biomass could be added or grown. Natural disturbances promote the plant biomass renewal while changing the level of standing biomass temporarily. Wild fires sweep the ground from time to time reducing the standing biomass to ashes, releasing CO_2 and H_2O back to nature. This cycle of natural growth and replacement keeps the plant biomass fluctuating below the saturation level. Therefore, not utilizing the plant biomass, in particular forest biomass, does not lead to an increase in the total amount of standing biomass on earth beyond its saturation level. Constantly harvesting the plant biomass at or below the rate at which it could be replenished has the same effect as if the plant biomass was left alone untouched. Sustaining the same or similar level of plant biomass on the Earth is achievable as Nature has taught us through natural disturbances. Therefore, harvesting and utilizing plant biomass, whether it be trees, forests, or grasses, do not automatically lead to any net change in the biomass coverage on earth. Forests and trees have the highest potential net energy benefit and standing quantity for a sustainable renewable chemical and energy development.

Example 15-4. A subtropical swamp area has been found to have a biomass carrying capacity of 2.0 kg · m^{-2} and productivity of 0.8 kg · m^{-2} · year^{-1}. Because of rising demands on energy resources, this swamp area is to be managed for biomass, which consisted of wetland grass and bushes. The cost of harvesting biomass can be approximated by

$$H_C = aX + b \tag{E15-4.1}$$

where a and b constants pending biomass species and terrain, and X is the biomass density. To harvest the biomass from the swamp, the coefficients are $a = \$0.02/\text{kg}$ and $b = \$1 \times 10^{-3} \cdot \text{m}^{-2}$.

Because of the high cost in harvesting swamp biomass and its low productivity, it is decided to replace the swamp with an algae field. The carrying capacity of algae under consideration is 0.09 $\text{kg} \cdot \text{m}^{-2}$ but has a higher productivity of 1.25 $\text{kg} \cdot \text{m}^{-2} \cdot \text{year}^{-1}$. The cost of harvesting algae is estimated by $a = \$0.01/\text{kg}$ and $b = \$4 \times 10^{-4} \cdot \text{m}^{-2}$. Determine the net benefit of converting the swamp to an algae field.

Solution. The conversion of the swamp to algae field causes a shift in sustainability from a diverse swamp (wetland system) to a single (biomass) species field. This is the significant change. Apart from this sustainability change, there is the change of productivity. We can estimate the productivity according to the data given. If the swamp remained as swamp, the frequency of harvesting is

$$0.8/2\,\text{year}^{-1} = 0.4\,\text{year}^{-1}$$

That is, we need to harvest 0.4 times a year. If the biomass is grown to 80% of full carrying capacity before harvesting, the cost of harvesting each year is given by

$$H_{CS} = \$(0.02 \times 0.8 \times 2 + 10^{-3}) \times 0.4/(\text{m}^2 \cdot \text{year}^{-1}) = \$0.0132\,\text{m}^{-2} \cdot \text{year}^{-1}$$

which translates to $\$0.0132/(0.8 \times 0.8)\ \text{kg}^{-1} = \$0.020625\ \text{kg}^{-1}$.

If the swamp was converted to an algae field, the frequency of harvesting is

$$1.25/0.09\,\text{year}^{-1} = 13.89\,\text{year}^{-1}$$

That is in every year, we need to harvest 13.89 times. If algae are grown to 80% of full capacity before harvesting, the cost of harvesting each year is given by

$$H_{CS} = \$(0.01 \times 0.8 \times 0.9 + 4 \times 10^{-4}) \times 13.89 = \$0.1056\,\text{m}^{-2} \times \text{year}^{-1}$$

which translates to $\$0.1056/(0.8 \times 1.25)\ \text{kg}^{-1} = \$0.10556\ \text{kg}^{-1}$.

Therefore, the conversion of swamp to algae increases biomass production by (1.25 – 0.8)/ 0.8 = 56.25%. However, the unit cost of biomass is increased by (0.10556 – 0.020625)/ 0.020625 = 411.8%. A combination of lower unit cost of harvesting and higher productivity does not make out to be beneficial in this case due to the much lower standing biomass of algae.

15.5. WOODY BIOMASS USE AND DESIRED SUSTAINABLE STATE

Low-carbon fuel standard (LCFS) is a rule enacted to reduce carbon intensity in transportation fuels. Its aim was to reduce the amount of fossil genic CO_2 into the atmosphere. This can be rather confusing as to how the LCFS carbon intensity can be measured for biomass. The plantation, harvesting, and processing of biomass all require energy input. Are the production and processing energy renewable? Even the conversion or change of land use indirectly affects the carbon emission scheme. On top of the confusion in splitting the source energy (or intended source of energy) used in production, processing, and transportation of the biomass fuel, there is still the net CO_2 emission in atmosphere.

Fossil energy source has higher energy density of available energy output per unit mass (and other known pollutant gases due to the composition of biomass). On the per carbon basis, however, the available energy output is similar to coal at room temperature (from energy regularity in section § 3.9) although still lower than hydrocarbons because of the oxygen (and hydrogen) content. When burning woody biomass and releasing effluent gas at high temperatures, the energy efficiency is reduced due to the extra water content resulted from the oxygen and hydrogen in woody biomass. Utilization of woody biomass for energy releases more CO_2 and H_2O into atmosphere than fossil use. Switching from fossil energy to woody biomass energy can thus cause a shift to higher CO_2 emission into atmosphere than continuing using fossil fuel. This phenomenon has fooled some people into believing woody biomass is worse than fossil energy source for the environment. In a short term (<32 years) after utilizing woody biomass, there is an increased amount of GHG over fossil fuel utilization as depicted by Fig. 15.12. The transition from fossil economy to woody biomass economy requires thus in excess of 32 years before seeing the same level of CO_2 in atmosphere.

In a sustainable or steady manner, renewable forest material is carbon neutral, i.e. utilizing forest material will not create a carbon imbalance over the life cycle of the forest, which is an extended 5–80-year time for managed forests as shown in Table 15.4. "*Catch and Release*" is the key in biomass utilization. Carbon dioxide is drawn from the atmosphere for plants to grow, while planting, management, conversion of biomass to bio-products, utilization and decomposition of bio-products will all produce carbon dioxide. In an optimal balanced operation, carbon dioxide is simply recycled during the life span of plant growth and

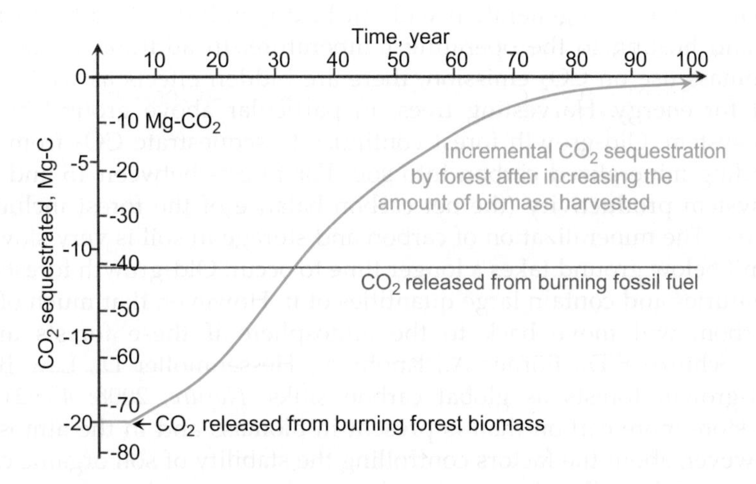

FIGURE 15.12 A schematic of incremental carbon storage after an extra 20 Mg-C (or 73.28 Mg-CO_2) harvested on the same stand above a traditional harvest (Redrawn based on Walker T, Cardellichio P, Colnes A, Gunn J, Kittler B, Perschel B, Recchia C, Saah D, "Biomass Sustainability and Carbon Policy Study", Commonwealth of Massachusetts Department of Energy Resources and Manomet Center for Conservation Sciences, June 2010.).

TABLE 15.5 Emission Specifications of Some Power Plants in the State of Massachusetts, USA

Power plant	Fuel type	CO_2, kg/GJ	NO_x, kg/GJ	Particulate matter, kg/GJ
Boardman (PGE)	Coal	287.5	0.107	0.019
Mount Tom Power Plant	Coal	227.3	0.189	0.025
Pioneer Valley Energy Center	Natural gas	99.3	0.007	0.004
Russell	Biomass wood	400.9	0.124	0.054
Pioneer Renewable Energy	Biomass wood	358.7	0.110	0.034
Palmer Renewable Energy (planned but dropped for greenwood instead)	Construction and demolition debris	393.7	0.112	0.022

bio-products. The net effect is that solar energy and atmospheric carbon dioxide are converted to energy and materials that are utilized by humans.

Utilization of forest materials imparts a price or impact on the environment. A change in sustainable state is expected. CO_2 is CO_2, whether it is from fossil or biogenic. Fossil energy sources are dense in energy content. Table 15.5 shows some environmental factors of energy production (electricity generation by burning fuel) from fossil source and woody biomass. Both the higher efficiency and denser energy content of the raw materials have contributed to much lower CO_2 emission of fossil than wood. There is the appearance of much higher carbon dioxide emission from woody biomass (nominally CH_2O) use due in part to the H_2O generation without heat gain but with a heat drain for H_2O evaporation and heating to the operating temperature. In addition to the clear impact of woody biomass use on CO_2 emission, there are hidden effects as well. Trees need to be harvested for energy. Harvesting trees, in particular above ground biomass, affect the forest ecosystem. Old-growth forest continues to sequestrate CO_2 from atmosphere, decaying sending mineralized carbon into soil. For forests between 15 and 800 years of age, net ecosystem productivity (the net carbon balance of the forest including soils) is usually positive. The mineralization of carbon and storage in soil is very slow and carbon saturation limit below ground takes a longer time to occur. Old-growth forests accumulate carbon for centuries and contain large quantities of it. However, that much of this carbon, even soil carbon, will move back to the atmosphere if these forests are disturbed (Luyssaert S., Schulze E-D., Börner A., Knohl A., Hessenmöller D., Law B.E., Ciais P., Grace J. Old-growth forests as global carbon sinks. *Nature*, 2008; 455:213–215). The world's soils store more carbon than is present in biomass and in the atmosphere. Little is known, however, about the factors controlling the stability of soil organic carbon stocks and the response of the soil carbon pool to climate change remains uncertain. The supply of fresh plant-derived carbon to the subsoil (0.6–0.8 m/depth) stimulates the microbial mineralization of 2567 ± 226 year-old carbon. In the absence of fresh organic carbon, an essential source of energy for soil microbes, the stability of organic carbon in deep soil layers is maintained, may prevent the decomposition of the organic carbon pool in deep soil layers in response to future changes in temperature. Any change in land use and agricultural practices that increases the distribution of fresh carbon along the soil profile could however stimulate the loss of ancient buried carbon (Fontaine S, Barot S, Barre P, Bdioui N, Mary B, Rumpel C. Stability of organic carbon in deep soil layers controlled by fresh carbon supply. *Nature*, 2007; 450: 277-U10). Managed forest stands on 80-year rotations stored only half the carbon of old-growth forests (Janisch JE and Harmon ME. Successional changes in live and dead wood carbon stores: implications for net ecosystem productivity. *Tree Physiology.* 2002; 22:77–89.). Therefore, if all the forests were converted to productive woody biomass field, there would be a net CO_2 input into the atmosphere (if the ocean and open land did not take in the then available excess CO_2). A well-managed woody biomass land will have a net CO_2 contribution to atmosphere if it was converted from natural forest. Still the net CO_2 contribution to the atmosphere would be the lowest when steady state (biomass harvesting rate equal to growth rate) was reached than other crop operations simply because of its unparallel high standing mass. When steady state is reached (80 years into the future for an 80-year rotation forest scheme), woody biomass becomes truly carbon neutral, although the CO_2 level in the atmosphere will be higher than what we know today. The consequence of not starting using woody biomass today would be simply increasing the CO_2 in the atmosphere to an even higher level.

Fig. 15.12 shows that the initial ***carbon debt*** (of 9 tons or 9 Mg) due to the use of woody biomass instead of fossil energy is shown as the difference between the total carbon harvested for biomass (20 Mg-C) and the carbon released by fossil fuel burning (11 Mg-C) that produces an equivalent amount of energy. The ***carbon dividend*** is defined as the portion of the fossil fuel emissions (11 Mg-C) that are offset by forest growth at a particular point in time. After the 9 Mg-C biomass carbon debt is recovered by forest growth (year 32), atmospheric GHG levels fall below what they would have been had an equivalent amount of energy been generated from fossil fuels. This is the point at which the benefits of burning biomass begin to accrue, rising over time as the forest sequesters greater amounts of carbon relative to the typical harvest.

Fig. 15.12 shows that zero net CO_2 emission would not occur after 100 years if one wishes the biomass to grow to its original level before harvesting. Fig. 15.11 (and Fig. 15.12) shows that biomass incremental growth is slow initially, very rapid in the middle of the biomass life span, and then slows down dramatically when saturation biomass is nearly reached. Is it economical or beneficial to harvest the woody biomass when saturation biomass has reached? If we choose this route, the productivity of the forest would be very low (incremental growth realized is nearly zero or negligible). This would be the scenario that woody biomass would not be renewable. A healthy woody biomass industry would be one that maximizes the productivity of the forest (if other parameters are fixed). This would not be corresponding to the case of near zero incremental growth. Referring in Fig. 15.12, harvesting at year 70, for example, would maintain a high-biomass productivity for the stand. However, either increased size of the stand or more biomass removal at harvest must be employed to receive the amount of woody biomass needed to generate that the extra 20 Mg-C required for the given amount of energy.

For a uniform stand of trees on a lot with uniform soil moisture and nutrients and constant atmospheric CO_2, the specific growth rate can be represented by

$$\mu_G = \mu_{max}\left(1 - \frac{X}{X_\infty}\right)^n \tag{15.8}$$

where specific biomass growth rate μ_G is that normalized by the standing biomass density or the amount of standing biomass over the area of the stand X; μ_{max} is the maximum specific biomass growth rate; and X_∞ is the maximum amount of standing biomass achievable or the carrying capacity. Both μ_{max} and X_∞ are functions of growth conditions and their relations to the biomass species. When $n = 1$, the growth rate is reduced to the logistic rate. The growth is proportional to the amount of live standing biomass when the tree is "young". As the tree ages or biomass increases, the specific growth rate decreases. When the saturation biomass level or carrying capacity is reached, the specific growth rate is zero. Therefore, the biomass growth is dependent on both the amount of biomass and the population distribution.

Mass balance over a stand leads to

$$\frac{dX}{dt} = r_X = \mu_G X \tag{15.9}$$

which describes the relationship of the standing biomass as a function of the growth time.

The Maximum amount of sustainable biomass available would be the maximum woody biomass production on site. The biomass production rate for a cycle time t is given by

$$P_X = \frac{X - X_0}{t} \tag{15.10}$$

where X_0 is the standing biomass of seedlings (or at time $t = 0$). At maximum sustainable rate

$$0 = \left.\frac{dP_X}{dt}\right|_{t_{max}} = \frac{t_{max}\left.\frac{dX}{dt}\right|_{t_{max}} - (X_{max} - X_0)}{t_{max}^2} \tag{15.11}$$

which leads to

$$P_{Xmax} = r_X|_{t=t_{max}} = \frac{X_{max} - X_0}{t_{max}} \tag{15.12}$$

Here t_{max} is the recycle time for maximum biomass production P_{Xmax}, and X_{max} is the standing biomass at time t_{max}.

Therefore, how the harvest is conducted is directly affecting the maximum amount of biomass available at a sustainably renewable level. The optimum and sustainable production rate of a biomass stand is the one that with final incremental growth rate at harvest equal to the average overall growth yield.

Example 15-5. Pinch line and optimum sustainable biomass production.

For a biomass growth curve shown in Fig. 15.12, what is the optimum recycle time, biomass yield, and production rate?

Solution. Since the growth curve is given as biomass changing with time, graphical method can be applied to solve the problem. Eqn (15.12) is the principle behind a simple graphical solution scheme.

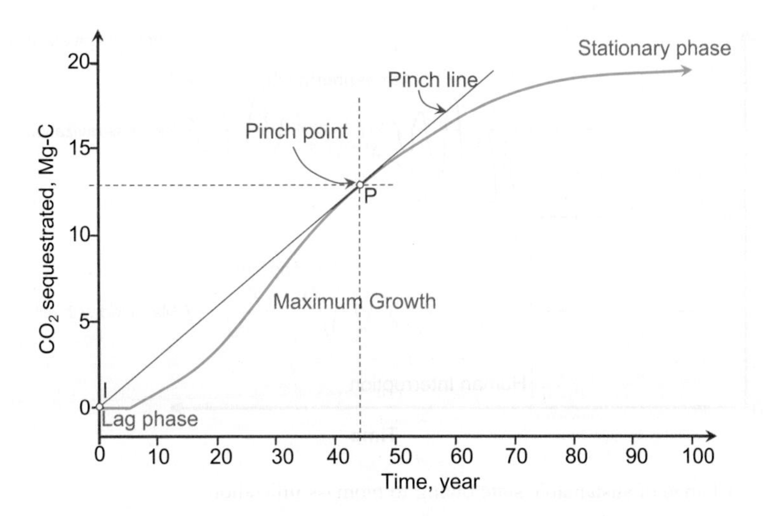

FIGURE E15-5.1 Finding the optimum biomass production from a growth curve.

To solve the problem graphically, we first plot the growth curve (X, t). Locate the starting (or initial) point of growth (after harvest and on new batch of growth) I, in this case is $t = 0$ and $X = 0$ Mg-C. Starting from point I, plot a straight line that only touch the growth curve once at a time after the growth started ($t > 0$). We call this line the Pinch Line. The pinch point P is the intercept of the pinch line and the growth curve.

We can read from Fig. E15-5.1 that the pinch point P is at 44.2 years, when the CO_2 sequestrated is 12.88 Mg-C. That is, the optimum point of harvest is at a 7.12 Mg-C deficiency as compared with the initial harvest (of 20 Mg–C). The biomass production rate is given by

$$P_{X\max} = \frac{X_{\max} - X_0}{t_{\max}} = \frac{12.88 - 0}{44.2}\text{Mg-C/year} = 0.2914\ \text{Mg-C/year}$$

Therefore, the optimum biomass yield on the given lot is to harvest the biomass at a 44.2-year cycle, which produces 12.88 Mg-C biomass each cycle, and the biomass production rate is 0.2914 Mg-C/year.

Example 15-5 shows that the optimum harvesting time is not near the time when the maximum standing biomass or saturation biomass level is reached. In this case, the biomass yield at optimum harvesting time is only about 65% of the saturation biomass or the biomass carrying capacity. The optimum utilization of woody biomass will result in a reduced level of standing biomass on the ground.

Fig. 15.13 illustrates the effect of biomass utilization as compared with fossil utilization. If there is no human disturbance, the level of CO_2 in the atmosphere and the standing biomass are stable or at a sustainable value as shown on the left portion of the Fig. 15.13. When fossil is used for energy by mankind, the atmospheric CO_2 increases monotonously with time (as shown also in Fig. 15.9). When biomass is used for energy, there is a higher rate of increase of CO_2 in the atmosphere initially (than using fossil for energy instead). There is also a decrease in the standing biomass at short times. However, when a longer time is elapsed, the atmospheric CO_2 is stabilized to a constant (or sustainable) level, which is higher than if

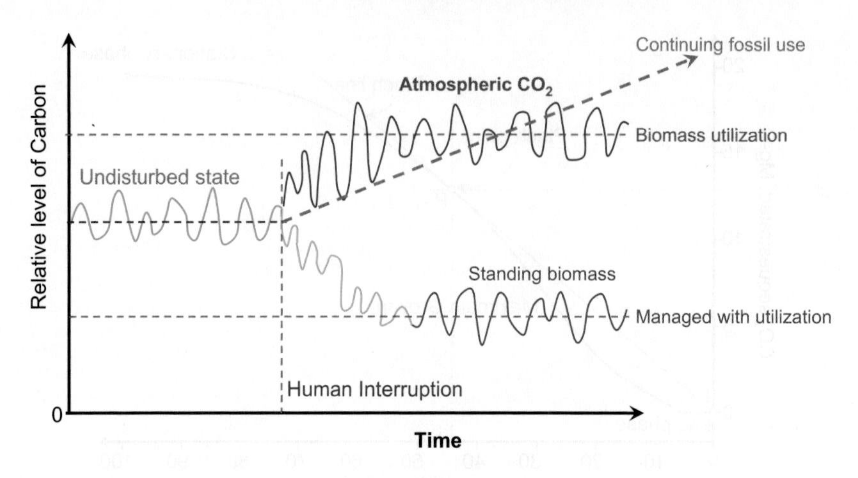

FIGURE 15.13 Change of sustainable state owing to biomass utilization.

no human interruption at all. Nevertheless, there is a new sustainable state. This is also reflected on the standing biomass. New sustainable states are foreseeable for biomass utilization, whereas fossil utilization does not lead to a sustainable state. Therefore, despite the changes caused by biomass utilization (true for all human interruptions), woody biomass use is sustainable.

The effect of biomass harvesting and utilization on the CO_2 concentration in atmosphere and storage depends not only on the standing biomass change (about 35% decrease for optimum biomass yield as shown in Example 15-5) but also depends on the life span of the harvested biomass and their derived products. If the harvested biomass was burnt for energy, the life span is very short. The net effect of biomass utilization is the difference of total biomass storage between a mature undisturbed forest and the managed forest should a mature forest is converted to a biomass producing forest. For a mature undisturbed forest, the total biomass storage is maximal at approximately the same as the carrying capacity, i.e.

$$X_{SU} = X_{\infty} \tag{15.13}$$

where X_{SU} is the total biomass storage for a mature undisturbed forest.

For a managed forest, the average standing biomass can be computed by

$$X_{av} = \frac{1}{t_H}\int_0^{t_H} X dt \tag{15.14}$$

where X_{av} is the average standing biomass, t_H is the harvesting time or the time between harvestings. For harvesting occurring at exponential growth, when $t \le t_L$, $X = X_0$ (lag phase) and when $t_L \le t \le t_H$, $X = X_0 \exp[\mu_G(t - t_L)]$ with $\mu_G =$ constant. Eqn (15.14) can be integrated to yield

$$X_{av} = X_0\frac{t_L}{t_H} + \frac{X_0\exp[\mu_G(t_H - t_L)] - X_0}{\mu_G t_H} \tag{15.15}$$

Let

$$X_H = X_0 \exp[\mu_G (t_H - t_L)] \tag{15.16}$$

be the standing biomass at harvest, then

$$\mu_G = \frac{1}{t_H - t_L} \ln \frac{X_H}{X_0} \tag{15.17}$$

Thus, the average standing biomass for a managed forest is given by

$$X_{av} = X_0 \frac{t_L}{t_H} + \frac{X_H - X_0}{\ln(X_H/X_0)} \left(1 - \frac{t_L}{t_H}\right) \tag{15.18}$$

Let the average life span of the biomass harvested and their derived products together be t_{PS} before degraded to CO_2 and emitted to the atmosphere. The total "biomass storage" for an optimally managed forest is then

$$X_{ST} = X_{av} + P_X t_{PS} = X_0 \frac{t_L}{t_{max}} + \frac{X_{max} - X_0}{\ln(X_{max}/X_0)} \left(1 - \frac{t_L}{t_{max}}\right) + \frac{X_{max} - X_0}{t_{max}} t_{PS} \tag{15.19}$$

If the growth follows the logistic growth rate, the average standing biomass for a managed forest is given by

$$X_{av} = X_0 \frac{t_L}{t_H} + \frac{X_\infty}{1 + \dfrac{\ln(X_H/X_0)}{\ln[(X_\infty - X_0)/(X_\infty - X_H)]}} \left(1 - \frac{t_L}{t_H}\right) \tag{15.20}$$

and the total "biomass storage" for an optimally managed forest is

$$X_{ST} = X_0 \frac{t_L}{t_{max}} + X_\infty \frac{X_{max} - X_0}{1 + \dfrac{\ln(X_{max}/X_0)}{\ln[(X_\infty - X_0)/(X_\infty - X_{max})]}} \left(1 - \frac{t_L}{t_{max}}\right) + \frac{X_{max} - X_0}{t_{max}} t_{PS} \tag{15.21}$$

Depending on the life span of the final product, the effect of forest biomass management on the carbon storage can be either positive or negative as compared with an unmanaged undisturbed forest. For longer product life span or CO_2 capture and storage after biomass conversion, a managed forest for biomass can turn the forest into a net CO_2 sink.

The biomass storage beneath the ground (i.e. roots) is dependent on the biomass species, location, climate, and harvesting frequencies and methods. For trees, the roots or beneath ground biomass is usually proportional to the above ground biomass. If new shoots and/or new trees can be restarted from harvested stump and/or roots, the reduction in the beneath ground biomass storage is small after harvest. In some species, however, the complete unit will die after the above ground biomass is removed, resulting in the decomposition of beneath ground biomass (after certain time). There is thus a great loss of biomass storage after harvesting. The softwood species commonly belong to this category. For hardwood, the loss of beneath ground biomass is minimal after harvesting the above ground biomass if the disturbance is not extensive enough to cause the whole system to die.

Therefore, in general as depicted by Fig. 15.13, the carbon storage will decrease and CO_2 in the atmosphere will increase when we start to manage forest for energy, chemicals, and materials. The net increase in the CO_2 in atmosphere is due to a combination of the short average life span of the harvest biomass before converted to CO_2 and the decrease in the amount of standing biomass. Burning of biomass for electricity and/or heat emits CO_2 shortly after harvesting. If one focuses on some special cases of applications, for example long-lasting materials, the net effect can be the opposite: a net capture of CO_2 from atmosphere.

For the same token, converting grassland to forest can dramatically increase the CO_2 capture from atmosphere to be stored as standing biomass. The net storage of biomass by grass and agricultural crops is negligible as compared with forest or trees. For example, the CO_2 storage due to forest growth in China and the developed world is substantial when compared with their pre-industrialized past due to the shifting of low-productive agriculture crop land to forest.

15.6. SOLAR ENERGY

Energy source sustainability and environmental impacts are two key factors in evaluating the benefits of energy source exploitation. Fig. 15.14 shows a schematic of the major energy flow to meet the needs of human society today. One can imagine that only energy originated from the sun may be considered as renewable on the planet. While nuclear energy could be lost if not harvested for human use, its deposit is limited and will run out long before the sun's ray. Nevertheless, nuclear energy use is a positive step toward energy sustainability transitioning out of fossil energy use. Geothermal energy refers to the energy available based on the temperature difference between atmosphere and that deep underneath the earth or deep in water. Exploiting the high temperature deep under the earth surface is the worst choice for energy production as promoting the temperature change inside the planet can lead to irreversible damage to the whole ecological system. Like nuclear energy, geothermal energy use does not contribute directly to CO_2 emission. However, removing thermal energy from the earth core is an act that cannot be reversed. The earth core is cooling slowly. Maintaining slow decaying in the temperature gradient along the radius of the earth is the ultimate sustainability goal toward long-time survival of the ecological systems we can envision today. Petroleum, gas, and coal, even if they were formed from biomass, are limited in their deposits and their recycle is at best questionable.

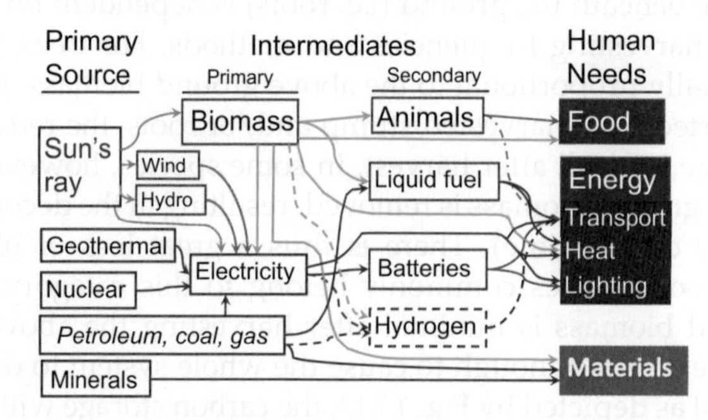

FIGURE 15.14 A schematic of major pathways of energy flow to meet human needs.

The radiation energy from the sun powers the ecological systems on earth. Fig. 15.15 shows the distribution of thermal radiation energy on earth. The thermal radiation can be quantified by

$$E = \varepsilon \sigma A_S T^4 \tag{15.22}$$

where ε is the emissivity of the body, σ is Stefan–Boltzmann constant or 5.6704×10^{-8} W·m^{-2}·K^{-4}, A_S is the surface area of the body, and T is the surface temperature of the emitting body. For thermal radiation absorption, A_S is the surface area of the body that receiving the radiation energy. The thermal radiation absorptivity has the same value as the emissivity.

As shown in Fig. 15.15, 174 PW or 174×10^{15} W of solar radiation reaches the earth's atmosphere, only about half of which (89 PW) is absorbed via earth surface (land and oceans). Not surprisingly, nearly half of the radiation reached to earth surface (40 PW) results in the evaporation of water, powering the water cycle on earth (Fig. 15.5). In total, there are 122 PW of solar radiation actively powering the ecosystems on earth, before the energy is radiated into the space. Partially intercepting the solar radiation beamed to earth surface to power directly the human society can be beneficial to the ecosystems as a whole on earth.

Solar energy has been harnessed by humans since ancient times using a range of ever-evolving technologies. Solar radiation, along with secondary solar-powered resources such as wind and wave power, hydroelectricity and biomass, accounts for most of the available renewable energy on earth. Only a minuscule fraction of the available solar energy is used.

Solar-powered electrical generation relies on heat engines (indirect conversion) and PVs (direct conversion). Solar energy's uses are limited only by human ingenuity. Indirect conversion of solar energy to meet the needs of humans is easier to implement. A partial list of solar applications includes space heating and cooling through solar architecture, potable water via distillation and disinfection, daylighting, solar hot water, solar cooking, and high

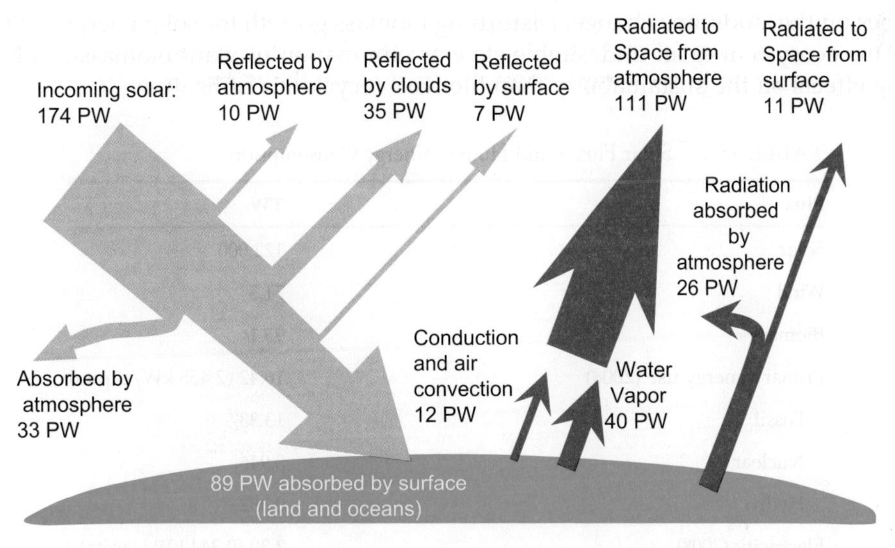

FIGURE 15.15 A schematic of major pathways of energy flow to around earth.

temperature process heat for industrial purposes. To harvest the solar energy, the most common way is to use solar panels.

Solar technologies are broadly characterized as either passive solar or active solar depending on the way they capture, convert, and distribute solar energy. Active solar techniques include the use of PV panels and solar thermal collectors to harness the energy. Passive solar techniques include orienting a building to the Sun, selecting materials with favorable thermal mass or light dispersing properties, and designing spaces that naturally circulate air.

Earth's land surface, oceans, and atmosphere absorb solar radiation, and this raises their temperature. Warm air containing evaporated water from the oceans rises, causing atmospheric circulation or convection. When the air reaches a high altitude, where the temperature is low, water vapor condenses into clouds, which rain onto the Earth's surface, completing the water cycle. The latent heat of water condensation amplifies convection, producing atmospheric phenomena such as wind, cyclones, and anti-cyclones. Sunlight absorbed by the oceans and landmasses keeps the surface at an average temperature of 14 °C. By photosynthesis, green plants convert solar energy into chemical energy, which produces food, wood, and the biomass from which fossil fuels are derived.

The total solar energy absorbed by Earth's atmosphere, oceans, and landmasses is approximately 122 PW or 122,000 TW as one can infer from Fig. 15.7. The energy reached the planet in 1 hour is more than the world used in 1 year in 2010. Photosynthesis captures approximately 95.1 TW in biomass. The amount of solar energy reaching the surface of the planet is so vast that in 1 year it is about twice as much as will ever be obtained from all of the Earth's nonrenewable resources of coal, oil, natural gas, and mined uranium combined.

From Table 15.6, it would appear that solar, wind, or biomass would be sufficient to supply all of our energy needs, however, the increased use of biomass has had a negative effect on global warming and dramatically increased food prices by diverting forests and crops into biofuel production. As intermittent resources, solar and wind energy need to be used along with a more reliable source. The major restriction on complete shifting to solar energy utilization lies on the landscape change. Disturbing biomass growth for solar energy capture can change the ecosystem to an undesirable state as elimination of plant biomass can have far-reaching effects on the sustainability than biomass recycle via utilization.

TABLE 15.6 Solar Fluxes and Human Energy Consumption

Flux	TW
Solar	122,000
Wind	71.3
Biomass	95.1
Primary energy use (2008)	16.42 (2.455 kW/capita)
Fossil	13.337
Nuclear	0.946
Hydro	0.352
Electricity (2008)	2.30 (0.344 kW/capita)

Solar energy can be harnessed in different levels around the world. Depending on a geographical location the closer to the equator the more "potential" solar energy is available. Plant biomass coverage on the ground is a key factor is whether or how the solar energy should be captured.

Solar technologies are broadly characterized as either passive or active depending on the way they capture, convert, and distribute sunlight. Active solar techniques use PV panels, pumps, and fans to convert sunlight into useful outputs. Passive solar techniques include selecting materials with favorable thermal properties, designing spaces that naturally circulate air, and referencing the position of a building to the Sun. Active solar technologies increase the supply of energy and are considered supply-side technologies, while passive solar technologies reduce the need for alternate resources and are generally considered demand-side technologies.

Solar power is the conversion of sunlight into electricity, either directly using PVs or indirectly using concentrated solar power (CSP). CSP systems use heliostats (lenses or mirrors) and tracking systems to focus a large area (via hundreds of movable mirrors or heliostats) of sunlight into a small beam. At the central location (focal point), heat engine is employed to convert the radiant heat into electricity. PV converts light into electric current using the photoelectric effect.

Commercial CSP plants were first developed in the 1980s, and the 354 MW SEGS CSP installation is the largest solar power plant in the world and is located in the Mojave Desert of California. Other large CSP plants include the Solnova Solar Power Station (150 MW) and the Andasol solar power station (100 MW), both in Spain. The 80 MW Sarnia Photovoltaic Power Plant in Canada is the world's largest PV plant.

Commercial solar water heaters began appearing in the United States in the 1890s. These systems saw increasing use until the 1920s but were gradually replaced by cheaper and more reliable heating fuels. As with PVs, solar water heating attracted renewed attention as a result of the oil crises in the 1970s but interest subsided in the 1980s due to falling petroleum prices. Development in the solar water heating sector progressed steadily throughout the 1990s and growth rates have averaged 20% per year since 1999. Although generally underestimated, solar water heating and cooling is by far the most widely deployed solar technology with an estimated capacity of 154 GW as of 2007.

15.7. GEOTHERMAL ENERGY

The Earth's core is very hot. Soil and rock have very low thermal conductivity. As the earth surface cooled for millions of years, it is the low thermal conductivity of rocks and soil that kept the earth's core hot. The sustainability of earth relies on the slow heat removal process to keep the earth warm. Therefore, deliberate drawing down the thermal energy stored deep underneath the earth is not a responsible action to the ecosystem.

Geothermal energy is thermal energy generated and stored in the Earth. Earth's geothermal energy originates from the original formation of the planet, from radioactive decay of minerals, from volcanic activity, and from solar energy absorbed at the surface. The geothermal gradient, which is the difference in temperature between the core of the planet and its surface, drives a continuous conduction of thermal energy in the form of heat from the core to the surface.

From hot springs, geothermal energy has been used for bathing since Paleolithic times and for space heating since ancient Roman times, but it is now better known for electricity generation. Worldwide, about 10,715 MW of geothermal power is online in 24 countries. An additional 28 GW of direct geothermal heating capacity is installed for district heating, space heating, spas, industrial processes, desalination, and agricultural applications.

Geothermal energy is not protected. Taking geothermal power has very low cost. Geothermal energy is reliable, and has very low gas emissions, but has historically been limited to areas near tectonic plate boundaries. Unfortunately, recent technological advances have dramatically expanded the range and size of viable resources, especially for applications such as home heating, opening a potential for widespread exploitation. Geothermal wells release GHGs trapped deep within the earth, but these emissions are much lower per energy unit than those of fossil fuels. As a result, geothermal power was viewed to be of potential to help in a short-term scale mitigates global warming if widely deployed in place of fossil fuels.

The Earth's geothermal resources are theoretically vast. There is no comparison between geothermal and fossil energy in terms of storage. However, geothermal energy is still finite, although the time scale to deplete geothermal resources is very long. Removing thermal energy from earth core cannot be reversed. Once the earth's core was cooled, the very ecosystem we enjoy today would not be there. Therefore, geothermal energy is not a sustainable energy for humanity to actively exploit. Depleting geothermal energy is even more dangerous than utilizing fossil energy.

15.8. SUMMARY

Sustainability is the capacity to endure in ecological terms. In more general scientific term, sustainability is the ability to continue without termination. Therefore, a sustainable system is one that has a "stable" "end" state. Monotonously increasing or decreasing of a given physical parameter is an indication of the system is not sustainable. In bioprocesses, sustainability is compatible with steady state.

The Sun's energy powers the entire ecosystem on earth: water cycle and biomass cycle. Energy stored by plants (primary producers) during photosynthesis, passes through the food chain to other organisms to ultimately power all living processes. Since the industrial revolution, the concentrated energy of the Sun stored in fossilized plants as fossil fuels has been a major driver of technology which, in turn, has been the source of both economic and political power. A discussion on sustainability must involve the chain of energy from the Sun to the two major cycles on the planet.

The water cycle provides opportunity for hydroelectric power development. Hydroelectricity eliminates the flue gas emissions from fossil fuel combustion, including pollutants such as sulfur dioxide, nitric oxide, carbon monoxide, dust, and mercury in the coal. Hydroelectricity also avoids the hazards of coal mining and the indirect health effects of coal emissions. Compared to nuclear power, hydroelectricity generates no nuclear waste, has none of the dangers associated with uranium mining, nor nuclear leaks. Unlike uranium, hydroelectricity is also a renewable energy source.

While both hydroelectricity and wind electricity are renewable and sustainable, hydroelectricity power plants have a more predictable load factor. If the project has a storage reservoir, it can be dispatched to generate power when needed. Hydroelectric plants can be easily regulated to follow variations in power demand. The water storage reservoirs can have a stabilizing effect on the "local climate", improving biomass cycles in otherwise arid areas.

Unlike fossil-fueled combustion turbines, construction of a hydroelectric plant requires a long lead time for site studies, hydrological studies, and environmental impact assessment. Hydrological data up to 50 years or more are usually required to determine the best sites and operating regimes for a large hydroelectric plant. Unlike plants operated by fuel, such as fossil or nuclear energy, the number of sites that can be economically developed for hydroelectric production is limited; in many areas, the most cost effective sites have already been exploited. New hydro sites tend to be far from population centers and require extensive transmission lines. Hydroelectric generation depends on rainfall in the watershed and may be significantly reduced in years of low rainfall or snowmelt. Long-term energy yield may be affected by climate change. Utilities that primarily use hydroelectric power may spend additional capital to build extra capacity to ensure sufficient power is available in low water years. The most serious industrial accidents of all are also the water storage reservoirs or the failure of the dams that forming the water storage reservoirs.

Biomass utilization also brings sustainable state change. Biomass has lower energy density than fossils. Switching from fossil energy use to biomass use will see an increase in carbon dioxide emission into the atmosphere. The increase in CO_2 emission is permanent. However, there is a new sustainable state (or CO_2 level) that is reachable with biomass use. This is in direct contrast to fossil energy use, where CO_2 emission is monotonous or a one-way traffic from ground to atmosphere. There is no sustainable state in sight if fossil was continuously been used. Apart from the sustainability impact, the depletion of fossil has made it imperative to move away from its utilization.

Wood or forest biomass has the highest saturation standing biomass, while algae have the highest production rate. Biomass production can be maximized by

$$P_{X\max} = r_X|_{t=t_{\max}} = \frac{X_{\max} - X_0}{t_{\max}} \tag{15.12}$$

i.e. the line originated from the initial point of standing biomass pinch at the accumulative biomass growth (or standing biomass) curve. The maximum biomass production (harvestable) rate is at a much lower standing biomass level than saturation biomass. Biomass utilization requires the gathering of biomass for processing. Denser or higher biomass capacity at harvesting provides more opportunities and easier access to commercial processing facilities. Therefore, high saturation biomass species are more advantageous than low saturation biomass species due to the collection and transportation restrictions. The lower standing biomass than saturation biomass also leads to more CO_2 staying in the atmosphere when biomass is managed for utilization. Utilization of biomass does lead to a sustainable state change.

Depending on the life span of the final product, the effect of forest biomass management on the carbon storage can be either positive or negative as compared with an unmanaged undisturbed forest. For longer product life span or CO_2 capture and storage after biomass conversion, a managed forest for biomass can turn the forest into a net CO_2 sink.

For a mature undisturbed forest, the total biomass storage is maximal at approximately the same as the carrying capacity, i.e.

$$X_{SU} = X_{\infty} \tag{15.13}$$

where X_{SU} is the total biomass storage for a mature undisturbed forest. The total "biomass storage" for an optimally managed forest where harvesting is within the exponential growth regime is given by

$$X_{ST} = X_{av} + P_X t_{PS} = X_0 \frac{t_L}{t_{max}} + \frac{X_{max} - X_0}{\ln (X_{max}/X_0)} \left(1 - \frac{t_L}{t_{max}}\right) + \frac{X_{max} - X_0}{t_{max}} t_{PS} \tag{15.19}$$

where X_{ST} is the total biomass storage for an optimal managed forest, X_0 is the standing biomass right after a harvest, t_L is the lag time from the last harvest to the exponential growth start, X_{max} is the standing biomass at optimal harvest time t_{max}, and t_{PS} is the average life span of the harvested biomass from the time of harvest to the emission of CO_2 into the atmosphere.

If the growth follows the logistic growth rate between the end of the lag phase and harvesting point, the average standing biomass for a managed forest is given by

$$X_{av} = X_0 \frac{t_L}{t_H} + \frac{X_{\infty}}{1 + \dfrac{\ln(X_H/X_0)}{\ln[(X_{\infty} - X_0)/(X_{\infty} - X_H)]}} \left(1 - \frac{t_L}{t_H}\right) \tag{15.20}$$

and the total "biomass storage" for an optimally managed logistic growth forest is

$$X_{ST} = X_0 \frac{t_L}{t_{max}} + X_{\infty} \frac{X_{max} - X_0}{1 + \dfrac{\ln(X_{max}/X_0)}{\ln[(X_{\infty} - X_0)/(X_{\infty} - X_{max})]}} \left(1 - \frac{t_L}{t_{max}}\right) + \frac{X_{max} - X_0}{t_{max}} t_{PS} \tag{15.21}$$

Therefore, in general as depicted by Fig. 15.13, the carbon storage will decrease and CO_2 in the atmosphere will increase when we start to manage forest for energy, chemicals, and materials. The net increase in the CO_2 in atmosphere is due to the short average life span of the harvested biomass before converted to CO_2. Burning of biomass for electricity and/or heat emits CO_2 shortly after harvesting. If one focuses on some special cases of applications, for example long-lasting materials, the net effect can be the opposite: a net capture of CO_2 from atmosphere.

Converting grassland to forest can dramatically increase the CO_2 capture from atmosphere to be stored as standing biomass. The net storage of biomass by grass and agricultural crops is negligible as compared with forest or trees. For example, the CO_2 storage due to forest growth in China and the developed world is substantial when compared with their pre-industrialized past due to the shifting of low productive agriculture crop land to forest.

Solar energy is vastly available and solar energy use appears to be less disturbing to the ecosystems. It is clear that in the direct solar energy utilization cycle (other than the construction of the facility), there is no water, carbon dioxide, or any other substance emission involvement. Efficient capture of solar energy is the key for sustainable exploitation. However, solar energy capture cannot interfere with plant biomass growth, for its impact would be far worse than biomass utilization.

Geothermal energy is most reliable as it is stored deep underneath the earth. It can be exploited from any point on the earth surface by deep drilling into the rocks. However, geothermal energy is neither sustainable nor renewable. Just because there is vast amount of geothermal energy is not the reason for us to exploit. It is a more desperate resource than anything else on earth.

Further Reading

Adams, W.M., Jeanrenaud, S.J., 2008. *Transition to Sustainability: Towards a Humane and Diverse World.* Gland, Switzerland: IUCN.

Blackburn, W.R., 2007. *The Sustainability Handbook.* London: Earthscan.

Blewitt, J., 2008. *Understanding Sustainable Development.* London: Earthscan.

Bras, R.L., 1990. Hydrology: *An Introduction to Hydrologic Science.* Addison-Wesley, Reading, Mass.

Christopherson, R.W., 2005. *Geosystems: An Introduction to Physical Geography.* 5th ed. Prentice Hall, Upper Saddle River, New Jersey.

Costanza, R., Graumlich, L.J. Steffen, W. (Eds.), 2007. *Sustainability or Collapse? An Integrated History and Future of People on Earth.* Cambridge, MA.: MIT Press.

Davie, T., 2002. *Fundamentals of Hydrology.* Routledge Publishing.

Klass, D., 1998. *Biomass for Renewable Energy, Fuels, and Chemicals.* New York, Academic Press.

Norton, B., 2005. *Sustainability, a Philosophy of Adaptive Ecosystem Management.* Chicago: The University of Chicago Press.

Smil, V., 2000. *Cycles of Life.* New York: Scientific American Library.

Soederbaum, P., 2008. *Understanding Sustainability Economics.* London: Earthscan.

Strahler, Alan H., Arthur Strahler., 2003. *Physical Geography: Science and Systems of the Human Environment.* 2nd ed. John Wiley and Sons, New York.

Sumner, G.N., 2000. Precipitation: Process and Analysis. Wiley, New York.

Watson, I., Burnett, A.D., Watson, A.D., 1993. *Hydrology: An Environmental Approach.* Lewis Publishers.

Wilson, E.O., 2002. *The Future of Life.* New York: Knopf.

Wright, R., 2004. *A Short History of Progress.* Toronto: Anansi.

PROBLEMS

15.1. A small mountainous community is relying on the water supply from a glacier lake. The water is being collected by the lake in the 4 months of summer (125 days) at a rate of 1 m^3/s. The average evaporation loss of water from the lake surface is 0.001 m^3/s. Determine the amount of sustainable water supply the community can rely on daily.

15.2. Solar energy is the source of renewable energy. Direct utilizing solar energy is therefore renewable. There is a certain group in the population that is strongly against the use of biomass: gas emission and particulate emission. It is decided that solar panels are to be built to cover an existing forest to produce electricity for a nearby city. Briefly describe

(a) If the outcome is sustainable based on sustainability concept.

(b) Is this a favorable decision as compared with the use of forest biomass?

15.3. The planet earth's core is so hot that the middle layer (mantle) is consisting of liquid ion. The surface of the earth has been cooled down millions of years of ago. Therefore, geothermal energy or the thermal energy inside the earth can be harvested without seasonal limitation (thus reliable). Using sustainability concept and briefly describe
(a) Is geothermal energy is renewable?
(b) Is geothermal energy sustainable?

15.4. Evaporation from water body regulates/buffers the temperature nearby. For a water body covering an area of 10^8 m^2, how much thermal energy is removed by evaporation? Assume an average water temperature of 290 K and evaporation rate of 1 $g/(m^2 \cdot s)$.

15.5. Water is the common solvent used by humanity. In chemical processes, there are more efficient solvents that can improve the economic benefits. For example, ethanol has been proposed to replace water in pulp production. Using sustainability concept and briefly describe
(a) Is ethanol use is renewable?
(b) Is ethanol use sustainable?
(c) Is ethanol use more sustainable than water use?

15.6. A hydroelectricity facility was built below a mountainous area. Owing to the seasonal weather changes from wet to dry, the available water flow changes significantly. In 1 year, the water flow rate in a low day was just 8% of that in a high flow "wet" day. Determine the change in the available electricity generation possible if a reservoir is built to maintain the water level.

15.7. A forested area has been found to have a biomass carrying capacity of 15 $kg \cdot m^{-2}$ and productivity of 0.3 $kg \cdot m^{-2} \cdot year^{-1}$. Because of rising demands on energy resources, the 50-year rotation of the forest is regarded as too long. This area is to be cleared to plant a perennial crop: switchgrass. It will take a couple of years to establish, but the annual productivity is expected to be at 1 $kg \cdot m^{-2} \cdot year^{-1}$. Discuss the pros and cons of such a change.

15.8. A large area of farm land has become less productive and farmers starting to move out of agricultural cropping tendering. Some area has turned into grassland due to inactivity. A forest product company has started to rent the idle farm land to grow Aspen trees. Since the land is loaned from farmers, the forest product company is forced to manage the growth and harvest of the trees at maximum output while keeping the cost minimum. Discuss the benefit of managing a "forest" land as comparing to managing a grassland for biomass production.

15.9. Competition of biofuel with food has generated another imbalance among the general population. Food could be diverted to produce biofuel and thus takes away the food that is available to certain groups of people. It is decided to switch from corn-based ethanol to cellulosic ethanol. To ensure this process to be successful, it is decided to turn the current corn crop land to switchgrass. Switchgrass can produce nearly the same amount of biomass, but at much lower fertilizer use and less energy input for cultivation. Briefly describe the sustainability impact and if the conflict was resolved in a sustainable manner.

15.10. A typical forest growth curve after the seedlings are fully established in the Northeast USA is shown in Fig. P15.10. When new seedlings are planted, it takes 5 years to

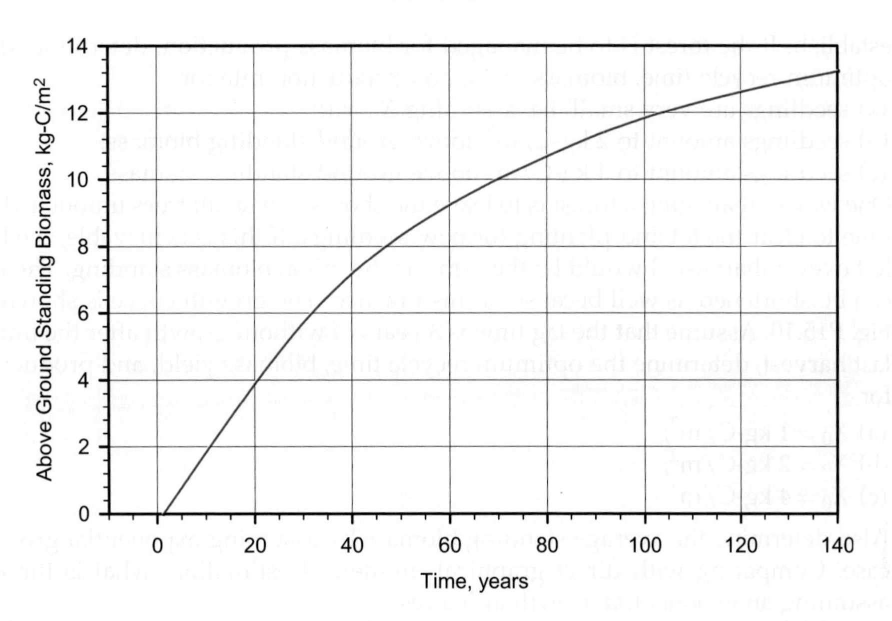

FIGURE P15.10

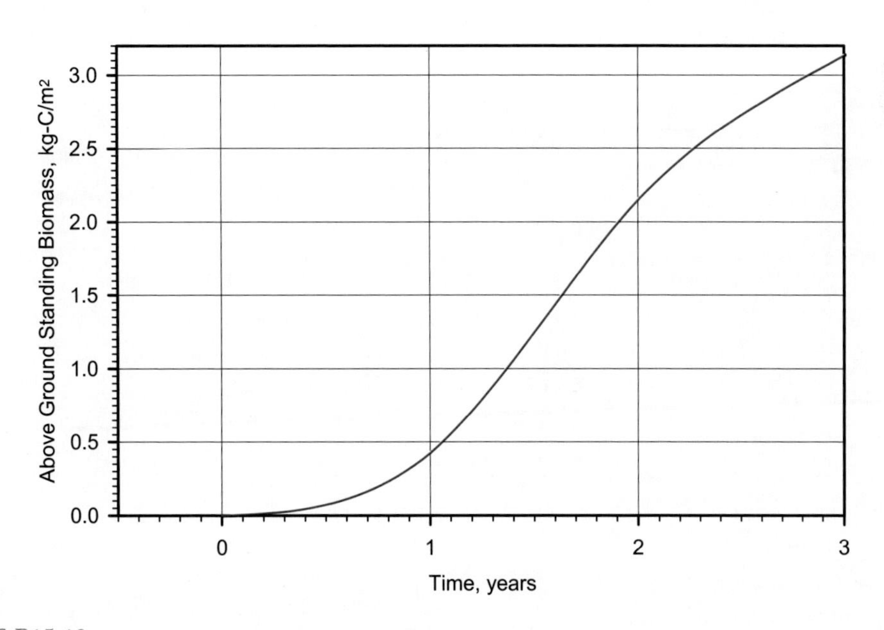

FIGURE P15.12

establish. If the forest is to be managed for biomass production, determine the optimum recycle time, biomass yield, and production rate for
(a) seedlings are very small, i.e. assuming $X_0 \approx 0$;
(b) seedlings amount to 2 kg-C/m^2 above ground standing biomass;
(c) seedlings amount to 4 kg-C/m^2 above ground standing biomass.

15.11. One way of managing a forest is to leave the shoots and small trees untouched, saving time to clear the lot and planting for new seedlings. If this is achievable, the biomass left over unharvested would be the same as the initial biomass standing. The lag time can be shortened as well because of this practice. The growth curve is shown in Fig. P15.10. Assume that the lag time is 3 years of without growth after the immediate last harvest, determine the optimum recycle time, biomass yield, and production rate for

(a) $X_0 = 1$ kg-C/m^2;
(b) $X_0 = 2$ kg-C/m^2;
(c) $X_0 = 4$ kg-C/m^2.

Also determine the average standing biomass by assuming exponential growth each case. Comparing with direct graphical–numerical estimation, what is the error of assuming an exponential growth at harvest?

15.12. Fig. P15.12 shows one of the best set of data from a cut-back study on short-rotation willow crop grown in Canastota, NY (courtesy of Dr Timothy Volk, SUNY ESF). The willow is cut to the ground and the growth rate on each harvest and then it regrows from the stamp. There is no lag time during cut-backs. Determine the optimum recycle time, biomass yield, and production rate. How does these numbers compare with forest biomass?

CHAPTER

16

Sustainability and Stability

OUTLINE

During the operations, a reactor can be operated under steady continuous conditions or unsteady conditions (such as a batch reactor). Steady continuous operation is desirable as the product quality can be maintained and controlled easily due to the everlasting

Bioprocess Engineering
http://dx.doi.org/10.1016/B978-0-444-59525-6.00016-0

operation without fluctuation in reaction conditions. In practice, especially in mass-production facilities, steady continuous operations are preferred. The steady continuous operation may also be termed *sustainable* operation, although a sustainable system need not be (strictly) stable. During steady operations, the feed conditions, reactor temperature, pressure, the extent of reaction, and yield are all invariant with time or vary only slightly with time within a narrow margin of fluctuation. This "narrow" margin of fluctuation is ideally very small in most chemical and biochemical process operations. However, in ecosystems (nature) and waste treatment facilities, the margin of fluctuations could be "big." To study the formation and maintenance of steady (sustainable) operation conditions in a reactor, the steady state and the stability are two important concepts.

Steady state refers to the equilibrium state of a bioprocess system, where all the parameters are invariant with time. One can imagine that the steady states are the positions that the ball can be placed along the path shown in Fig. 16.1. Of course, the strict steady state does not exist in reality due to fluctuations external to the system. We usually refer steady state to a bioprocess system where all the measurable parameters of interest are invariant on a given timescale and a given space volume scale (i.e. on an average sense). More precisely, steady state is a sustainable state. This is much the same as the continuum scale concept for a fluid. For example, we say a fluid is continuous, which is only valid if the timescale is "long" enough and the volume scale is "large" enough. When timescale is too short and/or volume scale is too small, molecules are individual objects that move about all the time, whereby continuum concept is void. For a continuous flow reactor, the steady state refers to the state where the material (including individual species) flow and energy flow are constant. When a catalyst is involved, the activity of the catalyst remains constant under the timescale of observation.

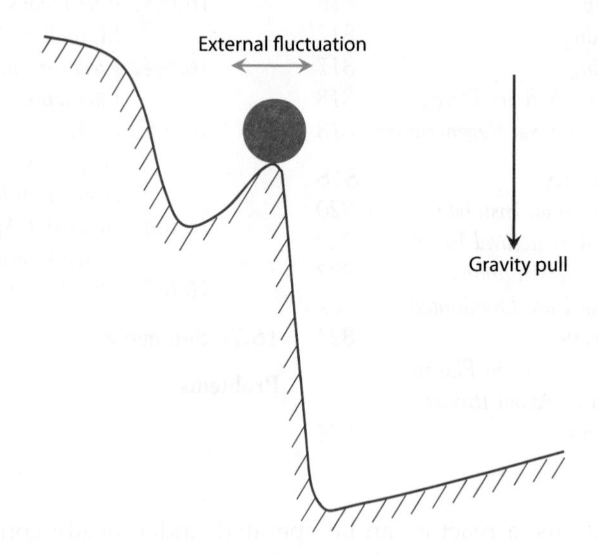

FIGURE 16.1 Equilibrium positions (steady states) of a ball on a curvy path.

Stability for a bioprocess system refers to the ability to dampen the "movements" effected by external disturbances to the bioprocess system. For example, there are two steady states for a normal person: either standing up or lying down. Clearly, lying down is a more stable state than standing up. When a person is lying down, the body center of mass is very close to the surface and there is more contacting area with the surface. At standing position, the center of mass is farther away from the surface and there are only two contacting spots (feet) with the surface. To maintain standing, a person must be constantly adjusting the center of mass to be directly vertical above and between the two feet. If one is weak, he/she may fall as ones' body is not able to adjust against sudden pushes (such as wind) exhibited fluctuations. For a steady reactor operation, one must maintain the reactor inlet (feed) conditions, surroundings (for example, temperature and air movement), and effluent rates constant. However, strict constant is not practical as fluctuations always exist. Fluctuation is stochastic and unexpected. If a reactor is able to self-adjust to return all the system parameters back to the steady state before fluctuation disturbances exerted, the reactor can maintain the set steady-state operations. In this case, the reactor is stable. If a reactor runs away from a set steady-state operation point when experiences fluctuations, then the reactor is not stable. For example, explosive gaseous reaction and genetic transformation caused by environmental fluctuations are two unstable bioprocess systems. Referring to Fig. 16.1, the location of the ball is not a stable steady state as any fluctuation would force the ball change the location and not able to return. Commonly, stability issues occur when multiple steady states (MSS) exist. Yet, there are cases where "instability" is associated with a single desirable or possible steady state.

One of the important aspects of reactor design is to seek desirable stable steady-state reaction conditions as reactor set point. Only stable steady state can be operated such that the bioprocess system will not runaway when fluctuations are encountered. As such, the quality of the product can be maintained. Normally, a bioprocess system is operated such that the output fluctuations are small, and it gradually returns to the desired set point when a fluctuation is expired. Therefore, bioprocess system stability is an important topic for bioprocess system (reactor) design and operations.

16.1. FEED STABILITY OF A CSTR

Let us first consider the simplest case of steady-state operations of a continuous-flow stirred tank reactor (commonly known as CSTR for chemical transformations, or chemostat for biotransformations) in which a single reaction is taking place under isothermal conditions:

$$\text{A} \rightarrow \text{Products}$$

We do not eliminate the possibility of multiple reactants and/or multiple products.

Fig. 16.2 shows a schematic of jacketed CSTR where the heat generated in the reactor is removed via a saturated liquid–vapor mixture, so that the reactor is maintained at a constant temperature T. The variability in operation is controlled so that only fluctuations can come in from the feed.

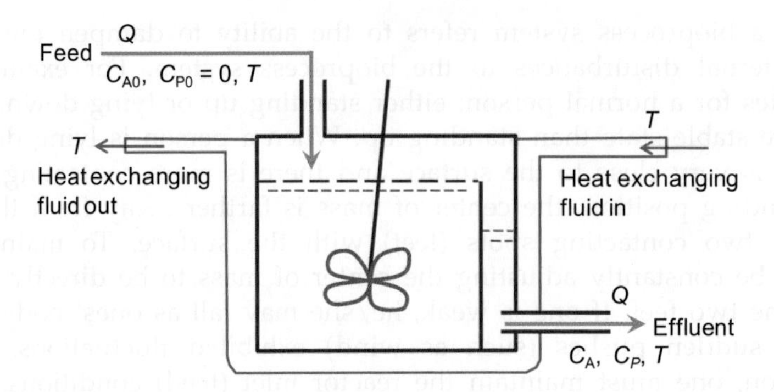

FIGURE 16.2 A schematic of isothermal CSTR/chemostat.

16.1.1. Multiple Steady States

As we have learned in Chapter 5, to solve an isothermal CSTR problem, only one equation needed, which is the mass balance equation. For a constant fluid level in the CSTR, the mole balance of reactant A leads to [see also Eqn (5.35)]

$$QC_{A0} - QC_A + r_A V = \frac{d(VC_A)}{dt} = V\frac{dC_A}{dt} \tag{16.1}$$

where V is the volume of the fluid in the reactor. Since the fluid level is constant, the volume remains constant all times. Substituting the reaction rate and dividing the volumetric flow rate Q throughout Eqn (16.1), we obtain

$$D(C_{A0} - C_A) + \nu_A r = \frac{dC_A}{dt} \tag{16.2}$$

where D is the dilution rate of the reaction mixture in the reactor.

$$D = \frac{Q}{V} \tag{16.3}$$

which is equivalent to the space velocity.

At steady state, Eqn (16.2) is reduced to

$$D(C_{A0} - C_A) = -\nu_A r \tag{16.4}$$

which is the molar (or mass) change rate of A in a CSTR per reactor volume. One can observe that the left-hand side is the molar (or mass) rate of A fed subtracted the molar (or mass) rate of A letting out of the reactor, divided by the reactor volume. Thus, one can refer the left-hand side as the molar (or mass) supply rate per reactor volume or simply molar (or mass) supply rate. That is

$$MS_A = D(C_{A0} - C_A) \tag{16.5}$$

which can be rearranged to give

$$MS_A = DC_{A0} f_A \tag{16.6}$$

Therefore, the mass rate supply of A to a CSTR is linearly related to the conversion and/or concentration, Eqn (16.6) or Eqn (16.5).

Let us now look at the right-hand side in the context of molar (or mass) balance. It is the molar (mass) consumption rate (or negative molar generation rate) of A. That is

$$\mathrm{MC_A} = -r_\mathrm{A} \tag{16.7}$$

The mass balance equation can thus be expressed as the mass supply rate of A to the reactor ($\mathrm{MS_A}$) equals to the mass consumption rate of A ($\mathrm{MC_A}$) in the reactor. The solution of a CSTR problem is thus visually illustrated in Fig. 16.3: on the plane of "mass change rate of A" versus "concentration of A" (or "fractional conversion of A"), the steady-state solution is the intercept between the "mass supply rate line" and the "mass consumption rate curve". That is

$$\mathrm{MC_A} = \mathrm{MS_A} \tag{16.8}$$

The steady-state solutions are characterized by the intercepts of the mass consumption curve and the mass supply line. In the schematic diagram shown in Fig. 16.3, there are three steady-state solutions. The number of steady-state solutions in this case is determined by the shape of mass consumption curve as one can infer from Fig. 16.3. MSS solutions exist if there are values of the independent variable ($C_\mathrm{A} > 0$ or $0 < f_\mathrm{A} < 1$) exists such that Eqn (16.8) and

$$\frac{\mathrm{dMC_A}}{\mathrm{d}C_\mathrm{A}} = \frac{\mathrm{dMS_A}}{\mathrm{d}C_\mathrm{A}} \tag{16.9a}$$

or

$$\frac{\mathrm{dMC_A}}{\mathrm{d}f_\mathrm{A}} = \frac{\mathrm{dMS_A}}{\mathrm{d}f_\mathrm{A}} \tag{16.9b}$$

hold true for some values of C_A or f_A by varying feed concentration C_{A0} or dilution rate D as illustrated in Figs. 16.4 and 16.5. The locations (or values of $C_{\mathrm{A0}} = C^*_{\mathrm{A0}}$ or $D = D^*$) at which

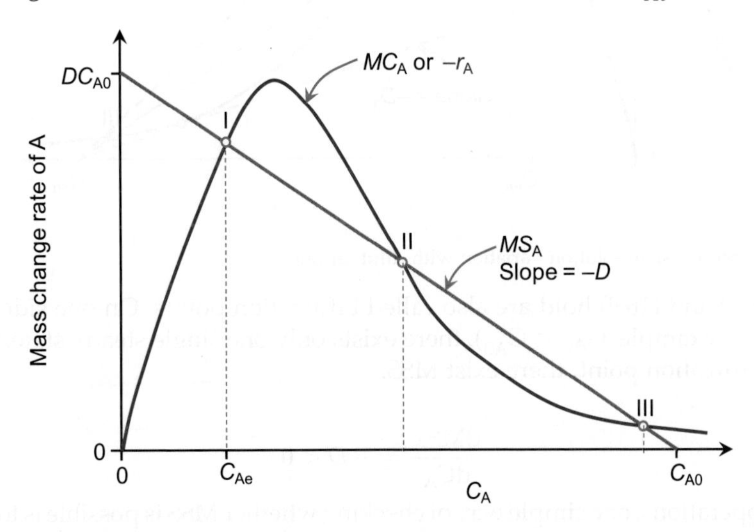

FIGURE 16.3 Schematic mass balances in a chemostat or CSTR. The mass consumption rate of A, $\mathrm{MC_A}$, is identical to the rate of reaction of A, $-r_\mathrm{A}$, in the CSTR operating conditions, whereas the mass supply rate of A (feed rate of A subtract the rate of A letting out of the CSTR), $\mathrm{MS_A}$, depends linearly on the concentration (for a constant density reactor).

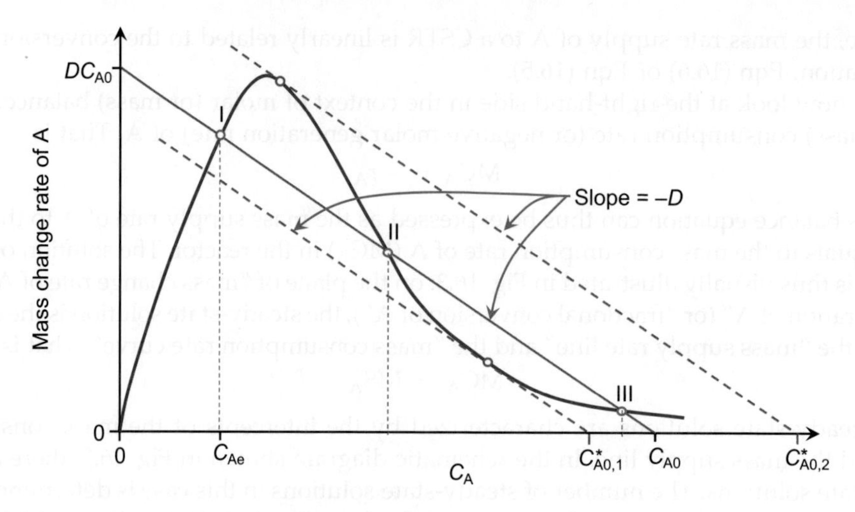

FIGURE 16.4 Steady-state solutions change with feed concentration C_{A0}.

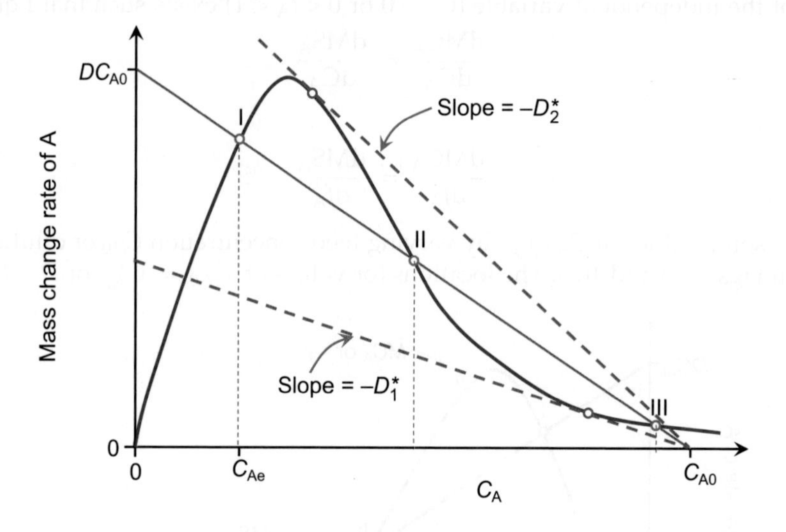

FIGURE 16.5 Steady-state solution variation with dilution rate.

both Eqns (16.8) and (16.9) hold are also called bifurcation points. On one side of the bifurcation point (for example $C_{A0} < C^*_{A0}$), there exists only one single steady state. On the other side of this bifurcation point, there exist MSS.

Since

$$\frac{\mathrm{dMS_A}}{\mathrm{d}C_A} = -D < 0 \tag{16.10}$$

For all CSTR operations, one simple way of checking whether MSS is possible is to determine if

$$\frac{\mathrm{dMC_A}}{\mathrm{d}C_A} = \frac{\mathrm{d}(-r_A)}{\mathrm{d}C_A} < 0 \tag{16.10}$$

since we have learned that the reaction rate normally increases with the concentrations of reactants. Therefore, if there is a region where an increase in the concentration of A can lead to a decrease in the rate of reaction, MSS is possible. Recall the kinetics we have learned so far, this type of rate law is possible for at least three cases: 1) surface reaction with adsorbed A decomposing requiring an additional free active site; 2) enzymatic reaction with substrate inhibition; and 3) cell growth with substrate inhibition. Figs. 16.3 through 16.5 are based on the kinetics given by case 1) and case 2) with no loss of enzyme from the reactor.

16.1.2. Stability of Steady State

Fig. 16.3 shows that there is at least one intercept between the mass consumption rate of A and mass supply rate of A, and there could be three intercepts. When more than one intercepts exist, we call this system MSS system. Although, there are MSS solutions, not all the steady states are stable that could be operated at. Points I, II, and III all satisfy steady-state conditions: $MC_A = MS_A$. The operating characteristics of each point are different.

1) CSTR operating at I

When the system is experienced with a fluctuation from feed, the CSTR could be upset in two ways. If the feed fluctuation caused the concentration in the reactor to shift left (i.e. lower) and then the fluctuation stopped, the mass consumption rate of A is decreased while the mass supply rate of A is increased: $MC_A < MS_A$. The net effect is an increase in the availability of A in the reactor and thus the reactor-operating conditions shift gradually back to point I. If the feed fluctuation caused the concentration in the reactor to shift right (i.e. higher) and then the fluctuation stopped, the mass consumption rate of A is increased while the mass supply rate of A is decreased: $MC_A > MS_A$. The net effect is a decrease in the availability of A in the reactor and thus the reactor-operating conditions shift gradually back to point I. Therefore, CSTR operated at point I has the ability to dampen the feed fluctuation caused steady-state shift. This is a stable-steady state.

2) CSTR operating at II

When the system is experienced with a fluctuation from feed, the CSTR could be upset also in two ways. If the feed fluctuation caused the concentration in the reactor to shift left (i.e. lower) and then the fluctuation stopped, the mass consumption rate of A is increased while the mass supply rate of A is increased less: $MC_A > MS_A$. The net effect is a decrease in the availability of A in the reactor and thus the reactor-operating conditions shift toward lower C_A and away from point II. On the other hand, if the feed fluctuation caused the concentration in the reactor to shift right (i.e. higher) and then the fluctuation stopped, the mass consumption rate of A is decreased while the mass supply rate of A is decreased less: $MC_A < MS_A$. The net effect is an increase in the availability of A in the reactor and thus the reactor-operating conditions shift toward higher C_A which is again as from point II. Therefore, CSTR operated at point II is not able to sustain any feed fluctuations. In other words, the CSTR cannot be operated at point II, although $MC_A = MS_A$ at point II. This is an unstable steady state.

3) CSTR operating at III

When the system is experienced with a fluctuation from feed, the CSTR could be upset in two ways. If the feed fluctuation caused the concentration in the reactor to shift left (i.e. lower) and then the fluctuation stopped, the mass consumption rate of A is increased slightly while the mass supply rate of A is increased more: $MC_A < MS_A$. The net effect is an increase in the availability of A in the reactor and thus the reactor-operating conditions shift gradually back to point III. If the feed fluctuation caused the concentration in the reactor to shift right (i.e. higher) and then the fluctuation stopped, the mass consumption rate of A is decreased slightly while the mass supply rate of A is decreased more: $MC_A > MS_A$. The net effect is a decrease in the availability of A in the reactor and thus the reactor-operating conditions shift gradually back to point III. Therefore, CSTR operated at point III has the ability to dampen the feed fluctuation caused steady-state shift. This is a stable steady state. This is a stable steady state that is not desirable in most industrial operations as the conversion is very low.

From Fig. 16.3, we observe that

$$\left.\frac{dMC_A}{dC_A}\right|_I > \left.\frac{dMS_A}{dC_A}\right|_I; \quad \left.\frac{dMC_A}{dC_A}\right|_{II} < \left.\frac{dMS_A}{dC_A}\right|_{II}; \quad \left.\frac{dMC_A}{dC_A}\right|_{III} > \left.\frac{dMS_A}{dC_A}\right|_{III}$$

Thus, the stable steady states satisfy Eqn (16.8) and

$$\frac{dMC_A}{dC_A} > \frac{dMS_A}{dC_A} \tag{16.10}$$

Inequality (16.10) indicates that the slope of the mass consumption rate curve is greater that the slope of mass supply rate line. Inequality (16.10) is referred to as the slope condition for CSTR feed stability.

If the working concentration we have chosen is not a reactant, rather a product is chosen, then the stability condition is changed to

$$MG_j = MR_j \tag{16.11}$$

and

$$\frac{dMG_j}{dC_A} > \frac{dMR_j}{dC_A} \tag{16.12}$$

where MG_j is the molar generation rate of (product) species j and MR_j is the molar removal rate of (product) species j.

16.1.3. Effect of Feed Parameters on MSS

Let us now continue on the discussion in Section 16.11. MSS exist if the rate low gives lower reaction rates at very high-feed reactant concentrations (than that at lower reactant concentrations). Feed conditions also affect whether MSS exits or not. In this section, we shall focus on the effect of feed conditions on the steady-state operations.

From Figs. 16.4 and 16.5, one can observe that there are two bifurcation points. When the feed parameter (C_{A0} or D) is set between the two bifurcation points, there are three solutions possible; otherwise there is only one steady-state solution. To illustrate clearly, this

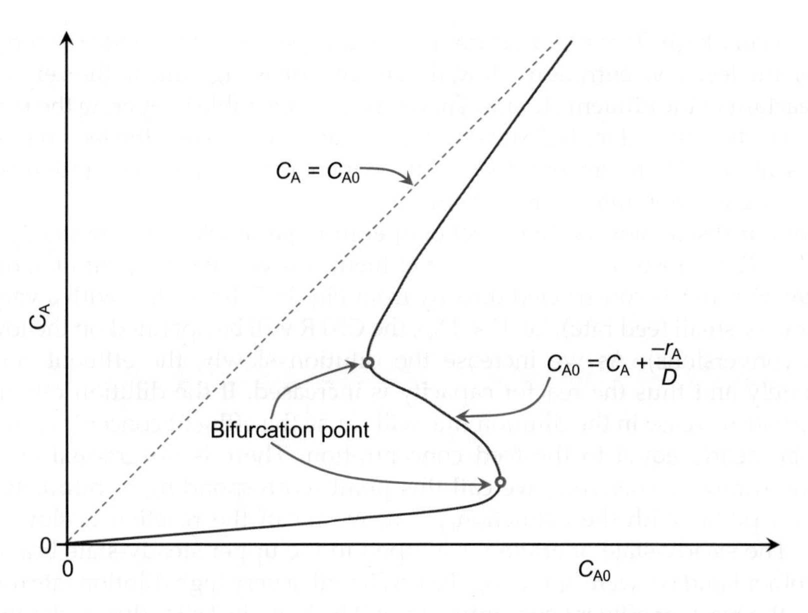

FIGURE 16.6 Steady-state solution of C_A as a function of feed concentration C_{A0} for a fixed dilution rate D.

bifurcation phenomenon, Figs. 16.6 and 16.7 show the variation of the steady-state solution (C_A) as a function of the feed parameters.

Fig. 16.6 shows that there are three values of C_A when the feed concentration C_{A0} is set between the two bifurcation points. Therefore, there are three branches of the steady solution: upper, middle, and lower branches. Based on our discussions in §16.1.2, both upper and lower branches are stable, while the middle branch is not stable. Therefore, the middle branch is not observable experimentally as any fluctuations would lead the operating point to shift away to a new location. We can observe from Fig. 16.6 that when the feed concentration is very high with a fixed dilution rate, the concentration of the reactant coming out of the

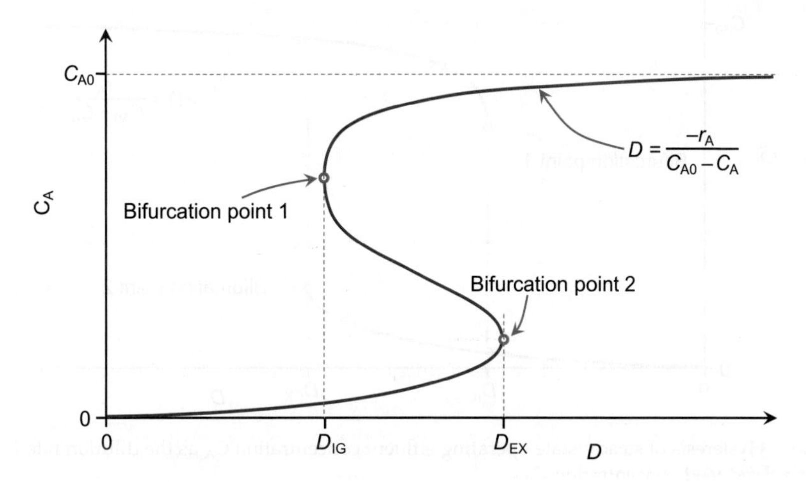

FIGURE 16.7 Steady-state solution of C_A as a function of dilution rate D for a fixed feed concentration C_{A0}.

reactor is also very high. This is not desirable operating strategy in practice as the conversion is low. When the feed concentration is low, the conversion is high due to the very low concentration of reactant in the effluent stream. Therefore, it is desirable to operate the reactor on the lower branch of the curve. Fig. 16.7 shows similar phenomena when the feed parameter dilution rate D is altered. Therefore, our discussion on increasing feed concentration is applicable to the increasing dilution rate (or feed rate).

To further our discussions on the effect of operating parameters on the steady-state operations of a CSTR, we focus on the change of effluent concentration C_A with the dilution rate (or feed rate). Fig. 16.8 is constructed directly from Fig. 16.7. If we start with a very low dilution rate (or very small feed rate), i.e. $D < D_{IG}$, the CSTR will be operated on the lower branch (with high conversions). As we increase the dilution slowly, the effluent concentration increases barely and thus the reactor capacity is increased. If the dilution rate increases to D_{EX}, any further increase in the dilution rate will cause the effluent concentration to increase sharply to be nearly equal to the feed concentration. There is no gradual change in the effluent concentration. Therefore, we call this point (corresponding to bifurcation point 2) the extinction point. With the extinction point, we mean the reaction is slowed down to a near stop. The steady-state operation is jumped to the upper steady-state branch.

If on the other hand we were operating the CSTR with a very high dilution rate (or feed rate), i.e. $D > D_{EX}$, the reactant effluent concentration will be high (just slightly smaller than the feed concentration). This indicates that the reactor capacity is low and decrease the feed rate (or dilution rate) is desired. Decreasing the dilution rate slowly, we do not observe any significant changes until $D = D_{IG}$. Further decrease the dilution rate to pass D_{IG}, we observe as sudden drop in the reactant effluent concentration. The CSTR steady operation jumped down to the lower branch from the upper branch. The reactor operation is favorable as high capacity is experienced. This shift point correspond to the bifurcation point 1, which is different from the bifurcation point 2 for increasing dilution rate. We call this bifurcation point the ignition point, meaning the reactor is started if we decrease the dilution rate from this point downward.

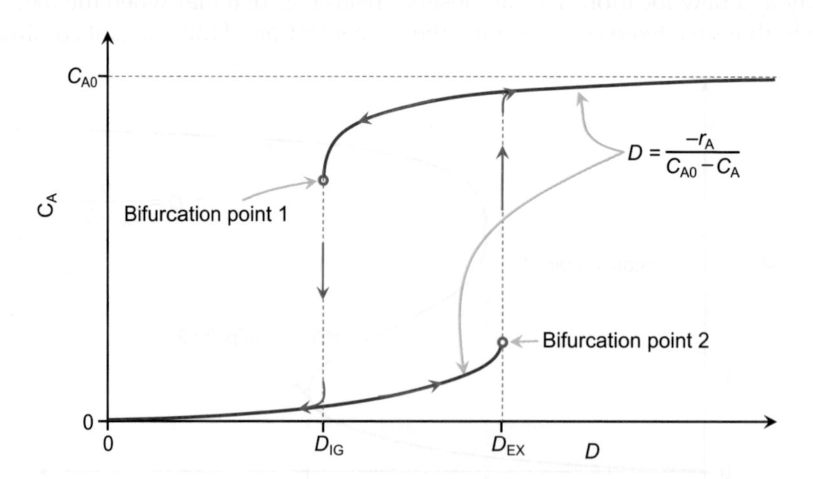

FIGURE 16.8 Hysteresis of steady-state operating effluent concentration C_A as the dilution rate D (or feed rate) is changed for a fixed feed concentration C_{A0}.

From Fig. 16.8, we observe that the CSTR operating conditions show a hysteresis when the dilution rate is increased and then decreased, or decreased and then increased. The cause of the hysteresis is due to the fact that the middle steady-state branch is not stable and cannot be operated on. Therefore, the path for increasing the dilution rate does not follow the reverse of decreasing the dilution rate. From Fig. 16.8, we also learned that how to operate the CSTR to achieve high conversions.

Example 16-1. Multiple steady states. The oxidation of carbon monoxide is carried out in a "fluidized" CSTR containing catalyst particles impregnated with platinum:

$$CO + \frac{1}{2}O_2 \overset{Pt}{\rightarrow} CO_2, \quad r = \frac{k_S K_A K_B^{1/2} C_A C_B^{1/2}}{(1 + K_A C_A + K_B^{1/2} C_B^{1/2})^2}$$

where C_A is the concentration of carbon monoxide and C_B is the concentration of oxygen. When the oxygen is in excess, the rate law can be reduced to

$$r = \frac{kC_A}{(1 + KC_A)^2} \tag{E16-1.2}$$

Determine the region (values of feed concentration C_{A0} and space time τ) where MSS exits.

Solution. A schematic of the fluidized bed reactor is shown in Fig. E16-1.1. Since oxygen is in excess, the concentration change of oxygen is negligible. Mole balance

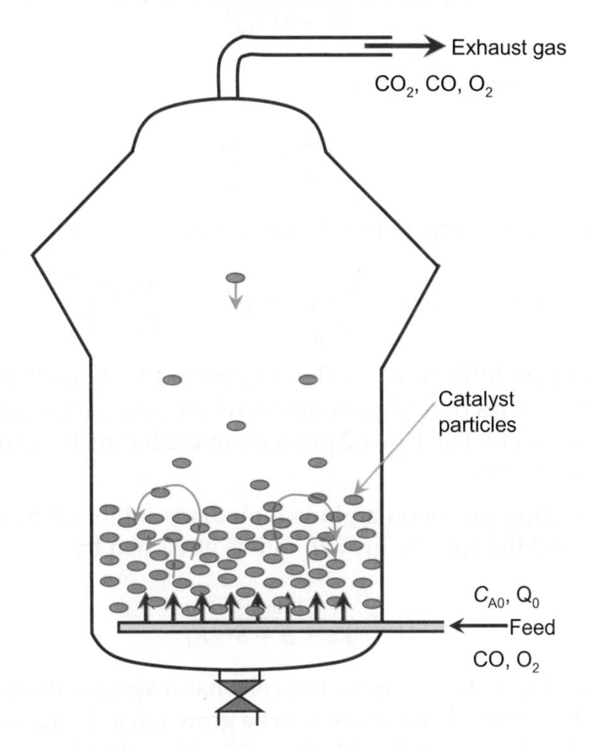

FIGURE E16-1.1 A schematic of fluidized bed CO converter.

on carbon monoxide over the entire reactor (assuming well mixed and at steady state) leads to

$$Q_0C_{A0} - QC_A + r_AV = \frac{d(VC_A)}{dt} = 0 \qquad \text{(E16-1.2)}$$

Furthermore, we assume that the volumetric rate remains constant. Eqn (E16-1.2) is reduced to

$$C_{A0} - C_A + r_A\tau = 0 \qquad \text{(E16-1.3)}$$

Substituting in the rate law, we obtain

$$C_{A0} - C_A - k\tau\frac{C_A}{(1+KC_A)^2} = 0 \qquad \text{(E16-1.4)}$$

In Eqn (E16-1.4), we have two feed parameters that can vary, τ and C_{A0}. In order for MSS to exist, there exist bifurcation points in the solution for C_A. That is, the derivative of Eqn (E16-1.4) with respect to C_A also holds,

$$C_{A0} - C_A^* - k\tau\frac{C_A^*}{(1+KC_A^*)^2} = 0 \qquad \text{(E16-1.5)}$$

$$-1 - k\tau\frac{1+KC_A^* - 2KC_A^*}{(1+KC_A^*)^3} = 0 \qquad \text{(E16-1.6)}$$

Eqn (E16-1.6) can be rearranged to give

$$k\tau = \frac{(KC_A^*+1)^3}{KC_A^*-1} \qquad \text{(E16-1.7)}$$

Substitute Eqn (E16-1.7) into Eqn (E16-1.5), we obtain

$$KC_{A0} = KC_A^* + \frac{KC_A^*+1}{KC_A^*-1}KC_A^* = \frac{2(KC_A^*)^2}{KC_A^*-1} \qquad \text{(E16-1.8)}$$

Therefore, the region where MSS exists can be determined by Eqns (E16-1.7) and (E16-1.8). Table E16-1.1 shows the values of feed parameters where bifurcation points exit (computed from Eqns E16-1.7 andE16-1.8). Fig. E16-1.2 plotted out the bifurcation points (solid line) and mapped out the region of MSS.

Example 16-2. A cell culture grows on a glucose media is inhibited by the substrate under isothermal conditions and the specific growth rate is governed by

$$\mu_G = \frac{\mu_{max}S}{K_S + S + S^2/K_I} \qquad \text{(E16-2.1)}$$

with $\mu_{max} = 0.1/\text{h}$, $K_S = 2$ g/L, $K_I = 25$ g/L. The cells has a specific death rate of $k_d = 0.01/\text{h}$ and a yield factor of $YF_{X/S} = 0.8$. The culture is to be grown in a chemostat with a sterile feed containing $S_0 = 100$ g/L substrate and a dilution rate of $D = 0.04/\text{h}$. Determine

TABLE E16-1.1 Feed Parameters Showing Bifurcation Points

KC_A^*	$k\tau$	KC_{A0}
1	∞	∞
1.010153	800	201.0051
1.02	412.1204	104.04
1.03	278.8476	70.72667
1.04	212.2416	54.08
1.05	172.3025	44.1
1.06	145.6969	37.45333
1.075	119.1223	30.81667
1.1	92.61	24.2
1.15	66.25583	17.63333
1.2	53.24	14.4
1.3	40.55667	11.26667
1.4	34.56	9.8
1.6	29.29333	8.533333
1.8	27.44	8.1
2	**27**	**8**
2.25	27.4625	8.1
2.5	28.58333	8.333333
3	32	9
5	54	12.5
6	68.6	14.4
8	104.1429	18.28571
10	147.8889	22.22222
14	259.6154	30.15385
18	403.4706	38.11765
22.5	603.6221	47.09302
26.22557	800	54.53043

(a) The steady-state solutions;
(b) Which steady-state solutions in a) can be operated, and which one is desired, and why?
(c) How should you start the reactor if the desired operating conditions are to be met?

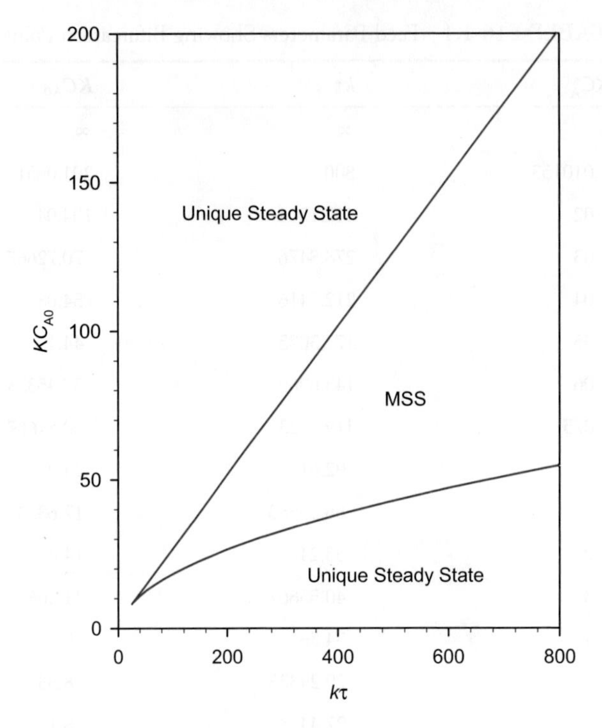

FIGURE E16-1.2 Feed parameter region where MSS exists.

Solution. Fig. E16-2.1 shows a schematic of the reactor operation.

(a) Mass balance on substrate (glucose) leads to

$$QS_0 - QS + r_S V = \frac{d(SV)}{dt} = 0 \tag{E16-2.2}$$

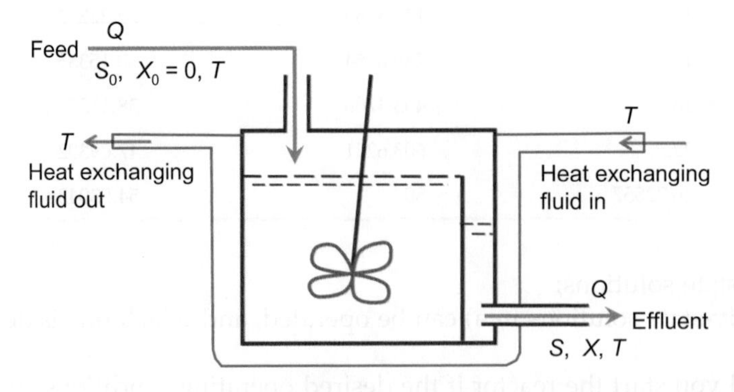

FIGURE E16-2.1 A schematic of a chemostat operation.

which can be reduced to

$$D(S_0 - S) = -r_S \tag{E16-2.3}$$

The rate of consumption of substrate is given by

$$r_S = -\frac{r_X|_{total}}{YF_{X/S}} = -\frac{\mu_G X}{YF_{X/S}} \tag{E16-2.4}$$

Thus, mass balance on substrate leads to

$$D(S_0 - S) = \frac{\mu_G X}{YF_{X/S}} \tag{E16-2.5a}$$

or

$$D(S_0 - S) = \frac{X}{YF_{X/S}} \times \frac{\mu_{max} S}{K_S + S + S^2/K_I} \tag{E16-2.5b}$$

which is equivalent to $MS_S = MC_S$. However, the right-hand side still contains an unknown quantity X that needs to be determined. Therefore, we cannot solve this equation alone.

Mass balance on biomass leads to

$$QX_0 - QX + r_X|_{net} V = \frac{d(XV)}{dt} = 0 \tag{E16-2.6}$$

Since the feed is sterile and substitute the net growth rate in Eqn (E16-2.6), we obtain

$$-QX + (\mu_G - k_d)XV = 0 \tag{E16-2.7}$$

which can be reduced to

$$D = \mu_G - k_d \tag{E16-2.8}$$

If $X \neq 0$. One should note that $X = 0$ is also a solution for Eqn (E16-2.7), which corresponds to the wash out conditions.

Eqn (16-2.8) can also rearranged to give

$$D + k_d = \mu_G \tag{E16-2.9}$$

which is in direct analogy to what we have learned so far:

$$SMR_X = SMG_X \tag{E16-2.10}$$

i.e. specific mass removal rate of biomass (by reactor effluent and cell death) = specific mass generation rate of biomass (by growth). This equation contains only one unknown and thus can be solved directly.

Substituting Eqn (E16-2.1) into Eqn (E16-2.9), we obtain

$$D + k_d = \frac{\mu_{max} S}{K_S + S + S^2/K_I} \tag{E16-2.11}$$

which can be reduced to a quadratic equation:

$$K_S + \left(1 - \frac{\mu_{max}}{D + k_d}\right) S + S^2/K_I = 0 \tag{E16-2.12}$$

Two roots can be obtained from Eqn (E16-2.12):

$$S = \frac{K_I}{2}\left(\frac{\mu_{max}}{D + k_d} - 1\right) \pm \sqrt{\frac{K_I^2}{4}\left(\frac{\mu_{max}}{D + k_d} - 1\right)^2 - K_S K_I} \tag{E16-2.13}$$

To determine the value of biomass concentration, we substitute Eqn (16-2.9) into (E16-2.5a) to yield

$$X = \frac{YF_{X/S}D}{D + k_d}(S_0 - S) \tag{E16-2.14}$$

Therefore, we have obtained three solutions:

(1) $X = 0$, $S = S_0 = 100$ g/L;
(2) $S = 2.1922$ g/L, $X = 62.597$ g-X/L; and
(3) $S = 22.8077$ g/L, $X = 49.403$ g-X/L.

Fig. E16-2.2 shows an illustration of the steady-state solutions. There are two intercepts of the specific mass removal rate line with the specific mass growth rate curve for $S < S_0$. Therefore, both intercepts are steady-state solutions; their corresponding substrate concentration values are given above.

(b) Steady states 1) and 2) can be operated on as they are stable steady states. One can imagine steady state 1) being stable as when cells are washed out and not introduced

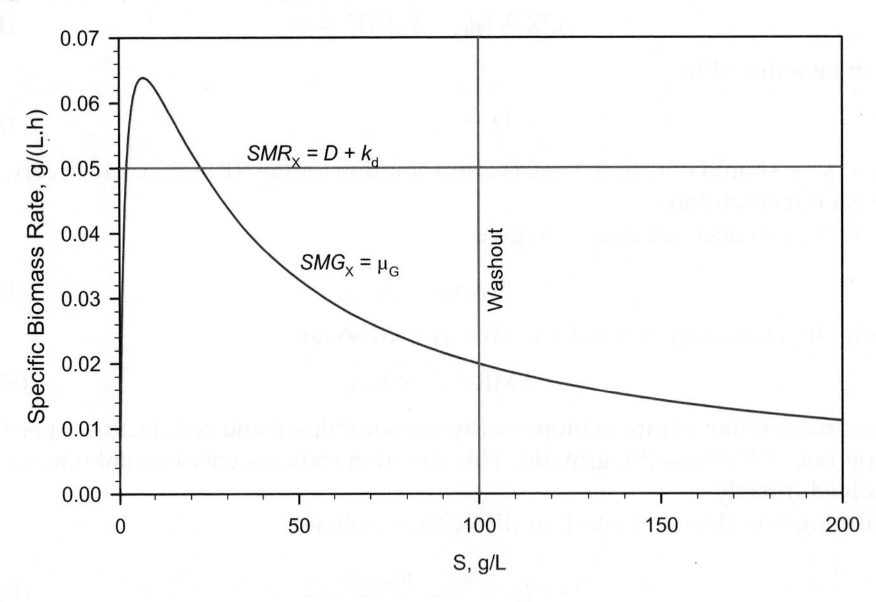

FIGURE E16-2.2 Graphic interpretation of the steady-state solution.

back in, they will remain out and no biomass would be produced. Steady state 2) is stable can be explained based on Fig. E16-2.2, or based on the fact that

$$\frac{dMR_X}{dS} - \frac{dMG_X}{dS} = X\left(\frac{dSMR_X}{dS} - \frac{dSMG_X}{dS}\right) + (SMR_X - SMG_X)\frac{dX}{dS} \tag{E16-2.15}$$

At steady-state locations,

$$\frac{dMR_X}{dS} - \frac{dMG_X}{dS} = X\left(\frac{dSMR_X}{dS} - \frac{dSMG_X}{dS}\right) \tag{E16-2.16}$$

Therefore, if $X > 0$, the above equation indicates that Eqn (16.12) is equivalent to

$$\frac{dSMR_X}{dS} < \frac{dSMG_X}{dS} \tag{E16-2.17}$$

That is, the steady state is stable if the slope of the specific mass removal rate of biomass (which is zero in Fig. E16-2.2) is smaller than the slope of the specific mass generation rate of biomass [which is positive at the location represented by solution 2)]. Thus steady state 2) is stable. Steady state 3) does meet this condition (E16-2.17).

Steady solution 2) is the desired operating point as the yield of biomass is the highest and the substrate concentration is the lowest in the reactor effluent.

(c) You can start the reactor with a seed culture, first as a batch. Do not leave the culture to grow for too long. However, make sure $S < 22.8$ g/L before gradually start with very small dilution rate, then gradually increase to $D = 0.04$/h.

16.2. THERMAL STABILITY OF A CSTR

Based on the discussions in Section 16.1, MSS exist if the reaction rate could be lower at high reactant concentrations (or at reactor inlet conditions). For an exothermic reaction operated under nonisothermal conditions, the reaction rate at the reactor inlet conditions can be lower than that in the reactor. Therefore, stability issue as we discussed earlier could apply to thermal stability in a CSTR for any exothermic reactions with any kinetics. For simplicity in discussion, let us consider the steady-state operations of a CSTR in which a single reaction is taking place:

$$A \rightarrow \text{Products}$$

We do not eliminate the possibility of multiple reactants and/or multiple products. For simplicity, we shall assume just one single reaction, although the analyses here are easily to extend to multiple reactions.

Fig. 16.9 shows a schematic of jacketed CSTR where the heat generated in the reactor is removed via a saturated liquid–vapor mixture. The simplification of using saturated liquid–vapor mixture is that the temperature of the heat transfer fluid can be assumed constant, and the heat transfer coefficient is usually high, ideal for industrial operations. However, this setup can be varied, and our discussions will still be valid with modifications in the heat-transfer term.

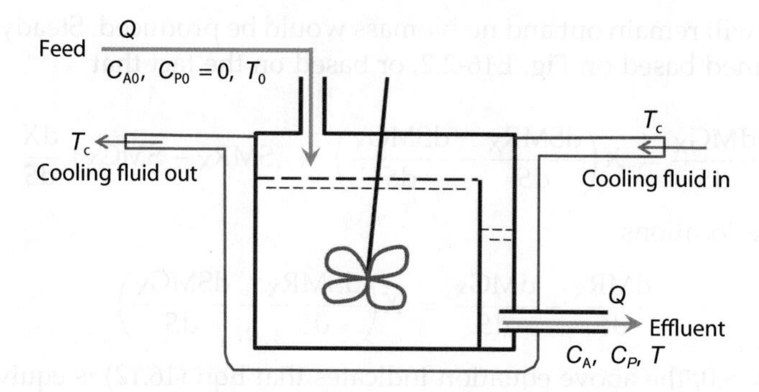

FIGURE 16.9 A jacketed CSTR with a saturated vapor–liquid fluid coolant.

As we have learned, to solve a nonisothermal reactor problem, two equations are needed: mass balance and energy balance. For a constant fluid level in the CSTR, the mole balance of reactant A leads to [see also eqn (5.35)]

$$QC_{A0} - QC_A + r_A V = \frac{d(VC_A)}{dt} = V\frac{dC_A}{dt} \tag{16.1}$$

Substituting the reaction rate and dividing the reactor volume V throughout Eqn (16.1), we obtain

$$D(C_{A0} - C_A) - r = \frac{dC_A}{dt} \tag{16.13}$$

where D is the dilution rate.

We next look at energy balance for the reaction mixture. Noting that the volume and pressure in the reactor are constant, we obtain from the first law of thermodynamics [see eqn (3.113)],

$$\sum_{j=1}^{N_S} QC_{j0}(H_j - H_{j0}) + Vr\Delta H_R + \sum_{j=1}^{N_S} C_{Pj}VC_j\frac{dT}{dt} = \dot{Q} - \dot{W}_s \tag{16.14}$$

The energy of stirring is dissipated into the reaction mixture, $\dot{W}_s \le 0$. Heat transfer into the reactor is accomplished by the jacket:

$$\dot{Q} = UA_H(T_c - T) \tag{16.15}$$

Assuming that the heat capacities are constant, we have

$$H_j - H_{j0} = C_{Pj}(T - T_0) \tag{16.16}$$

Letting

$$\begin{aligned} H_R &= \frac{UA_H}{V}(T - T_C) + (T - T_0)D\sum_{j=1}^{N_S} C_{j0}C_{Pj} - \frac{-\dot{W}_s}{V} \\ &= \left(\frac{UA_H}{V} + D\sum_{j=1}^{N_S} C_{j0}C_{Pj}\right)T - T_0 D\sum_{j=1}^{N_S} C_{j0}C_{Pj} - \frac{UA_H T_c - \dot{W}_s}{V} \end{aligned} \tag{16.17}$$

and

$$H_G = r(-\Delta H_R) \tag{16.18}$$

Eqn (16.14) can be reduced to

$$\frac{dT}{dt} = \frac{H_G - H_R}{\sum_{j=1}^{N_S} C_j C_{Pj}} \tag{16.19}$$

The way we regrouped to H_R and H_G are such that H_R is the heat of removal from the reactor (via the heat exchanger jacket and the reaction mixture flowing out, subtracted by the energy input due to the stirrer) and H_G is the heat generated in the reactor due to the reaction. Noting from Eqn (16.18), H_R is linearly related to reactor temperature T (straight line), while H_G is directly proportional to reaction rate in the reactor based on Eqn (16.8) and constant ΔH_R. If we normalize H_G and H_R with $(-\Delta H_R)$, then $H'_G = H_G/(-\Delta H_R)$ is equivalent to the rate of reaction in the reactor while $H'_R = H_R/(-\Delta H_R)$ is still linearly related to T.

At steady state, Eqn (16.19) is reduced to

$$H_R = H_G \tag{16.20}$$

And Eqn (16.13) is reduced to

$$DC_A + r = DC_{A0} \tag{16.21}$$

For a given kinetics, $r = f(T, C_A)$, the steady-state solutions can be obtained by two visual ways, depending which of the two Eqns (16.20) and (16.21) is solved first.

The first approach is solving the energy balance Eqn (16.20) first to render r and/or T as a function of reactant concentration in the reactor C_A only for a given heat-exchanging capacities, τ, and C_{A0}. Combining with the mole balance Eqn (16.21), we can completely solve the steady states of the CSTR. In this case, the solution procedure and qualities have been discussed in Section 16.1, except the influence of feed temperature, and heat-exchanging capacities. Nevertheless, we already learned how to approach the problem.

The second way is solving the mole balance Eqn (16.21) first to render r and/or C_A as a function of reactor temperature T only for a given τ and C_{A0}. Table 16.1 shows the solutions for some simple kinetic models. Combining with the energy balance Eqn (16.20), we can completely solve the steady states of the CSTR. Fig. 16.10 illustrates graphically how Eqn (16.20) is used to solve for the steady-state reactor operating temperature T. For the convenience of discussion, we further lump the operating parameters such that the heat of removal, Eqn (16.17), is reduced to

$$H_R = C_{HV}(T - T_H) \tag{16.22}$$

where

$$C_{HV} = \frac{UA_H}{V} + D\sum_{j=1}^{N_S} C_{j0} C_{Pj} \tag{16.23}$$

TABLE 16.1 Steady-state solutions of reactions in a CSTR with simple kinetic expressions. $\tau D = 1$.

(1) Zero order: A → Products, $r = k$

$$C_A = \max[C_{A0} - k\tau,\ 0];\ r = k$$

(2) Half-order: A → Products, $r = kC_A^{1/2}$

$$C_A = \frac{k^2\tau^2 + 2C_{A0} - k\tau\sqrt{k^2\tau^2 + 4C_{A0}}}{2};\ r = \frac{k}{2}\left(\sqrt{k^2\tau^2 + 4C_{A0}} - k\tau\right)$$

(3) First-order: A → Products, $r = k\,C_A$

$$C_A = \frac{C_{A0}}{1 + k\tau};\ r = \frac{kC_{A0}}{1 + k\tau};$$

(4) Second-order: A → Products, $r = kC_A^2$

$$C_A = \frac{\sqrt{1 + 4k\tau C_{A0}} - 1}{2k\tau};\ r = \frac{1 + 2k\tau C_{A0} - \sqrt{1 + 4k\tau C_{A0}}}{2k\tau^2};$$

(5) Second-order: A + B → Products, $r = k\,C_A C_B$

$$C_A = \frac{\sqrt{[1 - k\tau(C_{A0} - C_{B0})]^2 + 4k\tau C_{A0}} - 1 + k\tau(C_{A0} - C_{B0})}{2k\tau};\ C_B = C_{B0} - C_{A0} + C_A$$

$$r = \frac{1 + k\tau(C_{A0} + C_{B0}) - \sqrt{[1 - k\tau(C_{A0} - C_{B0})]^2 + 4k\tau C_{A0}}}{2k\tau^2};$$

(6) Autocatalytic: A + R → 2R + Products, $r = k\,C_A C_R$

$$C_A = \frac{1 + k\tau(C_{A0} + C_{R0}) - \sqrt{[1 + k\tau(C_{A0} + C_{R0})]^2 - 4k\tau C_{A0}}}{2k\tau};\ C_R = C_{R0} + C_{A0} - C_A$$

$$r = \frac{-1 + k\tau(C_{A0} - C_{R0}) + \sqrt{[1 + k\tau(C_{A0} + C_{R0})]^2 - 4k\tau C_{A0}}}{2k\tau^2};$$

(7) Unimolecular catalytic: A → Products, $r = \dfrac{kC_A}{K_A + C_A}$

$$C_A = \frac{\sqrt{(K_A - C_{A0} + k\tau)^2 + 4K_AC_{A0}} - K_A + C_{A0} - k\tau}{2};\; r = \frac{K_A + C_{A0} + k\tau - \sqrt{(K_A - C_{A0} + k\tau)^2 + 4K_AC_{A0}}}{2\tau};$$

(8) Unimolecular: A → Products, $r = \dfrac{kC_A^2}{K_A + C_A}$

$$C_A = \frac{\sqrt{K_A^2 + 4(1 + k\tau)C_{A0}} - K_A}{2(1 + k\tau)};\; r = \frac{K_A + 2C_{A0}(1 + k\tau) - \sqrt{K_A^2 + 4C_{A0}(1 + k\tau)}}{2(1 + k\tau)\tau}$$

(9) First-order reversible: A ⇄ P, $r = k_f C_A - k_b C_P$

$$C_A = \frac{C_{A0} + k_b\tau(C_{A0} + C_{P0})}{1 + (k_f + k_b)\tau};\; r = \frac{k_fC_{A0} - k_bC_{P0}}{1 + (k_f + k_b)\tau};$$

(10) First-order reversible catalytic: A ⇄ B, $r = \dfrac{k(C_A - C_B/K_C)}{1 + K_AC_A + K_BC_B}$

$$C_A = \frac{\sqrt{[1 + K_B(2C_{A0} + C_{B0}) + k\tau(1 + 1/K_C) - K_AC_{A0}]^2 - 4(K_A - K_B)[C_{A0} + (C_{A0} + C_{B0})(K_BC_{A0} + k\tau/K_C)]} - 1 - K_B(2C_{A0} + C_{B0}) - k\tau(1 + 1/K_C) + K_AC_{A0}}{2(K_A - K_B)};$$

$$C_A = \frac{C_{A0} + (C_{A0} + C_{B0})(K_BC_{A0} + k\tau/K_C)}{1 + K_B(2C_{A0} + C_{B0}) + k\tau(1 + 1/K_C) - K_AC_{A0}} \text{ if } K_A = K_B$$

(11) Second-order reversible: A ⇄ B + C, $r = k_f C_A - k_b C_BC_C$

$$C_A = \frac{1 + k_f\tau + k_b\tau(C_{B0} + C_{C0} + 2C_{A0}) - \sqrt{[1 + k_f\tau + k_b\tau(C_{B0} + C_{C0} + 2C_{A0})]^2 - 4k_b\tau[C_{A0} + k_b\tau(C_{B0} + C_{A0})(C_{C0} + C_{A0})]}}{2k_b\tau};$$

(Continued)

TABLE 16.1 Steady-state solutions of reactions in a CSTR with simple kinetic expressions. $\tau D = 1$.—*Cont'd*

(12) Second-order reversible: $A + B \leftrightarrows R$, $r = k_f C_A C_B - k_b C_R$

$$C_A = \frac{\sqrt{[1 - k_f\tau(C_{A0} - C_{B0}) + k_b\tau]^2 + 4k_f\tau[C_{A0} + k_b\tau(C_{A0} + C_{R0})]} - 1 + k_f\tau(C_{A0} - C_{B0}) - k_b\tau}{2k_f\tau}$$

$$r = \frac{1 + k_f\tau(C_{A0} + C_{B0}) + k_b\tau - \sqrt{[1 - k_f\tau(C_{A0} - C_{B0}) + k_b\tau]^2 + 4k_f\tau[C_{A0} + k_b\tau(C_{A0} + C_{R0})]}}{2k_f\tau^2}$$

(13) Second-order reversible: $A + B \rightarrow C + D$, $r = k_f C_A C_B - k_b C_C C_D$

$$C_A = \frac{\sqrt{[1 - k_f\tau(C_{A0} - C_{B0}) + k_b\tau(C_{C0} + C_{D0} + 2C_{A0})]^2 + 4(k_f - k_b)\tau[C_{A0} + k_b\tau(C_{A0} + C_{C0})(C_{A0} + C_{D0})]} - 1 + k_f\tau(C_{A0} - C_{B0}) + k_b\tau(C_{C0} + C_{D0} + 2C_{A0})}{2(k_f - k_b)\tau};$$

$$C_A = \frac{C_{A0} + k_b\tau(C_{A0} + C_{D0})(C_{A0} + C_{D0})}{1 - k_f\tau(C_{A0} - C_{B0}) + k_b\tau(C_{C0} + C_{D0} + 2C_{A0})} \text{ if } k_f = b_b$$

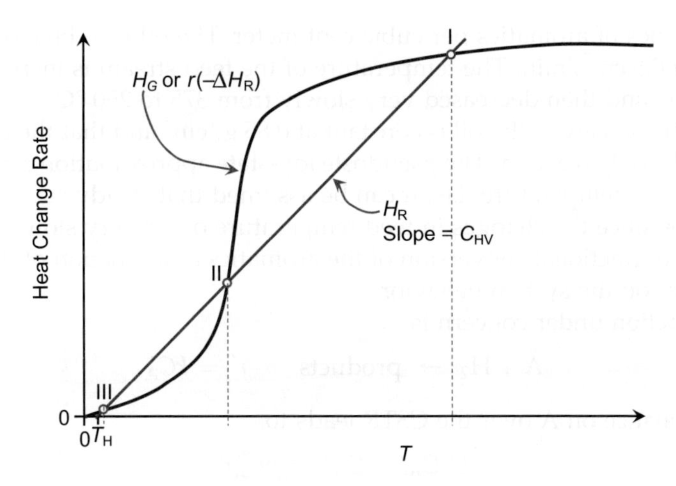

FIGURE 16.10 Heat of generation and heat of removal in a nonisothermal CSTR.

and

$$T_H = \frac{T_0 D \sum_{j=1}^{N_S} C_{j0} C_{Pj} + \dfrac{UA_H T_c - \dot{W}_s}{V}}{\dfrac{UA_H}{V} + D \sum_{j=1}^{N_S} C_{j0} C_{Pj}} \tag{16.24}$$

Now that the similarity of Figs. 16.8 and 16.3 clearly indicates that the solution procedure and qualitative behaviors of the steady solutions are similar. In this nonisothermal CSTR case, we have more feed parameters: feed concentration, feed temperature, feed rate, heat-exchange capacity (heat-exchange area and heat-exchange coefficient), heat-exchange fluid temperature, and stirrer energy input. All these parameters can be lumped to three parameters: D, C_{HV}, and T_H. The feed parameters change will alter one or more among D, C_{HV}, and T_H differently. Furthermore, the dilution rate affects the heat of generation (via r, see Table 16.1). If we leave the heat of generation curve alone (assuming constant), then the feed parameters can be reduced to two lumped parameters: C_{HV} and T_H. Feed concentrations, dilution rate, and heat-exchange capacity will have a dominant effect on C_{HV}, while feed temperature, heat-exchange fluid temperature, and stirrer energy input have a dominant effect on T_H.

Example 16-3 Thermal hysteresis: ignition/extinction curve.

The hydrogenation of aromatics (A) in an oil is to be carried out in a continuous well-mixed tank reactor at a constant hydrogen pressure. The reactor contains 20 g of catalyst and is operated adiabatically. The feed oil contains 30 wt% of A and the average molecular mass is 210. The average heat capacity is 1.75 J/(g·K) and the heat of reaction for hydrogenation of aromatics (A) is -2.0×10^5 J/mol. The rate function is

$$-r'_A = 1.3 \times 10^{11} e^{-16300/T} C_A \text{ moles-A/(h·g-cat)}$$

where C_A is in moles of aromatics per cubic centimeter. The oil is to be fed to the reactor at a constant rate of 0.5 cm^3/min. The temperature of the feed stream is increased very slowly from 250 to 375 °C and then decreased very slowly from 375 to 250 °C.

Assume that the density of the oil is constant at 0.85 g/cm^3 and that the hydrogenation of the aromatics is the only reaction. The pseudosteady-state approximation can be made for the slow changes in feed temperature, i.e., it can be assumed that steady state is achieved at all feed temperatures since the changes in feed temperature occur very slowly.

Prepare a plot of fractional conversion of the aromatics as a function of the feed temperature and comment on the system behavior.

Solution. The reaction under concern is

$$A + H_2 \rightarrow \text{products} \qquad r' = kC_A$$

Steady mole balance on A over the CSTR leads to

$$Q(C_{A0} - C_A) = m_{cat}r' \tag{E16-3.1}$$

where m_{cat} is the mass of the catalyst in the reactor. The left-hand side of Eqn (E16-3.1) represents the mass supplying rate of A (MS_A), while the right-hand side represents the mass consumption rates of A (MC_A). The general energy balance:

$$\sum_{j=1}^{N_S} F_{j0}(H_j - H_{j0}) + V\sum_{i=1}^{N_R} r_i\Delta H_{Ri} + \sum_{j=1}^{N_S} C_{Pj}n_j\frac{dT}{dt} - \frac{d(pV)}{dt} = \dot{Q} - \dot{W}_s \tag{3.133}$$

can be reduced for a steady CSTR with negligible stirrer work input and adiabatic operation to

$$Q\rho C_P(T - T_0) = m_{cat}(-\Delta H_R)r' \tag{E16-3.2}$$

The left-hand side of Eqn (E16-3.2) is the heat of removal (H_R) from the reactor, while the right-hand side is the heat of generation in the reactor (H_G).

To obtain the steady-state solutions, one is required to solve both the mass balance Eqn (E16-3.1) and energy balance Eqn (E16-3.2) for a nonisothermal reactor operation: $MS_A = MC_A$ and $H_R = H_G$. Eqn (E16-3.2) ÷ (E16-3.1) yields

$$\frac{T - T_0}{C_{A0} - C_A} = \frac{-\Delta H_R}{\rho C_P} \tag{E16-3.3}$$

which can be rearranged to give

$$T = T_0 + \frac{-\Delta H_R}{\rho C_P}C_{A0}f_A \tag{E16-3.4}$$

Substituting the rate expression and conversion in Eqn (E16-3.1), we obtain

$$QC_{A0}f_A = m_{cat}k_0 C_{A0}(1 - f_A)\exp\left(-\frac{E}{RT}\right) \tag{E16-3.5}$$

That is

$$T = \frac{-E/R}{\ln\left[\dfrac{f_A}{1 - f_A}\dfrac{Q}{m_{cat}k_0}\right]} \tag{E16-3.6}$$

Substituting Eqn (E16-3.6) into Eqn (E16-3.4), we obtain

$$T_0 = \frac{E/R}{\ln\left[\frac{1-f_A}{f_A}\frac{m_{cat}k_0}{Q}\right]} - \frac{-\Delta H_R}{\rho C_P} C_{A0} f_A \tag{E16-3.7}$$

Eqn (E16-3.7) is the mathematical description of the ignition–extinction curve (for conversion versus the feed temperature). We now find the parameters:

$$C_{A0} = \frac{\rho_{A0}}{M_A} = \frac{\omega_A}{M_A}\rho_0 = \frac{0.3}{210 \text{ g/mol}} \times 0.85 \text{ g/cm}^3 = 1.214 \times 10^{-3} \text{mol/cm}^3$$

$$\frac{-\Delta H_R}{\rho C_P} C_{A0} = \frac{2.0 \times 10^5 \text{ J/mol}}{1.75 \text{ J/(g·K)} \times 0.85 \text{ g/cm}^3} \times 1.214 \times 10^{-3} \text{ mol/cm}^3 = 163.26 \text{ K}$$

$$\frac{m_{cat}k_0}{Q} = \frac{1.3 \times 10^{11} \text{ cm}^3/(\text{h·g-cat}) \times 20 \text{ g-cat}}{0.5 \text{ cm}^3/\text{min} \times 60 \text{ min/h}} = 8.666 \times 10^{10}$$

Substituting these know parameters into Eqn (E16-3.7), we obtain

$$T_0 = \frac{16,300}{25.1853 + \ln\frac{1-f_A}{f_A}} - 163.26\, f_A \tag{E16-3.8}$$

which has a unit of Kelvin.

Eqn (E16-3.8) is plotted in Fig. E16-3.1 (by varying f_A between 0 and 1, we computed values of T_0, and then graphing the data out to yield Fig. E16-3.1). One can observe that there are multiple values of conversion f_A for some given values of feed temperature T_0 (between 554.10 and 581.12 K).

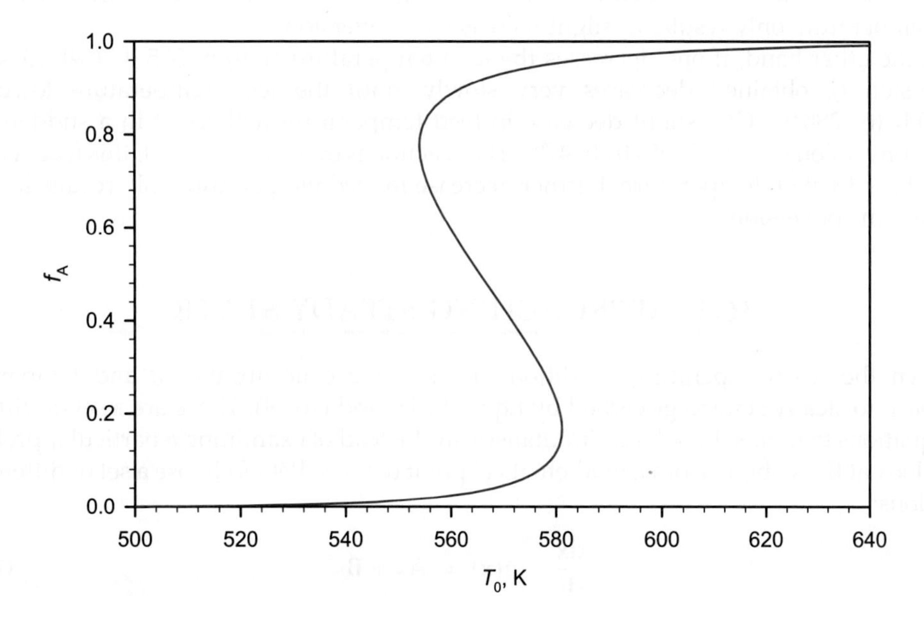

FIGURE E16-3.1 Variation of conversion with feed temperature.

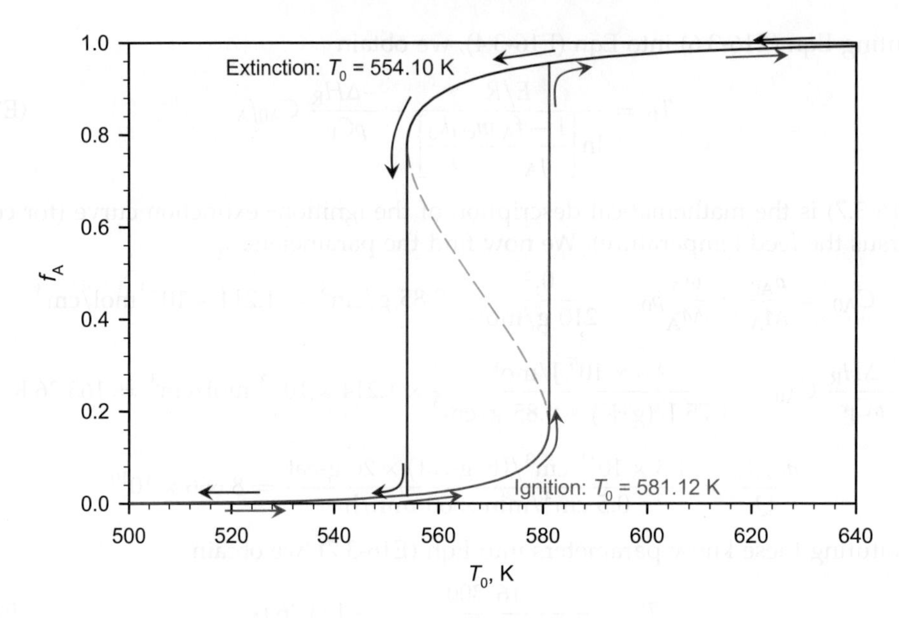

FIGURE E16-3.2 Ignitionextinction curve.

Fig. E16-3.2 shows the change in conversion achieved while varying the feed temperature. As one increases the feed temperature T_0 from 250 °C (523.15 K), the conversion f_A obtained increases very slowly, until the feed temperature reaches 581.12 K (or 307.97 °C) a slight increase in feed temperature will result in a sudden jump in the conversion f_A from 16.7% to over 95.58%. We call this feed temperature the ignition temperature. Further increase in feed temperature only results in slight increase in conversion.

On the other hand, if one decreases the feed temperature T_0 from 375 °C (648.15 K), the conversion f_A obtained decreases very slowly, until the feed temperature lowers to 554.10 K (or 280.95 °C) a slight decrease in feed temperature will result in a sudden drop in the conversion f_A from 77.5% to 16.47%. The reaction is quenched. We call this feed temperature the extinction temperature. Further decrease in feed temperature only results in slight decrease in conversion.

16.3. APPROACHING STEADY STATE

When the reactor-operating conditions are set, the concentration(s) and temperature approach to steady state as governed by Eqns (16.11) and (16.19). These are a set of differential equations that must be solved simultaneously. Instead of examining a particular problem, let us look at the stability from a mathematical point of view. Let us choose a set of differential equations:

$$\frac{d\mathbf{x}}{dt} = \mathbf{f}(\mathbf{x}) = \mathbf{A}\mathbf{x} + \mathbf{B} \tag{16.25}$$

and $\mathbf{x} = \mathbf{x}_0$ satisfies

$$0 = \mathbf{Ax} + \mathbf{B} \tag{16.26}$$

ie, $\mathbf{x}_0$ is the steady-state solution of (16.25). The initial condition is given as

$$t = 0, \ \ \mathbf{x} = \mathbf{x}_\mathrm{I} \tag{16.27}$$

which defines the state the system is at when time t is zero.

The solution to the set of differential equations is stable if for any give finitely small numbers ε and δ, with the norm of the difference between the initial conditions and the steady state solutions to be less than δ or $\|\mathbf{x}_\mathrm{I} - \mathbf{x}_0\| < \delta$,

$$\|\mathbf{x} - \mathbf{x}_0\| < \varepsilon \tag{16.28}$$

holds for any t. That is, if the solution is bounded to be of finite values, the system is stable. Furthermore, we say the (steady state) solution $\mathbf{x}_0$ is asymptotically stable if for a given value of $\delta_0 > 0$,

$$\|\mathbf{x}_\mathrm{I} - \mathbf{x}_0\| < \delta_0 \tag{16.29}$$

the following condition holds

$$\lim_{t \to \infty} (\mathbf{x} - \mathbf{x}_0) = 0 \tag{16.30}$$

Whether the solution to the set of differential equations is stable or not, the coefficient matrix $\mathbf{A}$ plays a key role. In particular, the real part of all the Eigen values of $\mathbf{A}$ must be < 0, i.e. $\mathrm{Re}(\lambda) < 0$. The Eigen values (λ's) can be determined by setting

$$\det(\mathbf{A} - \lambda \mathbf{E}) = 0 \tag{16.31}$$

For example, for a set of two differential equations, there are two Eigen values. The characteristics of the Eigen values determine how the solution approaches the steady-state solution. Fig. 16.11 shows the trajectories to the steady-state solution for different combinations of Eigen values. On the (x_1, x_2) plane, we have plotted the lines for steady-state behaviors ($f_1 = 0$ and $f_2 = 0$). One can observe that if the two Eigen values are real, the solution approaches the steady-state solution (x_{10}, x_{20}) only when both Eigen values are less than zero. Even then, the values of x_1 and x_2 can oscillate around the steady-state values (causing overshoot). If the two Eigen values are of conjugate imaginary values, the solution only approaches the steady-state solution when the real part of the Eigen values is less than zero. The oscillation is more pronounced when the Eigen values are not of real values.

Example 16-4 A cell culture grows on a glucose media is inhibited by the substrate under isothermal conditions and the specific growth rate is governed by

$$\mu_\mathrm{G} = \frac{\mu_\mathrm{max} S}{K_\mathrm{S} + S + S^2/K_\mathrm{I}} \tag{E16-4.1}$$

with $\mu_\mathrm{max} = 0.1\ \mathrm{h}^{-1}$, $K_\mathrm{S} = 2$ g/L, $K_\mathrm{I} = 25$ g/L. The cells has a specific death rate of $k_\mathrm{d} = 0.01$/h and a yield factor of $YF_{X/S} = 0.8$. The culture is grown in a chemostat with a dilution rate of $D = 0.04\ \mathrm{h}^{-1}$. Initially, the feed was sterile containing $S_{0\mathrm{I}} = 100$ g/L substrate (Example 16-2).

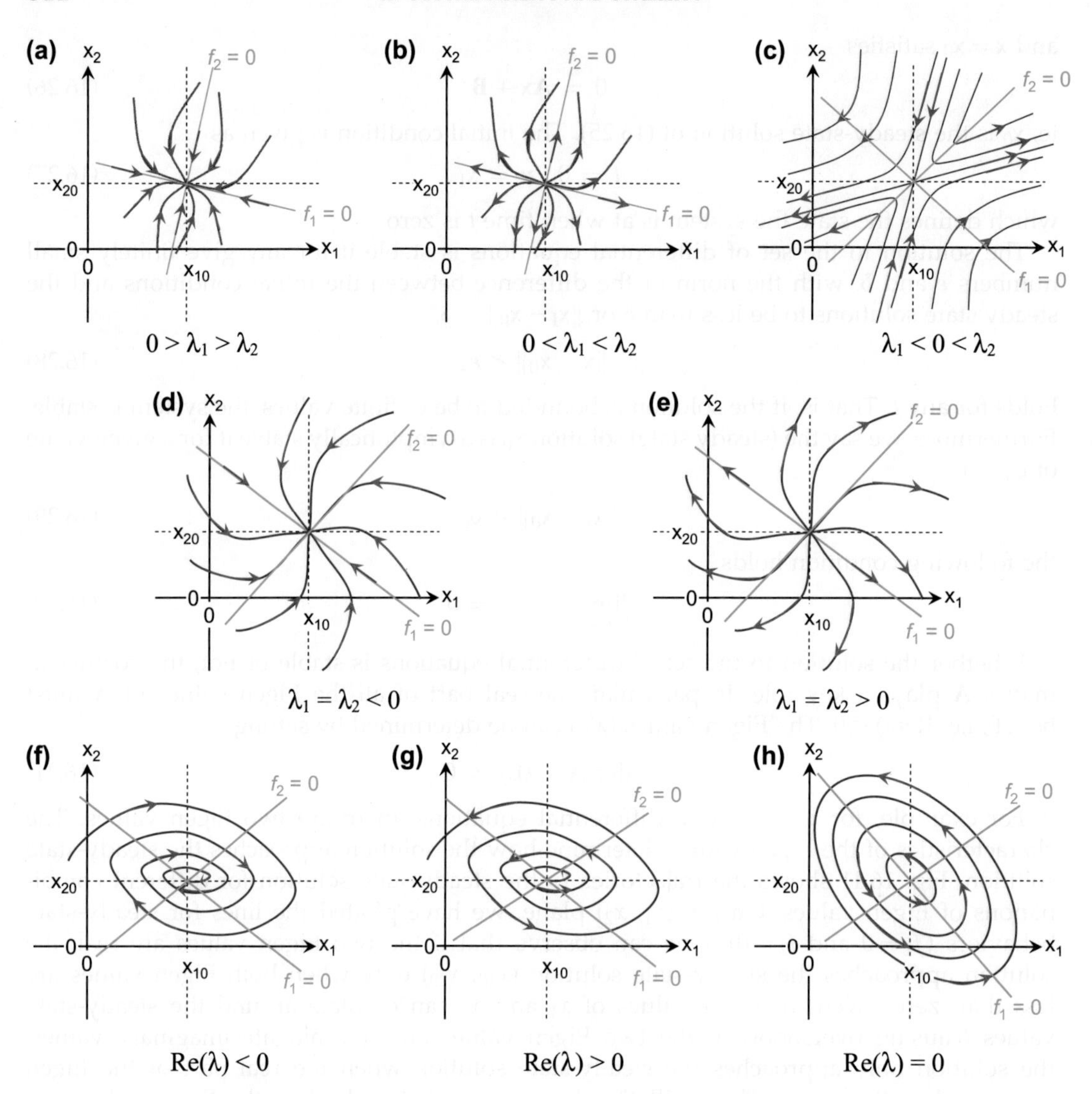

FIGURE 16.11 Schematics of trajectories to steady state solution for differential equations with different Eigen values. While systems (a), (d), (f), and (h) are sustainable, only (a), (d), and (f) are strictly stable.

However, the feed was unexpectedly diluted to $S_0 = 60$ g/L while all other operating parameters remained identical. Determine

(a) The new steady-state solutions;
(b) Which steady state is achieved when the system is left alone for a long time? How long that time is if both the substrate and the biomass concentrations are within 99% of the final steady state?
(c) Plot out the trajectory of b) on (S, X) plane.

(d) How is the trajectory look like when the conditions are reversed, i.e. from the steady state for $S_0 = 60$ g/L back to the case where the feed concentration is $S_0 = 100$ g/L with all other conditions remain the same.

Solution. The flow schematic is shown in Fig. E16-2.1.

(a) Mass balance on substrate (glucose) leads to

$$QS_0 - QS + r_S V = \frac{d(SV)}{dt} = 0 \tag{E16-4.2}$$

Since $V = \text{constant}$, Eqn (16-3.2) can be reduced to

$$\frac{dS}{dt} = D(S_0 - S) + r_S \tag{E16-4.3}$$

Substituting the rate

$$r_S = -\frac{r_X|_{\text{total}}}{YF_{X/S}} = -\frac{\mu_G X}{YF_{X/S}} \tag{E16-4.4}$$

We obtain

$$\frac{dS}{dt} = D(S_0 - S) - \frac{\mu_G X}{YF_{X/S}} = \text{MS}_S - \text{MC}_S \tag{E16-4.5}$$

At steady state, Eqn (16-4.5) is reduced to $\text{MS}_S = \text{MC}_S$.
Mass balance on biomass leads to

$$QX_0 - QX + r_X|_{\text{net}} V = \frac{d(XV)}{dt} \tag{E16-4.6}$$

Since the feed is sterile and substitute the net growth rate in Eqn (E16-4.6), we obtain

$$\frac{dX}{dt} = -DX + (\mu_G - k_d)X \tag{E16-4.7}$$

which can be rewritten as

$$\begin{array}{c} \underbrace{\mu_G - k_d X}_{\Downarrow} - \underbrace{DX}_{\Downarrow} \\ \dfrac{dX}{dt} = \text{MG}_X - \text{MR}_X \end{array} \tag{E16-4.8a}$$

or

$$\frac{dX}{dt} = X(\text{SMG}_X - \text{SMR}_X) \tag{E16-4.8b}$$

At steady state, Eqn (E16-4.8) is reduced to

$$D = \mu_G - k_d \qquad \text{(E16-4.9)}$$

If $X \neq 0$. Substituting Eqn (E16-4.1) into Eqn (E16-4.9), we obtain

$$D + k_d = \frac{\mu_{max} S}{K_S + S + S^2/K_I} \qquad \text{(E16-4.10)}$$

which can be solved to render two roots:

$$S = \frac{K_I}{2}\left(\frac{\mu_{max}}{D + k_d} - 1\right) \pm \sqrt{\frac{K_I^2}{4}\left(\frac{\mu_{max}}{D + k_d} - 1\right)^2 - K_S K_I} \qquad \text{(E16-4.11)}$$

To determine the value of steady-state biomass concentration, we substitute Eqn (16-4.9) into (E16-4.5) and setting $\frac{dS}{dt} = 0$ to yield

$$X = \frac{YF_{X/S} D}{D + k_d}(S_0 - S) \qquad \text{(E16-4.12)}$$

Therefore, we have obtained three solutions:

(1) $X = 0$, $S = S_0 = 60$ g/L;
(2) $S = 2.1922$ g/L, $X = 36.997$ g-X/L; and
(3) $S = 22.8077$ g/L, $X = 23.803$ g-X/L.

(b) The new steady state is $S = 2.1922$ g/L, $X = 36.997$ g-X/L. This new steady state can be identified without solving the differential equations since it is a stable steady state. The other stable steady state is the washout condition and it should not occur as the starting biomass concentration is much higher than that of the intended steady state.

To examine how quick the steady state can be reached, we must solve the two differential Eqns (E16-4.5) and (E16-4.8) simultaneously. The initial conditions for the two equations are at $t = 0$: $S = 2.1922$ g/L, $X = 62.597$ g-X/L. Fig. E16-4.1 shows the time evolutions of the biomass and substrate concentrations. We arrived at the solutions with OdexLims. The biomass concentration reached to 99% within the new steady state at 85.327 h, while the substrate concentration took longer at 103.099 h to reach within 99% of the final steady-state value.

(c) The trajectory of how the steady-state solution is approached. We plotted the solution obtained on the (S, X) plane. We also added the lines for setting $f_1 = MS_S - MC_S = 0$ and $f_2 = MG_X - MR_X = 0$. Along the curve of $f_1 = 0$, we also indicated the direction at which the value of f_2 is increasing, and vice versa. One can observe that the trajectory of the solution moves along a curved path clockwise. Initially, the mass balance on biomass was satisfied. However, it moved away from there and overshot the mass balance on substrate. The approaching to steady state was then slow.

(d) The trajectory for approaching steady state from a lower biomass concentration. We resolved the problem by simply altering the parameters for the initial state and the feed concentration (reverse of that shown in Fig. E16-4.2). Fig. E16-4.3 shows that the

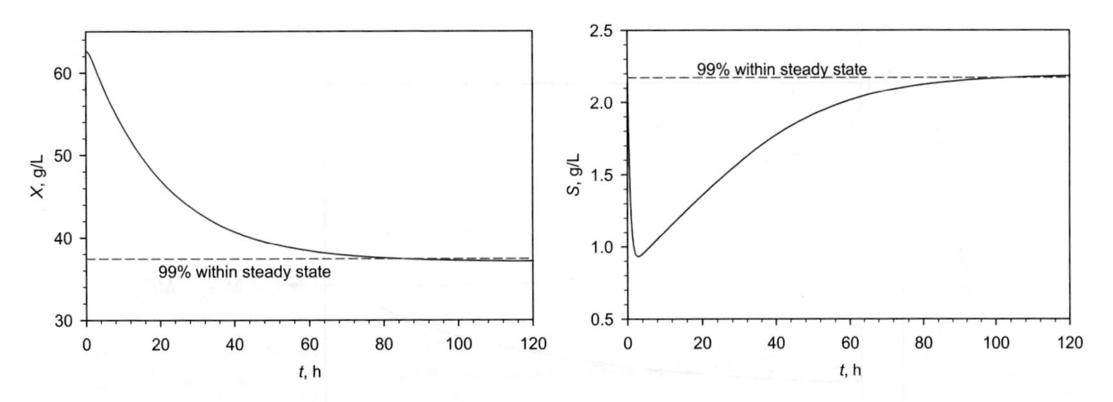

FIGURE E16-4.1 Variations of biomass concentration and substrate concentration with time to the new steady state. One can observe that it takes a long time to reach steady state.

trajectory is also a curved path (also following a clockwise), a new path than that shown in Fig. E16-4.2. It is not a path reversal of Fig. E16-4.2.

16.4. CATALYST INSTABILITY

Catalysts cannot be operated on indefinitely. Catalyst deactivate as its service is prolonged as we have learned in Chapter 9. Catalyst can be deactivated or catalytic activity can be lost

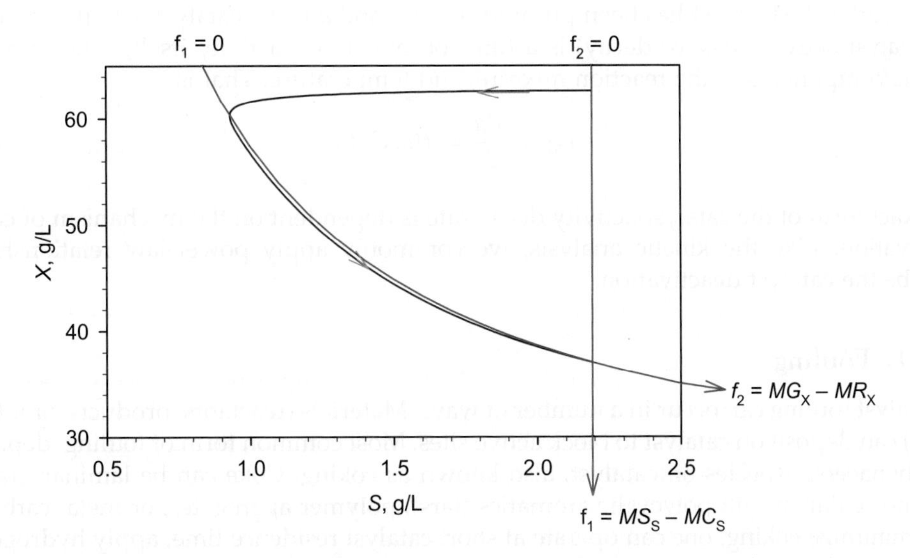

FIGURE E16-4.2 The trajectory from ($S = 2.1922$ g/L, $X = 62.597$ g-X/L) to the new steady state ($S = 2.1922$ g/L, $X = 36.997$ g-X/L) on (S, X) plane (with f_1 and f_2 indicated).

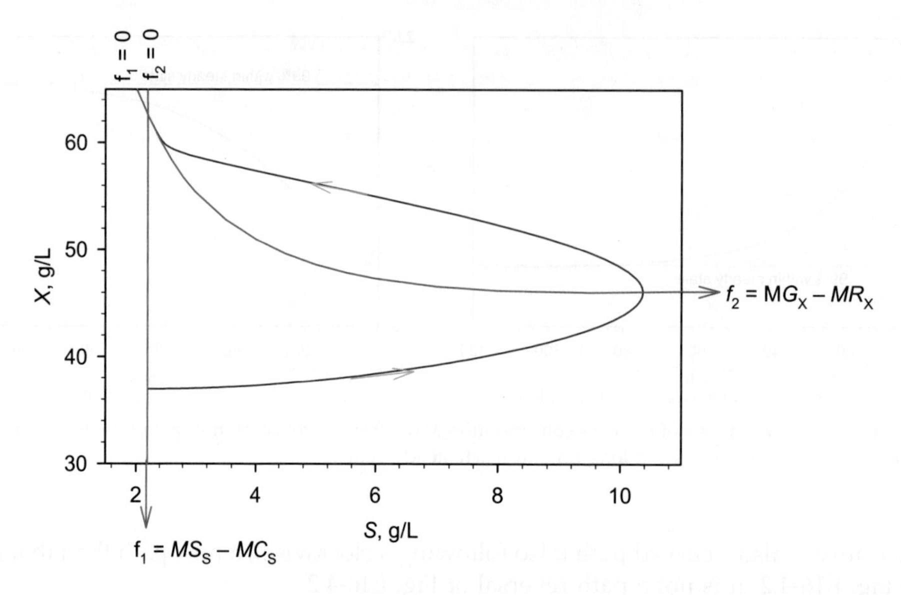

FIGURE E16-4.3 The trajectory from ($S = 2.1922$ g/L, $X = 36.997$ g-X/L) to the new steady state ($S = 2.1922$ g/L, $X = 62.597$ g-X/L) on (S, X) plane (with f_1 and f_2 indicated). The conditions are reversed from those of Fig. E16-4.2.

by fouling, poisoning, and sintering due to heat and pressure. The catalyst activity is defined based on the effective reaction rate as

$$r_{\text{eff}} = ar \tag{16.32}$$

where r is the rate of reaction with fresh catalyst (zero service time), r_{eff} is the observed rate of reaction after the catalyst has been put into service, and a is the catalyst activity. In general, the catalyst activity loss (or decay) is a function of catalyst activity itself, concentration of various components in the reaction mixture, and temperature. That is

$$r_{\text{cd}} = \frac{\text{d}a}{\text{d}t} = f(a, C, T) \tag{16.33}$$

The exact form of the catalyst activity decay rate is dependent on the mechanism of catalyst deactivation. Like the kinetic analysis, we commonly apply power-law relationships to describe the catalyst deactivation.

16.4.1. Fouling

Catalyst fouling can occur in a number of ways. Materials (reactants, products, or intermediates) can deposit on catalyst to block active sites. Most common form of fouling: deposition of carbonaceous species on catalyst, also known as coking. Coke can be laminar graphite, high-molecular-weight polycyclic aromatics (tars), polymer aggregates, or metal carbides.

To minimize coking, one can operate at short catalyst residence time; apply hydrogen gas to eliminate has phase carbon; and minimize temperature upstream (to prevent gas phase carbon from forming).

Fouling can cause catalyst pore blocking and catalyst particles agglomerate together. Pressure drop increase or throughput decrease; Increase internal mass transfer effect, i.e. lower effectiveness factor.

Catalyst activity can be modeled as an inverse function of foul concentration, which increases with increasing catalyst residence time.

16.4.2. Poisoning

Chemisorption of otherwise inert compounds in the process stream can make the active sites inaccessible to reactants. The poison may even modify the catalyst and/or active sites. The toxicity depends on the energy well of the adsorbed state.

For reversible adsorption of poison, the active site modification can be characterized by the addition of a competitive adsorbate. For example,

$$\theta_P = \frac{K_P C_P}{1 + K_A C_A + K_P C_P} \tag{16.34}$$

where P is the poisonous compound that is not participating in the desired reaction. When K_P is small (bond is weak), equilibrium may be reached in the process and the poison is regarded as reversible. If K_P is very big (bond is very strong), equilibrium may not be reached in the process and the poison is regarded as irreversible (as when equilibrium is reached, most of the active sites would be covered by the poison). Poison can either be impurities in the process stream or the product itself. There are three main types of poisons:

(1) Molecules with reactive heteroatoms (e.g. sulfur);
(2) Molecules with multiple bonds between atoms (e.g. unsaturated hydrocarbons);
(3) Metallic compounds or metal ions (e.g. Hg, Pd, Bi, Sn, Cu, Fe).

Poisons can be eliminated by physical separation, a dummy bed (for adsorption). Poison types 1) and 2) can be converted to nontoxic compounds by chemical treatment. If a product is poisonous, selectively remove it during the process can be exercised.

16.4.3. Sintering

Sintering is caused by growth or agglomeration of small crystals with make up the catalyst or its support. Structural rearrangement (sintering) leads to a decrease in surface area and/or effective number active sites. Sintering occurs when temperature exceeds

(1) $^1/_2\, T_m$ (i.e. half of its melting temperature) if "dry";
(2) $^1/_3\, T_m$ if steam is present as steam facilitates reorganization of many metals, alumina, and silica. Table 16.2 shows the sintering temperature for some common metals.

TABLE 16.2 Sintering Temperature for Common Metals

Metal	Cu	Fe	Ni	Pt	Pd
$^1/_3\, T_m$, °C	360	500	500	570	500

To prevent sintering, catalysts may be doped with stabilizers (high melting temperature and preventing agglomeration of small crystals) such as chromia, alumina, and magnesia. For platinum catalysts, adding trace amount of chlorinated compounds in the process stream. Chlorine increases the activation energy for the sintering process of Pt and thus reduces the sintering rate for platinum catalysts.

16.4.4. Catalyst Activity Decay

Deactivation by sintering (aging) can usually be modeled as a second-order decay in catalyst activity:

$$r_{cd} = k_{cd}a^2 = -\frac{da}{dt} \Rightarrow a = \frac{1}{1+k_{cd}t} \quad \& \quad k_{cd} = k_{cd0}\exp\left(-\frac{E_{cd}}{RT}\right) \tag{16.35}$$

Deactivation by coking is usually modeled with:

$$C_{Coke} = At^n \quad a = \frac{1}{1+\alpha_2 C_{Coke}} \quad \text{or} \quad a = \exp(-\alpha_1 C_{Coke}) \tag{16.36}$$

And deactivation by poisoning is commonly modeled with a power-law kinetics,

$$r_{cd} = k_{cd}C_P^m a^n = -\frac{da}{dt} \tag{16.37}$$

where P is the poison compound to the catalyst. It can either be a reactant or just an inert substance in the reaction mixture.

16.4.5. Spent Catalyst Regeneration

Sintered catalysts are usually not regenerated on site. Catalyst structural changes are not easy to recover and will required remaking.

Fouled catalysts can normally be regenerated by "burning." However, temperature must be controlled to minimize sintering.

Poisoned catalysts can be regenerated by 1) Desorption (with poison free stream) and 2) Steam treatment at high temperature (however, sintering can be a problem). For example:

$$Ni{-}S + H_2O \rightarrow NiO + H_2S$$

$$H_2S + 2H_2O \rightarrow SO_2 + 3H_2$$

16.5. GENETIC INSTABILITY

Genetic instability is part of the evolution process. The change of microorganisms subject to hostile environment has been exploited for bioprocesses as well, for example adaptation microorganisms to environments that they are not commonly in and productive. However, in this section, we focus more on the negative effects of genetic instability. Microorganism instability is an issue in particular for genetically altered or genetically

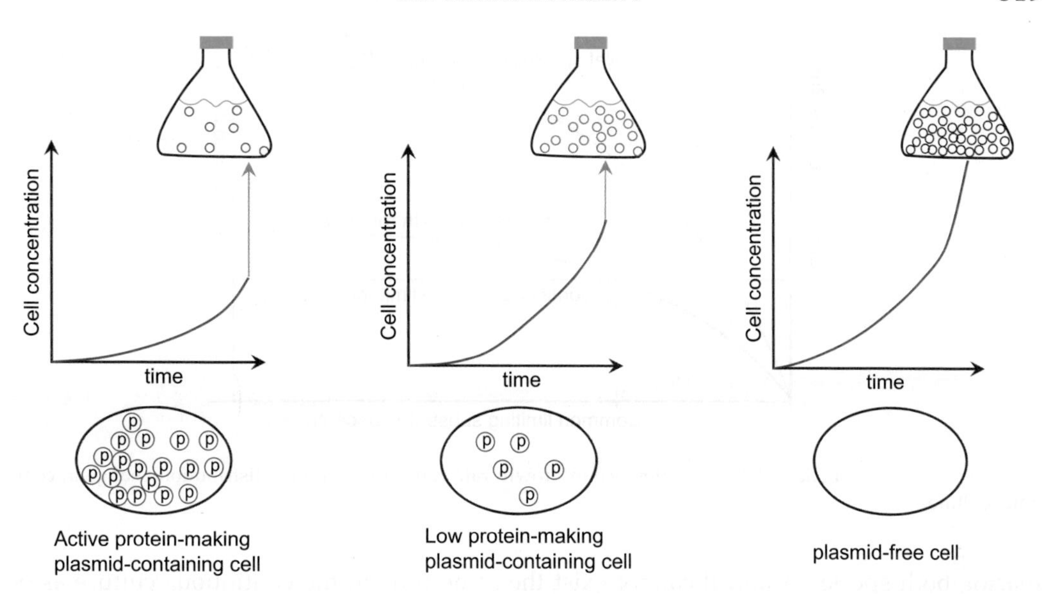

FIGURE 16.12 Genetic instability: cells contain active protein-making plasmids, ⓟ, must direct their cellular resources away from growth and hence more-plasmid containing cells grow slower; plasmid-free cells grow the fastest.

engineered organisms. There is a tension between the goal of maximal target-protein production and the maintenance of a vigorous culture. The formation of foreign protein takes away the cellular resources otherwise for natural growth. In addition, the formation of large amounts of foreign protein is always detrimental to the host cell, often lethal. Fig. 16.12 shows a schematic of the growth comparison among cells with different active protein–plasmid levels. Cells that lose the capacity to make the target protein often grow much more quickly and can displace the original, more productive strain. This leads to *genetic instability*: some cells could loose the plasmid, and the genetic differences grow with time as the plasmid-free cells grows much faster than the genetically engineered cells with active protein-making plasmid. Genetic instability can occur due to *segregational loss, structural instability, host cell regulatory mutations*, and the *growth-rate ratio* of plasmid-free or altered cells to plasmid-containing unaltered cells. Genetic instability can occur in any expression system. Fig. 16.12 illustrates this problem by considering gene expression from plasmids in bacteria.

Genetic instability is illustrated in Fig. 16.13 for continuous culture. In continuous culture as demonstrated in Example 16-2, Fig. E16-2.2, the steady state corresponds to the intercept of the specific biomass growth rate (intrinsic to cells) and the dilution rate (intrinsic to reactor operation or culture environment). In the simplistic case of two uninteracting species, the mere difference in the specific growth rates leads to the elimination of one species as shown in Fig. 16.13. The specific growth rate of A is lower than the specific growth rate of species B at a given (but same) common limiting substrate concentration. When the culture conditions are fixed, the final (steady-state) substrate concentration is determined by the amount of biomass grown in the reactor. Since only one substrate concentration can be realized in the

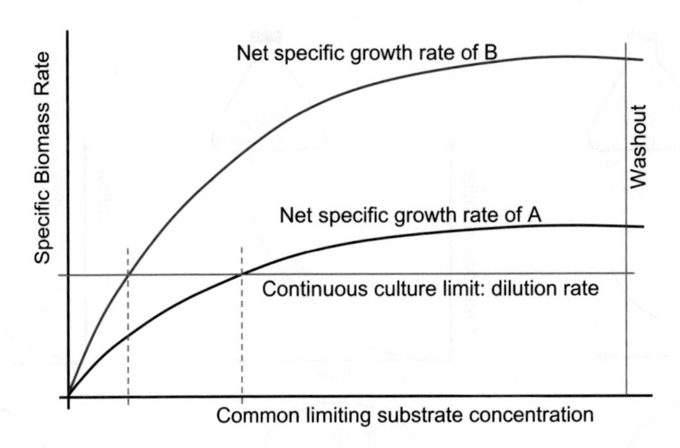

FIGURE 16.13 Genetic instability: difference in growth rate cause the cell type distribution change in continuous culture.

reactor, both species A and B cannot exist the same time in the continuous culture as one requires to maintain a higher substrate concentration (slow growth species A) while the other maintaining a lower substrate concentration (faster growth species B). At the right level of substrate concentration for faster growth species B, slower growth species A is "starved" (or grows slower than dilution rate). As a result, the faster growth species remains in the continuous culture.

16.5.1. Segregational Instability

Segregational loss occurs when a cell divides such that one of the daughter cells receives no plasmids, which is rare, but could occur as illustrated in Fig. 16.14. If the distribution of plasmids at division is random, the probability of forming a plasmid-free cell is given by

$$P = 2^{1-P_R} \tag{16.38}$$

where P_R is the number of plasmid replicative units. Plasmids can be described as *high-copy-number plasmids* ($P_R > 20$ copies per cell) and *low-copy-number plasmids* (sometimes as low as one or two copies per cell). Low-copy-number plasmids usually have specific mechanisms to ensure their equal distribution among daughter cells. High-copy-number plasmids are usually distributed randomly (or nearly randomly) among daughter cells following a binomial distribution. For high-copy numbers, almost all the daughter cells receive some plasmids, but even if the possibility of forming a plasmid-free cell is low (one per million cell divisions), a large reactor contains so many cells that some plasmid-free cells will be present (e.g. 1000 l with 10^{12} cells/l yields 10^{15} cells and 10^9 plasmid-free cells being formed every cell generation).

The segregational loss of plasmid can be influenced by many environmental factors, such as dissolved oxygen, temperature, medium composition, and dilution rate in a chemostat. Many plasmids will also form *multimers*, which are multiple copies of the same plasmid

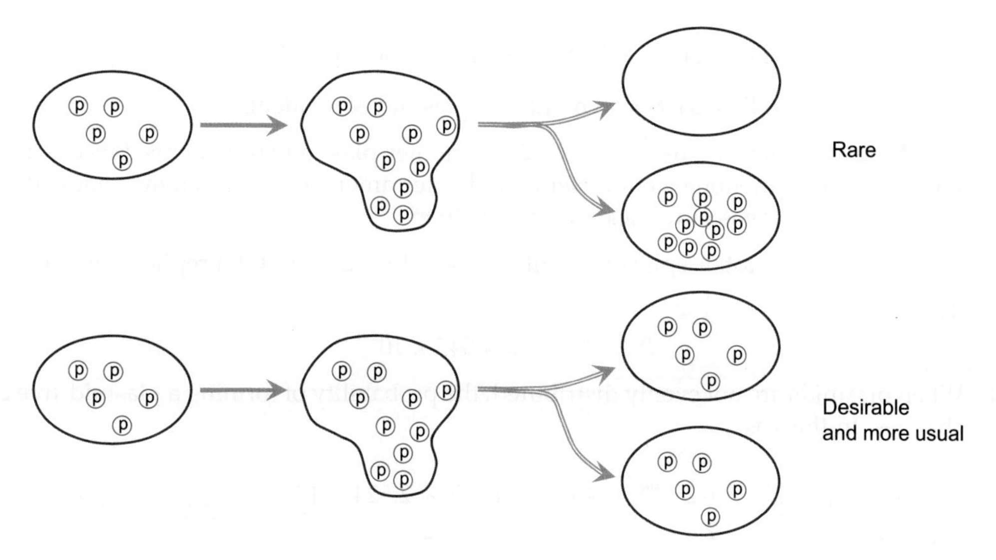

FIGURE 16.14 Segregational instability: a dividing cell donates all its active protein-making plasmids (p) to one progeny and none to the other.

attached to each other to form a single unit. The process of multimerization involves using host cell recombination systems. A *dimer* is a replicative unit in which two separate plasmids have been joined, and a *tetramer* is a single unit consisting of four separate monomers fused together.

Example 16-5 Segregational loss

What fraction of the cells undergoing division will generate a plasmid-free cell if:

(a) All cells have 64 plasmids at division?

(b) All cells have enough plasmid DNA for 64 copies, but one-half of the plasmid DNA is in the form of dimers and one-eighth in the form of tetramers?

(c) Half of the cells have 32 copies of the plasmid and half have 96 copies (the average copy number is 64 as in case a)?

Solution

(a) If we assume a random distribution at division, the probability of forming a plasmid-free cell is given by Eqn (16.38) or

$$P = 2^{1-P_R}$$

For $P_R = 64$ and $P = 1.084 \times 10^{-19}$ plasmid-free cells per division.

(b) If the total amount of plasmid DNA is equivalent to 50 single copies, we can determine the plasmid distribution from

$$M + D + T = 64 \text{ monomer plasmid equivalents}$$

$$D = 64/2 = 32 \text{ monomer plasmid equivalents}$$

$$T = 64/8 = 8 \text{ monomer plasmid equivalents}$$

which implies that $M = 64 - 32 - 8 = 24$ monomer plasmid equivalents. Since a dimer consists of two monomer equivalents and a tetramer of four monomer equivalents, the number of copies of replicative units is then

$$M + D/2 + T/4 = \text{total replicative units} = 24 + 16 + 2 = 42 \text{ total replicative units}$$

Thus,

$$P = 2^{1-42} = 4.547 \times 10^{-13}$$

(c) When plasmids are not evenly distributed, the probability of forming a plasmid-free cell changes. In this case,

$$\frac{P_{32} + P_{96}}{2} = \frac{2^{1-32} + 2^{1-96}}{2} = \frac{4.657 \times 10^{-10} + 2.524 \times 10^{-29}}{2} = 2.328 \times 10^{-10}$$

Note that although this population has the same average copy number as case a), the probability of forming a plasmid-free cell is 2.147×10^9 greater.

16.5.2. Plasmid Structural Instability

In addition to the problems of segregational instability, some cells retain plasmids but alter the plasmid so as to reduce its harmful effects on the cell (structural instability). For example, the plasmid may encode both for antibiotic resistance and for a foreign protein. The foreign protein drains cellular resources away from growth toward an end product of no benefit to the cell. However, if the investigator has added antibiotics to the medium, the cell will benefit from retaining the gene encoding the antibiotic resistance. Normal mutations will result in some altered plasmids that retain the capacity to encode for desirable functions (for example, antibiotic resistance) while no longer making the foreign protein. In other cases, cellular recombination systems will integrate the gene for antibiotic resistance into the chromosome. Cells containing structurally altered plasmids can normally grow much more quickly than cells with the original plasmids. A culture having undergone a change in which the population is dominated by cells with an altered plasmid has undergone structural instability.

16.5.3. Host Cell Mutations

Mutations in host cells can also occur that make them far less useful as production systems for a given product. These mutations often alter cellular regulation and result in reduced target-protein synthesis. For example, if the promoter controlling expression of the foreign protein utilizes a host cell factor (e.g. a repressor), then modification of the host cell factor may greatly modulate the level of production of the desired plasmid-encoded protein. The lac promoter (see our discussion in Chapter 10 of the lac operon) can be induced by adding chemicals; for a lac promoter, lactose or a chemical analog of lactose (e.g. isopropyl-β-D-thiogalactoside) can be used. Such promoters are often used in plasmid construction to control the synthesis of a plasmid-encoded protein. If induction of plasmid-encoded protein synthesis from this promoter reduces cellular growth rates, then a mutation that inactivates lac permease would prevent protein induction in that mutant cell. The lac permease protein is necessary for the rapid uptake of the inducer. Thus, the mutant cell would grow faster than the desired strain. Alternatively, a host cell mutation in the repressor, so that it would not recognize the inducer, would make induction impossible.

The key feature of this category of genetic instability is that a host cell mutation imparts a growth advantage to the mutant, so that it will eventually dominate the culture. In this case, the mutant cell will contain unaltered plasmids but will make very little of the target, plasmid-encoded protein.

16.5.4. Growth-Rate-Dominated Instability

The importance of all three of these factors (segregational loss of plasmid, structural alterations of the plasmid, and host cell mutations) depends on the growth-rate differential of the changed cell–plasmid system to the original host–vector system. If the altered host–vector system has a distinct growth advantage over the original host–vector system, the altered system will eventually dominate (i.e. genetic instability will occur).

The terms used to describe the cause of genetic instability are based on fairly subtle distinctions. For example, if genetic instability is due to segregational instability, we would infer that the rate of formation of plasmid-free cells is high. In this case, the number of plasmid-free cells would be high irrespective of whether the plasmid-free cells had a growth-rate advantage. If, on the other hand, we claimed that the genetic instability is growth-rate dependent, we would imply that the rate of formation of plasmid-free cells is low, but the plasmid-free cells have such a large growth-rate advantage that they outgrow the original host–vector system. In most cases, growth-rate dependent instability and one of the other factors (segregational loss, structural changes in the plasmid, or host cell mutations) are important.

The growth-rate ratio can be manipulated to some extent by the choice of medium (e.g. the use of *selective pressure* such as antibiotic supplementation to kill plasmid-free cells) and the use of production systems that do not allow significant target-protein production during most of the culture period. For example, an inducible promoter can be turned on only at the end of a batch growth cycle when only one or two more cell doublings may normally occur. Before induction, the *metabolic burden* imposed by the formation of the target protein is nil, and the growth ratio of the altered to the original host–vector system is close to 1 (or less if selective pressure is also applied). This *two-phase fermentation* can be done as a modified batch system, or a multistage chemostat could be used. In a two-stage system, the first stage is optimized to produce viable plasmid-containing cells, and production formation is induced in the second stage. The continual resupply of fresh cells to the second stage ensures that many unaltered cells will be present.

The problem of genetic instability is more significant in commercial operations than in laboratory-scale experiments. The primary reason is that the culture must go through many more generations to reach a density of 10^{13} cells/l in a 10,000 l tank than in a shake flask with 25 ml. Also, the use of antibiotics as selective agents may not be desirable in the large-scale system, owing either to cost or to regulatory constraints on product quality.

In the next section, we will discuss some implications of these process constraints on plasmid design. In the section following, we will discuss how simple mathematical models of genetic instability can be constructed.

16.5.5. Considerations in Plasmid Design to Avoid Process Problems

When we design vectors for genetic engineering, we are concerned with elements that control plasmid copy number, the level of target-gene expression, and the nature of the gene product, and we must also allow for the application of selective pressure (e.g. antibiotic resistance). The vector must also be designed to be compatible with the host cell.

Different *origins of replication* exist for various plasmids. The origin often contains transcripts that regulate copy number. Different mutations in these regulatory transcripts will yield greatly different copy numbers. In some cases, these transcripts have temperature sensitive mutations, and temperature shifts can lead to *runaway replication* in which plasmid copy number increases until cell death occurs.

Total protein production depends on both the number of gene copies (e.g. the number of plasmids) and the strength of the promoter used to control transcription from these promoters. Increasing copy number while maintaining a fixed promoter strength increases protein production in a saturated manner. Typically, doubling copy numbers from 25 to 50 will double the protein production, but an increase from 50 to 100 will increase protein production less than doubling. If the number of replicating units is above 50, pure segregational plasmid loss is fairly minimal. Most useful cloning vectors in *Escherichia coli* have stable copy numbers from 25 to 250.

Many promoters exist. Some of the important ones for use in *E. coli* are listed in Table 16.3. An ideal promoter would be both very strong and tightly regulated. A zero basal level of protein production is desirable, particularly if the target protein is toxic to the host cell. A rapid response to induction is desirable, and the inducer should be cheap and safe. Although temperature induction is often used on a small scale, thermal lags in a large fermentation vessel can be problematic. Increased temperatures may also activate a heat-shock response and increased levels of proteolytic enzymes. Many chemical inducers are expensive or might cause health concerns if not removed from the product. Some promoters respond to starvation for a nutrient (e.g. phosphate, oxygen, and energy), but the control of induction with such promoters can be difficult to do precisely. The recent isolation of a promoter induced by oxygen depletion may prove useful because oxygen levels can be controlled relatively easily in fermenters.

Anytime a strong promoter is used, a strong transcriptional terminator should be used in the construction. Recall from Chapter 10 that a terminator facilitates the release of RNA polymerase after a gene or operon is read. Without a strong terminator, the RNA polymerase may not disengage. If the RNA polymerase reads through, it may transcribe undesirable genes or may disturb the elements controlling plasmid copy numbers. In extreme cases, this might cause runaway replication and cell death.

The nature of the protein and its localization are important considerations in achieving a good process. To prevent proteolytic destruction of the target protein, a hybrid gene for

TABLE 16.3 Strong *Escherichia coli* Promoters

Promoter	Induction Method	Characteristics'
lacUV5	Addition of isopropyl-β-D-thiogalactoside	(About 5%)
tac	As above	Induction results in cell death (>30%)
Ipp-OmpA	As above	Suitable for secreted proteins (20%)
Ipp^P-5	As above	Strongest *E. coli* promoter (47%)
trp	Tryptophan starvation	Relatively weak (around 10%)
λp_L	Growth at 42 °C	See text (>30%)
$\lambda p_L/cl_{up}$	Addition of tryptophan	Easily inducible in large-scale production (24%)
att-nutL-p-att-N	10-Min incubation at 42 °C	No product is synthesized before induction (on/off promoter)
T7 promoter	Addition of isopropyl-β-D-thiogalactoside or viral infection	As above (>35%), low basal levels
T4 promoter	Viral infection	Method of induction inhibits product degradation
phoA	Phosphate starvation	Induction in large-scale production is complicated

Typical values of accumulated product as a percent of the total protein of induced cells are given in parentheses.
Source: G. Georgiou, AIChE J. *34:1233 (1988).*

the production of a fusion protein can be made. Typically, a small part of a protein native to the host cell is fused to the sequence for the target protein with a linkage that can be easily cleaved during downstream processing. Also, fusion proteins may be constructed to facilitate downstream recovery by providing a "handle" or "tail" that adheres easily to a particular chromatographic medium.

Another approach to preventing intracellular proteolysis is to develop a secretion vector in which a signal sequence is coupled to the target protein. If the protein is secreted in one host, it will usually be excreted in another, at least if the right signal sequence is used. Replacement of the protein's natural signal sequence (e.g. from a eukaryotic protein) with a host-specific signal sequence can often improve secretion. The secretion process is complicated, and the fusion of a signal sequence with a normally nonsecreted protein (e.g. cytoplasmic) does not ensure secretion, although several cases of secretion of normally cytoplasmic proteins have been reported. Apparently, the mature form of the protein contains the "information" necessary in the secretion process, but no general rules are available to specify when coupling a signal sequence to a normally cytoplasmic protein will lead to secretion.

To ensure the genetic stability of any construct and to aid in the selection of the desired host–vector combination, the vector should be developed to survive under selective growth conditions. The most common strategy is to include genes for antibiotic resistance. The common cloning plasmid, pBR322, contains both ampicillin and tetracycline resistance.

Multiple resistance genes are an aid in selecting for human-designed modifications of the plasmid.

Another strategy for selection is to place on the vector the genes necessary to make an essential metabolite (e.g. an amino acid). If the vector is placed in a host that is auxotrophic for that amino acid, then the vector complements the host (as an auxotrophic mutant would not be able to synthesize an essential compound on its own). In a medium without that amino acid, only plasmid-containing cells should be able to grow. Because the genes for the synthesis of the auxotrophic factors can be integrated into the chromosome or because of reversions on the parental chromosome, double auxotrophs are often used to reduce the probability of nonplasmid-containing cells outgrowing the desired construction.

One weakness in both of these strategies is that, even when the cell loses the plasmid, the plasmid-free cell will retain for several divisions enough gene product to provide antibiotic resistance or the production of an auxotrophic factor (see Fig. 16.15). Thus, cells that will not form viable colonies on selective plates (about 25 generations are required to form a colony) can still be present and dividing in a large-scale system. These plasmid-free cells consume resources without making product.

Another related problem, particularly in large-scale systems, is that plasmid-containing cells may protect plasmid-free cells from the selective agent. For example, auxotrophic cells

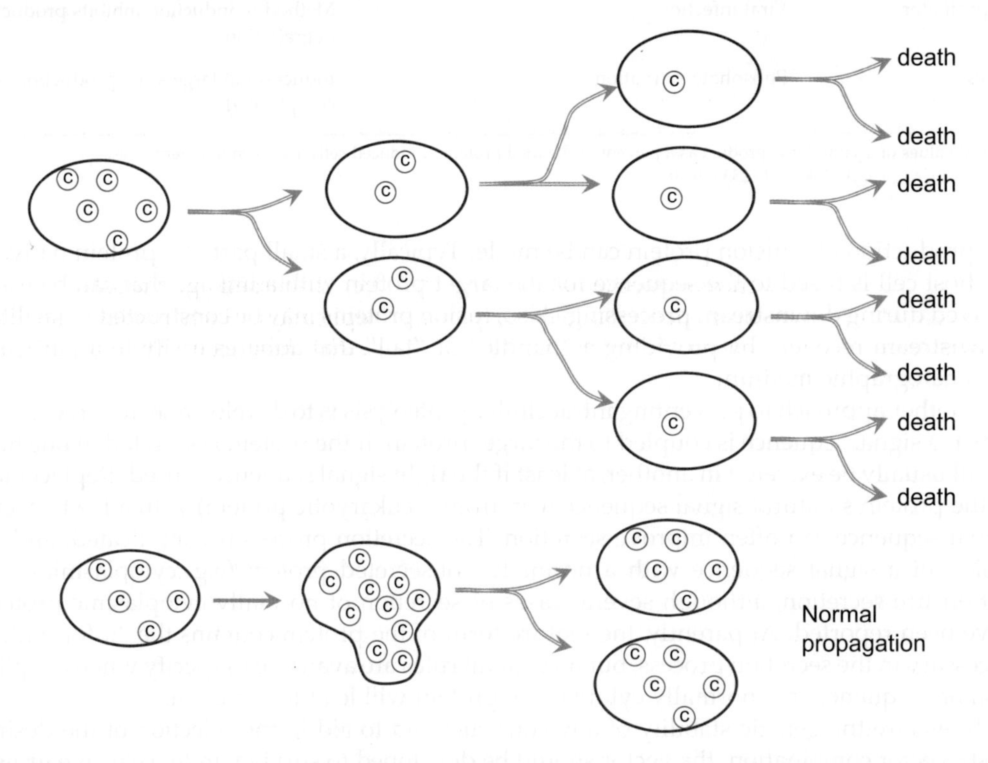

FIGURE 16.15 Newly born plasmid-free cells usually contain sufficient complementing factor © to withstanding killing by a selective agent or starvation from the lack of a growth factor. In this case, the plasmid-free cell undergoes three divisions before the complementing factor is reduced to an insufficient level leading to death.

with a plasmid may leak sufficient levels of the auxotrophic factor that plasmid-free cells can grow. With an antibiotic, the enzyme responsible for antibiotic degradation may leak into the medium. Also, the enzyme may be so effective, even when retained intracellularly, that all the antibiotics are destroyed quickly in a high-density culture, reducing the extracellular concentration to zero. Although genes allowing the placement of selective pressure on a culture are essential in vector development, the engineer should be aware of the limitations of selective pressure in commercial-scale systems.

The other useful addition to plasmid construction is the addition of elements that improve plasmid segregation. Examples are the so-called *par* and *cer* loci. These elements act positively to ensure more even distribution of plasmids. The mechanisms behind these elements are incompletely understood, although they may involve promoting plasmid membrane complexes (the *par* locus) or decreasing the net level of multimerization (the *cer* locus). Recall from Example 16.4 that multimerization decreases the number of independent, inheritable units, thus increasing the probability of forming a plasmid-free cell.

Any choice of vector construction must consider host cell characteristics. Proteolytic degradation may not be critical if the host cell has been mutated to inactivate all known proteases. Multimerization can be reduced by choosing a host with a defective recombination system. However, host cells with a defective recombination system tend to grow poorly. Many other possible host cell modifications enter into considerations of how to best construct a vector for a commercial operation.

These qualitative ideas allow us to anticipate to some extent what problems may arise in the maintenance of genetic stability and net protein expression. However, a good deal of research has been done on predicting genetic instability.

16.5.6. Host—Vector Interactions and Genetic Instability

Many of the structured mathematical models we discussed previously can be extended to include component models for plasmid replication. Such models can then predict how plasmid-encoded functions interact with the host cell. The quantitative prediction of the growth-rate ratio and the development of plasmid-free cells due to segregational losses can be readily made. The most sophisticated models will predict the distribution of plasmids within a population and even the effects of multimerization on genetic stability.

These models are too complex to warrant discussion in an introductory course. We will consider some simple models that mimic many of the characteristics we discussed with models of mixed cultures. A number of simple models for plasmid-bearing cells have been proposed. The key parameters in such models are the relative growth rates of plasmid-free and plasmid-containing cells and the rate of generation of plasmid-free cells (i.e. segregational loss). These parameters can be determined experimentally or even predicted for more sophisticated models of host—vector interactions.

Let us consider how a simple model may be constructed and how the parameters of interest may be determined experimentally.

The simplest model would be to consider only two cell types: plasmid free (X_-) and plasmid containing (X_+). Furthermore, we assume that all plasmid-containing cells are identical in growth rate and in the probability of plasmid loss. This assumption is the same as assuming that all cells have exactly the same copy number. As we showed in Example 16-4, the actual distribution of copy numbers can make a significant difference on plasmid loss. Also, plasmid-encoded protein production is not a linear function of copy number, so assuming that all cells have the same copy number may lead to incorrect estimates of the growth rate of plasmid-bearing cells. The assumption of a single type of plasmid-bearing cell is a weak assumption, but other assumptions would result in more differential equations to solve (and thus OdexLims or other numerical integrator will definitely come in handy).

Let us further restrict our initial considerations to a single-stage chemostat as illustrated in Fig. 16.16. Mass balances of the three species (plasmid-containing cells, plasmid-free cells, and substrate) lead to

$$-QX_+ + \mu_{G+}X_+V - r_{-/+}V = \frac{d(X_+V)}{dt} \tag{16.39}$$

$$-QX_- + \mu_{G-}X_-V + r_{-/+}V = \frac{d(X_-V)}{dt} \tag{16.40}$$

$$Q(S_0 - S) - \frac{\mu_{G+}X_+}{YF_{+/S}}V - \frac{\mu_{G-}X_-}{YF_{-/S}}V = \frac{d(SV)}{dt} \tag{16.41}$$

where

$$r_{-/+} = P_{-/+}\mu_{G+}X_+ \qquad 16.42$$

is the rate of generation of plasmid-free cells from plasmid-containing cells. $P_{-/+}$ is the probability of forming a plasmid-free cell. $YF_{+/S}$ and $YF_{-/S}$ are yield factors for the plasmid-containing cells and plasmid-fee cells, respectively.

$P_{-/+}$ can be estimated by Eqn (16.38) if the copy number is known or can be predicted with a more sophisticated structured segregated model. A value for $P_{-/+}$ could be estimated from an experimentally determined copy-number distribution as in Example 16-4c, which would be more realistic than assuming a monocopy number. As we will soon see, $P_{-/+}$ can be determined experimentally without a knowledge of copy number.

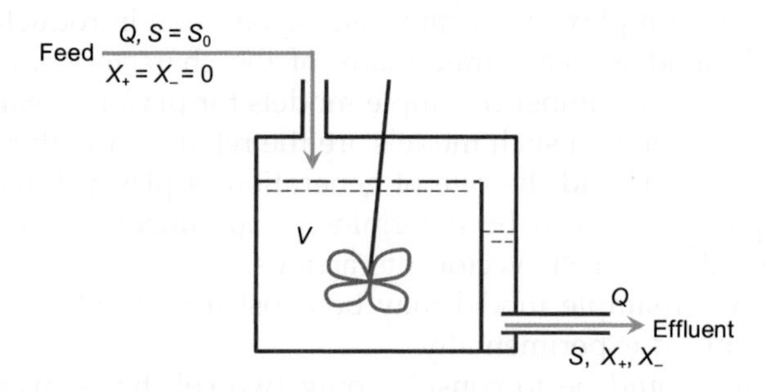

FIGURE 16.16 A schematic of chemostat cell culture.

Eqns (16.39) through (16.42) assume only simple competition between plasmid-containing and plasmid-free cells. No selective agents are present, and the production of complementing factors from the plasmid is neglected. The simplest assumption for cellular kinetics is that Monod equation holds for both plasmid-containing and plasmid-free cells,

$$\mu_{G+} = \frac{\mu_{+max} S}{K_{S+} + S} \tag{16.43a}$$

$$\mu_{G-} = \frac{\mu_{-max} S}{K_{S-} + S} \tag{16.43b}$$

Since the cultural volume is constant, Eqns (16.39) through (16.42) can be reduced to

$$-(D - \mu_{G+} + P_{-/+}\mu_{G+})X_+ = \frac{dX_+}{dt} \tag{16.44}$$

$$-(D - \mu_{G-})X_- + P_{-/+}\mu_{G+}X_+ = \frac{dX_-}{dt} \tag{16.45}$$

$$D(S_0 - S) - \frac{\mu_{G+}X_+}{YF_{+/S}} - \frac{\mu_{G-}X_-}{YF_{-/S}} = \frac{dS}{dt} \tag{16.46}$$

If we did choose to model the plasmid-containing cells by a multiple individual species, we would have (similar to Eqns 16.44 and 16.45) more differential equations to deal with than just these above three. The problem is further simplified if we assume that substrate reached steady state, i.e., the concentration of substrate does not change with time. This not only takes away on differential Eqn (16.46), but leads to constant specific growth rates as well.

Integrating Eqn (16.44), we obtain

$$X_+ = X_{+0} \exp[-(D - \mu_{G+} + P_{-/+}\mu_{G+})t] \tag{16.47}$$

where X_{+0} is the concentration of the plasmid-containing cells in the chemostat at time $t = 0$. Substituting Eqn (16.47) into Eqn (16.45) and multiplying $\exp[(D - \mu_{G-})t]\, dt$ on both sides, we obtain

$$\begin{aligned} &-(D - \mu_{G-})X_- \exp[(D - \mu_{G-})t]dt + P_{-/+}\mu_{G+}X_{+0} \exp[-(\mu_{G-} - \mu_{G+} + P_{-/+}\mu_{G+})t]dt \\ &= \exp[(D - \mu_{G-})t]dX_- \end{aligned} \tag{16.48}$$

Integrating Eqn (16.48), we obtain

$$X_- = X_{-0} \exp[(\mu_{G-} - D)t] - P_{-/+}\mu_{G+}X_{+0} \frac{\exp[(\mu_{G+} - P_{-/+}\mu_{G+} - D)t] - \exp[(\mu_{G-} - D)t]}{\mu_{G-} - \mu_{G+} + P_{-/+}\mu_{G+}} \tag{16.49}$$

Based on Eqns (16.48) and (16.49), we can determine the ratio of plasmid-free cells as

$$y_- = \frac{X_-}{X_+ + X_-}$$

$$= \frac{\left[\dfrac{y_{-0}}{y_{+0}}(\mu_{G-} - \mu_{G+} + P_{-/+}\mu_{G+}) + P_{-/+}\mu_{G+}\right]\exp[(\mu_{G-} - \mu_{G+} + P_{-/+}\mu_{G+})t] - P_{-/+}\mu_{G+}}{\mu_{G-} - \mu_{G+} + \left[\dfrac{y_{-0}}{y_{+0}}(\mu_{G-} - \mu_{G+} + P_{-/+}\mu_{G+}) + P_{-/+}\mu_{G+}\right]\exp[(\mu_{G-} - \mu_{G+} + P_{-/+}\mu_{G+})t]} \tag{16.50}$$

If we let

$$\mu_{-/+} = P_{-/+}\mu_{G+} \tag{16.51a}$$

$$\Delta\mu = \mu_{G-} - \mu_{G+} + P_{-/+}\mu_{G+} \tag{16.51b}$$

The Eqn (16.50) can be simplified to yield

$$y_- = \frac{\dfrac{y_{-0}}{1 - y_{-0}}\Delta\mu + \mu_{-/+} - \mu_{-/+}\exp(-t\Delta\mu)}{\dfrac{y_{-0}}{1 - y_{-0}}\Delta\mu + \mu_{-/+} + (\Delta\mu - \mu_{-/+})\exp(-t\Delta\mu)} \tag{16.52}$$

Eqn (16.52) can be applied directly to determine the specific rates and probability of loosing plasmid if a series of experimental data are available. Fig. 16.17 illustrates the instability profile for three limiting cases:

(1) $\mu_{G-} - \mu_{G+} >> P_{-/+}\,\mu_{G+}$ growth-rate-dependent instability dominant
(2) $\mu_{G-} - \mu_{G+} \le P_{-/+}\,\mu_{G+}$ segregational instability dominant
(3) $\mu_{G+} >> \mu_{G-} + P_{-/+}\,\mu_{G+}$ effective selective pressure

The difference in specific growth rates can be altered by medium and host–vector design.

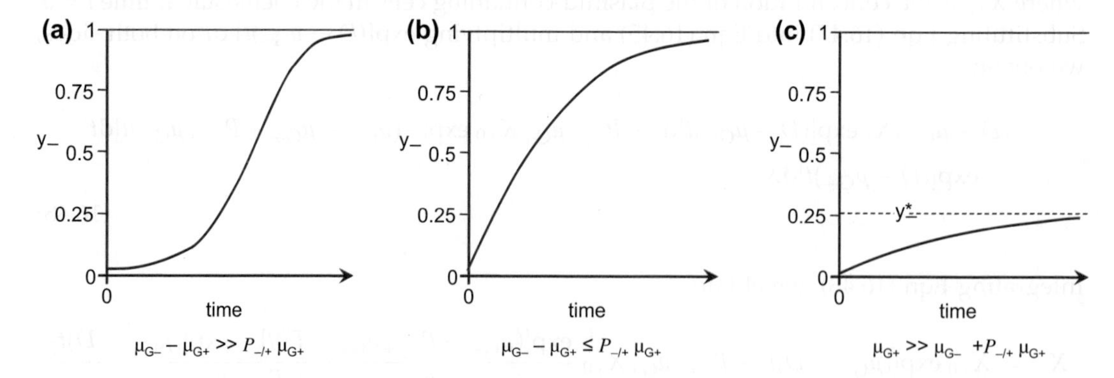

FIGURE 16.17 The shape of plasmid-free cell fraction versus time for three limiting cases of specific growth rates.

Example 16-6. Genetic instability of a continuous culture

The data in Table E16-6.1 were obtained for *E. coli* B/r-pDW17 at two different dilution rates in glucose-limited chemostats. The average plasmid copy number for pDW17 is about 40−50 copies per cell. About 12% of the total protein synthesized is due to the plasmid. The proteins are retained intracellularly in soluble form. Use these data to estimate $\Delta\mu$, $\mu_{-/+}$, μ_{G+}, μ_{G-}, and $P_{-/+}$.

Solution. Note that data on plasmid stability are usually given in terms of the number of generations, which is a nondimensionless time based on $(\ln 2)/D = 1$ generation. To estimate the growth parameters, the easiest way to do is use a spreadsheet program such as Excel to fit the experimental data with the model, Eqn (16.52). As one can observe from Eqn (16.52), there are two parameters can be obtained from the plasmid-free cell fractions versus time data: $\Delta\mu$ and $\mu_{-/+}$. Other parameters would need to be obtained from other data. For example, the growth rate for the plasmid-free cells can be determined by the dilution rate in this case.

TABLE E16-6.1 Experimental Values for Plasmid Stability of *Escherichia coli* B/r-pDW17 in a Glucose-Limited Chemostat

D = 0.30/h			D = 0.67/h		
Time, h	**No. of generations**	y_-	**Time, h**	**No. of generations**	y_-
0	0	≤0.002	0	0	≤0.002
11.6	5	0.010	10.3	10	0.010
23.1	10	0.030	20.7	20	0.035
46.2	20	0.13	31.0	30	0.15
57.8	25	0.22	41.4	40	0.34
69.3	30	0.39	51.7	50	0.65
80.9	35	0.76	62.1	60	0.81
92.4	40	0.88	72.4	70	0.93
104.0	45	0.97	82.8	80	0.98
116.5	50	1.00	93.1	90	1.0
138.6	60	1.00	103.5	100	1.0

Data source: Shuler & Kargi 2006.

Table E16-6.2 shows the least-square fit of the experimental data with Eqn (16.52). The variance between the computed values of y_- and those of experimental data are shown in the last row. One can observe that the fit for the higher dilution rate is better than that for the lower dilution rate. The results are plotted in Fig. E16-6. One can observe that the sigmoidal curves captured the data quite well. For $D = 0.3/\text{h}$, $\frac{y_{-0}}{y_{+0}} = 9.58 \times 10^{-4}$; $\Delta\mu = 0.09733/\text{h}$; $\mu_{-/+} < 10^{-8}/\text{h}$. Since at steady state, the dilution rate equals the specific growth rate, that is

$$\mu_{G-} = D = 0.3/\text{h}$$

TABLE E16-6.2 Spreadsheet Calculations of Least-Square Fit to Eqn (16.52)

$\frac{y_{-0}}{y_{+0}} = 9.58 \times 10^{-4}$; $\Delta\mu = 0.09733$/h; $\mu_{-/+} < 10^{-8}$/h; $D = 0.30$/h				$\frac{y_{-0}}{y_{+0}} < 10^{-8}$; $\Delta\mu = 0.1072$/h; $\mu_{-/+} = 6.93 \times 10^{-4}$/h; $D = 0.67$/h			
Time, h	y_-	$y_{-\text{computed}}$	Δy_-^2	**Time, h**	y_-	$y_{-\text{computed}}$	Δy_-^2
0	<0.002	0.000958		0	<0.002	1×10^{-8}	
11.6	0.01	0.002956	4.96×10^{-5}	10.3	0.01	0.012864	8.2×10^{-6}
23.1	0.03	0.008998	0.00044	20.7	0.035	0.050319	0.00024
46.2	0.13	0.079197	0.00258	31	0.15	0.147408	6.72×10^{-6}
57.8	0.22	0.210111	9.78×10^{-5}	41.4	0.34	0.350863	0.00012
69.3	0.39	0.448946	0.00348	51.7	0.65	0.621757	0.00080
80.9	0.76	0.715881	0.00195	62.1	0.81	0.83406	0.00058
92.4	0.88	0.885284	2.79×10^{-5}	72.4	0.93	0.938187	6.7×10^{-5}
104	0.97	0.959786	0.00010	82.8	0.98	0.978859	1.3×10^{-6}
116.5	1	0.986505	0.00018	93.1	1	0.992893	5.05×10^{-5}
138.6	1	0.998558	2.08×10^{-6}	103.5	1	0.997658	5.48×10^{-6}
			$\sigma = 0.03146$				$\sigma = 0.01441$

The value of other growth parameters can be computed as

$$\mu_{G+} = \mu_{G-} - \Delta\mu + \mu_{-/+} = 0.3 - 0.09733/\text{h} = 0.20267/\text{h}$$

$$P_{-/+} = \mu_{-/+} / \mu_{G+} < 5 \times 10^{-8}$$

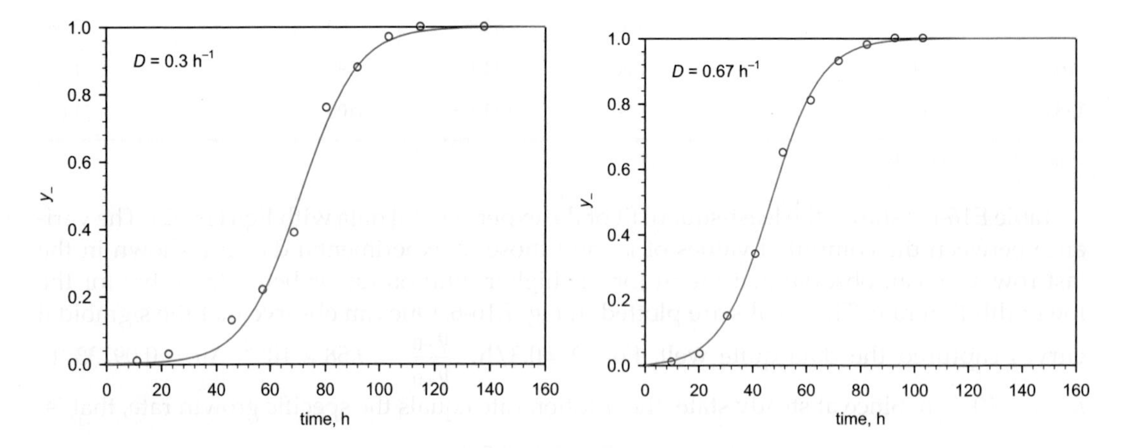

FIGURE E16-6 Plasmid instability of *Escherichia coli* B/r-pDW17 in a chemostat.

For $D = 0.67/\text{h}$, $\frac{y_{-0}}{y_{+0}} < 10^{-8}$; $\Delta\mu = 0.1072/\text{h}$; $\mu_{-/+} = 6.93 \times 10^{-4}/\text{h}$. Again at steady state, the dilution rate equals the specific growth rate,

$$\mu_{G-} = D = 0.67/\text{h}$$

The value of other growth parameters can be computed as

$$\mu_{G+} = \mu_{G-} - \Delta\mu + \mu_{-/+} = 0.67 - 0.1072 + 6.93 \times 10^{-4}/\text{h} = 0.5035/\text{h}$$

$$P_{-/+} = \mu_{-/+}/\mu_{G+} = 1.229 \times 10^{-3}$$

Consider Eqn (16.38) for the random formation of plasmid-free cells,

$$P = 2^{1-P_R} \tag{16.38}$$

where P_R is the number of plasmid replicative units. Since the average plasmid copy number for pDW17 is about 40–50, one can expect that $P_R \leq 40$. For $P_R = 40$,

$$P = 2^{1-40} = 1.82 \times 10^{-12}$$

Therefore, the data are consistent with the expectation. The observed probability is higher due to the fact that not all the replicative units consist of single plasmid copies (as demonstrated in Example 16-5).

Our discussion and example so far have been for continuous reactors. For most industrial applications involving genetically engineered organisms, batch or fed-batch operations are preferred. While continuous reactors are particularly sensitive to genetic instability, genetic instability can be a significant limitation for batch systems. As we have seen that time evolution is required even for continuous systems, fed-batch or batch systems would not add any complexity to the solution.

For a batch reactor, the mass balances on the cells yield:

$$\mu_{G+}X_+ - P_{-/+}\mu_{G+}X_+ = \frac{dX_+}{dt} \tag{16.53}$$

$$\mu_{G-}X_- + P_{-/+}\mu_{G+}X_+ = \frac{dX_-}{dt} \tag{16.54}$$

with initial conditions of $t = 0$, $X_+ = X_{+0}$, and $X_- = 0$. Assuming exponential growth (i.e. substrate sufficient), Eqn (16.53) can be integrated to yield

$$X_+ = X_{+0} \exp[(1 - P_{-/+})\mu_{G+}t] \tag{16.55}$$

Substituting Eqn (16.55) into Eqn (16.54) and integrating, we obtain

$$X_- = \frac{P_{-/+}\mu_{G+}X_{+0}}{(1 - P_{-/+})\mu_{G+} - \mu_{G-}} \{\exp[(1 - P_{-/+})\mu_{G+}t] - \exp(\mu_{G-}t)\} \tag{16.56}$$

From Eqns (16.55) and (16.56), we obtain

$$y_+ = \frac{X_+}{X_+ + X_-} = \frac{1}{1 + \dfrac{1 - \exp[(\mu_{G-} + P_{-/+}\mu_{G+} - \mu_{G+})t]}{(1 - P_{-/+})\mu_{G+} - \mu_{G-}} P_{-/+}\mu_{G+}} \tag{16.57}$$

Eqn (16.57) is usually recast in terms of number of generations of plasmid-containing cells (n_g), a dimensionless growth-rate ratio (α), and the probability of forming a plasmid-free cell upon division of a plasmid-containing cell ($P_{-/+}$). The mathematical definitions of n_g and α are:

$$n_g = \frac{\mu_{G+}t}{\ln 2} \tag{16.58}$$

$$\alpha = \frac{\mu_{G-}}{\mu_{G+}} \tag{16.59}$$

With these definitions, Eqn (16.57) becomes

$$y_+ = \frac{1 - \alpha - P_{-/+}}{1 - \alpha - P_{-/+} \times 2^{n_g(\alpha + P_{-/+} - 1)}} \tag{16.60}$$

16.6. MIXED CULTURES

As discussed in the previous section, stability issue comes into play when more than one species exist in a continuous culture. The dynamics of mixed cultures are important considerations in some commercial fermentations. They are critical to understanding the response of many ecological systems to stress. The use of organisms with recombinant DNA has added another dimension to our consideration of how cells within a population interact with each other. Some members of the population will lose or modify the inserted gene (often carried on a plasmid). Although a single species is present, the formation of mutant or plasmid-free cells leads to a distinct subpopulation. The interaction of the subpopulation with the original population follows the principles we will develop for mixed populations.

Multiple interacting species can give rise to a very complex dynamic behavior. In some cases, coexistence of species is prohibited; in others, complex sustained oscillatory behavior may be observed.

Many food fermentations, such as cheese manufacture, depend on multiple interacting species. The biological treatment of wastewaters relies on an undefined complex mixture of microorganisms. The ratio of various species in the treatment process is critical; sudden shifts in the composition of the population can lead to failure of the unit to meet its objectives.

16.6.1. Major Classes of Interactions in Mixed Cultures

The major interactions between two organisms in a mixed culture are competition, neutralism, mutualism, commensalism, amensalism, and prey–predator interactions.

Competition is an indirect interaction between two populations that has negative effects on both. In competition, each population competes for the same substrate. Two populations or microorganisms with similar nutrient requirements usually compete for a number of common, required nutrients when grown together. The outcome of competition between two species for the *same growth-limiting substrate* in an open system (e.g. a chemostat) is determined by the specific growth-rate limiting substrate concentration relationship. Two different cases can be distinguished in a mixed culture of two competing species A and B:

(1) μ_A is always greater than μ_B. 'The organisms with the fastest growth rate will displace the others from the culture. This is known as the *exclusion principle*.

(2) Crossover in $\mu_{net}-S$ relationship. In this case, the faster growing organism is determined by the dilution rate. Depending on the dilution rate, three different cases may be identified:

  (a) At the crossover point $D = \mu_X - k_d$; $S = S_X$, two species could be maintained in a chemostat at $D = \mu_X - k_d$. However, this is an unstable operating point.

  (b) If $D > \mu_X - k_d$, then $\mu_A - k_{dA} > \mu_B - k_{dB}$, and B will be washed out; A will dominate.

  (c) If $D < \mu_X - k_d$, then $\mu_B - k_{dB} > \mu_A - k_{dA}$, and A will be washed out; B will dominate.

In a batch system, both species would exist in culture media. The ratio of number density of species at a given time will be determined by the relative magnitudes of the specific growth rates and the initial concentrations of cells.

Neutralism is an interaction where neither population is affected by the presence of the other. That is, there is no change in the growth rate of either organism due to the presence of the other. Neutralism is relatively rare. One example of neutralism is the growth of yogurt starter strains of *Streptococcus* and *Lactobacillus* in a chemostat. The total counts of these two species at a dilution rate of 0.4/h are quite similar whether the populations are cultured separately or together. Neutralism may occur in special environments where each species consumes different limiting substrates and neither species is affected by the end products of the other.

Mutualism and *protocooperation* are more common than neutralism and may involve different mechanisms. In both cases, the presence of each population has a positive effect on the other. For mutualism, the interaction is essential to the survival of both species. In protocol operation, the interaction is nonessential. One mechanism is the mutual exchange of required substances or the removal of toxic end products by each organism.

The metabolisms of partner populations must be complementary to yield a mutualistic interaction. An example is the growth of a phenylalanine-requiring strain of *Lactobacillus* and a folic-acid-requiring strain of *Streptococcus* in a mixed culture. Exchange of the growth factors phenylalanine and folic acid produced by partner organisms helps each organism to grow in a mixed culture, while separate pure cultures exhibit no growth.

Another example of mutualistic interaction exists between aerobic bacteria and photosynthetic algae. Bacteria use oxygen and carbohydrate for growth and produce CO_2 and H_2O. The algae convert CO_2 to carbohydrates and liberate oxygen in the presence of sunlight.

One should note that *symbiosis* and mutualism are not the same. Symbiosis implies a relationship when two organisms live together. A symbiotic relationship may be mutualistic, but it may also be neutralistic, parasitic, commensalistic, and so on.

Commensalism is an interaction in which one population is positively affected by the presence of the other. However, the second population is not affected by the presence of the first population. Various mechanisms may yield a commensal interaction. Two common mechanisms are the following:

(1) The second population produces a required nutrient or growth factor for the first population.
(2) The second population removes a substance from the medium that is toxic to the first population.

An example of the first type of commensal interaction is the production of H_2S by Desulfovibrio (through the reduction of SO_4^{2-}), which is used as an energy source by sulfur bacteria.

$$H_2S \underset{\substack{\text{Desulfovibrio}\\ \text{(anaerobic)}}}{\overset{\substack{\text{Sulfur bacteria}\\ \text{(aerobic)}}}{\rightleftarrows}} SO_4^{2-}$$

An example of the second type of commensal interaction is the removal of lactic acid by the fungus *Geotrichium candidum*, which allows the growth of *Streptococcus lactis*. This interaction is utilized in cheese making using *S. lactis*. Lactic acid produced by *S. lactis* inhibits the growth of the bacteria. The fungus metabolizes lactic acid and improves the growth conditions for *S. lactis*.

Amensalism is the opposite of commensalism. In amensalism, population A is negatively affected by the presence of the other population (B). However, population B is not affected by the presence of population A. Various amensal interaction mechanisms are possible. Two common mechanisms are the following:

(1) Population B produces a toxic substance that inhibits the growth of population A.
(2) Population B removes essential nutrients from the media, thus negatively affecting the growth of population A.

One example of the first type of amensal interaction is the production of antibiotics by certain molds to inhibit the growth of others. Some microbes excrete enzymes that decompose cell-wall polymers. Such organisms destroy their competitors and also utilize the nutrients released by the lysed cells. The microbial synthesis of organic acids reduces pH and inhibits the growth of other organisms.

Predation and *parasitism* are interactions in which one population benefits at the expense of the other. These two interactions are distinguished by the relative size of organisms and the mechanisms involved. Predation involves the ingestion of prey by the predator organism. A good example of prey–predator interaction is the ingestion of bacteria by protozoa. This interaction is common in aerobic waste-treatment reactors such as activated sludge units. In parasitism, the host, which is usually the larger organism, is damaged by the parasite. The parasite benefits from utilization of nutrients from the host.

A common example of parasitism is the destruction of microorganisms by microphages. Although the physical mechanisms in predation and parasitism differ, these two phenomena have many common features in their conceptual and mathematical descriptions. In an open system, such as a chemostat where predator–prey interactions take place, the populations of predator and prey do not necessarily reach steady state but can oscillate at certain dilution rates. At the beginning of the operation prey concentration is high, but predator concentration is low. As the predators consume prey, the number of predators increases and the prey concentration decreases. After a while, a small prey population cannot support the large predator population, and the predator population decreases while prey population increases. Depending on the dilution rate and feed substrate concentration, these oscillations may be sustained or damped or may not exist.

Finally, note that these interactions can, and often do, exist in combination. For example, A and B may compete for glucose as a nutrient, but A requires a growth factor from B to grow. In such a case, both competition and commensalism would be present.

16.6.2. Interactions of Two Species Fed on the Same Limiting Substrate

Competition of two species for the same growth-rate-limiting substrate is common. The two organisms may stably coexist in a chemostat if both A and B follow Monod kinetics.

Fig. 16.18 shows a schematic of a chemostat with two competing species. Mass balances of species A and B, as well as the common growth-limiting substrate:

$$Q(0 - X_j) + r_j V = \frac{d(X_j V)}{dt} \tag{16.61}$$

$$Q(S_0 - S) + r_S V = \frac{d(SV)}{dt} \tag{16.62}$$

where $j = \text{A}$ or $j = \text{B}$. Noting that the growth rate follows Monod equation, i.e.

$$\mu_j = \frac{\mu_{j\max} S}{K_j + S} \tag{16.63}$$

and

$$r_j = (\mu_j - k_{dj}) X_j \tag{16.64}$$

$$-r_S = \frac{\mu_A X_A}{YF_{A/S}} + \frac{\mu_B X_B}{YF_{B/S}} \tag{16.65}$$

At steady state, there is no time variation of any quantity. Eqns (16.61) and (16.62) are reduced to

$$-\frac{Q}{V} X_j + (\mu_j - k_{dj}) X_j = 0 \tag{16.66}$$

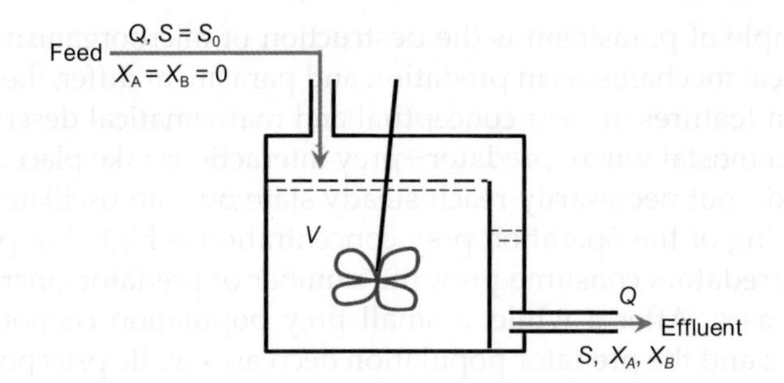

FIGURE 16.18 A mixed culture of A and B feeding on one common growth-rate-limiting substrate S in a chemostat.

$$\frac{Q}{V}(S_0 - S) - \left(\frac{\mu_A X_A}{Y_{A/S}} + \frac{\mu_B X_B}{Y_{B/S}}\right) = 0 \tag{16.67}$$

If both A and B coexist, that requires Eqn (16.66) be satisfied for both species A and B. Thus,

$$D = \frac{Q}{V} = \mu_j - k_{dj} = \mu_A - k_{dA} = \mu_B - k_{dB} \tag{16.68}$$

Substituting Eqn (16.63) into Eqn (16.68), we obtain

$$D = \frac{\mu_{Amax} S}{K_A + S} - k_{dA} = \frac{\mu_{Bmax} S}{K_B + S} - k_{dB} \tag{16.69}$$

Solving for the substrate concentration S, we obtain

$$S = b \pm \sqrt{b^2 + \frac{K_A K_B (k_{dA} - k_{dB})}{\mu_{Amax} - \mu_{Bmax} - k_{dA} + k_{dB}}} \tag{16.70}$$

where

$$b = \frac{\mu_{Bmax} K_A - \mu_{Amax} K_B + (K_A + K_B)(k_{dA} - k_{dB})}{2(\mu_{Amax} - \mu_{Bmax} - k_{dA} + k_{dB})} \tag{16.71}$$

Eqn (16.68) is meaningful only if S is real and $S \geq 0$, or positive real solution exists for Eqn (16.70). Consider the cases in Fig. 16.19 for different growth parameters. Coexistence is only possible at the point where both species exhibit the same net specific growth rate at the same substrate concentration. Fig. 16.19a shows that when $\mu_{Amax} > \mu_{Bmax}$ and $k_{dA} \leq k_{dB}$, cross-over of net specific growth curves occur only if $K_{SA} >> K_{SB}$, consequently, coexistence is possible only if $K_{SA} >> K_{SB}$. In Fig. 16.19b, when $\mu_{Amax} > \mu_{Bmax}$ and $k_{dA} > k_{dB}$, however, a value of S can be found from Eqn (16.70) that will allow both populations to coexist. The corresponding D for the crossover point is D_c.

Although this coexistence is mathematically obtainable, it is not a sustainable or stable solution. Thus, the coexistence is not physically attainable in real systems. In real systems, the dilution rate will vary slightly with time, and, in fact, the variation will show a bias. Using an analysis more sophisticated than appropriate for this text, it can be demonstrated that one competitor will be excluded from the chemostat if the intensity of the "noise" (random fluctuations) in D and the bias of the mean of D away from D_C are not both zero. Also, it is possible for either competitor to be excluded, depending on how D varies.

Two competitors can coexist if we modify the conditions of the experiments. Examples of such modifications include allowing spatial heterogeneity (the system is no longer well mixed or wall growth is present) or another level of interaction is added (e.g. adding a predator or interchange of metabolites). Also, operation of the chemostat in a dynamic mode (D is a function of time) can sometimes lead to coexistence. It is also interesting to note that the use of other rate expressions (e.g. substrate inhibition) can lead to multiple crossover points and potentially MSS.

Example 16-7. Mixed cultures (more than one distinct microbial species) are common in nature. Using two otherwise noninterfering species of different growth kinetics for feeding on the same substrate as an example, discuss the continuous culturing (chemostat) outcome. The two species are A and B. The kinetic relationships are $\mu_{Amax} = 1.5\ \mu_{Bmax}$ and $K_{SA} = 3K_{SB}$. The death rates are negligible to both species.

(a) Is it possible to maintain both species A and B in the chemostat? Determine the corresponding dilution rate.
(b) For a given high substrate feed rate or dilution rate (see $D > 0.8\ \mu_{Bmax}$), which species would survive?
(c) For a given low substrate feed rate (see $D < 0.6\ \mu_{Bmax}$), which species would survive?
(d) Is the solution in a) sustainable?

Solution. The two species have different growth rates. At high substrate concentrations, species A grows faster than species B. However, at low-substrate concentrations, species B could grow faster than species A because of its much lower saturation constant. Fig. E16-7 shows a sketch of the growth kinetics in a chemostat.

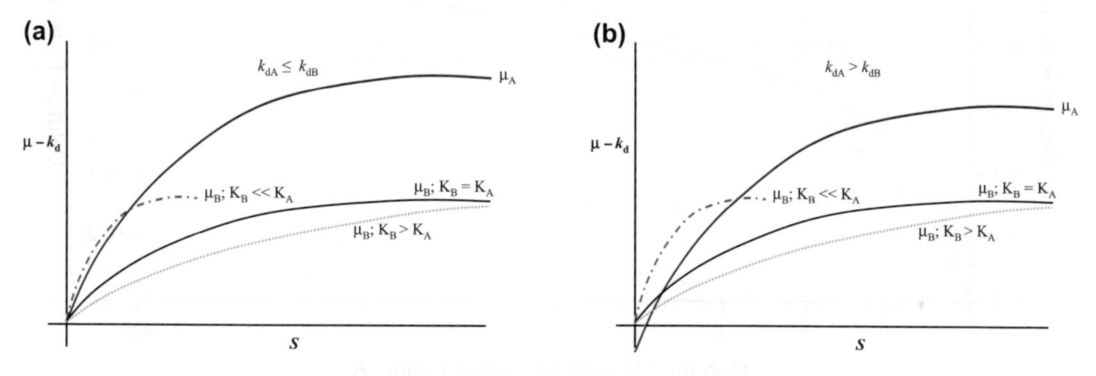

FIGURE 16.19 μ_{net}–S relationship for two competing species (A and B) in a mixed culture. (a) $\mu_{Amax} > \mu_{Bmax}$ and $k_{dA} \le k_{dB}$ (b) $\mu_{Amax} > \mu_{Bmax}$ and $k_{dA} > k_{dB}$

(a) Both species can coexist if there is a common substrate concentration at which both growth rate of A and growth rate of B are equal, and equal to the dilution rate. That is,

$$D = \mu_A = \mu_B \tag{E16-7.1}$$

The growth rates are given by

$$\mu_A = \frac{\mu_{Amax} S}{K_{SA} + S} = \frac{1.5 \mu_{Bmax} S}{3K_{SB} + S} \tag{E16-7.2}$$

and

$$\mu_B = \frac{\mu_{Bmax} S}{K_{SB} + S} \tag{E16-7.3}$$

Solving Eqns (E16-7.1) through (E16-7.3), we obtain

$$S = 3\,K_{SB} \quad \text{and} \quad D = \mu_A = \mu_B = 0.75\,\mu_{Bmax}$$

Therefore, there is a solution to the coexistence problem. It is possible to maintain both species in the reactor. A sketch of the solution is shown in Fig. E16-7.

(b) Refer to Fig. E16-7, because species A has high growth rate that species B, only species A will survive. At the same dilution rate, the substrate concentration will be driven lower than species B can survive,

(c) Refer to Fig. E16-7, because species B has higher growth rate at low substrate concentrations, species B will remain in the reactor.

(d) The coexistence point cannot be maintained sustainably as it is not a stable solution. It is clear than when the dilution rate fluctuates away from 0.75 μ_{Bmax}, one of the

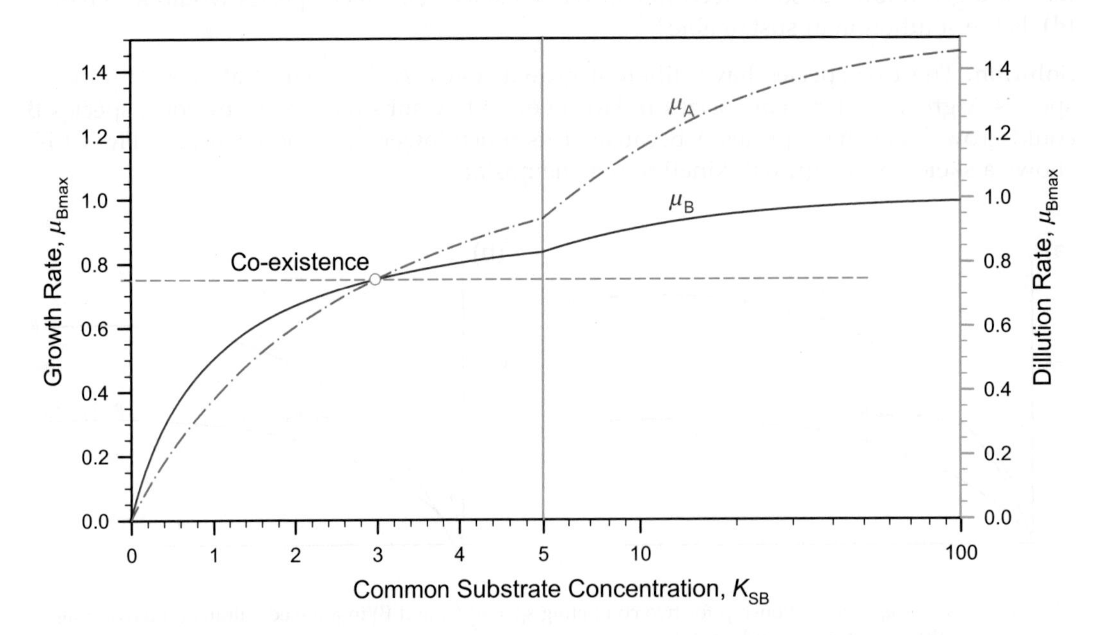

FIGURE E16-7

species would be washed out as one can infer from Fig. E16-7. Therefore, only one species would survive. As a result, the coexistence point is not realizable in operations.

16.6.3. Interactions of Two Mutualistic Species

Species A produces P_A as a by-product of growth, while species B produces P_B. Organism B requires P_A to grow, while A requires P_B. The feed to a chemostat contains all essential nutrients except for P_A and P_B and A and B may compete for substrate, S, in the feed as shown in Fig. 16.20.

Mass balances of species A and B, as well as the common growth-limiting substrate:

$$Q(0 - X_j) + r_j V = \frac{d(X_j V)}{dt} \tag{16.69}$$

$$Q(0 - P_j) + r_{Pj} V = \frac{d(P_j V)}{dt} \tag{16.70}$$

$$Q(S_0 - S) + r_S V = \frac{d(SV)}{dt} \tag{16.71}$$

Noting that

$$r_j = (\mu_j - k_{dj})X_j \tag{16.72}$$

$$r_{PA} = YF_{P_A}\mu_A X_A - \frac{\mu_B X_B}{YF_{B/P_A}} \tag{16.73}$$

$$r_{PB} = YF_{P_B}\mu_B X_B - \frac{\mu_A X_A}{YF_{A/P_B}} \tag{16.74}$$

$$r_S = -\frac{\mu_A X_A}{YF_{A/S}} - \frac{\mu_B X_B}{YF_{B/S}} \tag{16.75}$$

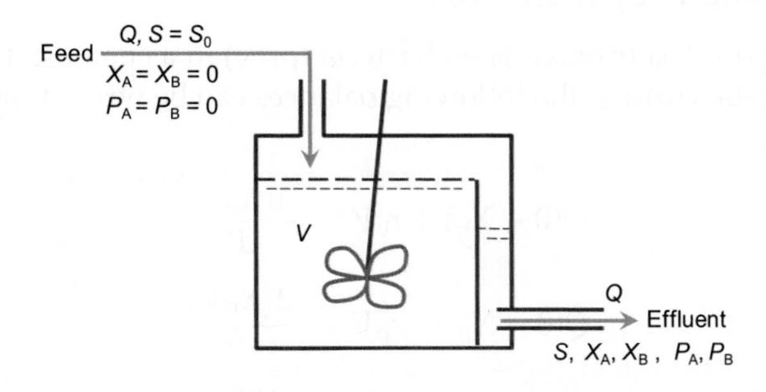

FIGURE 16.20 A mixed culture of A and B feeding on one common growth-rate-limiting substrate S in a chemostat; A also feeds on the by-product produced by B while B feeds on the by-product produced by A.

Note that YF_{B/P_A} is the biomass yield factor that requiring P_A as one of its substrates, and YF_{P_A} is the amount of P_A made per unit mass of A. Similar definitions apply to YF_{A/P_B} and YF_{P_B} If we consider the pure mutualistic state, then we ignore Eqn (16.71). For a coexistent state to exist, $D = \mu_A - k_{dA} = \mu_B - k_{dB}$. It is also clear that the rate of production of P_A and P_B must exceed their consumption (by the other species). Thus,

$$r_{PA} > 0 \Rightarrow YF_{P_A}\mu_A X_A > \frac{\mu_B X_B}{YF_{B/P_A}} \tag{16.76}$$

$$r_{PB} > 0 \Rightarrow YF_{P_B}\mu_B X_B > \frac{\mu_A X_A}{YF_{A/P_B}} \tag{16.77}$$

Since all the quantities in the equalities (16.76) and (16.77) are greater than zero, left-hand side multiply by left-hand side and right-hand side multiply by right-hand side leads to

$$YF_{P_A}\mu_A X_A YF_{P_B}\mu_B X_B > \frac{\mu_A X_A}{YF_{A/P_B}} \frac{\mu_B X_B}{YF_{B/P_A}} \tag{16.78}$$

Eliminating the identical terms, we obtain

$$YF_{P_A} Y_{P_B} > \frac{1}{YF_{A/P_B} YF_{B/P_A}} \tag{16.79}$$

It is also clear that the specific growth rates are less than their maximum values, that is

$$D < \min\left(\mu_{A\max} - k_{dA}, \mu_{B\max} - k_{dB}\right) \tag{16.80}$$

Eqns (16.79) and (16.80) determine whether Eqns (16.69) to (16.71) allow the potential existence of a purely mutualistic steady state. The stability of such a coexistent state has been examined, where μ_A and μ_B were represented by various growth functions. Using a linear stability analysis, it can be shown that this pure mutualistic state results in a saddle point (Fig. 16.11c), and the system is unstable for all physically accessible values of D. If, however, the growth-rate-limiting substrate for either A or B is S, then a stable coexistent state can be found.

16.6.4. Predator and Prey Interactions

The growth of a protozoa (predator) on bacteria (prey) in a chemostat is a classic stability problem. In a chemostat culture, the following balances can be written for substrate (S), prey (b), and predator (p).

$$Q(0 - X_b) + r_b V = \frac{d(X_b V)}{dt} \tag{16.81}$$

$$Q(0 - X_p) + r_p V = \frac{d(X_p V)}{dt} \tag{16.82}$$

$$Q(S_0 - S) + r_S V = \frac{d(SV)}{dt} \tag{16.83}$$

Noting that

$$r_{\mathrm{p}} = (\mu_{\mathrm{p}} - k_{\mathrm{dp}})X_{\mathrm{p}} = \frac{\mu_{\mathrm{pmax}} X_{\mathrm{b}}}{K_{\mathrm{p}} + X_{\mathrm{b}}} X_{\mathrm{p}} - k_{\mathrm{dp}} X_{\mathrm{p}} \tag{16.84}$$

$$r_{\mathrm{b}} = \mu_{\mathrm{b}} X_{\mathrm{b}} = (\mu_{\mathrm{bG}} - \mu_{\mathrm{b}k_{\mathrm{d}}})X_{\mathrm{b}} = \frac{\mu_{\mathrm{bmax}} S}{K_{\mathrm{b}} + S} X_{\mathrm{b}} - \frac{1}{YF_{p/b}} \frac{\mu_{\mathrm{pmax}} X_{\mathrm{p}}}{K_{\mathrm{p}} + X_{\mathrm{b}}} X_{\mathrm{b}} \tag{16.85}$$

$$r_{\mathrm{S}} = -\frac{1}{YF_{\mathrm{b/S}}} \mu_{\mathrm{bG}} X_{\mathrm{b}} = -\frac{1}{YF_{\mathrm{b/S}}} \frac{\mu_{\mathrm{bmax}} S}{K_{\mathrm{b}} + S} X_{\mathrm{b}} \tag{16.86}$$

where $YF_{\mathrm{b/S}}$ and $YF_{\mathrm{p/b}}$ are the yield coefficients for the growth of prey on substrate and the growth of predator on prey, respectively. Eqns (16.81) through (16.83) can be reduced to

$$\frac{\mathrm{d}X_{\mathrm{p}}}{\mathrm{d}t} = -(D - k_{\mathrm{dp}})X_{\mathrm{p}} + \frac{\mu_{\mathrm{pmax}} X_{\mathrm{b}}}{K_{\mathrm{p}} + X_{\mathrm{b}}} X_{\mathrm{p}} \tag{16.87}$$

$$\frac{\mathrm{d}X_{\mathrm{b}}}{\mathrm{d}t} = -DX_{\mathrm{b}} + \frac{\mu_{\mathrm{bmax}} S}{K_{\mathrm{b}} + S} X_{\mathrm{b}} - \frac{1}{YF_{\mathrm{p/b}}} \frac{\mu_{\mathrm{pmax}} X_{\mathrm{p}}}{K_{\mathrm{p}} + X_{\mathrm{b}}} X_{\mathrm{b}} \tag{16.88}$$

$$\frac{\mathrm{d}S}{\mathrm{d}t} = D(S_0 - S) - \frac{1}{YF_{\mathrm{b/S}}} \frac{\mu_{\mathrm{bmax}} S}{K_{\mathrm{b}} + S} X_{\mathrm{b}} \tag{16.89}$$

Eqns (16.87) through (16.89) govern the substrate−prey−predator concentration change with time in a continuous culture. This model was used to describe the behavior of *Dictyostelium discoideum* and *E. coli* in a chemostat culture and was found to predict experimental results quite well (Fig. 16.21). Fig. 16.21 shows that the prey and predator system is not stable, but marginally sustainable. Substrate (glucose), prey, and predator concentrations are oscillatory with a clear phase shift as expected. When prey concentration (population) is high, nearly all the substrates are consumed. High prey concentration is then followed by the increase in predator concentration (population), in turn causing the prey concentration to drop. When the prey concentration is low, predator population decrease is followed with a short delay while the substrate concentration gains. This trend is shown in Fig. 16.21 from both the predictions based Eqns (16.87) though (16.89) and the experimental measurements.

The washing out conditions can be obtained by examining Eqns (16.87) and (16.88). Eqn (16.87) indicates that if predator is starting to wash out $\frac{\mathrm{d}X_{\mathrm{p}}}{\mathrm{d}t} < 0$,

$$D - k_{\mathrm{dp}} > \frac{\mu_{\mathrm{pmax}} X_{\mathrm{b}}}{K_{\mathrm{p}} + X_{\mathrm{b}}} \tag{16.90}$$

if $X_{\mathrm{p}} > 0$. The maximum value of X_{b} is at which $X_{\mathrm{p}} = 0$ (predator already washed out):

$$X_{\mathrm{b}} \le YF_{\mathrm{b/S}}(S_0 - S) < YF_{\mathrm{b/S}} S_0 \tag{16.91}$$

Therefore, the washout condition for the predator (while prey is not washed out) is

$$D \geq k_{dp} + \frac{\mu_{pmax} YF_{b/S} S_0}{K_p + YF_{b/S} S_0} \tag{16.92}$$

All washout (both prey and predator are washed out) condition can be obtained by first setting $X_p = 0$ (prey washed out). Eqn (16.88) indicates that if prey is also being washed out $\frac{dX_b}{dt} < 0$,

$$D > \frac{\mu_{bmax} S}{K_b + S} \tag{16.93}$$

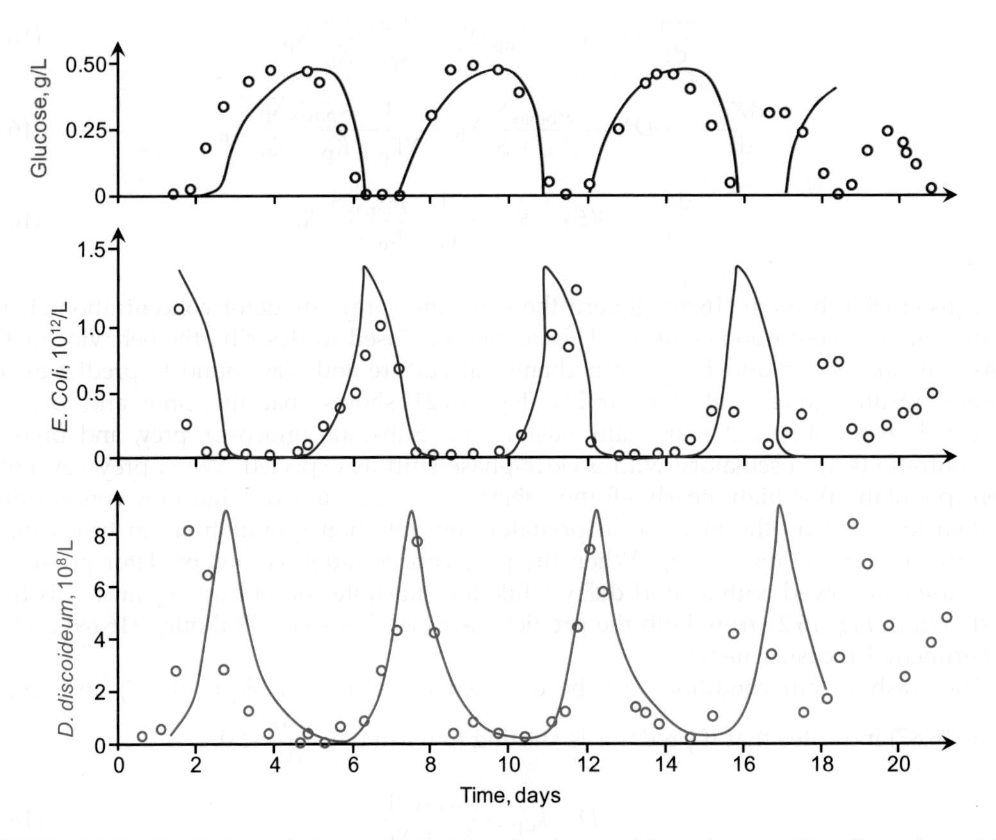

FIGURE 16.21 Oscillations of the concentrations of substrate (glucose), prey (*E. coli*), and predator (*D. discotideum*) with time in a continuous culture. Predictions based on Eqns (16.87) through (16.89) (lines), superimposed on experimental data (symbols), for continuous culture with a residence time of 16 h or $D = 0.0625$/h at 25 °C. The kinetic parameters are given by $k_{dp} = 0$, $\mu_{pmax} = 0.24$/h, $K_p = 4 \times 10^{11}$ *E. coli*/L, $\mu_{bmax} = 0.25$/h, $K_b = 5 \times 10^{-4}$ g/L, $YF_{p/b} = 7.14 \times 10^{-4}$ *D. discoideum*/*E. coli*, $YF_{b/S} = 3 \times 10^{12}$ *E. coli*/g. *Replotted from H. M. Tsuchiya, J. F. Drake, J. L. Jost, and A. G. Fredrickson, "Predator-Prey Interactions of* Dictyostelium discoideum *and* E. coli *in Continuous Culture", J. Bacteriology. 110(3): 1147-1153, 1972.*

The maximum value of substrate concentration in the chemostat culture is the feed concentration (prey washed out). Therefore, all washout condition is given by

$$D \geq \frac{\mu_{bmax} S_0}{K_b + S_0} \tag{16.94}$$

Fig. 16.22 shows the steady-state operating regions of the prey–predator system. A variety of types of dynamic coexistence behavior have been revealed by stability analysis for this prey–predator interaction. When both prey and predator coexist in the reactor, there is no stable solution as all the steady states are unstable. The trajectories to steady state are governed by Eqns (16.87) through (16.89). The Eigen values of the Jacobian determine the nature of the trajectories (Fig. 16.11); there are three Eigen values when both predator and prey are present, or when

$$D < k_{dp} + \frac{\mu_{pmax} YF_{b/S} S_0}{K_p + YF_{b/S} S_0} \tag{16.95}$$

The real Eigen value is positive. Therefore, there are no stable steady solutions. However, the solutions are sustainable as there is a bound or limit on the variations.

16.6.5. Lokka–Volterra Model—A Simplified Predator–Prey Interaction Model

A classical model that describes oscillations in a prey–predator system is the Lotka–Volterra model, which assumes $K_b \ll S$ (substrate is unlimited) and $K_p \gg X_b$ (prey population is very small). Eqns (16.87) through (16.89) are reduced to:

$$\frac{dX_b}{dt} = \mu'_b X_b - \frac{\mu'_p X_b X_p}{YF_{p/b}} \tag{16.96}$$

$$\frac{dX_p}{dt} = -k'_{dp} X_p + \mu'_p X_b X_p \tag{16.97}$$

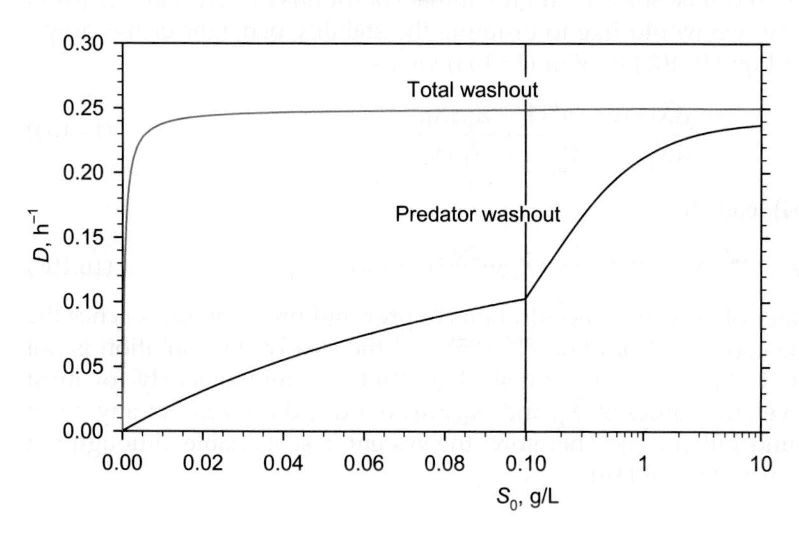

FIGURE 16.22 Steady-state operating regions of prey–predator model with Monod growth. The kinetic parameters are given by: $k_{dp} = 0$, $\mu_{pmax} = 0.24$/h, $K_p = 4 \times 10^{11}$ *E. coli*/L, $\mu_{bmax} = 0.25$/h, $K_b = 5 \times 10^{-4}$ g/L, $YF_{p/b} = 7.14 \times 10^{-4}$ *D. discoideum*/*E. coli*, $YF_{b/S} = 3 \times 10^{12}$ *E. coli*/g.

The first term in Eqn (16.96) describes the growth of prey on substrate and the second the consumption of prey by predators. The first and second terms in Eqn (16.97) describe the death of predator in the absence of prey and the growth of predator on prey, respectively. $YF_{p/b}$ is the yield of predators on prey (g/g), $\mu_b' = \mu_b - D$ is the net specific growth rate of prey on a soluble substrate, per hour, $\mu_p' = \mu_p$ is the specific growth rate of predator on prey, 1/(g-h), and $k_{dp}' = k_{dp} + D$ is the apparent specific removal rate of the predator, per hour.

Eqns (16.96) and (16.97) allow a steady-state solution for either batch growth ($D = 0$) or continuous culture ($D > 0$), where $\frac{dX_b}{dt} = 0$ and $\frac{dX_p}{dt} = 0$. Under these conditions

$$X_{bF} = \frac{k_{dp}'}{\mu_p'} = \frac{k_{dp} + D}{\mu_p} \tag{16.98}$$

$$X_{pF} = \frac{\mu_b' YF_{p/b}}{\mu_p'} = \frac{\mu_b - D}{\mu_p} YF_{p/b} \tag{16.99}$$

Let

$$\overline{X}_b = \frac{X_b}{X_{bF}} \tag{16.100}$$

$$\overline{X}_p = \frac{X_p}{X_{pF}} \tag{16.101}$$

Eqns (16.96) and (16.97) can be rearranged to give

$$\frac{d\overline{X}_b}{dt} = \mu_b'(1 - \overline{X}_p)\overline{X}_b \tag{16.102}$$

$$\frac{d\overline{X}_p}{dt} = -k_{dp}'(1 - \overline{X}_b)\overline{X}_p \tag{16.103}$$

Eqns (16.102) and (16.103) can be solved with the initial conditions of $X_b(t = 0) = X_{b0}$ and $X_p(t = 0) = X_{p0}$. In this case, we would like to examine the stability behavior of the prey–predator model. Dividing Eqn (16.102) by Eqn (16.103) yields

$$\frac{d\overline{X}_b}{d\overline{X}_p} = -\frac{\mu_b'(1 - \overline{X}_p)\overline{X}_b}{k_{dp}'(1 - \overline{X}_b)\overline{X}_p} \tag{16.104}$$

Integration of Eqn (16.104) leads to

$$(\overline{X}_p e^{-\overline{X}_p})^{\mu_b'}(\overline{X}_b e^{-\overline{X}_b})^{k_{dp}'} = (\overline{X}_{p0} e^{-\overline{X}_{p0}})^{\mu_b'}(\overline{X}_{b0} e^{-\overline{X}_{b0}})^{k_{dp}'} \tag{16.105}$$

which governs the trajectory of how the concentrations of prey and predator approaches the steady-state solution. One can infer from Eqn (16.105) that the steady-state solution is not achievable as $\overline{X}_p = 1$ and $\overline{X}_b = 1$ do not satisfy Eqn (16.105) simultaneously for most μ_b' and k_{dp}' values. However, the values of $\overline{X}_p$ and $\overline{X}_b$ are bound and not zero for any given set of non trivial and bound initial data. Therefore, the system is sustainable although not stable. This is a case similar to Fig. 16.11h).

The phase-plane analysis of the system can be made using Eqn (16.105). Fig. 16.23a describes the limit cycles (oscillatory trajectories) of prey–predator populations for different initial population levels. The Lotka–Volterra model considers the exponential growth of prey species in the absence of predator and neglects the utilization of substrate by prey species according to Monod form. The Lotka–Volterra oscillations depend on initial conditions and change their amplitude and frequency in the presence of an external disturbance. These types of oscillation are called soft oscillations.

Eqns (16.87)–(16.89) explain the more stable and sustained oscillations observed in nature, which are independent of initial conditions (that is, hard oscillations). A differential equation integrator (such as Odexlims used in this text) can be employed to obtain the solutions from the set of Eqns (16.87)–(16.89), and the phase–plane data are shown in Fig. 16.23b. Fig. 16.23b shows that the trajectory depends on the initial conditions, whereas the limit cycle (oscillation) is not dependent on the initial conditions. The dynamic solution does not approach the steady-state value; however, the populations are bound and nonzero. Even when the initial populations correspond to those of the steady-state solution (point F in Fig. 16.23b), minor fluctuations cause the dynamic populations to shift away and eventually confirm to the limit cycle (solid line). A 3D plot of the trajectory toward sustainable state and corresponding phase-plane trajectories on substrate versus prey population are shown in Fig. 16.24. Therefore, the system is sustainable, although not stable as the single-point/value steady-state solution cannot be maintained.

16.6.6. Industrial Applications of Mixed Cultures

Growth behavior differences and cell–cell interactions are the main causes of instabilities in mixed cultures as we have learned. Industrial applications are designed such instabilities are minimized to maintain process integrity and/or product quality.

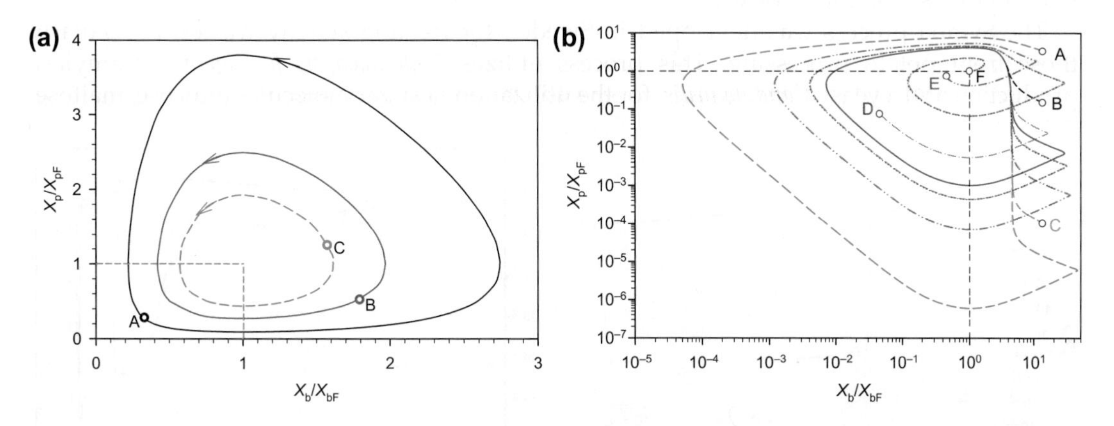

FIGURE 16.23 Phase-plane trajectories for prey–predator interactions. (a) Limit cycles predicted by Lotka–Volterra, Eqn (16.105), with $k'_{dp} = \frac{1}{2}\mu'_b$. (b) Trajectories when the substrate limitation and Monod predator growth rate are used: $D = 0.6\ \mu_{bmax}$, $\mu_{pmax} = 0.96\ \mu_{bmax}$, $k_{dp} = 0$, $K_b = 5 - 10^{-4}\ S_0$, $YF_{p/b} = 7.14 - 10^{-4}$, $YF_{b/S}\ S_0 = 3\ X_{b0}$, $K_p = 0.4\ X_{b0}$. The predicted steady-state point is defined by X_{pF} and X_{bF}. A, B, and C (and D, E, and F) represent different initial conditions.

Mixed microbial populations are commonly used in cheese making, a good example of using mixed cultures in food production. Cheeses of various types are produced by inoculating pasteurized fresh milk with appropriate lactic acid organisms. The bacteria used for lactic acid production are various species of *Streptococcus* and *Lactobacillus* in a mixed culture. Other organisms are used to develop flavor and aroma. Among these are *Brevibacterium linens, Propionibacterium shermanii, Leuconostoc* sp., and *Streptococcus diacetilactis*. After inoculation of pasteurized milk, a protein-rich curd is precipitated by the acidity of the medium, and the liquid is drained off. The precipitated curd is allowed to age by action of bacteria or mold. Some molds used in cheese making are *Penicillum camemberti* and *Penicillum roqueforti*.

Lactic acid bacteria are also used in whiskey manufacture. *Lactobacillus* added to the yeast reduces pH and, therefore, the chance of contamination. *Lactobacillus* also contributes to the flavor and aroma of whiskey. Lactic acid and ethanol react forming ethyl lactate which gives an aroma. A favorable interaction between yeast and lactic acid bacteria exists in ginger-beer fermentation.

The types of mixed cultures vary among applications. Food processing involves largely defined mixed culture and with batch operations, which represents one extreme of the mixed culture applications. Another extreme is the wastewater treatment process, where continuous operation is warranted for mass processing needs and undefined (may even be unknown) microbial cultures is typical and unavoidable. The low value (or zero value) of the product and a desire of minimum cost to destroy the substrate(s), both contributed to complex mixer of microbial cultures applied in wastewater treatment.

Wastewater treatment constitutes one of the largest scale uses of bioprocesses. Mixed cultures are also utilized in the anaerobic digestion of waste materials. Cellulase producers, acid formers, and methane producers are typical organisms involved in the anaerobic digestion of cellulosic wastes. However, attempts to encourage the growth of a particular species on waste materials are commonly made to maximize waste treatment rate and/or particular final products (valoration of wastes).

The Symba process was developed in Sweden for treating starchy wastes, particularly those from potato processing. This process utilizes *Endomycopsis fibuligera* for amylase production and a yeast, *Candida utilis*, for the utilization of sugar molecules (glucose, maltose,

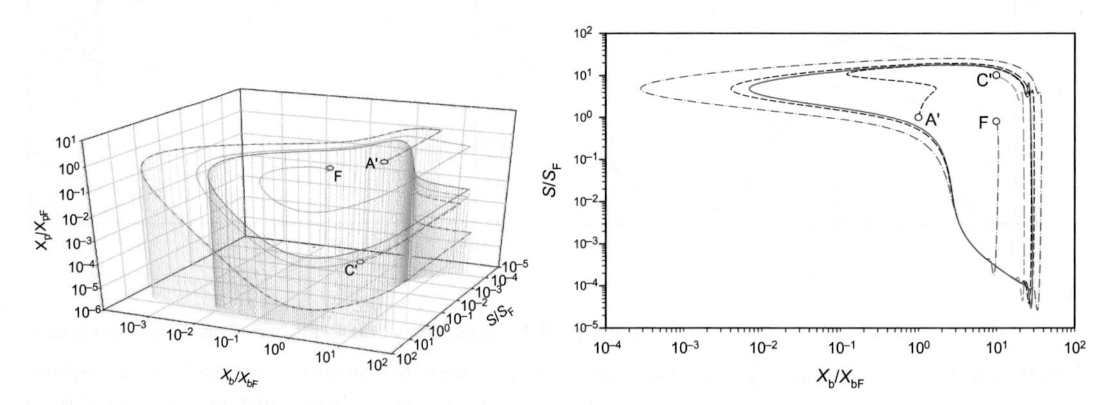

FIGURE 16.24 Phase trajectories for prey–predator interactions: $D = 0.6\ \mu_{bmax}$, $\mu_{pmax} = 0.96\ \mu_{bmax}$, $k_{dp} = 0$, $K_b = 5 \times 10^{-4}\ S_0$, $YF_{p/b} = 7.14 \times 10^{-4}$, $YF_{b/S}\ S_0 = 3\ X_{b0}$, $K_p = 0.4\ X_{b0}$.

etc.) produced from the hydrolysis of starch. Single-cell protein (SCP) is produced simultaneously with potato waste treatment.

Corn and pea wastes are also treated by a mixed culture of *Trichoderma viride* and *Geotrichium* sp. *Trichoderma viride* produces cellulase to break down cellulose into glucose, and *Geotrichium* produces amylases to break down starch into glucose. Both organisms utilize glucose for growth.

A mixed culture of *Candida lipolytica* and *Candida tropicalis* has been grown on hydrocarbons, *n*-paraffins, or gas oil for SCP production purposes in both laboratory and pilot-scale operations. The utilization of a mixed culture of yeasts was proved to yield better product quality as compared to pure yeast strains.

Gaseous hydrocarbon substrates like methane can be utilized by certain bacteria to produce SCP. Several experimental studies have shown that mixed cultures of methane utilizing organisms grow faster than pure cultures.

Certain methane-utilizing species of *Pseudomonas oxidize* methane to methanol. However, *Pseudomonas* is inhibited by methanol. Inclusion of a methanol-utilizing bacteria such as *Hyphomicrobium* into the growth medium eliminates the problem of methanol inhibition. This relationship is mutualistic in the sense that *Pseudomonas* supplies carbon source (CH_3OH) for *Hyphomicrobium*, and *Hyphomicrobium* removes the growth inhibitor (methanol) of *Pseudomonas*.

$$CH_4 \xrightarrow{Pseudomonas} CH_3OH \xrightarrow{Hyphomicrobium} CO_2 + H_2O \tag{16.106}$$

Feedback inhibition

A schematic of a typical wastewater treatment flowsheet is shown in Fig. 12.8 and redrawn in Fig. 16.25. *Activated-sludge* processes include a well-agitated and aerated continuous-flow reactor and a settling tank. Depending on the physical design of the tank and how feed is introduced into the tank, it may approximate either a PFR (plug flow reactor) or CSTR. A long narrow tank with single-feed approaches PFR behavior: circular tanks approach CSTR. The concentrated cells from the settling tank are recycled back to the stirred-tank reactor. Usually, a mixed culture of organisms is utilized in the bioreactor. Some of these organisms may produce polymeric materials (polysaccharides), which help the organisms to agglomerate. Floc formation is a common phenomenon encountered in activated-sludge processes, which may impose some mass transfer limitations on the biological oxidation of soluble organics; but good floc formation is essential to good performance of the system, since large dense floes are required in the sedimentation step. Cell recycle from the sedimentation unit improves the volumetric rate of biological oxidation (i.e. high-density culture) and therefore reduces the residence time or volume of the sludge reactor for a given feed rate. The recycle maintains the integrity of biocatalysts (microbials) in the process in case of minor upsets or fluctuations. The recycle ratio needs to be controlled to maximize BOD (biological oxygen demand) removal rate.

16.6.7. Mixed Culture in Nature

Mixed cultures of *organisms* are common in natural ecological systems. Microorganisms are involved in the natural cycles of most elements (e.g. carbon, hydrogen, nitrogen, oxygen, and sulfur). Simplified diagrams of the carbon and oxygen cycles are presented in Fig. 15.1 or

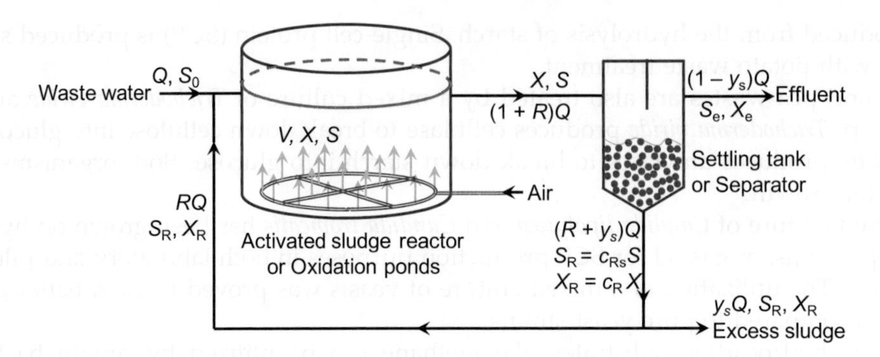

FIGURE 16.25 Schematic diagram of a typical wastewater processing unit.

Fig. 16.26. Organisms living in soil and aquatic environments actively participate in carbon and nitrogen cycles. For example, certain organisms fix atmospheric CO_2 to form carbohydrates, while others degrade carbohydrates and release CO_2 into the atmosphere. Similarly, some organisms fix atmospheric nitrogen (N_2) to form ammonium and proteins, while others convert ammonium into nitrite and nitrate (nitrification), and others reduce nitrate into atmospheric nitrogen (denitrification). Sulfur-oxidizing organisms convert reduced sulfur compounds (sulfur and sulfide) into sulfate, and sulfate-reducing organisms reduce sulfate into hydrogen sulfide. These interactions among different species take place in natural systems in a more complicated manner. The sustainability of the ecosystem maintained by a balanced action of all the organisms involved in completing the cycles.

16.7. SUMMARY

One of the important aspects of reactor design is to seek desirable stable steady-state reaction conditions as the reactor set point. Stable steady state is a subset of sustainable states that the system operates at a single valued point. While a sustainable system can be weakly stable, exhibiting limit cycle or oscillation between bound and nonzero values, industrial bioprocesses are preferably to be strictly stable. Only stable steady state can be operated such that the bioprocess system will not runaway when fluctuations are encountered. As such the quality of the product can be maintained. A real bioprocess system is operated such that the output fluctuations are small and it gradually returns to the desired set point when a fluctuation is expired. Therefore, bioprocess system stability is an important topic for bioprocess system (reactor) design and operations.

Stability of a reactor operation is usually associated with the existence of MSS. MSS exist if the rate law is not monotonic or the rate could be lower at very high-feed reactant concentrations (than that at lower reactant concentrations). When back mixing is strong (for example, CSTR or chemostat), multiple states appears. Therefore, MSS could exist for nonisothermal exothermic reactions (of any kinetics) and isothermal substrate inhibited systems in a CSTR. Feed conditions also affect whether MSS exits or not.

Catalyst stability or rather instability is another important issue. Catalyst deactivation is affected by the reaction mixture, temperature, and flow conditions.

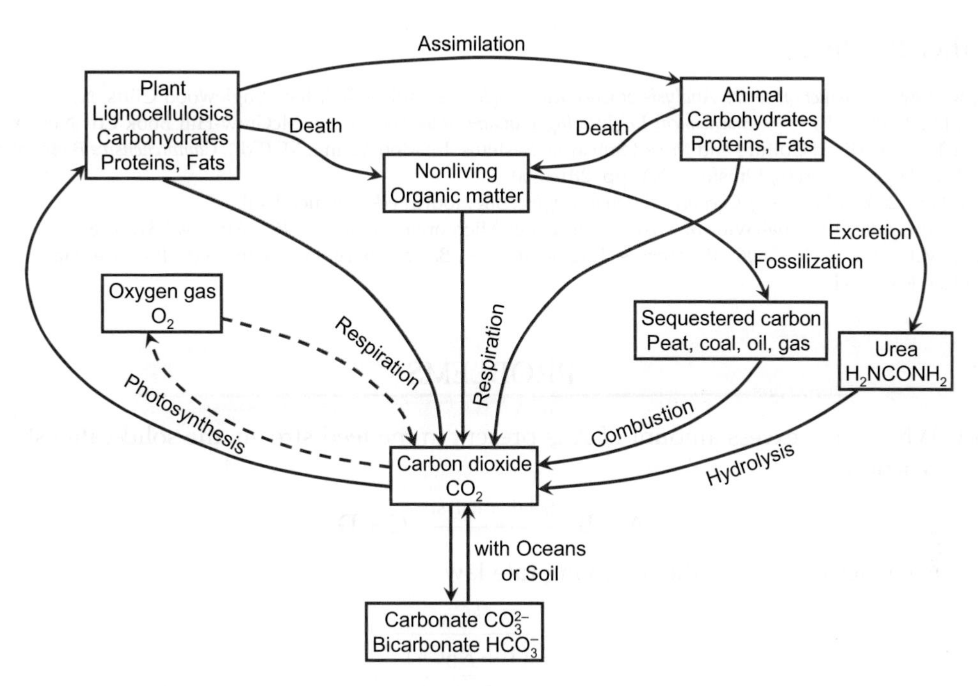

FIGURE 16.26 Simplified schematic of the carbon and major oxygen cycles.

The simplistic root for bioinstability is the difference in specific growth rate and mutation. Biostability is of concern for genetically engineered cells. Genetically engineered cells for industrial applications are commonly exploiting the cells to produce protein or products that are not generic to the host cells. As a result, the growth characteristics are altered as compared with the host cells. Genetic evolution back to the generic cell function looses the desired traits imposed to the cells. The genetic evolution can be modeled quite accurately with kinetic considerations.

Populations containing multiple species are important in natural ecosystems, well-defined processes, wastewater treatment, and systems using genetically modified cells. Some examples of interactions among these species are competition, neutralism, mutualism, protocooperation, commensalism, amensalism, predation, and parasitism. In real systems, several modes of interaction may be present. Mathematical analyses can be used to show that neither pure competition nor pure mutualism gives a stable steady state in a chemostat. Predator and prey model shows that while there are no stable steady states, the bioprocess can be sustainable and the final prey and predator populations oscillate in a confined cycle. Continuous culture can be employed to screen organisms of certain traits based on the growth instability. Spatial heterogeneity, dynamic fluctuations, and the addition of other interactions can lead to the sustained coexistence of species with competitive or mutualistic interactions.

One of the major process uses of mixed cultures is wastewater treatment. The activated-sludge system is commonly employed in treating wastewaters. Such a system can be considered a chemostat with cell recycle under aerobic conditions.

Further Reading

Aris, R., 1965. *Introduction to the Analysis of Chemical Reactors*, Prentice-Hall, Inc., Englewood Cliffs, NJ.
Bailey, J.E., Ollis, D.F., 1986. *Biochemical Engineering Fundamentals*, second ed. McGraw-Hill Book Co.: New York.
Bull, A.T., 1985. Mixed Culture and Mixed Substrate Systems. In: Moo-Young, M. (Ed.), *Comprehensive Biotechnology*, vol. 1, Pergamon Press, Elmsford, NY, pp. 281–300.
Fogler, H.S., 2006. *Elements of Chemical Reaction Engineering*, fourth ed. Prentice-Hall.
Fredrickson, A.G., 1977. Behavior of Mixed Cultures of Microorganisms, *Ann. Rev. Microbial* 31, 63-87.
Shuler, M.L., Kargi, F., 2006. Bioprocess Engineering – Basic Concepts, second ed. Prentice Hall, Upper Saddle River, NJ.

PROBLEMS

16.1. When large excess amount of A is present in the feed stream, the solid-catalyst reaction

$$A + B \xrightarrow{\text{Solid-catalyst}} C + D$$

is suggested to obey the following rate law

$$r' = \frac{kC_B}{(1 + K_B C_B)^2}$$

and experimental data on the reaction rate is shown in Fig. P16.1. A fluidized CSTR that can have 56 kg-catalyst loaded is available to use. A feed stream, of 2.4 m^3/min, containing 2.8 mol-B/m^3 solution in A is to be treated using the reactor.

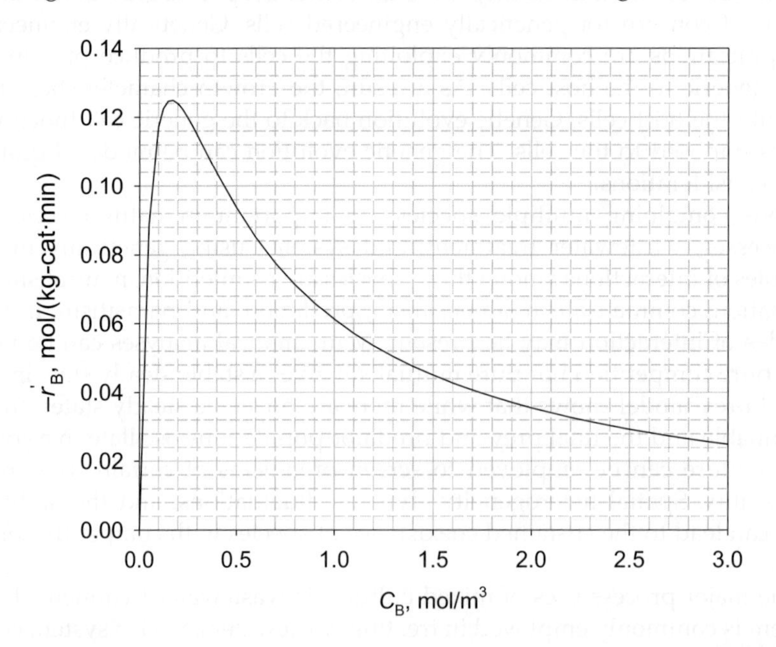

FIGURE P16.1 Experimental reaction rate as a function of concentration c_B when excess amount of A is present.

(a) Perform a steady-state mole balance on B.
(b) Plot the mole balance equation on the Fig. P16.1.
(c) Determine the possible steady-state conversion or conversions in the effluent stream.
(d) Comment on the stability of the solution or solutions obtained in part c).

16.2. A cell culture grows on a glucose media is inhibited by the substrate under isothermal conditions and the growth rate is governed

$$\mu_G = \frac{\mu_{max} S}{K_S + S + S^2/K_I}$$

with $\mu_{max} = 0.1\ h^{-1}$, $K_S = 0.1$ g/L, and $K_I = 10$ g/L. The cells have a specific death rate of $k_d = 0.005\ h^{-1}$ and a yield factor of $YF_{X/S} = 0.75$. The culture is to be grown in a chemostat with a sterile feed containing $S_0 = 80$ g/L substrate and a dilution rate of $D = 0.06\ h^{-1}$. Determine
(a) The steady-state solutions;
(b) Which steady-state solutions in a) can be operated, and which one is desired, and why?
(c) How should you start the reactor if the desired operating conditions are to be met?

16.3. A cell culture grows on a glucose media is inhibited by the substrate under isothermal conditions and the growth rate is governed

$$\mu_G = \frac{\mu_{max} S}{K_S + S + S^2/K_I} \quad \text{(P16.2-1)}$$

with $\mu_{max} = 0.8$/h, $K_S = 0.1$ g/L, $K_I = 10$ g/L. The cells has a specific death rate of $k_d = 0.01\ h^{-1}$ and a yield factor of $YF_{X/S} = 0.6$. The culture is to be grown in a chemostat with a sterile feed containing $S_0 = 80$ g/L substrate and a dilution rate of $D = 0.6\ h^{-1}$. Determine
(a) The steady-state solutions;
(b) Which steady-state solutions in a) can be operated, and which one is desired, and why?
(c) How should you start the reactor if the desired operating conditions are to be met?

16.4. A first-order homogeneous liquid reaction is carried out in a CSTR. The reactor initially contains 18 L of reactant (A) with a concentration of 3 mol/L. The initial temperature is 373 K and the reactor is well-insulated so that it can be assumed to be adiabatic. The feed rate is at 60 cm^3/s. The density of the liquid is 1000 kg/m^3 and the heat capacity is 4.182 kJ/(kg·K). $\Delta H_R = -2.09 \times 10^5$ J/mol-A. Feed concentration is 3 mol/L. The reaction rate is given by

$$-r_A = 4.48 \times 10^6 C_A \exp(-7554/T) \quad \text{mol/(L·s)}$$

(a) Determine whether MSS exist.
(b) Construct the ignition–extinction curve for the system.

(c) Calculate the steady temperature and concentration in effluent when the feed temperature is $T_0 = 298$ K.

(d) Plot T_e (effluent temperature) and f_A (total conversion in the effluent stream) as a function of time for the conditions set in part c). Determine the realized steady state.

16.5. A liquid-phase, exothermic first-order reaction (A → products) is to take place in a 4000 L CSTR. The Arrhenius parameters for the reacting systems are $k_0 = 2 \times 10^{13}\ \text{s}^{-1}$ and $E_a = 100\ \text{kJ} \cdot \text{mol}^{-1}$; the thermal parameters are $\Delta H_{RA} = -50\ \text{kJ} \cdot \text{mol}^{-1}$ and $C_P = 4\ \text{J} \cdot \text{g}^{-1} \cdot \text{K}^{-1}$; the density ($\rho$) is $1000\ \text{g} \cdot \text{L}^{-1}$.

(a) For a feed concentration (C_{A0}) of $4\ \text{mol} \cdot \text{L}^{-1}$, a feed rate ($Q_0$) of $5\ \text{L} \cdot \text{s}^{-1}$, and adiabatic operation, determine f_A and T at steady state, if the feed temperature (T_0) is (i) 290 K, (ii) 297 K, and (iii) 305 K;

(b) What is the minimum value of T_0 for autothermal behavior, and what are the corresponding values of f_A and T at steady state?

(c) For $T_0 = 305$ K as in a) (iii), explain, without doing any calculations, what would happen eventually if the feed rate (Q_0) were increased.

(d) If the result in c) is adverse, what change could be made to offset it at the higher throughput?

(e) Suppose the feed temperature (T_0) is 297 K, and it is desired to achieve a steady-state conversion (f_A) of 0.932 without any alternative possibility of steady-state operation in the "quench region." If a fluid stream is available at 360 K (T_c, assume constant) for use in a heat exchanger within the tank, what value of UA_H ($\text{J} \cdot \text{K}^{-1} \cdot \text{s}^{-1}$) would be required for the heat exchanger? Show that the "quench" region is avoided.

16.6. The exothermic gas-phase reaction

$$\text{A} \rightleftarrows \text{B} + \text{C} \quad r = k_f p_A - k_b p_B p_C$$

is to be carried out in a CSTR operating at a pressure of 50 bar. The required conversion is 22% with a pure A fed at 5 mol/s.

(a) Calculate the minimum reactor volume.

(b) Heat is removed from the reactor via cooling coils. What heat transfer area is required for steady operation if the overall heat transfer coefficient is $10\ \text{W}/(\text{m}^2 \cdot \text{K})$?

(c) Comment on the stability of the operating point.

The additional data are:

$$k_f = 0.435 \exp(-20,000/RT)\ \text{mol} \cdot \text{s}^{-1} \cdot \text{m}^{-3} \cdot \text{bar}^{-1}$$

$$k_b = 147 \exp(-60,000/RT)\ \text{mol} \cdot \text{s}^{-1} \cdot \text{m}^{-3} \cdot \text{bar}^{-2}$$

where RT is in J/mol. Feed temperature is 350 K; Coolant temperature is 400 K and mean heat capacities of A, B, and C are 30, 20, and 10 J/(mol K), respectively.

16.7. The gas-phase decomposing reaction

$$\text{A} \rightarrow \text{B} + \text{C} \quad r = kC_A$$

is to be carried out adiabatically in a flow reactor. The feed consists of pure A at a temperature of 298 K and a pressure of 1 bar. The feed rate is 0.1 mol/s. Neglect the pressure drop in the reactor.

(a) Calculate the operating temperature and conversion from a CSTR of volume 2 m^3. Indicate the stability of your solution.

(b) Calculate the volume of a PFR for a conversion of 0.99. Comment on your findings.

(c) Recalculate the volume of the PFR for a conversion of 0.99, but the feed to the reactor is preheated to 500 K.

The additional data are $k = 10^{11}\exp\left(-\frac{E}{RT}\right)\text{s}^{-1}$; $\frac{E}{R} = 18{,}000$ K; $\Delta H_R = -60$ kJ/mol-A; $\overline{C}_{PA} = 120$ J/(mol·K); $\overline{C}_{PB} = 80$ J/(mol·K); $\overline{C}_{PC} = 40$ J/(mol·K).

16.8. The elementary reversible liquid-phase reaction

$$A \rightleftarrows B$$

is to be carried out in a CSTR with a heat exchanger. Pure A enters the reactor at a molar flow rate of 10 mol/min. The inlet temperature is the same as the ambient temperature of the fluid in the heat exchanger, $T_0 = T_\infty = 320$ K. For your convenience, the fractional conversion of A is given as a function of the effluent temperature, T_e, in Fig. P16.8. Assume that the heat exchanger capacity, U_0A, can be changed at will. What is the value of U_0A required to obtain the maximum conversion, and what is the reactor temperature?

Additional data: $M_A = M_B = 58$ kg/kmol, $C_{PA} = C_{PB} = 167.4$ J/(mol·K), $\Delta H_R = -334.7$ kJ/mol at 400 K, $V = 10$ l and $Q_0 = 1$ L/min.

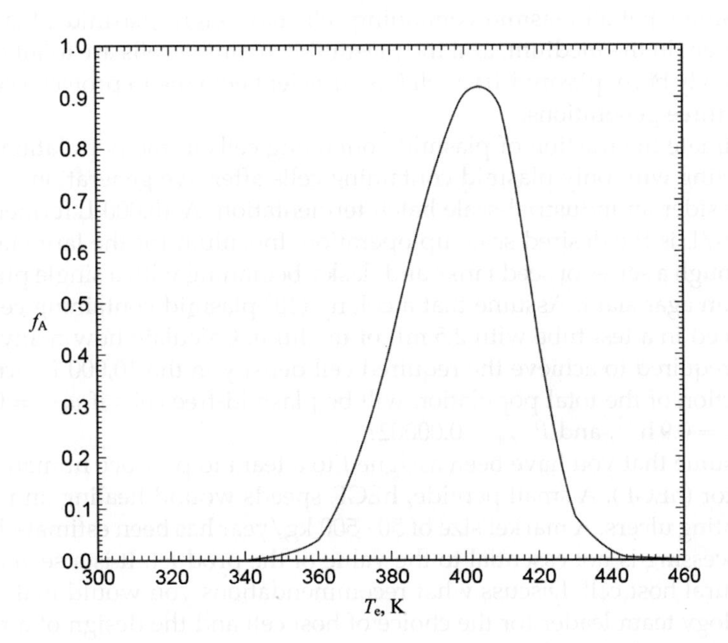

FIGURE P16.8

16.9. The liquid-phase reaction

$$A \rightleftarrows B \quad r = k_f C_A - K_b C_B$$

is to be carried out in a flow reactor. The rate constants are $k_f = \exp\left(13.18 - \frac{39,800}{RT}\right) \text{min}^{-1}$ and $k_b = \exp\left(24.78 - \frac{82,600}{RT}\right) \text{min}^{-1}$. The heat capacities are $\overline{C}_{PA} = \overline{C}_{PB} = 124\,\text{J}/(\text{mol}\cdot\text{K})$. The reactor can be operated between 290 and 500 K. The feed will be pure A.

For a CSTR capable of delivering a holding time of 1 min, what are the heat exchanger capability (UA_H) and start-up conditions required for a conversion of 0.62 if the feed and heat exchanging fluid are both at 290 K?

16.10. Given the following information, calculate the probability of forming a plasmid-free cell due to random segregation for a cell with 50 plasmid monomer equivalents:

(a) 40% of the total plasmid DNA is in dimers and 16% in tetramers.

(b) The distribution of copy numbers per cell is given in Table P16.10, assuming monomers only.

TABLE P16.10

Copy No. of plasmids	**≤3**	**4–8**	**9–13**	**14–18**	**19–23**	**24–28**	**29–33**	**34–38**	**≥39**
Population	0%	4%	10%	25%	25%	20%	12%	4%	0%

16.11. Assume that all plasmid-containing cells have eight plasmids; that an antibiotic is present in the medium, and the plasmid-containing cells are totally resistant; and that a newly born, plasmid-free cell has sufficient enzyme to protect a cell and its progeny for three generations.

Estimate the fraction of plasmid-containing cells in the population in a batch reactor starting with only plasmid-containing cells after five generations.

16.12. Consider an industrial-scale batch fermentation. A 10,000 L fermenter with 5×10^{13} cells/L is the desired scale-up operation. Inoculum for the large tank is brought through a series of seed tanks and flasks, beginning with a single pure colony growing on an agar slant. Assume that a colony (10^6 plasmid-containing cells) is picked and placed in a test tube with 2.5 mL of medium. Calculate how many generations will be required to achieve the required cell density in the 10,000 L fermenter. What fraction of the total population will be plasmid-free cells if $\mu_{G+} = 0.6\,\text{h}^{-1}$, $\mu_{G-} = 0.9\,\text{h}^{-1}$, and $P_{-/+} = 0.00002$?

16.13. Assume that you have been assigned to a team to produce human epidermal growth factor (hEGF). A small peptide, hEGF, speeds wound healing and may be useful in treating ulcers. A market size of 50–500 kg/year has been estimated. Posttranslational processing is not essential to the value of the product. It is a secreted product in the natural host cell. Discuss what recommendations you would make to the molecular biology team leader for the choice of host cell and the design of a reactor. Make your recommendations from the perspective of what is desirable to make an effective process. You should point out any potential problems with the solution you have proposed, as well as defend why your approach should be advantageous.

16.14. Develop a model to describe the stability of a continuous culture for a plasmid-containing culture. For some cultures, plasmids make a protein product (e.g. colicin in *E. coli*) that kills plasmid-free cells but does not act on plasmid-containing cells. Assume that the rate of killing by colicin is k_cCX_-, where k_c is the rate constant for the killing and C is the colicin concentration. Assume that the colicin production is first order with respect to X_+.

16.15. Consider the data in Table P16.15 for *E. coli* BIr-pDWI7 grown in a minimal medium supplemented with amino acids. Estimate $\Delta\mu$ and $\mu_{-/+}$. Compare the stability of this system to one with a glucose-minimal medium (Example 16-6).

TABLE P16.15

$D = 0.3\,h^{-1}$			$D = 0.67\,h^{-1}$		
Time, h	Generation	y_-	Time, h	Generation	y_-
0	0	0.003	0	0	0.003
4.6	2	0.010	5.2	5	0.010
11.5	5	0.04	10.3	10	0.015
16.0	7	0.08	16.5	15	0.05
23.1	10	0.30	20.6	20	0.13
27.7	12	0.43	31.0	30	0.34
34.7	15	0.55	41.4	40	0.68
46.2	20	0.96	51.7	50	0.95

16.16. It has been claimed that gel immobilization stabilizes a plasmid-containing population. A factor suggested to be responsible for the stabilization is compartmentalization of the population into very small pockets. For example, the pocket may start with an individual cell and grow to a level of 200 cells per cavity. Develop a mathematical formula to compare the number of plasmid-free cells in a gel to that in a large, well-mixed tank.

16.17. You must design an operating strategy to allow an *E. coli* fermentation to achieve a high cell density (> 50 g/L) in a continuous culturing system. You have access to an off-gas analyzer that will measure the pCO_2 in the exit gas. The glucose concentration must be less than 100 mg/L to avoid the formation of acetate and other inhibitory products. Develop an approach to control the glucose feed rate so as to maintain the glucose level at 100 ± 20 mg/L. What equations would you use and what assumptions would you make?

16.18. Develop a simple model for a population in which plasmids are present at division with copy numbers 2, 4, 8, 16, 32, or 64. You can assume that dividing cells either segregate plasmids perfectly or generate a plasmid-free cell.

16.19. Assume you have an inoculum with 98% plasmid-containing cells and 2% plasmid-free cells in a 2-L reactor with a total cell population of 2×10^{13} cells/L. You use this inoculum for a 1000-L reactor and achieve a final population of 4×10^{10} cells/mL. Assuming $\mu_{G+} = 0.5/\text{h}$, $\mu_{G-} = 0.8\ \text{h}^{-1}$, and $P_{-/+} = 0.000002$, predict the fraction of plasmid-containing cells.

16.20. Assume you scale up from 1 L of 1×10^{13} cells/L of 100% plasmid-containing cells to 27,000 L of 5×10^{12} cells/L, at which point overproduction of the target protein is induced. You harvest 6 h after induction. The value of P is 0.00004. Before induction $\mu_{G+} = 0.8\ \text{h}^{-1}$ and $\mu_{G-} = 0.9\ \text{h}^{-1}$. After induction μ_{G+} is $0.1\ \text{h}^{-1}$. What is the fraction of plasmid-containing cells at induction? What is the fraction of plasmid-containing cells at harvest?

16.21. A batch fermenter receives 1 L of medium with 5 g/L of glucose, which is the growth-rate-limiting nutrient for a mixed population of two bacteria (a strain of *E. coli* and *Azotobacter vinelandii*). *Azotobacter vinelandii* is five times larger than *E. coli*. The replication rate constants for the two organisms are: $\mu_{ECmax} = 1.0\ \text{h}^{-1}$, $k_{dEC} = 0.05\ \text{h}^{-1}$, $K_{SEC} = 0.01\ \text{gL}^{-1}$; $\mu_{AVmax} = 1.5\ \text{h}^{-1}$, $k_{dAV} = 0.10\ \text{h}^{-1}$, $K_{SAV} = 0.02$ g/L. The yield coefficients are $YF_{EC/S} = 0.5$ g-dw/g-glucose and $YF_{AV/S} = 0.35$ g-dw/g-glucose. The inoculum for the fermenter is 0.03 g-dw/L of *E. coli* (1×10^{11} cells/L) and 0.15 g-dw/L of *A. vinelandii* (1×10^{11} cells/L).

What will be the ratio of *A. vinelandii* to *E. coli* at the time when all of the glucose is consumed?

16.22. Mixed cultures (more than one distinct microbial species) are common in nature. Using two otherwise noninterfering species of different growth kinetics for feeding on the same substrate as an example, discuss the continuous culturing (chemostat) outcome. The two species are A and B. The kinetic relationships are: $\mu_{Amax} = 1.25\ \mu_{Bmax}$ and $K_{SA} = 2.5\ K_{SB}$. The death rates are negligible to both species.

(a) Is it possible to maintain both species A and B in the chemostat? Determine the corresponding dilution rate.

(b) For a given high substrate feed rate or dilution rate (see $D > 0.85\ \mu_{Bmax}$), which species would survive?

(c) For a given low substrate feed rate (see $D < 0.8\ \mu_{Bmax}$), which species would survive?

(d) Is the solution in a) sustainable?

16.23. We know that two bacteria competing for a single nutrient in a chemostat (well-mixed) could not coexist. Consider the situation where B can adhere to a surface but A cannot. Assume a is the surface area available per unit reactor volume and the rate of attachment is first order in X_B with a rate constant k_{aB}. The total sites available for attachment are $X_{BmaxAt}\, aV$. The attached cells can detach with a first-order dependence on the attached cell concentration X_{BAt} with a rate constant of k_{dB}. Attached cells grow with the same kinetics as suspended cells.

(a) Without mathematical proofs, do you think coexistence may be possible? Why or why not?

(b) Consider the specific case below and solve the appropriate balance equations for $D = 0.4\ \text{h}^{-1}$: $\mu_{Amax} = 1.0\ \text{h}^{-1}$; $\mu_{Bmax} = 0.5/\text{h}$, $K_{SA} = K_{SB} = 0.01\ \text{kg/m}^3$, $YF_{A/S} = YF_{B/S} = 0.5$ kg/kg, $S_0 = 5\ \text{kg/m}^3$, $a = 0.1\ \text{m}^2/\text{m}^3$, $X_{BmaxAt} = 1 \times 10^{-2}\ \text{kg/m}^2$, $k_{aB} = 1 \times 10^5\ \text{kg}^{-1}\cdot\text{m}^3\cdot\text{h}^{-1}$, $k_{dB} = 20\ \text{h}^{-1}$

16.24. Organism A grows on substrate S and produces product P, which is the only substrate that organism B can utilize. The batch kinetics gives rise to

$$\frac{dX_A}{dt} = \frac{\mu_{Amax}S}{K_S + S}X_A$$

$$\frac{dX_B}{dt} = \frac{\mu_{Bmax}P}{K_P + P}X_B$$

$$\frac{dP}{dt} = YF_{P/A}\frac{\mu_{Amax}S}{K_S + S}X_A - \frac{1}{YF_{B/P}}\frac{\mu_{Bmax}P}{K_P + P}X_B$$

$$\frac{dS}{dt} = \frac{1}{YF_{A/S}}\frac{\mu_{Amax}S}{K_S + S}X_A - \frac{YF_{P/A}}{YF_{P/S}}\frac{\mu_{Amax}S}{K_S + S}X_A$$

Assume the following parameter values:

$\mu_{Amax} = 0.18\,h^{-1}$; $\mu_{Bmax} = 0.29\,h^{-1}$, $K_S = 0.42$ g/L, $K_P = 0.30$ g/L, $YF_{A/S} = 0.30$ g/g, $YF_{B/S} = 0.5$ g/g, $YF_{P/S} = 1.0$ g/g, $YF_{P/A} = 4.0$ g/g, $S_0 = 10$ g/L.

Determine the behavior of these two organisms in a chemostat. Plot S, P, X_A, and X_B versus dilution rate. Discuss what happens to organism B as the dilution rate approaches the washout dilution rate for organism A.

16.25. An activated-sludge waste treatment system (Fig. P16.25) is required to reduce the amount of BOD_5 from 1 to 0.02 g/L at the exit. The sedimentation unit concentrates biomass by a factor of 3. Kinetic parameters are $\mu_{max} = 0.2\,h^{-1}$; $K_S = 0.08$ g/L, $YF_{X/S} =$ 0.50 g-MLVSS/g-BOD_5, $k_d = 0.01\,h^{-1}$. The flow of wastewater is 10,000 l/h and the size of the treatment basin is 50,000 L.

(a) What is the value of the net specific growth rate of cells, μ_{net}?

(b) What value of the recycle ratio must be used?

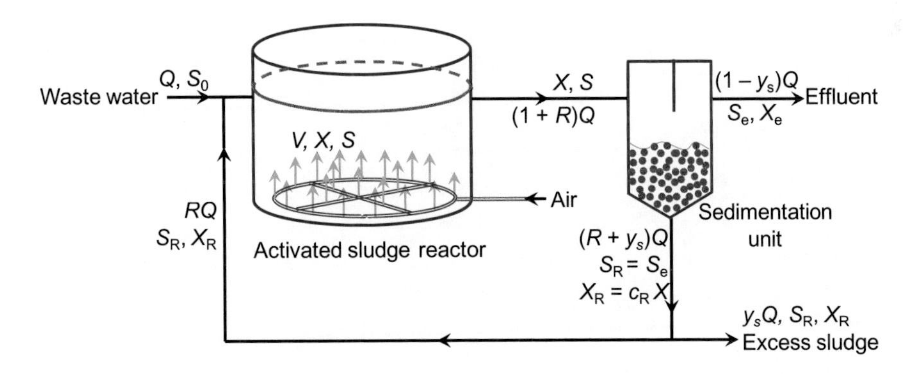

FIGURE P16.25 Schematic of an activated sludge waste treatment system.

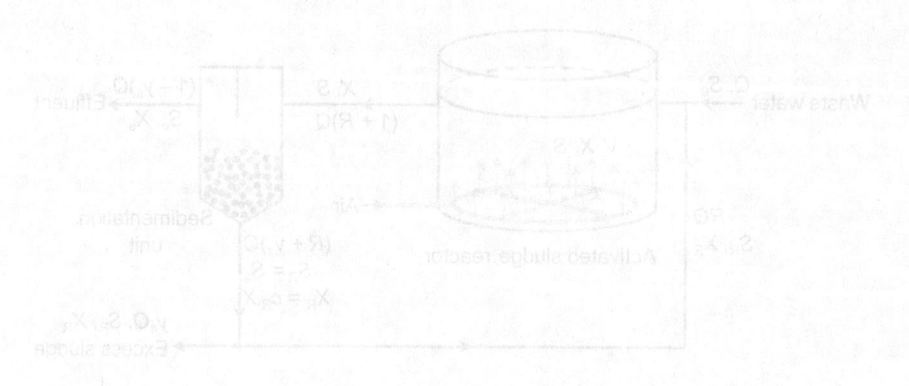

CHAPTER

17

Mass Transfer Effects: Immobilized and Heterogeneous Reaction Systems

OUTLINE

Bioprocess Engineering
http://dx.doi.org/10.1016/B978-0-444-59525-6.00017-2

With the exception of oxygen transfer, we have so far implicitly treated the bioreactions as homogeneous. In the case of multiphase systems, we have assumed that the phases are well mixed and there is no transport limitation between phases. Therefore, effectively, mass transfer effects have not been considered in our analyses other than oxygen transfer.

Ordinarily two phases are involved: gas/liquid, gas/solid, or liquid/solid. Bioreactions frequently involve three phases: gas/liquid/solid. For example, oxygen is supplied from gas phase, CO_2 produced is released into gas phase. The media are commonly liquid, or suspensions. Fermenting organisms may be viewed as solid (to be suspended into the media).

Heterogeneous catalytic reactions by nature involve a serial transport/reaction rate process, since the reaction species (substrates) must be transported to and removed from the surface site where the chemical transformation occurs. Therefore, mass transfer plays an important role in the reaction kinetics. In this chapter, we examine the effect of mass transfer on the overall rate of a reaction system.

17.1. MOLECULAR DIFFUSION AND MASS TRANSFER RATE

Mass transfer usually refers to any process in which diffusion of species plays a role. Diffusion of species is the spontaneous intermingling or mixing of atoms or molecules by random "thermal" motion. It gives rise to motion of the species relative to motion of the mixture as a whole. In the absence of other gradients (such as temperature, electric potential, pressure, or gravitational potential), molecules of a given species within a single phase will always diffuse from regions of higher concentrations to regions of lower concentrations due to the random motion of the molecules. This concentration gradient results in a molar flux of the species, which is described in general by the Fick's law,

$$\mathbf{J}_A = -D_A C \nabla x_A \tag{17.1}$$

where $\mathbf{J}_A$ is the diffusional flux of species A, D_A is the molecular diffusivity (against another species B: D_{AB} as in binary diffusion), C is the total concentration, and x_A is the volume fraction of species A in the mixture. Commonly, the volume fraction of A is understood as the same as the mole fraction, which hold true in gaseous phase.

Table 17.1 shows the magnitude of diffusivity in gaseous phase, liquid phase, and solid phase, and their relationships with respect to temperature and pressure. One can observe that the diffusivity is lowest in solid phase and highest in gas phase.

When flow-induced diffusion or dispersion is dominant, mass transfer is much faster than the molecular diffusion alone. Thermal random motion is limited by the system temperature.

TABLE 17.1 Diffusivity in Gaseous Phase, Liquid Phase, and Solid Phase

Phase	Order of magnitude, m²/s	Temperature (and pressure) dependence
Gas: bulk	10^{-5}	$D_{AB}(T,P) = D_{AB}(T_0,P_0)\dfrac{P_0}{P}\left(\dfrac{T}{T_0}\right)^{1.75}$
Gas: in fine capillaries (Knudsen diffusion)	10^{-6}	$D_A(T) = D_A(T_0)\left(\dfrac{T}{T_0}\right)^{\frac{1}{2}}$
Liquid	10^{-9}	$D_{AB}(T) = D_{AB}(T_0)\dfrac{T}{T_0}\exp\left(\dfrac{B_D}{T_0+C_D}-\dfrac{B_D}{T+C_D}\right)$
Solid	10^{-13}	$D_{AB}(T) = D_{AB}(T_0)\exp\left(\dfrac{E_D}{RT_0}-\dfrac{E_D}{RT}\right)$

Forced convection can generate much stronger fluid motion and thus induced mixing. To account for the flow-induced diffusion or dispersion, one usually resorts to mass transfer coefficient. That is,

$$N_A = k_c(C_{A1} - C_{A2}) \tag{17.2}$$

where N_A is the mass transfer flux in the direction from C_{A1} to C_{A2}. Mass transfer coefficient k_c is a function of flow, geometry, fluid, and mass transfer species.

Dwidevi PN and Upadhyay SN (*Ind. Eng. Chem. Process Des. Dev.* 1977, 16: 157) reviewed a number of mass transfer correlations for both fixed and fluidized beds and arrived at the following correlation for packed beds when $Re > 1$:

$$\varepsilon Sh = 0.4548 Sc^{1/3} Re^{0.5931} \tag{17.3}$$

where ε is the voidage or volume fraction/ratio of nonparticles in the bed, Sh is Sherwood number, Re is the Reynolds number, Sc is the Schmidt number. The dimensionless numbers are defined by

$$Sh = \frac{k_c d_p}{D_{AB}} \tag{17.4a}$$

$$Sc = \frac{\mu_f}{\rho_f D_{AB}} \tag{17.4b}$$

$$Re = \frac{d_p \rho_f U}{\mu_f} \tag{17.4c}$$

TABLE 17.2 Mass Transfer Coefficient in Gaseous and Liquid Phases, to or from Particles of Diameter d_p

Phase	Temperature (and pressure) dependence
Gas	$k_C \propto \dfrac{U^{0.5931} T^{0.777}}{(d_p P)^{0.4069}}$
Liquid	$k_C \propto \dfrac{U^{0.5931} T^{2/3}}{d_p^{0.4069}}$

where d_p is the particle diameter, μ_f is the dynamic viscosity of the fluid (liquid or gas phase), ρ_f is the density of the fluid, and U is the superficial fluid flow velocity (i.e. computed as if solid particles were absent in the bed: volumetric flow rate divided by cross-sectional area of flow). Mass transfer coefficient is thus a function of temperature, pressure, flow rate, and particle size (Table 17.2). The effect of transporting species only enters through the diffusivity D_{AB}.

17.2. EXTERNAL MASS TRANSFER

When reaction is catalyzed by solid catalyst (or enzyme or cells), the reaction is not occurring inside the bulk fluid phase. In this case, the reaction rate is only a function of the reactant concentrations right on the surface of the catalyst. The average concentration in the bulk fluid phase, C_{Ab} for species A, and that on the catalyst surface, C_{AS} for species A, are different in general due to the consumption of reactants (or generation of products). Fig. 17.1 shows a schematic of the reaction system. The solid catalyst is represented by a sphere with a radius of $d_p/2$, surface area of S and a volume of V. When pseudo-steady state is reached, the reaction rate and the mass transfer rate between the bulk and the catalyst surface must be equal. This is understood by a mass balance enclosing the catalyst (sphere) only:

$$N_A S - 0 + r_{AS} V = \frac{dn_A}{dt} \tag{17.5}$$

where n_A is number of moles of species A inside the catalyst particles, and r_{AS} is the rate of generation of A as evaluated by the concentrations on the surface of the catalyst (based on the volume of the catalyst). Since species A is not able to penetrate the solid, it is not able to accumulate inside the catalyst. Thus, the right-hand side is zero. Eqn (17.5) is thus reduced to

$$k_c a (C_{Ab} - C_{AS}) = -r_{AS} \tag{17.6}$$

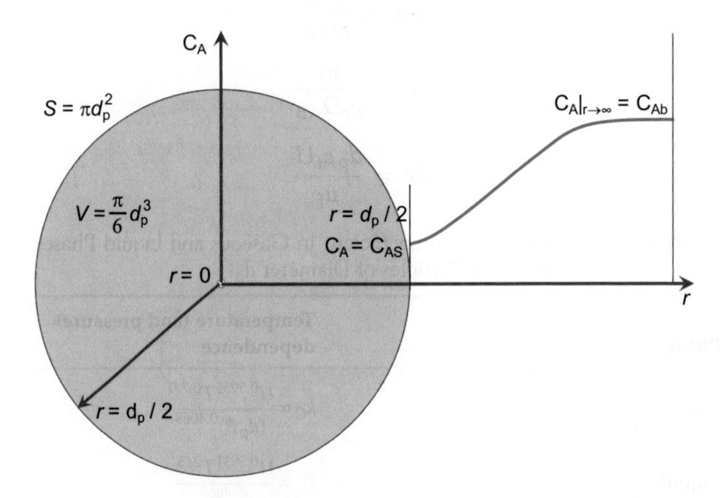

FIGURE 17.1 A schematic of a solid spherical particle and concentration of A in variation with the radial direction of the sphere.

where

$$a = \frac{S}{V} \tag{17.7}$$

is the specific external surface area of the catalyst particles.

One can infer from Chapters 8, 9, and 11 that the catalytic reaction rates are usually of the Langmuir form. For simplicity, let use the following rate form

$$-r_A = \frac{r_{max} C_A}{K_A + C_A} \tag{17.8}$$

as the base of our discussions. Here, $-r_A$ is the rate of disappearance of A based on the total volume of catalysts, and C_A is the concentration of A in the fluid phase. Eqn (17.8) can be unimolecular catalytic reaction rate, Michaelis–Menten equation, or Monod equation. When different kinetics is involved, one can replace the rate form and follow with the analyses as we will proceed.

In our analyses prior to this chapter, we have been assuming that the reaction rates can be calculated with the concentration in the bulk fluid phase. This can be true if only the mass transfer effect is negligible. There is a difference between the convenient rate form (based on the bulk fluid phase concentration) and the intrinsic kinetic rate form. Let us define an external effectiveness factor

$$\eta_e = \frac{r_{AS}}{r_A} \tag{17.9}$$

where r_{AS} is the rate calculated based on the concentrations available to the reaction (i.e. at the catalyst surface) and r_A is the rate calculated based on the bulk concentrations. It is thus intuitive that if mass transfer effects are negligible, the effectiveness factor η should be unity.

Let us consider the kinetics as given by Eqn (17.8), the effectiveness factor can be obtained if we know the value of C_{AS} for a given value of bulk concentration C_{Ab}. Substituting Eqn (17.8) into Eqn (17.6), we obtain

$$k_c a (C_{Ab} - C_{AS}) = -r_{AS} = \frac{r_{max} C_{AS}}{K_A + C_{AS}} \tag{17.10}$$

which can be reduced to a quadratic equation. There are two roots or solutions for the concentration at the surface. However, only one of them is physical, i.e. greater than zero and less than the bulk concentration. The reactant concentration of A on the catalyst surface can be solved to give

$$C_{AS} = \frac{1}{2}\left(C_{Ab} - K_A - \frac{r_{max}}{k_c a}\right) + \sqrt{\frac{1}{4}\left(C_{Ab} - K_A - \frac{r_{max}}{k_c a}\right)^2 + C_{Ab} K_A} \tag{17.11}$$

The effectiveness factor can be computed by

$$\eta_e = \frac{r_{AS}}{r_A} = \frac{k_c a(C_{Ab} - C_{AS})}{\dfrac{r_{max} C_{Ab}}{K_A + C_{Ab}}} = \frac{k_c a C_{Ab}}{r_{max}}\left(1 + \frac{K_A}{C_{Ab}}\right)\left(1 - \frac{C_{AS}}{C_{Ab}}\right)$$

$$= \frac{k_c a C_{Ab}}{r_{max}}\left(1 + \frac{K_A}{C_{Ab}}\right)\left[\frac{1}{2}\left(1 + \frac{K_A}{C_{Ab}} + \frac{r_{max}}{k_c a C_{Ab}}\right) - \sqrt{\frac{1}{4}\left(1 - \frac{K_A}{C_{Ab}} - \frac{r_{max}}{k_c a C_{Ab}}\right)^2 + \frac{K_A}{C_{Ab}}}\right] \tag{17.12}$$

If we define the external mass transfer Thiele modulus as the ratio of the reaction rate evaluated at fluid phase bulk conditions to the maximum possible mass transfer rate,

$$\phi_e = \frac{-r_{A,b}}{k_c a C_{Ab}} = \frac{\dfrac{r_{max} C_{Ab}}{K_A + C_{Ab}}}{k_c a C_{Ab}} = \frac{r_{max}}{(k_c a)(K_A + C_{Ab})} \tag{17.13}$$

Eqn (17.12) is then reduced to

$$\eta_e = \frac{1}{\phi_e}\left\{\frac{1 + \phi_e}{2}\left(1 + \frac{K_A}{C_{Ab}}\right) - \sqrt{\frac{1}{4}\left[1 - \phi_e - (1 + \phi_e)\frac{K_A}{C_{Ab}}\right]^2 + \frac{K_A}{C_{Ab}}}\right\}$$
$$= \frac{1 + \phi_e}{2\phi_e}\left(1 + \frac{K_A}{C_{Ab}}\right)\left[1 - \sqrt{1 - \frac{4\phi_e}{(1 + \phi_e)^2}\left(1 + \frac{K_A}{C_{Ab}}\right)^{-1}}\right] \tag{17.14}$$

Fig. 17.2 shows the effectiveness factor as computed by Eqn (17.14). The horizontal axis is a function of the mass transfer coefficient,

$$\phi_e^{-1} = \frac{k_c a(K_A + C_{Ab})}{r_{max}} \propto \frac{U^{0.5931}}{d_p^{0.4069}} \tag{17.15}$$

which is obtained based on the fact that r_{max} is proportional to the surface area and the mass transfer coefficient k_c is found in Table 17.2. Thus, Fig. 17.2 indicates that if one plots the effectiveness factor (or the apparent reaction rate) against $U^{0.5931}/d_p^{0.4069}$, it increases initially and finally levels off. If the apparent reaction rate is not increasing with increasing flow rate or decreasing catalyst particle size, the external mass transfer effects are negligible.

When the flow rate is low (or low agitation) and/or catalyst particle size is large, external mass transfer effects dominate the reaction system. When external mass transfer is limiting, the concentration of A on the catalyst surface becomes negligible, and

$$-r_A = \eta_e(-r_{A,b}) = k_c a(C_{Ab} - C_{AS}) \approx k_c a C_{Ab} \tag{17.16}$$

If we replot the effectiveness factor on a log-scale, Fig. 17.3 appears better at smaller mass transfer rates. When external mass transfer is dominant in the reaction system, the apparent reaction rate is of first order, irrespective of the intrinsic kinetics. For the limiting cases, Eqn (17.14) is reduced to

$$\eta_e = \min\left\{\frac{1}{\phi_e},\ 1\right\}, \text{ for } K_A = 0 \tag{17.17a}$$

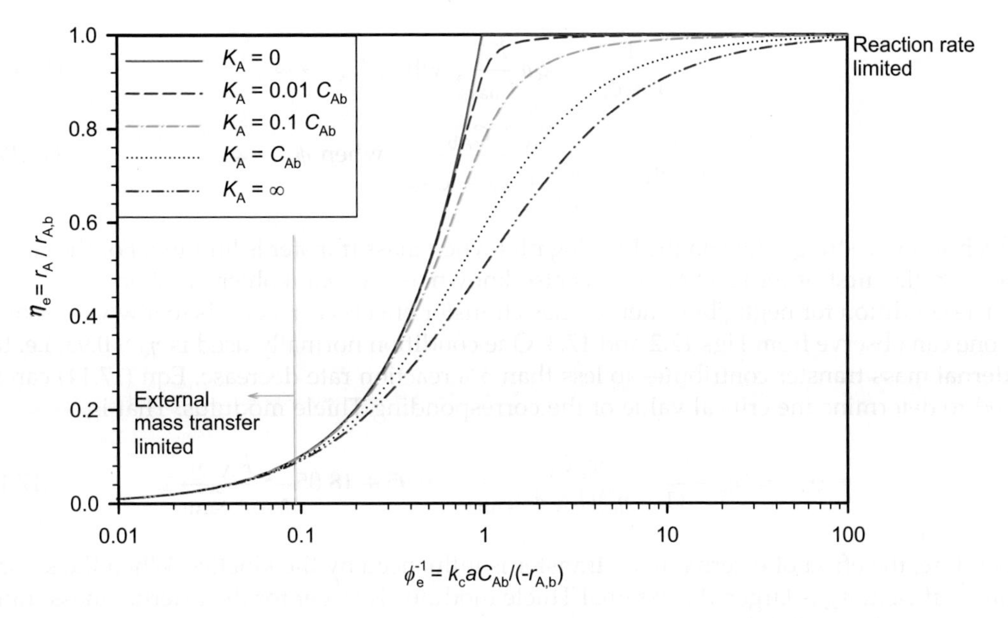

FIGURE 17.2 Effect of mass transfer coefficient on the rate of reaction.

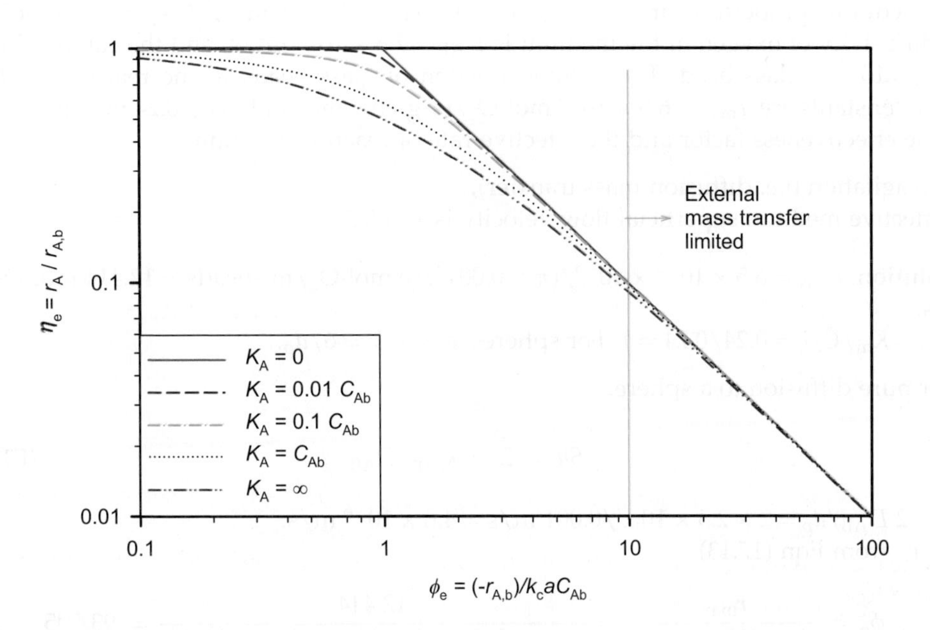

FIGURE 17.3 Effect of mass transfer coefficient on the rate of reaction on a log–log scale.

$$\eta_e = \frac{1}{1+\phi_e} = k_c a \frac{K_A}{r_{max}}, \text{ when } K_A \to \infty \tag{17.17b}$$

$$\eta_e = \frac{1}{1+\phi_e} = \frac{K_A + C_{Ab}}{\frac{r_{max}}{k_c a} + K_A + C_{Ab}}, \text{ when } \phi_e \to \infty \tag{17.17c}$$

which shows a straight line on the log–log plot when mass transfer is limiting. For the case of $K_A \to \infty$ (i.e. first-order reactions), ϕ_e is also known as the Damköhler number.

The condition for negligible external mass transfer effects corresponds to low values of ϕ_e as one can observe from Figs 17.2 and 17.3. One condition normally used is $\eta_e > 0.95$, i.e. the external mass transfer contributes to less than 5% reaction rate decrease. Eqn (17.14) can be used to determine the critical value of the corresponding Thiele modulus. That is,

$$\phi_e^{-1} = \eta_e + \frac{\eta_e^2 K_A}{(1-\eta_e)(K_A + C_{Ab})} > 0.95 + 18.05 \frac{K_A}{K_A + C_{Ab}} \tag{17.18}$$

Therefore, the effect of external mass transfer is influenced by the kinetics. When the saturation coefficient K_A is larger, the external Thiele modulus is larger for the external mass transfer effects to be negligible.

Example 17-1 Glucose oxidase catalyzes the oxidation of glucose. When glucose is present in excess, oxygen can be considered the limiting substrate. Michaelis–Menten kinetics may be applied to describe the oxygen-limited reaction rate. The enzyme is immobilized on the surface of nonporous glass beads. The particles are of $d_p = 0.001$ m, $\rho_s = 2762$ kg/m^3. The medium properties are: $\mu = 0.001$ Pa·s, $\rho_L = 1000$ kg·m^{-3}, $C_{O_2b} = 0.24$ mol·m^{-3}. The diffusivity of oxygen in the medium is $D_{AB} = 2.3 \times 10^{-9}$ m^2/s, and the catalyst loading is $[E]_0 = 10^{-6}$ g/glass bead. The volume fraction of glass beads in the reactor is 0.4. The kinetic constants are: $r_{max} = 6.5 \times 10^{-3}$ mol-O_2/(s·g-enzyme) and $K_m = 0.24$ mol·m^{-3}. Calculate the effectiveness factor and the effective rate of reaction assuming

1. no agitation (i.e. diffusion mass transfer);
2. effective medium superficial flow velocity is 1 m/s.

Solution. $r_{max} = 6.5 \times 10^{-3} \times 10^{-6}/(\pi \times 0.001^3/6)$ mol-O_2/m^3-beads $= 12.414$ mol-O_2/m^3-beads.

$K_{\beta b} = K_m/C_{Ab} = 0.24/0.24 = 1$. For spheres, $a = S/V = 6/d_p$.

1. For pure diffusion to a sphere:

$$Sh = 2 = k_c d_p / D_{AB} \tag{E17-1.1}$$

$k_c = 2\, D_{AB}/d_p = 2 \times 2.3 \times 10^{-9}/0.001$ m/s $= 4.6 \times 10^{-6}$ m/s.
Thus, from Eqn (17.13)

$$\phi_e = \frac{r_{max}}{(k_c a)\,(K_m + C_{Ab})} = \frac{12.414}{4.6 \times 10^{-6} \times (6/0.001) \times (0.24 + 0.24)} = 937.05$$

which is clearly mass transfer limiting. Eqn (17.17c) leads to

$$\eta_e = \frac{1}{1+\phi_e} = \frac{1}{1+937.05} = 1.066 \times 10^{-3}$$

The effective reaction rate is

$$-r_{A,obs} = \eta_e(-r_{Ab}) = 1.066 \times 10^{-3} \times \frac{12.414 \times 0.24}{0.24 + 0.24} \text{mol-O}_2/\text{m}^3\text{-beads}$$

$$= 6.617 \times 10^{-3} \text{mol-O}_2/\text{m}^3\text{-beads}$$

2. $U = 1$ m/s, $\text{Re} = d_p U \rho_L / \mu = 0.001 \times 1 \times 1000/0.001 = 1000$

$\varepsilon = 1 - 0.4 = 0.6$, $\text{Sc} = \mu/(\rho_L \times D_{AB}) = 0.001/(1000 \times 2.3 \times 10^{-9}) = 434.78$.

Eqn (17.3) leads to

$$Sh = \frac{0.4548 Sc^{1/3} \text{Re}^{0.5931}}{\varepsilon} = \frac{k_c d_p}{D_{AB}} \tag{E17-1.2}$$

Thus,

$$k_c = \frac{0.4548 Sc^{1/3} \text{Re}^{0.5931}}{\varepsilon d_p} D_{AB}$$

$$= 2.3 \times 10^{-9} \frac{0.4548 \times 434.78^{1/3} \times 1000^{0.5931}}{0.6 \times 0.001} \text{ m}^2/\text{s}$$

$$= 7.945 \times 10^{-4} \text{m}^2/\text{s}$$

From Eqn (17.13)

$$\phi_e = \frac{r_{max}}{(k_c a)(K_m + C_{Ab})} = \frac{12.414}{7.945 \times 10^{-6} \times (6/0.001) \times (0.24 + 0.24)} = 5.425$$

Applying Eqn (17.14), we obtain

$$\eta_e = \frac{1}{\phi_e}\left\{\frac{1+\phi_e}{2}\left(1+\frac{K_A}{C_{Ab}}\right) - \sqrt{\frac{1}{4}\left[1-\phi_e-(1+\phi_e)\frac{K_A}{C_{Ab}}\right]^2 + \frac{K_A}{C_{Ab}}}\right\}$$

$$= \frac{1}{5.425}\left\{\frac{1+5.425}{2}(1+1) - \sqrt{\frac{1}{4}[1-5.425-(1+5.425)\times 1]^2 + 1}\right\}$$

$$= 0.16748$$

The effective reaction rate is

$$-r_{A,obs} = \eta_e(-r_{Ab}) = 0.16748 \times 10^{-3} \times \frac{12.414 \times 0.24}{0.24 + 0.24} \text{mol-O}_2/\text{m}^3\text{-beads}$$

$$= 1.0396 \text{ mol-O}_2/\text{m}^3\text{-beads}$$

Therefore, increasing agitation or flow in the reactor leads to a significant increase in the effective reaction rate.

Example 17-2. Maneuvering a Space Satellite. Hydrazine has been studied extensively for use in monopropellant thrusters for space flights of long duration. Thrusters are used for altitude control of communication satellites. Here, the decomposition of hydrazine over a packed bed of alumina-supported iridium catalyst is of interest (Smith O.I. and Solomon W.C. *Ind. Eng. Chem. Fund.* 21: 374, 1982). In a proposed study, a 5% hydrazine in 95% helium mixture is to be passed over a packed bed of cylindrical particles 2.54 mm in diameter and 5.08 mm in length at a gas-phase superficial velocity of 10 m/s and a temperature of 750 K. The kinematic viscosity of helium at this temperature is 4.5×10^{-4} m^2/s. The hydrazine decomposition reaction is believed to be external mass transfer limited under these conditions. If the packed bed is 0.0508 m in length, what conversion can be expected? The bed porosity is 35% and the diffusivity of hydrazine in helium is 6.9×10^{-5} m^2/s at 298 K. Assume isothermal operation.

Solution. Hydrazine (A) decomposition reaction is represented by

$$N_2H_4 \rightarrow N_2 + 2H_2$$

which is highly exothermic and thus suitable as rock fuel. The reaction is carried out isothermally in a packed bed reactor. As a first approximation, we assume that the reactor can be characterized as a plug flow reactor or PFR (i.e. neglect the back-mixing caused by dispersion in the bed). A schematic of the reactor is shown in Fig. E17-2.1 below,

Mole balance of A (hydrazine) in the differential volume (between z and $z + \mathrm{d}z$) leads to

$$A_c U C_A|_z - A_c U C_A|_{z+\mathrm{d}z} + r_A A_c \mathrm{d}z = 0 \tag{E17-2.1}$$

where A_c is the cross-sectional area of the bed and U is the superficial flow velocity. Dividing Eqn (17-2.1) by $A_c\mathrm{d}z$ and letting $\mathrm{d}z \rightarrow 0$ and assuming U and A_c are constant, we obtain

$$-U\frac{\mathrm{d}C_A}{\mathrm{d}z} + r_A = 0 \tag{E17-2.2}$$

The reaction occurs only on the catalyst surface with catalyst not moving,

$$(-r_A)A_c\mathrm{d}z = k_c(C_A - C_{AS})a_c A_c \mathrm{d}z \tag{E17-2.3}$$

where C_{AS} is the concentration of A on the catalyst surface at axial location z and a_c is the specific surface area of the particles in the bed,

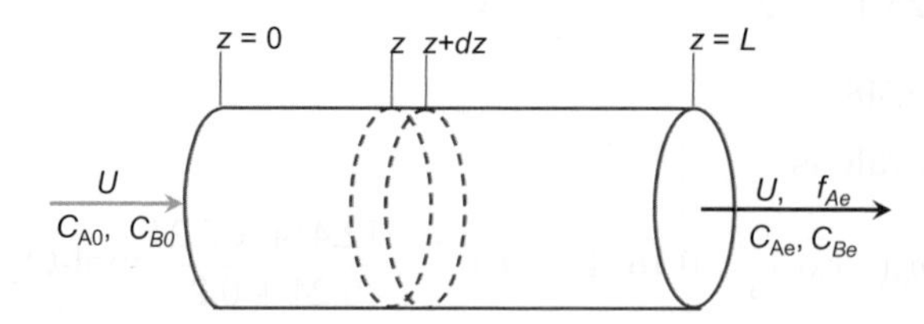

FIGURE E17-2.1 A schematic of a PFR.

$$a_c = \frac{\text{total surface of the particles}}{\text{bed volume}}$$

$$= \frac{\text{total surface of the particles}}{\text{total volume of the particles}} \times \frac{\text{total volume of the particles}}{\text{bed volume}} \tag{E17-2.4}$$

$$= \frac{2 \times \frac{1}{4}\pi d_c^2 + \pi d_c h_c}{\frac{1}{4}\pi d_c^2 h_c}(1-\varepsilon) = \frac{2d_c + 4h_c}{d_c h_c}(1-\varepsilon)$$

Here d_c is the diameter of the cylindrical particle, h_c is the length of the cylindrical particle, and ε is the bed porosity.

Since mass transfer is limiting, the concentration of A on the catalyst surface is very small as compared with the bulk concentration.

$$C_{AS} \approx 0 \tag{E17-2.5}$$

Substituting Eqns (E17-2.3) and (E17-2.5) into Eqn (E17-2.2), we obtain

$$U\frac{dC_A}{dz} + k_c a_c C_A = 0 \tag{E17-2.6}$$

Integrating with the limit $C_A = C_{A0}$ at $z = 0$, we obtain

$$\frac{C_A}{C_{A0}} = \exp\left(-\frac{k_c a_c}{U}z\right) = 0 \tag{E17-2.7}$$

The conversion of A at the end of the reactor is given by

$$f_{Ae} = \frac{C_{A0} - C_A}{C_{A0}} = 1 - \exp\left(-\frac{k_c a_c}{U}L\right) \tag{E17-2.8}$$

Now we need to evaluate the mass transfer coefficient k_c. Correlations can be found in references, for example, Perry's Chemical Engineers' Handbook. In this case, we can also use Eqn (17.3).

The particle diameter may be computed via volume average, that is,

$$d_p = \left[\frac{6}{\pi} \times \frac{1}{4}\pi d_c^2 h_c\right]^{\frac{1}{3}} = \left[\frac{3}{2}d_c^2 h_c\right]^{\frac{1}{3}} = 3.663 \times 10^{-3} \text{ mm}$$

The Reynolds number

$$\text{Re} = \frac{d_p \rho U}{\mu} = \frac{d_p U}{\nu} = \frac{3.663 \times 10^{-3} \times 10}{4.5 \times 10^{-4}} = 81.407$$

The diffusivity needs to be corrected for temperature effects,

$$D_{AB} = D_{AB,0}\left(\frac{T}{T_0}\right)^{1.75} = 6.9 \times 10^{-5}\left(\frac{750}{298}\right)^{1.75} \text{m}^2/\text{s} = 3.47 \times 10^{-4} \text{ m}^2/\text{s}$$

The Schmidt number

$$Sc = \frac{\mu}{\rho D_{AB}} = \frac{\nu}{D_{AB}} = \frac{4.5 \times 10^{-4}}{3.47 \times 10^{-4}} = 1.297$$

From Eqn (17.3), we obtain

$$k_c = \frac{D_{AB}}{d_p} Sh = \frac{D_{AB}}{\varepsilon d_p} \times 0.4548 Sc^{1/3} Re^{0.5931}$$

$$= \frac{3.47 \times 10^{-4}}{0.35 \times 3.663 \times 10^{-3}} \times 0.4548 \times 1.297^{1/3} \times 81.4^{0.5931} \text{ m/s}$$

$$= 1.824 \text{ m/s}$$

The specific surface area from Eqn (E17-2.4),

$$a_c = \frac{2d_c + 4h_c}{d_c h_c}(1-\varepsilon) = \frac{2 \times 2.54 + 4 \times 5.08}{2.54 \times 5.08} \times (1 - 0.35) \text{ mm}^{-1} = 1.280 \times 10^3 \text{ m}^{-1}$$

From Eqn (E17-2.8),

$$f_{Ae} = 1 - \exp\left(-\frac{k_c a_c}{U} L\right) = 1 - \exp\left(-\frac{1.824 \times 1.280 \times 10^3}{10} \times 0.0508\right)$$

$$= 1 - 7.06 \times 10^{-6} \approx 1$$

That is, near complete conversion.

17.3. REACTIONS IN ISOTHERMAL POROUS CATALYSTS

When active reaction sites are also available inside porous particles in addition to the external (outer) surface, one needs to account for the reaction occurring inside the particles. In solid catalysis, catalyst is supported by a solid matrix and the active sites are distributed on the surfaces inside the pores of the catalyst. In reactions catalyzed by biocatalysts, one commonly constrains biocatalyst in capsules (spherical particles), growing biocatalysts into a "thin" film, or by attaching on surfaces (slabs). In these cases, the catalytic reaction is not just occurring on the external surfaces but inside the "porous solid particles" as well. Especially in the case of encapsulation, the reaction is negligible on the external surface of the particle itself. Reaction and diffusion occur in the same time inside the particles. Therefore, internal (intraparticle) diffusion and reaction can be dominant in most heterogeneous reaction systems.

Fig. 17.4 shows two commonly encountered geometries of catalysts. The concentration of reactant A is highest in the bulk fluid phase. Mass transfer takes species from the bulk fluid phase to the solid (catalyst) external surface. Reactant A diffuses into the porous catalyst and reacted away. When it reaches the farthest side of catalyst, the concentration of A is the lowest, and no mass flow passing the farthest side.

Fig. 17.5 shows a schematic of a porous catalyst layer, which is a simplification and generalization from Fig. 17.4a and b. Other than the side marked as "outer surface" at $x = \delta_p$, all the surfaces are either impermeable (solid wall) or symmetrical conditions (i.e. zero normal

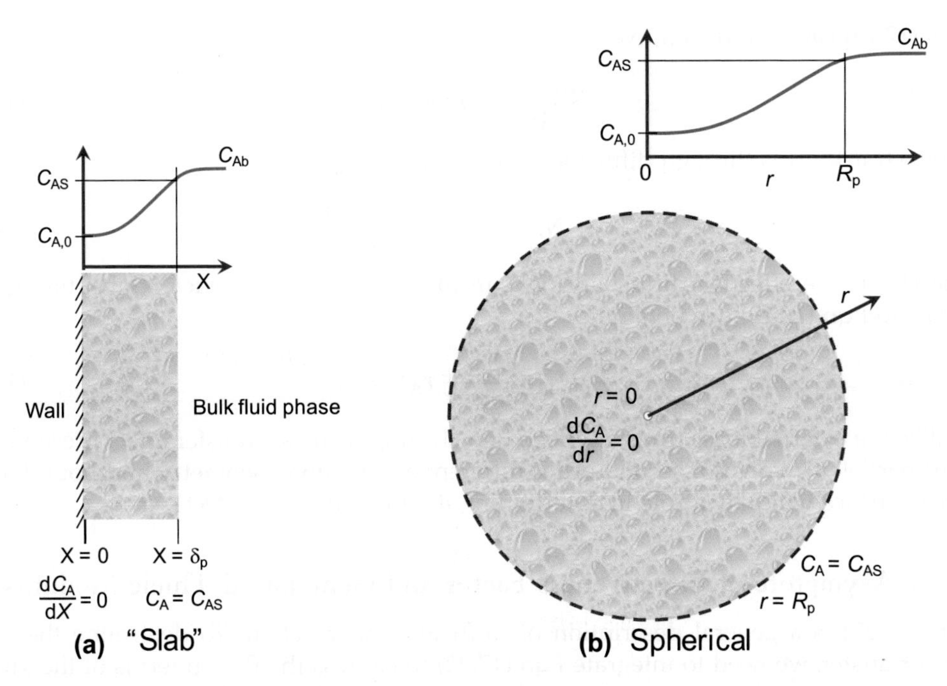

FIGURE 17.4 Schematic of mass transfer and reaction geometries for (a) an infinite slab and (b) a spherical particle.

concentration gradient) hold. Therefore, along the direction of x, one can effectively think of A is the transporting though a conduit centered along the x-axis. The cross-sectional area of the conduit may not be constant (as in the case of Fig. 17.4b). Mass balance at pseudo-steady state inside the particle, Fig. 17.5 with mass transfer flux N_A from $x + dx$ to x, leads to

$$N_A S|_{x+dx} - N_A S|_x + r_A S dx = \frac{dn_A}{dt} = 0 \tag{17.19}$$

where n_A is the number of moles of A in the differential volume (between x and $x + dx$) of particle, S is the cross-sectional area perpendicular to the path of diffusion/transport x.

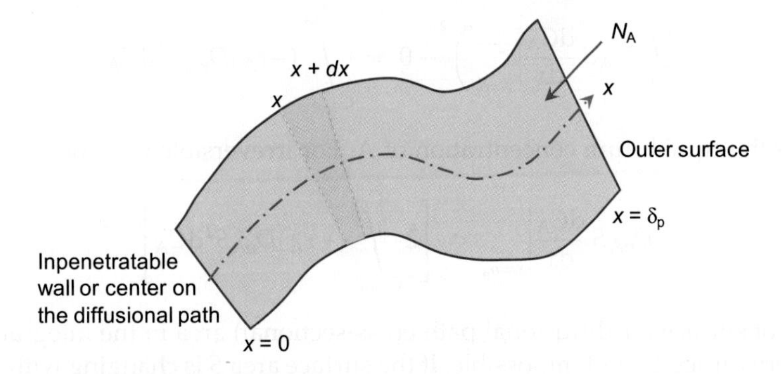

FIGURE 17.5 Diffusion and reaction along a curved path with variable cross-sectional area.

Eqn (17.19) can be reduced to

$$\frac{d(N_A S)}{dx} + r_A S = 0 \tag{17.20}$$

Since the transport is through diffusion only, we have

$$N_A = D_{eA}\frac{dC_A}{dx} \tag{17.21}$$

where D_{eA} is the effective diffusivity of A inside the "porous" particle. Substituting Eqn (17.21) into Eqn (17.19), we obtain

$$\frac{d}{dx} D_{eA} S \frac{dC_A}{dx} + r_A S = 0 \tag{17.22}$$

Unlike the external mass transfer effect, Eqn (17.10), the mass transfer effect presented by porous particles involves a second-order differential equation. Geometry and boundary or external surface will play a role in determining the mass transfer effects.

17.3.1. Asymptote of Effectiveness Factor and Generalized Thiele Modulus

Eqn (17.22) is a general description of diffusion and reaction. To determine the effect of mass transfer, we need to integrate Eqn (17.22) to express the flux in terms of the known parameters, such as the concentration at the outer surface. Eqn (17.22) can be rewritten as

$$\frac{dC_A}{dx} d\left(D_{eA} S \frac{dC_A}{dx}\right) = -r_A S dC_A \tag{17.23}$$

To integrate this equation, we need to identify reasonable boundary conditions. To find the asymptotic behavior of the effectiveness factor, we would like to make sure that when the mass transfer is limiting, geometry and reaction kinetics do not deviate the computational procedure. When mass transfer is limited, the concentration of A at the wall opposite to the outer surface (or the center of the particle if no wall) is minimum (either zero or the equilibrium concentration) and the flux of A is zero. Integration of this equation gives

$$\frac{1}{2}\left(D_{eA} S \frac{dC_A}{dx}\bigg|_{x=\delta_p}\right)^2 - 0 = \int_{C_{Ae,0}}^{C_{AS}} (-r_A) D_{eA} S^2 dC_A \tag{17.24}$$

where $C_{Ae,0}$ is the equilibrium concentration of A. For irreversible reactions, $C_{Ae,0} = 0$. Thus,

$$D_{eA} S \frac{dC_A}{dx}\bigg|_{x=\delta_p} = \left[2 \int_{C_{Ae,0}}^{C_{AS}} (-r_A) D_{eA} S^2 dC_A\right]^{\frac{1}{2}} \tag{17.25}$$

The presence of surface (or diffusional path cross-sectional) area in the integrand makes the integration very difficult if not impossible. If the surface area S is changing with x, we need to know how C_A is changing with x before the change of S with C_A can be determined.

Therefore, while Eqn (17.25) is very general, it is of very limited use. At the extreme case of mass transfer limitation, the diffusion of A into the catalyst occurs only on the thin layer of the catalyst next to the external surface and thus the cross-sectional area along the diffusion path can be assumed constant (not changing). Since we are looking for the asymptotic behavior, this is not a bad assumption to make. Therefore,

$$D_{eA}\frac{dC_A}{dx}\bigg|_{x=\delta_p} = \left[2\int_{C_{Ae,0}}^{C_{AS}}(-r_A)D_{eA}dC_A\right]^{\frac{1}{2}} \tag{17.26}$$

The overall reaction rate is balanced by the diffusion flux into the catalyst particle. Thus, the effectiveness factor can be computed by

$$\eta = \frac{r_{A,obs}}{r_{AS}} = \frac{D_{eA}S\frac{dC_A}{dx}\Big|_{x=\delta_p}}{(-r_{AS})V} = \frac{a}{-r_{AS}}\left[2\int_{C_{Ae,0}}^{C_{AS}}(-r_A)D_{eA}dC_A\right]^{\frac{1}{2}} \tag{17.27}$$

where V is the volume of the catalyst particle or a catalyst layer attached on the wall. At this point, we have determined the asymptotic behavior of the effectiveness factor. One can observe that the right-hand side of Eqn (17.27) is only a function of concentration at the outer surface, particle size, and reaction rate and diffusivity parameters. Eqn (17.27) can be rewritten as

$$\eta|_{\phi\to\infty} = \frac{1}{\phi} \tag{17.28}$$

where ϕ is called the generalized Thiele modulus. The generalized Thiele modulus is defined as

$$\phi = \frac{(-r_{AS})}{a}\left[2\int_{C_{Ae,0}}^{C_{AS}}(-r_A)D_{eA}dC_A\right]^{-\frac{1}{2}} \tag{17.29}$$

From this discussion, one can expect that when mass transfer limitation is extremely strong or the generalized Thiele modulus ϕ is large, the effectiveness factor can be computed through Eqns (17.28) and (17.29) for any reaction kinetics and any geometry. When the Thiele modulus is small, one can expect that the effectiveness factor is a function of catalyst particle geometry and a weak function of the kinetics. The effect of particle geometry is obvious as indicated by Eqn (17.24). The effect of reaction kinetics comes from the fact that the value of C_A at which the flux is zero inside the catalyst is a function of the reaction kinetics.

For the convenience of discussion, we shall define a dimensionless parameter:

$$K_\beta = \frac{K_A}{C_{AS}} \tag{17.30}$$

When $K_\beta = 0$, Eqn (17.8) reduces to a zeroth-order kinetics. When $K_\beta \to \infty$, Eqn (17.8) reduces to a first-order kinetics. In most bioreactions, the value of K_β is small. We next examine the effectiveness factor at these two extreme conditions.

With kinetics given by Eqn (17.8), the generalized Thiele modulus is given by

$$\phi = \frac{1}{a}\sqrt{\frac{r_{max}}{2D_{eA}C_{AS}}}\frac{[1 - K_\beta \ln(1 + K_\beta^{-1})]^{-\frac{1}{2}}}{1 + K_\beta} \tag{17.31}$$

17.3.2. Isothermal Effectiveness Factor for $K_A = 0$

When $K_\beta \rightarrow 0$, the reaction rate becomes constant and Eqn (17.18) can be integrated more easily. Although the reaction rate is constant, one must be aware that the reaction rate would be zero if there were no reactants available to react.

17.3.2.1. Effectiveness Factor for a Zeroth-Order Reaction in an Isothermal Porous Slab

For a slab (Fig. 17.4a), or catalyst grown (or attached) to a flat wall, Eqn (17.22) can be integrated to give

$$\int_0^{D_{eA}\frac{dC_A}{dx}} dD_{eA}\frac{dC_A}{dx} = \int_{x_0}^{x} r_{max}dx \tag{17.32}$$

which yields

$$D_{eA}\frac{dC_A}{dx} = r_{max}(x - x_0) \tag{17.33}$$

Integrate once more

$$\int_0^{C_A} D_{eA}dC_A = \int_{x_0}^{x} r_{max}(x - x_0)dx \tag{17.34}$$

Thus, the concentration inside the porous catalyst is given by

$$C_A = \frac{r_{max}}{2D_{eA}}(x - x_0)^2 \tag{17.35}$$

At the outer surface, the concentration is known and

$$C_{AS} = \frac{r_{max}}{2D_{eA}}(\delta_p - x_0)^2 \tag{17.36}$$

which can be solved to obtain the value of x_0. There are two roots, but only one of them is physical (i.e. less than δ_p):

$$x_0 = \delta_p - \sqrt{\frac{2D_{eA}C_{AS}}{r_{max}}} \tag{17.37}$$

Clearly, when $x_0 = 0$, the effectiveness factor is unit (no mass transfer effect). Because the reaction rate is constant, the effectiveness factor can be computed from the ratio of the active portion of the catalyst. That is,

$$\eta = 1, \text{ for } \phi \leq 1 \tag{17.38a}$$

$$\eta = \frac{(\delta - x_0)S}{\delta S} = \sqrt{\frac{2D_{eA}C_{AS}}{r_{max}\delta_p^2}} = \frac{1}{\phi}, \text{ for } \phi = 1 \tag{17.38b}$$

Therefore, the asymptotic behavior is the same as the effectiveness factor when $\phi \geq 1$.

17.3.2.2. Effectiveness Factor for a Zeroth-Order Reaction in an Isothermal Porous Sphere

For a spherical geometry (Fig. 17.4b), we can proceed in the same manner as for the slab. The difference is that the cross-sectional area along the diffusion path is a function of the radius. Integrating Eqn (17.22) between outer surface and inside the sphere where reactant just depleted (at $r = r_0$) gives

$$\int_0^{D_{eA}r^2\frac{dC_A}{dx}} dD_{eA}r^2\frac{dC_A}{dr} = \int_{r_0}^{r} r_{max}r^2 dr \tag{17.39}$$

which yields

$$D_{eA}r^2\frac{dC_A}{dx} = \frac{1}{3}r_{max}(r^3 - r_0^3) \tag{17.40}$$

Divide both sides by r^2 and integrate once more,

$$\int_0^{C_A} D_{eA}dC_A = \int_{r_0}^{r} \frac{1}{3}r_{max}(r - r_0^3 r^{-2})dr \tag{17.41}$$

Thus, the concentration is given by

$$C_A = \frac{r_{max}}{6D_{eA}}(r^2 - 3r_0^2 + 2r_0^3 r^{-1}) \tag{17.42}$$

At the outer surface, the concentration is given by

$$C_{AS} = \frac{r_{max}}{6D_{eA}}(R_p^2 - 3r_0^2 + 2r_0^3 R_p^{-1}) \tag{17.43}$$

which can be solved to obtain the value of r_0. There are three roots (for method of solution, see Chapter 18), but only one of them is physical (i.e. greater than 0 and less than R_p):

$$\frac{r_0}{R_p} = \frac{1}{2} + \cos\left[\frac{4\pi}{3} + \frac{1}{3}\arccos\left(\frac{12D_{eA}C_{AS}}{r_{max}R_p^2} - 1\right)\right] \tag{17.44}$$

The other two solutions are such that $\frac{4\pi}{3}$ in Eqn (17.44) is replaced by either 0 or $\frac{2\pi}{3}$. Clearly, when $r_0 = 0$, the effectiveness factor is unit (no mass transfer effect). Because the reaction rate is constant, the effectiveness factor can be computed from the ratio of the active portion of the catalyst. That is,

$$\eta = \frac{R_\mathrm{p}^3 - r_0^3}{R_\mathrm{p}^3} = 1 - \left(\frac{r_0}{R_\mathrm{p}}\right)^3 \tag{17.45}$$

For a spherical coordinate, the generalized Thiele modulus is given by

$$\phi = \lim_{K_\beta \to 0} \frac{1}{a}\sqrt{\frac{r_{\max}}{2D_{\mathrm{eA}}C_{\mathrm{AS}}}}\frac{[1 - K_\beta \ln(1 + K_\beta^{-1})]^{-\frac{1}{2}}}{1 + K_\beta} = \frac{R_\mathrm{p}}{3}\sqrt{\frac{r_{\max}}{2D_{\mathrm{eA}}C_{\mathrm{AS}}}} \tag{17.46}$$

Thus, the effectiveness factor for spherical particles is given by

$$\eta = 1, \text{ for } \phi \le \frac{\sqrt{3}}{3} \tag{17.47a}$$

$$\eta = 1 - \left\{\frac{1}{2} + \cos\left[\frac{4\pi}{3} + \frac{1}{3}\arccos\left(\frac{2}{3\phi^2} - 1\right)\right]\right\}^3, \text{ for } \phi > \frac{\sqrt{3}}{3} \tag{17.47b}$$

17.3.3. Isothermal Effectiveness Factor for $K_A \to \infty$

When $K_\beta \to \infty$, the reaction rate becomes first order (with a rate constant being $r_{\max}/K_A$) and Eqn (17.22) is a linear differential equation. The linear differential equation can be solved analytically to obtain closed form expressions.

The generalized Thiele modulus is given by

$$\phi = \lim_{K_\beta \to \infty} \frac{1}{a}\sqrt{\frac{r_{\max}}{2D_{\mathrm{eA}}C_{\mathrm{AS}}}}\frac{[1 - K_\beta \ln(1 + K_\beta^{-1})]^{-\frac{1}{2}}}{1 + K_\beta} = \frac{1}{a}\sqrt{\frac{r_{\max}}{D_{\mathrm{eA}}K_\mathrm{A}}} \tag{17.48}$$

In this case, the value of $r_{\max}/K_A$ is finite, representing the rate constant for the first-order reaction.

17.3.3.1. Effectiveness Factor for a First-Order Reaction in an Isothermal Porous Slab

For a slab geometry, the solution to Eqn (17.22) is given by

$$\frac{C_\mathrm{A}}{C_{\mathrm{AS}}} = \frac{\cosh(x\sqrt{r_{\max}/K_\mathrm{A}/D_{\mathrm{eA}}})}{\sinh(\delta_\mathrm{p}\sqrt{r_{\max}/K_\mathrm{A}/D_{\mathrm{eA}}})} = \frac{\cosh(x\phi/\delta_\mathrm{p})}{\sinh(\phi)} \tag{17.49}$$

and the effectiveness factor is given by

$$\eta = \frac{\tanh\phi}{\phi} \tag{17.50}$$

17.3.3.2. Effectiveness Factor for a First-Order Reaction in an Isothermal Porous Sphere

For a spherical geometry, the solution to Eqn (17.22) is given by

$$\frac{C_A}{C_{AS}} = \frac{R}{r}\frac{\sinh(r\sqrt{r_{max}/K_A/D_{eA}})}{\sinh(R_P\sqrt{r_{max}/K_A/D_{eA}})} = \frac{R_P}{r}\frac{\sinh(3\phi r/R_P)}{\sinh(3\phi)} \tag{17.51}$$

and the effectiveness factor is given by

$$\eta = \frac{\phi\coth(3\phi) - 1/3}{\phi^2} \tag{17.52}$$

17.3.4. Effectiveness Factor for Isothermal Porous Catalyst

In the previous sections, we have learned that the effectiveness factor can be determined fairly easily for slab and spherical geometries at the extreme values of K_A. For a finite value of K_A, Eqn (17.22) is nonlinear and closed form solution is not as easy to obtain. Therefore, numerical solution is generally used.

17.3.4.1. Isothermal Effectiveness Factor in a Porous Slab

For "thin" film and surface attachment geometries as shown in Fig. 17.4a, Eqn (17.22) is reduced to

$$D_{eA}\frac{d^2C_A}{dx^2} + r_A = 0 \tag{17.53}$$

since the cross-sectional area perpendicular to the mass transport is constant and so is the diffusivity. Again, let us consider the kinetics described by Eqn (17.8), i.e.,

$$D_{eA}\frac{d^2C_A}{dx^2} - r_{max}\frac{C_A}{K_A + C_A} = 0 \tag{17.54}$$

Letting $C_{A+} = C_A/C_{AS}$ and $x_+ = x/\delta_P$, one can reduce Eqn (17.54) to give

$$\frac{d^2C_{A+}}{dx_+^2} - 2\phi^2(1+K_\beta)^2[1 - K_\beta\ln(1+K_\beta^{-1})]\frac{C_{A+}}{K_\beta + C_{A+}} = 0 \tag{17.55}$$

Central difference scheme can be applied to solve Eqn (17.55) efficiently. The effectiveness factor can be obtained by integrating the reaction rate over the porous catalyst,

$$\eta = \frac{r_{A,obs}}{r_{AS}} = \frac{D_{eA}S\left.\dfrac{dC_A}{dx}\right|_{x=\delta}}{(-r_{AS})V} = \frac{1}{(-r_{AS})V}\int_0^\delta(-r_A)S\,dx = \frac{\int_0^1(-r_A)dx_+}{-r_{AS}} \tag{17.56}$$

Integration can be obtained via either the Trapezoidal or the Simpson's rule. Because central difference method as well as the Trapezoidal rule or Simpson's rule all have symmetrical error sequences, an extrapolation technique can be employed to speedup the convergence. Table 17.3 shows the converged solutions obtained from Excel.

The convergence of the numerical solution is fast. Still, one may not be willing to solve Eqn (17.8) every time when it is needed. Fig. 17.6 shows the effectiveness factor as a function of the Thiele modulus and K_β. One can observe that the curves in Fig. 17.6 are of the same shapes as those in Fig. 17.3. In other words, the effectiveness factor for internal mass transfer limitation is similar to that of external mass transfer limitation.

Reading numbers from tables or graphs is extremely inconvenient. At this point, we do know the closed form solutions for the two extreme cases: $K_\beta = 0$ and $K_\beta \to \infty$. It becomes natural to look for interpolation of the effectiveness factor. For example, Moo-Young M and Kobayashi T (Effectiveness factors for immobilized enzyme reactions. *Can. J. Chem. Eng.* 1972, 50:162–167):

$$\eta = \frac{\eta_0' + K_\beta \eta_1'}{1 + K_\beta} \tag{17.57}$$

where η_0' is the effectiveness factor for $K_\beta = 0$ (or for zeroth-order kinetics) with ϕ evaluated by setting $K_\beta = 0$, and η_1' is the effectiveness factor for $K_\beta \to \infty$ (or for first-order kinetics) with ϕ evaluated by assuming $K_\beta \to \infty$. For slab geometry, the maximum error is about 10% and occurs at $\phi = 1$ and $K_\beta = 0.2$.

An easier way to compute the effectiveness factor is to use the same ϕ values (of finite K_β) with the two extreme cases,

$$\eta = \frac{\eta_0[0.15\,K_\beta^{-1} + 0.3\ln(1 + K_\beta^{-1})] + \eta_1}{1 + 0.15\,K_\beta^{-1} + 0.3\ln(1 + K_\beta^{-1})} \tag{17.58}$$

with η_0 the effectiveness factor for $K_\beta = 0$ and η_1 is the effectiveness factor for $K_\beta \to \infty$. The maximum error from Eqn (17.58) is within 3%.

17.3.4.2. *Isothermal Effectiveness Factor in a Porous Sphere*

For spherical particles (Fig. 17.4b), Eqn (17.22) is reduced to

$$\frac{\mathrm{d}}{\mathrm{d}r} D_{eA} 4\pi r^2 \frac{\mathrm{d}C_A}{\mathrm{d}r} + r_A 4\pi r^2 = 0 \tag{17.59}$$

since the cross-sectional area perpendicular to the mass transport is the surface area of a sphere with a radius of r. Again, let us consider the kinetics described by Eqn (17.8), i.e.,

$$D_{eA} \frac{\mathrm{d}}{\mathrm{d}r} r^2 \frac{\mathrm{d}C_A}{\mathrm{d}r} - r_{max} \frac{C_A}{K_A + C_A} r^2 = 0 \tag{17.60}$$

Let us define the dimensionless radius and concentration by

$$r_+ = \frac{r}{R_p}, \quad \text{and} \quad C_{A+} = \frac{C_A}{C_{AS}} \tag{17.61}$$

TABLE 17.3 Numerical Solutions of the Effectiveness Factor as a Function of Thiele Modulus ϕ and Saturation Coefficient K_β for a Slab Geometry

$\phi \backslash K_\beta$	∞	10	2	1	0.5	0.1	0.01	0.001	0.0001
0.01	0.999967	0.999969	0.999975	0.999980	0.999985	0.999995	0.999999	1.000000	1.000000
0.0125	0.999948	0.999951	0.999961	0.999968	0.999977	0.999992	0.999999	1.000000	1.000000
0.015	0.999925	0.999930	0.999943	0.999954	0.999966	0.999989	0.999999	1.000000	1.000000
0.0175	0.999898	0.999904	0.999923	0.999937	0.999954	0.999984	0.999998	1.000000	1.000000
0.02	0.999867	0.999875	0.999899	0.999918	0.999940	0.999980	0.999997	1.000000	1.000000
0.0225	0.999831	0.999842	0.999872	0.999896	0.999924	0.999974	0.999997	1.000000	1.000000
0.025	0.999792	0.999805	0.999842	0.999872	0.999906	0.999968	0.999996	1.000000	1.000000
0.0275	0.999748	0.999764	0.999809	0.999845	0.999886	0.999962	0.999995	0.999999	1.000000
0.03	0.999700	0.999719	0.999773	0.999816	0.999865	0.999954	0.999994	0.999999	1.000000
0.0325	0.999648	0.999670	0.999734	0.999784	0.999841	0.999946	0.999993	0.999999	1.000000
0.035	0.999592	0.999617	0.999691	0.999749	0.999816	0.999938	0.999992	0.999999	1.000000
0.0375	0.999532	0.999561	0.999646	0.999712	0.999789	0.999929	0.999991	0.999999	1.000000
0.04	0.999467	0.999500	0.999597	0.999673	0.999760	0.999919	0.999990	0.999999	1.000000
0.045	0.999326	0.999367	0.999490	0.999586	0.999696	0.999897	0.999987	0.999999	1.000000
0.05	0.999167	0.999219	0.999370	0.999489	0.999624	0.999873	0.999984	0.999998	1.000000
0.055	0.998993	0.999055	0.999238	0.999381	0.999545	0.999846	0.999981	0.999998	1.000000
0.06	0.998802	0.998876	0.999093	0.999264	0.999459	0.999817	0.999977	0.999998	1.000000
0.065	0.998594	0.998681	0.998936	0.999136	0.999365	0.999785	0.999973	0.999997	1.000000
0.07	0.998370	0.998470	0.998766	0.998998	0.999263	0.999751	0.999969	0.999997	1.000000
0.08	0.997872	0.998003	0.998388	0.998691	0.999037	0.999674	0.999959	0.999996	1.000000
0.09	0.997309	0.997474	0.997961	0.998343	0.998781	0.999588	0.999948	0.999995	0.999999
0.1	0.996680	0.996884	0.997483	0.997954	0.998495	0.999490	0.999936	0.999993	0.999999
0.125	0.994824	0.995140	0.996070	0.996804	0.997646	0.999201	0.999899	0.999990	0.999999
0.15	0.992567	0.993018	0.994347	0.995397	0.996606	0.998845	0.999854	0.999985	0.999998
0.175	0.989915	0.990523	0.992315	0.993735	0.995374	0.998421	0.999801	0.999979	0.999998
0.2	0.986876	0.987661	0.989978	0.991818	0.993948	0.997927	0.999738	0.999973	0.999997
0.225	0.983460	0.984438	0.987336	0.989645	0.992326	0.997361	0.999665	0.999965	0.999996
0.25	0.979674	0.980864	0.984394	0.987217	0.990506	0.996720	0.999583	0.999956	0.999996
0.275	0.975531	0.976946	0.981156	0.984535	0.988486	0.996002	0.999490	0.999947	0.999995
0.3	0.971042	0.972693	0.977624	0.981598	0.986263	0.995203	0.999386	0.999936	0.999994

(Continued)

TABLE 17.3 Numerical Solutions of the Effectiveness Factor as a Function of Thiele Modulus ϕ and Saturation Coefficient K_β for a Slab Geometry—*Cont'd*

$\phi \backslash K_\beta$	∞	10	2	1	0.5	0.1	0.01	0.001	0.0001
0.325	0.966218	0.968117	0.973804	0.978407	0.983835	0.994319	0.999270	0.999924	0.999992
0.35	0.961072	0.963228	0.969701	0.974963	0.981199	0.993347	0.999141	0.999910	0.999991
0.375	0.955619	0.958036	0.965318	0.971267	0.978352	0.992281	0.998999	0.999895	0.999989
0.4	0.949872	0.952554	0.960663	0.967320	0.975290	0.991117	0.998841	0.999878	0.999988
0.43	0.942607	0.945609	0.954725	0.962254	0.971329	0.989581	0.998631	0.999856	0.999986
0.46	0.934965	0.938286	0.948413	0.956831	0.967049	0.987882	0.998395	0.999831	0.999983
0.49	0.926971	0.930607	0.941741	0.951055	0.962444	0.986008	0.998130	0.999803	0.999980
0.52	0.918653	0.922594	0.934720	0.944930	0.957509	0.983942	0.997831	0.999771	0.999977
0.55	0.910036	0.914273	0.927365	0.938462	0.952238	0.981667	0.997494	0.999735	0.999973
0.57735	0.901942	0.906437	0.920380	0.932270	0.947136	0.979395	0.997149	0.999697	0.999969
0.6	0.895081	0.899781	0.914403	0.926933	0.942693	0.977357	0.996832	0.999663	0.999966
0.65	0.879491	0.884605	0.900626	0.914501	0.932179	0.972298	0.996008	0.999572	0.999957
0.7	0.863381	0.868855	0.886112	0.901206	0.920683	0.966350	0.994966	0.999456	0.999945
0.75	0.846864	0.852638	0.870943	0.887100	0.908199	0.959340	0.993614	0.999301	0.999929
0.8	0.830044	0.836056	0.855205	0.872243	0.894734	0.951054	0.991799	0.999085	0.999907
0.85	0.813021	0.819207	0.838988	0.856706	0.880310	0.941235	0.989240	0.998761	0.999873
0.9	0.795885	0.802183	0.822382	0.840565	0.864965	0.929589	0.985371	0.998212	0.999815
0.95	0.778717	0.785068	0.805476	0.823909	0.848761	0.915808	0.978892	0.997009	0.999681
1	0.761592	0.767941	0.788359	0.806827	0.831777	0.899618	0.966528	0.991126	0.997888
1.25	0.678625	0.684325	0.702435	0.718440	0.739252	0.785859	0.799970	0.800000	0.800000
1.5	0.603430	0.607929	0.621711	0.633079	0.646287	0.665224	0.666667	0.666667	0.666667
1.75	0.537927	0.541192	0.550675	0.557753	0.564801	0.571283	0.571429	0.571429	0.571429
2	0.482012	0.484254	0.490369	0.494432	0.497852	0.499985	0.500000	0.500000	0.500000
2.25	0.434677	0.436160	0.439942	0.442164	0.443743	0.444443	0.444444	0.444444	0.444444
2.5	0.394644	0.395602	0.397878	0.399058	0.399769	0.400000	0.400000	0.400000	0.400000
2.75	0.360675	0.361282	0.362629	0.363244	0.363559	0.363636	0.363636	0.363636	0.363636
3	0.331684	0.332064	0.332851	0.333169	0.333307	0.333333	0.333333	0.333333	0.333333
3.25	0.306768	0.307004	0.307460	0.307623	0.307684	0.307692	0.307692	0.307692	0.307692
3.5	0.285193	0.285339	0.285602	0.285685	0.285711	0.285714	0.285714	0.285714	0.285714
3.75	0.266371	0.266461	0.266612	0.266654	0.266666	0.266667	0.266667	0.266667	0.266667

TABLE 17.3 Numerical Solutions of the Effectiveness Factor as a Function of Thiele Modulus ϕ and Saturation Coefficient K_β for a Slab Geometry—*Cont'd*

$\phi \backslash K_\beta$	∞	10	2	1	0.5	0.1	0.01	0.001	0.0001
4	0.249832	0.249886	0.249973	0.249995	0.250000	0.250000	0.250000	0.250000	0.250000
4.5	0.222167	0.222187	0.222216	0.222221	0.222222	0.222222	0.222222	0.222222	0.222222
5	0.199982	0.199989	0.199998	0.200000	0.200000	0.200000	0.200000	0.200000	0.200000
5.5	0.181812	0.181815	0.181818	0.181818	0.181818	0.181818	0.181818	0.181818	0.181818
6	0.166665	0.166666	0.166667	0.166667	0.166667	0.166667	0.166667	0.166667	0.166667
6.5	0.153845	0.153846	0.153846	0.153846	0.153846	0.153846	0.153846	0.153846	0.153846
7	0.142857	0.142857	0.142857	0.142857	0.142857	0.142857	0.142857	0.142857	0.142857
8	0.125000	0.125000	0.125000	0.125000	0.125000	0.125000	0.125000	0.125000	0.125000
9	0.111111	0.111111	0.111111	0.111111	0.111111	0.111111	0.111111	0.111111	0.111111
10	0.100000	0.100000	0.100000	0.100000	0.100000	0.100000	0.100000	0.100000	0.100000
20	0.050000	0.050000	0.050000	0.050000	0.050000	0.050000	0.050000	0.050000	0.050000
40	0.025000	0.025000	0.025000	0.025000	0.025000	0.025000	0.025000	0.025000	0.025000
50	0.020000	0.020000	0.020000	0.020000	0.020000	0.020000	0.020000	0.020000	0.020000
100	0.010000	0.010000	0.010000	0.010000	0.010000	0.010000	0.010000	0.010000	0.010000

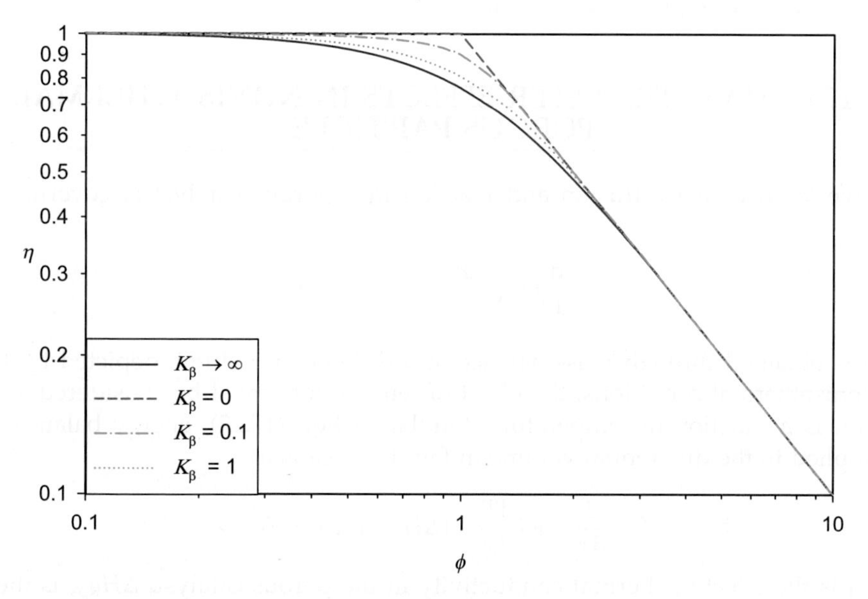

FIGURE 17.6 Effect of effectiveness factor for a slab geometry.

Eqn (17.60) can be rewritten as

$$\frac{d}{dr_+} r_+^2 \frac{dC_{A+}}{dr_+} - 3\phi^2(1+K_\beta)^2[1-K_\beta \ln(1+K_\beta^{-1})] \frac{C_{A+}}{K_\beta + C_{A+}} r_+^2 = 0 \tag{17.62}$$

Again, central difference scheme can be applied to solve Eqn (17.62) efficiently. The effectiveness factor can be obtained by integrating the reaction rate over the porous catalyst,

$$\eta = \frac{r_{A,obs}}{r_{AS}} = \frac{D_{eA} S \left.\frac{dC_A}{dx}\right|_{x=\delta_p}}{(-r_{AS})V} = \frac{1}{(-r_{AS})V} \int_0^{R_p} (-r_A) S dr = \frac{3 \int_0^1 (-r_A) r_+^2 dr_+}{-r_{AS}} \tag{17.63}$$

Integration can be obtained via either the Trapezoidal or the Simpson's rule. Because central difference method as well as the Trapezoidal rule or Simpson's rule all have symmetrical error sequences, an extrapolation technique can be employed to speedup the convergence. Table 17.4 shows the converged solutions obtained from Excel.

Fig. 17.7 shows the variation of the effectiveness factor with Thiele modulus for diffusion and reaction inside porous spheres. One can observe that the overall behavior in a spherical geometry is quite similar to that in a porous slab.

Similar to Eqn (17.58), the effectiveness factor for a sphere can be computed by,

$$\eta = \frac{\eta_0 [0.186 K_\beta^{-1} + 0.306 \ln(1+K_\beta^{-1})] + \eta_1}{1 + 0.186 K_\beta^{-1} + 0.306 \ln(1+K_\beta^{-1})} \tag{17.64}$$

with η_0 the effectiveness factor for $K_\beta = 0$ and η_1 is the effectiveness factor for $K_\beta \to \infty$. The maximum error from Eqn (17.64) is within 1%.

17.4. MASS TRANSFER EFFECTS IN NONISOTHERMAL POROUS PARTICLES

We have learned that diffusion and reaction in a porous catalyst is governed by Eqn (17.22),

$$\frac{d}{dx} D_{eA} S \frac{dC_A}{dx} + r_A S = 0 \tag{17.22}$$

which was obtained through mass balance in a differential volume depicted by Fig. 17.5. Under nonisothermal conditions, the effect of temperature must be considered as the rate of reaction is a function of temperature. Similar to Eqn (17.22), energy balance, i.e. Eqn (3.113) applied to the differential volume in Fig. 17.5, leads to

$$\frac{d}{dx} k_{eT} S \frac{dT}{dx} + (\Delta H_{R,A}) r_A S = 0 \tag{17.65}$$

where k_{eT} is the effective thermal conductivity in the porous catalyst, $\Delta H_{R,A}$ is the heat of reaction per unit amount of A (consumed).

TABLE 17.4 Numerical Solutions of the Effectiveness Factor as a Function of Thiele Modulus ϕ and Saturation Coefficient K_β for a Spherical Particle

$\phi \backslash K_\beta$	∞	100	10	1	0.5	0.1	0.01	0.001
0.01	0.999940	0.999940	0.999944	0.999963	0.999973	0.999991	0.999999	1.000000
0.0125	0.999906	0.999907	0.999912	0.999942	0.999958	0.999986	0.999998	1.000000
0.015	0.999865	0.999866	0.999873	0.999917	0.999939	0.999979	0.999997	1.000000
0.0175	0.999816	0.999818	0.999828	0.999887	0.999917	0.999972	0.999996	1.000000
0.02	0.999760	0.999762	0.999775	0.999853	0.999892	0.999963	0.999995	1.000000
0.0225	0.999696	0.999698	0.999715	0.999814	0.999863	0.999954	0.999994	0.999999
0.025	0.999625	0.999628	0.999648	0.999770	0.999831	0.999943	0.999993	0.999999
0.0275	0.999547	0.999550	0.999575	0.999722	0.999795	0.999931	0.999991	0.999999
0.03	0.999460	0.999464	0.999494	0.999669	0.999757	0.999918	0.999990	0.999999
0.0325	0.999367	0.999371	0.999406	0.999611	0.999714	0.999904	0.999988	0.999999
0.035	0.999266	0.999271	0.999311	0.999549	0.999669	0.999888	0.999986	0.999999
0.0375	0.999157	0.999163	0.999209	0.999482	0.999620	0.999872	0.999984	0.999998
0.04	0.999041	0.999048	0.999101	0.999411	0.999567	0.999854	0.999982	0.999998
0.045	0.998787	0.998795	0.998862	0.999254	0.999452	0.999815	0.999977	0.999998
0.05	0.998503	0.998513	0.998596	0.999079	0.999323	0.999771	0.999971	0.999997
0.055	0.998190	0.998202	0.998301	0.998886	0.999181	0.999723	0.999965	0.999996
0.06	0.997847	0.997861	0.997979	0.998674	0.999025	0.999670	0.999959	0.999996
0.065	0.997474	0.997491	0.997630	0.998444	0.998856	0.999613	0.999951	0.999995
0.07	0.997072	0.997091	0.997252	0.998196	0.998672	0.999550	0.999943	0.999994
0.08	0.996181	0.996206	0.996415	0.997643	0.998265	0.999412	0.999926	0.999992
0.09	0.995173	0.995205	0.995468	0.997017	0.997803	0.999254	0.999906	0.999990
0.1	0.994051	0.994090	0.994413	0.996318	0.997285	0.999077	0.999884	0.999988
0.125	0.990749	0.990808	0.991305	0.994247	0.995749	0.998548	0.999816	0.999981
0.15	0.986755	0.986839	0.987541	0.991716	0.993863	0.997892	0.999733	0.999972
0.175	0.982094	0.982206	0.983139	0.988726	0.991622	0.997102	0.999631	0.999961
0.2	0.976794	0.976936	0.978124	0.985278	0.989019	0.996171	0.999510	0.999949
0.225	0.970886	0.971059	0.972519	0.981373	0.986047	0.995089	0.999368	0.999934
0.25	0.964402	0.964609	0.966354	0.977012	0.982700	0.993846	0.999203	0.999916
0.275	0.957379	0.957620	0.959658	0.972200	0.978970	0.992427	0.999011	0.999896
0.3	0.949854	0.950130	0.952462	0.966939	0.974847	0.990816	0.998789	0.999873

(Continued)

TABLE 17.4 Numerical Solutions of the Effectiveness Factor as a Function of Thiele Modulus ϕ and Saturation Coefficient K_β for a Spherical Particle—*Cont'd*

$\phi \backslash K_\beta$	∞	**100**	**10**	**1**	**0.5**	**0.1**	**0.01**	**0.001**
0.325	0.941865	0.942175	0.944801	0.961233	0.970323	0.988994	0.998532	0.999845
0.35	0.933452	0.933796	0.936709	0.955091	0.965390	0.986937	0.998234	0.999813
0.375	0.924654	0.925030	0.928221	0.948518	0.960039	0.984618	0.997888	0.999776
0.4	0.915511	0.915917	0.919372	0.941525	0.954262	0.982003	0.997481	0.999732
0.43	0.904137	0.904579	0.908328	0.932594	0.946759	0.978419	0.996893	0.999667
0.46	0.892389	0.892861	0.896878	0.923098	0.938626	0.974266	0.996157	0.999584
0.49	0.880328	0.880828	0.885081	0.913064	0.929858	0.969440	0.995207	0.999474
0.52	0.868016	0.868539	0.872997	0.902525	0.920459	0.963811	0.993924	0.999316
0.55	0.855510	0.856053	0.860682	0.891520	0.910440	0.957224	0.992053	0.999057
0.5773503	0.843985	0.844542	0.849298	0.881115	0.900781	0.950236	0.989282	0.998457
0.6	0.834378	0.834945	0.839786	0.872256	0.892420	0.943638	0.985152	0.994165
0.65	0.813076	0.813658	0.818621	0.852034	0.872890	0.926155	0.966071	0.973093
0.7	0.791796	0.792382	0.797390	0.831095	0.852090	0.904634	0.939551	0.945454
0.75	0.770698	0.771281	0.776264	0.809691	0.830329	0.879998	0.910216	0.915300
0.8	0.749912	0.750486	0.755388	0.788067	0.807955	0.853701	0.880080	0.884520
0.85	0.729543	0.730103	0.734879	0.766453	0.785319	0.826924	0.850189	0.854108
0.9	0.709671	0.710213	0.714830	0.745048	0.762740	0.800411	0.821107	0.824595
0.95	0.690355	0.690876	0.695311	0.724019	0.740480	0.774586	0.793131	0.796257
1	0.671636	0.672135	0.676373	0.703495	0.718738	0.749683	0.766403	0.769222
1.25	0.587552	0.587935	0.591165	0.610819	0.621116	0.641131	0.651821	0.653623
1.5	0.518683	0.518971	0.521385	0.535646	0.542907	0.556878	0.564307	0.565559
1.75	0.462617	0.462836	0.464669	0.475347	0.480724	0.491026	0.496489	0.497410
2	0.416673	0.416844	0.418272	0.426533	0.430673	0.438582	0.442769	0.443474
2.25	0.378602	0.378739	0.379879	0.386452	0.389737	0.396000	0.399310	0.399868
2.5	0.346667	0.346778	0.347709	0.353061	0.355730	0.360812	0.363495	0.363947
2.75	0.319559	0.319652	0.320425	0.324867	0.327078	0.331284	0.333502	0.333876
3	0.296296	0.296375	0.297027	0.300772	0.302634	0.306172	0.308037	0.308351
3.25	0.276134	0.276201	0.276759	0.279958	0.281548	0.284565	0.286155	0.286423
3.5	0.258503	0.258561	0.259044	0.261809	0.263181	0.265785	0.267157	0.267388
3.75	0.242963	0.243014	0.243435	0.245848	0.247045	0.249316	0.250510	0.250712

TABLE 17.4 Numerical Solutions of the Effectiveness Factor as a Function of Thiele Modulus ϕ and Saturation Coefficient K_β for a Spherical Particle—*Cont'd*

$\phi\backslash K_\beta$	∞	100	10	1	0.5	0.1	0.01	0.001
4	0.229167	0.229211	0.229582	0.231707	0.232760	0.234757	0.235807	0.235984
4.5	0.205761	0.205797	0.206091	0.207774	0.208608	0.210187	0.211018	0.211158
5	0.186667	0.186695	0.186935	0.188301	0.188977	0.190258	0.190930	0.191044
5.5	0.170799	0.170823	0.171021	0.172152	0.172712	0.173770	0.174327	0.174420
6	0.157407	0.157427	0.157594	0.158546	0.159017	0.159907	0.160374	0.160453
6.5	0.145957	0.145974	0.146116	0.146928	0.147330	0.148088	0.148487	0.148554
7	0.136054	0.136069	0.136192	0.136893	0.137239	0.137894	0.138238	0.138295
7.5	0.127407	0.127420	0.127527	0.128139	0.128440	0.129011	0.129310	0.129361
8	0.119792	0.119803	0.119897	0.120435	0.120700	0.121202	0.121465	0.121509
8.5	0.113033	0.113043	0.113127	0.113604	0.113839	0.114283	0.114516	0.114556
9	0.106996	0.107005	0.107079	0.107505	0.107715	0.108111	0.108319	0.108354
9.5	0.101570	0.101578	0.101645	0.102027	0.102215	0.102571	0.102758	0.102789
10	0.096667	0.096674	0.096734	0.097079	0.097249	0.097571	0.097739	0.097768
12.5	0.077867	0.077871	0.077910	0.078131	0.078240	0.078446	0.078554	0.078572
15	0.065185	0.065188	0.065215	0.065369	0.065445	0.065588	0.065663	0.065675
17.5	0.056054	0.056057	0.056077	0.056190	0.056245	0.056350	0.056406	0.056415
20	0.049167	0.049168	0.049184	0.049270	0.049313	0.049393	0.049436	0.049443
22.5	0.043786	0.043787	0.043799	0.043868	0.043902	0.043965	0.043999	0.044004
25	0.039467	0.039468	0.039478	0.039533	0.039560	0.039612	0.039639	0.039643
27.5	0.035923	0.035924	0.035932	0.035978	0.036000	0.036043	0.036065	0.036069
30	0.032963	0.032964	0.032971	0.033009	0.033028	0.033064	0.033083	0.033086
35	0.028299	0.028300	0.028305	0.028333	0.028347	0.028373	0.028387	0.028390
40	0.024792	0.024792	0.024796	0.024818	0.024828	0.024848	0.024859	0.024861
45	0.022058	0.022058	0.022061	0.022078	0.022087	0.022102	0.022111	0.022112
50	0.019867	0.019867	0.019869	0.019883	0.019890	0.019903	0.019910	0.019911
55	0.018072	0.018072	0.018074	0.018085	0.018091	0.018102	0.018107	0.018108
60	0.016574	0.016574	0.016576	0.016586	0.016590	0.016599	0.016604	0.016605
70	0.014218	0.014218	0.014219	0.014226	0.014230	0.014236	0.014240	0.014240
80	0.012448	0.012448	0.012449	0.012454	0.012457	0.012462	0.012465	0.012465
90	0.011070	0.011070	0.011071	0.011075	0.011077	0.011081	0.011083	0.011084
100	0.009967	0.009967	0.009967	0.009971	0.009973	0.009976	0.009977	0.009978

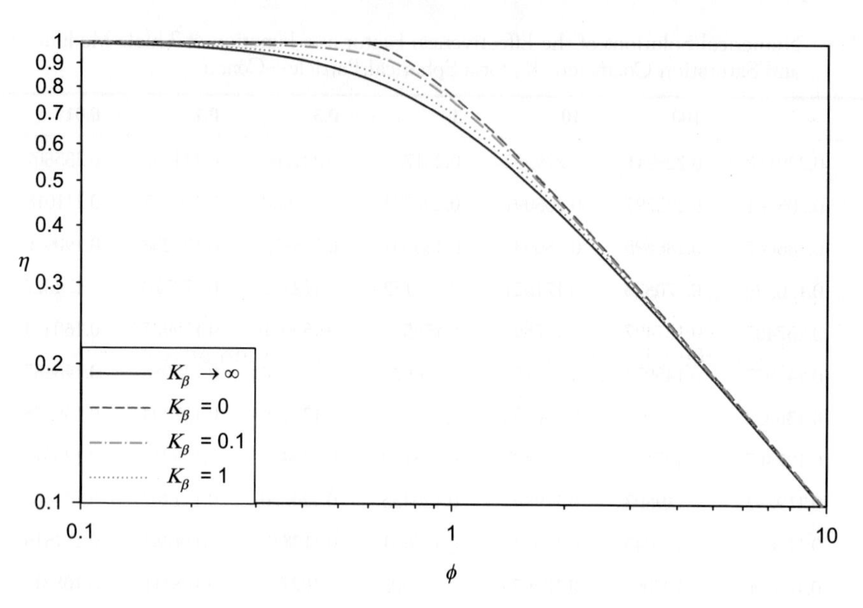

FIGURE 17.7 Effect of effectiveness factor for spherical geometry.

Instead of having one differential equation (for isothermal cases), we now have two differential Eqns (17.22) and (17.65). If the heat of reaction is constant, i.e. not a function of temperature (and pressure, or concentration), Eqn (17.65) – $(\Delta H_{R,A}) \times$ Eqn (17.22) yield,

$$\frac{d}{dx} k_{eT} S \frac{dT}{dx} - (\Delta H_{R,A}) \frac{d}{dx} D_{eA} S \frac{dC_A}{dx} = 0 \tag{17.66}$$

Integrate (17.66) once, we obtain

$$k_{eT} S \frac{dT}{dx} - (\Delta H_{R,A}) D_{eA} S \frac{dC_A}{dx} = \left[k_{eT} S \frac{dT}{dx} - (\Delta H_{R,A}) D_{eA} S \frac{dC_A}{dx} \right]_{x=0} \tag{17.67}$$

When $x = 0$ or $C_A = 0$ (i.e. the deepest location inside the porous catalyst the reactant diffuses to), both heat flux and mass transfer flux are zero. Therefore, the right-hand side of Eqn (17.67) is zero. Dividing through by S and integrating the resultant equation, we obtain

$$k_{eT} T - (\Delta H_{R,A}) D_{eA} C_A = k_{eT} T_S - (\Delta H_{R,A}) D_{eA} C_{AS} \tag{17.68}$$

where T_S is the temperature on the external surface of the catalyst. We have assumed constant k_{eT} and D_{eA} to arrive at Eqn (17.68). Rearranging Eqn (17.68), we obtain

$$T = T_S + \frac{(-\Delta H_{R,A}) D_{eA}}{k_{eT}} (C_{AS} - C_A) \tag{17.69}$$

Therefore, the temperature is linearly related to the concentration and thus the internal effectiveness factor can be evaluated by solving one differential Eqn (17.22) with temperature given by Eqn (17.69). This significantly reduced the computing power needed.

Let,

$$\beta = \frac{(-\Delta H_{R,A}) D_{eA} C_{AS}}{k_{eT} T_S} \tag{17.70}$$

Eqn (17.69) is reduced to

$$\frac{T}{T_S} = 1 + \beta\left[1 - \frac{C_A}{C_{AS}}\right] = 1 + \beta(1 - C_{A+}) \tag{17.71}$$

The parameter β can be viewed as the ratio of maximum possible temperature difference divided by the external surface temperature. Since the maximum temperature deviation from the external surface is at the location where concentration of A is zero. That is,

$$\frac{T_{max}}{T_S} = 1 + \beta[1 - 0] \tag{17.72}$$

or

$$\beta = \frac{T_{max} - T_S}{T_S} = \frac{\Delta T_{max}}{T_S} \tag{17.73}$$

Because the rate of reaction usually increases with temperature (if catalyst is not denatured or thermally destabilized), one can thus expect the effectiveness factor to be greater than 1 if the reaction is exothermic ($\Delta H_{R,A} < 0$). For kinetics given by Eqn (17.8), there are two parameters, r_{max} and K_A, and both changes with temperature. For simplicity, let us assume that K_A changes with temperature weakly and thus nearly a constant. Arrhenius law renders

$$r_{max} = r_{max,0} \exp\left(-\frac{E_a}{RT}\right) \tag{17.74}$$

where E_a is the activation energy. Let

$$\gamma = \frac{E_a}{RT_S} \tag{17.75}$$

Eqn (17.8) is reduced to

$$-r_A = \frac{r_{max,0} C_A}{K_A + C_A} \exp\left(-\frac{T_S}{T}\gamma\right) = \frac{r_{max,0} C_{A+}}{K_\beta + C_{A+}} \exp\left[-\frac{\gamma}{1 + \beta - \beta C_{A+}}\right] \tag{17.76}$$

Thus, the asymptotic behavior can be obtained via the generalized Thiele modulus, Eqn (17.29), or

$$\phi = \frac{-r_{AS}}{a}\left[2\int_{C_{Ae,0}}^{C_{AS}} (-r_A) D_{eA} \mathrm{d}C_A\right]^{-\frac{1}{2}} \tag{17.29}$$

which yields

$$\phi = \sqrt{\frac{r_{max,0}}{2 D_{eA} C_{AS}}} \frac{e^{-\gamma}}{1 + K_\beta} \frac{1}{a}\left[\int_0^1 \frac{C_{A+}}{K_\beta + C_{A+}} \exp\left(-\frac{\gamma}{1 + \beta - \beta C_{A+}}\right) \mathrm{d}C_{A+}\right]^{-\frac{1}{2}} \tag{17.77}$$

The nonisothermal effects for internal diffusion limited cases can be quantified by

$$\frac{\phi_{\beta=0}^2}{\phi^2} = e^{\gamma} \frac{\int_0^1 \frac{C_{A+}}{K_\beta + C_{A+}} \exp\left(-\frac{\gamma}{1+\beta-\beta C_{A+}}\right) dC_{A+}}{1 - K_\beta \ln(1 + K_\beta^{-1})} \tag{17.78}$$

Therefore, the impact of nonisothermal effects can be significant. Higher effectiveness factor is obtained for higher β.

Table 17.5 shows the thermal parameters for some exothermic catalytic reaction systems. One can observe that the value of β is commonly less than 0.2 and the range of γ is between 10 and 30.

Fig. 17.8 shows the internal effectiveness factor with thermal effects for diffusion and reaction in a "porous" sphere. The solid curves are numerical solutions, whereas the dashed lines are the asymptotic solutions as given

$$\eta = \frac{1}{\phi} = a(1 + K_\beta) e^{\gamma} \sqrt{\frac{2 D_{eA} C_{AS}}{r_{max,0}}} \left[\int_0^1 \frac{C_{A+}}{K_\beta + C_{A+}} \exp\left(-\frac{\gamma}{1+\beta-\beta C_{A+}}\right) dC_{A+} \right]^{\frac{1}{2}} \tag{17.79}$$

One can observe that the effectiveness factor can be greater than 1 for exothermic reactions ($\beta > 0$) and multiple steady states can exist at small Thiele modulus for highly exothermic reactions.

Example 17-3. Particle size effect. A decomposition reaction is carried out on a solid catalyst

$$A \rightarrow B + C$$

over two different pellet sizes. The pellets were contained in a differential reactor that has sufficient turbulence such that the external mass transfer effects are negligible. We know that the adsorption coverage of A on the catalyst site is minimal and thus $K_A \rightarrow \infty$. The

TABLE 17.5 Thermal Parameters for Some Exothermic Catalytic Reactions

Reaction system	β	γ
Ammonia synthesis	6.1×10^{-5}	29.4
Methanol oxidation	1.1×10^{-2}	16.0
Ethylene hydrogenation	6.6×10^{-2}	23.3
Benzene hydrogenation	1.2×10^{-1}	14.2
Sulfur dioxide oxidation	1.2×10^{-2}	14.8

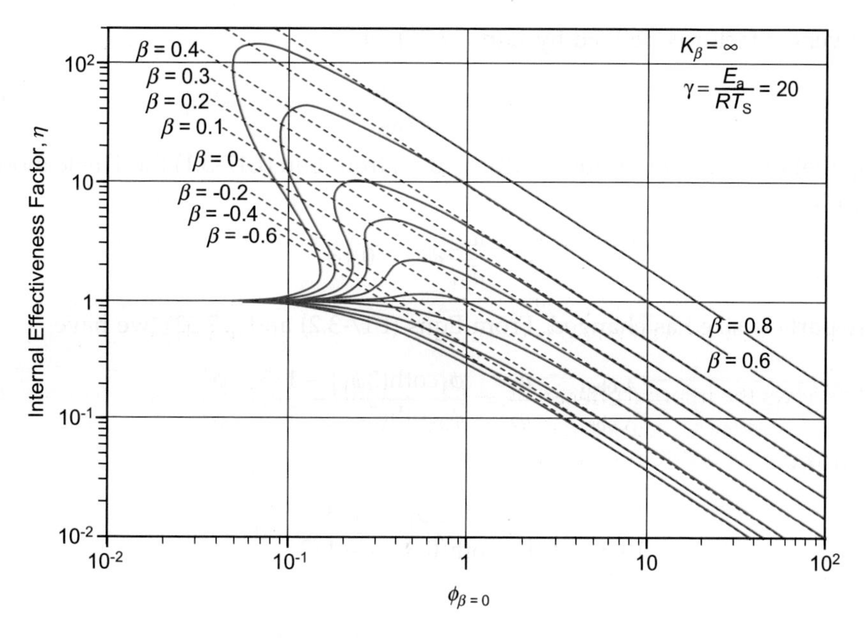

FIGURE 17.8 Thermal effect on the effectiveness factor for spherical geometry.

reaction on the catalyst surface is thus virtually first order. The results of two experimental runs made under identical conditions are as shown in Table E17-3.1. Estimate the Thiele modulus and effectiveness factor for each pellet. How small should the pellets be made to virtually eliminate all internal diffusion effects on the overall reaction kinetics?

TABLE E17-3.1

	Pellet size, mm	Measured Rate, mol-A/(g-cat·s)
Run 1	2.54	2.00
Run 2	0.254	10.5

Solution. When $K_A \to \infty$, the Thiele modulus is defined by Eqn (17.48), or

$$\phi = \frac{d_p}{6}\sqrt{\frac{r_{max}}{D_{eA}K_A}} \tag{E17-3.1}$$

and the effectiveness factor is given by Eqn (17.52),

$$\eta = \frac{\phi \coth(3\phi) - 1/3}{\phi^2} \tag{17.52}$$

The effectiveness factor is defined by Eqn (17.27), or

$$\eta = \frac{-r_{A,obs}}{-r_{AS}} \tag{E17-3.2}$$

Assuming that the Thiele modulus for Run 1 is ϕ_1, from Eqn (E17-3.1) the Thiele modulus for Run 2 is given by

$$\phi_2 = \frac{d_{p2}}{d_{p1}}\phi_1 = 0.1\phi_1 \tag{E17-3.3}$$

since only particle size has changed. From Eqns (E17-3.2) and (17.52), we have

$$\frac{-r_{A,obs1}}{-r_{A,obs2}} = \frac{\eta_1}{\eta_2} = \frac{\phi_1 \coth(3\phi_1) - 1/3}{\phi_2 \coth(3\phi_2) - 1/3} \times \frac{\phi_2^2}{\phi_1^2} \tag{E17-3.4}$$

which leads to

$$\frac{2.00}{10.5} = \frac{\phi_1 \coth(3\phi_1) - 1/3}{0.1\phi_1 \coth(0.3\phi_1) - 1/3} \times 0.01$$

or

$$0.0525 = \frac{0.1\phi_1 \coth(0.3\phi_1) - 1/3}{\phi_1 \coth(\phi_1) - 1/3} \tag{E17-3.5}$$

This equation can be solved to give $\phi_1 = 5.9103$. Therefore, we can compute

$\eta_1 = 0.15965$ by using Eqn (17.52);
$\phi_2 = 0.59103$ by using Eqn (E17-3.3);
$\eta_2 = 0.83188$ by using Eqn (17.52).

For negligible intraparticle diffusion effects, we set $\eta_3 > 0.95$. From Eqn (17.52), we obtain $\phi_3 < 0.299529$.

From Eqn (E17-3.1), $\frac{\phi_3}{\phi_1} = \frac{d_{p3}}{d_{p1}}$. Thus, $d_{p3} = \frac{\phi_3}{\phi_1} d_{p1} < \frac{0.299529}{5.9103} \times 2.54\,\text{mm} = 0.1287\,\text{mm}$.

Therefore, when the pellet size is smaller than 0.1287 mm, the internal diffusion effects are virtually eliminated.

Example 17-4. Isothermal internal effectiveness factor for different kinetics. We have discussed the internal kinetics using a particular example, Eqn (17.8), which is an irreversible rate equation. What happens if different kinetics is observed? The least we can be sure is that the procedure we have learned can be applied to any kinetics. In some cases, the results can even be directly used. Here is an example: reaction

$$A \rightleftarrows B \tag{E17-4.1}$$

occurs on a single site solid catalyst. LHHW kinetics is given by

$$-r_A = \frac{k'(C_A - C_B/K_C)}{1 + K'_A C_A + K'_B C_B} \tag{E17-4.2}$$

which is identical to Eqn (9.88) except we have used primes here for the kinetic constants. In the reaction mixture (bulk fluid phase), the concentration of A and B together are $C_0 = C_A + C_B$. Derive the effectiveness factor for this reaction system.

Solution. This is a reversible kinetics case. From stoichiometry, we obtain

$$C_A + C_B = C_0 = \text{constant} \tag{E17-4.3}$$

and this is valid anywhere inside the catalyst when pseudo-steady state has established. Thus, Eqn (E17-4.2) can be written in terms of C_A only by making use of this stoichiometry relation, Eqn (E17-4.3). That is,

$$-r_A = \frac{k'[C_A - (C_0 - C_A)/K_C]}{1 + K'_A C_A + K'_B(C_0 - C_A)} \tag{E17-4.4}$$

Let

$$C'_A = C_A - \frac{C_0}{1 + K_C} \tag{E17-4.5}$$

Eqn (E17-4.4) can be further reduced to

$$-r_A = \left(1 + \frac{1}{K_C}\right) \frac{k'}{K'_A - K'_B} \frac{C'_A}{\dfrac{1 + (K'_A + K_C K'_B)C_0/(1 + K_C)}{K'_A - K'_B} + C'_A} \tag{E17-4.6}$$

which can be reduced to

$$-r_A = \frac{r_{max} C'_A}{K_A + C'_A} \tag{E17-4.7}$$

where

$$r_{max} = \left(1 + \frac{1}{K_C}\right) \frac{k'}{K'_A - K'_B} = \frac{(1 + K_C)k'}{K_C(K'_A - K'_B)} \tag{E17-4.8a}$$

$$K_A = \frac{1 + (K'_A + K_C K'_B)C_0/(1 + K_C)}{K'_A - K'_B} \tag{E17-4.8b}$$

Therefore, this reversible kinetics is reduced to the same form as the irreversible kinetics given by Eqn (17.8) with the exception that the concentration of A is replaced by the difference of concentration of A from the equilibrium concentration of A as given by Eqn (E17-4.5). Since the equilibrium concentration is constant, and from Eqn (17.22)

$$\frac{d}{dx} D_{eA} S \frac{dC_A}{dx} + r_A S = 0 \tag{17.22}$$

we obtain the governing equation inside the porous catalyst as

$$\frac{d}{dx} D_{eA} S \frac{dC'_A}{dx} + r_A S = 0 \tag{E17-4.9}$$

That is, the solution we obtained so far is directly applicable since the derivative of a constant is zero. By definition, the generalized Thiele modulus is given by

$$\phi = \frac{(-r_{AS})}{a}\left[2\int_{C_{Ae,0}}^{C_{AS}}(-r_A)D_{eA}dC_A\right]^{-\frac{1}{2}} \tag{17.29}$$

Noting that

$$C'_{Ae,0} = C_{Ae,0} - \frac{C_0}{1+K_C} = 0 \tag{E17-4.10a}$$

$$C_{Ae,0} = \frac{C_0}{1+K_C} \tag{E17-4.10b}$$

Eqn (17.29) is integrated out to give

$$\phi = \frac{1}{a}\sqrt{\frac{r_{max}}{2D_{eA}C'_{AS}}}\frac{[1-K_\beta \ln(1+K_\beta^{-1})]^{-\frac{1}{2}}}{1+K_\beta} \tag{E17-4.11}$$

with K_β given by Eqn (17.30), r_{max} and K_A given by Eqn (E17-4.8), and

$$C'_{AS} = C_{AS} - \frac{C_0}{1+K_C} \tag{E17-4.12}$$

Indeed, the equation for the Thiele modulus is directly applicable, Eqn (E17-4.11) is identical to (17.31).

This last example shows that when different kinetics is observed, the same approach to effectiveness factor can be applied. The key to the analysis is to convert all the dependent variables (i.e. concentrations) into one single dependent variable (concentration). While the final forms of equations may or may not the same, one can solve the equations in the same manner. We also learned in this section that nonisothermal reaction systems can be treated in the same way, with one additional (energy balance) equation.

17.5. EXTERNAL AND INTERNAL MASS TRANSFER EFFECTS

When both internal and external mass transfer effects are important, the rate of the reaction system is governed by

$$k_c a(C_{Ab} - C_{AS}) = aN_A|_{\text{To surface}} = -D_{eA}a\left.\frac{dC_A}{dx}\right|_{\text{at surface}} = (-r_{AS})\eta \tag{17.79}$$

That is, mass transfer from the bulk fluid phase to the external catalyst surface is the same as the mass transfer flux into the catalyst particle and the same as the observed reaction rate (or effective reaction rate).

The overall effectiveness factor can be defined as

$$\eta_o = \frac{r_{A,obs}}{r_{A,b}} = \eta_e \eta \tag{17.80}$$

Thus, the combined effect of internal mass transfer (and nonisothermal effects) and the external mass transfer effects can be determined from the analyses of the previous sections. Iterative solutions may be needed as the surface concentration needs to be determined in the same time as the effectiveness factor η is determined.

Example 17-5. Nitrate in groundwater is becoming more of a problem. In addition to measures aiming at applying lower loads of fertilizers, the need for effective treatment procedures is increasing. One of the alternatives investigated is removal of nitrate by conversion to gaseous N_2 using denitrifying bacteria immobilized in gel beads. Calculate the required size of an ideally mixed bioreactor treating 100 m^3/h of groundwater. The concentration of nitrate in the groundwater is 50 g/m^3 and the treated water contains 1 g/m^3 nitrate. The load of gel beads in the reactor is 0.2 m^3-gel/m^3-reaction mixture. The diameter of the gel beads is 1.5 mm, the diffusivity of nitrate inside the gel is 10^{-10} m^2/s. Mass transfer coefficient of nitrate in the reactor is 10^{-5} m/s. The kinetic constant are given by $r_{max} = 0.4$ g/(s·m^3-gel) and $K_m = 2$ g·m^{-3}.

Solution: The bioreactor is ideally well-mixed (or CSTR, as shown in Fig. E17-5.1); thus the concentration of nitrate in the reactor is equal to the concentration in the effluent, i.e. $C_{Ab} = 1$ g·m^{-3}. Mass balance of A (nitrate) over the CSTR gives

$$QC_{A0} - QC_{Ab} + r_A V = 0 \tag{E17-5.1}$$

The reaction occurs inside the gel (particle), and nitrate must diffuse from the bulk solution to the gel surface. Thus,

$$\begin{aligned}(-r_A)V &= \eta(-r_{AS})V_{gel} \\ &= k_c a_c V(C_{Ab} - C_{AS})\end{aligned} \tag{E17-5.2}$$

where V_{gel} is the total volume of gel particles, r_{AS} is the rate of reaction based on the gel volume and concentration of A on the external surface of gel particle, a_c is the specific area of gel external surface area (over the reactor volume), and η is the internal effectiveness factor.

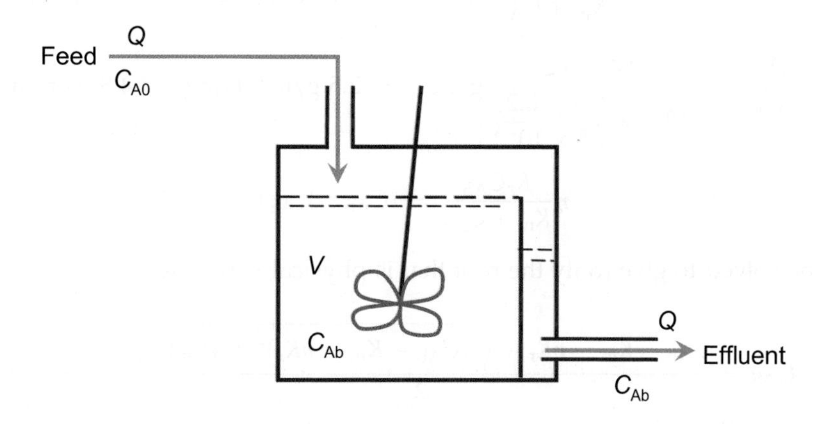

FIGURE E17-5.1 A schematic of the CSTR water treatment system.

The rate of reaction can be expressed as

$$r_A = \frac{r_{max} C_A}{K_m + C_A} \tag{E17-4.3}$$

when the reaction rate and concentration of A are evaluated based on the gel volume. The kinetic parameters are given by $r_{max} = 0.4$ g/(s/m^3-gel) and $K_m = 2$ g/m^3-gel. To compute the effectiveness factor, we need both K_β and ϕ. From the saturation constant,

$$K_\beta = \frac{K_m}{C_{AS}} \tag{E17-4.4}$$

and the Thiele modulus can be computed by Eqn (17.31) or

$$\phi = \frac{d_p}{6}\sqrt{\frac{r_{max}}{2D_{eA}C_{AS}}}\,\frac{[1 - K_\beta \ln(1 + K_\beta^{-1})]^{-1/2}}{1 + K_\beta} \tag{E17-4.5}$$

Both K_β and ϕ require C_{AS}, which is an unknown that needs to be determined from Eqn (E17-4.2). Therefore, iterative scheme is needed to solve the problem.

Since $C_{AS} < C_{Ab} = 1$ g/m^3, we know from Eqn (E17-4.4) that $K_\beta > 2$. We can start the iterative solution by assuming $K_\beta \to \infty$. Eqn (E17-4.5) leads to

$$\phi|_{K_\beta \to \infty} = \frac{d_p}{6}\sqrt{\frac{r_{max}}{D_{eA}K_m}} \tag{E17-4.6}$$

$\phi_{K_\beta} \to \infty = 11.18$. From Eqn (17.52),

$$\eta_1 = \frac{\phi \coth(3\phi) - 1/3}{\phi^2} \tag{E17-4.7}$$

$\eta = 0.08678$. With a value of η, we can solve for concentration of nitrate on the gel surface through Eqn (E17-4.2), or

$$\eta \frac{r_{max} C_{AS}}{K_m + C_{AS}} V_{gel} = k_c a_c V (C_{Ab} - C_{AS}) \tag{E17-4.8}$$

Let $K_r = \dfrac{r_{max} V_{gel}}{k_c a_c V} = \dfrac{0.4 \times 0.2}{10^{-5} \times \dfrac{6(1-0.2)}{1.5 \times 10^{-3}}}$ g/m^3 $= 2.5$ g/m^3. Eqn (E17-4.8) is reduced to

$$\eta \frac{K_r C_{AS}}{K_m + C_{AS}} = (C_{Ab} - C_{AS}) \tag{E17-4.8}$$

which can be solved to give (only the root that is physical is retained):

$$C_{AS} = \frac{C_{Ab} - K_m - \eta K_r + \sqrt{(C_{Ab} - K_m - \eta K_r)^2 + 4K_m C_{Ab}}}{2} \tag{E17-4.9}$$

That is, $C_{AS} = 0.93108$ g/m^3.

Now if we assume $C_{AS} = 0.93108\ \text{g/m}^3$: Eqn (E17-4.4) gives $K_\beta = 2.148$; $\phi = 8.700$; Eqn (E17-4.7) gives $\eta_1 = 0.11054$; Eqn (17.47b) gives $\eta_0 = 0.1120$; Eqn (17.64) gives $\eta = 0.11078$. Eqn (E17-4.9) gives $C_{AS} = 0.91318\ \text{g/m}^3$, which is slightly different from our first calculated value.

To get a converged solution, we use Excel solver continuing on the iterations (toward C_{AS} not changing), we obtain $C_{AS} = 0.91349\ \text{g/m}^3$, $\eta = 0.11036$. This solution is very close to that from our second iteration.

Eqns (E17-4.1) and (E17-4.2) gives

$$V = Q\frac{C_{A0} - C_{Ab}}{-r_A} = Q\frac{C_{A0} - C_{Ab}}{\eta(-r_{AS})V_{gel}/V} = Q\frac{C_{A0} - C_{Ab}}{\eta\dfrac{r_{max}C_{AS}}{(K_m + C_{AS})}(1-\varepsilon)} \tag{E17-4.10}$$

Thus,

$$V = Q\frac{C_{A0} - C_{Ab}}{\eta\dfrac{r_{max}C_{AS}}{(K_m + C_{AS})}(1-\varepsilon)} = \frac{100}{3600} \times \frac{50 - 1}{0.11036 \times \dfrac{0.4 \times 0.91249}{2 + 0.91249} \times 0.2}\ \text{m}^3$$

$$= 491.7\ \text{m}^3$$

The required working volume of the reactor is $491.7\ \text{m}^3$.

17.6. ENCAPSULATION IMMOBILIZATION

When enzymes or other biocatalysts are immobilized via encapsulation, there is no reaction occurring outside of the "porous particle." A schematic of the geometry is shown in Fig. 17.9. Substrate is transferred from the bulk fluid phase to the outer shell (external surface) of the particle and then permeates through the shell, reaching the biocatalyst. That is,

$$k_c S_O(C_{Ab} - C_{Ai}) = \frac{k_P}{\delta_S} S_O(C_{Ai} - C_{AS}) = -D_{eA} S \left.\frac{dC_A}{dx}\right|_{\text{at inner surface}} = (-r_{Ai})\eta \tag{17.81}$$

where S_O is the surface area of the outer shell, k_p is the permeability of A through the capsule shell, δ_S is the thickness of the capsule shell, C_{Ai} is the concentration of the A at the outer surface (interface), and C_{AS} is the concentration of A at the inner shell surface of the capsule.

There are three parameters one can control, in addition to the particle size. These parameters are: enzyme of biocatalyst loading (inside the capsule), capsule shell material, or permeability and the capsule shell thickness. When permeability k_p is increased and/or the shell thickness is decreased, mass transfer rate increases and thus favorable to the reaction system as whole, However, there is a limitation on the capsule shell material: containing the biocatalyst inside the shell while sustaining the reaction environment. Therefore, the capsule shell is physically limiting the reaction system. Particle size effect follows the same trend as solid catalyzed systems: smaller particle size leads to higher mass transfer rate and higher effectiveness factor.

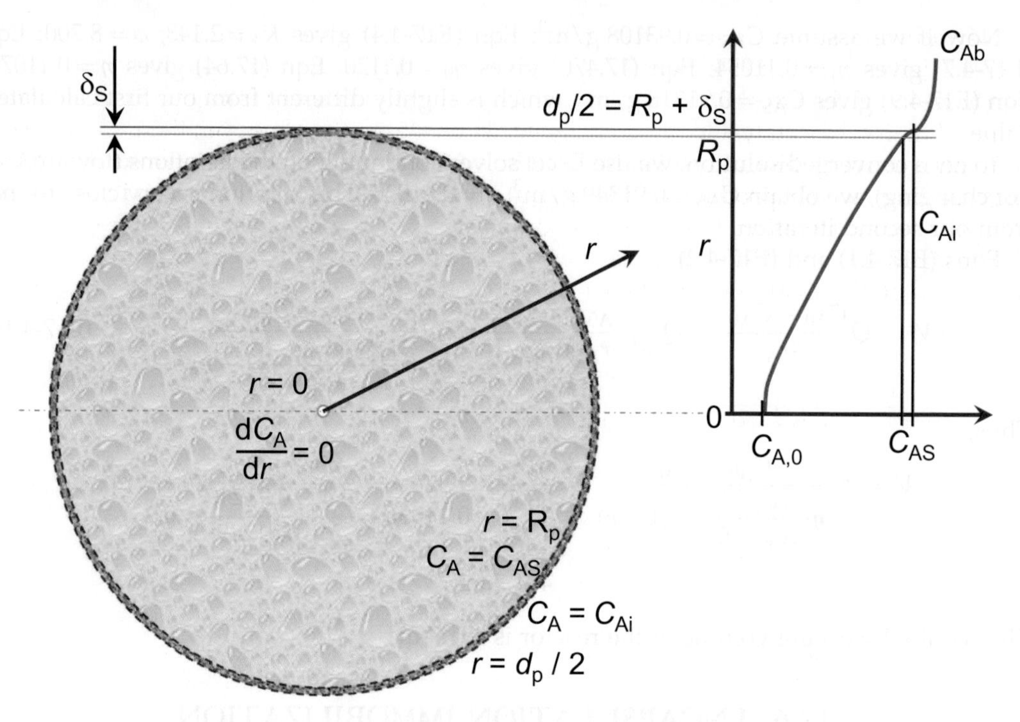

FIGURE 17.9 A schematic of diffusion and reaction in a spherical capsule.

For enzyme (or biocatalyst) loading, the situation can be more complicated. Enzyme loading affects maximum rate r_{max} as well as the diffusivity inside the shell D_{eA}. Since maximum reaction rate is proportional to the enzyme loading, higher biocatalyst loading leads to higher maximum rate. Higher biocatalyst loading decreases the effective diffusivity. Therefore, higher biocatalyst loading results in a higher Thiele modulus and lower effectiveness factor. The Thiele modulus is defined by

$$\phi = \frac{-r_{AS}}{a}\left[2\int_{C_{Ae,0}}^{C_{AS}}(-r_A)D_{eA}\mathrm{d}C_A\right]^{-\frac{1}{2}} \tag{17.29}$$

Thus, the changing of biocatalyst loading results in the change of Thiele modulus by

$$\phi = \phi_0\sqrt{\frac{r_{max}D_{eA}(E_0)}{r_{max0}D_{eA}(E)}} = \phi_0\sqrt{\frac{ED_{eA}(E_0)}{E_0D_{eA}(E)}} \tag{17.82}$$

where E_0 is the biocatalyst loading initially, at which the Thiele modulus is ϕ_0. When diffusion is limiting at least after increasing the biocatalyst loading,

$$\eta\times(-r_{Ai}) = \eta_0\times(-r_{Ai0})\times\frac{r_{max}\phi_0}{r_{max0}\phi} = \eta_0\times(-r_{Ai0})\sqrt{\frac{ED_{eA}(E)}{E_0D_{eA}(E_0)}} \tag{17.83}$$

If the diffusion is not limiting, the effectiveness factor remains unchanged and thus the increase in the overall net is clearer.

Therefore, if the effect of biocatalyst loading on the diffusivity is negligible, the overall effect of higher biocatalyst loading is higher net reaction rate. However, there is a physical limit on how much biocatalyst loading can be achieved. One can observe from Eqn (17.83) that as long as the product of biocatalyst loading and effective diffusivity does not decrease with increasing biocatalyst loading, increasing biocatalyst load is beneficial to the reaction system. However, there is a cost associated with biocatalyst loading and also the stability issue of biocatalyst at high loading, there is an optimum biocatalyst loading.

17.7. EXTERNAL AND INTERNAL SURFACE EFFECTS

When the external surface area of the catalyst is significant as compared with the internal surface area, one needs to consider the external surface area separately. The surface area of porous particles can be expressed as

$$a_c = a_e + a_i \tag{17.84}$$

where a_c is the total surface area (internal and external) per unit volume of the porous particle, a_i is the internal surface area per unit volume of the catalyst, and a_e is the external surface area per unit volume. For spherical particles,

$$a_e = 6\frac{1-\varepsilon_p}{d_p} \tag{17.85}$$

where d_p is the particle size and ε_p is the internal catalyst porosity. Let us define the ratio of external to internal surface areas by

$$a_r = \frac{a_e}{a_i} \tag{17.86}$$

The rate of the reaction system is governed by

$$k_c a(C_{Ab} - C_{AS}) = aN_A|_{\text{To surface}} + (-r'_{AS})a_e = -D_{eA}a\frac{dC_A}{dx}\bigg|_{\text{at surface}} + (-r'_{AS})a_e \tag{17.87}$$

Based on our earlier definition for internal mass transfer effects:

$$aN_A|_{\text{To surface}} = -D_{eA}a\frac{dC_A}{dx}\bigg|_{\text{at surface}} = (-r'_{AS})a_i\eta \tag{17.88}$$

Let us now define an overall effectiveness factor for the total surface area, i.e.,

$$\eta_s = \frac{SN_A|_{\text{To surface}} + (-r'_{AS})a_e V}{(-r'_{AS})a_c V} = \frac{aN_A|_{\text{To surface}} + (-r'_{AS})a_e}{(-r'_{AS})a_c} \tag{17.89}$$

which is reduced to

$$\eta_s = \frac{(-r'_{AS})a_i\eta + (-r'_{AS})a_e}{(-r'_{AS})a_c} = \frac{a_i\eta + a_e}{a_c} \tag{17.90}$$

That is, the overall surface effectiveness factor is given by

$$\eta_s = \frac{\eta + \dfrac{a_e}{a_i}}{1 + \dfrac{a_e}{a_i}} = \frac{\eta + a_r}{1 + a_r} \tag{17.91}$$

If the external surface area to the internal surface area ratio is known, the overall surface effectiveness factor can be determined through Eqn (17.91). Eqn (17.91) indicates that the effectiveness factor with higher fraction of external surface area (or small particle sizes) gives rise to higher values.

The overall effectiveness factor can then be defined as

$$\eta_o = \frac{r_{A,obs}}{r_{A,b}} = \eta_e\eta_s = \eta_e\frac{\eta + a_r}{1 + a_r} \tag{17.92}$$

The external surface area can be more important in solid catalysis, especially when particle size is small.

17.8. THE SHRINKING CORE MODEL

The shrinking core model as it states that deals with available reactants leaving the solid particle and thus causing the solid particle to "shrink." Fig. 17.10 shows a schematic of the "shrinking" solid in a porous matrix. The shrinking core model is applicable in areas ranging from pharmacokinetics (e.g. dissolution of pills in the stomach), to biomass gasification (solid to gas phase), to biomass extraction (solid to liquid phase), to porous catalyst regeneration (solid to gas phase), to coal particle combustion (solid to gas phase), to pulping and bleaching of fibers (solid to liquid phase), to pyrolysis.

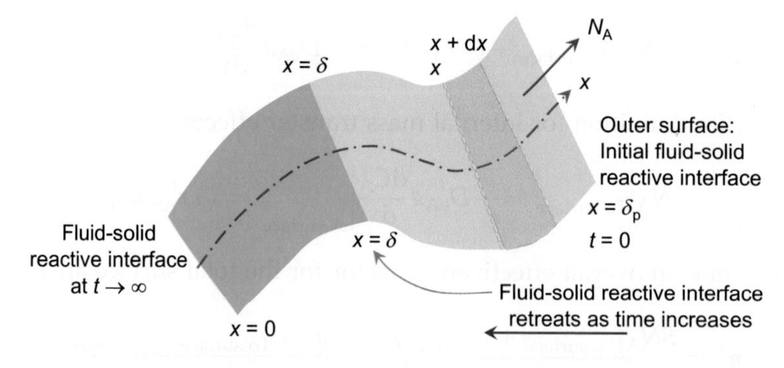

FIGURE 17.10 A schematic of a retreating fluid–solid reactive interface in a porous matrix.

Mass balance at pseudo-steady state above the retreating fluid–solid reactive interface inside the porous matrix leads to

$$N_A S|_x - N_A S|_{x+dx} + r_A S dx = \frac{dn_A}{dt} = 0 \tag{17.93}$$

where n_A is the number of moles of A in the differential volume (between x and $x + dx$) of particle, S is the cross-sectional area perpendicular to the path of diffusion/transport x.

Since there is no reaction occurring as the reactive interface is not included inside the volume of mass balance, Eqn (17.93) leads to

$$\frac{d(N_A S)}{dx} = 0 \tag{17.94}$$

That is,

$$N_A S = N_A S|_{x=\delta} \tag{17.95}$$

where $x = \delta$ is the reactive interface. At the reactive interface, A is being produced for the fluid phase.

$$N_A S|_{x=\delta} = r''_A S_\delta \tag{17.96}$$

where r''_A is the rate of formation of A per unit reactive fluid–solid interface area, and S_δ is the solid surface area at time t.

Since the transport is through diffusion only, we have

$$N_A = -D_{eA} \frac{dC_A}{dx} \tag{17.97}$$

where D_{eA} is the effective diffusivity of A. Substituting Eqns (17.95) and (17.96) into Eqn (17.97), we obtain

$$-D_{eA} S \frac{dC_A}{dx} = r''_A S_\delta \tag{17.98}$$

Noting that reaction rate is evaluated at the retreating interface and thus not a function of the C_A on the left-hand side of Eqn (17.98). Separation of variables and integration lead to

$$-\int_{C_{A\delta}}^{C_{AS}} D_{eA} dC_A = r''_A S_\delta \int_{\delta}^{\delta_p} \frac{dx}{S} \tag{17.99}$$

where $C_{A\delta}$ is the concentration of A in the fluid phase right at the retreating reactive fluid–solid interface ($x = \delta$) and C_{AS} is the concentration of A in the fluid phase at the initial solid surface ($x = \delta_p$). Integration in Eqn (17.99) requires the knowledge of how the cross-sectional area S changes along the path of diffusion. In practical applications, two cases are common: diffusion out of spherical particle (catalysts are commonly made spherical) and linear (woodchips, for example, may be regarded as slab or linear in each way you observe).

Solution of (Eqn 17.99) depends on the geometry as the cross-sectional area perpendicular to the transport path may change along the transport path. Solution of (Eqn 17.99) is to ensure that the mass transport flux N_A can be determined by the difference in concentrations $C_{A\delta} - C_{AS}$. Once the flux relationship is found, mass balance

$$r''_A S_\delta = N_A S = k_c S_{\delta_p}(C_{AS} - C_{Ab}) \tag{17.100}$$

can be applied to solve for the concentrations at the intermediate location ($x = \delta_p$) and thus relate the reaction rate and/or mass transfer rate to concentrations at the interface and/or the bulk fluid phase. If there is no porous matrix, the diffusion term (middle of Eqn 17.100) is not needed. However, the mass transfer coefficient k_c would be changing with the shrinking core (or a function of δ).

17.8.1. Time Required to Completely Dissolve a Porous Slab Full of Fast-Reactive Materials

For linear or rectangular particles, $S = \text{constant}$ and Eqn (17.99) is integrated to yield

$$D_{eA}(C_{A\delta} - C_{AS}) = r''_A(\delta_p - \delta) \tag{17.101}$$

which renders the mass transfer flux

$$N_A = D_{eA}\frac{C_{A\delta} - C_{AS}}{\delta_p - \delta} = r''_A \tag{17.102}$$

Assuming that the reaction on the retreating interface is very fast, the concentration of A at this interface is then the equilibrium concentration of A, C_{Ae}. Combining Eqn (17.102) with Eqn (17.100), we obtain

$$N_A = D_{eA}\frac{C_{Ae} - C_{AS}}{\delta_p - \delta} = k_c(C_{AS} - C_{Ab}) \tag{17.103}$$

Solving for C_{AS}, we obtain from Eqn (17.103)

$$C_{AS} = \frac{D_{eA}C_{Ae} + k_c(\delta_p - \delta)C_{Ab}}{D_{eA} + k_c(\delta_p - \delta)} \tag{17.104}$$

Substitute Eqn (17.104) into (17.105), we obtain the mass transfer flux or dissolution/reaction rate at the retreating interface

$$N_A = \frac{D_{eA}k_c(C_{Ae} - C_{Ab})}{D_{eA} + k_c(\delta_p - \delta)} \tag{17.105}$$

Mass balance of the total dissoluble materials in the porous matrix leads to

$$-C_{Ae}\phi_A S d\delta = N_A S dt \tag{17.106}$$

where C_{Ae} is the total concentration of equivalent A (pure), which is the same as the equilibrium concentration of A at the retreating surface, and ϕ_A is the volume fraction of the dissoluble solids in the porous matrix.

Substituting Eqn (17.105) into (17.106) and rearranging, we obtain

$$-C_{Ae}\phi_A[D_{eA} + k_c(\delta_p - \delta)]d\delta = D_{eA}k_c(C_{Ae} - C_{Ab})dt \tag{17.107}$$

Integration of Eqn (17.107) between ($t = 0$, $\delta = \delta_p$) and ($t = t_f$, $\delta = 0$), we obtain the time required for complete dissolution of the porous slab as

$$t_f = \frac{C_{Ae}\phi_A\delta_p(2D_{eA} + k_c\delta_p)}{2D_{eA}k_c(C_{Ae} - C_{Ab})} \tag{17.108}$$

If external mass transfer is also very fast, i.e. $k_c \to \infty$, Eqn (17.108) is reduced to

$$t_f = \frac{C_{Ae}\phi_A\delta_p^2}{2D_{eA}(C_{Ae} - C_{Ab})} \tag{17.109}$$

17.8.2. Time Required to Completely Dissolve a Porous Sphere Full of Fast-Reactive Materials

For spherical particles, $S = 4\pi r^2$ with $x \equiv r$, and Eqn (17.99) is reduced to

$$D_{eA}(C_{A\delta} - C_{AS}) = r''_A\left(\delta - \frac{\delta^2}{R_p}\right) \tag{17.110}$$

which renders the mass transfer flux

$$N_AS = 4\pi D_{eA}\frac{C_{A\delta} - C_{AS}}{R_p - \delta}R_p\delta = 4\pi r''_A\delta^2 \tag{17.111}$$

Assuming that the reaction on the retreating interface is very fast, the concentration of A at this interface is then the equilibrium concentration of A, C_{Ae}. Combining Eqn (17.111) with Eqn (17.100), we obtain

$$N_AS = 4\pi D_{eA}\frac{C_{Ae} - C_{AS}}{R_p - \delta}R_p\delta = 4\pi R_p^2k_c(C_{AS} - C_{Ab}) \tag{17.112}$$

Solving for C_{AS}, we obtain from Eqn (17.112)

$$C_{AS} = \frac{D_{eA}\delta C_{Ae} + k_cR_p(R_p - \delta)C_{Ab}}{D_{eA}\delta + k_cR_p(R_p - \delta)} \tag{17.113}$$

Substitute Eqn (17.113) into Eqn (17.112), we obtain the mass transfer flux or dissolution/reaction rate at the retreating interface

$$N_AS = 4\pi R_p^2\frac{D_{eA}k_c\delta(C_{Ae} - C_{Ab})}{D_{eA}\delta + k_cR_p(R_p - \delta)} \tag{17.114}$$

Mass balance of the total dissoluble materials in the porous matrix leads to

$$-C_{Ae}\phi_A4\pi\delta^2d\delta = N_ASdt \tag{17.115}$$

where C_{Ae} is the total concentration of equivalent A (pure), which is the same as the equilibrium concentration of A at the retreating surface, and ϕ_A is the volume fraction of the dissoluble solids in the porous matrix.

Substituting Eqn (17.114) into (17.115) and rearranging, we obtain

$$-C_{Ae}\phi_A\delta[D_{eA}\delta + k_c R_p(R_p - \delta)]d\delta = D_{eA}k_c R_p^2(C_{Ae} - C_{Ab})dt \tag{17.116}$$

Integration of Eqn (17.116) between ($t = 0$, $\delta = R_p$) and ($t = t_f$, $\delta = 0$), we obtain the time required for complete dissolution of the porous slab as

$$t_f = \frac{C_{Ae}\phi_A R_p(2D_{eA} + k_c R_p)}{6D_{eA}k_c(C_{Ae} - C_{Ab})} \tag{17.117}$$

If external mass transfer is also very fast, i.e. $k_c \to \infty$, Eqn (17.117) is reduced to

$$t_f = \frac{C_{Ae}\phi_A R_p^2}{6D_{eA}(C_{Ae} - C_{Ab})} \tag{17.118}$$

17.9. SUMMARY

The reaction rate expression used in the analysis in this chapter is given by

$$-r_A = \frac{r_{max}C_A}{K_A + C_A} \tag{17.8}$$

where C_A is the concentration of A in the fluid phase and $-r_A$ is the rate of disappearance of A based on the total volume of the body of the catalyst (not the fluid phase or the mixture). When reaction kinetics is different, the same procedures can be followed to evaluate the mass transfer effects.

The effectiveness factor for external mass transfer is defined as

$$\eta_e = \frac{r_{AS}}{r_{A,b}} \tag{17.9}$$

where r_{AS} is the rate of A evaluated with the particle external surface conditions (i.e. $C_A = C_{AS}$ and $T = T_S$) and $r_{A,b}$ is the rate of A evaluated with the bulk fluid phase conditions (i.e. $C_A = C_{Ab}$ and $T = T_b$).

The Thiele modulus for external mass transfer is defined for an intrinsic reaction rate given by Eqn (17.8),

$$\phi_e = \frac{-r_{A,b}}{k_c a C_{Ab}} = \frac{r_{max}}{(k_c a)(K_A + C_{Ab})} \tag{17.13}$$

and the external mass transfer effectiveness factor is given by

$$\eta_e = \frac{1 + \phi_e}{2\phi_e}\left(1 + \frac{K_A}{C_{Ab}}\right)\left[1 - \sqrt{1 - \frac{4\phi_e}{(1 + \phi_e)^2}\left(1 + \frac{K_A}{C_{Ab}}\right)^{-1}}\,\right] \tag{17.14}$$

The external Thiele modulus is a function of the mass transfer coefficient and is a function of the flow rate and particle size. Noting that r_{max} is proportional to the surface area of the particle, we obtain

$$\phi_e^{-1} = \frac{k_c a C_{Ab}}{-r_{A,b}} \propto \frac{U^{0.5931}}{d_p^{0.4069}} \tag{17.15}$$

A condition for negligible external mass transfer effects, i.e. $\eta_e > 0.95$, is given by

$$\phi_e^{-1} = \eta_e + \frac{\eta_e^2 K_A}{(1-\eta_e)(K_A + C_{Ab})} > 0.95 + 18.05\frac{K_A}{K_A + C_{Ab}} \tag{17.18}$$

Therefore, the effect of external mass transfer is influenced by the reaction kinetics. When the saturation coefficient K_A is larger, the external Thiele modulus is larger for the external mass transfer effects to be negligible.

The internal mass transfer effectiveness factor is defined by

$$\eta = \frac{r_{A,obs}}{r_{AS}} \tag{17.27}$$

and the Thiele modulus is defined based on asymptotic behavior of η by Eqn (17.29),

$$\phi = \frac{-r_{AS}}{a}\left[2\int_{C_{Ae,0}}^{C_{AS}} (-r_A) D_{eA} \mathrm{d}C_A\right]^{-\frac{1}{2}} \tag{17.29}$$

where a is the specific "outer surface" area of the particle, S/V. Here the "outer surface" area S is the area of the particle including solid surface and "pore" cross-sectional area at the fluid–particle interface. K_β is defined as a dimensionless saturation constant:

$$K_\beta = \frac{K_A}{C_{AS}} \tag{17.30}$$

When $K_\beta = 0$, Eqn (17.8) reduces to a zeroth-order kinetics. When $K_\beta \to \infty$, Eqn (17.8) reduces to a first-order kinetics. In most bioreactions, the value of K_β is small.

With kinetics given by Eqn (17.8), the generalized Thiele modulus is given by

$$\phi = \frac{1}{a}\sqrt{\frac{r_{max}}{2D_{eA}C_{AS}}}\,\frac{[1 - K_\beta \ln(1 + K_\beta^{-1})]^{-\frac{1}{2}}}{1 + K_\beta} \tag{17.31}$$

For isothermal systems, the use of the generalized Thiele modulus unifies all the particle shapes and reaction kinetics when the Thiele modulus is large. When Thiele modulus is small, both particle shape and reaction kinetics play a role in the effectiveness factor. Table 17.6 shows a summary of the internal mass transfer effects on the reaction kinetics and catalyst particle shape: slab and sphere.

For nonisothermal reaction systems, two new parameters are added even in the case where the saturation constant K_A is assumed not temperature dependent:

$$\beta = \frac{(-\Delta H_{R,A}) D_{eA} C_{AS}}{k_{eT} T_S} \tag{17.70}$$

TABLE 17.6 Internal Mass Transfer Effectiveness Factor

Geometry	Slab	Sphere
Thiele modulus, ϕ	$\phi = \sqrt{\frac{r_{max}\delta_P^2}{2D_{eA}C_{AS}}}\frac{[1-K_\beta \ln(1+K_\beta^{-1})]^{-\frac{1}{2}}}{1+K_\beta}$	$\phi = \frac{R_P}{3}\sqrt{\frac{r_{max}}{2D_{eA}C_{AS}}}\frac{[1-K_\beta \ln(1+K_\beta^{-1})]^{-\frac{1}{2}}}{1+K_\beta}$
η_0	$\eta_0 = 1$, for $\phi \le 1$	$\eta_0 = 1$, for $\phi \le \frac{\sqrt{3}}{3}$
	$\eta_0 = \frac{1}{\phi}$, for $\phi \ge 1$	$\eta_0 = 1 - \left\{\frac{1}{2} + \cos\left[\frac{4\pi}{3} + \frac{1}{3}\arccos\left(\frac{2}{3\phi^2} - 1\right)\right]\right\}^3$, for $\phi \le \frac{\sqrt{3}}{3}$
η_1	$\eta_1 = \frac{\tanh\phi}{\phi}$	$\eta_1 = \frac{\phi\coth(3\phi) - 1/3}{\phi^2}$
η	$\eta = \frac{\eta_0[0.15K_\beta^{-1} + 0.3\ln(1+K_\beta^{-1})] + \eta_1}{1 + 0.15K_\beta^{-1} + 0.3\ln(1+K_\beta^{-1})}$	$\eta = \frac{\eta_0[0.186K_\beta^{-1} + 0.306\ln(1+K_\beta^{-1})] + \eta_1}{1 + 0.186K_\beta^{-1} + 0.306\ln(1+K_\beta^{-1})}$
$\eta > 0.95$	$\phi^{-1} > 0.95 + \frac{1.553K_\beta}{0.52 + K_\beta - 0.16K_\beta\ln(1+K_\beta^{-1})}$	$\phi^{-1} > 1.442 + \frac{1.897K_\beta}{0.605 + K_\beta - 0.193K_\beta\ln(1+K_\beta^{-1})}$

and

$$\gamma = \frac{E_a}{RT_S} \tag{17.75}$$

where $\Delta H_{R,A}$ is the heat of reaction per unit A reacted, k_{eT} is the effective thermal conductivity in the particle, T_S is the temperature at the external surface, E_a is the activation energy (governing r_{max}). The temperature change is linearly related to the concentration change if the parameter β is constant. That is,

$$\frac{T}{T_S} = 1 + \beta\left[1 - \frac{C_A}{C_{AS}}\right] = 1 + \beta(1 - C_{A+}) \tag{17.71}$$

The parameter β can be viewed as the ratio of maximum possible temperature difference divided by the external surface temperature. Since the maximum temperature deviation from the external surface is at the location where concentration of A is zero. The rate of reaction for a nonisothermal system is given by

$$-r_A = \frac{r_{max,0}C_A}{K_A + C_A}\exp\left(-\frac{T_S}{T}\gamma\right) = \frac{r_{max,0}C_{A+}}{K_\beta + C_{A+}}\exp\left[-\frac{\gamma}{1 + \beta - \beta C_{A+}}\right] \tag{17.76}$$

Thus, the asymptotic behavior can be obtained via the generalized Thiele modulus,

$$\phi = \sqrt{\frac{r_{\max,0}}{2D_{eA}C_{AS}}} \frac{e^{-\gamma}}{1+K_\beta}\frac{1}{a}\left[\int_0^1 \frac{C_{A+}}{K_\beta + C_{A+}} \exp\left(-\frac{\gamma}{1+\beta-\beta C_{A+}}\right) dC_{A+}\right]^{-\frac{1}{2}} \tag{17.77}$$

For exothermic reactions, the effectiveness factor can be greater than unity due to the higher reaction rate at internal sites due to the slow heat removal.

Overall effectiveness factor

$$\eta_o = \frac{r_{A,obs}}{r_{A,b}} = \eta_e \eta \tag{17.80}$$

The use of $r_{A,b}$ to define the overall effectiveness factor is for the convenience of reactor design calculations. Since the bulk phase concentrations are easily obtained and/or measured, reaction rate based on bulk concentrations are preferred.

For biocatalyst immobilized system via encapsulation, capsule size, biocatalyst loading (inside the capsule), capsule shell material or permeability, and the capsule shell thickness, all play important roles on the reaction system as a whole. Smaller (capsule) particle size leads to higher mass transfer rate and higher effectiveness factor. When capsule shell permeability k_p is increased and/or the shell thickness is decreased, mass transfer rate increases and thus favorable to the reaction system as whole, however, there is a limitation on the capsule shell material: containing the biocatalyst inside the shell while sustaining the reaction environment.

For enzyme (or biocatalyst) loading, the situation can be more complicated. Enzyme loading affects maximum rate r_{max} as well as the diffusivity inside the shell D_{eA}. Since maximum reaction rate is proportional to the enzyme loading, higher biocatalyst loading leads to higher maximum rate. Higher biocatalyst loading decreases the effective diffusivity. Therefore, higher biocatalyst loading results in a higher Thiele modulus and lower effectiveness factor. If the effect of biocatalyst loading on the diffusivity is negligible, the overall effect of higher biocatalyst loading is higher net reaction rate. However, there is a physical limit on how much biocatalyst loading can be achieved.

When external surface area is important, the overall surface effectiveness factor is given by

$$\eta_s = \frac{\eta + \frac{a_e}{a_i}}{1 + \frac{a_e}{a_i}} = \frac{\eta + a_r}{1 + a_r} \tag{17.91}$$

which can employed to substitute the effectiveness factor for internal mass transfer as if there is no external surface area.

The overall effectiveness factor with internal and external surface area effects can then be defined as

$$\eta_o = \frac{r_{A,obs}}{r_{A,b}} = \eta_e \eta_s = \eta_e \frac{\eta + a_r}{1 + a_r} \tag{17.92}$$

where a_r is the ratio of external surface area to the internal surface area.

In general, iterative solutions are necessary when both internal and external mass transfer effects are important. Reactor analysis including the mass transfer effects can be incorporated by including the effectiveness factor with the reaction rate as one would.

The shrinking core model is applicable in areas ranging from pharmacokinetics (e.g. dissolution of pills in the stomach), to biomass gasification (solid to gas phase), to biomass extraction (solid to liquid phase), to porous catalyst regeneration (solid to gas phase), to coal particle combustion (solid to gas phase), to pulping and bleaching of fibers (solid to liquid phase), to pyrolysis. Mass transfer, especially diffusion in the solid matrix is often the rate-limiting step in biomass conversion processes.

Further Reading

Aris, R., 1975. The Mathematical Theory of Diffusion and Reaction in Permeable Catalysts, Oxford, England: Clarendon Press.

Blanch, H.W., Clark, D.S., 1996. Biochemical Engineering, New York: Marcel Dekker, Inc.

Doran, P.M., 1995. Bioprocess Engineering Principles, New York: Academic Press.

Fogler, H.S., 1999. Elements of Chemical Reaction Engineering, 3rd ed. Upper Saddle River, NJ: Prentice Hall.

Frank-Kamenetskii, D.A., 1969. Diffusion and Heat Transfer in Chemical Kinetics, 2nd ed. New York: Plenum Press.

Nielsen, J., Villadsen, J., Lidén, G., 2003. Bioreaction Engineering Principles, 2nd ed. New York: Kluwer Academic/Plenum Publishers.

Satterfield, C.N., 1970. Mass Transfer in Heterogeneous Catalysis. Cambridge, MA: MIT Press.

vant't Riet, K., Tramper, J., 1991. Basic Bioreactor Design, New York: Marcel Dekker, Inc.

PROBLEMS

17.1. Glucose oxidase catalyzes the oxidation of glucose. When glucose is present in excess, oxygen can be considered the limiting substrate. Michaelis–Menten kinetics may be applied to describe the oxygen-limited reaction rate. The enzyme is immobilized on the surface of nonporous glass beads. The particles are of $d_p = 0.12$ mm, $\rho_s = 2762\ \text{kg} \cdot \text{m}^{-3}$. The medium properties are: $\mu = 0.001$ Pa, $\rho_L = 1000\ \text{kg} \cdot \text{m}^{-3}$, $C_{O_2b} = 0.18\ \text{mol} \cdot \text{m}^{-3}$. The diffusivity of oxygen in the medium is $D_{AB} = 2.1 \times 10^{-9}\ \text{m}^2/\text{s}$, and the catalyst loading is $[E]_0 = 2 \times 10^{-8}$ g per glass bead. The volume fraction of beads is 0.4 in the reactor. The kinetic constants are: $r_{max} = 5.8 \times 10^{-2}$ mol-O_2/(s·g-enzyme), and $K_m = 0.1\ \text{mol} \cdot \text{m}^{-3}$. Calculate the effectiveness factor and the effective rate of reaction assuming

(a) no agitation (i.e. diffusion mass transfer);

(b) effective medium flow velocity is 0.5 m/s.

17.2. Consider a system where a flat sheet of polymer coated with enzyme is placed in a stirred beaker. Michaelis–Menten kinetics is applicable to this enzyme. The intrinsic maximum reaction rate r_{max} of the enzyme is 5×10^{-3} mol/(s·g-enzyme). The enzyme loading on the surface has been determined as 1.2×10^{-5} g-enzyme/m^2-support. In solution, the value of saturation constant K_m has been determined to be 2×10^{-3} mol/L. The mass transfer coefficient has been estimated as $k_L = 5.8 \times 10^{-4}$ m/s. What is the effective reaction rate if a) the bulk concentration is 5×10^{-3} mol/L; b) the bulk concentration is 0.2 mol/L.

17.3. Assume that for an enzyme immobilized on the surface of a nonporous support material the external mass transfer resistance for substrate is not negligible as compared to the reaction rate. The enzyme is subject to substrate inhibition.

(a) Are multiple states possible?

(b) Could the effectiveness factor be greater than one?

17.4. Hydrazine has been studied extensively for use in monopropellant thrusters for space flights of long duration. Thrusters are used for altitude control of communication satellites. Here the decomposition of hydrazine over a packed bed of alumina-supported iridium catalyst is of interest (Smith O.I. and Solomon W.C. *Ind. Eng. Chem. Fund*. 21: 374, 1982). In a proposed study, a 2% hydrazine in 98% helium mixture is to be passed over a packed bed of cylindrical particles 2 mm in diameter and 5 mm in length at a gas-phase superficial velocity of 5 m/s and a temperature of 700 K. The kinematic viscosity of helium at this temperature is 4.0×10^{-4} m^2/s. The hydrazine decomposition reaction is believed to be external mass transfer-limited under these conditions. If the packed bed is 0.05 m in length, what conversion can be expected? The bed porosity is 28% and the diffusivity of hydrazine in helium is 6.9×10^{-5} m^2/s at 298 K. Assume isothermal operation.

17.5. **(a)** Weetall H.H. and Havewala N.B. (*Biotechnol. Bioeng. Symp*. No. 3, Wiley, New York, pp. 241–266, 1972) report the following data (Table P17.5-1) for the production of dextrose from com starch using both soluble and immobilized (azo-glass beads) glucoamylase in a fully agitated CSTR system.

TABLE P17.5-1

	Product concentration, g-dextrose/L	
Time, min	**Soluble**	**Immobilized**
0	12	18.4
15	40	135
30	76.5	200
45	94.3	236
60	120	260
75	135.5	258
90	151.2	262
105	150.4	266
120	155.7	278
135	160.1	300
150	164.9	310
165	170	306
225		316
415		320

1. Soluble data: $T = 60$ °C, $[S]_0 = 168$ g-starch/L, $[E]_0 = 11{,}600$ units, volume = 1000 mL.

2. Immobilized data: $T = 60\ ^\circ C$, $[S]_0 = 336$ g-starch/L, $[E]_0 = 46{,}400$ units, volume = 1000 mL.

   Determine the maximum reaction velocity, r_{max} (g/min/unit of enzyme) and the saturation constant, K_m ($g \cdot L^{-1}$).

(b) The same authors studied the effect of temperature on the maximum rate of the hydrolysis of corn starch by glucoamylase. The results are tabulated in Table P17.5-2. Determine the activation energy (E_a, cal/mole) for the soluble and immobilized enzyme reaction.

TABLE P17.5-2

	r_{max}, 10^{-9} mol · min^{-1} · unit enzyme^{-1}	
T, °C	Soluble	Azo-immobilized
25	0.62	0.80
35	1.42	1.40
45	3.60	3.00
55	8.0	6.2
65	16.0	11.0

(c) Using these results, determine if immobilized enzyme is diffusion limited.

17.6. The decomposition of cyclohexane to benzene and hydrogen is mass transfer limited at high temperatures. The reaction is carried out in a 50-mm-i.d. pipe 20 m in length packed with spherical pellets 5 mm in diameter. The pellets are coated with the catalyst only on the outside. The bed porosity is 40%. The entering volumetric flow rate is 60 L/min.

(a) Calculate the number of pipes necessary to achieve 99.9% conversion of cyclohexane from an entering gas stream of 5% cyclohexane and 95% H_2 at 2 atm and 500 °C.

(b) How much would your answer change if the pellet diameter were each cut in half?

(c) How would your answer to part (a) change if the feed were pure cyclohexane?

17.7. In a certain chemical plant, a reversible fluid-phase isomerization

$$A \rightleftarrows B$$

is carried out over a solid catalyst in a tubular packed-bed reactor. If the reaction is so rapid that mass transfer between the catalyst surface and the bulk fluid is rate limiting, show that the kinetics are described in terms of the bulk concentrations C_A and C_B by

$$-r_A = \frac{k_B(C_A - C_B/K_C)}{1/K_C + k_B/k_A}$$

where $-r_A$ = moles of A reacting per unit area of catalyst per unit time, k_A and k_B are the mass transfer coefficients for A and B, and K_C is the reaction equilibrium constant.

It is desired to double the capacity of the existing plant by processing twice the feed of reactant A while maintaining the same fractional conversion of A to B in the reactor. How much larger a reactor, in terms of catalyst weight, would be required if all other operating variables are held constant? Describe the effects of the flow rate, temperature, and particle size at conversion.

17.8. You are working for company A and you join a research group working on immobilized enzymes. Harry, the head of the lab, claims that immobilization improves the stability of the enzyme. His proof is that the enzyme has a half-life of 10 days in free solution but under identical conditions of temperature, pH, and medium composition, the measured half-life of a packed column is 30 days. The enzyme is immobilized in a porous sphere of 5 mm in diameter. Is Harry's reasoning right? Do you agree with him and Why?

17.9. A decomposition reaction is carried out on a solid catalyst

$$A \rightarrow B$$

over two different pellet sizes. The pellets were contained in a differential reactor that has sufficient turbulence such that the external mass transfer effects are negligible. We know that the adsorption coverage of A on the catalyst site is minimal and thus $K_A \rightarrow \infty$. The reaction on the catalyst surface is thus virtually first order. The results of two experimental runs made under identical conditions are as shown in Table P17.9-1. Estimate the Thiele modulus and effectiveness factor for each pellet. How small should the pellets be made to virtually eliminate all internal diffusion effects on the overall reaction kinetics?

TABLE P17.9-1

	Pellet size, mm	**Measured rate, mol-A/(g-cat·s)**
Run 1	2.00	3.80
Run 2	0.200	20.0

17.10. A decomposition reaction is carried out on a solid catalyst

$$A \rightarrow B + C$$

over two different pellet sizes. The pellets were contained in a differential reactor that has sufficient turbulence such that the external mass transfer effects are negligible. We know that the adsorption coverage of A on the catalyst site is very strong and thus $K_A \rightarrow 0$. The reaction on the catalyst surface is thus virtually zeroth order. The results of two experimental runs made under identical conditions are as shown in Table P17.10-1. Estimate the Thiele modulus and effectiveness factor for each pellet. How small should the pellets be made to virtually eliminate all internal diffusion effects on the overall reaction kinetics?

TABLE P17.10-1

	Pellet size, mm	Measured rate, mol-A/(g-cat·s)
Run 1	10.0	5.00
Run 2	1.00	10.0

17.11. The enzyme, urease, is immobilized in Ca-alginate beads 2 mm in diameter. The maximum intrinsic rate of urea hydrolysis is $r_{max} = 0.5$ mol/(L·h) for the particular enzyme loading is suspended media. Diffusivity of urea in Ca-alginate beads is $De = 1.5 \times 10^{-9}$ m^2/s, and the intrinsic saturation constant for the enzyme is $K_m = 0.2$ mmol/L. By neglecting the liquid film and Ca-alginate shell resistances on the beads, determine the following when the urea concentration in the bulk liquid is 0.5 mmol/L:

(a) Observed rate of hydrolysis r, Thiele modulus, and effectiveness factor.

(b) Observed rate of hydrolysis r, Thiele modulus, and effectiveness factor for a particle size of $d_p = 4$ mm.

17.12. The enzyme, urease, is immobilized in Ca-alginate beads 2 mm in diameter. When the urea concentration in the bulk liquid is 0.5 mmol/L, the rate of urea hydrolysis is $r = 0.01$ mol/(L·h). Diffusivity of urea in Ca-alginate beads is $De = 1.5 \times 10^{-9}$ m^2/s, and the intrinsic saturation constant for the enzyme is $K_m = 0.2$ mmol/L. By neglecting the liquid film and Ca-alginate shell resistances on the beads,

(a) Determine the maximum rate of hydrolysis r_{max}, Thiele modulus, and effectiveness factor.

(b) What would be the values of r_{max}, Thiele modulus, and effectiveness factor for a particle size of $d_p = 4$ mm?

17.13. Uric acid is degraded by uricase enzyme immobilized in porous Ca-alginate beads. Experiments conducted with different bead sizes result in the following rate data:

TABLE P17.13-1

Bead diameter d_p, mm	1	2	3	4	5	6	7	8
Rate, mg/(L · h)	200	198	180	140	100	70	50	30

(a) Determine the effectiveness factor for particle sizes $d_p = 5$ mm and $d_p = 7$ mm.

(b) The following data (Table P17.13-2) were obtained for $d_p = 5$ mm at different bulk uric acid concentrations.

TABLE 17.13-2

S_b, mg/L	10	25	50	100	200	250
r, mg/(L·h)	10	20	30	40	45	46

Assuming negligible liquid film and Ca-alginate shell resistances, calculate r_{max} and K_m for the enzyme. Assume no substrate or product inhibition.

17.14. Urea dissolved in aqueous solution is degraded to ammonia and CO_2 by the enzyme urease immobilized on surfaces of nonporous polymeric beads. Conversion rate is controlled by transfer of urea to the surface of the beads through liquid film, and the conversion takes place on the surfaces of the beads. The following parameters are given for the system:
$k_L = 0.2$ cm/s; $K_m = 0.2$ g/L
$r_{max} = 0.01$ g-urea/m^2-support surface
$S_b = 1$ g-urea/L
(a) Determine the surface concentration of urea.
(b) Determine the rate of urea degradation under mass transfer-controlled conditions.

17.15. The bioconversion of glucose to ethanol is carried out in a packed-bed, immobilized-cell bioreactor containing yeast cells entrapped in Ca-alginate beads. The diffusivity of glucose inside the alginate beads is 10^{-10} m^2/s. The rate-limiting substrate is glucose, and its concentration in the feed bulk liquid phase is $S_0 = 5$ g/L. The nutrient flow rate is $Q = 2$ L/min. The particle size of Ca-alginate beads is $d_p = 5$ mm. The Michaelis–Menten rate constants for this conversion are: $r_{max} = 100$ g-S/(L·h) and $K_m = 10^{-3}$ g/L. The surface area of the alginate beads per unit volume of the reactor is $a_c = 2500$ m^2/m^3, and the cross-sectional area of the bed is 0.01 m^2. The external mass transfer resistance and the diffusional resistance through the alginate shell are negligible. Determine the required height for 80% conversion of glucose to ethanol at the exit stream.

17.16. A effectively first-order (i.e. $K_A \to \infty$, due to the low coverage of A on the catalyst) heterogeneous irreversible reaction is taking place within a spherical catalyst pellet that is plated with platinum throughout the pellet. The reactant concentration halfway between the external surface and the center of the pellet (i.e. $r = R/2$) is equal to one-tenth the concentration of the pellet's external surface. The concentration at the external surface is 0.001 mol/L, the pellet diameter is 2.0×10^{-5} m, and the diffusion coefficient is 0.1 cm^2/s.

$$A \to B$$

(a) What is the concentration of reactant at a distance of 3×10^{-6} m inward from the external pellet surface?
(b) To what diameter should the pellet be reduced if the effectiveness factor is to be 0.8?
(c) If the catalyst support were not yet plated with platinum, how would you suggest that the catalyst support be plated *after* it had been reduced by grinding?

17.17. Nitrate in groundwater is becoming more of a problem. In addition to measures aiming at applying lower loads of fertilizers, the need for effective treatment procedures is increasing. One of the alternatives investigated is removal of nitrate by conversion to gaseous N_2 using denitrifying bacteria immobilized in gel beads. Calculate the content of an ideally mixed bioreactor treating 150 m^3/h of groundwater. The concentration of nitrate in the groundwater is 45 g/m^3 and the treated water contains 0.8 g/m^3 nitrate. The load of gel beads in the reactor is 0.25 m^3-gel/m^3-reaction mixture. The diameter of the gel beads is 2 mm, the diffusivity of nitrate inside the gel is 10^{-10} m^2/s. Mass transfer coefficient of nitrate in the reactor is 10^{-5} m/s. The kinetic constant are given by $r_{max} = 0.5$ g/(s m^3-gel) and $K_m = 1$ g · m^{-3}.

17.18. Invertase catalyzes the hydrolysis of sucrose to glucose and fructose (invert sugars). The reaction follows Michaelis–Menten kinetics with $r_{max} = 2 \times 10^{-4}$ mol · L^{-1} · s^{-1} and $K_m = 0.001$ mol/L. It is decided to carry out the reaction in a PFR packed with particles immobilized invertase at 50% in volume fraction. The catalyst particles are 3.5 mm in diameter and the effective diffusivity of sucrose inside the particle is 0.2×10^{-9} m^2/s. The available sucrose stream has a concentration of 350 g/L and we need to produce 35 Mg invert sugar per day with 99% conversion. Compute the amount of catalyst or volume of reactor required. Neglect the external mass transfer effects.

17.19. In Table P17.19, the oxygen-18 data were obtained from soil samples taken at different depths in Ontario, Canada. Assuming that all the ^{18}O was laid down during the last glacial age and that the transport of ^{18}O to the surface takes place by molecular diffusion, estimate the number of years since the last glacial age from the data. Independent measurements give by diffusivity of ^{18}O in soil as 2.64×10^{-10} m^2/s.

TABLE P17.19

Depth from surface, m	0	3	6	9	12	18	21	24
^{18}O concentration ratio	0	0.35	0.65	0.83	0.94	1.00	1.00	1.00

17.20. If disposal of industrial liquid wastes by incineration is to be a feasible process, it is important that the toxic chemicals be completely decomposed into harmless substances. Table P17.20 shows the data for the burning of liquid droplets. What can you learn from these data?

TABLE P17.20

Time, s	20	40	50	70	90	110
Droplet size, μm	9.7	8.8	8.4	7.1	5.6	4.0

CHAPTER

18

Bioreactor Design and Operation

OUTLINE

Bioprocess Engineering
http://dx.doi.org/10.1016/B978-0-444-59525-6.00018-4

"Commit your blunders on a small scale and make your profits on a large scale"

Leo Hendrik Baekeland, the inventor of Bakelit, 1916

Design of reactors depends on numerous factors such as product throughput, quality control requirement, substrate consistency, type and properties of biocatalyst, regulatory constraints, etc. Table 18.1 shows some of the more obvious characteristics of bioreactors in scale. Understanding the capabilities and limits of different designs is critical in successfully producing the desired product. Utilizing a bioreactor designed for microbial fermentation for cell culture products could have disastrous results as metabolic and microkinetic control mechanism may differ greatly. Discussions will be made on design features for bioreactors and scale-up/scale-down considerations that need to be taken into consideration when implementing bioreactor systems. Bioinstrumentation and controls utilized in process systems are important in reactor design and operation. Another aspect that dominates the design of bioreactor system is sterilization. Being able to produce a pure culture is of the utmost importance in producing the desired product. Undesired organisms not only consume raw materials intended for producing the desired product, they often produce undesired contaminants which may not be able to be separated from the desired product. We will identify some sterilization design considerations and techniques for maintaining pure cultures.

18.1. BIOREACTOR SELECTION

There are numerous designs for reactor systems. As we have discussed in Chapter 5, there are two basic types of ideal flow reactors: plug flow reactor (PFR) and continuous stirred-tank reactor (CSTR). Selection of PFR is favored for homogeneous reaction systems, non-catalytic systems, non-autocatalytic (including heat) systems, and/or immolized catalytic systems. Tubular membrane and packed bed reactors can normally be approximated as PFR's (with different feeding and/or withdrawing patterns). Well-mixed reactors, either batch or CSTR, are more flexible in handling bioreactions and will be the focus of this chapter.

Bioreaction processes have occurred for thousands years as fermentations have converted sugars to wine and beer back to the Roman age. The function of bioreactor includes: containment (insurance of sterility), introduction of gaseous reactants (e.g. oxygen), introduction of liquid reactants (e.g. carbon source), removal of gaseous products (e.g. carbon dioxide), control of the physical environment (e.g. temperature, shear rate, and pH), suspension (e.g. cells, particulate matter), and dispersion (two-phase systems). In this section, we will

TABLE 18.1 Characteristics of Scale in Bioreactor Operations

Parameter	Lab scale	Production scale
Cash flow	Negative	Positive
Volume	5–15 L	30 m^3
Oxygen transfer rate (OTR)	300–500 mmol/(L · h)	100 mmol/(L · h)
Heat transfer	40–70 kW/m^3	<20 kW/m^3
Power input	15–30 kW/m^3	1–3 kW/m^3

learn some of the basic types of bioreactors: 1) reactors with internal mechanism, 2) bubble columns, and 3) loop reactors. All three types of reactors are invariably concerned with three-phase reactions (gas-liquid-solid). Prediction of reactor performance is difficult due to the complex fluid mechanics coupled with the complex nature of cells.

The traditional fermentor utilizes a stirred-tank vessel, either be batch or continuous. The stirred-tank fermentor employs internal baffles and agitator to obtain needed mixing. These bioreactors are highly flexible and can provide high K_La (volumetric mass transfer coefficient) values for gas transfer. Gas under pressure is applied through subsurface spargers to provide gases needed for cellular metabolism. The size of the gas bubbles and dispersion through the reactor vessel are critical to the performance of the bioreactor. Fig. 18.1 shows a typical stirred-tank fermentor.

Gas dispersion is mainly the function of the impeller (oxygen transfer into the culture). The impeller must provide sufficient agitation to disperse the gas bubbles throughout the vessel and increase their residence time. The desire for rapid gas dispersion must however be balanced with the impact on the culture. High shear impellers are generally utilized on microbial systems, where high-gas transfer rates and cellular growth require rapid dispersion and mass transfer through the vessel. For eukaryotic cells, a high shear environment can be detrimental.

Fig. 18.2 shows the variation of growth rate with shear rate for an animal cell culture. One can observe that mammalian cell cultures are very sensitive to shear. At low shear rates (low agitation rates), the growth rate of mammalian cells remains relatively unchanged with changing shear rates. As the integrated shear, $\frac{2\pi\omega D_i}{D_R - D_i}$, is increased beyond 17 s^{-1}, any further increase in agitation speed ω or impeller diameter D_i will result in a sharp decrease in the growth rate of the animal cell FS-4.

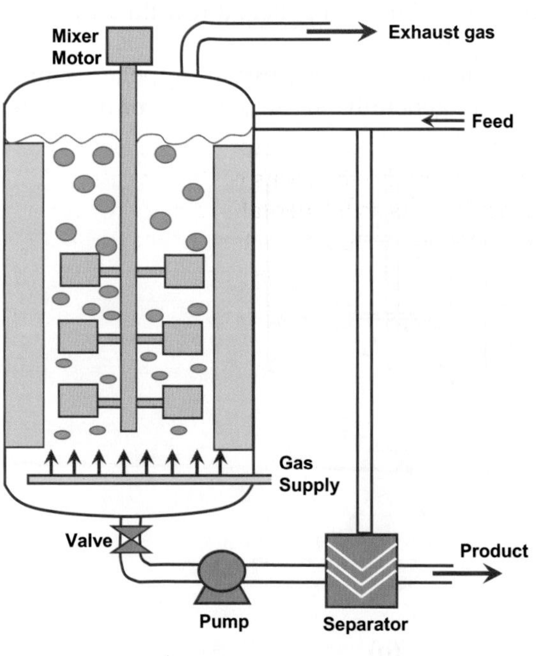

FIGURE 18.1 Stirred-tank fermentor.

Agitation also provides the mixing actions which facilitate heat transfer from the bioreactor. Agitation of the vessel is desired to achieve homogenous conditions within the bioreactor. In large bioreactors, homogeneity is extremely difficult to achieve. There are two main types of impellers used for stirred-tank bioreactors—disc and turbine and marine style impellers. Fig. 18.3 provides an example of each. Fig. 18.3a shows the schematic of a disc and turbine style impeller and its impact on the flow patterns inside the reactor. Radial flow dominates in a vessel with disc and turbine impellers. Compartments of fluids are possible around the impeller.

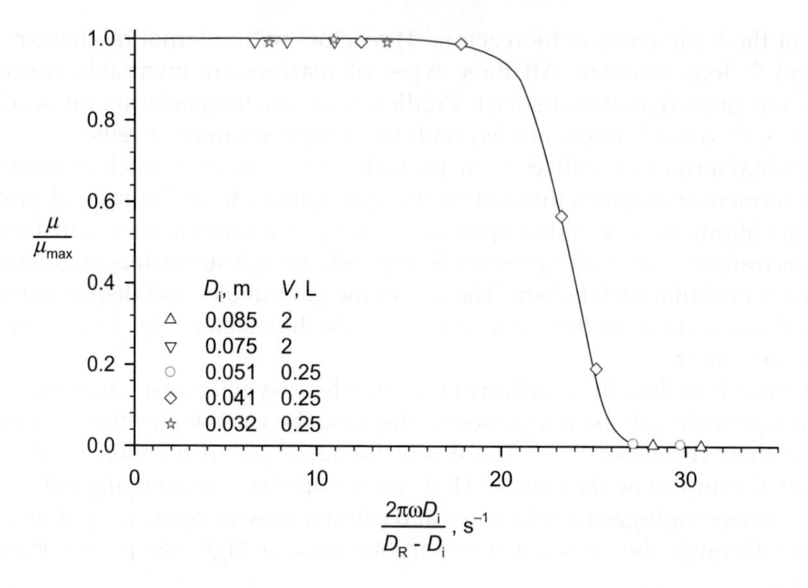

FIGURE 18.2 Relative growth rate of FS-4 animal cells on microcarriers as a function of the integrated shear factor (data from Croughan MS, Sayre ES, and Wang DIC. "Viscous reduction of turbulent damage in animal cell culture", Biotechnol. Bioeng. 33:862, 1989). D_R is the reactor vessel diameter, D_i is the impeller diameter, V is the volume of the reactor, and ω is the rotation rate of the impellers.

Fig. 18.3b shows a schematic of marine style impellers. Marine impellers throw fluid upward and thus causing top and bottom mixing to occur more easily.

Table 18.2 shows some criteria for the impeller selection. Disc and turbine impellers pump fluids in radial flow in the vessel. The impellers are generally 30–40% of reactor diameter.

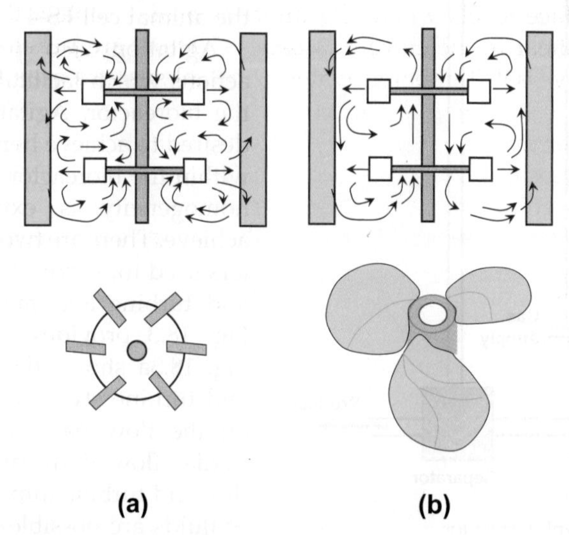

FIGURE 18.3 Disc and turbine impeller (a) and marine style impeller (b).

TABLE 18.2 Characteristics of Propeller and Disk Turbine

Characteristics	Propeller	Disk turbine
Flow direction	Axial	Radial
Gassing	Less suitable	Highly suitable
Dispersing	Less suitable	Highly suitable
Suspending	Highly suitable	Less suitable
Blending	Highly suitable	Suitable

The impellers provide high shear and high dispersion. Marine style impellers pump fluids in axial flow through the vessel. These impellers are generally 40–50% of reactor diameter. Axial flow systems induce less shearing and utilize less energy as compared to radial systems. They also break up the compartmentalization often observed in radial systems.

To augment mixing and gas dispersion, baffles are used to increase the disruption in the vessel and minimize vortex. Typically four baffles are used and are 8–10% of reactor diameter. Animal cell cultures do not typically use baffles due to shear concerns.

Bioreactors are mainly constructed with 316 SS wetted parts. With animal cell cultures, 316L SS is common. Non-product contact surfaces are generally constructed of 304 SS. Geometric dimensions greatly impact bioreactor performance. Microbial cultures generally have a height to diameter ratio (H/D_R) of 2–3:1. This is mainly due to the high-gas transfer requirements for the fast growing cells. Animal cell cultures are typically designed to an H/D_R ratio of 1:1. The location of the agitator impellers can be an important parameter. The number and location of impellers are often dictated by gas transfer requirements. For processes where media are fed to the bioreactor, thus increasing the vessel volume, interface levels where the impeller blades contact the liquid surface can produce significant shear to the culture. Most bioreactors are jacketed vessels to provide heat transfer for the vessel. Tempered water or glycol systems are utilized to control the bioreactor temperature. Internal heat transfer coils are also utilized; however, efficiencies gained in heat transfer are often lost due to fouling of the coils by microbial growth. The bioreactor jacket can also be used to assist sterilization of the vessel.

Foaming is also a significant consideration for bioreactor systems. If foaming escapes the bioreactor, it can wet the vent filters, increasing the venting pressure drop, reducing the gas flow to the bioreactor. Of greater concern, the wetted filter can become a pathway for contamination. The extent of foaming can effectively reduce the operating level of the bioreactor, as space is needed for gas to disengage from liquid, and ultimately reduce the vessel's throughput. Foaming challenges are often minimized by two methods: 1) mechanical foam breaker and 2) surface-active chemical agent. Although chemicals may be very effective in controlling foam, they usually lower K_La. They also can be detrimental to the cellular growth.

Sterility is of primary concern when designing all bioreactor systems. The desire for the bioreactor is to produce a pure culture, which is a culture where only the desired organism is detectably present. Openings to the vessel should be minimized to what is essential. A balance needs to be completed between the number of probes needed for process control

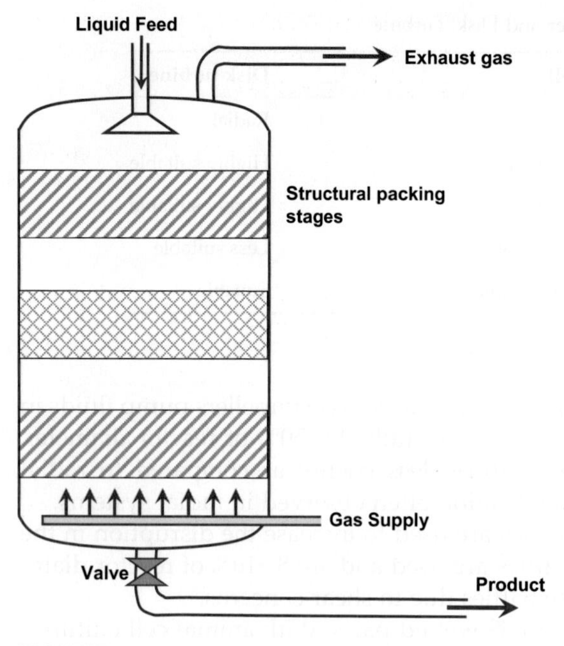

FIGURE 18.4 Bubble column reactor.

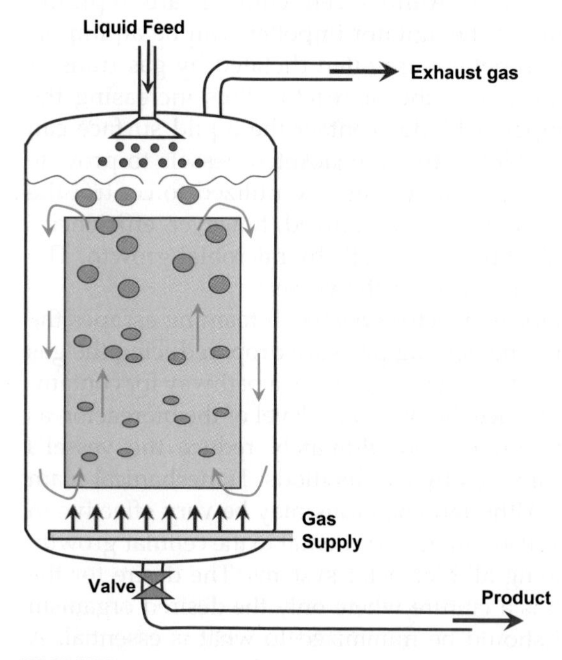

FIGURE 18.5 Internal airlift loop reactor.

and minimizing the number of openings which improves the chances for maintaining sterility. All surfaces within the vessel must be smooth and are often electropolished. O-rings are used for small openings, typically for probes used in process control. Gaskets are used for larger openings such are piping connections to the tank and the agitator mounting flanges. Agitators are equipped with seals to provide integrity between the vessel and outside environment. Double mechanical seals, with steam quench, are often utilized on microbial and animal cell culture applications. Vessels are designed to be free draining and cleanable. And ultimately, bioreactor systems must be designed to be steamable in place. Bioreactors are designed to be steamable from the top, down, so condensate cannot collect and compromise the heat kill or organisms.

Fig. 18.4 illustrates a bubble column reactor which provides a low shear environment for the culture. These columns are suitable for low viscosity Newtonian broths. The structural packing (of high porosity) can provide high contact area, keeping bubbles small or breaking the bubbles. They have higher energy efficiencies than agitated vessels in terms of the amount of gas transfer per unit power. However, bubble column reactors may be limited by foaming and bubble coalescence and are generally less flexible than stirred-tank bioreactors. The multistage arrangement (separated by structural packing) alleviates the bubble coalescence problem, further increasing mass transfer efficiency.

Fig. 18.5 shows a concentric draught-tube bioreactor with annular liquid down flow (loop reactor or airlift reactor). Loop reactors have intermediate characteristics between bubble columns and stirred-tank bioreactors. The fast upflowing air in the center draught tube carries medium and cells upward. At the top, bubbles break out of the medium, dropping cells and liquid medium. Cells and liquid medium flows down from the annulus on the side and then being carried upward from the center region (draught tube). Loop reactors can handle more viscous fluids than bubble columns and applied to situation where bubble coalescence is generally not a problem.

18.2. REACTOR OPERATIONAL MODE SELECTION

There are three general operation modes for a stirred-tank reactor: batch, continuous (or CSTR or chemostat), and fed-batch. The features of these (ideal) reactors have been discussed in Chapters 3, 4, 5, 11, 12, and 13. A summary of the reactor performance features is given in Table 18.3. A batch reactor has nearly an identical flow contact pattern as a PFR. There

TABLE 18.3 A Summary of Reactor Operational Modes for a Stirred-Tank or Well-Mixed Reactor

Operational model	Batch	CSTR	Fed-batch
Substrate	Highest concentration in the reactor, concentration decreases with residence time inside the reactor,	Lowest concentration in the reactor; constant and controllable concentration in the reactor	Start-up period similar to batch, and the bulk of the operation could mimic a CSTR
Desired product	Lowest concentration in the reactor, concentration increases with residence time in the reactor	Highest concentration in the reactor. Ability to promote the desired product selectivity by controlling the substrate concentration	Above
By-product	Reduced opportunity for degradation product(s) from desired product(s)	Reduced opportunity for side-product formation with a controlled substrate concentration	Above
Catalyst and/or cells	Residence time of catalyst is controllable and uniform; catalysts/cells are selected; complete catalysts replaceable at each batch	Residence time of suspended catalysts/cells is not uniform in the reactor; selection favors fast growth cells; fractional catalysts/cells replacement can be implemented	Same as batch operation
Flexibility	Distinctive batches, quality ensured at each batch level, easy to change operations	High throughput, easy to control, consistent quality, difficult to change operations	Distinctive batches, moderate throughput, quality controllable at each batch, easy to change operations
Applications	Small quantity production, high value substrate/product, multiple products/substrates/processes on demand; catalyst instability (mutation)	Large quantity production; high demand; consistent substrate supply and product quality demand; stable catalyst or controllable through feed	Process requiring strict product quality control while flexible operation is required or catalyst unstable with long duration of operations

is no "back-mixing" of the reactant stream with product stream. Reactants are loaded initially and the products are unloaded at the end of the reaction. A batch reactor is characterized by no input into or output from the reactor during the course of the reaction, eliminating the potential of external contamination. The substrate concentration remains highest inside the reactor, while the product concentration remains the lowest possible in the reactor. The reactor operation is terminated when reaction is completed as desired. A CSTR is characterized by a steady feed of substrate(s) into and effluent out of the reactor. The substrate concentration can be controlled to a given value and is the lowest in the reactor. The product concentration in the reactor is the highest. The reactor operation is not to be terminated frequently (by design). A fed-batch reactor is a mode between batch and CSTR operation. It can be designed to capture the qualities of a CSTR operation (and more), while maintaining the flexibility of a batch reactor operation.

The primary form of continuous culture is a steady-state CSTR or *chemostat*. A chemostat ensures a time-invariant chemical environment for the cell cultivation. The net-specific growth rate is equal to the dilution rate, which is determined by the flow rate to the chemostat. Thus, the growth rate can be manipulated by the investigator. This is a typical method of controlling the cell growth (and/or production formation rate). A constant dilution rate gives rise to a constant specific growth rate, which is equivalent to a fixed exponential growth rate. Another benefit is the control of substrate concentration in the reactor at a given value, which can promote a desired product formation. A *cytostat* (or *turbidostat*) adjusts flow rate to maintain a constant cell density (via turbidity). Cell density control via adjusting flow rate is not effective except at high flow rates. A turbidostat operates well at high flow rates (near the washout point) and is useful in selecting cellular subpopulations that have adapted to a particular stress.

Continuous culturing is more productive than batch culturing. The productivity of chemostat increases with increasing dilution rate to a maximum before sharply decreases near the washout limit. There is a maximum cell biomass concentration near the washout limit.

The growth and/or product formation patterns can be different between batch and continuous cultivations. In a batch system, lag phase is commonly observed which is absent in a continuous system. On the other hand, Crabtree effect can be observed with changing flow rates in a continuous system, which is absent in a batch cultivation curve since the change occurs when the substrate is nearly completely consumed.

Bioreactors using suspended cells can be operated in many modes intermediate between a batch reactor and a single-stage chemostat. Although a chemostat has potential productivity advantages for primary products, considerations of genetic instability, process flexibility, low quantities of product demand, and process reliability (such as biocontamination and biostability) have greatly limited the use of chemostat units. The use of cell recycle with a CSTR increases volumetric productivity and has found use in large-volume, consistent production demand and low-product value processes (e.g. waste treatment and fuel-grade ethanol production).

Multistage continuous systems improve the potential usefulness of continuous processes for the production of secondary metabolites and for the use of genetically unstable cells. The perfusion system is another option that is particularly attractive for animal cells.

Batch operations are not controllable as all the substrate is added into the reactor at the start. Fed-batch reactor is based on feeding of a growth-limiting nutrient substrate to a culture. Cell growth and fermentation can be controlled by the feeding strategy. The fed-batch strategy is typically used in bio-industrial processes to reach a high cell density in the bioreactor. Mostly, the feed solution is highly concentrated to avoid dilution of the bioreactor. In essence, fed-batch reactor is applied in such a fashion that a chemstat or CSTR is simulated with a seemingly batch operation. The controlled addition of the nutrient directly affects the growth rate of the culture and allows avoiding overflow metabolism (formation of side metabolites, such as acetate for *Escherichia coli*, lactic acid in cell cultures, ethanol in *Saccharomyces cerevisiae*), oxygen limitation (anaerobiosis).

Substrate limitation offers the possibility to control the reaction rates to avoid technological limitations connected to the cooling of the reactor and oxygen transfer. Substrate limitation also allows the metabolic control, to avoid osmotic effects, catabolite repression, and overflow metabolism of side products. Therefore, there are different operation strategies for fed-batch: 1) constant feed rate or constant growth/fermentation rate; 2) exponential feed rate or constant specific growth rate. The exponential growth with fed-batch operation can be at any rate, up to the maximum rate in the exponential growth phase of a batch growth. This is the case that closely resembles a chemostat operation. Usually, maximum growth rate is not wanted for undesired by-product production which can be high at maximum growth.

18.3. AERATION, AGITATION, AND HEAT TRANSFER

For industrial-scale fermentors, oxygen supply and heat removal are key design limitations. The severity of the oxygen requirement is a function of the organism. The oxygen uptake ratio (OUR) can be written:

$$\mathrm{OUR} = X\mu_{O_2} \tag{18.1}$$

where μ_{O_2}—specific uptake rate of oxygen and X is the biomass concentration. Typical values of μ_{O_2} are shown in Table 18.4.

OUR represents the consumption rate of oxygen, which is the demand from the cells. OUR is balanced by the OTR when pseudo steady state is reached. OTR is given by

$$\mathrm{OTR} = K_L a\,(C^* - C_L) \tag{18.2}$$

where C^*—oxygen solubility, C_L—actual dissolved oxygen (DO), and $K_L a$ is the volumetric mass transfer coefficient.

The value of $K_L a$ can be estimated by:

$$K_L a = k(P_0/V)^{0.4}(v_s)^{0.5}\omega^{0.5} \tag{18.3}$$

where k—empirical constant, P_0—power requirement, V—bioreactor volume, v_S—superficial gas velocity, and ω—agitator rotation rate.

The value of P_0 can be estimated from other correlations, such as

$$P_0 = k'\left(\frac{P_u^2\omega D_i^2}{Q^{0.56}}\right)^{0.45} \tag{18.4}$$

TABLE 18.4 Typical Respiration Rates of Microbes and Cells in Culture

Organism	μ_{O_2}, mmol-O_2/(g-dw h)
Bacteria	
E. coli	10–12
Azotobacter sp.	30–90
Streptomyces sp.	2–4
Yeast	
S. cerevisiae	8
Molds	
Penicillium sp.	3–4
Aspergillus niger	ca. 3
Plant cells	
Acer pseudoplatanus (sycamore)	0.3
Saccharum (sugar cane)	1–3
Animal cells	
HeLa	0.4×10^{-12} mol-O_2/(h·cell)
Diploid embryo WI-38	0.15×10^{-12} mol-O_2/(h·cell)

where P_u is the power requirement for ungassed vessel (i.e. in the absence of aeration or airflow into the reactor).

K_La is dependent on the media, salts, surfactants, pressure, and temperature making it difficult to predict. K_La is however measurable. Four approaches are generally used to measure K_La: unsteady state, steady state, dynamic, and sulfite test. The reactor is filled with water or medium and sparged with nitrogen to remove oxygen. The air is introduced and DO is monitored until the bioreactor is nearly saturated.

In the case of no consumption of oxygen in the reactor, mass balance of oxygen in the reactor leads to

$$\frac{dC_L}{dt} = K_La(C^* - C_L) \tag{18.5a}$$

which can be integrated to yield

$$C_L = C^* - (C^* - C_{L0})\exp(-K_La \cdot t) \tag{18.5b}$$

The DO changes exponentially with time for unsteady-state accumulation of oxygen. This is the theoretical basis for unsteady-state method of measuring the oxygen transfer coefficient. It is the simplest and easiest one to implement.

The sulfite method is conducted in the presence of Cu^{2+}, where sulfite (SO_3^{2-}) is oxidized to sulfate (SO_4^{2-}) in a zero order reaction. The reaction is very rapid and consequently C_L approaches zero. The rate of sulfate formation is monitored and is proportional to O_2 consumption (½ mol O_2 consumed to produce 1 mol of SO_4^{2-}). Mass balance of oxygen in the reactor leads to:

$$\frac{1}{2}\frac{dC_{SO_4^{2-}}}{dt} = K_L a \cdot (C^* - 0) \tag{18.6a}$$

$$K_L a = \frac{1}{2C^*}\frac{dC_{SO_4^{2-}}}{dt} \tag{18.6b}$$

where $C_{SO_4^{2-}}$ is the concentration of sulfate (SO_4^{2-}) and C^* is a constant dependent on the medium composition, pressure, and temperature and can be measured separately.

The steady-state method uses a fermentor with active cells and may be the best method to determine $K_L a$. This method requires accurate measurement of O_2 in all gas exit streams and reliable measurement of C_L. Mass balance on O_2 in the gas allows rate of O_2 uptake, OUR according to the following equation:

$$K_L a = \frac{OUR}{C^* - C_L} \tag{18.7}$$

OUR can be estimated with off-line measurements of a sample in a respirometer, but information from the actual fermentor is ideal. C^* is proportional to pO_2 which depends on the total pressure and fraction of the gas that is O_2. At sparger point, pO_2 is significantly higher than at exit due to higher pressure and consumption in the bioreactor. Knowledge of residence time distribution of gas bubbles is necessary to estimate a volume-averaged value of C^*.

The final method is the dynamic method. This method is a simpler method that only requires the measurement of DO and can be used under actual fermentation conditions. Mass balance on oxygen in the reactor leads to

$$\frac{dC_L}{dt} = OTR - OUR \tag{18.8a}$$

or

$$\frac{dC_L}{dt} = K_L a(C^* - C_L) - \mu_{O_2} X \tag{18.8b}$$

This method requires the air supply to be shut off for a short period (<5 min) then turned back on. With the gas supply off, $K_L a$ will be zero, and the slope of the descending curve will give the OUR or $-\mu_{O_2} X$:

$$\frac{dC_L}{dt} = -\mu_{O_2} X \tag{18.9}$$

Fig. 18.6 provides an example of the response of DO in a bioreactor when stopping and restarting airflow. The DO is kept at a relatively high level when air is continuous sparged into the reactor. When air sparging is stopped, the continuous consumption of oxygen by

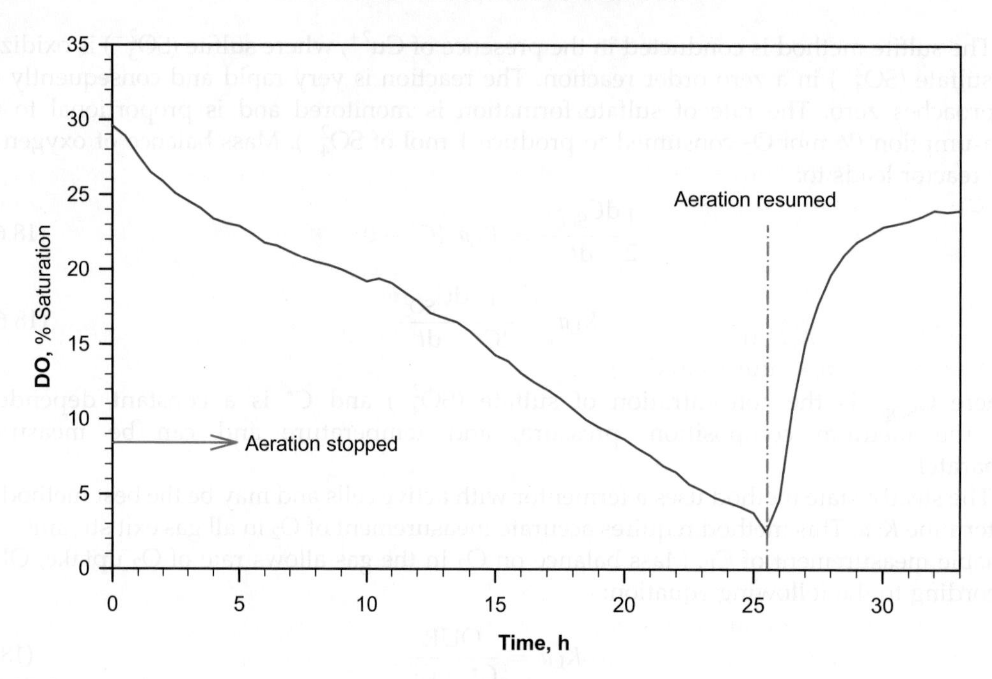

FIGURE 18.6 DO variation during the exponential growth period of *Burkholderia cepacia* in wood extract hydrolysate, while aeration is changed in a 1.3 L bioflo 110 fermentor.

the cells causes the DO level to decrease steadily as there is no supply to make up the oxygen consumption. The lowest value of C_L must be above the critical O_2 concentration so μ_{O_2} is independent of C_L. The relatively constant slope of DO decrease is an indication of constant oxygen consumption rate. The descending curve is caused by the oxygen consumption, thus the mass transfer can be decoupled. When air sparging is resumed, the DO increases due to the mass transfer rate being higher the consumption rate. The ascending curve is a combination of mass transfer and consumption.

Once K_La is established, it can be used to estimate the rate of metabolic heat generation and the total amount of cooling surface required. When oxygen is the rate-limiting step, the rate of oxygen consumption is equal to the rate of oxygen transfer. If the maintenance requirement of O_2 is negligible compared to growth, then:

$$\frac{\mu_G X}{YF_{X/O_2}} = K_La(C^* - C_L) \tag{18.10}$$

or

$$\mu_G X = YF_{X/O_2} K_La(C^* - C_L) \tag{18.11}$$

The heat generated during microbial growth can be calculated using the heat of combustion of the substrate and of cellular material. The heat of combustion of the substrate is equal to the sum of the metabolic heat and heat of combustion of the cellular material.

$$\frac{\Delta H_{c,S}}{YF_{X/S}} = \Delta H_{c,X} + YF_{H/X} \tag{18.12}$$

Where ΔH_S is the heat of combustion of the substrate, $YF_{X/S}$ is the substrate yield factor, $\Delta H_{c,X}$ is the heat of combustion of the cells, and $YF_{H/X}$ is the metabolic heat evolved per gram of cells produced. The equation can be rearranged to yield:

$$YF_{H/X} = \frac{\Delta H_{c,S}}{YF_{X/S}} - YF_{X/S}\Delta H_{c,S} \tag{18.13}$$

The bioreactor heat transfer surface area required can then be calculated given the heat transfer fluid temperature and design flow rates.

18.4. SCALE-UP

The preceding sections have discussed the complexities of design parameters for bioreactors. This section will consider how the complexities impact scaling for bioreactors. If the height to diameter ratio remains constant, surface to volume ratio dramatically decreases during scale-up. This changes the contribution of surface aeration and dissolved carbon dioxide removal in comparison to the contribution from sparging. Physical conditions in a large fermentor cannot exactly duplicate those in a small fermentor if geometric similarity is maintained. When changes alter the distribution of chemical species in a reactor or destroy or injure cells, the metabolic response of the culture will differ from one scale to another. Table 18.5 demonstrates the interdependence of scale-up parameters. In this example, a stirred-tank diameter has been scale-up by a factor of 5. The height to diameter ratio remained constant. Comparison of four common scale-up approaches is shown: constant power-to-volume ratios (P_0/V), constant K_La, constant tip speed (ωD_i, or impeller rotation rate ω times impeller diameter D_i), and constant Reynolds Number (Re).

Different scale-up rules can give very different results. Scale-up problems are all related to transport processes. Relative timescales for mixing and reaction are important in determining degree of heterogeneity. Scale-up may move from a system where microkinetics control the system at small scale to one where transport limitations control the system response at large scale. When a change in the controlling regime takes place, the results for the small-scale experiments become unreliable in predicting large-scale performance. One approach to predicting reactor limitations is the use of characteristic time constants for conversion and transport processes. Typical time constants are: the residence time or V/Q for flow system, diffusion time scale L^2/D_e, mixing time $4V/(1.5\omega D_R^3)$ for stirred vessel, conversion time C_A/r, etc. Processes with time constants that are small compared to the main processes appear to be essentially at equilibrium. For example, if $(K_La)^{-1} \ll t_{O_2}$ conversion, then the broth would be saturated with O_2 because O_2 supply is much more rapid than the conversion. Conversely, if the O_2 consumption is of the same order of magnitude as O_2 supply $[(K_La)^{-1} \approx t_{O_2}$ conversion], the dissolved O_2 concentration may be very low. Experimental measurements of DO have shown great variability in O_2 concentration with some values at zero. This means that cells pass periodically

TABLE 18.5 Scale-Up Comparison from 75 to 10,000 L Bioreactor with Impeller Size to Fermentor D_i/D_R and Fermentor Shape Factor H/D_R Remaining Constant

Scale-up criterion	Notation	Small fermentor, 75 L	Production fermentor, 10,000 L			
			Constant P_0/V	Constant ω	Constant ωD_i	Constant Re
Energy Input	$P_0 \propto \omega^3 D_i^5$	1	133.3333	3479.8823	26.0991	0.1957
Energy input/volume	$P_0/V \propto \omega^3 D_i^2$	1	1	26.0991	0.1957	0.0015
Impeller rotation number	ω	1	0.3371	1	0.1957	0.0383
Impeller diameter	D_i	1	5.1087	5.1087	5.1087	5.1087
Pump rate of impeller	$Q \propto \omega D_i^3$	1	44.9500	133.3333	26.0991	5.1087
Pump rate of impeller/volume	$Q/V \propto \omega$	1	0.3371	1	0.1957	0.0383
Maximum impeller speed (shear rate)	ωD_i	1	1.7223	5.1087	1	0.1957
Reynolds number	$Re = \omega D_i^2 \rho/\mu$	1	8.7987	26.0991	5.1087	1

through anaerobic regions. Since many cells have regulatory circuits to respond to changes from aerobic to anaerobic conditions, these may be constantly altering cellular metabolism.

Scale-up traditionally is highly empirical and must have no change in the controlling regime during scale-up, particularly if the system is only reaction or only transport controlled. Common scale-up rules are the maintenance of: (1) constant power-to-volume ratios (P_o/V), (2) constant K_La, (3) constant stirrer lade tip speed (ωD_i), (4) combination of mixing time and Reynolds Number, or (5) constant substrate or product level (usually DO). Each approach has resulted in successful and unsuccessful examples. Failure of the rules is related to changes in the controlling regime upon scale-up. The nature of the practical operating boundaries for an aerated, agitated fermentor can be summarized in Fig. 18.7. The boundaries are fuzzy but must be appreciated for the existence of such constraints.

Example 18-1. Consider scale-up from a lab fermentor of 1 L working volume to a 30,000 gal vessel. The small fermentor has a height to diameter ratio of 2.5. The impeller diameter is 30% of the inside tank diameter. Agitator speed is 400 rpm and Rushton impellers are used. Determine the dimensions of the large fermentor and agitator speed for:

(a) constant P_0/V;
(b) constant impeller tip speed;
(c) constant Reynolds number.

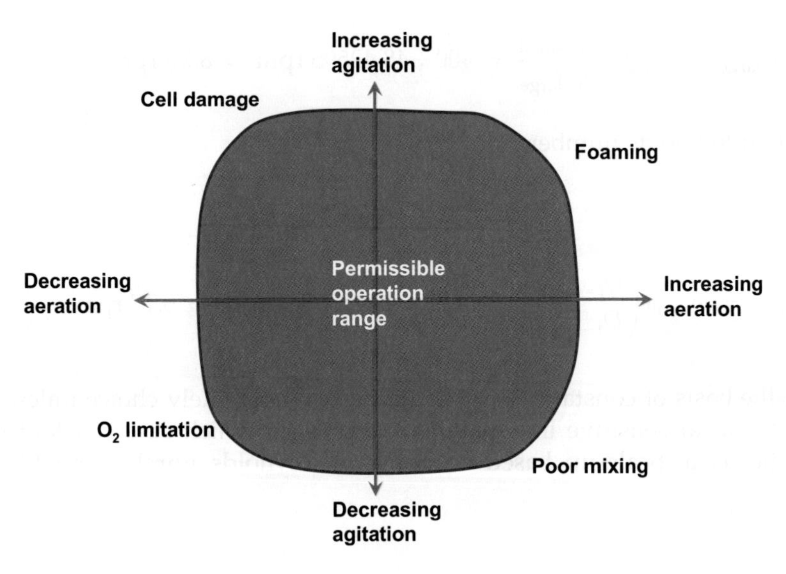

FIGURE 18.7 Practical operating boundaries for aerated, agitated fermentor.

Solution. Assume geometric similarity and the reactor are cylindrical. The dimensions of the small reactor can then be obtained as follows:

$$V = \frac{\pi}{4}D_R^2 H = \frac{\pi}{4}D_R^2 \times 2.5D_R = \frac{5\pi}{8}D_R^3 \tag{E18-1.1}$$

$$D_R = \left(\frac{8V}{5\pi}\right)^{\frac{1}{3}} \tag{E18-1.2}$$

$D_R = 0.07986$ m; $H = 0.19965$ m; $D_i = 0.3$ m; $D_R = 0.02396$ m.

The large reactor is of 30,000 gal and geometrically similar to the small reactor. Therefore, the scale factor in reactor dimensions is the cubic root of the volume ratio. That is $(30{,}000 \times 3.785412 \div 1)^{1/3} = 48.42595$. Therefore, the dimensions of the large reactor are

$D_R = 3.867$ m; $H = 9.668$ m; $D_i = 1.1602$ m.

(a) For constant P_0/V;

$$(\omega^3 D_i^2)_{\text{small}} = (\omega^3 D_i^2)_{\text{large}} \tag{E18-1.3}$$

$$\omega_{\text{large}} = \omega_{\text{small}}\left(\frac{D_{\text{i-small}}}{D_{\text{i-large}}}\right)^{\frac{2}{3}} = 400 \times 48.42595^{-\frac{2}{3}}\ \text{rpm} = 30.1 \tag{E18-1.4}$$

(b) For constant impeller tip speed;

$$(\omega D_i)_{\text{small}} = (\omega D_i)_{\text{large}} \tag{E18-1.5}$$

$$\omega_{\text{large}} = \omega_{\text{small}} \frac{D_{\text{i-small}}}{D_{\text{i-large}}} = 400 \div 48.42595 \text{ rpm} = 8.26 \text{ rpm} \tag{E18-1.6}$$

(c) For constant Reynolds number.

$$(\omega D_{\text{i}}^2)_{\text{small}} = (\omega D_{\text{i}}^2)_{\text{large}} \tag{E18-1.7}$$

$$\omega_{\text{large}} = \omega_{\text{small}} \left(\frac{D_{\text{i-small}}}{D_{\text{i-large}}} \right)^2 = 400 \times 48.42595^{-2} \text{ rpm} = 0.17 \text{ rpm} \tag{E18-1.8}$$

Scale-up on the basis of constant P_0/V would be the most likely choice unless the culture was unusually shear sensitive like mammalian cells, in which case constant impeller tip speed may be used. Scale-up based on constant Reynolds number would usually not be used.

18.5. SCALE-DOWN

Scale-down models provide a small-scale experimental system that duplicates exactly the same heterogeneity in environment that exists at the larger scale. At the smaller scale, many parameters can be tested more quickly and less expensively than at the production scale. Scale-down models are also used to demonstrate proof of process during technology transfers. In many cases, scale-up will require using existing production facilities, so it is important to replicate the production facilities at a smaller scale. They can be used to evaluate proposed process changes for an existing operating process and can be used to estimate the system's response (growth rate, product formation, formation of contaminating by-products) to changes in medium composition (new supplier of raw materials), introduction of modified production strains, use of different inoculum preparation, new antifoam agents, and for testing for O_2 and CO_2 tolerances.

18.6. BIOINSTRUMENTATION AND CONTROLS

The maintenance of optimal conditions for product formation in the complex operating environment of a bioreactor requires the control and measurement of at least a few parameters. Almost all fermentors have pH, temperature, and DO control. In addition, fermentor pressure control is also common. A balance of functional benefit of control versus a significant increase in the probability of contamination must be achieved. Instrumentation must be sterilizable, preferably with steam. They must be able to withstand high temperatures (121 °C) in the presence of high humidity (100%). Chemical sterilization may be used to allow for temperature-sensitive devices but is less desirable. Instrumentation must be compatible with the designed limitation of sterility. In addition to the instrumentation identified above, the following parameters are also monitored and controlled for the

TABLE 18.6 Approaches to Monitoring and Control of the Chemical Environment

Approach	Measuring devices and compounds monitored
1. Insertable probes	pH electrode; H^+
	Redox electrodes; redox potential
	Ion selective electrodes; NH_3, NH_4^+, Br^-, Cd^{2+}, Hg^{2+}, Ca^{2+}, Cl^-, Cu^{2+}, CN^-, SCN^-, F^-, BF_4^-, I^-, Pb^{2+}, NO_3^-, ClO_4^-, K^+, Ag^+, Na^+, S^{2-}, SO_4^{2-}
	O_2 probes (galvanic or polarographic; pO_2
	CO_2 probes; activity of dissolved CO_2, pCO_2
	Fluorescence probes; NADH
	Biosensors; wide range of compounds potentially detectable
2. Exit gas analyzers	Paramagnetic analyzer (O_2); thermal conductivity or long-path infrared analyzers (CO_2)
	Flame ionization detector; low levels of organically bound carbon, especially useful for volatile organics such as ethanol or methanol
	Mass spectrometer; O_2, CO_2, volatile substances (can also be used on liquid streams)
	Semiconductor gas sensors; flammable or reducing gases or organic vapors
3. Measurements from liquid slipstreams	HPLC; dissolved organics, particularly useful for proteins—auto analyzer
	Mass spectrometer; dissolved compounds that can be volatilized
	Enzymatic methods; potentially wide range, but glucose has received most attention

physical environment: 1) agitator shaft power, 2) foam, 3) gas flow rate, 4) liquid flow rate, 5) liquid level, 6) viscosity, and 7) turbidity.

On-line measurements of concentrations beyond pH and DO are difficult, but progress is being made. Table 18.6 summarizes techniques that have been considered for determining concentration of key components.

Since many fermentation processes require extensive periods for completion, there is a need to worry about replacement of insertable probes in addition to the probe performance. Mechanical design may dictate placement of the probes, even though heterogeneity in a large fermentor may be position dependent. Because of potential probe fouling, probes need to be installed with sufficient turbulence to help keep them clean. Due to extensive periods for fermentation completion, it is important that probe response be stable for extended periods. Probe fouling in an extended fermentation is a significant challenge. Probe drift can be a problem and in situ recalibration is not always possible.

Advancement in exit gas instruments at lower costs (mass spectrometer) has made this more attractive. These devices can be installed for use on several fermentors. The main limitation is that only volatile components can be monitored. On-line HPLC is powerful for measuring levels of dissolved solutes, particularly proteins from genetically engineered cells. These devices require using liquid slipstream and sample preparation, usually micro or ultra filtration. HPLC instruments also require significant time delays associated with sampling. Nuclear magnetic resonance (NMR) can provide important information on intracellular metabolism for off-line or small-scale growth experiments. In summary, current instrumentation to monitor fermentors online is very limited.

Having the physical characteristics of the bioreactor presents the next challenge—what to do with it. Current fermentor design and control techniques are limited. Computer-controlled fermentors are common, particularly at pilot plant scale. Typical computerized control applications are for data logging, i.e. data historian. Computerized control systems also provide regulatory control to open/close valves or turn on/off motors. Control loops for DO, temperature, pH, and pressure control are also common. Automation of recipe driven activities such as Clean-in-Place (CIP) or Steam-in-Place (SIP) is common, although control based on cellular activity is limited.

One application involves control based on CO_2 in the off-gas, coupled with substrate concentration in the feed and nutrient flow rates, allowing the glucose feed rate to be manipulated to maintain glucose concentrations at an optimal level. This control strategy depends on mass balances and gateway sensor concept. If glucose sensing is available, glucose control can be accomplished with a feedback control system.

Good process control for fermentation awaits improved models of cultures, more sophisticated sensors, and advances in nonlinear control theory.

18.7. STERILIZATION OF PROCESS FLUIDS

Sterility is an absolute concept. A system is never partially or almost sterile. On a practical basis, sterility means the absence of any detectable viable organism. In a pure culture, only the desired organism is detectably present. The cost of contamination for a bioreactor can be high. For example, undesired organisms can cause the waste of substrate or generation of waste products, while bacteriophage can cause the decay of fermentative organisms. The biocontaminant can be bacteria, fungi, yeast, viruses, etc. In majority of the bioprocesses, elimination of biocontaminants is essential for the success of the operation. In animal cell cultures, one often demands pure culture. The presence of undesired organisms is often the basis for rejection of the batch. Disinfection differs from sterilization in that a disinfectant reduces the number of viable organism to a low, but nonzero number. Fluid streams can be sterilized in two ways: 1) physical removal of cells and viruses (filtration) and 2) inactivation of living particles by heat, radiation, or chemicals.

Sterilization of process fluids can be implemented batchwise or continuously. Batch sterilization is suitable for batch operations and for sterilization of process equipment. For continuous operations, continuous sterilization of process fluids (liquid medium, gas, and suspensions) is more advantageous.

18.7.1. Batch Thermal Sterilization

Death is considered the failure of the cell, spore, or virus to reproduce or germinate when placed in a favorable environment. The probability of extinction of the total population, $P_0(t)$, is

$$P_0(t) = [1 - p(t)]^{N_0} \tag{18.14}$$

where $p(t)$ is the probability that an individual will still be viable at time, t, and N_0 is the number of individuals initially present. The expected value of individuals present at time, t, $E[N(t)]$ is

$$E[N(t)] = N_0 p(t) \tag{18.15}$$

While the variance of this expected value, $V[N(t)]$ is

$$V[N(t)] = N_0 p(t)[1 - p(t)] \tag{18.16}$$

The specific death rate, k_d is

$$k_d = \frac{1}{-E[N(t)]}\frac{d}{dt}E[N(t)] = -\frac{d}{dt}\ln p(t) \tag{18.17}$$

So far in modeling cell death rate, we have been assuming a first order rate or a constant specific death rate. When this first-order death model in which k_d is constant is applied:

$$p(t) = \exp(-k_d t) \tag{18.18}$$

which is equivalent to

$$E[N(t)] = N_0 \exp(-k_d t) \tag{18.19}$$

Decimal reduction time, t_{DR}, is the time for number of viable cells to reduce by 10 fold. That is

$$0.1 = \exp(-k_d t_{DR}) \tag{18.20}$$

$$t_{DR} = \frac{\ln 10}{k_d} \tag{18.21}$$

Fig. 18.8 is a plot of $N(t)/N_0$, strictly speaking $E[N(t)]/N_0$, versus time, which is called a survival curve. The survival curve can be applied to indicate the relative sterility as $E[N(t)]/N_0$ is the probability of surviving cells relative to the total cells initially. We often drop $E[*]$ notation with an understanding that the number of cells need not be an integer in computing the number of survived cells statistically. In practice, of course, there is no such thing as 1.1 or 0.2 cells alive. To ensure the sterility of the culture, one must ensure a low number (a small fraction of a cell) survival in absolute terms. Even one live spore can repopulate in the reactor. When the number of cells present initially is high, the survival ratio must even be smaller for sterility.

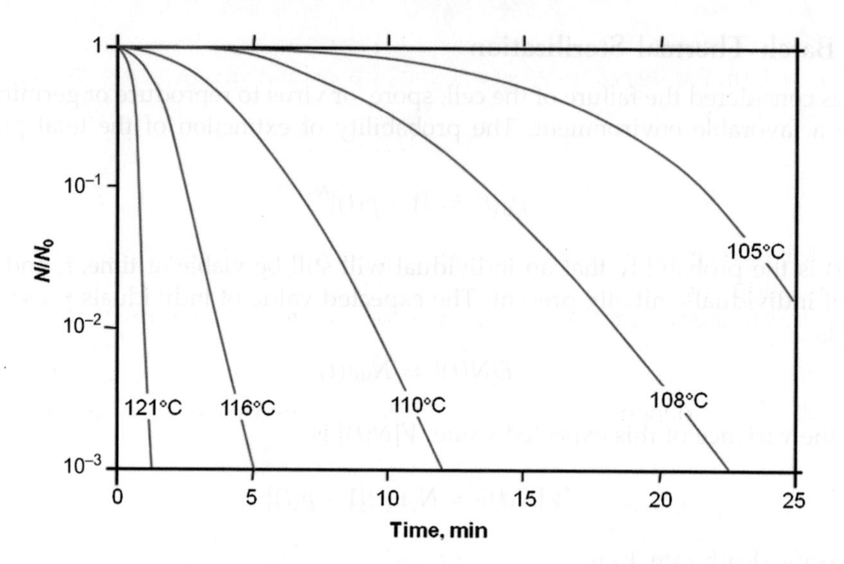

FIGURE 18.8 Typical survival curve (depicting cell death) for spores of *Bacillus stearothermophilus* Fs7954 in distilled water.

Most microbe populations are not homogeneous. Often a subgroup is more resistant to the sterilization method chosen. Also, organisms growing in flocs tend to be more resistant to death. These factors are important in processing. Especially in stringent safety required systems, prudent investigation of the potential "hard-to-kill" pollution is needed.

As we have discussed earlier that survival curve or ratio is not appropriate for ensuring sterility of the medium, we need to use a more absolute reference to sterility. Therefore, the probability of one cell surviving in the entire fermentation medium of concern is a good indicator to use. The probability of the entire population not vanishing during the sterilization process can be calculated based on Eqns (18.14) and (18.18),

$$P_1(t) = 1 - P_0(t) = 1 - [1 - p(t)]^{N_0} = 1 - (1 - e^{-k_d t})^{N_0} \tag{18.22}$$

For most applications, we want to ensure that $P_1(t)$ is very small to ensure that no cells in the entire population surviving during sterilization. Computationally, this can be challenging as N_0 can be large in large vessels. In the literature, numerical charts or graphs were frequently used, but they are not convenient and not compatible with modern convenience of superior computing powers. Eqn (18.22) can be expanded to give

$$\begin{aligned} P_1(t) &= 1 - (1 - e^{-k_d t})^{N_0} \\ &= N_0 e^{-k_d t} - \frac{N_0(N_0 - 1)}{2} e^{-2k_d t} + \frac{N_0(N_0 - 1)(N_0 - 2)}{6} e^{-3k_d t} \\ &\quad - \frac{N_0(N_0 - 1)(N_0 - 2)(N_0 - 3)}{24} e^{-4k_d t} + \ldots + \frac{(-1)^n N_0!}{n!(N_0 - n)!} e^{-nk_d t} + \ldots \end{aligned} \tag{18.23}$$

which is a fast convergent series for the cases we are interested in, i.e. long enough time to sterilize the system. For fast estimation, one can approximate the probability of unsuccessful fermentation $P_1(t)$ by

$$P_1(t) \approx \frac{N_0 e^{-k_d t}}{1 + \frac{N_0 - 1}{2} e^{-k_d t}} \tag{18.24}$$

Therefore, for the same level of sterilization, the time and/or temperature requirement is different for different size of reactors. The dimensionless sterilization time that can be employed to examine the sterilization of any given reactor can be estimated by

$$t_S = k_d t - \ln N_0 \tag{18.25}$$

Specific death rate dependence on temperature is given by Arrhenius equation:

$$k_d = k_{d0} \exp(-E_{ad}/RT) \tag{18.26}$$

where E_{ad} is the activation energy for the death of the organism and k_{d0} is the pre-exponential specific death rate constant. Values of E_{ad} range from 250 to 650 kJ/mol. Bacterial spores are typically more thermal resistant than vegetative forms of bacteria or yeast. At 121 °C, for example, the specific death rate k_d for vegetative cells may range up to 10^{10}/min, while k_d for spores is 0.5–5.0 min^{-1}. Mold spores are 2–10 times more resistant to vegetative forms of bacteria, viruses and bacteriophage are 1–5 times more resistant. Therefore, sterilization design is usually based on destruction of bacterial spores.

For typical spores of *B. stearothermophilus*, $k_{d0} = 8.236 \times 10^{37}$ min^{-1} and $E_{ad} = 283$ kJ/mol, while for *E. coli*, $E_{ad} \approx 530$ kJ/mol. Typically sterilizations occur at 121 °C. For most spores, k_d falls very rapidly with temperatures. There is a 10-fold decrease of death rate at $T = 110$ °C rather than 121 °C. The sterilization is accomplished by increase the temperature to a set temperature, commonly 121 °C, for a period of time and then cool down to working temperature (Fig. 18.9). For each heat sterilization, the dimensionless sterilization time can be computed by

$$t_S = k_{d0} \int_0^t e^{-\frac{E_{ad}}{RT}} dt - \ln N_0 \tag{18.27}$$

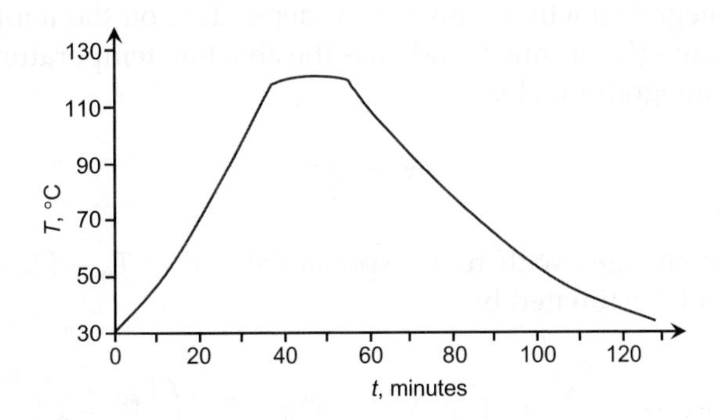

FIGURE 18.9 Typical sterilization temperature profile.

TABLE 18.7 General Equations for Temperature Change with Time During Heating and Cooling Periods in Batch Sterilizations. T_O Is the Initial Temperature of the Medium; T_S Is the Temperature of the Isothermal (Saturated) Steam; T_{ci} Is the Temperature of Water Entering the Jacket; b's Are Constants Changing Only with the Properties of Medium and Heat Transfer Fluid; as well as Heat Transfer Coefficient or Heating rate (for Electrical Heating)

Heat transfer method	Temperature–time profile	Integral function: $E(x)$
Direct sparging with steam	$T = T_O\left(1+\frac{b_1 t}{1+b_O t}\right)$	Eqn (18.33)
Electrical heating	$T = T_O(1+bt)$	Eqn (18.34)
Heating from isothermal steam in jacket	$T = T_S\left(1+\frac{T_O - T_S}{T_S}e^{-bt}\right)$	Eqn (18.31)
Cooling with cold water in jacket	$T = T_{ci}\left(1+\frac{T_O - T_{ci}}{T_{ci}}e^{-bt}\right)$	Eqn (18.31)

as temperature is a function of time. The total number of cells can be computed by

$$N_O = VC_{XO} \tag{18.28}$$

with V being the reactor volume and C_{XO} being the number concentration of cells initially present in the reactor.

The temperature change in the vessel is a function of the heating/cooling methods. Table 18.7 shows some of the functional forms of temperature change during the heating up and cooling down periods of the sterilization process. In Chapter 4, we have learned how to integrate Eqn (18.27), i.e. H-Factor. Commonly, there are three types of time–temperature profiles: linear (electrical heating), exponential (noncontact heat exchanger), and hyperbolic (direct mixing/contact with another fluid stream). The integral in Eqn (18.27) can be represented by

$$\int_0^t e^{-\frac{E_{ad}}{RT}} dt = ET\left(\frac{E_{ad}}{RT}\right) - ET\left(\frac{E_{ad}}{RT_O}\right) \tag{18.29}$$

where $ET(x)$ is the integral function with a form dependent on the temperature profile, T is the absolute temperature (K) at time t, and T_O is the absolute temperature at time $t = 0$ or the starting point of the integration. Here

$$x = \frac{E_{ad}}{RT} \tag{18.30}$$

If the temperature changes with time exponentially $T = T_\alpha + (T_O - T_\alpha)e^{-bt}$, the corresponding integral can be estimated by

$$ET(x) = \frac{E_{ad}}{bRT_\alpha}\exp(-x)\left[\sum_{i=0}^{n}(-1)^i i! \sum_{m=0}^{i}(-1)^m x^{-i+m-1}\left(\frac{E_{ad}}{RT_\alpha} - x\right)^{-m-1} + \cdots\right] \tag{18.31}$$

Since Eqn (18.30) is an asymptotic series, it diverges if too many terms are taken. At small value of n, increasing the number of terms (n) leading to convergent value for $ET(x)$. The value of n is taken such that

$$n!\sum_{m=0}^{n}(-1)^m x^{-n+m-1}\left(\frac{E_{\text{ad}}}{RT_\alpha}-x\right)^{-m-1} \geq (n+1)!\sum_{m=0}^{n+1}(-1)^m x^{-n+m-2}\left(\frac{E_{\text{ad}}}{RT_\alpha}-x\right)^{-m-1} \quad (18.32)$$

i.e. maintaining a converging trend of the series. We stop the series before it starts to diverge.

If the temperature is a hyperbolic function of time, $T = T_0\left(1+\frac{b_1 t}{1+b_0 t}\right)$, then the integral is given by

$$ET(x) = \frac{(2b_0-b_1)E_{\text{ad}}}{(b_1-b_0)^2 RT_0}\exp(-x)\left[\sum_{i=0}^{n}(-1)^i(i+1)!\left(x-\frac{E_{\text{ad}}}{RT_0}\frac{b_0}{b_1-b_0}\right)^{-i-2}+\cdots\right] \quad (18.33)$$

which is also an asymptotic series. Restriction on the number of terms to monotonously decreasing value of successive terms applies.

If the temperature changes with time linearly, $T = T_0(1+bt)$, the integral can be estimated by

$$ET(x) \approx -\frac{E_{\text{ad}}}{RbT_0}\exp(-x)x^{-2}\left[1-2x^{-1}+\ldots+(-1)^n(n+1)!x^{-n}\right] \quad n < x \quad (18.34)$$

Thus, the dimensionless time can be computed if the temperature profile is known.

The higher t_S is, the more likelihood of being successful in a fermentation. For example, a dimensionless time t_S of 4.605 yields one unsuccessful fermentation in 100 fermentations, whereas doubling the dimensionless time t_S to 9.21 yields one unsuccessful fermentation in 10,000 fermentations. Therefore, a dimensionless time of 10 should be sufficient for most applications.

18.7.2. Continuous Thermal Sterilization

Like reactor operations, the sterilization can be operated resembling those of PFR and CSTR operations.

18.7.2.1. Thermal Sterilization in a CSTR

Fig. 18.10 shows a sketch of a well-mixed sterilizer. Viable cell balance in the CSTR leads to

$$QC_{X0} - QC_X - k_d C_X V = \frac{d(C_X V)}{dt} = 0 \quad (18.35)$$

Therefore, the probability of a microorganism surviving the heat treatment in a CSTR is

$$p(\tau) = \frac{C_X}{C_{X0}} = \frac{1}{1+k_d\tau} \quad (18.36)$$

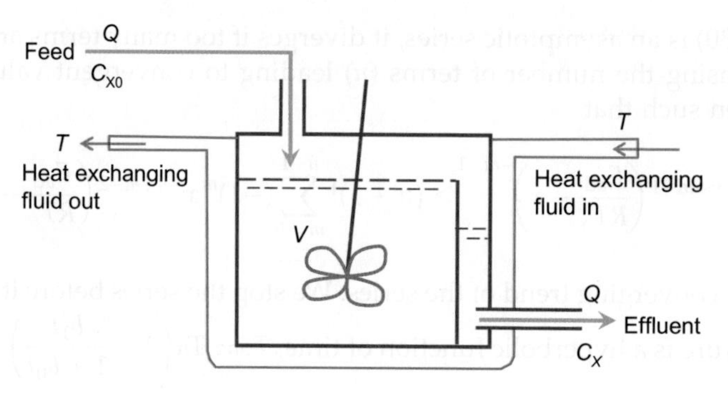

FIGURE 18.10 Sterilization in a well-mixed reactor.

where τ is the space time of the process fluid spent in the heat treatment zone, $\tau = \frac{V}{Q}$. The probability of the entire population in one reactor-full process fluid (or in one dilution) not vanishing from the heat treatment is

$$P_1(\tau) = 1 - P_0(\tau) = 1 - [1 - p(t)]^{C_{X0}V} = 1 - \left(\frac{k_d\tau}{1 + k_d\tau}\right)^{C_{X0}V} \tag{18.37}$$

which corresponds to the dimensionless sterilization time of

$$t_S = \ln(1 + k_d\tau) - \ln(C_{X0}V) \tag{18.38}$$

Comparing Eqns (18.38) and (18.25), the value of dimensionless sterilization time from Eqn (18.38) is much smaller than the batch sterilization if the residence time for the CSTR is kept the same as the batch. To make sure a small value of $P_1(\tau)$, we need a large stirred tank to ensure large value of $k_d\tau$. Complete backmixing of the process fluid making the viable cells at the effluent identical to everywhere in the reactor. Because of the fresh supply of viable cells, the probability of the entire population in the reactor to vanish is at its minimum. Therefore, the CSTR option is not attractive for continuous sterilization operations. It is ineffective for heat sterilization in a CSTR.

18.7.2.2. Thermal Sterilization in a PFR

We next examine a PFR option for continuous sterilization. Fig. 18.11 shows a diagram of a tubular sterilizer. Viable cell balance in the differential volume between x and $x + dx$ along the tubular axis gives

$$QC_X|_x - QC_X|_{x+dx} - k_d C_X A_{cr} dx = \frac{\partial(C_X A_{cr} dx)}{\partial t} = 0 \tag{18.39}$$

where x is the tube length coordinate (from the feed point) and A_{cr} is the cross-sectional area of the tube. Divide Eqn (18.39) by dx and letting $dx \to 0$, we obtain

$$k_d C_X A_{cr} + \frac{d(QC_X)}{dx} = 0 \tag{18.40}$$

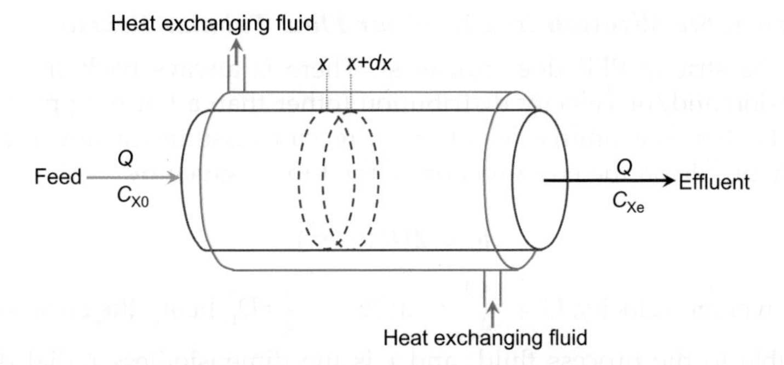

FIGURE 18.11 Sterilization in a well-mixed reactor.

Integrating Eqn (18.40), we obtain the probability of a contaminant cell surviving the heat treatment

$$p(\tau) = \frac{C_X}{C_{X0}} = e^{-k_d \tau} \tag{18.41}$$

where τ is the space time of the fluid medium through the whole length of the sterilization section L, that is

$$\tau = \frac{A_{cr} L}{Q} \tag{18.42}$$

Therefore sterilization in a PFR is quite similar to that of the batch process. The probability of the entire population in one reactor-full process fluid (of volume V) not vanishing from the heat treatment is

$$P_1(\tau) = 1 - P_0(\tau) = 1 - [1 - p(\tau)]^{C_{X0} V} = 1 - (1 - e^{-k_d \tau})^{C_{X0} V} \approx \frac{C_{X0} V e^{-k_d \tau}}{1 + \frac{C_{X0} V - 1}{2} e^{-k_d \tau}} \tag{18.43}$$

which corresponds to the dimensionless sterilization time of

$$t_S = k_d \tau - \ln(C_{X0} V) \tag{18.44}$$

Eqn (18.44) is nearly identical to Eqn (18.25). Thus, sterilization in a PFR is just as sterilization in a batch reactor. However, the heating up and cooling down requirements are not as stringent as batch sterilization.

Continuous sterilization in a PFR set-up, particularly a high-temperature short-exposure time process, can significantly reduce damage to medium ingredients while achieving high levels of cell destruction. Other advantages include improved steam economy and more reliable scale-up. The amount of steam needed for continuous tube flow sterilization is 20–25% that used in batch processes. The time required is also significantly reduced because heating and cooling are virtually instantaneous. Therefore, for sterilizing process fluids, it is advantageous to design the sterilization in a PFR setting.

18.7.2.3. Thermal Sterilization in a Laminar Flow Tubular Reactor

In practice, the strictly PFR does not exist. There is always backmixing due to flow-induced dispersion and/or velocity distribution (other than a flat plug profile). Let us first look at the sterilization in a laminar flow tubular reactor. Assume the flow is fully developed and the velocity profile on the cross-section of the tube is given by

$$u = 2U(1 - r^2) \tag{18.45}$$

where U is the average velocity, $U = \frac{Q}{A_{cr}}$ with $A_{cr} = \frac{1}{4}\pi D_R^2$ being the cross-sectional area of the tube available to the process fluid, and r is the dimensionless radial distance (radial distance divided by the tube radius) from tube center. If we neglect the transverse diffusion/dispersion, the cells would follow the streamline. The cells in the center of the tube will spend less time in the sterilization zone than those near the tube wall. Therefore, the overall probability of a cell surviving the sterilization is

$$\begin{aligned} p(\tau) &= \int_0^1 2r\frac{u}{U}\frac{C_X}{C_{X0}}dr = \int_0^1 4r\,(1-r^2)\exp\left[-\frac{k_d\tau}{2\,(1-r^2)}\right]dr \\ &\overset{y=\frac{k_d\tau}{2(1-r^2)}}{=\!=\!=\!=} \frac{1}{2}(k_d\tau)^2\int_{\frac{k_d\tau}{2}}^{\infty}\frac{e^{-y}}{y^3}dy \end{aligned} \tag{18.46}$$

where τ is the space time and defined by Eqn (18.42). Since $k_d\tau$ is greater than 2 for meaningful sterilization operations, integration of Eqn (18.46) leads to

$$\begin{aligned} p(\tau) &= -(k_d\tau)^2\frac{e^{-y}}{2y^3}\left[1 - 3y^{-1} + 12y^{-2} - \cdots + (-1)^n\frac{(n+2)!}{2}y^{-n}\right]\Bigg|_{\frac{k_d\tau}{2}}^{\infty} \\ &\quad - (-1)^n\frac{(n+3)!}{4}(k_d\tau)^2\int_{\frac{k_d\tau}{2}}^{\infty}\frac{e^{-y}}{y^{n+1}}dy \approx \frac{4(k_d\tau+2)}{k_d\tau(k_d\tau+8)}\exp\left(-\frac{k_d\tau}{2}\right) \end{aligned} \tag{18.47}$$

Comparing Eqn (18.47) with Eqn (18.41), one can infer that sterilization in laminar flow reactor is less effective than that in a PFR of the same space time. However, it is much more effective than in a CSTR as described by Eqn (18.36). The probability of the entire population in one reactor-full process fluid of volume V not vanishing from the laminar flow heat treatment is

$$P_1(\tau) = 1 - P_0(\tau) = 1 - [1 - p(\tau)]^{C_{X0}V} \approx \frac{C_{X0}V\dfrac{4(k_d\tau+2)}{k_d\tau\,(k_d\tau+8)}\exp\left(-\dfrac{1}{2}k_d\tau\right)}{1+\dfrac{2(C_{X0}V-1)\,(k_d\tau+2)}{k_d\tau\,(k_d\tau+8)}\exp\left(-\dfrac{1}{2}k_d\tau\right)} \tag{18.48}$$

which corresponding to the dimensionless sterilization time of

$$t_S = \frac{1}{2}k_d\tau - \ln\frac{4(k_d\tau + 2)}{k_d\tau(k_d\tau + 8)} - \ln(C_{X0}V) \tag{18.49}$$

Therefore, the effectiveness of a laminar flow sterilizer is about half of that of a PFR.

18.7.2.4. Thermal Sterilization in a Turbulent Flow Tubular Reactor

Let us now visit the tubular flow reactor analysis by incorporating the backmixing into the cell balance. Along the axis (x) of the tube, mass balance in a differential volume (Fig. 18.11) at steady state yields

$$\left.\left(QC_X - D_{\text{eff}}A_{\text{cr}}\frac{dC_X}{dx}\right)\right|_x - \left.\left(QC_X - D_{\text{eff}}A_{\text{cr}}\frac{dC_X}{dx}\right)\right|_{x+dx} - k_dC_XA_{\text{cr}}dx = 0 \tag{18.50}$$

where D_{eff} is the dispersion coefficient (or flow-induced diffusion coefficient), and A_{cr} is the cross-sectional area of the tube. Divide Eqn (18.50) by dx and letting $dx \to 0$, we obtain

$$k_dA_{\text{cr}}C_X + \frac{d}{dx}\left[QC_X - D_{\text{eff}}A_{\text{cr}}\frac{dC_X}{dx}\right] = 0 \tag{18.51}$$

There are two Eigen values for this differential equation:

$$\lambda_{1,2} = \frac{Q \pm \sqrt{Q^2 + 4D_{\text{eff}}A_{\text{cr}}^2k_d}}{2D_{\text{eff}}A_{\text{cr}}} \tag{18.52}$$

We therefore need two boundary conditions to fully specify the system (well-posedness). Physically, we know that the exit condition does not affect the progress of sterilization inside the tubular reactor. Backward dispersion of contaminant cells is not important for evaluating the sterilization operations. When $D_{\text{eff}} \to 0$,

$$\begin{aligned}\lim_{D_{\text{eff}}\to 0}\lambda_{1,2} &= \lim_{D_{\text{eff}}\to 0}\frac{Q \pm \sqrt{Q^2 + 4D_{\text{eff}}A_{\text{cr}}^2k_d}}{2D_{\text{eff}}A_{\text{cr}}} \\ &= +\infty, -\frac{k_dA_c}{Q}\end{aligned} \tag{18.53}$$

With the negative sign in Eqn (18.53), the solution for PFR is recovered. Therefore, only one mode is physical and that mode should be the monotonous decay mode. We neglect the positive Eigenvalue. The solution is thus given by

$$p(\tau) = \frac{C_X}{C_{X0}} = \exp\left(\frac{Q - \sqrt{Q^2 + 4D_{\text{eff}}A_{\text{cr}}^2k_d}}{2D_{\text{eff}}A_{\text{cr}}}x\right) \tag{18.54}$$

The dispersion coefficient may be written as,

$$D_{\text{eff}} = a_{\text{d}} \frac{Q}{A_{\text{cr}}} D_{\text{R}} \tag{18.55}$$

where a_{d} is a constant, varies only with the flow conditions. For turbulent flows in a pipe,

$$a_{\text{d}} = 3 \times 10^7 \text{Re}^{-2.1} + 1.35\,\text{Re}^{-0.125} \tag{18.56}$$

which is valid for $\text{Re} = \frac{D_{\text{R}} \rho Q}{\mu_{\text{v}} A_{\text{cr}}} = \frac{4 \rho Q}{\pi \mu_{\text{v}} D_{\text{R}}} > 2000$. Here μ_{v} is the viscosity of the liquid medium.

For a tube of constant diameter of D_{R} and length L, Eqn (18.51) is reduced to

$$p(\tau) = \exp\left(\frac{1 - \sqrt{1 + 4 a_{\text{d}} D_{\text{R}} L^{-1} k_{\text{d}} \tau}}{2 a_{\text{d}} D_{\text{R}}} L\right) \tag{18.57}$$

The probability of the entire population in one reactor-full process fluid of volume V not vanishing from the heat treatment is

$$P_1(\tau) = 1 - P_0(\tau) = 1 - [1 - p(\tau)]^{C_{X0} V} \approx \frac{C_{X0} V \exp\left(\frac{1 - \sqrt{1 + 4 a_{\text{d}} D_{\text{R}} L^{-1} k_{\text{d}} \tau}}{2 a_{\text{d}} D_{\text{R}}} L\right)}{1 + \frac{C_{X0} V - 1}{2} \exp\left(\frac{1 - \sqrt{1 + 4 a_{\text{d}} D_{\text{R}} L^{-1} k_{\text{d}} \tau}}{2 a_{\text{d}} D_{\text{R}}} L\right)} \tag{18.58}$$

which corresponds to the dimensionless sterilization time of

$$t_{\text{S}} = \frac{\sqrt{1 + 4 a_{\text{d}} D_{\text{R}} L^{-1} k_{\text{d}} \tau} - 1}{2 a_{\text{d}} D_{\text{R}}} L - \ln(C_{X0} V) \tag{18.59}$$

Example 18-2. Holding time and tube length requirement for a continuous sterilizer.

Medium at a flow rate of 3.6 m^3/h is to be sterilized by heat exchange with steam in a continuous sterilizer. The liquid contains bacterial spores at a concentration of $2 \times 10^{12}\ \text{m}^{-3}$. The sterilization temperature is to be conducted at 121 °C, at which the death rate of the bacterial spores is $k_{\text{d}} = 400\ \text{h}^{-1}$. The sterilizer tube has an inner diameter of 0.1 m; the density of the medium is 1000 kg/m^3 and the viscosity is 0.001 Pa s. How long of the tube is needed to sterilize the medium for a risk of 0.001 for fermentation of each sterilizer full of medium?

Solution: $Q = 3.6\ \text{m}^3/\text{h} = 0.001\ \text{m}^3/\text{s}$; $\text{Re} = \frac{4 \rho Q}{\pi \mu_{\text{v}} D_{\text{R}}} = \frac{4 \times 1000 \times 0.001}{\pi \times 0.001 \times 0.1} = 12732 > 2000$

$$a_{\text{d}} = 3 \times 10^7 \text{Re}^{-2.1} + 1.35\,\text{Re}^{-0.125} = 0.486$$

$C_{X0} = 2 \times 10^{12}$; $P_1(\tau) \leq 0.001$; $V = \frac{\pi}{4} D_{\text{R}}^2 L$; $\tau = V/Q$. Solving Eqn (18.55) with Excel,

$$P_1(\tau) \approx \frac{C_{X0} V \exp\left(\frac{1 - \sqrt{1 + 4 a_{\text{d}} D_{\text{R}} L^{-1} k_{\text{d}} \tau}}{2 a_{\text{d}} D_{\text{R}}} L\right)}{1 + \frac{C_{X0} V - 1}{2} \exp\left(\frac{1 - \sqrt{1 + 4 a_{\text{d}} D_{\text{R}} L^{-1} k_{\text{d}} \tau}}{2 a_{\text{d}} D_{\text{R}}} L\right)}$$

We obtain $L = 49.1$ m. Therefore, a 50-m long section of sterilization can meet the needs.

Example 18-3. Continuous sterilizer.

A fermentor of 10 m^3 is to be used to carry out the bioprocess. Medium at a flow rate of 1.2 m^3/h is to be sterilized by heat exchange with steam in a continuous sterilizer. The liquid contains bacterial spores at a concentration of 2.5×10^{11} m^{-3}. The sterilization temperature is to be conducted at 125 °C, at which the death rate of the bacterial spores is $k_d = 500/h$. The sterilizer tube has an inner diameter of 1.2 m; the density of the medium is 1100 kg/m^3 and the viscosity is 0.00125 Pa · s. How long of the tube is needed to sterilize the medium for a risk of one viable cell contamination in 6 months? What is the required dimensionless sterilization time?

Solution: Before we answer the question, we need to decide what the question asks us to do. A risk of one viable cell contamination in 6 months seems to imply that

$$p(\tau) = \frac{1}{C_{X0}Qt} = \frac{1}{2.5 \times 10^{11} \times 1.2 \times 6 \times 30.5 \times 24} = 7.59 \times 10^{-16}$$

which is a relative condition for sterilization. In the problem statement, we were told the volume of the fermentor $V = 10$ m^3 but not whether the fermentation is continuous or batch. One can also use a more stringent (absolute) condition, that is, the probability of unsuccessful fermentation

$$P_1(\tau) = \frac{VC_{X0}}{C_{X0}Qt} = \frac{10 \times 2.5 \times 10^{11}}{2.5 \times 10^{11} \times 1.2 \times 6 \times 30.5 \times 24} = 0.001897$$

for each reactor full of medium. We shall compare both cases.

The sterilization process is continuous in a tubular reactor. The flow conditions are

$Q = 1.2\ m^3/h = 3.333 \times 10^{-4}\ m^3/s$; $\quad \mathrm{Re} = \dfrac{4\rho Q}{\pi \mu_v D_R} = \dfrac{4 \times 1100 \times 3.333 \times 10^{-4}}{\pi \times 0.00125 \times 1.2} = 311.24 <$ 2000, i.e. laminar flow. Therefore, Eqns (18.47) through (18.49) apply.

$$p(\tau) \approx \frac{4(k_d\tau + 2)}{k_d\tau(k_d\tau + 8)} \exp\left(-\frac{k_d\tau}{2}\right) \tag{18.47}$$

$$P_1(\tau) \approx \frac{C_{X0}V \dfrac{4\,(k_d\tau + 2)}{k_d\tau\,(k_d\tau + 8)} \exp\left(-\dfrac{1}{2}k_d\tau\right)}{1 + \dfrac{2\,(C_{X0}V - 1)\,(k_d\tau + 2)}{k_d\tau\,(k_d\tau + 8)} \exp\left(-\dfrac{1}{2}k_d\tau\right)} \tag{18.48}$$

and

$$t_S = \frac{1}{2}k_d\tau - \ln\frac{4(k_d\tau + 2)}{k_d\tau(k_d\tau + 8)} - \ln(C_{X0}V) \tag{18.49}$$

The kinetic condition to use with these equations is given by

$$k_d\tau = k_d\frac{\pi}{4Q}D_R^2L = \frac{500}{3600} \times \frac{\pi}{4 \times 3.333 \times 10^{-4}} \times 1.2^2L = 471.24\,L$$

with the tube length L being in meters.

(a) Setting $p(\tau) = 7.59 \times 10^{-16}$ for Eqn (18.47), we can solve with Excel for $k_d\tau = 63.91$. Therefore, $L = 0.1356$ m. A short section of the tube will be sufficient to meet the requirement.

$$t_S = \frac{1}{2}k_d\tau - \ln\frac{4(k_d\tau + 2)}{k_d\tau\,(k_d\tau + 8)} - \ln(C_{X0}V)$$
$$= \frac{63.91}{2} - \ln\frac{4(63.91 + 2)}{63.91 \times (63.91 + 8)} - \ln(2.5 \times 10^{11} \times 10) = 6.267$$

(b) Setting $P_1(\tau) = 0.001897$ for Eqn (18.48), we can solve with Excel for $k_d\tau = 63.91$. Therefore, $L = 0.1356$ m. We arrived practically at the same answer as that for setting $p(\tau) = 7.59 \times 10^{-16}$.

18.7.3. Sterilization of Liquids

Thermal inactivation is preferred for large-scale sterilization of equipment and liquids. It is the most reliable method of sterilization.

Sterile filtration is often used where elevated temperatures can be detrimental to the process fluid. Liquid streams are steam or filter sterilized. Filtration with 0.2–0.45 μm membrane filter can be used to remove microbial components. The membrane filter itself must be sterilized before use, via thermal sterilization. The use of membrane between 0.2 μm and 0.45 μm is to ensure microorganism not passing through the membrane (needing finer pore sizes) while maintaining high throughput (for larger pore sizes). Sterile filtration is described in further detail for gases. Materials of construction for the filter membranes are application dependent. Liquid media filtration is generally not as effective or reliable as heat or thermal sterilization. Viruses and mycoplasma are able to pass through membrane filters. Care must be taken to prevent holes or tears (leaks) in the membrane. Usually, filter-sterilized medium is incubated for a period of time before use to ensure its sterility.

Heat-sensitive equipment can be sterilized with chemical agents or radiation. Chemical agent for sterilization must leave no residue that would be toxic to the culture or otherwise adulterate the product. Typical chemical agents used are: ethylene oxide, 70% ethanol water acidified to pH 2 with HCl, formaldehyde, 3% sodium hypochlorite.

Radiation sterilization can be applied to equipment surfaces as well as processing liquids. Radiation sterilization is usually used for sterilization of filtration equipment but not commonly used for large equipment due to operational difficulties involving applying radiation to large areas. The radiation sources can be applied include γ-ray, electron beam, or UV light. γ-radiation has better penetration into materials but is much more dangerous to work with. Electron beam systems are not commonly used for sterilizing the insides of fermentors but are becoming more prevalent in the sterilization of presterilized components such as filters. UV light is the simplest of the radiations to be used, as it can be provided by basic UV light bulbs. These are often encased in quartz tubes to protect them, as glass is insufficiently transparent in the UV range. UV can sterilize surfaces but cannot penetrate fluids easily.

18.7.4. Sterilization of Gases

Filtration methods are almost always used when sterilizing process gases. Depth or surface filters can be used, but surface membrane cartridge filters are predominantly used. Membrane filters utilize sieving for particle removal. With both depth and surface filters, pressure drop is critical. Increased operating pressures for utility gas systems significantly increased the cost of operation. Membrane filters are manufactured with uniformly small pores to prevent passage of particles with a radius larger than the pore radius. These filters can be steam sterilized many times. Condensate formed on non-sterile side cannot pass into the sterile side. Filters used on gas services are generally hydrophobic, not allowing liquids to pass through. All sterile filters require testing for integrity, usually before and after each use. At bubble point, diffusion testing is commonly utilized to conduct integrity test sterile filters. As indicated earlier, there is a significant need to minimize pressure drop.

18.7.5. Ensuring Sterility

Thermal sterilization is the most common techniques applied in the industry. Temperature and time are to be selected based on the thermal stability of medium, as well as the thermal stability of the potential undesirable microorganisms present. Usually, tests need to be conducted to verify sterile conditions. For sterilizing known microorganisms, one must take into account subcultures that are more thermal stable. Although the population might be small, these more thermal stable subcultures could have much lower activation energies (of deactivation).

One particularly resistant undesired biocontaminant is prions or infectious proteins. Commonly, infectious particles possessing nucleic acid are dependent upon it to direct their continued replication. Prions, however, are infectious by their effect on normal versions (or desired folding forms) of the protein. Prions induce normal proteins to re-fold and to be added (*grow*) to prions. Sterilizing prions therefore require the denaturation of the protein to a state where the molecule is no longer able to induce the abnormal folding of normal proteins. Prions are generally quite resistant to proteases, heat, radiation, and formalin treatments, although their infectivity can be reduced by such treatments. Effective prion decontamination relies upon protein hydrolysis or reduction or destruction of protein tertiary structure. Examples include bleach, caustic soda, and strongly acidic detergents. Prion is very thermal resistant. In a pressurized steam autoclave, 134 °C (274 °F) for 18 min may not be enough to deactivate the agent of disease. Ozone sterilization is being studied as a potential method for prion denaturation and deactivation. Partially denatured prions can be renatured to an infective status under certain artificial conditions.

The World Health Organization recommends any of the following three procedures for the sterilization of all heat-resistant surgical instruments to ensure that they are not contaminated with prions:

(1) Immerse in a pan containing 1 mol/L NaOH and heat in a gravity-displacement autoclave at 121 °C for 30 min; clean; rinse in water; and then perform routine sterilization processes.

(2) Immerse in 1 mol/L NaOH or sodium hypochlorite (2% available chlorine) for 1 h; transfer instruments to water; heat in a gravity-displacement autoclave at 121 °C for 1 h; clean; and then perform routine sterilization processes.

(3) Immerse in 1 mol/L NaOH or sodium hypochlorite (2% available chlorine) for 1 h; remove and rinse in water, then transfer to an open pan and heat in a gravity-displacement (121 °C) or in a porous-load (134 °C) autoclave for 1 h; clean; and then perform routine sterilization processes.

18.8. ASEPTIC OPERATIONS AND PRACTICAL CONSIDERATIONS FOR BIOREACTOR SYSTEM CONSTRUCTION

Sterilization as described in section §18.6 ensures the sterility of the entering process fluids during operations. To maintain a sterile operation, one must also ensure the sterility of the equipment at the start of operation and consider the potential of biocontaminants accumulation and/or unintended entrapment especially. Aseptic operations are achieved by a combination of sterile system at the start and elimination of the potential of biocontaminants during the operations. A good example of the failure caused by the negligence of aseptic operation (around fermentors) was that of the former North East Biofuels, Fulton, New York. The project was a $200 million retrofit from a closed brewery to 110 million gal/year capacity ethanol facility. It operated for 6 months before going bankrupt and was sold to Sunoco for $8.5 million.

Industrial bioreactors for sterile operation are usually designed as steel pressure vessels capable of withstanding full vacuum up to about 3 atm positive pressure at 150–180 °C. A manhole is provided on large vessels to allow workers entry into the tank for cleaning and maintenance; on smaller vessels the top is removable.

For pressure vessels, spherical (or round) structure is most stable, while cubic or flat structures are weak. Cylindrical reactors are commonly constructed to save space and material use. Flat head plates are commonly used with laboratory-scale fermentors; for larger vessels, a domed construction is preferred for lower material cost. Large fermentors are equipped with a lighted vertical sight glass for inspecting the contents of the reactor.

Nozzles for medium, antifoam, acid and alkali addition, air-exhaust pipes, pressure gauge, and a rupture disc for emergency pressure release are normally located on the head plate. Side ports for pH, temperature, and DO sensors are required at minimum; a steam-sterilizable sample outlet should also be provided. The vessel must be fully drainable via a harvest nozzle located at the lowest point of the reactor. If the vessel is mechanically agitated, either a top- or bottom-entering stirrer is installed.

18.8.1. Equipment, Medium Transfer, and Flow Control

Bioprocess operations outside of the food and beverage industry are commonly carried out utilizing pure (most cases single) cultures. Aseptic conditions must be maintained to ensure the efficiency of these bioprocesses. Keeping the reactor free of foreign organisms is especially important for slow-growing cultures which can be quickly overrun by contamination. Fermentors must be capable of operating aseptically for a number of days, sometimes months.

Typically, 3–5% of fermentations in an industrial plant are lost due to failure in sterilization. However, the frequency and causes of contamination vary considerably from process to process. For example, the nature of the product in antibiotic fermentations presents some protection from contamination; fewer than 2% of production-scale antibiotic fermentations are lost through contamination by microorganisms or phage. In contrast, a contamination rate of 17% was reported for industrial-scale production of β-interferon from human fibroblasts cultured in 50-L bioreactors (Morandi M and Valeri A 1988 Industrial Scale Production of β-interferon. Adv. Biochem. Eng./Biotechnol. 37, 57–72).

Industrial fermentors and associated pipings are designed for in situ steam sterilization under pressure or SIP. The use of saturated steam is common and advantageous over other hot fluids. As steam is applied to a vessel or pipe, the hot steam transfers its energy (heat) to the wall of the pipe or vessel, raising its temperature. The transfer of heat from the steam decreases the enthalpy of the saturated water vapor, causing it to condense at constant temperature. This condensation decreases the volume of the water by a factor of 815 for steam at 121 °C. This results in a pumping action (pressure drop when water vapor condenses), drawing more steam to the areas of greatest consumption, i.e. the areas that are the coldest. This provides a more even temperature profile and makes the heating process less likely to result in cold spots and dead legs. As a result, the sterilization is uniform.

The vessel should have a minimum number of internal structures, ports, nozzles, connections, and other attachments to ensure that steam reaches all parts of the equipment. For effective sterilization, all air in the vessel and pipe connections must be displaced by steam. The reactor should be free of crevices and potential stagnant areas where liquid or solids can accumulate; polished welded joints could use in preference to other coupling methods. Small cracks or gaps in joints and fine fissures in welds are prone to harboring microbial contaminants and are avoided in bioreactor system construction whenever possible. After sterilization, all nutrient medium and air entering the fermentor must be sterile. As soon as flow of steam entering the fermentor is stopped, sterile air is introduced to maintain a slight positive pressure in the vessel. The positive pressure in the vessel prevents entry of air-borne contaminants. Filters preventing passage of microorganisms are fitted to exhaust gas lines; this serves to contain the culture inside the fermentor and ensures against contamination should there be a drop in operating pressure.

Flow of liquids to and from the fermentor is controlled using valves. Because valves are a potential entry point for contaminants, their construction must be suitable for aseptic operation. Common designs such as simple gate and globe valves have a tendency to leak around the valve stem and accumulate broth solids in the closing mechanism. Although used in the fermentation industry, they are unsuitable if a high level of sterility is required. Values should be constructed such that no openings out of the pipe even if the valve stem is removed by accident. This can be achieved by constructing an inner wall with expandable materials to seal the entire valve section. Fig. 18.12 shows a sketch of a pinch valve where flexible material is used to build an inner tubing. Flexible sleeves and/or diaphragms are the common choices for the closing mechanism to be isolated from the contents of the pipe and there are no dead spaces in the valve structure. Rubber or neoprene capable of withstanding repeated sterilization cycles is used to construct the valve closure; the main drawback is that these components must be checked regularly for wear to avoid valve failure. To minimize costs, ball and plug valves are also used in fermentor construction.

18.8.2. Stirrer Shaft

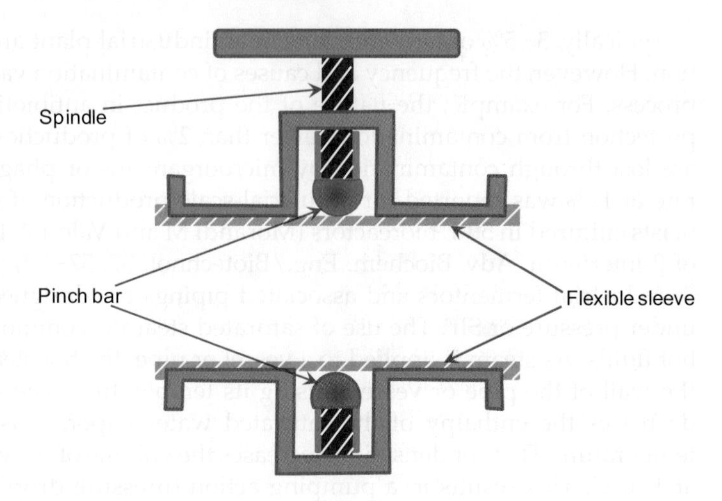

FIGURE 18.12 A schematic of a pinch valve.

With stirred reactors, the "opening" where stirrer shaft enters the vessel is a potential entry point for contamination. The gap between the rotating stirrer shaft and the fermentor body must be sealed. If the fermentor is operated for long periods, wear at the seal opens the way for air-borne contaminants. Several types of stirrer seal have been developed to prevent contamination. On large fermentors, mechanical seals are commonly used. One part of the assembly is stationary while the other rotates on the shaft; the precision-machined surfaces of the two components are pressed together by springs or expanding bellows and cooled and lubricated with water. Mechanical seals with running surfaces of silicon carbide paired with tungsten carbide are often specified for fermentor application. Stirrer seals are especially critical if the reactor is designed with a bottom-entering stirrer; double mechanical seals may be installed to prevent fluid leakage. On smaller vessels, magnetic drives can be used to couple the stirrer shaft with the motor; with these devices, the shaft does not pierce the fermentor body. A magnet in a housing on the outside of the fermentor is driven by the stirrer motor; inside, another magnet is attached to the end of the stirrer shaft and held in place by bearings. Sufficient power can be transmitted using magnetic drives to agitate vessels up to at least 800 L in size (Chisti Y. 1992 Assure Bioreactor Sterility. Chem. Eng. Prog. 88, 80–95). However, the suitability of magnetic drives for viscous broths, especially when high oxygen transfer rates are required, is limited.

18.8.3. Fermentor Inoculation and Sampling

To prevent contamination during inocula transfer operations, both vessels are maintained under positive air pressure. The simplest aseptic transfer method is to pressurize the inoculum vessel using sterile air; culture is then effectively blown into the larger fermentor through a connecting pipe. The fermentor and its piping and the inoculum tank and its piping including valves are sterilized separately before culture is added to the inoculum tank. Because these connectors were open prior to being joined, they must be sterilized before the inoculum tank is opened.

Sampling ports are commonly fitted to fermentors to allow for removal of broth intermittently. The sampling ports must be constructed such that the outside (i.e. away from the fermentor vessel) is sterilizable with steam before sample withdraw and can maintain high temperature on the pipe to fend off foreign microorganisms to enter the fermentor vessel.

18.8.4. Materials of Construction

Fermentors are constructed from materials that can withstand repeated steam sterilization and cleaning cycles. Materials contacting the fermentation medium and broth should also be nonreactive and nonabsorptive. Glass is used to construct fermentors up to about 30-L capacity. The advantages of glass are that it is smooth, non-toxic, corrosion-proof, and transparent for easy inspection of the vessel contents. Because entry ports are required for medium, inoculum, air, and instruments, such as pH and temperature sensors, glass fermentors are usually equipped with stainless steel head plates containing many screw fittings.

Most pilot- and large-scale fermentors are made of corrosion-resistant stainless steel, although mild steel with stainless steel cladding has also been used. Cheaper grades of stainless steel may be used for the jacket and other surfaces isolated from the broth. Copper and copper-containing materials must be avoided in all parts of the fermentor contacting the culture because of its toxic effect on cells. Interior steel surfaces are polished to a bright "mirror" finish to facilitate cleaning and sterilization of the reactor; welds on the interior of the vessel are ground flush before polishing. Electropolishing is preferred over mechanical polishing, as mechanical polishing leaves tiny ridges and grooves in the metal to accumulate dirt and microorganisms.

18.8.5. Sparger Design

The sparger, impeller, and baffles determine the effectiveness of mixing and oxygen transfer in stirred-tank bioreactors. Three types of sparger are commonly used in bioreactors: porous, orifice, and nozzle. Porous spargers of sintered metal, glass, or ceramic are used mainly in small-scale applications. Gas throughput is limited because the porous sparger poses a high resistance to flow. Cells growing through the fine holes and blocking the sparger can also be a problem. Orifice sparger also known as perforated pipes are constructed by making small holes in piping which is then fashioned into a ring or cross and placed at the base of the reactor; individual holes must be large enough to minimize blockages. Orifice spargers have been used to a limited extent for production of yeast and single-cell protein and in waste treatment. *Nozzle spargers* are used in many agitated fermentors from laboratory to production scale. These spargers consist of a single open or partially closed pipe providing a stream of air bubbles; advantages compared with other sparger designs include low resistance to gas flow and small risk of blockage. Other sparger designs have also been developed. In *two-phase ejector injector*, gas and liquid are pumped concurrently through a nozzle to produce tiny bubbles; in *combined sparger agitator* designs for smaller fermentors, a hollow stirrer shaft is used for delivery of air. Irrespective of sparger design, provision should be made for in-place cleaning of the interior of the pipe.

18.8.6. Evaporation Control

Aerobic cultures are continuously sparged with air. Most components of air are inert and leave directly through the exhaust gas line. If air entering the fermentor is dry, water is continually stripped from the medium and leaves the reactor as vapor. Over time, evaporative water loss can be significant. Water loss is more pronounced in a bubble reactor because the gas flow rate required for good mixing and mass transfer is generally higher than in a stirred reactor.

To combat evaporation problems, air sparged into fermentors may be pre-humidified by bubbling through columns of water outside the fermentor; humid air entering the fermentor has less capacity for evaporation than dry air.

Fermentors are also equipped with water-cooled condensers to return to the broth any vapors carried by the exit gas. Evaporation can be a particular problem when products or substrates are more volatile than water. For example, *Acetobacter* species are used to produce acetic acid from ethanol in a highly aerobic process requiring large quantities of air. It has been reported for stirred-tank reactors operated at air flow rates between 0.5 and 1.0 L-air/min/L-broth^{-1} that from a starting alcohol concentration of 5%, 30–50% of the substrate is lost within 48 h due to evaporation (Akiba T. and Fukimbara, 1973 Fermentation of volatile substrate in a tower-type fermentor with a gas entrainment process. J. Ferment. Technol. 51. 134–141.).

18.9. EFFECT OF IMPERFECT MIXING

So far, we have been based on our analysis on ideal reactors: well mixed in batch and CSTR for example. This perfect mixing can never be achieved in reality, but it does give us a convenient tool in reactor analysis and design. When scaling reactor up or down, the degree of mixing can have a significant effect, especially for microbes.

One method of examining non-ideal contacting in reactors is through residence time distribution. While residence time distribution is a useful tool in detecting possible mixing behaviors, it is of little use in terms of reactor performance analysis. Different contacting schemes, for example a PFR followed by a well-mixed flow reactor, have the combined residence time distribution as that if the order of the two reactors is reversed. However, the effluents out of the last reactor can be different if the reaction kinetics is not of first order.

Ideally, one would solve the Navier–Stokes equation (momentum balance and overall mass balance), together with mass balance equations, and the reaction kinetics, for a real reactor. This has the potential of correctly predicting the behavior in a reactor. While we are in the reach of computational capabilities, still the computational effort is significant. Traditionally, empirical methods are used at least for fast estimation.

There are two classic approaches to model the non-ideality of mixing in mixed flow reactors: 1) surface adhesion of cells and 2) compartments of different flow conditions, including dead zones. Fig. 18.13 shows a schematic of natural compartmentalization of culture in a chemostat. The mixing flow pattern of stirrers can generate semi segregation of regions of cultures, in turn the reactor behaviors are affected by the semi-separated region formation.

18.9.1. Compartment Model

Compartmentalization can occur due to non-ideal mixing. Different parts of the reactor may behave as if they are isolated from the other parts. Refer to Fig. 18.13, mass balances in the top compartment with Monod growth model lead to

$$\frac{dX_1}{dt} = k_{LX}a(X_2 - X_1) - (1 + \alpha_1)DX_1 + \left(\frac{\mu_{max}S_1}{K_S + S_1} - k_d\right)X_1 \tag{18.60}$$

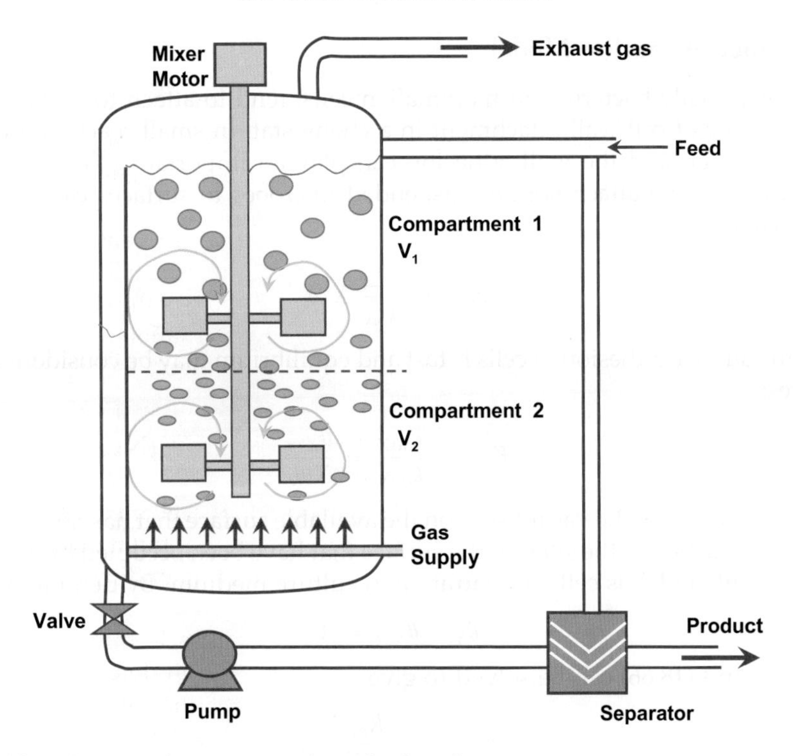

FIGURE 18.13 Schematic of compartment formation in a chemostat.

$$\frac{dS_1}{dt} = k_{LS}a(S_2 - S_1) + (1 + \alpha_1)D(S_0 - S_1) - \frac{1}{YF_{X/S}}\frac{\mu_{max}S_1}{K_S + S_1}X_1 \tag{18.61}$$

where α_1 is the volumetric ratio of the lower compartment to the top compartment, the volumetric mass transfer coefficients ($k_{LX}a$ and $k_{LS}a$) are based on the top compartment and the dilution rate (D) is based on the total reactor volume. In strongly mixed flow reactors (high Reynolds number), the mass transfer coefficients are nearly the same for all species (as molecular diffusion is negligible compared to flow-induced diffusion or dispersion), either be (fine) solid particles (like microbes) or soluble molecules (like sugar substrates).

Mass balances in the lower compartment with Monod growth model lead to

$$\frac{dX_2}{dt} = \frac{k_{LX}a}{\alpha_1}(X_1 - X_2) + \left(\frac{\mu_{max}S_2}{K_S + S_2} - k_d\right)X_2 \tag{18.62}$$

$$\frac{dS_2}{dt} = \frac{k_{LS}a}{\alpha_1}(S_1 - S_2) - \frac{1}{YF_{X/S}}\frac{\mu_{max}S_2}{K_S + S_2}X_2 \tag{18.63}$$

For steady-state operations, none of the concentrations would be changing with time. Therefore, Eqns (18.60) through (18.63) are reduced to a set of algebraic equations as usual for the continuous cultures.

18.9.2. Surface Adhesion Model

Microbes, especially bacteria and mammalian cells, tend to attach to surfaces. Fig. 18.14 shows a schematic of cell wall attachment in a chemostat. In small reactors, the surface to volume ratio is high and the wall adhesion can play an important role especially at low cell concentrations. The attachment of suspended microbes to surfaces can be modeled as adsorption. That is

$$X + \sigma \underset{k_{deX}}{\overset{k_{adX}}{\rightleftarrows}} X \cdot \sigma \tag{18.64}$$

Assume the surface adhesion of cells is fast and equilibrium may be considered for continuous cultures:

$$K_{\sigma X} = \frac{k_{adX}}{k_{deX}} = \frac{\theta_{X \cdot \sigma}}{X \theta_V} \tag{18.65}$$

where θ_V is the fraction of the vacant sites on the available surface that has no cells attached to them, $\theta_{X \cdot \sigma}$ is the fraction of the sites on the surface that have been occupied by cells, $K_{\sigma X}$ is the adhesion constant, and X is cell concentration in culture medium. By definition:

$$\theta_V + \theta_{X \cdot \sigma} = 1 \tag{18.66}$$

Eqns (18.65) and (18.66) can be solved to give

$$\theta_{X \cdot \sigma} = \frac{K_{\sigma X} X}{1 + K_{\sigma X} X} \tag{18.67}$$

Therefore, the total viable concentration of cells in the reactor is given by

$$X_T = X + C_\sigma \theta_{X \cdot \sigma} = X + C_\sigma \frac{K_{\sigma X} X}{1 + K_{\sigma X} X} \tag{18.68}$$

where C_σ is the concentration of total available adhesion sites on surfaces in the reactor. In some cases, the adhesion of cells on the solid surface can be regarded as irreversible, i.e. $K_{\sigma X} \to \infty$. Eqn (18.68) is then reduced to

$$X_T = X + C_\sigma \tag{18.69}$$

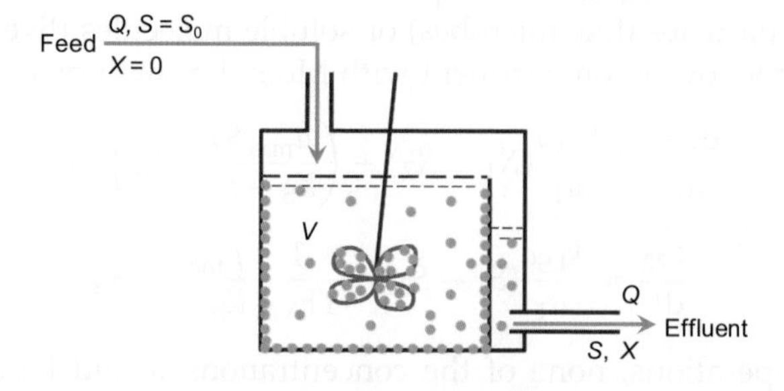

FIGURE 18.14 A schematic of a continuous culture with both suspended cells (X) and surface attached cells. The suspended cells are subject to removal by flow, whereas the surface attached cells are less affected by the flow.

Mass balances over the reactor (with Monod growth model) lead to

$$\frac{dX_T}{dt} = -DX + \left(\frac{\mu_{max}S}{K_S + S} - k_d\right)X_T \tag{18.70}$$

$$\frac{dS}{dt} = D(S_0 - S) - \frac{1}{YF_{X/S}}\frac{\mu_{max}S}{K_S + S}X_T \tag{18.71}$$

Note that cell growth and death are based on the total viable cells in the reactor, whereas the cell removal from the reactor only occurs for the suspended cells.

At steady state, variation with time is zero. Eqns (18.69), (18.70) and (18.71) give

$$-DX + \left(\frac{\mu_{max}S}{K_S + S} - k_d\right)\left(X + C_\sigma \frac{K_{\sigma X}X}{1 + K_{\sigma X}X}\right) = 0 \tag{18.72}$$

$$D(S_0 - S) - \frac{1}{YF_{X/S}}\frac{\mu_{max}S}{K_S + S}\left(X + C_\sigma \frac{K_{\sigma X}X}{1 + K_{\sigma X}X}\right) = 0 \tag{18.73}$$

Furthermore, we are looking for nontrivial solutions as $X = 0$ is the washout condition. Eliminating the trivial solution from Eqn (18.72), we obtain

$$-D + \left(\frac{\mu_{max}S}{K_S + S} - k_d\right)\left(1 + C_\sigma \frac{K_{\sigma X}}{1 + K_{\sigma X}X}\right) = 0 \tag{18.74}$$

If $C_\sigma = 0$ (i.e. no surface attachment), Eqn (18.74) gives

$$S = \frac{(D + k_d)K_S}{\mu_{max} - D - k_d} \tag{18.75}$$

which is a unique solution (apart from the trivial solution $S = S_0$). Therefore, there are only one two-steady states for Monod growth culture without wall attachment.

Eqns (18.73) and (18.74) can be solved to obtain nontrivial steady-state solution(s) for chemostat with wall attachment. Numerical solutions can be achieved for example, by trial and error or with Excel. Substituting Eqn (18.74) into Eqn (18.73) and solving for X, we obtain

$$X = YF_{X/S}(S_0 - S)\left(1 - \frac{K_S + S}{\mu_{max}S}k_d\right) \tag{18.76}$$

which can be substituted into Eqn (18.74) to reduce the number of variables to one (just the substrate concentration, S). Close form (or exact) solutions can also be obtained via Cardano procedure by substituting Eqns (18.76) and (18.74) to give

$$a_3S^3 - a_2S^2 + a_1S - a_0 = 0 \tag{18.77}$$

where

$$a_3 = K_{\sigma X}YF_{X/S}(\mu_{max} - D - k_d)(\mu_{max} - k_d) \tag{18.78a}$$

$$a_2 = K_{\sigma X}YF_{X/S}S_0(\mu_{max} - D - k_d)(\mu_{max} - k_d) + K_{\sigma X}YF_{X/S}K_S[(D + 2k_d)(\mu_{max} - k_d) - Dk_d] + \mu_{max}[(\mu_{max} - k_d)(1 + K_{\sigma X}C_\sigma) - D] \quad (18.78b)$$

$$a_1 = K_{\sigma X}YF_{X/S}S_0K_S[(D + 2k_d)(\mu_{max} - k_d) - Dk_d] + K_{\sigma X}YF_{X/S}K_S^2k_d(D + k_d) + K_Sk_d\mu_{max}(1+K_{\sigma X}C_\sigma) + D\mu_{max}K_S \quad (18.78c)$$

$$a_0 = K_{\sigma X}YF_{X/S}K_S^2k_d\, S_0(D + k_d) \quad (18.78d)$$

Let

$$S = y + \frac{a_2}{3a_3} \quad (18.79)$$

Eqn (18.77) is reduced to

$$y^3 + 3a_5y - 2a_4 = 0 \quad (18.80)$$

where

$$a_5 = \frac{a_1}{3a_3} - \frac{a_2^2}{9a_3^2} \quad (18.81a)$$

$$a_4 = \frac{a_0}{2a_3} - \frac{a_1a_2}{6a_3^2} + \frac{a_2^3}{27a_3^3} \quad (18.81b)$$

The solution to Eqn (18.79) can be obtained by letting

$$y = x + \frac{\alpha}{x} = x - \frac{a_5}{x} \quad (18.82)$$

The substitution by Eqn (18.82) can reduce Eqn (18.80) into a quadratic equation, which can be solved easily to give two roots

$$x^3 = a_4 \pm a_6 \quad (18.83)$$

where

$$a_6 = \sqrt{a_4^2 + a_5^3} \quad (18.84)$$

These two roots give identical values to y in Eqn (18.82). Therefore, one of the roots can be used. The next step is to take the cubic roots from Eqn (18.83), which yields three roots: one real and one pair of conjugate complex roots (if $a_4 + a_6$ is real). Substituting back to S, we obtain the solutions to Eqn (18.77):

$$S_1 = y_1 + \frac{a_2}{3a_3} = x_1 - \frac{a_5}{x_1} + \frac{a_2}{3a_3} = \frac{a_2}{3a_3} + \sqrt[3]{a_4 + a_6} + \sqrt[3]{a_4 - a_6} \quad (18.85a)$$

$$S_2 = y_2 + \frac{a_2}{3a_3} = x_2 - \frac{a_5}{x_2} + \frac{a_2}{3a_3} = \frac{a_2}{3a_3} + \frac{-1 + \sqrt{3}i}{2}\sqrt[3]{a_4 + a_6} + \frac{-1 - \sqrt{3}i}{2}\sqrt[3]{a_4 - a_6} \quad (18.85b)$$

$$S_3 = y_3 + \frac{a_2}{3a_3} = x_3 - \frac{a_5}{x_3} + \frac{a_2}{3a_3} = \frac{a_2}{3a_3} + \frac{-1-\sqrt{3}i}{2}\sqrt[3]{a_4 + a_6} + \frac{-1+\sqrt{3}i}{2}\sqrt[3]{a_4 - a_6} \quad (18.85c)$$

where i is the imaginary unit,

$$i = \sqrt{-1} \quad (18.85e)$$

All three roots (S_1, S_2, S_3) can be real if $a_6^2 \leq 0$ or at least S_1 is of real value. There can be multiple steady-state solutions besides the trivial solution. Also, there are regions where realistic steady-state solution does not exist at all. For example, when D is in the neighborhood of μ_{max}—k_d the right-hand side of Eqn (18.70) would be able to equal to 0. There is also potential for coexistence of microbes in continuous culture because of the added flexibility in wall attachment.

Fig. 18.15 shows the steady-state solutions of a continuous *Enterobacter cloacae* (formerly *Aerobacter cloacae*) culture in a chemostat. The symbols are experimental data, while the lines are drawn with surface adhesion of cells. There are three real solutions for the substrate concentrations and only one has a value between 0 and S_0. One can observe that the washout region has a long trail before the biomass concentration drops to zero and the substrate increases to feed concentration.

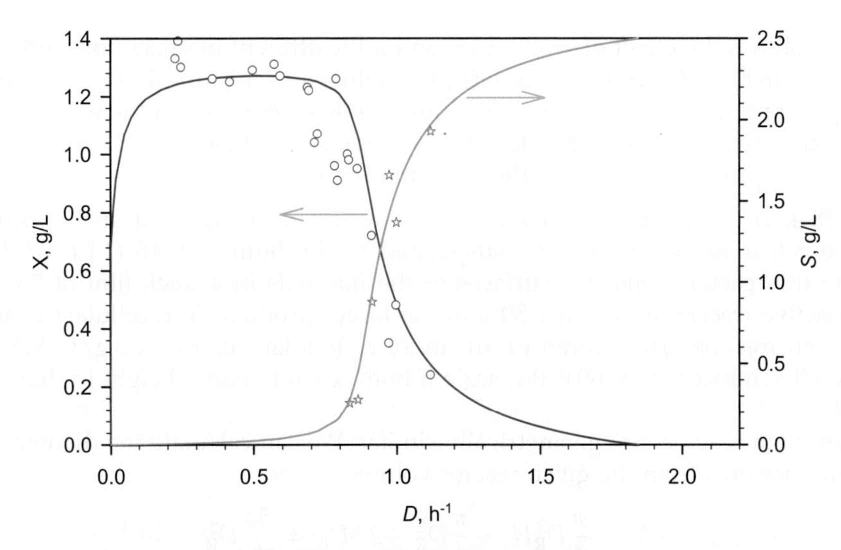

FIGURE 18.15 Effect of surface adhesion of cells on the continuous culture of *E. cloacae* (formerly *A. cloacae*). The parameters used for the lines are:

S_0, g/L	μ_{max}, h^{-1}	k_d, h^{-1}	$YF_{X/S}$, g/g	K_S, g/L	$K_{\sigma X}$, L/g	C_σ, g/L
2.5	0.8	0.014	0.53	0.018	7.7	0.1786

Data from Herbert D, Elsworth R, and Telling R. C., "The Continuous Culture of Bacteria; a Theoretical and Experimental Study", J. Gen. Microbiol. 14, 601–622 (1956).

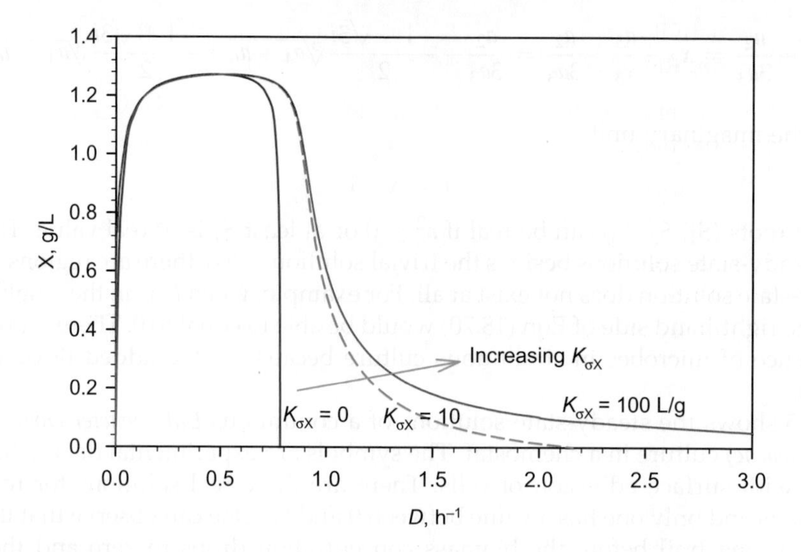

FIGURE 18.16 Effect of surface adhesion of cells on the continuous culture on the effluent biomass concentration from a chemostat.

Fig. 18.16 shows the effect of wall adhesion on the effluent biomass concentration with parameters from Fig. 18.15. One can observe that when no wall adhesion exists, the biomass concentration rapidly drops to zero as the dilution rate increases near the washout limit. As the adhesion isotherm constant $K_{\sigma X}$ is increased, the tail elongates or the biomass concentration decreases much slower at higher dilution rates.

Example 18-4. After a batch fermentation, the system is dismantled and approximately 75% of the cell mass is found to be suspended in the liquid phase (1 L), while 25% is attached to the reactor walls and surfaces of the internals in a thick film of 3 mm. Work with radioactive tracers shows that 50% of the target product (intracellular) is associated with each cell fraction. The overall productivity of this lab reactor is 5 g/L. What would be the overall productivity at 60,000-L scale if both reactors had a height to diameter ratio of 2.5 to 1?

Solution. Both reactors are geometrically similar. We can calculate the diameter and the resulting surface area from the given reactor volume.

$$V = \frac{\pi}{4} D_R^2 H = \frac{\pi}{4} D_R^2 \times 2.5 D_R = \frac{5\pi}{8} D_R^3 \tag{E18-4.1}$$

$$S_R = \pi D_R H = 2.5\pi D_R^2 = 2.5\pi \left(\frac{8V}{5\pi}\right)^{\frac{2}{3}} = 2(5\pi)^{\frac{1}{3}} V^{\frac{2}{3}} \tag{E18-4.2}$$

For the 1-L lab reactor, the productivity is from two sources:

(1) Suspended cells, $5 \times 1 \times \frac{1}{2}$ g = 2.5 g.
(2) Surface attached cells, 2.5 g = $X_S \times 2(5\pi)^{1/3} 1^{2/3}$.

Thus, the productivity per unit surface area, $X_S = 1.25 \div (5\pi)^{1/3}$ g/dm^2.
For the large reactor, the productivity is then

(1) from suspended cells, $5 \times 60{,}000 \times ½$ g = 150 kg
(2) from surface attached cells, $[1.25 \div (5\pi)^{1/3}] \times 2(5\pi)^{1/3} \times 60{,}000^{2/3}$ g $= 2.5 \times 60{,}000^{2/3}$ g $= 3.8315$ kg

Thus, the total productivity from the 60,000-L reactor is 153.8315 kg.

If no wall growth had been present (but with the same level of productivity in the lab reactor), the 60,000-L reactor would have yielded 300-kg target product. Thus, wall growth, if present, can seriously alter the productivity of a large-scale reactor. Scale-up option should also be adjusted.

18.10. SUMMARY

For a well-mixed reactor, there are three common operational modes: batch, CSTR, and fed-batch. The selection of the operational modes depends on the catalyst stability, substrate supply, product demand, and regulatory requirements. A summary of the effect of operational mode on bioreactor operation is listed in Table 18.3. Batch operation has the best flexibility (at each batch of operation), while CSTR has the highest productivity. CSTR has the effect of screening for fast growth cells and in general not suited for fermentation with genetically modified cells.

There are three basic reactor types for aerobic cultivation of suspended cells: (1) systems with internal mixing mechanisms, (2) bubble columns, and (3) loop reactors. While bubble and loop reactors offer advantages of higher efficiency and lower shear, the traditional stirred-tank reactor is more flexible and can handle broths that become highly viscous. Design of a bioreactor is a balance of productivity and sterility. The desired product is to produce a pure culture where only the desired organism is detectably present.

For industrial-scale fermentors, oxygen supply and heat removal are key design limitations. K_La is dependent on the media, salts, surfactants, pressure, and temperature making it difficult to predict. K_La is however measurable. Once K_La is established, it can be used to estimate the rate of metabolic heat generation and the total amount of cooling surface required.

Scale-up is difficult because conditions in a large vessel are more heterogeneous than in a small vessel. Scale-up problems are all related to transport processes. If geometrically similar vessels are used, it is impossible to maintain shear, mixing times, and K_La identically in both large and small vessels. Scale-down techniques are useful in identifying the controlling regime at the smaller scale, where many parameters can be tested more quickly and less expensively than at the production scale.

Bioreactor instrumentation and control are less advanced than in the petrochemical industry. Improvements in sensor technology and the dynamical models of bioreactors are critical to improvements in control technology.

Sterilization is the removal of biocontaminants or foreign organisms for a fermentation system and the surrounding equipment. Scientists and engineers who are familiar with biological testing, as in a fermentation laboratory, will be familiar with autoclaves. These systems apply steam to an internal vessel at 121 °C, usually for 15 min. Instruments, samples, fermentation media, and even fermentor components can all be sterilized by placing them inside of the autoclave vessel. Many surgical instruments are sterilized through the use of very high temperatures, usually in excess of 150 °C, to rapidly remove any contamination. Prepackaged medical instruments are often sterilized through the use of ethylene oxide or formaldehyde vapors applied over a period of few hours. Biological contamination of paper machines, water systems, and even pots and pans is often removed through use of commercially available biocide solutions or material such as ozone or chlorine. All of these are potentially viable methods for the sterilization of fermentation systems.

Industrial fermentors and associated pipings are designed for in situ steam sterilization under pressure or SIP. The use of saturated steam is common and advantageous over other hot fluids. As steam is applied to a vessel or pipe, the hot steam transfers its energy (heat) to the wall of the pipe or vessel, raising its temperature. The transfer of heat from the steam decreases the enthalpy of the saturated water vapor, causing it to condense at constant temperature. This condensation decreases the volume of the water by a factor of 815 for steam at 121 °C. This results in a pumping action (pressure drop when water vapor condenses), drawing more steam to the areas of greatest consumption, i.e. the areas that are the coldest. This provides a more even temperature profile and makes the heating process less likely to result in cold spots and dead legs. As a result, the sterilization is uniform.

Sterilization of process fluids is dependent on the expectation of probability of successful fermentations. While relative measures (ratio of surviving cells in the initial cells) have been used, more valid measure is the absolute sterility or rather the probability of one single cell surviving in a given fermentation medium. Therefore, the sterility measure is a function of the medium size. Stringent requirement leads to a longer reduced or dimensionless sterilization time t_S. In a batch sterilization,

$$t_S = k_{d0} \int_0^t e^{-\frac{E_{ad}}{RT}} dt - \ln N_0 \tag{18.27}$$

The integral can be computed numerically as shown in Table 18.7 for commonly seen time–temperature profiles. If the temperature is constant, Eqn (18.27) is reduced to

$$t_S = k_d t - \ln N_0 \tag{18.25}$$

Bacterial spores are known to be more thermal resistant than vegetative forms of yeast, bacteria, and bacteriophages. Usually, sterilization is designed based on bacterial spores. For typical spores of *B. stearothermophilus*, $k_{d0} = 8.236 \times 10^{37}$/min and $E_{ad} = 283$ kJ/mol.

Larger reactor vessel requires longer sterilization time (or higher temperature) as the number of unwanted cells, N_0, is higher in a larger vessel. The same sterilization level can be maintained with the same t_S value. Large-scale bioreactors also place heavy demands on processes to sterilize fluids entering the bioreactor. A dimensionless sterilization time of $t_S = 4.6$ yields one unsuccessful fermentation per 100 fermentations, whereas $t_S = 9.2$ yields one unsuccessful fermentation per 10,000 fermentations.

It is desirable to sterilize process fluid continuously as it is more reliable and requires less steam. In this case, CSTR or stirred-tank sterilization is not recommended, whereas tubular sterilizers are highly desirable. For continuous sterilization in laminar flow regime, the probability of microorganisms surviving the thermal sterilization is given by

$$p(\tau) \approx \frac{4(k_d\tau + 2)}{k_d\tau(k_d\tau + 8)} \exp\left(-\frac{k_d\tau}{2}\right) \tag{18.47}$$

where τ is the space time of the sterilizing fluid in the sterilization zone. The probability of the entire population in one reactor-full process fluid not vanishing from the laminar flow heat treatment is

$$P_1(\tau) \approx \frac{C_{X0} V \dfrac{4\,(k_d\tau + 2)}{k_d\tau\,(k_d\tau + 8)} \exp\left(-\dfrac{1}{2} k_d\tau\right)}{1 + \dfrac{2\,(C_{X0}V - 1)\,(k_d\tau + 2)}{k_d\tau\,(k_d\tau + 8)} \exp\left(-\dfrac{1}{2} k_d\tau\right)} \tag{18.48}$$

which corresponds to the characteristic sterilization time of

$$t_S = \frac{1}{2} k_d\tau - \ln \frac{4\,(k_d\tau + 2)}{k_d\tau\,(k_d\tau + 8)} - \ln(C_{X0}V) \tag{18.49}$$

where C_{X0} is the estimated cell concentration in the sterilizing fluid and V is the volume of fluid of basis for sterilization. The sterility can be measured by the probability of unsuccessful fermentations or contamination in a certain time period of fermentation (1 day of operation, 1 week of operation, or 1 month of operation). Thus, the volume V depends on the basis of sterility. If one fermentor volume full of medium is considered as the basis and then V is the volume of the fermentor.

For continuous sterilization with a tube of length L and diameter D_R in the turbulent flow regime, the probability of microorganisms surviving the thermal sterilization is given by

$$p(\tau) = \exp\left(\frac{1 - \sqrt{1 + 4a_d D_R L^{-1} k_d\tau}}{2a_d D_R} L\right) \tag{18.57}$$

where the dispersion constant a_d is given by,

$$a_d = 3 \times 10^7 \mathrm{Re}^{-2.1} + 1.35\mathrm{Re}^{-0.125} \tag{18.56}$$

The probability of the entire population in one reactor-full process fluid not vanishing from the heat treatment is

$$P_1(\tau) \approx \frac{C_{X0} V \exp\left(\dfrac{1 - \sqrt{1 + 4a_d D_R L^{-1} k_d\tau}}{2a_d D_R} L\right)}{1 + \dfrac{C_{X0}V - 1}{2} \exp\left(\dfrac{1 - \sqrt{1 + 4a_d D_R L^{-1} k_d\tau}}{2a_d D_R} L\right)} \tag{18.58}$$

which corresponds to the dimensionless sterilization time of

$$t_S = \frac{\sqrt{1 + 4a_d D_R L^{-1} k_d \tau} - 1}{2a_d D_R} L - \ln (C_{X0} V) \tag{18.59}$$

where D_R is the diameter of tube and L is the length of the tube in the sterilization zone.

Liquid streams are steam or filter sterilized. Steam sterilization is preferred, but the sterilization process cannot damage the ability of the medium to support growth. Filtration methods are almost always used when sterilizing process gases. Depth or surface filters can be used, but surface membrane cartridge filters are predominantly used.

Thermal sterilization is the most common techniques applied in the industry. Temperature and time are to be selected based on the thermal stability of medium, as well as the thermal stability of the potential undesirable microorganisms present. Usually, tests need to be conducted to verify sterile conditions. For sterilizing known microorganisms, one must take into account subcultures that are more thermal stable. Although the population might be small, these more thermal stable subcultures could have much lower activation energies (of deactivation).

Industrial bioreactors for sterile operation are usually designed as steel pressure vessels capable of withstanding full vacuum up to about 3 atm positive pressure at 150–180 °C. Nozzles for medium, antifoam, acid and alkali addition, air-exhaust pipes, pressure gauge, and a rupture disc for emergency pressure release, are normally located on the head-plate. Side ports for pH, temperature, and DO sensors are required at minimum; a steam-sterilizable sample outlet should also be provided. The vessel must be fully drainable via a harvest nozzle located at the lowest point of the reactor. If the vessel is mechanically agitated, either a top- or bottom-entering stirrer is installed. To maintain aseptic operations, special considerations are needed for sealing the opening where stirrer shaft entering the vessel, control valves, and sampling ports.

One particularly resistant undesired biocontaminant is prions or infectious proteins. Commonly, infectious particles possessing nucleic acid are dependent upon it to direct their continued replication. Prions, however, are infectious by their effect on normal versions (or desired folding forms) of the protein. Prions induce normal proteins to refold and to be added (*grow*) to prions. Sterilizing prions therefore require the denaturation of the protein to a state where the molecule is no longer able to induce the abnormal folding of normal proteins. Prions are generally quite resistant to proteases, heat, radiation, and formalin treatments, effective prion decontamination relies upon protein hydrolysis or reduction or destruction of protein tertiary structure.

Microbes, especially shear-sensitive bacteria and mammalian cells, tend to attach to surfaces. The attachment of suspended microbes to surfaces can be modeled as adsorption. That is

$$X + \sigma \underset{k_{deX}}{\overset{k_{adX}}{\rightleftarrows}} X \cdot \sigma \tag{18.64}$$

Therefore, the total viable concentration of cells in the reactor is given by

$$X_T = X + C_\sigma \theta_{X \cdot \sigma} = X + C_\sigma \frac{K_{\sigma X} X}{1 + K_{\sigma X} X} \tag{18.68}$$

where C_σ is the concentration of total available adhesion sites on surfaces in the reactor and $K_{\sigma X}$ is the surface adhesion coefficient.

Surface adhesion delays washout in a chemostat. The cells adhered on the vessel surfaces are less likely to be taken out of the reactor by the outflowing stream. However, the adhesion–desorption balance eventually leads to the washout if the flow rate exceeds the critical limit. The washout is more gradual if cells adhere to the vessel surfaces, and a log tail could exist if the adhesion is strong.

Further Reading

Aiba, S., Humphrey, A.E., Mills, N.F., 1973. *Biochemical Engineering*. 2nd ed. Academic Press, New York.

Bailey, J.E., Ollis, D.F., 1986. *Biochemical Engineering Fundamentals*, 2nd ed. McGraw-Hill Book Co., New York.

Blanch, H.W., Clark, D.S., 1966. *Biochemical Engineering*. Marcel Dekker. Inc. New York.

Butt, J.B., 1999. *Reaction Kinetics and Reactor Design*, 2nd ed. Marcel Dekker, Inc., New York.

Doran, P.M., 1995. *Bioprocess Engineering Principles*, Academic Press. San Diego.

Prave, P., and others. 1987. *Fundamentals of Biotechnology*, VCH Verlagsgesellschaft, Weinheim, Germany.

Shuler, M.L., Kargi, F., 2006 *Bioprocess Engineering Basic Concepts*, 2nd ed. Prentice Hall.

Stephanopoulose, G. (Ed.), 1993. *Bioprocessing* (vol. 3 of *Biotechnology.* 2nd ed. H.-J. Rehm and G. Reed. (Eds).), VCH, New York.

Williams, J.A., 2002. "Keys to bioreactor selections." *Chemical Engineering Progress*, **98**(3), 34–41.

PROBLEMS

18.1. The k_La of a small bubble column has been measured as 20 h^{-1} at an airflow of 4 L/min. If the rate of oxygen uptake by a culture of *Catharathus roseus* is 0.2 mmol-O_2/(g-cell h), and if the critical oxygen concentration must be above 10% of saturation (about 8 mg/L) for this plant cell culture, what is the maximum concentration of cells that can be maintained in this reactor?

18.2. A value of $k_La = 30\ h^{-1}$ has been determined for a fermentor at its maximum practical agitator rotational speed and with air being sparged at 0.5 L-gas/(L-reactor volume · min). *Escherichia coli* with a μ_{O_2} of 10 mmol-O_2/(g-X h) is to be cultured. The critical DO concentration is 0.2 mg/L. The solubility of oxygen from air in the fermentation broth is 7.3 mg/L at 30 °C.

(a) What maximum concentration of *E. coli* can be sustained in this fermentor under aerobic conditions?

(b) What concentration could be maintained if pure oxygen was used to sparge the reactor?

18.3. A continuous culture system is being constructed. The fermentation tank is to be 50,000 L in size and the residence time is to be 2 h. A continuous sterilizer is to be used. The unsterilized medium contains 10^4 spores/L. The value of k_d has been determined to be 1 min^{-1} at 121 °C and 61 min^{-1} at 140 °C. For each temperature (121 °C and 140 °C), determine the required residence time in the holding section so as to ensure that 99% of the time 4 weeks of continuous operation can be obtained without contamination (due to contaminants in the liquid medium).

18.4. A medium containing a vitamin is to be sterilized. Assume that the number of spores initially present is 10^5/L. The values of the pre-Arrhenius exponential factor and E_{ad} for the spores are $k_{d0} = 10^{36}\ \text{min}^{-1}$ and $E_{ad} = 270$ kJ/mol. For the inactivation of the vitamin, the values of E_{ad} and k_{d0} are 40 kJ/mol and $10^4\ \text{min}^{-1}$. The initial concentration of the vitamin is 30 mg/L. Compare the amount of active vitamin in the sterilized medium for 10-L and 10,000-L fermentors when both are sterilized at 121 °C when we require in both cases that the probability of an unsuccessful fermentation be 0.001. Ignore the effects of the heat-up and cool-down periods.

18.5. Consider the data given in Table P18.5 on the temperature changes in a 10,000-L fermentor, which includes the heat-up and cool-down periods. Use the values for the Arrhenius parameters given in Problem 18.4 and assume an initial spore concentration of 10^5/L and a vitamin concentration of 30 mg/L.

TABLE P18.5

Time, min	0	10	20	30	40	50	55	60	65	70	90	100	120	140
Temperature, °C	30	40	54	70	95	121	121	121	106	98	75	64	46	32

(a) What is the probability of a successful sterilization?
(b) What fraction of the vitamin remains undegraded?
(c) What fraction of the vitamin is degraded in the sterilization period?
(d) What fraction of the vitamin is degraded in the heat-up and cool-down periods?
(e) What is the fraction of spores deactivated in the heat-up and cool-down cycles?

18.6. *E. coli* has a maximum respiration rate, $\mu_{O_2 max}$ of about 240 mg-O_2/(g-cell·h). It is desired to achieve a cell mass of 20 g/cell. The $k_L a$ is 120 h^{-1} in a 1000-L reactor (800-L working volume). A gas stream enriched in oxygen is used (i.e. 80% O_2) which gives a value of $C^* = 28$ mg/L. If oxygen becomes limiting, growth and respiration slow; for example,

$$\mu_{O_2} = \frac{\mu_{O_2 max} C_L}{0.2\text{mg/L} + C_L}$$

where C_L is the DO concentration in the fermentor. What is C_L when the cell mass is at 20 g/L?

18.7. The temperature history of the heating and cooling of a 40,000-L tank during sterilization of medium is: 0–15 min, $T = 85$ °C; 15–40 min, $T = 121$ °C; 40–50 min, $T = 85$ °C; 50–60 min, $T = 55$ °C; >60 min, $T = 30$ °C. The medium contains vitamins, the most fragile of the vitamins has an activation energy for destruction of 40 kJ/mol, and the value of k_{d0} is $1 \times 10^4\ \text{min}^{-1}$. Assume vitamin destruction is first order and the initial concentration is 50 mg/L. R is 8.314 J/(mol·K). The medium contains 2.5×10^3 spores/L. The spores have an $E_{ad} = 270$ kJ/mol, and k_d at 121 °C is 1.02 min^{-1}. Estimate:

(a) the probability of a successful sterilization and
(b) what fraction of the vitamin remains active?

18.8. In cultivation of baker's yeast in a stirred and aerated tank, lethal agents are added to the fermentation medium to kill the organisms immediately. Increase in DO concentration upon addition of lethal agents is followed with the aid of a DO analyzer and a recorder. Using the data in Table P18.8, determine the oxygen transfer coefficient, $k_L a$, for the reactor. Saturation DO concentration is $C^* = 9$ mg/L.

TABLE P18.8

Time, min	1	2	2.5	3	4	5
DO, mg/L	1	3	4	5	6.5	7.2

18.9. A stirred-tank reactor is to be scaled down from 10 to 0.1 m^3. The dimensions of the large tank are: $D_R = 2$ m; $D_i = 0.5$ m; $\omega = 100$ rpm.
(a) Determine the dimensions of the small tank (D_R, D_i, H) by using geometric similarity.
(b) What would be the required rotational speed of the impeller in the small tank if the following criteria were used?
(1) Constant tip speed
(2) Constant impeller Re number

18.10. An autoclave malfunctions, and the temperature reaches only 119.5 °C. The sterilization time at the maximum temperature was 20 min. The jar contains 10 L of complex medium that has 10^5 spores/L. At 121 °C, $k_d = 1.0$/min and $E_{ad} = 380$ kJ/mol. What is the probability that the medium was sterile?

18.11. A 10 m^3 chemostat is operated with a dilution rate of 0.1 h^{-1}. A continuous sterilizer with steam injection and flash cooling is to be designed to deliver sterilized medium to the fermentor. Medium in the holding section of the sterilizer is maintained at 125 °C. The concentration of contaminants in the raw medium is 5×10^{12} m^{-3}; an acceptable contamination risk is 0.01 on a weekly basis. The activation energy and pre-exponential factor of the cell thermal death rate are estimated at 300 kJ/mol and 2.3×10^{36} s^{-1}. The sterilizer tube inner diameter is 0.15 m. The liquid medium density is 1000 kg/m^3, and viscosity is 0.9×10^{-3} Pa·s.
(a) Determine the length of the holding section and space time required;
(b) Determine the length of the holding section and space time if the inner tube diameter is 1 m instead.

18.12. A 12-m^3 fermentor is available to carry out the fermentation. The medium stream of 1.5 m^3/h is to be sterilized continuously. Medium in the holding section of the sterilizer is maintained at 121 °C. The concentration of contaminants in the raw medium is 2.5×10^{12} m^{-3}; an acceptable contamination risk is 0.1 on a monthly basis. The activation energy and pre-exponential factor of the cell thermal death rate are estimated at 300 kJ/mol and 2.3×10^{36} s^{-1}. The sterilizer tube inner diameter is 1.5 m. The liquid medium density is 1200 kg/m^3, and viscosity is 1.5×10^{-3} Pa·s.
(a) Determine the length of the holding section and space time required;
(b) Determine the dimensionless time required.

18.13. You wish to produce active retrovirus, and you are investigating the effect of temperature on the process. Active virus is subject to decay with a rate constant, $k_d = 2.2\ \text{day}^{-1}$ at 37 °C and 0.76/day at 31 °C. The rate of virus production from a packaging cell line is $k_p = 3.5$ virus · cell^{-1} · day^{-1} at 37 °C and 3.0 virus · cell^{-1} · day^{-1} at 31 °C. Assume that there are 5×10^6 cells and the volume of the liquid medium is 5 mL. The initial number of virus in solution is zero. How many viruses are there in 1 mL solution 1 day after initiation of virus production if the temperature is maintained at 35 °C?

18.14. What value of k_La must be achieved to sustain a population of 5×10^9 cells/L when the oxygen consumption is 0.1×10^{-12} mol-O_2/(h cell)?

18.15. Hybridoma cells immobilized on surfaces of Sephadex beads are used in a packed column for production of monoclonoal antibodies (Mab). Hybridoma concentration (*X*) is approximately 5 g/L in the bed (total bed volume). The flow rate of the synthetic medium and glucose concentration are: $Q = 2$ L/h and $S_0 = 40$ g/L, respectively. The specific rate constant for glucose consumption is 1 L/(g-X·day). Assume that there are no diffusion limitations and glucose is the rate-limiting nutrient. Determine

(a) the volume and the packed bed height for 95% glucose conversion. Bed diameter is $D_R = 0.2$ m. Neglect the growth of the hybridomas and assume first-order kinetics.

(b) the effluent Mab concentration and overall productivity if $YF_{P/S} = 4$ mg-Mab/g-S.

18.16. A small laboratory reactor is used to obtain data on the growth of *E. coli* on glucose. The vessel is cylindrical with a liquid volume of 1 L and is 0.1 m in diameter. The walls and the base of the vessel are covered with a film of *E. coli*, which *grows* to a concentration of 10^5 cells/m^2. The reactor is operated as a chemostat, with an inlet substrate concentration of 2.0 g/L glucose. The yield coefficient for *E. coli* may be taken to be 10^7 cells/g-glucose, and the maximum specific growth rate is 0.8 h^{-1}. The Monod constant K_S is 100 mg glucose/L.

The vessel is to be used to collect data on the kinetics of *E. coli* growth under glucose limitation. How would the observed yield coefficient vary with dilution rate under these conditions of wall growth? Plot $X/(S_0 - S)$ a function of *D*. What fraction of the substrate is consumed by cells attached to the wall? In determining the kinetics parameters, only the bulk cell and substrate concentrations are measured, and the contribution by cells attached to the wall is ignored. The cells on the wall consume substrate at a rate described by the Monod equation with the kinetic constants given above. Their number remains constant due to the combined effects of cell growth and cell lysis.

If a washout experiment is performed (*D* is set at a value greater than the maximum growth rate and the cell concentration in the exit stream is monitored with time) what is the behavior you would expect in the presence and absence of wall growth? Plot the cell concentration as a function of time for both cases.

Index

Note: Page numbers with "f" denote figures; "t" denote tables.

C

D

E

K

L

M

N

O

Q

R

S

T